Textbook of
## BASIC NURSING

# Textbook of
# BASIC NURSING

## Second Edition

**Ella M. Thompson, R.N., B.S.**

Formerly Field Consultant and Associate Executive Director,
National Association for Practical Nurse Education and Service;
formerly Member, Job Analysis Committee and Chairman, Production
Committee of the Curriculum Committee, United States Office of Education.

**Caroline Bunker Rosdahl, R.N., M.A.**

Coordinator of Health Occupations Education, Technical Education Center,
Anoka, Minnesota; Instructor, Industrial Education Department,
University of Minnesota.

## J. B. LIPPINCOTT COMPANY

*Philadelphia / Toronto*

SECOND EDITION

COPYRIGHT © 1973 BY J. B. LIPPINCOTT COMPANY

Distributed in Great Britain by
Blackwell Scientific Publications
Oxford, London, and Edinburgh

ISBN 0-397-54146-5

Printed in the United States of America

Cover and text design by Joseph B. Crossen

5  7  9  8  6

*Library of Congress Cataloging in Publication Data*

Thompson, Ella M
    Textbook of basic nursing.

    Includes bibliography

    1. Practical nursing.    I. Rosdahl, Caroline Bunker,
joint author.    II. Title.    [DNLM: 1. Nursing, Practical.    WY 195 T469t 1973]

RT62.T5   1973                610.73              73-5989

ISBN 0-397-54146-5

# Preface

The second edition of *Textbook of Basic Nursing* is a thorough revision of one of the most respected single-volume textbooks designed for students of practical nursing and practitioners. Several features have been added.

**Behavioral Objectives.** Behavioral objectives are included at the beginning of each chapter. These objectives serve several purposes:

*General Overview of the Chapter.* By reading the objectives the teacher or student can identify, at a glance, the major content of the chapter. Nothing is included in the objectives which is not discussed in the chapter.

*Formulation of Lessons or Teaching Strategies.* The instructor, by scanning the objectives, can plan her teaching; if manipulative tasks are identified, the instructor will know that she must plan a clinical-type teaching method, as well as a procedural-type evaluation of the student's progress; if cognitive material is identified, the instructor will often be able to present the material via lecture, films, or other information-giving methods.

*Built-in Evaluative Criteria.* The objectives are behavioral—that is, the student must be able to *do something;* she must be able to demonstrate that learning has taken place by performing an activity, whether that activity be describing, identifying, or performing a manipulative or clinical skill correctly. The instructor need simply to use the objectives in evaluation—Can the student do this particular task—yes or no? Evaluation will consist of not only paper-and-pencil evaluations, but of clinical and other performance as well.

*Student Self-Evaluation.* The student, by reading the objectives, can determine for herself whether or not she meets the criteria for successfully completing the chapter's goals.

The student need merely ask herself, after reading each objective, "Can I do that—yes or no?" In this way, the student will be able to more effectively pace her own learning. Students may also wish to use the objectives to test each other or to study together.

*Student Pre-test.* In a situation where challenge examinations are available, the objectives can be used as a guide for allowing a student to be exempt from a particular portion of the material.

*The Instructor as a Facilitator.* The use of behavioral objectives allows the instructor to spend more time in assisting those students who are moving more slowly. Thus, the instructor becomes a facilitator of learning, rather than a "giver of all information." This is not to imply that any student can become a practical nurse simply by reading a book; neither does it imply that the role of the instructor is easier. To the contrary, the instructor will find her job more challenging than ever before, since she must now meet the specific needs of each individual student, as well as the needs of the student group as a whole.

*Special Note About Objectives.* Some of the behavioral objectives may not be attained simply by reading the chapter; however, by the end of the entire practical nursing program, the student should be able to meet each and every objective stated in the book.

**Additional Content.** This book is a complete practical nursing text, with a great deal more depth than the previous edition. It could be used as the basic text for any practical nursing program. Of particular note is the addition of expanded chapters dealing with maternal and child care, placing more emphasis on obstetrical and pediatric nursing than in the previous edition. The medical-surgical content has been updated and presented in greater depth.

**Levels-of-Learning Materials.** Some of the introductory chapters could be used for nursing-assistant courses, with the student progressing at her own rate in meeting the objectives. The more advanced student could then continue through the book and pursue a practical nursing program, with the appropriate clinical and classroom instruction.

**General Considerations.** The 5 general considerations used in planning the first edition were followed and expanded in this revision.

*Approaching the patient as a person with psychological as well as physical needs, with emphasis on total patient care.* It no longer suffices for the nurse to be able to make the patient physically comfortable; she must also be able to make him psychologically comfortable in his environment, an aspect of care that goes beyond the "illness and cure" approach.

In this edition, much more emphasis is given to the total concept of basic human needs—the basic needs of *all people,* whether nurse or patient, old or young. Nursing is, in fact, assisting people to meet their basic needs or those special needs which they are unable to meet because of illness or age.

*Presenting accurate scientific data and the application of scientific principles to nursing practice.* Although the authors have followed the current trend in emphasizing the psychosocial approach to nursing care, they are aware that in order to practice efficiently, the practical nurse must be well-grounded in basic scientific principles, signs and symptoms, treatment, nursing care and complications of illness conditions. Pharmacology, diet therapy, rehabilitation, and mental health are discussed as they apply to each condition, even though each is covered in a separate chapter. In order to better understand the cause and the control of disease, a separate chapter is devoted to the study of microbiology.

The scientific content has been considerably expanded and updated in this edition.

*Considering the normal condition before the abnormal and proceeding from the simple to the more complex situation.* The necessity for a sound working knowledge of normal body function and structure becomes increasingly important as the practical nurse assumes more responsibility for assisting with the care of the acutely ill patient. In addition to treating each body system in a separate chapter, one chapter is devoted to describing the normal body as an integrated whole. Elementary principles of chemistry and physics as they apply to body function are discussed here. Clinical applications are made in order to introduce the student to the concept of understanding illness and disease as a deviation from normal.

The entire book has been reorganized to follow not only the concept of *simple to complex,* but also to follow the normal life span of people. Thus, the normal scientific foundations and basic nursing skills are presented first; then, the book follows the normal life span through pregnancy, childhood, and adulthood and into the aging process. The final chapters of the book are designed to assist the student to competently make the transition from student to graduate practical nurse.

*Incorporating the sociological implications and community health aspects of nursing, with preventive as well as restorative care.* A full chapter is devoted to community health, while the broad concept of the family as a unit and the nurse-patient-family relationship forms the core of Unit 3. Developmental tasks of the healthy child at various age levels are discussed, and considerable attention is given to the adolescent, an age often neglected in student texts. The role of the father as an integral part of the family group is incorporated into the unit on Maternal and Child Care.

The mental health section of the book has been expanded to include not only more material on psychosocial disabilities in general but also an entire new chapter on chemical dependency, written by a leading expert in the field, Arthur James Morgan, M.D.

*Including content which the student will find applicable from the time of her (or his) orientation, through the period of actual experience in clinical areas and later, as a graduate practitioner.* Several chapters have been devoted to the orientation of the student as an undergraduate and later, as a graduate practical nurse. Additional learning aids, such as an extensive glossary, a list of medical terms, and a bibliography are found at the back of the book.

Despite the massive revision of content and the addition of much relatively advanced material, the authors have striven to preserve this book's heritage of readability and informality of presentation, plus an approach that is essentially practical. They have not hesitated to include suggested methods and procedures wherever appropriate, recognizing the value of such in reinforcing the student's self-confidence besides providing a point of departure for action. In all such instances the authors have furnished the rationale of each step, with the object of promoting essential understanding and the flexibility of mind that goes with it. It is hoped that *Textbook of Basic Nursing,* with its immensely broadened base of theory from many disciplines coupled with a practical orientation, will help to develop in the student that coordination of head, hands and heart which is the touchstone of the superior bedside practitioner.

**Special Note:** The use of "she" to describe the practical nurse is not intended to imply that all practical nurses are women. Many men are entering the field of nursing as well. However, for convenience sake the use of the pronoun "she" will differentiate the nurse from the patient, who is often referred to as "he."

# Acknowledgments

The authors gratefully acknowledge all the people and agencies who assisted in the preparation of this revision.

Many public and private agencies contributed materials and illustrations. Special thanks go to several organizations in the Minneapolis-St. Paul area which provided illustrations, notably the Hennepin County General Hospital and the University of Minnesota Health Sciences Center. We also express appreciation to Mrs. Lyn Hubschman, Director, Social Services Department, Pennsylvania Hospital, Philadelphia, who contributed information regarding social service.

Special thanks are also due to the entire Health Occupations staff of the Technical Education Center in Anoka, Minnesota. Particular recognition is extended to the practical nursing faculty, especially, Donna Richardson, R.N., B.A. for her assistance with the medical-surgical portions of this text.

Thanks also are due to the editors of Lippincott for their undying and extensive efforts.

# Contents

**UNIT 1: PERSONAL AND VOCATIONAL RELATIONSHIPS**

1. Introduction and Orientation . . . . . . . . . . 3
2. Guides to Effective Learning . . . . . . . . . 11
3. Basic Needs of All People . . . . . . . . . 18

**UNIT 2: PERSONAL AND ENVIRONMENTAL HEALTH**

4. Over-All Health Aspects . . . . . . . . . 23
5. Personality and Health . . . . . . . . . 25
6. Community Health . . . . . . . . . 32
7. Microbes and Man . . . . . . . . . 37

**UNIT 3: THE FAMILY**

8. Growth and Development . . . . . . . . . 47
9. Adolescence . . . . . . . . . 59
10. Family Living . . . . . . . . . 65

**UNIT 4: THE LIVING BODY: NORMAL BODY STRUCTURE AND FUNCTION**

11. The Body as an Integrated Whole . . . . . . . . . 73
12. The Body's Cell Pattern: Tissues and Membranes . . . . . . . . . 85
13. The Musculoskeletal System . . . . . . . . . 89
14. The Nervous System . . . . . . . . . 106
15. The Circulatory System . . . . . . . . . 113
16. The Respiratory System . . . . . . . . . 125
17. The Digestive System . . . . . . . . . 130
18. The Urinary System . . . . . . . . . 139
19. How Life Begins: The Reproductive System . . . . . . . . . 143
20. The Endocrine System . . . . . . . . . 150
21. The Sensory System . . . . . . . . . 155

xii / *Contents*

## UNIT 5: MEETING THE NUTRITIONAL NEEDS OF PEOPLE

22. Food for Growth and Energy . . . . . . . . . . . . . . . 161
23. From Market to Meals . . . . . . . . . . . . . . . . . . 175
24. Special Diets to Meet Patients' Needs . . . . . . . . . . 177

## UNIT 6: DEVIATIONS FROM NORMAL

25. The Signs and the Symptoms of Illness . . . . . . . . . 185

## UNIT 7: FUNDAMENTAL NURSING SKILLS

26. The Patient in His Surroundings . . . . . . . . . . . . 193
27. Introducing the Patient to the Hospital . . . . . . . . . 203
28. Assisting the Physician . . . . . . . . . . . . . . . . . 223
29. Assisting the Patient to Meet Daily Needs . . . . . . . . 230
30. Nursing Treatments to Meet Special Patient Needs . . . . 267
31. The Patient With Special Oxygen Needs . . . . . . . . . 297
32. Nursing Care for Patients Having Surgery . . . . . . . . 310
33. Administering Selected Medications to the Patient . . . . 322
34. Rehabilitation . . . . . . . . . . . . . . . . . . . . . 374
35. First Aid and Care in Emergencies . . . . . . . . . . . 379

## UNIT 8: CARE OF THE MOTHER AND NEWBORN INFANT

36. The Beginning Family—Pregnancy as a Normal Process . . . 397
37. Assisting the Mother During Labor, Delivery, and Puerperium . . . 415
38. Care of the Neonate . . . . . . . . . . . . . . . . . . 426

## UNIT 9: ASSISTING THE CHILD WHO IS ILL

39. Fundamental Aspects of Pediatric Nursing . . . . . . . . 445
40. The Infant, the Toddler, and the Preschool Child . . . . 458
41. The School-Age Child and the Adolescent . . . . . . . . 492
42. The Handicapped Child . . . . . . . . . . . . . . . . . 499

## UNIT 10: ASSISTING THE ADULT WHO HAS IMPAIRED BODY STRUCTURE OR FUNCTION

43. The Patient With Cancer (Oncologic Nursing) . . . . . . 509
44. The Patient With a Skin Disorder . . . . . . . . . . . . 516
45. The Patient With Musculoskeletal Disease or Injury . . . 526

46. The Patient With a Disturbance of the Nervous System . . . . . . . . . . 543
47. The Patient With a Cardiovascular Disease or a Blood Disorder . . . . . . . 572
48. The Patient With a Respiratory Disorder . . . . . . . . . . . . . 596
49. The Patient With a Digestive Disorder . . . . . . . . . . . . . 624
50. The Patient With a Urinary Disorder . . . . . . . . . . . . . 656
51. The Patient With a Reproductive Disorder . . . . . . . . . . . . 670
52. The Patient With an Endocrine Disorder . . . . . . . . . . . . 691
53. The Patient With a Disorder of the Sensory System . . . . . . . . . 708
54. The Patient With an Allergy . . . . . . . . . . . . . . . . 726

## UNIT 11: SPECIAL NEEDS OF THE AGING PERSON

55. The Geriatric Patient . . . . . . . . . . . . . . . . . . 733

## UNIT 12: ASSISTING THE PATIENT WHO IS EXPERIENCING A PSYCHOLOGICAL DISORDER

56. The Person With a Psychiatric Problem . . . . . . . . . . . . 741
57. Drug Misuse (By Arthur James Morgan, M.D.) . . . . . . . . . . 760

## UNIT 13: BRIDGING THE GAP BETWEEN STUDENT AND GRADUATE

58. Career Opportunities in Practical Nursing . . . . . . . . . . . 779
59. The Legal Aspects of Practical Nursing . . . . . . . . . . . . 785
Glossary . . . . . . . . . . . . . . . . . . . . . . 789
Medical Terminology . . . . . . . . . . . . . . . . . . 801
Bibliography . . . . . . . . . . . . . . . . . . . . . 805
Index . . . . . . . . . . . . . . . . . . . . . . . 813

# Unit 1:
## Personal and Vocational Relationships

1. *Introduction and Orientation*
2. *Guides to Effective Learning*
3. *Basic Needs of All People*

# 1

# Introduction and Orientation

---

## BEHAVIORAL OBJECTIVES

*The student successfully attaining the goals of this chapter will be able to:*

- *identify some of the important historical events in the development of practical nursing.*
- *differentiate between practical nursing and professional nursing.*
- *describe how the role and functions of the practical nurse have changed over the years.*
- *define the specific role of the Licensed Practical Nurse today.*
- *describe practical nurse education as it exists today.*
- *discuss the meaning of the term approved school and state the reasons for attending only an approved school.*
- *describe the types of licensure laws which govern nursing in the United States and to find out which type of licensure exists in the student's home state.*
- *identify several nursing associations, state who is allowed to join, note the goals of the group, and discuss reasons why the practical nurse should belong to such an organization.*
- *list at least 10 ethical considerations in practical nursing and discuss each in terms of factors relating to the nurse personally and to the patient and his safety.*

---

## PRACTICAL NURSING AS A CAREER

### The Nature of Nursing

Nursing is a special kind of service that helps the patient, as a person, meet the daily needs of life which he cannot satisfy because of illness or injury. The assistance offered by the nurse should be provided in a supportive and positive fashion so that the patient's self-image as a worthy human being is maintained. By sincerely caring about her patient, the nurse strengthens his feelings of self-respect and dignity; this reinforcement helps him meet the various discomforts and problems associated with his illness.

### How It Is Today

How many practical nurses are there? We do not know exactly, but the number of licensed practical nurses (LPN's) is above 370,000. More than 200,000 practical nurses are working in hospitals alone. In addition, many thousands more, many of them not trained, are practicing in other situations. It gives you some idea of how many sick people there are when you know that we also have over 700,000 professional nurses, yet we still cannot provide a nurse for everybody who needs one. We need more professional nurses and trained practical nurses to give people the kind of care they need.

## The Title and The Job

The practical nurse has had a number of titles such as *trained attendant, nurses' aide* and *nursing attendant. Practical nurse* is the recognized title today because it is the title which people know best and which practical nurses themselves seem to prefer. (The exceptions are in California and Texas, where the word *vocational* is used instead of *practical*.) These titles also include the word *nurse* to indicate what this worker does. Do not confuse the person who is called a *nurses' aide* with the trained practical nurse. Today the *nurses' aide* or helper means a person who is taught on the job to do the work which makes good nursing possible.

The National Association for Practical Nurse Education and Service gives this definition for the practical nurse: *A trained practical nurse is a person prepared by an approved educational program to share in the care of the sick, in rehabilitation and in the prevention of illness, always under the direction of a licensed physician and/or a registered professional nurse.*

Trained practical nurses do many of the same things that professional nurses do for patients—the choice of nurse depends on how sick the patient is. For example, a patient might be so ill that a practical nurse would not even be able to make the bed or give the patient a bath; yet, we usually think that these are simple nursing procedures which people can learn to do without being nurses.

In a statement issued in 1970, the National Federation of Licensed Practical Nurses (NFLPN) described the expanding role of the LPN in today's health care system. The Federation said that the LPN, working under the direction of a qualified health professional, may give direct patient care to a patient whose condition is relatively stable and may perform nursing functions in various complex clinical situations.

The Federation also suggests that the LPN should plan to continue her education after graduation, and that in following a personal and professional code of ethics, she should practice within the limits of her capabilities and be willing to ask for guidance when it is needed.

The NFLPN statement continues: "The LPN participates in the planning, implementation and evaluation of nursing care in all settings where nursing takes place." Among the nursing skills needed by the practical nurse are: establishing effective human relationships, assisting the patient to meet his daily needs, and recognizing all aspects of the patient's needs, including emotional, psychological and religious needs. Sometimes the LPN will be asked to administer medications or to carry out specific nursing treatments. In certain situations, after receiving special training, the practical nurse may be asked to supervise other health personnel or to serve as team leader or charge nurse.

## What a Registered Nurse Does

Registered nurses spend from 2 to 5 years learning how to do the things they need to know. They may have special training that teaches them how to be public health nurses and how to be specialists in the care of psychiatric, tubercular, medical or surgical patients. They are responsible for the care of the acutely ill patients; they teach professional and practical nurse students; they direct nurses and other people who work in hospitals; and they are in charge of hospital wards. Professional nurses also perform many duties today that only doctors performed 25 years ago.

## Why We Need Practical Nurses

This is why we need practical nurses. In the first place, there are not enough professional nurses to go around. Secondly, we have learned that not everyone needs a professional nurse; trained practical nurses can take care of those patients who are not acutely ill. Thirdly, since medical science has lengthened life, people live longer than they did in our grandparents' day, so that many of the patients are older people. By 1980, we are told, 1 person out of every 10 will be 65 or older. This means that more people are going to need nursing care.

In any town there is a wide variety in the kinds of nursing needed. Sometimes patients must go to hospitals; sometimes they can be treated at home. Some illnesses are short; others last for months and even years. Hospitals discharge many patients who still need nursing care. Placement bureaus and doctors help people to decide whether they need a professional or a practical nurse.

## NURSING SCHOOLS

Professional nurses have always been taught that nursing is responsible work; many of them sincerely believed that only professional nurses could provide nursing care. The practical nurses they knew were not trained; some of them were obviously not fit to be nurses at all. Nobody seemed to realize that there were places for two kinds of nurses; no one thought of training the practical nurse for her work. Yet all the time people who needed nurses had to turn to anyone who was willing to help them. They knew that some practical nurses did very poor work, but they appreciated the good ones all the more. They did not realize how dangerous it might be to let an untrained person take care of sick people.

However, a few professional nurses believed there was a place for the practical nurse, too. They saw that there were not enough professional nurses to take care of the people who were sick at home. They knew how satisfactory a practical nurse could be if she were responsible and intelligent. They thought she should be trained, and they were sure intelligent women would rather be taught how to do their work properly.

Public-spirited citizens knew how hard it was to obtain care for a sick person; they agreed with these interested professional nurses and found the money to open the first practical nursing schools.

### The Pioneer Schools

**The Ballard School.** In 1893, the first of these schools was opened in New York City by the YWCA. It was one of several courses offered for women under the title of the Ballard School; Miss Lucinda Ballard, an interested New York woman, gave money for this venture. The practical nursing program was a 3-months' course to train women to give simple nursing care to people in their own homes.

**The Thompson Practical Nursing School.** The next school started with money that was given originally to help poor sewing women in Brattleboro, Vermont. Mr. Thomas Thompson, a wealthy man who lived there during the Civil War, was disturbed about the women who were making shirts for the Army at a dollar a dozen. The pay was wretched, but they had to support their families somehow while the men were away at war. He left money in his will to help them. Mr. Richard Bradley, the executor, was a public-spirited man who saw that Brattleboro citizens needed nursing service, too. He thought that women could be taught to do some of the nursing that people with moderate incomes needed and could pay for. Why not do two things—help needy women to earn a living and provide nursing care? So finally, in 1907, some of the money for the poor sewing women was used to open a practical nursing school.

**The Household Nursing School.** In Boston, a group of women were determined that something should be done to provide nursing care for people who were sick at home. They called on Mr. Bradley for advice; he was only too glad to tell them about the school in Brattleboro and encouraged them to follow Brattleboro's example. So, in 1918, the Household Nursing Association School of Attendant Nursing* was opened. The Brattleboro and the Boston schools are still in existence today. The Ballard School closed in 1949 because of YWCA reorganization plans.

These were the *pioneer practical nursing schools.* All of them have trained hundreds of women the community could not do without. Each school was quite different, but all were set up for the same thing—training practical nurses. They planned regular classwork and experience that would teach the practical nurse how to take care of her patients. They took an important step to give sick people safe nursing care.

### The Schools Today

We have come a long way since those early days. Today there are over 1250 approved practical nursing programs in different parts of the country—you notice that all 3 of the first schools were in the East. There have been

---

* Later renamed the Shepard-Gill School of Practical Nursing, in honor of Katherine Shepard Dodge, the first director, and Helen Z. Gill, her associate and successor.

other changes. The first schools were under private agencies. Schools today are also sponsored by hospitals and by local boards of education in the public schools—the latter group has increased rapidly. These courses are under the vocational education division of a school system and give qualified adults an opportunity for further education. The schools follow much the same pattern in the things they teach practical nurses, and the courses are approximately the same in length.

Education in a state vocational school is free or low in cost; in addition many loans and scholarships are available if needed. No one need leave a practical nursing program school because of lack of funds. Your guidance counselor can give you helpful information on these matters.

## Approved Schools

When you plan to be a practical nurse, you want to be sure you will learn what you need to know and how to do what will be required of you. Here is an important thing about nursing: since a nurse works with human beings we must be sure people are safe with her. You can learn to sew by reading a book. Your mistakes will not harm anybody; but you cannot afford to make mistakes with human lives. This is why we must have *approved* practical nursing schools.

When a school is on the approved list, it means that a nursing authority (usually the State Board of Nursing) has visited it and is satisfied that the students are receiving the kind of training they need. *Approved* tells you that a school (1) teaches the specific things a practical nurse must know; (2) provides experience with the kind of patients she will take care of when she is practicing nursing; (3) employs qualified instructors to teach and supervise the students' practice in the classroom and on the hospital wards; and (4) provides that the graduates will be eligible for examination and licensure as LPN's. It means, too, that the course is of the required minimum length, usually at least 9 months.

Students in these schools are selected carefully. They are men and women who range in age from 18 to over 50. Students must have good health and good grooming and must be responsible people. Schools may vary in some

of these requirements, but, in general, they follow the same pattern.

Most of the practical nursing courses are given in the daytime for 5 days a week. However, there are some approved courses in which the student attends classes in the evening. It will take her longer to complete this work, but it allows her to go on working in the daytime.

## GUIDE FOR TRAINING THE PRACTICAL NURSE

### Setting Up Standards

How do we know what a practical nurse should learn? In 1941, a small group of directors and instructors in the practical nursing schools, together with some interested citizens, organized the National Association for Practical Nurse Education (NAPNE), now called the National Association for Practical Nurse Education and Service (NAPNES). They wanted to improve the education of the practical nurse and to set up standards for her instruction and service. They were looking ahead to the time when the practical nurse could take her place in nursing with dignity and confidence.

### Practical Nursing Possibilities

In 1945, the U.S. Office of Education appointed a committee to study the possibilities of the practical nurse. Professional nurses, teachers, physicians, hospital administrators, vocational educators and a practical nurse worked together for 2 years to define the duties of the practical nurse. The result was a manual* which gave the schools something to go by in training practical nurses. A second committee produced further suggestions† to guide directors and instructors in planning a teaching program.

Many changes have been made since these guides were published, and there will be more. Every day we know more about what the trained practical nurse can learn and do, so of

---

* Practical Nursing—An Analysis of the Practical Nurse Occupation, U.S. Government Printing Office, 1947.

† Practical Nursing Curriculum, U.S. Government Printing Office, 1950.

course we must try to find the best ways to give her the best possible instruction—interested groups are working on this all the time.

## The Course Plan

The course has been planned carefully to give students the information they need to know about the human body, health, various illnesses and their treatment, and the nursing skills used in the care of patients. The importance of a pleasing personality and of the nurse's personal development is emphasized. Above all, the student learns to center her attention on doing what is best for the individual patient.

Early in the course the students begin to work with patients, at first for a limited time each week and in a limited way. Hospital practice gradually increases. Instructors are with the students, supervising their work and conducting classes planned to help them apply to the care of patients what they have learned. You can see why this is important—it protects the patients and helps each student. The student always has a teacher to guide her and correct her mistakes until she is efficient and the patients are safe with her.

## Continuing Education

Much discussion goes on today about whether practical nursing is an end in itself or whether the LPN should be given the opportunity of becoming a registered nurse and if so, how this should be carried out. Many schools are developing challenge examinations and other means of evaluation which will enable the practical nurse to progress to another level without repeating the material she already knows.

## LICENSING FOR NURSES

### What a License Means

Licensing for any group of workers is important. *Licensing laws* protect the public from unqualified workers; they establish standards for any profession or occupation. A license helps people to tell the difference between a qualified and an unqualified worker in any kind of work.

Both professional and practical nurses are licensed to practice nursing. Every state, as well as the District of Columbia, Puerto Rico, Guam, Samoa and the Virgin Islands, has a licensing law for practical nurses. When a student (professional or practical nurse) has been graduated from an approved school, she is eligible to take the state licensing examination set up for her group, and, if she passes, she can use the title RN or LPN.

## The Registered Nurse

The nurse who passes the examination and pays the required registration fee becomes licensed under the title *registered nurse,* or *R.N.* She may have an Associate Degree, a diploma or a Baccalaureate or higher degree.

## The Licensed Practical Nurse

The practical nurse who passes the examination and pays the required registration fee becomes licensed under the title *licensed pratical nurse,* or *LPN.* There are 2 exceptions—in California and Texas the legal title is *licensed vocational nurse,* or *L.V.N.*

## The Licensing Laws

There are some differences in the licensing laws from state to state. For instance, in some states it is illegal for any nurse to practice nursing for pay without a license. If she does, she can be prosecuted. This is a *mandatory* law. In some states this affects only professional nurses.

In other states the law does not forbid practicing nursing without a license but does forbid using the title "licensed practical nurse" if the nurse does not have a license.

Does this mean that you have a choice between being licensed or unlicensed? Not really, because today a license is the passport to employment as a reputable practical nurse. It tells any prospective employer that you are a qualified person. Naturally, you cannot afford to be without this important credential, and the time is sure to come when a license will be essential in order to work in any state.

Some states operate under the so-called "grandfather clause," whereby under certain circumstances it is possible to take the licensure examination without attending a practical nursing program. However, it is advisable to check all details thoroughly and to make sure that licensure by this method is recognized in all areas of work and in all states.

# NURSING ORGANIZATIONS

## The NAPNES, Inc.

The National Association for Practical Nurse Education and Service was the first national nursing organization to concentrate all its efforts on the development and the improvement of practical nurse education, together with advancing the interests of practical nurses themselves. It was organized in 1941, with 20 members—membership is now in excess of 25,000.

**Membership.** The NAPNES has 3 types of membership:

1. Individual—open to professional nurse instructors and directors of practical nursing schools, licensed practical nurses, representatives of hospital, health and education groups and citizens interested in helping practical nursing to grow and to improve.

2. Per capita—open to members of state practical nurse associations voting a per capita assessment of dues.

3. Future (student)—open to students in approved practical nursing schools on a divided payment basis while they are in the school. Full membership is continued for a year after graduation at no extra cost.

This national nursing association has helped practical nursing grow. These are some of the things it does: it has a national office in New York City that answers inquiries about practical nursing; it sends a consultant to a state or group to help set up a practical nursing school; it publishes helpful leaflets and booklets; it publishes a list of the approved schools; it approves practical nursing schools that meet NAPNES standards and wish to have national approval; it publishes the magazine, *The Journal of Practical Nursing,* every month. It has helped practical nurses to organize their own state associations. It has a convention every year with special sessions for practicing practical nurses and for students.

## The NFLPN, Inc.

The National Federation of Licensed Practical Nurses was organized in 1949. It is a national membership organization for licensed practical nurses in the United States; membership is open to licensed practical nurses who are members in the individual state associations. Provision is made also for individual and associate membership. The stated objectives of the NFLPN are:

To work actively with allied groups and the public to help meet the health needs of our country.

To continue to work for state laws which would provide mandatory licensure for all who nurse for hire.

To continue to work for licensed practical nurse representation on state boards of nursing.

To seek recognition in all employing agencies for the legal title "Licensed Practical Nurse" and the recognition of practical nursing as a distinct vocation separate from that of auxiliary personnel.

To encourage state associations to promote group insurance plans for their members to provide protection in cases of illness or disability.

To encourage all employing agencies to provide in-service programs for the licensed practical nurses.

To strive to increase the quality and the quantity of well-prepared licensed practical nurses.

To formulate a plan on public relations to interpret the field of practical nursing to allied groups and the lay public.

To strive to improve communications to every member.

To work to improve leadership within the organization.

The Federation works with the state practical nurse associations to help them in organizational matters through institutes and workshops; also, it holds an annual convention for its thousands of members. Its official bimonthly publication is *Bedside Nurse.*

## The NLN

The National League for Nursing has accepted practical nurses as members since 1952. In 1956 a consultant in practical nursing was employed, and in 1957 a Council on Practical Nursing was established. In 1961 the Council was replaced by the creation of the Department of Practical Nursing. The NLN, through its Department of Evaluation Service, has developed a number of tests which are used widely by the practical nursing schools. Among these tests are a pre-entrance test, used as one indication of an applicant's eligibility for admission, and achievement tests such as NIP and TUC (Nursing Including Pharmacology and Three Units of Content) to be used during the course and on its completion. The Evaluation Service has developed also the state licensing examination currently used by the majority of state boards of nursing.

## The ANA

The American Nurses' Association is an organization for registered nurses only. The practical nurse should be aware of this organization, since it publishes several periodicals and a great deal of literature. The ANA often sponsors workshops which the practical nurse may be eligible to attend.

## The State Practical Nurse Associations

Practical nurses can be very proud of the work that they have done in starting their state associations. There is a state association of practical nurses in every state, in the District of Columbia and in Puerto Rico and the Virgin Islands. Each state association conducts an annual convention; most of them publish their own magazine every month. They have worked to get licensing laws if none existed and to improve existing laws. They have promoted workshops for their members and have provided scholarships for attendance at summer courses for selected members to train for organizational leadership.

**Extension Courses.** One of the outstanding accomplishments of the state practical nurse associations has been the promotion of extension courses for their members, many of whom are licensed practical nurses without training. These extension courses are open only to licensed practical nurses who have been doing practical nursing; they are not open to men or women who have never done nursing. Thousands of people have taken the 64-hour course and progressed to the 240-hour Education Units course. The outlines for these courses

were prepared by the NAPNES; the teachers are professional nurses. The state associations promote and handle registration of classes, arrange for the instructors and classroom facilities and see that the essential records are on file in the state office.

## A CODE OF ETHICS

The LPN is expected to abide by a code of ethics. The word *ethics* may be defined as the conduct appropriate for all members of a group. Such a code might include these points:

1. To conserve life and alleviate suffering and to promote health and preserve life. The nurse does not have the right to make judgments as to the taking of a life. Part of the nurse's responsibility is to be adequately prepared to assist in an emergency or in the usual hospital situation in such a way as to protect the patient against injury or death. Negligence or inability to perform one's duties is as unethical as performing a wrongful act.

2. To give nursing care which is not influenced or altered by the personality of the patient, his race, social status or religion or by any other external factor. The care given to all patients must be of the same quality, regardless of any personal considerations of the patient or of the nurse.

3. To maintain high standards of personal ethics in her personal life.

4. To keep up to date with nursing so as to be adequately prepared to give the best possible care to the patient. This includes attending in-service education meetings and maintaining active membership in practical nursing organizations, as well as reading the current nursing journals.

5. To keep confidential all information regarding the patient. Although information contained in a patient's chart may be subpoenaed by a court of law, the nurse never voluntarily divulges information of a confidential nature unless the patient's best interests require this to be done.

In answer to the patient's statement, "I will tell you something if you promise not to tell anyone," the nurse can indicate that she will keep the confidence only if it will not be dangerous to the physical or mental health of the patient. In almost every case, the patient will divulge the information anyway—he brought it up because he wanted to discuss it. If the nurse promises not to tell anyone and then is given critical information, she places herself in a difficult situation.

6. To do no damage to the public good. This

means not using her position as a nurse or her nursing uniform in any advertising or selling scheme or as a means of obtaining favors.

7. To be a responsible member of society by upholding the laws of that society.

8. To make some decisions about nursing care. She must not delegate duties to anyone who is not qualified to perform these duties. The practical nurse must also remember that she is always under the supervision of the RN or doctor.

9. To report pertinent information as soon as possible after she learns of it, so the patient will receive the best possible care.

10. To know her own limitations and not hesitate to request assistance when necessary. If the nurse does not know how to "look it up" herself, she should know whom to ask.

11. *Never* to participate in any unethical procedure.

12. Never to prescribe treatments or medications or take harmful drugs herself.

13. To carry out orders with the greatest skill possible. The nurse is expected to abide by the individual rules and regulations of her place of employment. If these rules and regulations are not in accordance with her code of personal ethics, she should discuss this with her supervisor. The nurse is also obligated to report unethical practices on the part of a person or institution to the appropriate authorities. It is as unethical to *avoid* reporting an illegal or unethical practice as it is to participate in this practice. Examples of such conduct include charging a patient for services not rendered, personally using drugs prescribed for a patient, working while intoxicated and personally taking or using supplies assigned to a patient.

14. To serve her employer loyally, give proper notice of resignation and give support to the aims of the institution.

15. Not to accept tips or gifts from patients. In special situations, the instructor should be consulted for suggestions as to how to handle this situation.

# 2

# Guides to Effective Learning

## BEHAVIORAL OBJECTIVES

*The student successfully attaining the goals of this chapter will be able to:*

- *describe the basic essentials relating to effective study habits and demonstrate utilization of these study methods.*
- *read meaningfully, take useful and comprehensive notes in class, utilize teaching machines and auto-tutorial equipment, practice effective problem-solving, and take tests in such a way as to enhance, rather than hinder, learning.*
- *participate actively in class projects, discussions, clinical and classroom laboratory experiences, and other learning situations.*
- *communicate effectively and kindly with co-workers and with patients and their visitors, as demonstrated through written and oral means, as well as in nonverbal interactions.*
- *begin to write or present orally a comprehensive and interesting nursing care study, which will enhance the education of the student doing the writing, as well as that of other students.*
- *discuss some of the ways in which the nurse's own opinion of self and of others can influence patient care.*

## GETTING YOUR BEARINGS

Whether you have just graduated from high school or have been out of school for some time, you will want to do your best in your basic nursing program. In the months ahead you will be learning many things: the technics of nursing; scientific facts about the human body and how it behaves in health and illness; rules and regulations of a hospital; methods of observing the patients under your care, which includes noting the patient's behavior and appearance and the effects of treatments; and ways of getting along with people—to mention only a few.

### Get the Facts

A textbook gives you essential information, but your instructors will refer you to other books, pamphlets and magazine articles which will add to your knowledge. The school library and the local community library provide excellent information resources. Radio and TV programs may serve as additional sources of information. You can find other information sources, but how will you know that the information is reliable? First, look at the source of the information: an expert or a recognized organization in any field speaks with authority and usually has the latest information.

### Learn by Observation

Observation means understanding as well as seeing. You observe for a purpose—to note the effects of a medicine or a treatment or the patient's physical and mental reactions. To do this effectively, you must know why a medicine or a treatment is given and note whether or not it accomplishes its purpose, as well as observing any other effects that it may have. In addition to being a "seeing eye" you must have the knowledge you need to make correct judgments. The nurse's observations of a patient's reactions and behavior are important as signs of the patient's progress toward recovery and may indicate the need for changes in his medical and nursing treatment.

## Learn by Practice

You learn nursing skills by observing how the instructor demonstrates nursing procedures and then by practicing these procedures, first in the classroom with your fellow students and then with actual patients in the hospital —always under the helpful supervision of an instructor. At the same time, the instructor will be showing you how to apply what you are learning in every subject to the care of each individual patient. This means that you must constantly practice combining many different kinds of information.

## Learn by Listening

Your instructors give you much information in classroom lectures (see How To Take Notes, p. 13. To get the most out of a lecture, come to class with your lesson assignment completed. Put everything else out of your mind and concentrate on the subject being discussed. A class period is the give-and-take session between instructor and students. The instructor interprets information and adds to it; she highlights important points and puts them in the right order; she ties them in with other facts that you have learned. Class discussion provides an opportunity to get facts straight and to ask for an explanation of puzzling points.

## Aids to Learning

**The Field Trip.** A field trip shows you some process at work. It may be a market, a health department, milk pasteurization or physical therapy. You get a clearer impression by seeing an operation than you do by reading about it. To make the most of a field trip, you must have some information before you go. Then you must know what to look for or you may not get the information you need. **A Word About Films.** Films, too, give you clearer impressions than reading, by showing you people and action. Films also show you places and things that are too far away to visit or impossible to observe firsthand. You will need to know why a film is shown to you and what to look for. Like a field trip, a film strengthens impressions you already have.

**Teaching Machines.** The nursing student, especially one who has been out of school for a few years, may feel overwhelmed by the large number and variety of teaching machines which are now in use. However, these aids to learning are usually easy to operate and to use, and most students enjoy learning in this manner, once they have become familiar with the equipment. The tape recorder, the filmstrip projector, the slide projector, the continuous film loop cassette projector and the movie projector are some of the widely used mechanical aids to learning.

**Role Playing.** This is a method by which the student is allowed to test solutions to problems before actually working with a real patient. The students act out the roles of patient and nurse and try various approaches and solutions to nursing problems.

## Self-Study Programs

Some schools have arranged their courses so as to allow the student to progress at her own rate of speed. In these programs the learning materials are identified, the instructors are available, and the student sets the pace. This plan offers a tremendous advantage: the student can ask questions when she needs to, can spend whatever time she needs on a specific topic and can advance at the rate best suited to her ability.

## How To Study

**Study Time and Place.** You are going to have a very full schedule for the next few months, so you will have to plan to use your study time to the best advantage to avoid falling behind in your work.

If you have been out of school for some time and are no longer in the habit of studying, it may be a little difficult at first to re-establish the habit. Or if you live at home, it may be hard to find a quiet place away from the family. A suitable place is important. It should be well-lighted, with space to write and to spread your books out conveniently and quiet enough so that you will not be distracted by the radio or TV or easily interrupted by questions or audible conversations. Family and friends should not disturb you while you are studying.

Assemble everything you need to work with before you settle down. Try to keep your work area neat, by having only the necessary items at hand. Simple comforts, such as a straight chair and a cool room, will help you to stay alert and concentrate.

Plan ahead. Don't waste time! Finish one thing before starting another; it is very difficult to concentrate if you skip around in studying. Take time out for a "breather" now and then. Finally, remember that your mind can absorb only so much at one sitting. After 3 hours of concentrated reading, at the most, you will have "had it," so to speak, and the longer you go on after that, the less you will retain.

## How Do You Read?

**Reading for a Purpose.** Reading for pleasure and reading for information are quite different. You can read a murder mystery and hardly notice what is going on around you, but your anatomy lesson requires a different type of concentration. Beyond the moment, it is not important to remember how the murderer was caught but you *must* remember how the digestive system functions. Therefore, different reading methods are necessary according to your purpose. Technical material requires more time because you will have to look up and learn technical terms. You will also need to make notes of important points if you are reading to get additional information about an assigned topic.

The system you use for going over a topic is important too. You can (1) read it over quickly once, to get the general idea; (2) read it again, paying close attention to each part and asking yourself questions about it as you go along so as to make sure you understand it; and (3) make a brief summary of the whole in your own words. Do steps 2 and 3 several times until you have mastered the sense of the subject. It will stay in your memory longer if you space the last 2 combined steps over several days instead of depending on a "cram job" the night before an examination.

## How To Take Notes

You fix information more firmly in your mind by making notes during your reading. The most logical way to do this is to follow an outline form with main headings and notations under each heading. Except for definitions, try to put the main ideas in your own words. Some guides for taking reading notes are:

1. Put down the topic heading. Under it note the main points, using subheadings if necessary, with enough information about each point to explain it.
2. Write down the title and the page of the reference in case you desire to refer to it again. It is often helpful to file this type of information on file cards, so it can be retrieved or rearranged more easily.
3. Include additional information that you have not found in any other reference.
4. Make a note of anything that puzzles you; this will serve as a reminder to yourself to bring it up in class or to ask your instructor about it.
5. Look up unfamiliar words in the dictionary; use your medical dictionary for technical terms. You will also find a glossary of medical terms and a list of combining forms (prefixes and suffixes) in your textbook. Make a list of such words and their definitions and use it as a quiz for yourself.
6. Occasionally it may be useful to study with a friend. You can informally "test" each other.

You will also take notes in class lectures. Some guides for this type of note taking are:

1. Try to follow an organized outline by making notes of the topics and the important points under each one. Your instructor will make this easier for you by emphasizing them or by writing them on the chalkboard as she talks.
2. Try to take down the "sense" of what the instructor is saying. If you try to include every word you may miss the point entirely.
3. Put a question mark after anything that is not clear to you so you can ask about it before the class is over.
4. If necessary, rewrite your notes after taking them in class. This will help also to establish the information firmly in your mind.
5. Check your notes for usefulness. They should help you to review a subject and by that standard should give you correct information as well as enough information. They should be arranged in a logical order—a notebook full of disorganized writing is a waste of time.

## How To Solve a Problem

There are guides that you can use in solving a problem. The first one is to be sure that you *know exactly what the problem is.* Examine the facts critically and try to define the difficulty and its causes. Then think of all the *possible answers* and what each one holds for accomplishing your purpose. Try to determine which solution will be the most satisfactory with the least disturbance to anyone else. Use your reasoning powers and put your emotions aside. If another person is involved consider his side and try to imagine how each possible solution will affect others.

You must be wise enough also to know when you are confronted with a problem which you cannot handle alone. You may not have the necessary authority to carry out the solution, or there may be angles that you do not understand fully. It may be that you need the help of your head nurse or your instructor. At this point, you can take your problem to the proper person for assistance.

Remember, then, that it requires both logical thinking and imagination to solve a problem, using what you have learned from your past experience and being able to know when you cannot solve a particular problem without help.

## Tests and Examinations

**Objective Tests.** The most commonly used "pencil and paper" examination is the objective test which is answered with check marks or fill-ins. While this type of test requires very little writing, it calls for a great deal of thinking. It consists of various forms of questions or statements such as the following:

*Multiple choice*—you select the answer from a list of several, only one of which is correct.

*Example:* The recommended method for losing weight is to_____
1. Avoid eating breakfast.
2. Go on a banana diet.
3. Consult your doctor about a diet.
4. Limit your diet to 500 calories a day.

*True-false*—you are given a statement which you check as right or wrong.

*Example:* The pancreas is part of the urinary system. T__ F__

*Completion*—you fill in the missing word or words in a sentence to make it a true statement.

*Example:* The temperature of the water for a hot-water bag should not be higher than _____ degrees.

*Matching*—you are given 2 columns of words or phrases and asked to match each item in the first column with the related item in the second column.

These examples may not mean much now, since you do not have the information necessary to answer the questions, but they show you some of the types of examinations to expect.

**Essay Tests.** One other type of question should be mentioned—the essay. For example, you may be asked to write in a few sentences or in a paragraph how you would handle a certain nursing problem in a given situation. This type of question requires the ability to express ideas clearly and briefly. Plan your answers before you write—this will help relieve any tension or anxiety you may have about the test. Underline important points so the instructor will not miss them when she is grading your paper. Write legibly—the instructor will have difficulty understanding an answer which she cannot read. Also remember that the instructor would prefer to read a short, correct response, rather than sift through a mass of words to find the answer.

**The State Board Examination.** The state board examination is the test which you will take after graduation from an approved practical nursing program. If you successfully complete this examination, you will be legally allowed to use the title, Licensed Practical Nurse. To help give you practice in answering the kinds of questions asked in this examination, your school will probably include similar types of questions in the tests given throughout your course of study.

**Machine-Scored Answer Sheets.** If you have been out of school for a while, you may not have seen answer sheets which are scored by machine. The use of this method of scoring gives your instructors more time to assist you with problems in your school work, since they are freed from the tedious task of correcting by hand. Your instructor will show you how to take these tests.

**Clinical Evaluation.** In addition to taking written tests on your course work, you will be evaluated on your clinical work. Your clinical grade will be based on factors such as performance in carrying out nursing procedures, attitude, reactions to criticism, efforts to improve, ability to get along with people, appearance, health habits, punctuality, dependability, nursing ethics, and day-by-day responses in class. The final grade is based on a composite of all these ratings. Be thankful for tests and ratings! They are the checks and balances that steady you: they indicate strengths, weaknesses and areas where improvement is needed.

## PROCESSES USED IN LEARNING

### Communications

Communication means giving information and sharing thoughts and ideas. To be proficient in the art of communication means being able to convey to others what you mean so that it will be understood. It also means being sensitive to what others are trying to tell you, verbally or otherwise. We are apt to think of communication as mainly verbal, but a great deal of communication goes on by means of gestures, actions, manner and facial expressions.

A nurse needs to be especially sensitive to such communications from her patients or co-workers. For instance, a patient may not *say* anything when you explain a treatment you are about to give, yet his eyes may tell you he is afraid.

If you listen, observe and ask questions you will be an effective communicator. In most instances, you should *listen* rather than talk. One of your functions as a nurse is to record pertinent information about your patient; you cannot do this if you are doing all the talking.

### Effective Speech

Since we do depend on *speech* to a great extent to put an idea across, its effectiveness is influenced not only by *what* we say but also by *how* we say it. Try to answer a patient's questions or to explain a procedure in plain, everyday language, using as few technical terms as possible. Your medical and nursing

vocabulary will be unfamiliar to him. Your tone of voice is also very important. Never "talk down" to the patient.

Pay him the courtesy of addressing him as "Mr. Wright"—don't call him "grandpa" or "dear," even if he is 80 years old and seems like a dear old man to you. Above all, avoid the habit (which seems all too common) of phrasing your questions in the plural, such as "How are *we* feeling this morning?" or "*We* didn't eat all of *our* breakfast, did *we?*" Sound as if you are really interested in how the patient feels and in what he tells you. If you are hurried (as you easily may be), try not to let the pressure show in your voice or actions.

### Effective Writing

Writing is a means of communication you will use often in recording your observations of patients, in taking notes and in writing reports. Therefore, you must be able to say what you mean clearly and concisely. An adequate vocabulary and a command of simple English will help you here. Legible writing is a necessity, since you will be required to fill out forms and record your observations on patients' charts. Most hospitals have adopted printing as the acceptable form for keeping patients' records. Of course, correct spelling is a part of effective writing. Even a minor deviation from correct spelling in your charting may make a life-and-death difference to your patient. If you are unsure of the spelling or exact meaning of a word, "look it up." It is worth the extra time and effort to the health and well-being of your patient.

### How We Remember

The average person literally stores volumes of information in his brain. This is his *memory stock* which consists of lifetime or permanent memories, such as his name and address, the multiplication tables, rules of grammar, important events in his life and knowledge he uses every day in his job. He also has a short-term memory made up of passing bits of information, such as the name of someone he is introduced to casually, which he makes little or no effort to remember beyond the moment.

Opinions differ about how memory operates. One school of thought believes that every impression the brain receives makes a tiny pathway in the brain; another says chemistry or electricity enters into it. They believe that electrical impulses pass along a memory path from time to time, even when we are not trying to stimulate them, and help to strengthen the memory. Time, then, would also strengthen it. This could explain why elderly people often remember things that happened to them in childhood more clearly than they remember recent events. Whatever the process, we have reliable proof that everything we hear, see or experience leaves some sort of impression on the brain. The problem is how to get it off the shelf!

The situation is not hopeless—learning to remember is a skill, just as learning to write is a skill; like any skill it takes perseverance and practice to develop, but there are rules to help you. To begin with, your memory of anything depends largely on the strength of the impression it made on your brain. This, in turn, will depend on how interested you were in remembering it, how much you needed to remember it, the effect it had on your life or how striking or unusual it was. Any one of these conditions or a combination of them will tend to make the impression deep and lasting.

If we look at many ordinary things without really seeing them because we are not consciously observing them, the impression is not very strong. So the *first* rule is to observe carefully. The *second* rule is to pay attention to directions by looking at the person giving them and listening carefully. The *third* rule is to decide what is important to remember. We remember what we wish to remember. Deciding that something is important helps to fix it in the mind. The *fourth* rule has to do with repetition; the more you go over an idea, the better your memory of it will be. The best time for doing this is immediately after a new fact is presented because forgetting is also going on even as you learn.

Take into account the things that make you forget. If you are tired, worried or out-of-sorts, your memory lags—this is no time to study. People devise tricks to help themselves remember. This is permissible as long as the devices do not become so complicated that you cannot remember what they were supposed to remind you of!

## THE NURSING CARE STUDY

A nursing care study is a report about a selected patient with whom you have worked. It is the story of your observations of a person throughout his illness—it includes such things as treatments, tests, diet, medicines, x-rays and nursing care—and tells how they affected the patient. A nursing care study will show how well you understood the reasons for specific treatments or medications. It will also show how keenly you were aware of the patient as a person in trouble and how well you were able to identify and meet the patient's needs.

To begin with, give the patient a name. If you must invent one, avoid such old perennials as "Smith" or "Jones." Much of your information is taken from the patient's chart, and to really make him a person this information must be personalized and put into phrases and sentences, otherwise, he will seem like a robot, operated by push buttons. Compare these 2 beginnings for a nursing care study:
*This?*
"A male, aged 52, admitted by ambulance. Patient weak, pale, skin cold, pulse rapid, heat applied."
*Or This?*
"Mr. Daly, a 52-year-old farmer, was admitted to Ward D by ambulance, after falling from a ladder in his barn. He was unable to help himself in getting into bed; he was pale and his skin was cold; his pulse was 130 and slightly irregular. Hot-water bags and warm blankets were applied at once and he was given 1/6 gr. of morphine, since he was having a great deal of pain."

Which is the more interesting? Which sounds as if it were about a real person? The first example is an accurate record of the facts, and it might have been copied word for word from the chart, but it is the record of a faceless male. In the second example, the "male, aged 52," comes to life as "Mr. Daly." You can picture this middle-aged man. Perhaps you know someone like him; you are interested in what happens to him. You want to know how he felt—did he get warm, did his pulse slow down, was his pain relieved? Did the nurse have any problems in giving him nursing care and how did she handle them? Did he improve—slowly, rapidly or not at all? How long was he hospitalized? Who would look after him when he was discharged? Did this person have instructions about his care? From whom?

Finally, your nursing care study may be read by other nurses who hope to find in it some suggestions to help them in their care of patients. It is doubly important, then, that you make them want to read it and that you tell them the things they want to know. The surest way to do this is to make them feel that you are writing about a *person*.

Your instructor may give you an outline to use as a guide in writing a nursing care study. It might include such points as:

1. The patient's *background* (his age, occupation, family situation, economic status, past experience with illness)

2. His *present illness* (how it developed, the symptoms, treatments and medications and their effects, any complications that developed and what was done about them)

3. His *nursing care* (reassurance of the patient, problems that came up and how they were handled, restorative nursing measures used)

## INTERPERSONAL RELATIONSHIPS

### Understanding Yourself

Your success as a nurse (and as a person) will depend on your ability to get along with people; you begin to develop this ability by learning to understand your own behavior and the reasons for it. Take a good honest look at your actions and the motives behind them—it will help you to understand similar actions and motives in others. This is hard to do because it means being willing to admit your imperfections, no matter how much it makes you squirm. Then you must make up your mind you will change and set about doing it.

Patients are understandably apprehensive about what may happen to them; they want (and need) a nurse who is steadfast, kind and reassuring—one who appreciates their problems and is someone they can lean on and trust. This does not mean that you will agonize with the patient in his suffering, for if you become so emotionally involved that you suffer too much, you will be useless in helping him.

### The Patient's Point of View

Many of the services a nurse gives to a patient are highly personal; some of them might seem personally distasteful if you did not know that they are essential to his recovery and are a necessary part of nursing care. What about the patient? No doubt he is embarrassed and humiliated because you must bring him a bedpan and change his bed if he is incontinent. His distress is lessened when he sees that you do not seem to find such services distasteful. He will be grateful also for your consideration in dealing with handicaps. Your attitude toward the patient is reflected to the patient's family, who need the reassurance provided by your genuine interest in the patient and your skillful nursing care.

### Patients Are People

It is always a great temptation to place the blame on a patient or to label him "difficult" if he resists your efforts to carry out the orders prescribed for him. There are 2 sides to this picture. First of all, the patient is a person—illness is one more problem added to those he may have already. He may seem uncooperative, but he is doing only what seems natural to him. Think of the adjustments he is expected to make: to let himself be waited on, to change his eating habits, to put up with pain and discomfort. These are problems he must handle in addition to his personal worries—his job, the payments on the house or rent, the care of children, his new expenses—is it any wonder that he seems to be difficult?

Another thing—it is quite possible that the patient thinks that you are the one who is being difficult. You give him baths he does not want, bring him milk when he longs for beer, stick him with needles every day and interfere with his life in a dozen ways. Does he stop to think that you are only following the doctor's orders? On the contrary, it seems logical to him that you are to blame because you are the one who does the things that upset him, yet at the same time he must depend on you to help him. Or if there is a language problem, he might think it is your fault that he does not understand what you are saying.

# 3

# Basic Needs of All People

BEHAVIORAL OBJECTIVES

*The student successfully attaining the goals of this chapter will be able to:*
- *discuss the basic needs of all people and describe how the nurse may assist people to meet these basic needs or those special needs which result from illness or age.*
- *describe specific needs of the family and of the community in relation to health and illness.*

There are certain basic needs which must be met to maintain life. These basic needs are common to all people throughout the world, whether old or young, well or ill. And it is only after these needs have been met that the individual gives consideration to other non-essential needs. Of course factors such as age, emotional status, and illness may modify these needs. For example, Fred Whitehouse, a specialist dealing with the needs of the aged, defines the basic needs of this age group as:

*Not* to function is to die.
*Not* to be physically active brings atrophy.
*Not* to have purpose generates despair.

However, basic needs are generally defined in more specific terms. Dr. A. H. Maslow, a psychologist, has offered his definition of the hierarchy of basic needs. He states that "a need once fulfilled is no longer motivating." He goes on to say that the individual moves up the hierarchy of needs from bottom to top, first fulfilling physiological needs, such as obtaining food, shelter, oxygen, warmth and sleep, and then attempting to satisfy emotional needs such as the need for security, the need for belonging and being accepted, the need for self-esteem, the need to reach his creative potential and the need to know and to understand. At the top are the needs of the highest order: the needs for beauty, cleanliness and consistency of feeling and acting.

Stating Dr. Maslow's theory in different words—the person who is hungry will not be concerned about cleanliness or learning until he is fed; the person who is in pain will not be concerned about personal appearance until the pain is relieved; the preoperative patient will not be adequately prepared for his operation unless he feels safe and secure. This concept has implications for personal and family life, as well as for nursing.

This chapter will acquaint you with the basic needs of all people. Later chapters will discuss the special needs of the person who is ill.

## THE INDIVIDUAL'S NEEDS

**Physiological Needs.** Every person needs to have enough food and water to sustain life, as well as enough oxygen, rest and sleep. He must also be provided with shelter and body cover appropriate to his specific environment. Elimination of wastes from the body is necessary to maintain the balance of the body systems and to prevent disease or disorders caused by the accumulation of waste products. All body systems must be functioning in order to sustain life and to allow the pursuit of other needs.

**Sex Needs.** Sexual gratification must be obtained even if vicariously. Unlike other needs on this level, this need may be sublimated.

**Safety Needs.** One must feel secure, both physically and emotionally, before he can be comfortable enough within himself to move on to meet other needs.

**Social Needs.** Each person needs to feel accepted and loved by his family and friends.

**Ego Needs.** Each person must feel that he is worthwhile and important. He must possess "positive self-esteem." If this is not the case, serious personality disorders can result.

**Self-fulfillment Needs.** When a person is secure enough within himself and has met his physiological needs, he can begin to fulfill his creative needs, as already described.

**Cognitive Needs.** It also holds true that learning and understanding can begin to develop only after the physiological needs have been met.

**Esthetic and Consistency Needs.** Highest in the hierarchy are the *esthetic* needs—the need for beauty and order—and the *consistency* need—the need for a certain amount of sameness in daily living.

Many nonessential needs may be met in ways which differ more or less from those followed by most people. Some of these ways may be considered abnormal by most people. Everyone, however, tries to fulfill his needs insofar as he can.

## THE FAMILY'S NEEDS

The family has needs that differ from those of its individual members. The family unit should remain intact as far as possible; of course, this often cannot be done when one member is ill. By encouraging visitors, by assisting the patient to work out financial or child-care problems, and by assisting with referral to the proper hospital and community agencies, the nurse contributes to the integrity of the family unit.

Whenever possible, the members of the family should be included in the nursing care of the patient and should always be informed about his progress. In such ways, they are helped to feel a part of the patient's total care and rehabilitation.

## THE COMMUNITY'S NEEDS

The community has basic needs for the welfare of all its residents. Among these needs are public health measures (such as vaccination programs), access to health care, maintenance services (such as water and electricity), and emergency services (such as offered by firemen and the police).

## THE INDIVIDUAL'S RESPONSE TO ILLNESS

The purpose of this discussion about basic needs is to enable you to recognize and appreciate the special needs of the sick person. If you have ever been in the hospital, you know how it feels to surrender your clothes, your belongings and your individuality and to follow orders about when to eat, sleep and take a bath and even when to go to the bathroom. You can do much to prevent the patient's feeling dehumanized—whether you are giving care in the hospital, in his home or in the doctor's office. If you will always think of the patient as a person whose need for physical and emotional support is greater than normal because he is sick, and if you will emphasize his strengths rather than his weaknesses, you will do much toward aiding in his recovery.

# Unit 2:
# Personal and Environmental Health

4. *Over-all Health Aspects*
5. *Personality and Health*
6. *Community Health*
7. *Microbes and Man*

# Over-All Health Aspects

If Americans had to choose between health and money, they would choose health, although many of them do not know what health really is. Of course everybody wants bright eyes, firm muscles and that "on top of the world" feeling. These, however, are only the signs of health. Many people think that health is not being sick. Health education, on the other hand, teaches us what good health is and how to make the most of our individual possibilities. It is important to know what good health is before you begin to work with sick people; you can understand illness only by knowing first what being well is. This part of the book gives you information about health which you need as a citizen, a person and a nurse.

## A DEFINITION OF HEALTH

The World Health Organization was set up on the principle that the health of every nation is part of the foundation in building the kind of world we want. This is how it defines health:

Health is a state of complete physical, mental and social well-being and not merely the absence of disease or infirmity.

The enjoyment of the highest attainable standard of health is one of the fundamental rights of every human being without distinction of race, religion, political belief, economic or social condition.

The health of all people is fundamental to the attainment of peace and security and is dependent upon the fullest cooperation of individuals and states.

## HEALTH AND HEREDITY

Comparatively few diseases are known to be inherited. It is true that it is possible to inherit a susceptibility to disease of certain parts of the body, such as the lungs, kidneys or heart, or a predisposition to allergies.

Many community resources exist to help educate and care for persons with congenital and inherited health problems.

### Congenital Defects

Certain abnormalities and unusual conditions such as color blindness, deaf-mutism and Down's syndrome are known to be inherited.

It is well to point out here that some babies are born with defects that are not due to heredity but are the result of some interference with the baby's prenatal development. These congenital defects may be due to infectious diseases or injuries to the mother during pregnancy or to certain chemical substances taken during that time.

## Inherited Mental Ability

Mental ability is inherited, but if it is not used, it does not develop to its fullest extent. A person with a high degree of mental ability may not be as successful in life as his friend who works harder and so makes the most of a less brilliant mental inheritance.

## Total Health

Health is much more than brushing your teeth or taking baths and vitamins. It includes your thoughts and feelings, and it influences your efficiency and your relations with other people. This applies to your patients too. So we must consider health in its broadest meaning, or *total health,* which includes:

*Social Health:* A sense of responsibility for the health and welfare of others

*Physical Health:* Physical fitness—the body functioning at its best

*Mental Health:* A mind that grows, reasons and adjusts

*Emotional Health:* Feelings and actions that bring satisfaction

*Spiritual Health:* Inner peace and security in spiritual faith

## PSYCHOLOGY AND BEHAVIOR

Psychology is the study of the mental processes that direct behavior. Our mental and emotional health is measured by our behavior. Psychologists have taught us that a person uses both his conscious and his subconscious mind to direct his actions. By studying the ways people behave, it has been found that there are certain patterns people follow to satisfy essential basic needs of the body, mind and spirit.

## MENTAL ILLNESS

People with difficulties that affect the mind are sick people, as truly as if they had physical ailments. It is old-fashioned today to think that mental illness is mysterious and unusual. Thousands of people in the United States are in mental hospitals for special treatment; many of them recover and go back to normal lives. Modern medicine recognizes the difficulties that people meet and has devised ways of helping people to adjust to a complicated world. This special field of medicine is called *psychiatry.* The doctor is called a *psychiatrist.*

The *mind* is the part of us that makes decisions. People who are unable to make the decisions that help them to carry on as independent human beings and to fit into the world are mentally ill. There are different kinds of mental illness, many of which are related to physical disorders or conditions. Tumors and injuries destroy brain tissues; syphilis organisms have the same effect. As people age, brain tissue sometimes loses its normal qualities. During the menopause, disturbances of the hormone balance in the body may cause mental disorders.

## Effect of Emotions

Another type of mental illness is caused by emotional disturbances. The psychologist is concerned with finding the reasons for emotional difficulties, for when a person's behavior becomes so abnormal that he cannot lead a reasonably normal life or may injure other people, he is mentally ill. There are degrees of this kind of mental illness and many people we work with and know, while they are not ill, are not mentally healthy. Some of the people with poor mental health become mentally ill; others continue leading unsatisfactory lives. We need more psychiatrists to treat mentally ill patients. Most of us probably could improve our mental health—as we said before, the difference between poor mental health and mental illness is just a difference in the degree of satisfactory adjustment to life.

## POSITIVE HEALTH

Good health means that your body, your mind and your emotions are working efficiently, in proper balance. Doctors give a great deal of attention to the effects of mental and emotional attitudes on the body. They find that some people complain of pain which can be traced to emotional difficulties. A doctor's business is to keep the body in working order, but to correct physical difficulties, he must first discover their cause. This means that he must consider everything about the patient. This kind of treatment is not new, but it has a comparatively new name: *psychosomatic medicine.* (*Psycho* means mind, *somatic* means body.) Remember that this principle applies to nursing, too; so think of your patients as *people,* not as *cases.*

# 5

# Health and Personality

## BEHAVIORAL OBJECTIVES

*The student successfully attaining the goals of this chapter will be able to:*

- *describe what is meant by good personal health and exemplify a belief in this premise through the use of positive health habits and through good patient teaching in this area.*
- *demonstrate a knowledge of good posture and effective body mechanics when carrying out everyday activities and when giving nursing care.*
- *maintain good personal hygiene as demonstrated by cleanliness and proper care of the total body.*
- *trace the development of people's personality and use this study as a basis for evaluating and improving one's own personality and interpersonal relationships.*
- *show evidence of maturity and positive mental health in his or her everyday life, in the giving of helpful nursing care, and by healthy reactions to stress or to emergency situations.*

## HEALTH

You may think that already you have heard enough about personal health to last the rest of your life, but good health habits are worth emphasizing, even more so in a career like nursing where they can seriously affect your efficiency and the impression you create. They can help or hinder you physically—nursing is hard work; and they can also affect you mentally—you are sure to be upset if you do not make a good impression on the people whom you meet and with whom you work.

Health might be given more serious attention if people realized how much it affects the way they look. Admit it or not, everybody wants to be attractive. Personal attractiveness begins with good grooming, which is based on good health habits. The most expensive cosmetics will not offset the impression left by dull and dirty hair, greasy skin and slouching posture. Good health habits can help you to make the most of your assets—knowing that you look and feel your best will give you poise and confidence. It will also help to give others

confidence in you, for everyone likes to be with people who are well groomed. Attention to your health habits will pay dividends in popularity.

### Posture

The way you stand, sit or move affects your efficiency and the impression you create. Good posture improves your health—you breathe better, your circulation and muscle tone are improved, you save energy and prevent muscle strain. These are only part of the benefits. Good posture makes you look taller and slimmer, pulls you in at the waist, lifts your chest and keeps the parts of your body in balance. It gives you poise and grace; one of the first things a professional model learns is how to stand, sit and move gracefully and easily.

*Posture* is the position of your body—the way its parts are lined up when you stand, sit, move or when you are lying down. You use your muscles to keep your body in good alignment. Think of your spine as a set of building

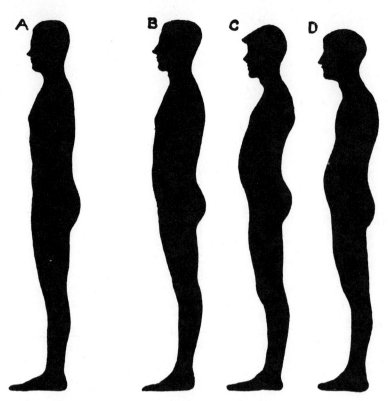

FIGURE 5-1. Posture. *A* shows the body in good posture; *B*, *C* and *D* in increasingly poorer posture. (Harvard University Chart)

blocks (*the vertebrae*) set one above the other and held together by strong bands of elastic tissue (*the muscles*) which can be made to stretch or contract to keep your body in line. Correct use of muscles is the secret of good posture. Nature has provided the appropriate muscles for every body movement, but the use you make of them is up to you. Poor posture overstrains some muscles and over-relaxes others. One authority compares good and poor posture in this way: (See Fig. 5-1.)

| Good Posture (Fig. A) | Poor Posture (Figs. B, C, D) |
|---|---|
| Head erect with chin drawn in | Head projecting forward |
| Chest lifted | Chest flat |
| Shoulders back resting on spine | Shoulders curved forward |
| Lower abdomen flat, upper abdomen full | Abdomen protruding |
| Natural curves of back | Exaggerated natural curves |
| Toes pointing straight ahead, weight on outer borders of feet | Weight carried on inner borders of feet, toes pointing too far inward or outward |

## The Way You Sit

To sit slouched in your seat, head down, chest collapsed, abdomen protruding, is very tiring. This position interferes with your breathing, strains your neck and back muscles and throws your weight on the end of your spine. Good posture is considerably more restful once it becomes a habit. Try sitting well back in your chair, with your spine straight, your head erect and your feet flat on the floor. Naturally, it will take time and perseverance to change a bad habit, but the improvement in the way you look and feel will be worth it.

## Bending and Sitting

Many nurses are not aware of how they look to others as they move about. When wearing a short skirt, you should bend at the knees rather than at the waist. When sitting, arrange your legs so that neither the tops of your hose nor the bottom of your girdle shows. It is often more comfortable to do nursing care in a pants uniform, if it is allowed.

## Body Mechanics

The human body is like a machine with many parts. To be efficient these parts must work together. The operation of this machine—the way you use your body in any activity—is equally important. Since you want to move with the least amount of strain, you must use your muscles effectively, making the longest and the strongest muscles do the work. For example, a look at the anatomy charts will tell you there are no long, strong muscles in the lower part of the back, but you do find such muscles in the arms and legs. Therefore, to avoid back strain you lift with your arms and legs.

## Lifting and Moving

Lifting, moving and carrying are daily activities that can be very tiring if we do not know how to save energy. Some methods are more effective than others because they are based on physical laws that never change. From these laws we learn that:

It is easier to pull, push or roll an object than it is to lift it.

*Reason: In lifting, you have to overcome the pull of gravity.*

It takes less effort to lift or move an object if you work as close to it as possible. Use your leg muscles as much as possible, and your back muscles as little as possible.

*Reason: This brings your center of gravity and that of the object closer together, and the stronger muscles are in the legs.*

Rocking backward or forward on your feet uses your body weight as a force for pulling or pushing.

*Reason: This lessens the strain on your arms and back.*

A nurse is expected to be able to help her patients to use good body mechanics. The first step is to practice good body mechanics herself.

## Food and Health

Food is important for health since life could not go on without it. In Chapter 22 of this book you will learn about essential foods and the use of food in the body. Study it carefully for it applies to you personally as well as to patients. You will learn that individual nutritional needs vary in some respects, depending upon body build, age or activity, and that people's eating habits (including your own) are affected by their work habits. In spite of these variations, everyone needs certain food materials to keep the body functioning and in good repair. Certainly, to work effectively and as a health teacher, a nurse should understand and practice good nutrition.

## Elimination Habits

Your intestinal tract works efficiently to get rid of waste if you cooperate. The intestine has to be stretched to start the motions that push out waste. The woody fibers in vegetables and fruits supply bulk, or roughage, so you need both vegetables and fruits in your diet. When the nerve impulses in the rectum indicate that waste is ready to be emptied, they should be heeded. The habit of emptying the rectum at a definite time every day helps to prevent constipation. There is nothing to worry about if you regularly do this as infrequently as every 2 or 3 days—some people's intestines move more slowly than others.

**Fluids.** You can help your kidneys to do their work efficiently by drinking enough fluids to keep up your body's water supply. Periodic health examinations, including urinalysis, are checkups to discover disturbances early enough to prevent serious damage. You should consult a doctor immediately if any symptoms of disturbance show in the urine itself or in connection with voiding. Unusual swelling in any part of the body, headaches, dizziness or sight disturbances or shortness of breath are danger signals that you should report to your doctor at once.

## DENTAL HEALTH

In spite of the advances in knowledge concerning the causes of dental health problems, dental services to correct or prevent such problems are not reaching many of the people who need them most. Young people, especially, seem to be the victims of dental neglect—the percentage of high school pupils with dental caries is far too high for comfort. School health programs should include dental examinations but many times do not.

## Water Fluoridation

The effects of fluorine in preventing tooth decay first became known in 1902, when a dentist in Colorado Springs became curious about the brown stains on the teeth of some of his patients. As he studied this condition of "mottled enamel," as he called it, he discovered that it was caused by excessive fluorine in the drinking water. However, the interesting thing was that he found also that the people with the brown stains had less tooth decay. As a result of his study and of other research, it has been proven also that a dilute solution of sodium fluoride swabbed on children's teeth aids resistance to tooth decay.

An important outcome of this discovery is the water fluoridation program. A community can test its water supply, and if it is deficient in fluorine, fluorides can be added. It is estimated that 1 part fluoride to a million parts of water is an effective amount. Fluorides are available in toothpaste, bottled water or in tablets. However, the cheapest and most effective way to supply them is by fluoridation of a community water supply.

**The Fluoridation Controversy.** Approximately 51 million Americans are now drinking fluoridated water. Fluoridation has been approved by such outstanding authorities as the U.S. Public Health Service, the American Public Health Association, the World Health Association, the American Medical Association and many more. However, its acceptance as desirable is far from unanimous. As a result many communities are still without fluoridated water.

## Effects of Diet on Teeth

Diet is very important when the teeth are forming. For the first 6 to 8 years of life, the minerals, calcium and phosphorus, and the vitamins A, C and D are essential to form normal teeth. Once the teeth are formed, starches and sugars are the only foods that have any effect on them—unfortunately, that effect is harmful. Diet also affects the gums and the jaws. If the vitamin and the mineral supply are inadequate, the jaw bones become porous and the teeth loosen; the gum tissues may become diseased.

In all age groups diet affects dental health. Nutrition for young children may be inade-quate in almost every type of family today. The enormous consumption of candy bars and other sweets interferes with nutrition in teen-age and older groups.

## YOUR OWN EYES

Two things are important: know the signs of eye difficulty and consult an eye specialist for help. He is an *ophthalmologist,* or *oculist,* a physician especially trained in the care of eye disorders and the correction of vision difficulties. Because he is a physician also, he considers eye problems in relation to the body as a whole. The *optician,* grinds lenses and fills prescriptions for glasses, and the *optometrist,* is qualified to test for and correct errors in refraction.

Danger signs that should send you to an eye specialist are: persistent headaches, painful, watery, inflamed eyes, eye discharges and visual disturbances. To take chances with your eyesight is to risk serious interference with your career.

Wash your hands before touching your eyes to avoid introducing infection. If something gets into your eye, do not rub it—you may only scratch your eyeball or embed a particle in the tissue. If tear secretions do not wash it out, consult a doctor. Oculists discourage the use of an eye cup because of the danger of infection; the preparations advertised as effective in brightening and rejuvenating the eyes are probably harmless in themselves. One danger in using eyewashes is that you may be harming your eyes by using them as a substitute for needed medical attention.

## YOUR UNIFORM

The patient's first impression of the nurse is usually based mainly on her appearance. A clean pressed uniform and polished shoes are important to that first impression. Full uniform should be worn when the nurse is on duty; this includes cap, watch and any accessories required by the school.

You should wear little or no jewelry while on duty. A ring might scratch a patient, collect bacteria and hinder effective handwashing. Dangling earrings are not professional-looking and distract from your appearance. Pierced earrings, if worn, should be very small.

## MENSTRUAL HEALTH HABITS

*Menstruation* is a normal process. During your menstrual period you should be able to exercise, take baths and live as you normally would. In fact, doctors recommend following the usual routine with special attention to cleanliness to prevent body odor. They also endorse using vaginal tampons (instead of pads), provided they are changed often enough to prevent irritation. As a rule, they do not recommend douches after menstruation as vaginal irrigation is not necessary for a normal, healthy vagina.

Try to relax when your menstrual period is due and avoid the "cramps" caused by tense muscles. Heat over the pelvic area often relieves minor discomforts. Of course it is possible for an anatomical or functional irregularity to cause menstrual difficulties. If pains or backache are persistent or severe enough to incapacitate you, consult a doctor for examination and advice.

### Consult a Doctor

Consult your doctor about any of the following irregularities:

1. Vaginal bleeding between periods.
2. Vaginal bleeding after the menopause.
3. Excessive menstrual flow.
4. Absence of menstruation before the usual time menopause would be expected. (Exceptions are during pregnancy and sometimes while breast-feeding a baby.)

And remember, after 20, a yearly gynecological examination should be routine for *every woman* for early discovery and treatment of actual or potential malignant conditions.

## EXERCISE AND REST

### Exercise

If body tissues are not used, they atrophy and die. One of the reasons for exercise is to maintain muscle tone so we need some variety in exercise to benefit muscles in different parts of the body. An individual's age, occupation and general condition help to determine the amount and kind of exercise that is best for him. Sports provide exercise and fun and relaxation at the same time. However, walking, gardening and household activities also exercise both large and small muscles. Nursing activities—bending, lifting, stretching, walking—provide exercise every day. A moderate amount of daily exercise is better than occasional spurts of strenuous activity. In general, we are told that up to 40, exercise should be enough to promote muscle growth, and after that enough to maintain muscle tone.

### Sleep, Rest and Relaxation

Everyone does not need the same amount of sleep. You can tell if you are getting enough if you wake up rested and ready to go. You can expect some fatigue after a healthy day's work, but it should be normally nothing that a good night's sleep will not cure. If you are chronically tired, something is wrong, and you need medical advice. Sometimes after a day's work, rest is needed rather than sleep. Try lying relaxed and letting your thoughts drift. A change of activity or watching television, listening to the radio or reading is also restful.

## PERSONALITY

Perhaps one of the reasons you gave for wanting to be a nurse is the desire to "work with people." Life is not easy, and people often are hard to understand, but you have to take both as you find them. When working with people, it is necessary to know how to get along with them. Why do some people succeed and others fail? Because the successful ones know how to make people feel comfortable, and the others do not. We all have to change to fit ourselves in. Your personality can help or hinder you.

### What Personality Is

Personality begins when a baby is conceived —the parents give a child physical characteristics and mental ability. Nature also has a part in it—a body defect, such as blindness, for example, will influence personality. As soon as the baby is born, he begins to shape his personality as he struggles with his small world. Food, illnesses, playmates, experiences at school and contacts with religion affect him all his life. His personality will show how successfully he has handled his problems. His home life and the personalities of his parents affect him more than anything else. He needs to be safe, with people who care about him, feed him and keep him comfortable and happy in a pleasant, friendly place where people like each other.

## What Maturity Is

As an adult you are expected to behave like one. Laws set an age when you are permitted to drive a car, get married or vote. This means it is taken for granted that people grow wiser as they grow older. However, *maturity* is not necessarily based upon chronological age. Maturity or grown-upness is showing judgment, keeping your head, taking the knocks with the boosts and settling your problems like an adult, not like a child.

## What Behavior Is

As we said before, life is full of problems. They become more complicated as we grow up; if we learn to handle them as we go along, we are ready to do what is expected of grown-up people. How, then, do people get on the wrong track? For a number of reasons: all of them are tied in with 3 needs—affection, security and success. Our ways of behaving grow out of trying to satisfy these needs. We try one thing, then another and another; sometimes we are successful and sometimes not. We do not like to fail—failure makes us feel tense and uncomfortable. You try to avoid these tense feelings and keep a good opinion of yourself. Here is what you may do: Dodge every responsibility—if you do not try you cannot fail! Keep away from people, then you will not have to wonder whether they like you. Try to get out of doing unpleasant things. However, will these methods work?

## Emotions

Emotions are feelings; emotions give you all your pleasant or unpleasant moments and are frequently expressed in your behavior. Feelings make life interesting and exciting, help you to get things done and give you individuality. In the process of growing, your body and its functions become full-grown; your mind learns more complicated things; you

learn to meet and associate with people. This is maturity or being grown-up. But you are not mature if you still express your emotions as a child or an adolescent. We try to work toward emotional maturity from childhood on, so we will gradually learn to control and direct our emotions to match our adult bodies and minds.

When a baby is hungry, or a pin sticks him, or he kicks off the covers, he expresses his feelings by movements or howls. He cannot wait; he wants attention *now*—he screams until someone makes him comfortable again. We put up with this kind of behavior in babies but not in grownups—we expect adults to control their feelings. Learning to do so is a gradual process. We learn to bear pain without screaming and to keep our tempers when we are crossed; we learn not to be afraid; we manage to keep from being always either depressed or wildly happy. A baby *demands* and *accepts*—he gives little or nothing in return. An adult *gives* and is not too greatly concerned about the return.

Of course, physical factors can also affect how we feel. The endocrine glands (the glands of internal secretion such as the thyroid) affect our emotions. If they are sluggish, we become dull or depressed; if they are overactive, we become restless or excitable.

## Stress

Stress is one of the factors which affect our behavior. Medical authorities recognize that the stress and the strain of modern life affect people's health and well-being and as a result, their behavior. It is the wear and tear that is part of being alive. We feel stress every day as we exert ourselves to get our work done, deal with our problems at home, attend classes or drive a car. A certain amount of stress is necessary and indispensable because it spurs us on to our best efforts and makes life more colorful and exciting. Increasing tension temporarily helps to get a job done, alerts the body's defenses against disease or danger and helps us to meet an emergency or a difficult situation. Stress becomes a problem only when we are unable to handle it constructively.

Stress may be due to physical pain, discomfort or to emotional pressures such as fear, anxiety, affection or hate. It creates tensions which may be harmful if they recur frequently or are allowed to persist. Prolonged tension affects both behavior and health. In caring for patients, it is important to know the kinds of tensions that are likely to develop and how to relieve them. Sick people are under physical stress, but often it is the emotional stress which is more discouraging. We help to relieve these pressures by explaining nursing procedures as we prepare to carry them out and by performing them efficiently with the least possible amount of discomfort. We help to prevent and reduce tensions also by letting a patient talk about his fears and worries, by placing his call signal within easy reach, by answering his signal promptly, by assuring privacy during nursing treatments and by encouraging him to help himself as much as possible.

Remember, though, that you too are under stress whether you are learning a new kind of work, taking on responsibilities, or adjusting to people and to new routines. Avoid letting stress affect the kind of person you are by having unnecessary tensions affect your work. Concentrate on doing one thing at a time instead of worrying about everything that has to be done. Do not waste time in rebelling against people or things that you cannot change. There is nothing abnormal about an occasional upset, but frequent "blow-ups" are danger signals of pressure build-ups. If things seem to be getting you down, try letting off steam by some physical activity. Take a brisk walk, go bowling, do your laundry. Take time for some recreation. A change gives you time for a new look at your problems. Talk over your problems with a sympathetic friend or member of your family. Keep physically fit. Your physical condition affects your attitude toward people and toward life. You must be able to handle your own tensions successfully before you can help patients to handle theirs.

## Good Manners Come First

First impressions are strong, and people feel kindly toward the person who is thoughtful and friendly. Courtesy means being thoughtful of other people—your patients, their families and your co-workers. Good manners tell you to come forward to speak to a doctor, your head nurse, your instructor or a visitor if they are in need of assistance. On a hospital ward or in your patient's room, you are more or less a hostess, as you would be in your own home. You will help bewildered visitors to find their way around; you will lend a helping hand to the people you work with. You will be tactful and make allowances for occasional sharp words and quick tempers. After all, you have known what it means to be rushed and worried.

# 6

# Community Health

## BEHAVIORAL OBJECTIVES

*The student successfully attaining the goals of this chapter will be able to:*
- *discuss at least 2 of the major public health problems which exist in the United States today, with special emphasis upon at least one local problem and the attempts at its solution.*
- *identify at least 2 federal agencies which work to protect the health of the public, describe some of their activities, and discuss how they relate to local and state agencies.*
- *compare and contrast the functions and organizational structures of government public health agencies and voluntary agencies.*
- *list communicable diseases for which immunization is available.*
- *define medical quackery and cite examples of its use and abuse.*
- *identify means used for protecting mothers and newborn babies, and describe some of the services and facilities available to the blind or partially-sighted.*

## HEALTH PROTECTION

Health problems are not exactly the same in every community. To begin with, they are related to the country, the climate, the food habits and the living standards of the people who live there. Some groups have large families and are accustomed to living in crowded quarters; others will eat only a few types of food. Others are influenced by superstitions and fears which lead to poor health habits and the wrong kind of medical care. In an industrial city, lay-offs and shut-downs increase health problems. Depressions, wars, housing shortages and rising costs of living also affect health.

### Health Agencies

Group action is the most effective way of dealing with health problems. In this country, as in every country, health problems increase with the population. This leads to a need to organize groups to deal with these problems by setting up measures for health protection. Today we have many such groups on national, state and local levels. Some of these groups, known as public health departments, are official agencies of the federal, state or municipal governments and are supported by public funds. Others are independent or voluntary agencies such as the American Heart Association or the American Cancer Society, supported by voluntary contributions from individuals and groups.

**Federal Agencies.** On the national level, the federal government agency concerned with health is the United States Public Health Service (USPHS), one of several agencies under the Department of Health, Education and Welfare. Some of the other agencies are the Food and Drug Administration, the Social Security Administration, the Office of Vocational Rehabilitation and the Office of Education.

The USPHS has many responsibilities for health protection, including the investigation and control of all diseases, protection from diseases carried by immigrants, control of sanitation on trains, ships and aircraft in interstate commerce, control of the manufacture and sale of biological products and the cooperation with state health departments in disease control. It is also responsible for publishing and distributing health information.

Many other departments of the federal government have a hand in health protection; for example, the Department of Agriculture through its various bureaus is concerned with the control of insect- and animal-borne diseases and with meat and other food inspection, while the Bureau of Internal Revenue enforces the antinarcotic laws.

**State Health Departments.** State health departments, through their divisions or bureaus, are responsible for health protection within a state. Their services are concerned with sanitation, food and water inspection, maternal and child health, public health nursing, laboratory services, vital statistics and other services. State health laws must conform to federal laws, but states also have the right to make their own health laws, as necessary, to protect the health of the people.

**City Health Departments.** City health departments are concerned with the health protection within a city. Sometimes this interest is extended to provide health services to the county as well—which makes more services possible for more people. Usually the health department operates under a Board of Health which sets up policies and regulations which are carried out under the direction of a health officer, preferably a doctor with public health training. A city health department provides services in relation to conditions that affect everyone: it inspects the places where food is sold and the people who handle food. It checks the water and milk supply, housing, sewage and other waste disposal facilities and provides services regarding air pollution. It provides school health services and health education, clinics and hospital and nursing care. Health protection in a large city is big business.

**Local Health Services.** Health protection in rural areas and in towns and villages is provided by county, district or local health units. Each unit has its own health department which aims to provide the same basic services as those supplied by a city health department. The state health department supervises and gives consultant services to health units.

## Ecology

The growing recognition that man is but one part of a complex system of life, that he is a part of the universe and dependent upon the balance of life and the growth and death of all living organisms on the planet earth, has awakened many concerned citizens to the need to preserve this balance. The study of the mutual relationships between living beings and their environment is called ecology. The task of preserving the ecological balance, so that man will have air to breathe, water to drink, and food to eat, is decidedly complicated. Technology has proved to be both a blessing and a curse. Today new sources of energy which will not pollute the air, land, or water are being sought. The nurse, as a member of the health team, will be called upon to know about and work for the kind of study and action which will contribute to a healthy environment. Her roles as citizen and nurse will grow in the over-all effort to make this a safe world.

## Air and Water Pollution

Air pollution is greatest in industrial areas, but every large city has some air pollution problems, even though it may have comparatively few industries, as is the case in Washington, D.C. A very great source of air pollution is the exhaust from automobiles. The smog situation in Los Angeles, for example, is the result of the combined action of fog, smoke and automobile exhaust gases which produce substances harmful to health. Smog also causes crop damage.

Air pollution has been shown to be responsible for increases in respiratory infections such as chronic bronchitis, asthmatic attacks and emphysema. Heavy air pollution will cause irritation of the eyes, nose and throat, and may possibly have further serious effects not yet known on health. Air pollution also damages plant growth and affects buildings.

Water pollution is a serious and increasing health hazard. A number of diseases are transmitted by contaminated water; typhoid fever, dysentery and infectious hepatitis are noted examples. Water pollution not only affects people, but it is also a menace to wildlife and fish and recreation areas. It is estimated that at least 45 million fish are killed in the United States each year by polluted water. Increasing demands on the national water supply make it necessary to reuse water, thereby requiring that waste water be treated to make it safe for reuse. In many areas this treatment is inadequate.

The federal government has a responsibility for insuring a safe water supply for the people in this country. Until recently, our national government had little or no authority to do this; it was left up to state and local governments. Legislation now gives the Public Health Service the authority and the funds to establish waste treatment projects.

## Drugs and Health

The Food and Drug Administration is the national agency charged with the responsibility of protecting the public from harmful drugs and from false claims about the efficiency of a drug. The first attempt at this kind of protection was the Federal Food, Drug and Cosmetic Act passed in 1938. In 1951 the law was amended to curb abuses in the use of additional dangerous drugs, such as sleeping pills, thyroid pills, sex hormones and antibiotics. The amendment required pharmaceutical companies to label all drugs that were considered potentially dangerous, with the caution to druggists that the drugs were not to be dispensed without a doctor's prescription.

**FDA Approval.** Since 1951, the many new discoveries in the treatment of disease have led to the production of a vast number of new drugs. It is estimated at more than 400 every year. Before the FDA approves a drug, it requires evidence that the drug does what it claims to do and that it has been clinically tested on a sufficient number of patients for an adequate length of time to prove it is safe for use.

**AMA Council on Drugs.** The American Medical Association's Council on Drugs gives information to doctors about drugs and releases an annual list of new drugs. The Council is also establishing a central registry in Chicago to provide up-to-date information about unfavorable effects of drugs and chemicals. It is estimated that approximately 1 million people suffer every year from the side effects of drugs they have taken to make them well.

**Worthless Remedies.** Unfortunately, the market is flooded with an endless number of worthless and unapproved remedies: they claim to bring sleep, remove pain, lengthen life and cure arthritis, cancer and dozens of other ailments ranging from dental caries to athlete's foot. One preparation listed 18 conditions for which it was effective. The fly-by-night companies that manufacture these products are interested only in making money, and, unfortunately, there are always people who are willing to furnish testimonials about the benefits they think they have received. The FDA frequently finds it necessary to file judgments against such companies for making false claims about their products. Why are so many people taken in by claims for a drug? For one thing, they do not know how to tell the difference between true and false claims. Also, as one victim remarked: "on your bed of pain, you will try anything, at any cost."

# HEALTH ENEMIES

## Controlling Communicable Diseases

In spite of precautions to prevent disease, people do get sick, so health authorities have another responsibility—they must keep disease from spreading. There are 2 ways of controlling communicable diseases: (1) state laws require physicians to report cases of specific diseases to the local health department, (2) the health department sees that persons with a communicable disease are isolated. It also puts persons exposed to a communicable disease under restrictions or quarantine for the length of time that it takes the disease to develop. *Quarantine* means that no one may enter or leave a house where there is a communicable disease; *isolation* means that no one enters the room of a sick person except the person who is taking care of him. Regulations are not identical for every disease. You will learn how to isolate a patient to protect others and yourself.

## Medical Quackery

Millions of people spend countless dollars every year on supposedly sure cures for every imaginable ailment. False claims for food supplements, drugs, treatments and various devices induce people to spend money which they may actually need for food. More serious still, some people turn to quacks for help instead of to reputable physicians, thereby running the risk of delaying vital treatment until it is too late. One study of people who had been admitted to a hospital after being in the hands of quacks showed that nearly half of those who died could have been saved by earlier medical treatment.

Cancer and arthritis "cures,"* machines purporting to give off healing "z" rays (there is no such thing as a "z" ray) and so-called electrotherapy treatments also entrap people with real or imaginary ailments. The sale of many of these devices has been made illegal, but new ones keep turning up. Although the Federal Trade Commission has the power to crack down on false advertising, there are ways of getting around such action. For example, there is no way to prevent books from advocating any practice in the name of health so long as they do not commercialize a specific product.

## HEALTH SERVICES

### Prenatal and Postnatal Health

Proper care of mothers before, during and after childbirth protects their health and helps to ensure healthy babies. As these babies grow up, they, in turn, need protection against disease and other conditions that harm growth; they need opportunities to become healthy, happy citizens, equipped with a good health heritage to pass on to their children. Governmental and private public health agencies provide information about prenatal and postnatal care; if necessary, they pay for medical and nursing services and provide food for the expectant mother and clothing for the baby. Classes for expectant mothers and fathers,

---

* Up to now, no cure for cancer or arthritis has been found.

such as those at the Maternity Center Association in New York City, teach prospective parents how to prepare for their baby and how to take care of him after he is born. The death rate for mothers and infants has gone down spectacularly in the last 30 years. Many hospitals sponsor their own prenatal classes. (See Chapter 36.)

The community is interested in protecting the child's health before he goes to school. Some communities have established well-child clinics to check on children's health and prevent disease before it occurs. Care in nurseries and nursery schools, immunization programs and training in good health habits lay the foundations for good citizenship. Most children are required to have physical, dental, and eye examinations before entering school. They must be up to date on diphtheria, tetanus, and whooping cough immunizations, as well as those against smallpox and measles. Sometimes mumps and polio immunizations are also required.

### Public Safety

The National Safety Council and the state councils promote safety by analyzing the causes of accidents and suggesting ways to prevent them. They distribute information about accident prevention in industry, in the home and on the public highways. Highway and traffic laws protect everyone by requiring inspection of motor vehicles, driving licenses, speed regulation and highway markings. All states now require seat belts and head rests as standard equipment for new motor vehicles. Building regulations and inspection reduce fire, accident and health hazards. Education programs, such as the Red Cross First Aid and Home Safety programs, teach people how to act in emergencies and how to prevent accidents and injuries in their homes.

### Peacetime Blood Banks

Blood is so important to life that doctors and hospital and health officials consider blood banks a public health necessity. In 1948, the Red Cross began a gigantic program to set up blood donation centers around the entire country. These centers are still operating in many states, and new ones are being opened as the need arises. They supply blood when it is needed in community emergencies, such as accidents and disasters, or for treatment in certain illnesses. This is a contribution of the American people to life and health. Nearly every drop of blood is donated and costs the recipient little. A donor may even have his donation of blood credited to another center.

## The American Red Cross

The American Red Cross is well-known to many Americans. It provides numerous services including aid to persons in time of disaster. The Practical Nurse can volunteer as a Red Cross Volunteer Nurse and serve on emergency first aid teams for public functions or as a nurse in time of an emergency.

## Help for the Blind

Approximately 500,000 persons in the United States are either totally blind or so nearly blind that they cannot carry on normal activities. About half of these people are 65 or older. Many of their sight difficulties are due to the effects of aging or to diseases which go with the older years, such as cataracts, arteriosclerosis (hardening of the blood vessels) or high blood pressure (hypertension). The other half of our blind population were either born blind or have lost their sight as the result of infectious disease or accidents.

The partially sighted are an in-between group, with special needs which are not the same as those of the blind, and this group often is not given the kind of attention that will be most helpful. For example, they may be able to read with special magnifying glasses and do not need to learn Braille. On the side of prevention, the National Society for the Prevention of Blindness works with many groups in planning sight-saving programs. We are stressing the use of every means for helping the blind or the partially sighted to live and work as members of the community and not as an isolated group. (See Chapter 53 for a further discussion of blindness.)

# 7

# Microbes and Man

## BEHAVIORAL OBJECTIVES

*The student successfully attaining the objectives of this chapter will be able to:*

- *trace the development of and define the sciences of microbiology and immunology.*
- *list the 6 vital functions of microorganisms and discuss each.*
- *discuss the various means of studying microorganisms.*
- *identify the conditions necessary for the growth of microorganisms.*
- *name the 6 classifications of organisms and define each.*
- *specifically identify the 3 general types of bacteria; compare and contrast pathogens and nonpathogens, spore-formers and nonspore-formers; describe how bacteria multiply and the effects of this multiplication; and give examples of diseases caused by each of the 3 types of pathogenic bacteria.*
- *define the term* communicable disease; *relate ways in which diseases are spread; and discuss means for preventing the spread of disease and ways of assisting the patient to kill the organism, once he has contracted the disease.*
- *discuss the factors affecting the virulence of the disease-producing organism, once it has entered the body.*
- *name at least 3 of the body's natural defenses against disease.*
- *define the term* immunity *and identify how it occurs; define the types of immunity and give examples of the situation in which each might occur.*

In addition to the visible world in which we live, there is another world around us which we cannot see by ordinary means. Plants, animals and as yet unclassified organisms flourish in our invisible surroundings. Because these living things cannot be seen without the aid of magnifying lenses, they are called *microorganisms,* or *microbes* (from the Greek *micros,* small; and *bios,* life). Men were puzzled for centuries by actions caused by microorganisms. Everyday happenings could not be explained: Where do living things originate? Why does food spoil and other matter decay? Why do wounds become inflamed? Why does pus appear? Why and how do diseases spread —sometimes across continents?

Thinkers in early days accepted the belief that living things created themselves or were made from nonliving matter. Flies were thought to originate from putrefying food and animal manure; people believed that lice came from dirty clothes and bed covers. Some accepted the idea that evil spirits entered the body, that sickness was a punishment for sin, or that the "humours" of the body were in mysterious imbalance. In spite of today's proofs that none of these things cause illness, you can still see signs of this kind of thinking. There are people who still wrap a soiled stocking around their neck to cure a sore throat, eat celery to improve their brains and eat bread crusts to make their hair curly.

## EARLY CONTRIBUTIONS

### Invention of the Microscope

Some scientists in earlier times believed that there were invisible living things, but they had no way of proving or disproving their theories since they had no tools for observation. However, with the growth of science in the 16th century, men began to experiment with glass magnifying lenses. *Anton van Leeuwenhoek* (1632–1723), a Dutch businessman, contributed to the early development of lenses. His hobby was grinding lenses and making simple microscopes. In the course of his investigations, Leeuwenhoek saw many types of living creatures invisible to the naked eye and excitedly wrote to the Royal Society of London of these discoveries of "little animals." He described and drew pictures of the 3 types of bacteria as well as of other microbes.

The early microscopes were crude and inadequate. During the early 1800's the compound microscope (containing several lenses) was developed and improved, and *microbiology,* the study of organisms too small to be seen without the aid of a microscope, began its golden age. Today, we have the powerful electron microscope, which utilizes an electron beam instead of light and provides an enlarged image of extremely small objects.

One of the outstanding scientists in the early days of microbiology was Louis Pasteur (1822–1895) who disproved the age-old theory of spontaneous generation and indicated, through his work on fermentation, that the causes for the spoilage of food and drink were microorganisms.

### Immunology

In addition to the aforementioned accomplishments, Pasteur further developed the science of *immunology,* popularized by Jenner and his cowpox *vaccine,* to form the foundation of the preventive medicine programs of today. Smallpox was a disease greatly feared; 200 years ago 1 out of every 10 deaths was caused by this scourge. Edward Jenner, a physician of the 1700's learned that dairy maids who contracted cowpox were free from the risk of infection of smallpox. In 1796 cowpox broke out on a farm near Jenner's home, and a dairy maid, Sarah Nelmes, was infected with the cowpox from her employer's cows. Jenner inoculated a healthy 8-year-old, James Phipps, with some of the material from a sore on Sarah's hand. After several days the sores from James Phipps' inoculation healed without mishap. In order to prove that the boy was protected against smallpox, Jenner later inoculated him several times with matter from a smallpox patient, but no symptoms of the disease occurred. We call this protection against smallpox "vaccination," from the Latin word *vacca,* meaning cow.

Robert Koch (1843–1910) developed a method for obtaining pure growths of microorganisms (cultures) and was then able to prove that a specific organism was the cause of a specific disease. Baron Joseph Lister (1827–1912) introduced antiseptic technics in surgery, greatly reducing wound infections.

### The Filtrable Viruses

These early scientists in the field of microbiology suspected the existence of other, much smaller microorganisms that were still invisible. Eventually their existence was proven, and they were called viruses. Because they passed through the finest laboratory filters, they were named the filtrable viruses. Not only were they invisible, but it was also impossible to culture them by commonly used means. Although many men worked on disease problems caused by the filtrable viruses and definitely established their presence, no one knew anything about the organisms themselves until it was found that they would grow only in living matter. Viruses were successfully cultured in living tissues and chick embryos. With the development of the powerful electron microscope, viruses were finally visible. Modern microbiology has made huge strides in the study of the virus. To give you an idea of the size of a virus, the electron microscope can see objects as small as 5 *angstroms.* (An angstrom is 1/250 millionth of an inch.)

## THEN AND NOW

Because of the work of these pioneers in the development of microbiology, modern medicine is now able to look for and find the cause of a disease, to treat its source rather than its symptoms, and to cure rather than to palliate. It is often possible to make a *culture* of an organism, determine what that organism is and then determine what drug will kill the organism. An understanding of the methods of transmission of disease has given us the modern concept of preventing disease before it starts by teaching good personal and community health practices to individuals, groups and entire nations.

## CHARACTERISTICS OF ORGANISMS

### Organisms Are Active

Each individual microorganism is able to carry out some or all of the following vital functions characteristic of living organisms: (1) metabolism, (2) growth, (3) reproduction, (4) irritability, (5) motion and (6) protection.

All living organisms take in oxygen, use it to burn food for energy and growth and then excrete the wastes—a total process called *metabolism.* The microbes have this ability as well as the ability to increase in size or grow and to produce new members of their species (under ideal conditions, a single bacterium will produce almost 17 million descendants in 12 hours).* They react in varying ways to changes in their environment, thus showing irritability or response to the stimulus of changing conditions. Many of the microorganisms are able to move under their own power, as animals do.

Of the thousands of species of microbes in existence, most of them are harmless, and many are directly beneficial to man. Man's "staff of life," the bread we eat daily, is raised by the action of the microorganisms, the gas-generating yeast cells, within it. Beer and wine are made with microorganisms that cause fermentation. The sharp pungent cheeses some people consider the most delicious owe their flavor to the molds. Many drugs, such as penicillin, are made from molds. The decomposition of animal and vegetative wastes is dependent on microbes. The soil would not be fertile without them. Thus all higher forms of life, ourselves included, could not exist without the microorganisms. Comparatively few types of microbes are harmful to man.

These are the *pathogens* (Greek *pathos,* disease and *gennan,* to produce), and are the ones we will be concerned with in nursing.

### How Microorganisms Are Studied

To facilitate the study of microorganisms, scientists have developed various methods for growing them within the laboratory. A growth of microorganisms for laboratory study is called a *culture.* The cultures are grown usually in test tubes or on small flat covered plates called petri dishes. The material on which the microbes are spread or planted is the culture medium. There are various types of culture media for different purposes. The earliest used was *agar,* a gelatin-like substance developed from seaweed.

To see and study the individual characteristics of microorganisms grown in cultures, a small amount of the material to be examined is placed on a clean oblong piece of glass called a *slide.* This slide is then prepared in one of several ways for viewing under the microscope. The organisms may be stained by drops of *dye* or viewed in their living, moving state in a drop of liquid culture placed in a hollow spot on a slide. Some forms are seen best in an arrangement in which they appear light against a dark background.

### How Microorganisms Grow

Certain factors in the environment promote the growth of microbes. These are darkness, warmth, moisture, food and a suitable oxygen supply. If you remove any one of these, the microbial population decreases. Here, then, is the beginning of the microbial control technics that are so important in nursing practice.

The green plants we see daily need light to grow because they contain the green pigment *chlorophyll.* The microorganisms, many of which are very low forms of plant life, do not contain chlorophyll. Thus they are colorless and grow well in darkness. Many microorganisms are killed when exposed to the ultraviolet rays of the sun. Moderately diffuse light, however, usually does not affect them.

The temperature at which a specific microorganism grows best is said to be its *optimum temperature.* Most of the microorganisms with which we are concerned grow best at temperatures ranging from that of a cool room to

---

* An experiment at the University of Nebraska indicated that underclothing worn for 6 days contained 10,000,000 bacteria *per square inch.*

slightly above normal human body temperature.

All microorganisms require water for growth. The matter in or on which they grow must contain available moisture (such as jellies) or may be an actual liquid (such as milk).

Since the microorganisms do not contain chlorophyll, they cannot manufacture their own food from raw materials and, therefore, must find it ready-made. Some organisms live within or at the expense of another living creature, called its *host*; these are the *parasites*. Others live on the dead remains of plants and animals; these are the *saprophytes*.

Some chemicals check the growth of microorganisms or kill them outright, by injuring the cell and thus interfering with the life processes. These are known as *antiseptics* and *disinfectants*. Generally speaking, antiseptics slow down the growth of microorganisms, but may or may not destroy them. Disinfectants are used in an attempt to destroy disease organisms.

## KINDS OF ORGANISMS

Just as we classify the plants and animals with which we are familiar into various groups, so do we differentiate the microorganisms. Because of their differences in form, size, rates of growth and other characteristics, we are able to classify them into the following general groups:

1. protozoa
2. fungi, including molds and yeasts
3. bacteria
4. rickettsiae
5. viruses
6. parasitic worms

Although strictly speaking parasitic worms are not microorganisms, they are generally included in the study of microbiology because they are microscopic in certain stages of their life cycles, and cannot be studied without the use of the microscope.

### Protozoa

*Protozoa* are 1-cell forms of animals. They are all able to move by various means. Some of the diseases in man caused by pathogenic protozoa are amoebic dysentery and malaria.

### Fungi

The *fungi* include the molds and yeasts, which are low forms of plant life. We are all familiar with the common *molds*: a fuzzy patch on jelly and fruits, a sooty appearance on breads, or the blue veins interspersed through sharp cheeses. They grow best at room temperature and have a characteristic musty smell. They send extensive threads or branches called *hyphae* throughout the material on or in which they are growing. Some of the hyphae extend beyond the surface of the host material and when mature produce at their tips rounded cases containing microscopic *spores*. The spores give the molds their characteristic colors. The spores are wafted about by the slightest currents of air and when they find suitable conditions, they attach themselves and begin another growth of mold. Ringworm and athletes foot are common fungus diseases. *Yeasts* reproduce by budding. Each parent cell grows or produces a bud (daughter cell) which eventually breaks off and grows in the same manner. Yeasts require sugars in solution as their food; as the yeasts use the sugar, a chemical change called *fermentation* occurs, during which the sugar is changed to alcohol and carbon dioxide. Many industries use controlled fermentation in the process of preparing their products. Thrush (moniliasis) is a disease caused by pathogenic yeasts.

### Bacteria

*Bacteria* are single-cell organisms considered to be microscopic, colorless plants (see Fig. 7-1). They are divided into 3 groups according to their form. If the bacterium is spherical, it is called a *coccus* (pl. cocci) from the Greek word meaning "berry"; if rod shaped, a *bacillus* (pl. bacilli) from the Latin word meaning "little stick"; and if curved, or spiral shaped, a *spirillum* (pl. spirilla). Some spirillum-like microorganisms are also called spirochetes.

**How Bacteria Multiply.** Most of the pathogenic bacteria are parasites. Bacteria reproduce by simply splitting into 2 parts. As each bacterium matures and reaches its maximum growth, it divides across the middle to form 2 new cells like the first. This type of reproduction is called *fission*. A very few types

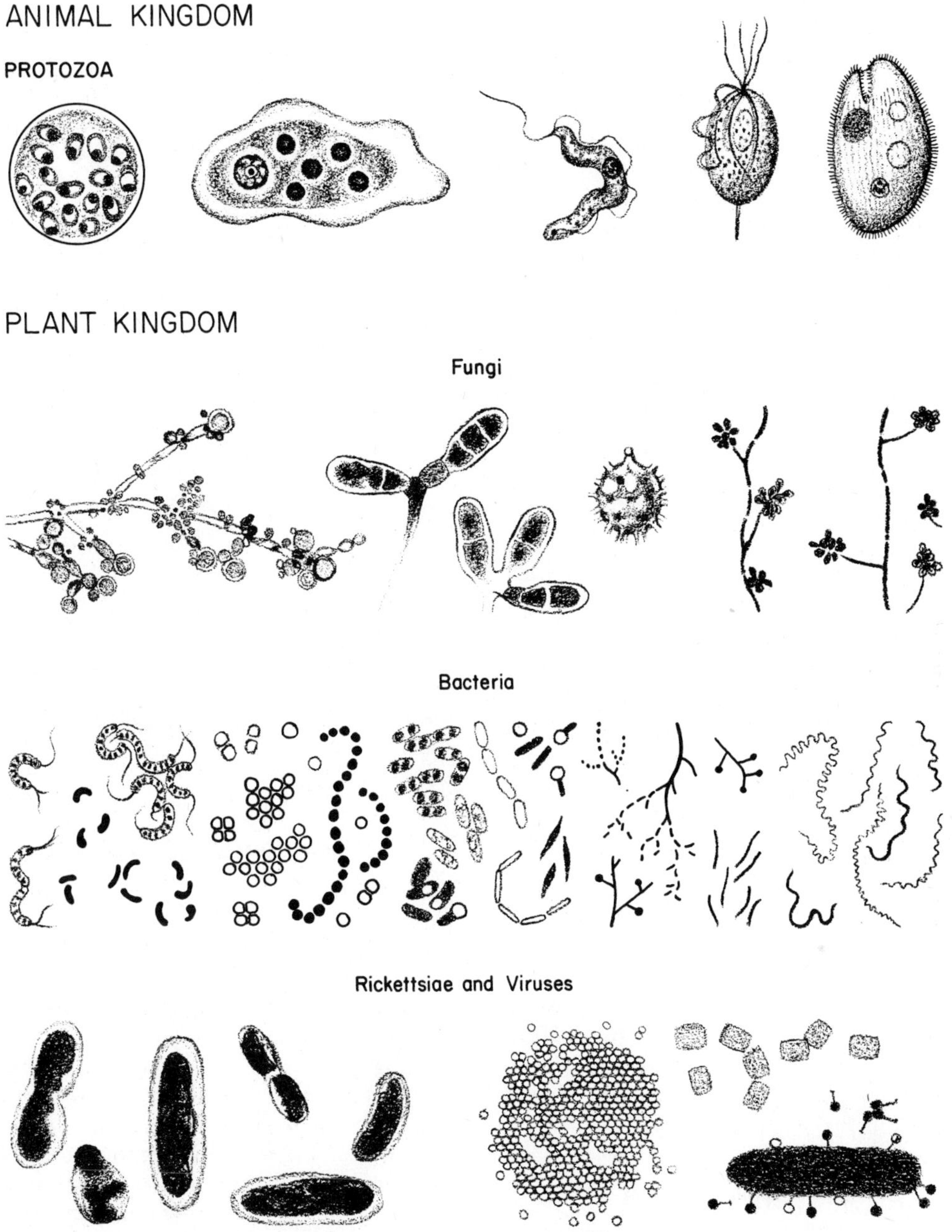

## ANIMAL KINGDOM

**PROTOZOA**

## PLANT KINGDOM

**Fungi**

**Bacteria**

**Rickettsiae and Viruses**

Figure 7-1. Representative types of microorganisms. Not drawn to scale. (Von Gremp, Z., and Broadwell, L.: Practical Nursing Study Guide and Review, ed. 2. Philadelphia, Lippincott, 1965)

of bacilli are spore-formers; that is, when conditions are unfavorable for their growth, a protective covering (spore) is developed and the bacillus goes into a nonactive phase. This spore is like a suit of armor; it survives light, drying, boiling, most chemicals and other ordinarily destructive conditions. When favorable conditions again develop, the spore will "sprout" or germinate. Because of their added protection, spore-forming pathogens are more difficult to control and destroy than any others.

Most bacteria move by means of one or more whip-like projections (flagella) which propel them through liquids. The cocci do not have flagella.

Different species of bacteria have their own optimal temperatures for growing; however, most pathogens grow best at human body temperature. All pathogens are killed at 212° F., the boiling point of water, *except* the spore-formers. The lowest temperature at which pathogenic bacteria can survive varies. To assure that certain articles used in the hospital are *sterile,* that is, free from the presence of any microorganisms including spore-formers, steam under pressure is used for sterilizing. This is provided in an apparatus called an *autoclave.* Some organisms cannot survive in the presence of oxygen. These are called *anaerobic* organisms (without oxygen). Examples of these are the organisms which cause gas gangrene and tetanus. Most organisms require oxygen for growth and are called *aerobic.*

**Bacteria and Disease.** Some of the infections caused by nonspore-forming species of bacteria include boils, streptococcal sore throats, and rheumatic fever. Examples of infections caused by spore-forming bacteria are tuberculosis, leprosy, and typhoid fever.

## Rickettsiae

*Rickettsiae* are microscopic forms of life in size between the bacteria and the virus. They are nonspore-forming and are readily killed by heat. Like the viruses, they can grow only in living tissue within the cells of their host. Rickettsiae are transmitted to man only through the bite of insects which carry them. The effects of the infection vary from minor discomfort to fatal disease. A typical rickettsial infection is Rocky Mountain spotted fever, transmitted by ticks.

## Viruses

Viruses are protein substances which show certain properties of living things and are too small to be seen with the ordinary microscope. The virus has no means of locomotion, it possesses no source of power and it cannot grow. It does, however, contain DNA and RNA (see Chapter 11) but cannot reproduce until it has taken over a living cell. The other cell then becomes a culture medium for the virus. It is very difficult to culture certain viruses, and our limited knowledge of them has been gained mostly since the early 1930's. The physiology of the virus cannot be studied by direct observation since they cannot be seen by usual laboratory methods, and most information about the virus has been gained by studying their effects, rather than by observing the virus itself. Most known methods of destroying viruses are not satisfactory, nor are drugs for control of virus infections very effective. The most satisfactory method for preventing such virus infections as smallpox and polio is by vaccination. Vaccines for other virus diseases are presently being developed; among the newest is a vaccine effective against measles.

## Worm Infestations

Worms are called by the more scientific name of *helminths.* Man is infested with worms by either eating food contaminated by larvae (immature, microscopic forms) or eggs of the helminths, or by being bitten by an insect that deposits the larvae at the site. Usually symptoms are not apparent unless the infestation is massive. Tapeworms and hookworms are examples of helminths that infest man.

## COMMUNICABLE DISEASES

Many diseases caused by the microorganisms are *communicable;* that is, they spread from one individual to another. Microbes have several avenues of spread (transmission), one of which is by direct contact. This means through touching or body contact, as in shaking hands, kissing or sexual relations. Another direct method of spread is by *droplet infection*—the spread of pathogens via microscopic drops of moisture expelled from the mouth or nose when a person talks, laughs, coughs or sneezes. Colds and other respiratory infections are easily spread by droplet infection in crowded places.

Indirect contact implies that there is an intermediary object which harbors the microbes from the infected person and carries the microorganisms to the new victim. Nonliving carriers of pathogens, such as water, food, air dust, soil and various objects, are called *fomites.* Living carriers of disease organisms (rats, fleas, lice, etc.) are *vectors.* A *human carrier* is a person who exhibits no signs or symptoms of a disease, but who carries disease pathogens in his body and transmits the disease to others. The carrier may transmit disease by direct or indirect contact.*

## Disease Prevention

Knowledge of how pathogens enter and leave the body is essential in preventing the spread of disease (prophylaxis). They enter through: (1) the respiratory system, (2) the gastrointestinal system, (3) the urinary and reproductive systems and (4) breaks in the skin or mucous membrane.

Microorganisms may leave the body in any of the natural body discharges—mucus, sputum, saliva, urine and feces, as well as in vomitus and exudate from surface lesions.

## INFECTION

Whether or not the pathogens will produce an active infection once they have gained entry to the body, depends both upon the infecting agent and upon the host. An *infection* is a condition in which the body is invaded by pathogens which then increase in number, causing injurious effects and their symptoms. Within the body, pathogenic microorganisms produce 2 possible effects: they either destroy the tissues in which they are living or produce substances that are poisonous. These poisons are called *toxins.* Some infections produce both effects. Whether or not the pathogen or the affected person is the victor in the battle that takes place when pathogens enter the body depends on several factors: (1) the route by which the pathogens enter the body, (2) the number of invading organisms, (3) the virulence (strength) of the invaders and (4) the resistance of the body, that is, the effectiveness of its defenses against disease organisms.

For specific microorganisms to cause disease within the body, they must enter by an effective route. The typhoid bacillus must enter the digestive tract; the meningococcus uses the nose as its chief portal of entry. Their presence in other systems of the body would produce no disease effects.

If the number of pathogens entering the

body is small, they are easily overcome by the natural defenses of the body. The greater the number of pathogens present, the greater their opportunity to set up a stronghold of disease within the body of the host.

The virulence or strength of the pathogens is subject to chance, sometimes for reasons unknown. If the microbes have been weakened, the body will overcome them before they produce disease. If the pathogen is extremely virulent, the defenses of the body may be overcome, at least temporarily. Strength is always the victor.

## The Body's Defenses

The body's natural defenses are many; it is well able to protect itself from the daily onslaughts of the pathogens. Intact skin covering the body surface and intact mucous membranes lining its cavities (those which open to the outside) serve as barriers against the microbes. In addition, the sticky mucus secreted by the mucous membranes in some cavities traps the organisms and prevents their journey further into the body.

The mucous membranes of the respiratory tract are covered with *cilia,* hairlike projections which are in constant motion. This wavelike motion, which resembles a soft breeze passing through tall grass, pushes a constant flow of mucus and the foreign particles trapped within it up and out of the lungs. If you consider the dust particles and other contaminants we inhale daily, you can appreciate the protection the cilia offer.

Some of the natural secretions of the body, in addition to their primary function, are also responsible for protection. Saliva, tears, gastric secretions and other secretions prove to be foes of the microbes. Tears and saliva are now believed to have antiseptic qualities and can "float away" or wash out microbes by purely mechanical means as well. The gastric secretions, particularly hydrochloric acid, are so potent that they easily destroy most ingested pathogens.

The white blood cells and the lymphatic system play a major part in the natural body defenses. When pathogenic microorganisms enter the body, the white blood cells (leukocytes) increase in number and engulf the invaders at or near their point of entry. Other microbes which have passed beyond the nor-

---

* A famous carrier was "Typhoid Mary," a cook who infected scores of people with typhoid fever without contracting the disease herself.

mal barricades of the body are shunted into the lymphatic vessels in the lymph and carried to the nodes where they are destroyed by *phagocytosis,* the process of engulfing (or ingesting) and destroying bacteria and other foreign particles. Body cells which have this ability are *phagocytes.*

The increase in body temperature (fever) in the presence of pathogens is an automatic defense. In most infections the higher temperature checks the growth of microbes until the more effective defenses of the body are marshalled. In certain circumstances it is not desirable to reduce elevated body temperature.

## Susceptibility to Infection

Many factors determine an individual's susceptibility to infection. The general state of health is important; chronic fatigue and poor nutrition weaken seriously the body's defenses. Age also plays a part; the normal degeneration processes of aging make a person more vulnerable to disease processes. Emotional factors, such as anxiety, may also influence the chance of developing illnesses by altering the body's physiology and metabolic balance.

We have already said that some microorganisms use our bodies as their natural home. These microbes are called the "normal flora" of the body and play a necessary role in resistance to disease. The ability of some species of microbes to live together is called *symbiosis.* An association in which one species of microorganisms prevents the growth of another or actually destroys members of another species is termed *antibiosis.* Many of the normal body flora have an antibiotic relationship to the enemy pathogens and contribute immeasurably to the maintenance of health.

**Antibiotics.** The process of antibiosis has given us numerous powerful weapons for treating infection—the drugs we call *antibiotics.* An antibiotic is a chemical substance that inhibits the growth of or destroys bacteria. (Antibiotics are discussed in more detail in Chapter 33.)

## Immunity

A person who cannot acquire a certain disease is said to be immune to it. Immunity is either *inborn* (inherited) or *acquired.* Inborn immunity is the resistance with which man has been endowed through inheritance from his forefathers. There is a difference in susceptibility of various species: man is *naturally* immune to the "hoof and mouth disease" of cattle. Different races have developed varying degrees of immunity to specific infections. For example, Negroes have a greater immunity to malaria than do white people.

Generally speaking, *inborn* immunity seems to depend on the general defense mechanisms of the human species. *Acquired* immunity results from the development of specific antibodies in the person's blood. Any foreign substance that gains entrance to the body and induces a specific immune response is called an *antigen.* The specific immune response which is formed is called an *antibody.* Antigens characteristically are substances derived from living matter, usually protein in nature. Since the body regards the antigen as an invader, you can assume that the resultant production of antibodies is a defense mechanism of the body—an attempt at protection.

Each antigen stimulates formation of its own antibodies, and each kind of antibody is specific for one type of antigen only. Because microorganisms are living matter, you will understand that every microorganism (or its toxic secretions) acts as an antigen. (The substance produced in reaction to microbial toxins is called an antitoxin.)

*Acquired* immunity is either active or passive.

*Active* immunity is resistance to disease as a result of the development of antibodies within the body of the individual. It is developed in several ways: (1) by the person actually having the disease or (2) by injections of vaccines, which are preparations consisting of attenuated living microbes, dead pathogens, or weakened toxins prepared from cultures of pathogens (*toxoids*).

*Passive* immunity occurs when a person is given a substance containing antibodies or antitoxins that have been developed in another person or animal. This substance is called either a *serum* or an *antitoxin.* The resultant immunity from a serum or antitoxin is said to be passive because the body of the recipient plays no active part in response to an antigen. Newborn babies have passive but temporary immunity from the antibodies of their mothers.

# Unit 3:
## The Family

8. *Growth and Development*
9. *Adolescence*
10. *Family Living*

# 8

# Growth and Development

## BEHAVIORAL OBJECTIVES

*The student successfully attaining the goals of this chapter will be able to:*

- *identify some of the basic needs and the special needs of every child, if he is to grow and develop into a well-functioning adult.*
- *discuss the concept of discipline and how it affects the psychosocial development of the child.*
- *discuss heredity and environment and their effects upon physical and psychosocial development.*
- *describe the usual patterns of each stage of child growth and development in terms of both physical and psychosocial characteristics. The student must be able to describe the average child at various ages.*
- *discuss differences between children of the same age and identify the point of difference at which the parents should become concerned.*
- *discuss special problems such as bed-wetting, physical or mental impairment, toilet training, masturbation, or thumb-sucking in terms of underlying influences and in the handling of the problem.*

Children are a country's stake in the future; as the adults of tomorrow, they will be its responsible citizens. Every ten years the President of the United States calls together key people for the White House Conference on Children. (Formerly called the White House Conference on Children and Youth, the first conference was called by President Theodore Roosevelt in 1909.) In the past, a single conference was held to discuss the special problems of children and youth. However, in 1970, it was decided to hold a Children's Conference (ages 0-13) in 1970 and a Youth Conference (ages 14-24) in 1971. The planners of the conferences believed that it was no longer realistic to hold a single conference for both groups.

In 1970, over 4,000 people came together for a week in the nation's capital, to discuss "the many related and overlapping problems affecting children."* The Conference dis-

*From the *Report to the President: White House Conference on Children, 1970.* U.S. Government Printing Office, Washington, D.C.

cussed such topics as Individuality; Learning; Health; Parents and Families; Communities and Environments; Laws, Rights, and Responsibilities; and Child Service Institutions.

Some of the specific goals of the Conference were stated in the Preamble. "This should be a Conference about love . . . about our need to love those to whom we have given birth . . . and those who are most helpless and in need . . . and those who give us a reason for being . . . and those who are most precious for themselves—for what they are and what they can become. Our children. . . . We want for our children a full opportunity for learning in an environment in which they can reach and grow and take pride in themselves . . . the right to be healthy . . . the right to have the respect of others . . . to live under laws that are fair and just . . . to love their country because their country has earned their love. . . . This we want for our children. Therefore this we must want for *all* children. There can be no exceptions."

Adults are responsible for preparing the child to take his place in the adult world, to make friends, to find and hold a job, and usually to marry and have a family. As a nurse, you will share responsibility for his health, but you must also be concerned about his personality. Unless you consider the whole of him, you may not help his body at all.

## THE NEEDS OF CHILDREN

### Parental Authority

What parents regard as "being bad" is often only the child's way of trying to meet his basic needs. We know that spanking will not cure wrong-doing and that bribes and threats and coaxings are only temporary tricks to persuade children to cooperate with us. There are 3 basic methods by which adults attempt to guide or teach children to act in a fashion acceptable for our society. As you can see from the following examples, the degree of success varies.

Dianne's father believes that his child should recognize and accept *authority* from the time she is able to understand the spoken word. His usual

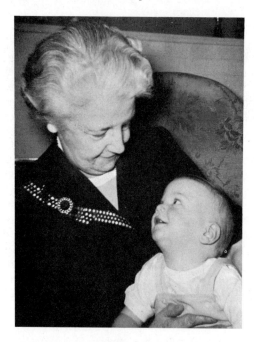

Figure 8-1. The child who is loved and knows it has the inner security to keep working on his developmental tasks.

answer to requests is "No," and he punishes his child with spankings and other physical measures. Dianne may be a well-behaved child in her family circle, but her rebellion is shown in many ways when she is outside her parents' reach.

Patrick's parents are *"permissive,"* with the result that he makes the majority of his own decisions. Sometimes Pat's decisions are satisfactory, and sometimes they are not. Occasionally, he wants to participate in activities that are beyond his abilities and development, and when he is unable to manage these experiences, he is frustrated and disappointed.

Tony's parents base his discipline and their "Yes" or "No" on his *developmental level.* They endeavor to understand his abilities and his lack of them and to adapt their disciplinary technics to this stage. At 2 years of age, Tony was not permitted to cross the street because he did not comprehend its dangers; during his fourth year, because he would soon be walking to kindergarten alone, he was taught safety measures that he could then understand and remember. This seems to be a reasonable compromise in discipline.

In order to apply their philosophy of discipline, parents need considerable knowledge and understanding of their child's behavior as he develops through various stages and ages. Their plan to motivate him toward the behavior they desire, to channel or discipline his actions concurrently with his growth cycles, is called *developmental technics,* and his achievements and subsequently his altered behavior are his personal *developmental tasks.*

## GROWING AND LEARNING

The nurse will often be called upon to care for children, both healthy and ill. She therefore needs to understand normal development. By knowing how most children can be expected to behave at certain ages, she will be better prepared to care for any child for whom she has responsibility. In caring for children, she also needs to understand normal behavior before she can understand abnormal behavior. It helps, for example, to know that during illness, a child may regress, that is, relive an earlier stage of his development.

### How Growth and Development Proceed

Growth and development, which are considered a single process, go on constantly, continuing through childhood and into adulthood.

*Growth* is defined as a change in body structure, while *development* is defined as a change in body function. They occur simultaneously and are interdependent. For example, the child cannot learn to control his bowel movements (development) until his muscles are strong enough (growth) and until he can understand what he is to do.

These changes in growth and development occur in an orderly sequence—one developmental task must be accomplished before another can be attempted. Thus, most children are able to do certain tasks at about the same age, although there are variations within the normal range.

In relation to the body, growth and development follows a cephalocaudal and a proximodistal direction.

*Cephalocaudal* means "from head to foot"; the baby can lift his head before he can sit up, he can make sounds before he can walk.

*Proximodistal* means "from the center to the outside"; the baby can roll over before he can pick up small objects.

Growth and development progresses from the *simple* to the *complex*; the baby learns to sit before he learns to walk, he learns to babble before he learns to speak. You can see how this idea applies to your own progress— you must learn principles and basic technics before you can master complex procedures.

Growth and development is also *inclusive,* that is, it involves the "whole" child, his family, and their culture.

**Heredity and Environment.** Both heredity and environment influence the newborn. Nobody knows for sure which one has a stronger influence or whether they are of approximately equal importance.

*Hereditary* characteristics refer to those characteristics a person inherits from his forbears —mother, father, grandparents, etc. These are often called *genetic* factors. Skin color, eye color, and body build are examples of inherited characteristics.

*Environment* is the sum total of all the conditions and factors that surround the newborn. The kind of housing, the presence of other children, and the amount of medical care available are examples of environmental elements. You can understand that the baby born into a wealthy family may develop differently from the one born into a poor family. Then too, religious practices, nationality, and even location of birth have a bearing on a child's development.

## Evaluating Growth and Development

Growth and development as a single process is divided into physical, physiological, motor, intellectual, emotional, and social aspects; the last three are often considered together as psychosocial development. All aspects of growth and development, however, are closely related and interdependent; walking is controlled by *motor* development; motor development depends on normal bone and muscle growth (*physical*); normal growth depends on adequate food and energy (*physiological*), while the nervous system exercises over-all control (*intellectual*). If the baby is neglected, his *emotional* development will suffer; or if the culture in which he lives is too protective, his *social* development will suffer.

## STAGES OF GROWTH

### The Normal Neonate

A newborn infant is a totally dependent creature with a wide range of characteristics. On the average he weighs about 7 pounds and is about 20 inches long. Although he may lose some of this weight during the first few days of life, he regains it quickly. He cries lustily (crying is the newborn's only way of communicating), kicks vigorously, wiggles and squirms, and sucks often, even when he is not eating. (Evidence indicates that some infants suck their thumbs before they are born.) For all the crying he does, he sheds no tears, because the lacrimal or tear glands are not yet functional. His favorite position is the fetal position, in which his head is tucked forward and his knees bent up to his chin. Indeed all of him is curled into a ball, even his tiny fists.

The nervous system with which a child is born is his for a lifetime; his reactions to internal and external sensations and stimuli help to shape him physically, intellectually, emotionally, and socially. While he cannot focus his eyes and sees very little, he does

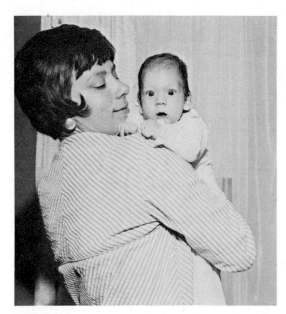

Figure 8-2. The 2-month-old child is able to hold his head steady and focus his eyes on his surroundings, although his back must be supported when he is held. He is able to smile, as he becomes a social being. He has gained 4 to 6 pounds and has grown about 2 to 4 inches since he was born. This marks the fastest postnatal growing period of his lifetime. (Photo by Sisson Studio, Buffalo, Minnesota)

respond to brightly colored objects. He hears well and is easily startled and sometimes is disturbed by loud noises. While his temperature regulating devices are not stable, he responds to heat and cold and therefore must be kept warm and comfortable.

Although the neonate's nervous system is not entirely developed at birth, he is equipped with certain reflexes (involuntary activities) which are necessary for his survival. The *sucking* reflex is vital to his obtaining nourishment; the *rooting* reflex enables him to search for and find the nipple; the *cough* or *gag* reflex prevents or helps to prevent choking, although the newborn chokes or gags often until this reflex is better developed; the *grasp* reflex causes the baby to grasp when something touches his palm. This last reflex disappears as the baby grows older and begins to gain conscious control over his movements.

## The Infant

By the time 4 weeks have passed, the baby has made such progress that he is "graduated"

to the rank of infant. He can now raise his head and turn his chin to the side, although his lack of head control is still marked. He can stare directly ahead for a short time and may be able to focus his eyes on a light. He cries to signal his needs and stops crying when comforted and satisfied. He has a preferred sleeping position, and although sleeping habits vary widely, he will probably sleep 18 to 20 hours a day.

At this stage, a baby's progress can almost be seen from day to day. When he is 6 weeks old, he begins to make purposeful movements. He stops crying when he is picked up—he is beginning to understand that someone will comfort him. As he becomes aware of his surroundings he smiles, babbles when spoken to, and follows lights within his view.

## General Development During the First Year

**Weight.** During the first 3 months of life, the baby has gained about 2 pounds per month and has grown about 1 to 2 inches. In the period from 3 months to 6 months, he will gain about 1 pound per month. Therefore, by the time he is 6 months old, the baby will have about doubled his birth weight. By the end of 1 year, he will weigh about 3 times his birth weight and be about half again as tall as at birth.

**Teeth.** Teeth begin to erupt at about 6 to 7 months of age. The first to erupt generally are the 2 lower central incisors, followed by the 4 top central incisors. By 1 year of age most babies generally have these 6 teeth. Since there is great variation in tooth eruption patterns, parents should not be alarmed if the usual pattern is not followed.

**Food.** The baby begins to eat solid food during the first year of life. Cereal is followed by meat, vegetables, and fruit. Although formula or breastmilk may still be given, most babies drink whole milk after the first few months.

**The 3-Month-Old.** At 3 months, the baby usually can reach for and grasp articles and is able to turn over.

**The 4-Month-Old.** The 4-month-old baby can sit with support and is beginning to coo and babble, especially when someone talks to him. His lacrimal glands have developed fully, so that he now sheds tears when he cries. He usually sleeps all night and takes 2 or 3 naps during the day.

**The 5-Month-Old.** The 5-month-old can hold his head steady, is able to recognize people, and tries to hold his bottle.

**The 6-Month-Old.** At this age the baby can now pull himself up and sit for a short time without support. He can also turn over in bed without help. Behavior differences associated with sex begin to show up now: the boy begins to assert himself and the girl becomes more passive. Psychologists differ as to whether this is the result of hereditary or environmental factors.

**The 9-Month-Old.** By this time, the baby has learned to crawl and is "all over the house" and "into everything."

**The 1-Year-Old.** By about 10 months of age, the baby can usually pull himself up and stand while holding onto something. He then learns to walk around furniture and to stand by himself. At about 1 year of age, he can probably take 1 or 2 steps alone.

The year-old child can feed himself finger foods, can hold his own bottle, and can also drink out of a cup without difficulty.

He knows his name and responds when spoken to. In turn he can say 2 or 3 simple words, such as "baby" and "bye-bye." He is very sociable and wants to play. He laughs aloud and loves games such as hide-and-seek.

## Success Balances Failure

Between the ages of 4 and 7 months, the infant undertakes many new activities (developmental tasks). The inevitable failures as he makes every effort to succeed in these new tasks lead to frustration. As he goes through these stages, as physical development hastens on, he begins to achieve success in many of his undertakings and becomes happy and satisfied. Gesell calls this "equilibrium"; the total personality is in balance. Temporarily at least, he is able to do the things he tries to do; his abilities are equal to his efforts, and he is generally pleased with his success. His growth, desires, emotions and accomplishments are balanced. At 7 months, a child can not only grasp the reached-for object but he can put it in his mouth. (This includes his own toes.) He is very pleased with his accomplishment of transferring objects from one hand to another and will happily entertain

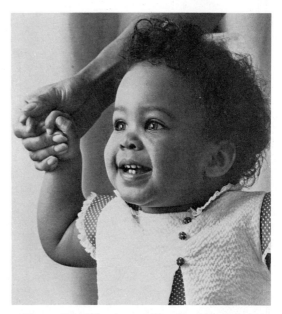

Figure 8-3. The 1-year-old takes her first shaky steps with assistance. Notice the normal tooth development for the 1-year-old child. She is bright-eyed and ready to conquer the world! (Gerber Products Company)

himself at this task. He also enjoys what is to him the purposeful activity of bouncing or banging. He makes many different sounds, and although he can amuse himself for long intervals, he enjoys the company of others and is very friendly.

# AGES 1 TO 10

## The Beginning of the Toddler Stage

**Age 1.** The happy mobile 1-year-old has passed through several peak stages of accomplishments (equilibrium) and several stages of frequent frustrations (disequilibrium). His growth rate is slowing, and his social, physiological and psychological functions have reached the point where they also advance at a slower rate. This does not mean that new skills do not appear; the creeping or beginning-to-walk 1-year-old is a dashing, climbing explorer at 15 months; but the peak periods of accomplishment are further apart.

The slowed physical growth is reflected by the fact that, between 1 and 4 years of age, the child gains only 4 to 6 pounds annually and grows only about 2 to 3 inches per year. How-

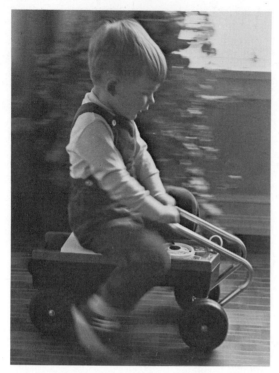

Figure 8-4. The 2-year-old likes toys that he can ride. He is a dynamo of constant activity; he never stops. He becomes very frustrated with toys which he cannot manage or with things he cannot do. His emotions are very close to the surface—he is extremely happy or very sad, seldom in between. He loves activity, noise, water, animals, and other people, as long as he gets his own way. He wants to be helpful and to be good, so that he is accepted by the family. (Mattel, Inc.)

ever, physical and motor skills show great strides; he can now fit simple shaped objects into appropriate holes and can build a tower of 2 or 3 blocks. Verbal skills also improve; the toddler has a speaking vocabulary of about 20 to 30 words, although he understands many more, as shown by his ability to follow directions.

His social contacts begin to broaden at this age as he shares his playtime with other children. However, he seems to play next to a playmate rather than with him. This so-called *parallel play* will continue until his social skills are better developed.

**Age 18 Months.** A day in the life of the 18-month-old (and of his parents) is far from smooth. At 1½ he is much more difficult to live with than when he was 1. Then, he was

sociable and cheerful and friendly most of the time; but by 1½, he is beginning to sense that he controls certain aspects of his environment, and he starts to take advantage of this to the fullest. He is a "no" creature in all respects and usually rejects all demands. He is a "now" creature who has no ability to wait. Sharing is beyond his comprehension, and he takes all to and for himself. He seems to derive his greatest consolation and pleasure from being the opposition in every situation.

**Age 2.** The change to the balance of the 2-year-old is very welcome in most households. He is good-natured, warmly affectionate, and easily pleased—a virtual joy to his family. As he learns to move with more sureness and safety, he begins to explore his surroundings with interest. However, since he is also accident-prone, definite limits must be set for him.

His neuromusclar coordination has increased to the point where he can put on and take off simple items of clothing, such as slip-on shirts; he can climb stairs without crawling, and can throw or kick a large ball. His tower of blocks is now 5 or 6 blocks high; he loves to knock it over and set it up again. He can string beads, scribble with crayons, and turn book pages, 1 or 2 at a time.

The vocabulary of the 2-year-old includes about 300 to 350 words, which he combines into simple sentences. He learns through playing word games and number games, through watching educational programs on television, and through doing simple wooden puzzles.

**Age 2½.** Parents should heed the warning that the charming, pleasant 2-year-old becomes the "Terrible Tommy" of 2½. When he decides to pour his milk from the large pitcher, no one may help; if he insists on putting on his own pants and ends up with both legs in one pant leg, it cannot be changed: he is the boss. If Mother kissed him twice before lifting him from his crib on Monday, she must kiss him twice on Tuesday—his routines are rigid! He resists any change, even in such details as demanding one specific glass or dish over and over. With all his rigidity, the child of this age is unable to make a choice. "I will —I won't" becomes a frequent and exasperating experience. However, patient parents find to their relief that the active, persistent, enthusiastic, ritualistic 2-year-old soon enters the balanced calm area of 3.

## The Preschool Age

**Age 3.** The child at this age is in a stage of happy conforming equilibrium. His "No" changes to "Yes," and his routines become more flexible. His increased motor and language skills enable him to accomplish the developmental tasks required at this age.

Physically, he now has a full set of baby teeth (deciduous), consisting of 10 upper and 10 lower teeth. He weighs about 30 to 35 pounds and is 30 to 36 inches tall. Although he has achieved about half his adult height, his physical development is slowing down. He will probably gain less than 6 pounds per year and about 3 inches annually, until he enters school. Physical skills, however, are more refined. He can dress and undress himself almost completely, can manage large buttons and zippers, can build high towers with blocks, can draw recognizable forms such as a square or a man, and can form objects with clay.

Intellectually, his growth has progressed to the point where he can count to 3 or higher, can identify objects in pictures, and can tell which of 2 or 3 objects are alike. His vocabulary numbers about 1,000 words, which he uses in incessant talk. His ability to use words also reflects his ability to reason. (Psychologists believe that the child of high verbal ability possesses greater reasoning ability, as measured by I.Q. tests.)

Emotionally, the child of 3 has a great desire to be independent and to do everything for himself; he can brush his teeth, put on most of his clothes, and feed himself. He also demonstrates better control over his emotions. He identifies with and imitates the parent of the same sex. During this *Oedipal* stage, when attention and interest focus on the parent of the opposite sex, he may feel competitive and jealous toward the other parent. A boy talks of marrying Mommy, and a girl of marrying Daddy.

Generally, the child tries hard to do what is expected of him and to be obedient and helpful. He is becoming sensitive to social interactions and is easily hurt by scolding.

Socially, the child of 3 or 4 is beginning to play *with* other children, as well as next to them. He can make up simple games and is learning to share and to wait his turn. Play differences between boys and girls begin to

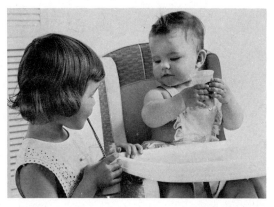

Figure 8-5. The girl of 4 or 5 delights in having a younger brother. She "takes care" of him and pretends that she is the mommy. She helps him in every way that she can. Here she encourages him to drink his milk. (Gerber Products Company)

develop. Girls show a preference for quiet games, such as card games, playing with dolls, and coloring. Boys prefer rough and loud games; they play with trucks, balls, hammers and other tools.

To briefly summarize, the play and growth activities of the 3-year-old proceed with ease and delight. His wants and his ability to carry out his desires are well balanced: he is pleased with himself and his associates. He is very friendly and willing to share. His friendliness and his interest in words and in sharing his thoughts and knowledge make him an enjoyable and entertaining companion.

**Age 3½.** At age 3½ there is a great alteration in behavior; again, disequilibrium appears in many phases. The smooth motor functions of 3 may be replaced by clumsy actions of falling. Children frequently stutter at this age; they may seem to be tense and insecure; they may suck their thumb more and seem to be jittery and whiny. This new, uncertain child is in continual need of the usually unreserved attention lavished on the affectionate 3-year-old.

**Age 4.** At 4, the pendulum swings to the opposite extreme. Uncertainty and insecurity are traded for the most brash self-confidence. He looks at a wider world (even if it does extend only to the corner of the block), and he is quite sure he can conquer it. It is hoped that his parents will be able to preserve some of this confidence while firmly controlling it. Ilg and Ames, authorities on child development, describe the 4-year-old as "out of bounds in most every direction. He breaks things . . . runs away . . . Laughter alternates with fits of rage . . . A terrible toughness seems to come over him . . . he swears, swaggers, boasts and brags."

As he leans toward 5, he again begins to assemble his abilities and control his skills. He is beginning to form concepts about abstract relationships, as indicated by his ability to remember what object is missing in a room and that "tomorrow" follows "today." He has a vocabulary of at least 2000 words, and can probably count to 10. He can usually print part of his name and can state his age and his full name.

In his social relationships he tries hard to be a friend and to get along with others. He will, however, engage in physical fighting, hitting, kicking, and biting in the process. Girls, on the other hand, are more likely to yell at each other in their disagreements.

At 4½ he likes to draw and build with a purpose in mind. He wants to be sure that things are "real" and enjoys talking about what he thinks and knows.

**Age 5.** Many parents find it difficult to believe that their frustrating 4-year-old could be transformed into their angel of 5. He is quite comfortable within himself and in his relations with others. He is satisfied with his world of home and family, although he may live in a land of make-believe, peopled by imaginary playmates and an imaginary family with fanciful names, which he insists on using. The developmental tasks which he has mastered are sufficient for the moment. He is a good child, temporarily pleased with the balance and the equilibrium of his interests and his skills.

## The School-Age Child

**Age 6.** "And now I am six and as clever as clever. I hope I'll be six now forever and ever" goes A. A. Milne's description of the psychology of the 6-year-old.

Parents and family have been ousted from first place; the 6-year-old thinks that he is the most important and the best. Because he always has to be first, he is difficult to live with. The eruption of the smooth behavior of the 5-year-old into the volcanic behavior of the 6-year-old is sometimes incomprehensible to parents. A squashy, squeezing "I love you" may be followed by "I hate you" 2 minutes later. (Gesell says "Six" is at his worst with his mother.) He recognizes no needs of others and demands that everyone give in to him.

The 6-year-old's saving grace is his eagerness to try new situations and his enthusiasm for learning and adventure. If his self-development and reaching out from the family can be accepted by parents as a big step forward, understanding will soften the difficulties.

The most important event in the life of the 6-year-old, is the beginning of school. As he enters a new world other than the world of home, he becomes increasingly independent. Since school occupies much of his waking hours, events at school begin to play a large part in his life. He is interested in everything, wants to learn, and is eager to please the teacher. He asks questions in a never-ending search for information.

In accordance with his entry into school, the child's reasoning and conceptual powers expand. He can tell time and can count to at least 40 or 50; often he is able to recognize the letters of the alphabet, the numbers from 1 to 10, and his own name. In fact, he may be able to read simple words. His speaking vocabulary, on the other hand, numbers at least 2500 words. As the year progresses, he will learn to count to about 100 and to subtract numbers up to 10.

As he approaches six, he begins to lose his deciduous teeth as the permanent teeth begin to erupt (see Fig. 17-2). From the time a child enters school, at about age 6, a slow, steady period of growth begins. He will gain about 5 to 7 pounds a year and will grow about 2½ inches a year until puberty (sexual maturity), when he will undergo a growth spurt. It now becomes difficult to identify an "average" because the variations among normal children are much wider.

**Age 7.** The child of this age is sensitive and presents a changed picture. He becomes quiet and thoughtful and tends to worry and daydream. Yet he craves adult approval and is very sensitive to criticism. He is described by some authorities as "moody." He observes, listens, reads—this is an age of learning. His sense of touch becomes a source of knowledge. He loves to feel things, to explore by touch-

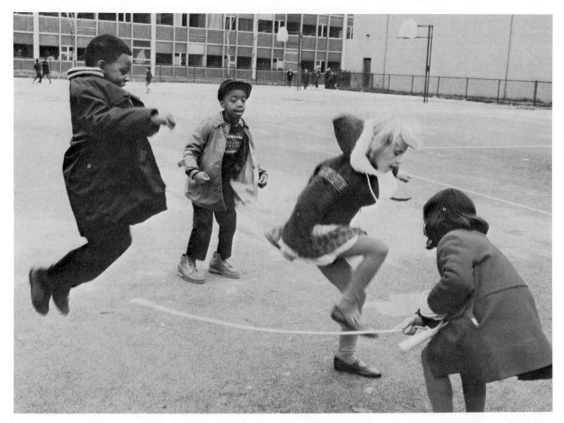

Figure 8-6. Eight-year-olds are exuberant and joyful and full of life and energy. Since they enjoy playing together, team games or sports are desirable. They accept each other without reservation and play together, without recognizing differences. From *Your Children's Health Day by Day*, National Dairy Council)

ing, rubbing, and crumbling. The 7-year-old girl has a reasonable enjoyment of life, but she seems to enjoy unhappiness: "You don't love me"; "I'm going to run away"; "You're mean to me." She wants a retreat of her own for "mooding."

Boys and girls of this age are aware of each other, but do not play together. In fact, they are usually antagonistic and may fight and call each other nasty names.

As the child nears eight, he gains in self-confidence and poise. As he becomes more stable, he is better able to cope with his world.

**Age 8.** If the 7-year-old is quiet and withdrawn, the 8-year-old bounces back into life. New facts and difficult tasks—these are joyful challenges for the child. He is extremely active, daring, and unaware of danger—hence he can easily be injured. His self-confidence is so great that he does not believe anything can happen to him. Enthusiasm and energy often cause the 8-year-old to undertake too much, and he recognizes his failures. Guidance is needed to prevent constant new projects from becoming repeated failures and to prevent overexertion. Fortunately, at this age, the child now appreciates how others treat him and also is concerned about how he affects them. A child of 8 is good for Mother's ego: although to the sensitive 7-year-old, his mother is a real trial, "Eight" enjoys, needs, and wants his mother's company.

However, the "gang" or friends occupy an important place in his life, and he will do almost anything for them. The members of the gang usually share secrets, including a favorite hangout, and they dislike girls so much at this point that they actually fight with them openly at times.

**Age 9.** The 9-year-old is a new story—independent and individual. At 7, he needed to investigate and to learn about himself. At 8, he needed to assure relationships with the outside world. "Nine" gives evidence of beginning to coordinate the developmental patterns of ages 7 and 8. Being self-reliant, he proves himself able to make most decisions pertaining to the usual activities. The family circle may seem to be too constricting and he tends to want to become involved in interests and activities outside the family. Much of his time is spent with friends, the "gang," or with other clubs and groups. In spite of all evidences of self-reliance, the 9-year-old worries a great deal and complains about developmental tasks in which he must assume responsibility—studies and home tasks alike.

However, he often works hard at learning—experimenting with a chemistry set and reading voraciously. He loves stories of adventure and imagination, and he searches endlessly for imaginary or real heroes whom he can emulate—for this is the age of "hero worship," when photographs and stories of some outstanding athlete or movie star are collected and cherished.

**Age 10.** At age 10 there is a great improvement—a more mature version of the delightful child of 5. The typical 5-year-old accepted himself and others and was pleased with his world. The typical 10-year-old is a satisfied child, also. He enjoys his family, his school, and life in general. He enjoys being obedient because it is reasonable and pleasing. He is friendly and realistic, and accepts himself and life as it comes. Never again will his mother and father enjoy such complete approval and acceptance of themselves as parents and people as that offered by their agreeable 10-year-old.

## Other Concerns

There are other areas of behavior which concern parents, such as discontinuing bottle feedings, toilet training, bed wetting, thumb sucking, rocking, and head banging. As in all decisions relating to child care, these "problems" must be handled on an individual basis. And, as in all things human, authorities differ about preferred methods. From 1911 to the present time, first at the Yale Clinic of Child Development and then at its successor, the Gesell Institute of Child Development, developmental research and studies have concentrated on the "analysis, interpretation, and management of relatively normal manifestations" of childhood. The results of these studies furnish a suggested middle-of-the-road solution for many of the concerns of parents and re-emphasize the need for recognizing the pace of development, as well as the ability of each child.

**Mountains From Molehills.** If the wide divergence in physical growth alone is considered—the rate of development of the various groups of muscles or the development of the nervous system—then the wise parents will be less disturbed about the child who hangs on to the habits which are mainly disturbing to them.

Many infants are ready to relinquish the bottle at the end of their first year. If a mother feels the child will not get enough milk, she may substitute custards, cheeses, ice cream, etc. Changing the color or style of the bottle or nipple at 15 months may encourage a child to drink from a pretty cup, but a reluctant child may want a bedtime bottle until he is 2 or 3 years old. It helps his active little body and mind to relax for sleep. As his third birthday draws near, he is usually willing to exchange it for a colorful toy beside his bed.

**Masturbation.** Even a year-old infant likes to touch things and handle them; he finds as he grows older that touching some parts of his body gives him pleasant sensations. The preschool child sometimes finds that handling his genitals relieves tensions rising from conflict with his parents. There is nothing abnormal or shameful about this; but if the child is shamed or threatened or punished it may have an injurious effect on his sexual expression later in life. The happy, busy child is not likely to seek comfort in masturbation.

**Fact and Fantasy.** The imaginative child may often confuse fact with fiction. Tommy's mother, reproving Tommy for what she thought was an untruth, asked him if he remembered what happened to Annanias and Sapphira. "Sure," he said, "They were struck dead for lying, and I saw them carried into the drug store." Quite likely at some time, he had seen some unconscious person carried into the drug store. Children try to make what is sense, for them, out of things they hear. Jean rushed home from Sunday School to report that Jesus is sneaking through Humboldt Park. This remarkable statement originated from the words of the hymn: "Jesus is seeking the humble heart."

**Toilet-Training.** Toilet-training is also an individual matter. Certainly we can see that nervous system development as well as muscular response and control are vital clues in this parental puzzle. Around 9 to 10 months, Kathy had established a fairly regular routine for bowel movements following her evening meal. Kathy's mother was overjoyed, for again it is mainly to the parent that early toilet-training is important. However, the problem here may be that Mother, not Kathy, has recognized the habit time, and Mother may be frustrated by irregular habit times in the future. As pointed out by Jeans, Wright and Blake, Mother must watch instead for "signs that indicate readiness to learn" rather than regularity. In many fortunate children, "readiness to learn" occurs around 2 years of age.

Bowel-training is usually accomplished with less effort than bladder-training, but this may not be true for some children (usually boys). Some perfectly normal children still do not have total conscious control by 5 years of age. Lane and Beauchamp in *Understanding Human Development* point out that "Under severe emotional strain or fatigue, children will loose control of their bladders for many years after they begin school." But, most parents are relieved to find that toilet-training, barring occasional accidents, is well under way by 3 years of age.

**Bed-Wetting.** Bed-wetting (enuresis) is another problem, usually for parents of boys. Most children who are unable to master this developmental task are unable to do so because of physiological immaturity. For example, Danny, at age 4, exhibits excellent bowel control as well as fairly good daytime bladder control. However, it can be observed that he urinates at frequent intervals and occasionally is not dry after a nap. He is often wet an hour after he is asleep at night.

Danny evidently has a very limited bladder capacity, and his parents will have to accept the fact that Danny may be wetting his bed for a long time. When Danny is a little older and can sleep 3 hours or more without wetting, perhaps getting him up during the night will furnish a better solution. Restricting fluids between the evening meal and bedtime sometimes helps.

If the bed-wetting persists (and physical and psychological problems have been eliminated), there are other measures that can be tried. Some children have an "irritable" bladder, a condition in which a small amount of urine in the bladder produces the desire to urinate. In this case, the physician may order a drug to decrease the irritability. The child also can be encouraged to withhold the urine voluntarily during the daytime. This gradually distends the bladder, increasing its size, and promoting retention. At the same time, a drug may be ordered to produce lighter sleep.

**Thumb-Sucking.** Thumb-sucking may begin around 3 or 4 months of age. Most infants are interested in popping everything into their mouths by the time they reach 7 months, and their thumb is a handy object. Usually by the time the child is 2 years of age, he sucks his thumb only when he is tired or hungry. The 3-year-old has a strong affection for his thumb and for his favorite blanket or soft toy. At 4 he is often ready to give up the blanket.

Many times parents have been told that thumb-sucking alters the shape of the mouth, with resultant "poor bite" and distorted teeth. But there is some disagreement about this. This controversy deprives the parent of a clear-cut guide to follow. However, most authorities agree that thumb-sucking does not affect the structure of the mouth and teeth *if* it is stopped before the second teeth appear.

**Rocking.** Rocking and head-banging are also habits that usually lose their usefulness to the child as other outlets become more available. If bed-rocking has not stopped by the time a child is 3 or 4, moving him to a bigger bed is usually an automatic cut-off. Head-banging sometimes causes bruises and, therefore, is worrisome to parents. Children who do this have many similar characteristics, such as sleeping restlessly, having strong likes and dislikes, and resisting if not permitted to have their own way. Spanking, scolding, and other punishments do not stop head-banging. Picking up the child will distract him momentarily. Since children usually enjoy music, a record player or radio played softly in their room will sometimes help them to relax.

## Parents Should Know

Parents will see that each one of their children differs from the others in the same behavior at the same age. But, most parents will enjoy the developmental progress of their children if they have a greater perception of the general direction of their growth. An understanding of a child's need to resist will not always relieve the stress and the distress of the moment but will greatly assist Mother and Dad in guiding him toward the next stage in which he usually yields to reason.

Parents are happier if they see changes in their children as signs of growth and progress. The instinctive curiosity of children, as well as their physical growth, carries them to new fields to conquer. C. Anderson Aldrich and Mary M. Aldrich in *Babies Are Human Beings* state: "The greatest educator of all time will be the person who shows us the way to conduct children through the preschool years so that this baby eagerness to learn is maintained."

Sincere concern for long-range development of their children leads many parents to seek knowledge which will foster greater understanding and happy parent-child relationships. This knowledge and understanding will not eliminate the need for parental discipline and guidance. Rather, it enhances it. It encourages a "mutual respect" approach to a balanced family relationship. Each family member can "practice the skills and preserve the satisfactions of his age level." Understanding the needs and the problems of children will supply parents with clues to more effective methods of control or discipline for each stage and age. It will offer support to both parent and children in working toward their mutual goal of increased abilities, skills, self-knowledge, and self-discipline: all signposts of maturity.

## The Nurse Should Know

If you know the physical and the psychological development characteristics of the different ages and stages, if you know what needs are stronger at one time than another, you will know what behavior is reasonable to expect. Through your knowledge of the child's possible and probable achievements and abilities, you will be able to establish a richer relationship with the children for whom you will be caring as a nurse. Remember that the child who is normally stable may regress when he becomes ill. He may find it a traumatic experience to be taken to the hospital and left there. Many children worry about their condition and feel that they are never going to get better. This is particularly difficult when the child *is* gravely ill or when he has a degenerative or fatal disease.

# 9

# Adolescence

---

## BEHAVIORAL OBJECTIVES

*The student successfully attaining the goals of this chapter will be able to:*

- *describe the specific developmental tasks which the preadolescent and adolescent must meet as he or she moves on toward adulthood.*
- *state characteristics which are shown by most young people at ages 10, 11, and 12, and during early, middle, and late adolescence.*
- *design a plan for presenting information relating to human sexuality to young people of 10, 11, and 12 years of age.*
- *discuss the need of the preadolescent or adolescent for discipline; describe the most effective methods of discipline and identify why these means are usually effective.*
- *describe the specific physical changes which take place between the ages of 10 and 18 in boys and in girls; and discuss the psychological implications of these changes.*

---

The study of adolescence is called ephebiatrics. This time of life is marked by a rapid spurt of growth, at the end of which the youth will have achieved his adult height. Although there is tremendous physical growth, emotional needs predominate during this period; the adolescent spends much of his time searching for meaning in life and for his own identity.

## THE STEP INTO PREADOLESCENCE

The slow swing to age 11 brings more indications of the progress to maturity (although parents find the intensive 11-year-old somewhat jarring after the casual 10-year-old). The often difficult and restless qualities of the child are not regressions to earlier stages. He is an "adolescent in the making." His negativeness is a form of self-assertion, a beginning step in the establishment of the mature "I." His unending talk and arguments, his seeming impudence and rudeness indicate his inexperience in mastering new developmental tasks.

Physically as well as psychologically, age 11 characterizes a state of change. Most boys at 11 do not show the changes of puberty. Only 25 per cent have started to grow more rapidly, but many appear to have a heavier or more marked skeletal structure. In girls there is a great variation in physical structure and sexual development. The average 11-year-old girl has reached a period of rapid growth and shows signs of impending sexual maturity. Interest and occasional embarrassment accompany awareness of female curves; only a few girls of 11 menstruate.

The child of 11 is a dynamo, physically and psychologically. Energy bursts forth at every seam. Even while apparently sitting still, he is in constant motion: he stretches, wiggles, jiggles, waves his arms, clicks his feet together and generally finds it impossible to remain still.

Rebellions against parents, noisy and fault-finding quarrels with brothers and sisters and constant evasion of helping at home are irritating to live with. Patience is necessary, and the child needs to be handled with understanding and firmness. Although many of his new undertakings are to test independence and self-reliance, he still needs strong support and guidance from parents. The fact that he behaves best away from home gives clues to his self-discipline and other possibilities in his future growth pattern.

## Shadows of Adult Potential

The gradual change to 12 shows improvement in meeting the challenges of maturity. The 12-year-old is more organized emotionally and is improved in his ability to see situations in total perspectives. He is not adult; but relative to his age, he indicates his positive capacities toward adulthood.

The psychological awareness of age 12 has broadened beyond self. He has gained more objectivity in his approval of self and others. This, plus his expanding sense of humor, makes his family associations much more pleasant.

Because the child of 12 is so enthusiastic, he brings spirit and buoyancy to all his undertakings. Extensive projects in school show initiative and effort. However, this high pitch of enthusiasm and initiative may get out of hand. Planned parties and social events need adult supervision, or the boisterous group activity of this age can wreck the party.

There is a slight improvement in attitude toward chores that he now regards as a necessity to be endured, but he still needs frequent reminding by parents, and he realizes it. As one 12-year-old wrote in an essay: "I think I should pick up my good clothes after church. I think parents should punish when necessary." At age 12, renewed interest is shown in working for money as a means to his extras.

Most girls at 12 are in a stage of rapid gains in both height and weight. Breast development is definite, and menstruation most commonly begins during the twelfth year. Early periods are frequently irregular.

Variation in physical growth is marked in 12-year-old boys; the average boy shows some incipient pubertal changes by the end of this year. Spontaneous erections without external cause occur and are confusing to the 12-year-old. It should be explained to him that this involuntary discharge of semen is a natural occurrence, as natural as the change in the

voice and the growth of a beard. Boys are often more interested in sex from the view of their own development rather than from the view of adult sexual activity.

Twelve-year-olds are often concerned about appearance. Style, color and fit of clothing are important. They also take baths with less resistance and may enjoy soaking in the tub. However, both boys and girls may soak for hours, only to emerge not much cleaner than before the bath—they just forgot to wash!

Following only gradually upon the imbalances of age 11, age 12 shows shadows of adult potentials. The enthusiasm, the occasional self-discipline, the humor, the intelligence and the self-knowledge are clues to the constitutional treats and cultural moldings which will mature within the coming decade.

Most young people have reached 90 per cent of their adult height by age 12 or 13. They have tripled in length and gained 20 times in weight since birth! The 13-year-old has all his permanent teeth except his wisdom teeth.

## The Over-all Needs of the Preadolescent

Although the middle years or preadolescent years of childhood show specific trends of their own, there are general characteristics which can be summarized. The need to be part of a group or gang emerges, as both an inclusive and an exclusive force. Boys are more tolerant and informal in groups, and at this stage their "gang" is broadly inclusive. Girls are more choosy.

Physical development is variable, but in all preadolescent children some signs of sexual growth appear, accompanied by a curiosity about biologic sex facts. If this information is provided by the right people, in the right way, then good attitudes about sex will be formed. If the parents, the teachers or the counselors do not give the information that the child seeks, he will find misinterpretation and unwholesome attitudes in jokes, stories, immoral books and perhaps the "wise" older teenager.

Because of the widened horizons of interest as well as the increase in physical growth, children in these years work at many new skills. Sports become a great interest. Cooking may appeal to both boys and girls. It is hoped that adults will give them room to grow.

Family relations may be delicate at this age. The attitude toward younger brothers and sisters is either protective or one of annoyance; the attitude toward parents is variable and extends from annoyance and criticism to genuine understanding. A wholesome family relationship at this time can influence lifetime interpersonal success, for it fosters respect of self and of others. The parents' respect for the child's need for self-assertion, privacy, information, recognition, acceptance, experimentation and growth in all developmental areas and for an understanding of adult imperfections furnishes a firm foundation for guidance and pleasure in coming years. At the same time the adolescent also wants guidance and reasonable rules. As stated by Lane and Beauchamp: "The cement of mental health is self-respect." Self-respect is nourished by respect for and from others.

**The Period of Reflection.** As in other stages of maturity, the 13-year-old develops many and new forms of behavior. In contrast with the open spirit of the middle years of childhood, the early adolescent shows tendencies to seclusion and moodiness.

Gesell and Ilg call worry the "cardinal maturity trait at this stage of adolescent development . . . the major key to the psychology of the 13-year-old." He has become aware of and takes pleasure in this emerging reasoning ability. He reflects on self and others and assesses new experiences. Appraisal of interaction between self and the world needs a place as well as time, so the young teenager tends to spend more time alone.

His measurings naturally include his family. His criticisms plus his withdrawal are often a source of puzzlement as well as hurt to parents. Both girls and boys have long associations with the mirror. They use the mirror as a prop for their role-playing, testing and measuring themselves in the situations they imagine.

By the completion of their thirteenth year, most girls have about reached their adult height and have established menstrual periods. Boys have begun their rapid growth and experience erections. Only about half have had nocturnal emissions (release of semen while sleeping), although most know about them.

**Social Awareness.** The child of 13 has taken further steps to maturity in the social area. Table manners are improved, and washing hands, taking baths and brushing teeth are becoming part of the routine. Appearance and selection of clothes are important, but care of clothing leaves much to be desired.

Authorities feel that at no other stage of development is there such need for conformity to the group, while at the same time, such development of individuality. Through this year and the remaining years of adolescence, the maturing teenager takes frequent flights of independence but has a strong need to return to the nest for guidance and encouragement.

As always in developmental progression, patterns are tempered and adjusted by individuality.

## ADOLESCENCE

### Coming to Terms With Reality

The introspection of age 13 permits the child of 14 to move forward with a relaxation of inner and outer tensions. Laughter is heard once more; he has achieved self-assurance. Glandular changes, alterations in body chemistry, the challenges of his age, plus the continuing unbelievable capacity to consume food, provide a great supply of energy.

The 14-year-old is more accepting of other people as individuals and is discriminatingly aware of personalities. His sense of humor releases tensions that previously have taxed family relationships. He is less critical and more tolerant of his parents, although he still has tendencies to regard them and their ideas as truly antique. He likes his brothers and sisters "more than he thought he did." "Talk, talk, talk, talk" is many an adult's version of this age. Authorities state this is a true growth characteristic and a developmental achievement of 14-year-olds. They show increased natural ability in perceiving more than one side of situations and are no longer frustrated by being unable to express or verbalize their own ideas. They are able to say what they think—a task of maturity.

**The Introduction of Sex Boundaries.** By the age of 14 most girls have the physical figure and appearance of young women. Few will add further height; breast and other secondary sex characteristics are adult.

Most boys grow more at 14 than at any other age. A strong muscular appearance and continued deepening of the voice add to the impression of maturity. Nocturnal emissions have begun for most; if the boys are properly informed, they accept it as a natural occurrence.

Further sex education is needed and accepted. Although dating may not yet be a routine practice, boys and girls are interested in each other. They need to know that controls are necessary and why the controls need to be developed. They seem to accept this information if presented accurately and forthrightly. They are not yet ready to make decisions on their own. Parents must help to establish reasonable and sensible boundaries. These are accepted best by the 14-year-old if he is forewarned and forearmed with knowledge and understanding.

## Toward Independence

These middle years of childhood are baffling to many adults. They have been described as the "phase when the nicest children behave in the most awful way." The physical alterations, the brash self-assertion, the preoccupation with self, the rapid change from streaks of independence to the dependent attitude of the child, the gay blithe spirit, the moody introspection—all are real challenges to the most interested and conscientious parent.

In the panorama of growth, these characteristics show that the child is growing away from childhood; and in accord with the orderly pattern this permits the advancement to the next stage of maturity—growth to adulthood.

Traces of the outgoing 14-year-old, friendly and enthusiastic, are sometimes difficult to find in sensitive, indifferent or resisting 15-year-olds. Fifteen-year-olds are afflicted with a development that a knowing mother called "sophomoritis." (The word is combined from *sophos* meaning wise and *moros* meaning foolish.) This perceptive mother also stated that the fifteenth year of each of her children was the "worst year in being a parent."

The teenager is pulling away from childhood. He feels that he should be self-reliant.

Although he values the dependencies of home and school, he feels a need to counterbalance these with independence. Since he is searching for a method of balance, his immaturity frequently produces withdrawal, belligerence or defiance. Because of the characteristics of 15, this may be an age of beginning juvenile delinquency. He views all parental directions as control and he sometimes seeks guidance away from home.

Fifteen has some ideas concerning his future; he has begun to plan for more than present interests and activities. His maturing has improved his relationship with brothers and sisters. Because he has vague ideas of marrying and of having a home and a career of his own, he scrutinizes home and parents closely. Parents may feel that they have been rejected because of their failure to meet the perfectionist standards of their observing 15-year-old.

In most girls, adult physical characteristics have already developed, and changes are concerned in bringing these characteristics toward the fuller blossom of womanhood. The menstrual cycle has become more regular.

Fifteen-year-old boys are approaching full growth. Reproductive organs are adult size; secondary sex characteristics are marked. Sexual response is more directed and less subject to stimuli such as fear. Authorities feel that masturbation increases at 15 and that calm reassurance from Father will help some boys to channel activities. These authorities suggest that keeping active does not reduce the tendency to masturbation but increases control.

Increased independence brings more interest and responsibility in self-care. Boys, especially, have huge appetites, but occasionally the 15-year-old loses or gains weight for a specific purpose. He also recognizes sleep needs and plans to "catch up" if he is tired. All continue to improve in cleanliness, and although boys may need reminders, girls are generally interested in baths, deodorants, shampoos and nail care.

At age 15, the adolescent likes to choose his own clothing and usually makes more purchases than in previous years. There is general improvement in the care of his clothes as well as in the care of his room. However, as part of the home relationship, the 15-year-old does not prove to be a good helper. Interest is shown in work away from home because it provides money. If the 15-year-old recognizes that his own money comes to him as a result of his own efforts, he may even become very interested in saving as well as earning.

## Independence Sprouts

The true actions and attitudes of maturity are beginning to be obvious in the middle teenager. In his interpersonal relations, he is friendly and self-confident. Gesell, Ilg and Ames state: "Wholesome *self-assurance* is his cardinal trait, and a symptom of his potentials." This may not have been true earlier in the teen years, when the youth often seemed to be dissatisfied, uncertain and even rebellious. "He then had a *spirit* of independence —now he has achieved, instead, a *sense* of independence."

The informal interest in people and awareness and acceptance of social responsibilities make the middle teen years a companionable age, one with many friendships of both sexes. Family relationships usually improve. The 15- or 16-year-old acts so much more grown-up that most parents automatically accept the attitude of independence from him. He has so many interests and associations outside home that time spent with the family is limited; but he often consults parents about problems (if parents are willing to discuss them at this adult level), and he likes to feel free to have home as a base for his friends.

Further physical development is not marked in girls. The girl of 14 to 16 is often ready to accept menstruation simply as part of adult biology. Most boys at this age have reached close to adult height. The finishing touches seem to be the smoothing and the toughening appearance of boys.

Many young people find it increasingly difficult to maintain sexual control. Since petting or "making-out" is more common, young people need to discuss some of the problems involved. With the availability of birth control means, venereal disease has become perhaps a greater threat than pregnancy. Young people need an opportunity to discuss these feelings with each other and with adults, so that they can make appropriate decisions in their lives.

## Toward Adulthood

The 16-year-old has made strides in maturing intellectually, as well as physically and emotionally. His judgment ability has been stimulated and developed through his accomplishing the tasks of the preceding years. He, as well as his peers, usually finds the ensuing years of adolescence happy and fruitful.

We can find reason to study the adolescent from the point of view of numbers alone, for the 1970 adolescent population was over 16 million. However, there are other more appealing reasons to interest us in the teenager. The cycles of growth can be seen in strong clarification: the realization of the possibility of further accomplishments; the curiosity, the challenge, the thrust, effort and frustration in this further development; and the enjoyment and the satisfactions of the achievement.

The next few years are those of further transition from adolescence through young adulthood, but there is no sharp area of demarcation to divide these years. They bring further progress to maturity. The natural progress and ultimate task of the adolescent is to "grow up." The attitude and the success of each child in his progress to maturity is determined by his heredity and environment, the culture in which he lives and the self-determination and perceptions of the individual child.

Various authorities define the components of achieving maturity in various ways but generally agree on certain important steps. Lane and Beauchamp define the developmental tasks of adolescents as achieving independence from home and developing satisfactory heterosexual relationships. They quote Frankwood Williams as follows: "He begins life entirely dependent, egocentric, irresponsible; he should become fully independent, altruistic, responsible. He has to pass from the completely filial to the completely parental attitude."*

Other authorities break the broad goals into more defined tasks, but all tasks ultimately involve independence from parental domination and the acceptance of individual responsi-

---

* Williams, F. E.: *in* Lane, H., and Beauchamp, M.: Understanding Adolescence, p. 313, Englewood Cliffs, N. J., Prentice-Hall, 1959.

bility. For instance, emancipation from parental ties is seen in the form of intellectual, emotional and economic independence. Further, in order to initiate and maintain satisfactory interpersonal relations with both sexes, the adult must have developed wholesome concepts of self-identity, self-respect and self-control. In assuring the adult's freedom to decide upon a course of action, the mature adult must develop and recognize the purpose of his action and be willing to accept personal responsibilities and social duties.

The contribution of a wholesome family life is strongly supported by evidence. Schneider states that the "adolescent's family is the most important single determination of his growth pattern, his mental health and his adjustments."

Homes are happy when family relationships are based on mutual respect and affection. Mutual respect recognizes the task of the parent to discipline the child and the task of the child to adjust to discipline. The gradual growth to independence demands the development of self-discipline in the mature adult; children agree themselves that they need firm disciplinary measures, fairly imposed according to their age and the extent of their mis-

behaviors. Many students of child behavior believe that strict "discipline for discipline's sake" stirs rebellion and undermines the child's self-respect.

The freedom of the child to use his home for his own friends and own activities, the use of family conferences for planning or for solving problems, wholesome companionship within the family and recognized moral standards all furnish guidelines for learning to respect one's self and others and to live with others.

"When the teen-ager is loved, accorded a measure of freedom and responsibility, disciplined in a sensible and respectful manner, encouraged to grow up and to achieve self-identity, he, in turn, will love and respect his parents, enjoy family life and achieve a healthy, mature adulthood. In this way, the circle of parent-child relationships is successfully completed, and the dynamics of the relationships oriented to a skillful and intelligent solution of the adolescent problem as well as the problems of adolescence."*

---

* Steimel, R. J., Ph.D., editor: Psychological Counseling of Adolescents, p. 79, Washington, D.C., Catholic University of America Press, 1962.

# 10

# Family Living

---

## BEHAVIORAL OBJECTIVES

*The student successfully attaining the goals of this chapter will be able to:*

- *discuss the influence and importance of the family unit upon any person; discuss the influence of the family upon the nurse as a person and upon the patient as a person.*
- *list some of the developmental tasks of the American family as originally stated by Duvall.*
- *trace the development of the family unit through its various stages; marriage and establishment, childbearing, childlaunching, and the aging process.*
- *discuss the concept of the patient as a member of the family unit and the adaptations which may take place within that family unit when a person is ill.*

---

You can use your own experience to understand how other people and patients feel about their homes and families. Successful relationships throughout your lifetime will depend in part on your ability and willingness to understand the other fellow. Your job begins with understanding people, extends to understanding the patient and includes helping him and his family adjust to his illness.

## THE FAMILY UNIT

All living centers around the home and the family. The family is the basic unit of successful society. The most primitive of people had rigid customs regarding the establishment of a family and rules for maintaining its integrity. History records that as family responsibility and relationships in great nations deteriorated and decayed, their civilizations crumbled from within.

The primary purpose of marriage, the socially approved relationship between the sexes, is the establishment of a family for the procreation and the education of children. The ideal family relationship is characterized by mutual affection and respect. This chapter will help to guide you to the realization that every patient is a person *before* he is a patient, that he has a home of some kind which is his base. You cannot separate him from this tie merely because he happens to be sick. Sometimes his home life is not satisfactory—he may be unhappy at home and not at all eager to go back. On the opposite side of the picture is the mother of a family who longs to return home and look after her children and her house as soon as possible. Either way, you can see that family life affects *everyone* and that home is an important place.

### Changes Within the Family

As an individual develops from infancy to maturity and eventually old age, so the development of the normal family can be similarly traced through various stages and cycles. As the child has ages and stages which demand effort and energy on his part, so too does the family have a developmental cycle of growth which passes through phases of greater and lesser effort and responsibility, through periods of hectic activity and times of relative calm, and times for doing tasks and duties compensated for by breathing spells to enjoy the fruits of the efforts. The rhythm of the family life cycle is almost as predictable as the rhythm of the tides.

Sociologists divide the family cycle into different phases, the number of phases varying from 2 to 22. However, generally speaking, the family starts with *marriage* and the *establishment period* and then moves into the *childbearing stage*. As the child grows, the family makes new adjustments, and the child responds; the coming of each new child makes new adjustments necessary. As the children mature and are allowed or encouraged to leave the family group, the family goes through another part of the cycle, the *child-launching stage*. Eventually, the family returns to its original size (a couple), and at this time further adjustments have to be made. Successful acceptance of the roles of the *aging family* is frequently the most difficult adjustment of all.

Each of the stages of family life has its own pleasures and rewards to compensate for its sacrifices and duties. Socially acceptable behavior in any area and aspect of life follows the belief or the philosophy that rights bring corresponding duties, and duties bring corresponding rights. If you are a loyal citizen, you not only enjoy the rights and the privileges of your citizenship, but you also accept the duties of obeying the laws and respecting others. Members of families who reap the benefits of living within the group solidify family relationships by assuming a share of the problem-solving responsibilities and the duties as well. The duties and the rewards of members of a family through the various phases of its cycle are called *developmental tasks*.

## What a Family Is

The family is a group of related people (by marriage, birth, or adoption) whose purpose is to establish and maintain a unit which promotes the total development of its members.

The family developmental tasks which have been defined as essential for growth and success of American families are basically as follows:*

---

* Freely adapted from Duvall, E. M.: Family Development, p. 149. Philadelphia, Lippincott, 1971.

1. Supplying a home, food, clothing and other physical needs such as health care.
2. Providing material requirements and facilities—as well as respect, affection and discipline—according to the needs of individual family members.
3. Dividing the responsibility for and assigning the work load within the family group.
4. Guiding and directing the desires of the members into socially acceptable channels in various areas related to eating, elimination, sex, interpersonal relations, and other matters.
5. Bearing or adopting children, including new members by marriage; allowing members of the family to leave the group.
6. Establishing standards for communication, affection, disagreement, etc., as well as sanctions or punishments for actions that are out of bounds.
7. Guiding members to establish healthful relationships in the community through the church, the school and other sources.
8. Maintaining motivation and morale by recognition, affection, encouragement and family loyalty.

Each person within a successful family must maintain his individuality, establish a contributing role in his relationship with each of its members and interact compatibly within the total group.

## Marriage and Establishment Stage

Some of the developmental tasks of the establishment phase include setting up a home, working out a system of finance and economy, and dividing the work and the routine chores which are a responsibility of family life. Where to live is usually one of the easier tasks for newlyweds. Typically, their first home is rented, close to their work and often near family and friends. The budget is not always as simple. The average young couple today is accustomed to the comforts of their parents' home, to the niceties for which parents have worked and sacrificed and enjoyed giving. Thus the couple is not used to "doing without" the extras. The constant sales enticements for the luxuries of living make them seem like necessities, and the average young married couple either makes tremendous sacrifices to live like the "Joneses" or wonders how the "Joneses" can manage all the extras when they cannot.

Traditionally, the duties of the roles of the husband and the wife were as explicitly "his" and "hers" as the embroidered towels. The husband "worked from sun to sun," and the wife's "work was never done." Today the trend to share responsibilities and to decide who will do what according to individual interests, abilities and time is more familiar to the majority of families. It is common today to find young couples doing the marketing together, buying household furnishings together and even sharing the responsibilities of cooking and cleaning.

This is not to say that this aspect of modern marriage is without problems. The person who said that we should choose our parents carefully was thinking about the effect of home life on the children. The husband may have emerged from a household where both parents felt that housework was totally women's work. Or perhaps in the wife's family the duties were shared, with the father preparing Sunday breakfast and often helping with household tasks, varying from waxing floors to doing the supper dishes.

Some developmental tasks which begin in the establishment phase carry over into following phases of marriage. These include: achieving an effective system of communication; building sexual relationships which are mutually satisfactory; forming understanding relationships with relatives; and developing a philosophy together which can recognize both individuality and "togetherness" in daily living and can give aim and purpose to married life. The task of problem-solving is usually divided into several steps which progress according to the following general pattern: recognizing the problem, analyzing its causes, developing possible solutions and applying the solutions in the order in which they seem to be most acceptable and effective until a satisfactory conclusion of the problem is reached.

## Childbearing Stage

There is seldom a relationship so fulfilling as that of parent to child. No matter what the couple felt about the initial certainty of pregnancy, the arrival of a first child is usually an occasion of wonder and joy. The father, done with the tensions of waiting, relaxes and exults. The mother, tired but relieved after the delivery, basks in a serene sense of accomplishment. Every day brings new pleasures to parenthood.

The wife is now faced with many additional duties. New and continuing parent responsibilities must be realized and accepted. The needs vary for children of different ages—providing space for each child, assuring clean bodies, clothes and surroundings and a balanced diet, reorganizing family routines to accommodate the infant and toddler, toilet training, being interested in and guiding the growth tasks of several children—all this, while maintaining a helpful satisfying relationship with her husband, relatives and community, is the wife's undertaking, one which sometimes becomes overwhelming. One survey concerned with fatigue in homemakers indicated that 70 per cent of tired housewives had toddlers. Another study showed that college athletes at the peak of their physical fitness were unable to duplicate the constant activities of the toddler or produce their continual energy output for 12 hours.

The father has new problems of his own. He finds financial demands ballooning while his income increases at a slower pace. Children's schedules destroy leisurely mealtime pleasures and sometimes menace sleep and rest as well. His job responsibilities and community contacts are usually increasing as well in this active time of life. Yet, he must find time to encourage the growth tasks of all members of his family and combine them into a family design or plan.

Communication between husband and wife, including sexual communication and recreational opportunities, may be sharply displaced as their family grows. Private conversation is difficult. Children are omnipresent; the baby jabbers, the preschooler talks loudly and endlessly; the school child has many confidences and jokes to be appreciated—who can think, let alone communicate in such confusion? However, at this stage of the family cycle, communication is a family developmental task for all members, and if the jabbers and jokes are enjoyed at least a good part of the time, it all contributes to a happy family life. Wise parents keep their avenues of communication as clear as possible, spread responsibilities for household tasks and arrange for some adult stimulation outside the home as well.

Families in the childbearing stage are sometimes so pressured that they need more than 24 hours in the day. The average family of today has 1 or 2 children. (In 1700, the average family included 7 or 8 children.) College graduates tend to have fewer children than noncollege graduates. The average girl marries at about age 20, as opposed to the high number of teenage marriages in the 1950's. (In 1967, only 15 per cent of all 18-year-old girls were married.) The average mother of today has her first child at 22 years of age, her last at 26 to 30. (Since the female college graduate is likely to marry later and is likely to have fewer children, she also has her last child between the age of 26 and 30.) The average mother is 27 or 28 when she enters her first child in school, and he becomes a teenager when she is 35. The first child marries when the mother is about 42 to 45. Before the mother is 50, her last child marries (earlier for daughters and later for sons), and she becomes a grandmother at about age 52. She now shares her childless home with her husband until she is widowed in her mid-60's. She lives as a widow for about 16 years.

The average father marries at 22, has his first child at 24 to 25 years of age, his last around 28 to 30. When he is about 38, his first child is a teenager. When he is in his mid 40's, he becomes father-of-the-bride (or groom) for the first time. His last child marries by the time he is 50. The father usually lives to about age 65.

## The Childlaunching Stage

As this stage of the family cycle begins, the family is at its maximum size. As each child leaves home for college, military service, a job, or to marry, the parental task is reorganization of the family from the household full of children (for some, one child is a full household) to the house again occupied by the parental couple alone.

As education has become more highly valued and as the unskilled occupations become fewer, both the family and the schools help to stimulate the interest of young men and women in college or vocational preparation. However, a realistic appraisal of the person's capabilities must be made. Aspirations beyond a possible achievement level can result in disappointment for both the parent and the child. However, most young people should be able to prepare themselves vocationally today when there are more than 50,000 vocations from which to choose.

As the children reach adulthood, the developmental tasks of other stages, such as financial obligations, budgeting and sharing work responsibilities continue. The philosophy of life which the parents have built through two or more decades of rearing their children will provide them with feelings of achievement.

As the older children marry, the new in-law relationships enter the picture, and the family development tasks go on. A major one is to accept, even if they do not always approve, and to appreciate the differences in ideals, habits and philosophies in the new generation. These changes in ways of living are inevitable.

The typical family picture shows the last child leaving home before his parents leave their 40's. This allows a "seventh inning stretch" for parents in their middle years.

## Life Goes On at 40

Failure to adjust to the "empty nest" can lead to unhappiness and depression. Habits of pressure—time, work, finances—may be so ingrained that leisure and recreation are difficult adjustments. In our present society the husband and father who has devoted himself entirely to progressing in business may be regarded by his peers as eminently successful; but his own opinion, as well as his family's opinion of his success may be less satisfactory than that of the man who has enjoyed closer involvement within the family group.

Couples find the middle years a comfortable and serene period; fewer demands allow more time for them to be together and to enjoy life. Financial projects for children shrink, and time for shared activities expands. Grandchildren provide pleasure; grandparents must help without interfering, must love without smothering, and must be available without being intrusive. The middle-aged man and wife find that the rewards of time allow them to come to terms with themselves, as well as to find satisfaction in opportunities still available. The middle years prove to be a fine time to plan for financial security in later years: the expense of childrearing is lifted; the husband's income is usually at its peak; the wife

TABLE 10–1. INCREASE OF THE MIDDLE-AGED AND OLDER
POPULATIONS IN THE UNITED STATES*

| Year | Total Population | Approximate Percentage of People, Aged 45-64 Years | 65+years |
|---|---|---|---|
| 1900 | 76 million | 7% male<br>7½% female<br>14½% of total population | 1⅔% male<br>1¾% female<br>3½% of total population |
| 1960 | 160 million | 10% male<br>11% female<br>21% of total population | 2¾% male<br>3% female<br>5¾% of total population |
| 1980 | 250 million (projected) | 9½% male<br>9% female<br>18½% of total population | 3% male<br>3½% female<br>6½% of total population |

* (Adapted from Tibbitts and Donahue. Aging in Today's Society, page 13. Englewood Cliffs, N.J. Prentice-Hall, 1960; and Duvall, E. M. Family Development, page 64, Philadelphia, J. B. Lippincott, 1971.)

may wish to work, as do about half the wives in the age group of 45 to 54.

Financial planning for the older years accepts the statistical fact that wives live longer than husbands; therefore, both husband and wife should be fully aware of the status of their finances.

## Age Is Relative

People who are growing older cannot be lumped together and treated alike any more than those of any other age. As in other phases of the life cycle, the husband and the wife, together and as individuals, must themselves undertake the developmental tasks of this period to make it successful.

Present society is too eager to estimate age in years instead of in a person's ability to make the most of any time of life. As Marie Dressler, an actress of former years, once said: "It's not how old you are but how you are old."

Another contemporary problem is that Americans are so determined to glorify youth and a pretty face that people are ashamed to admit their age. Beauty parlors prosper as women struggle to stop the clock. Men, too, resist the sands of time as they seek remedies for receding hairlines and enlarging waistlines. Many men are also faced with an employer's plan of enforced retirement which makes continued working impossible and decreased income inevitable.

Robert Browning said:

Grow old along with me!
The best is yet to be.
The last of life, for which the first was made . . .

According to the latest statistics, this is just what our population is doing—growing old. Ten per cent of our citizens are over 65 years of age (see Table 10-1). The average life span has increased 20 years since 1900. "The older American has nearly 18 million faces."* This aging population brings economic and social adaptations within the family group as well as in wider society. Those basic needs—security, affection and the need to be useful and wanted—still are important, and problems arise because many older people are denied these satisfactions.

Happily, some attempts are being made to use the valuable abilities of retired people. As an example, Hastings College of Law, affiliated with the University of California, will not hire anyone under 65 years of age. It has 17 faculty members who average 73 years of age with an average of 42 years in

* The Older American, p. 1, Washington, D.C., Superintendent of Documents, 1963.

teaching law. David Snodgrass, dean, reports: "We are extremely happy with our older faculty. They know their business and over the years have gotten rid of all their bad habits."

## THE PATIENT IS PART OF THE FAMILY

Now that you know the "person," you will begin to understand the "patient." Your first step in this cooperative job is important. You must try to see hospital patients as people who have homes, families and friends. Their likes and dislikes, their belongings and their visitors will tell you many things about them. You must remember first that no two people are exactly alike. What does the patient think about? One is the illness itself. Another is the family, especially if the patient is the one responsible for the housekeeping or child care. If the patient is the wage-earner, money will be a worry. If the illness is long and expensive, this can be a worry in itself.

With these things as a start, how do you fit in? First, as a nurse, of course, your job is to make your patient comfortable and to do what the physician prescribes. Next, you must remember that the patient will get well faster if he is contented. He will be relieved to know that you are interested in and aware of his family and his life with them. A referral to the hospital social worker may be helpful to the patient.

### You Work Together

If the patient is ill at home, you also might be stepping into the household as a manager to keep the household on an even keel and plan each day so that it will run smoothly. You should be able to help the family with the changes they need to make because there is a sick person in the house. You can accomplish this by making the family realize that this is a job to be done together. If the patient must have quiet, you can help with plans to keep the children amused or out of the way. Explain why they may not be allowed to see the patient or why visits must be short. This can be tricky, because people cannot always see how members of the family or friends could tire the patient or upset him. This can be especially difficult if one of the family was taking care of the patient before

you came. This person may not want to see you take over. Let her help in any way possible until she learns to have confidence in you.

### Illness Can Be Expensive

Discuss with the family the equipment which you will need for the patient. See what can be used from the home, and when purchases are necessary, explain what is needed and help the family to obtain them as economically as possible. For example, you would not recommend Monel metal basins and bedpans unless the family could afford them—you would suggest a less expensive type. You must be guided by the kind and the length of the illness as well as the family pocketbook when you choose or recommend specific equipment.

In many communities there are volunteer agencies which will supply equipment for the home patient at little or no cost. You can find out about these services through your Health and Welfare Council, your local Public Health Nurse, your local Red Cross chapter or from an agency directly concerned with your patients' illness, such as the Heart Association, the American Cancer Society or the National Society for Crippled Children and Adults.

### Conclusion

It is very important that you know much about the patient—his anatomy and physiology, his personality and his place in the family and the larger community. You must remember that the patient is an individual as well as an integral part of a family group. In helping the patient and his family during illness, you will get better results if you understand the influences that make them behave as they do. You will have more patience with children when you understand and appreciate their development patterns, their family background and their training. You will be more tolerant of older patients when you appreciate the economic and the emotional pressures that affect them, their nationality and religious backgrounds and the things they hold dear. The patient must always be considered in his family setting.

# Unit 4:

# The Living Body: Normal Body Structure and Function

11. *The Body as an Integrated Whole*
12. *The Body's Cell Pattern: Tissues and Membranes*
13. *The Musculoskeletal System*
14. *The Nervous System*
15. *The Circulatory System*
16. *The Respiratory System*
17. *The Digestive System*
18. *The Urinary System*
19. *How Life Begins: The Reproductive System*
20. *The Endocrine System*
21. *The Sensory System*

# 11

# The Body as
# an Integrated Whole

---

### BEHAVIORAL OBJECTIVES

*The student successfully attaining the goals of this chapter will be able to:*

- *define cell, protoplasm, matter, compound, physical change, chemical change, and mixture.*
- *list the characteristics of all cells, which differentiate living matter from nonliving matter.*
- *diagram a cell and label the cell membrane, cytoplasm, and nucleus; list the chief functions of each of these structures; describe the process of mitosis.*
- *describe the role and actions of chromosomes; briefly discuss the activities of RNA and DNA.*
- *discuss the concept of fluid and electrolyte balance, considering the influence of the cell membrane and electrolytes; discuss the effect of a disease process upon this fluid and electrolyte balance.*
- *list the types of tissues in the body and give an example of each.*
- *define the term tumor.*
- *describe the structural organization of the human body in terms of the structural units of cells, tissues, organs, and systems; give examples of each structural unit.*
- *identify which organs comprise the major body systems and identify the location of each organ on a body model or chart.*
- *correctly utilize the anatomical terms which apply to body positions, directions, and cavities.*
- *describe the relationship between systems of the body and the principle of homeostasis.*
- *define metabolism, catabolism, and anabolism.*

---

In recent years science has produced such a profusion of miracles that we have almost lost our capacity to wonder at them. Even so, anybody—even the most learned scientist—who looks within the human body continues to be awed by its marvels of engineering, architecture, efficiency, and economy. As we study the structure and the function of the body, we learn to appreciate even more the intricate patterns which enable each of us to perform as a miraculously integrated human being. This study is called *anatomy* (body structure) and *physiology* (body function). It constitutes an important part of the nurse's training, because in order to recognize deviations from the normal, the nurse must be familiar with the normal. Without this knowledge she could not understand the patient's needs and why he is not able to meet them without assistance.

## THE UNIT OF LIFE

In a brick building, the unit of structure is "one brick." The unit of structure and organization of the body is "one cell"—the building block of the body. This fact was first established by two German biologists, Schleiden and Schwann, and it has been the foundation from which all biological sciences have developed. *All* living things, plants and animals alike, are made up of cells. The smallest forms of life, the microorganisms, are composed of a single cell. The human body, on the other hand, is made up of millions of cells.

## PROTOPLASM

The cells of all living creatures are composed of a substance called protoplasm (meaning "original substance"). Protoplasm has been analyzed in the laboratory, and we know what chemicals it contains—ordinary materials that we see around us in varying forms every day. However, we have not been able to make protoplasm in the laboratory. Apparently, it is the organization of the material in the cells, and not some exclusive chemical, that gives it that property which we call life. Life can be defined in several ways. It is the interval between the birth, or conception, of an organism and its death. It is animate being—the quality that distinguishes a functional being from a dead body or purely chemical substance.

Although the *quality* of life remains elusive, the *"stuff"* of life is familiar—all part and parcel of that fixed reservoir of matter composing the interior of our planet, its surface and the atmosphere enveloping it.

## MATTER

Matter is said to be anything that occupies space and has weight. All the matter in the world, living and nonliving, can be broken down into slightly over 100 different elements. Elements are not *the* simplest form of matter, but only the simplest form obtainable by ordinary chemical means. Some common elements are carbon, iron, sulfur, copper, oxygen, hydrogen, and nitrogen.

The smallest unit of any element is the atom. Atoms in turn are composed of subatomic particles, which only rather recently have been subjected to intensive study. As far as we are concerned, the main subatomic particles are electrons, protons, and neutrons, which are arranged in relation to one another in somewhat the same manner as the earth and the other planets are arranged around the sun. An atom of one element differs from that of another element in the arrangement of its subatomic particles. For instance, a hydrogen atom has 1 proton with 1 electron whirling around it; an atom of oxygen has 8 electrons revolving about a central mass composed of 8 protons and 8 neutrons. Each element has its own characteristic atom.

### Compounds

Atoms of 2 or more elements can combine to form an enormous variety of substances called compounds. In every compound, the atoms of its elements combine in definite proportions. For example, the most common compound found on the surface of the earth is water. Water is formed when 2 atoms of hydrogen are combined with 1 atom of oxygen. In chemical shorthand, water is expressed as $H_2O$.

Suppose you were able to take a knifeblade and cut a drop of water in two, and then divide one of these halves. If you continued to divide each half into smaller and smaller fractions, finally you would come to a particle which you could not divide and still have water left. This single particle of water is called a *molecule,* which consists solely of the 2 hydrogen atoms and the 1 oxygen atom. Therefore, a molecule is the least quantity of atoms needed to form a particular compound.

### Physical and Chemical Changes

Water has a definite chemical structure, $H_2O$. Normally, it is a liquid. Freeze water, and it changes to a solid, ice; boil it, and it becomes water vapor, steam. The water has undergone a *physical* change—that is, a change in its outward properties. However, it is still water, $H_2O$, no matter which of these 3 states it is in. Its chemical structure remains unchanged. However, if you pass a direct electric current through a sample of water, a more fundamental change occurs. The water gradually disappears because the electric current breaks it down into the 2 invisible gases of which water is composed—hydrogen and oxygen. In this instance, the chemical structure of the water has been changed; the water molecules have been made to disintegrate into their respective elements. A *chemical* change has occurred. Familiar types of chemical change are the processes of burning (called combustion) and the rusting of iron. In all chemical changes, compounds are broken down into substances that no longer have the same chemical structure of the original compound. Completely rusted iron no longer has the same characteristics of iron; burned wood is no longer wood, but ashes and gases instead.

## Mixtures

Not all elements or compounds will combine chemically when brought together. A *mixture* is a class of matter in which 2 or more substances are mixed together without forming a new compound. Salt water is an example of a mixture. Both the salt and the water remain 2 separate compounds. They can be brought together in any proportion, and they can be separated by a physical change, such as boiling. In a true compound, the elements combine in definite proportions, and they cannot be separated except through a chemical change.

## Energy

Speaking practically, energy is the ability to do work. It takes many forms: light energy, heat energy, mechanical energy, chemical energy, etc. One type of energy can be converted into another. For instance, energy from the sun (heat, light, and other types of radiation) is stored in natural fuels such as oil and coal. These contain chemical energy, which is transformed into mechanical energy in engines. Engines can turn generators, producing electrical energy; electricity in turn can be transformed into light and heat.

The chemical combining of elements and compounds is called a *chemical reaction*. All chemical reactions are accomplished by a transfer of energy. For example, the cells of the body receive energy from food materials

(see p. 130). Chemical reactions that take place in protoplasm result in the release of heat energy, mechanical energy, and other forms of energy which are all a part of the so-called "life processes."

## LIVING MATTER

Protoplasm is a semiliquid substance which resembles the white of an egg. It is composed mostly of water (about 70%) and protein compounds, which "build up" the cell and supply it with energy when combined with oxygen. Protoplasm contains mineral elements (calcium, sodium, sulfur, etc.), carbohydrates (sugars and starches), and lipids (fats and fatty substances). Protoplasm in its simplest form has 5 general characteristics: irritability, motility, metabolism, growth, and reproduction. These 5 characteristics are used to distinguish living matter from nonliving matter.

*Irritability* means that protoplasm responds to a change in its environment; that is, it reacts in some way to a stimulus. An example of this is the action of a nerve cell of the body. When a nerve is stimulated, an electrical impulse is touched off and travels along the nerve as though a fuse had been lighted.

*Motility* is the ability to move. The protoplasm moves within the cells of both plants and animals. Sperm cells, the male reproductive cells, are capable of rapid self-propulsion. Some cells are capable of ameboid movement ("ameboid" referring to the tiny 1-celled animal called an ameba which can move about by itself). The protoplasm of these cells bulges out into footlike processes called pseudopodia ("false feet"), and then the entire cell follows the foot. An example of this type of cell is certain white blood cells which travel by ameboid movement through the blood vessel walls to sites of inflammation and infection in the body.

Another type of motion is contractility, which is the ability of a cell to become shorter and thicker in response to a signal sent out by a nerve. This property is most highly developed in cells that make up the muscles.

*Metabolism* is the process by which the cells build protein and produce energy. It is the sum total of all the physical and chemical processes that take place within a cell. Food and oxygen which enter the cell in dissolved forms react chemically (catabolism, the breaking-down process) and liberate the energy necessary for the cell to carry on its work (anabolism, the building-up process). At the same time, the cell uses some of the products of these reactions for its own nourishment, for the manufacture of more protoplasm and for certain specialized activities such as secreting. (A secretion is a cell-discharge useful to another body part.) Another phase of metabolism involves the removal of the waste products following the chemical reactions. The factors controlling the passage of food and oxygen into and the waste products out of the cell will be considered later in this chapter.

*Growth* and *reproduction* produce an increase in the total amount of protoplasm as a result of an increase in the number of cells. Through a complicated process called *mitosis,*

cells can divide into 2 parts and reproduce themselves. Each of the "daughter" cells is an exact genetic duplicate of the original or "mother" cell from which it came. If the body is thought of as a group of cells, mitosis is responsible for its growth as well as the repair and the replacement of injured and dead tissues. The speed with which cells reproduce varies, but many thousands are formed daily in the skin alone to compensate for those lost by shedding or destroyed by injury or disease. Reproduction also refers to division of the ovum (the egg cell) which is responsible for the creation of new individuals and the preservation of the species.

## THE CELL

Cells are too small to be seen without a microscope (the sole exception in the body is

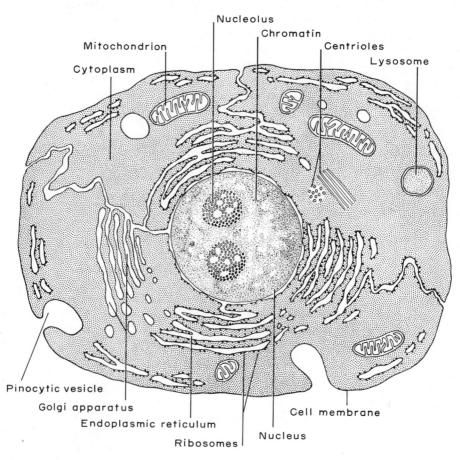

Figure 11-1. Diagram of a typical cell. (Chaffee, E. E., and Greisheimer, E. M.: Basic Physiology and Anatomy, ed. 2. Philadelphia, Lippincott, 1969)

the ovum). Although cells may be of different sizes, shapes, and types, having only a vague resemblance to each other, their general plan of structure is the same. They all have a *cell membrane* (also called the cell wall or plasma membrane) which is a firm boundary resembling a delicate film. Within the membrane is the *cytoplasm,* the material which makes up the body of the cell. Suspended in or near the center of the cell is the *nucleus* enveloped by its nuclear membrane. The nucleus is responsible for the reproduction (division) of the cell and the coordination of certain cell activities. The nucleus also contains a tiny globule known as the *nucleolus* which is particularly important in reproduction. In some cells, a secondary nucleolus is also present. Usually, the nucleus is filled with a network of fine strands (linen fibers) on and between which are globules of a material called *chromatin.* All of these structures, of course, are part of the protoplasm.

The cytoplasm is a miniature chemical laboratory involved in many complicated processes vital to the life of the cell. It is here that the work of the cell is carried on.

Two of the important structures in the cytoplasm are the *mitochondria,* rod-shaped bodies active in the production of power and energy, and granules of *ribonucleic acid* (RNA) related to the production of protein, the important constituent of all protoplasm. The *centrosomes* (centrioles) are small paired bodies also important in cell division. Many other less important structures have been identified in the cytoplasm, particularly since the invention of the electron microscope with its tremendous magnifying powers. A typical cell is seen in Figure 11-1.

Within the cell nucleus are small chromatin granules called *chromosomes* which contain the genes (Fig. 11-2). Although human reproductive cells are known to have 23 pairs of chromosomes (46 total), the genes are present in the thousands. Genes transmit specifications for the characteristics of a species. They determine whether a living organism is male or female, whether it has blue or brown eyes, whether it has light or dark skin. In other words, in human reproduction, the genes transfer from one generation to the next all the characteristics which are inherited. If there were no organization to this process of

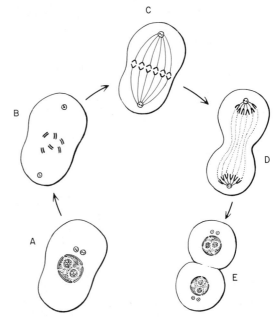

Figure 11-2. Diagram of a cell undergoing mitosis. (A) Typical cell. (B) The nuclear membrane disappears and the chromosomes come together in pairs. The centrosomes separate and are drawn towards opposite ends of the cell. (C) The chromosomes split, so that half move towards each centrosome. (D) The cell begins to elongate, thinning in the middle with the cell wall following the same shape. (E) The cell splits into 2 parts with half the cytoplasm, nuclear material and cell wall in each of the 2 new cells.

cell division, known as *mitosis,* each new cell would not have the same characteristics as the original. As it is, because of the genes, each of the 2 new cells is genetically identical with the original from which it was formed.

This amazing process of mitosis occurs as a result of a rearrangement of the particles in the nucleus. Briefly, what happens is that the centrosomes separate and are drawn toward opposite ends of the cell. The nuclear membrane then disappears, and the chromosomes split so that half move toward each centrosome. The cell then begins to elongate, thinning in the middle with the cell wall following the same shape. It finally splits into 2 parts with half the cytoplasm, the nuclear material, and the cell wall in each of the 2 new cells (see Fig. 11-2).

For years scientists have studied the process of cell division and the resulting duplication of cells. They found within the chromosomes

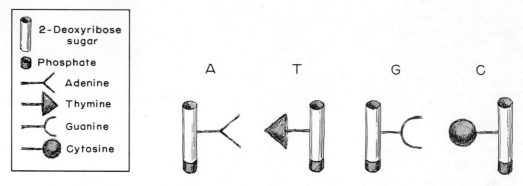

Figure 11-3. Structural units (nucleotides) of a DNA molecule. Each unit consists of a phosphate group and a sugar group to which is attached a nitrogenous base (adenine or thymine or guanine or cytosine). (Chaffee, E. E., and Greisheimer, E. M.: Basic Physiology and Anatomy, ed. 2. Philadelphia, Lippincott, 1969)

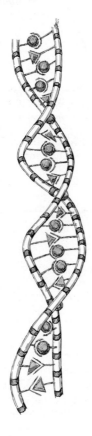

Figure 11-4. Schematic representation of the spiral ladder arrangement of repeating nucleotide units found in the DNA molecule. It is thought that anywhere from 500 to 1,000 of these rungs make up a single gene, and that there are over 1,000 genes in a single chromosome. (Chaffee, E. E., and Greisheimer, E. M.: Basic Physiology and Anatomy, ed. 2. Philadelphia, Lippincott, 1969)

a chemical compound called DNA (deoxyribonucleic acid) which plays an important part in the storing and transferring of genetic information. The following description of a DNA molecule and its function, taken from *Basic Physiology and Anatomy* by Chaffee and Greisheimer, will help you understand how genetic information is stored in a chemical compound and then precisely duplicated.

In 1953, Dr. James Watson and Dr. Francis Crick first introduced the concept that a DNA molecule resembles a spiral ladder. The sides of the ladder are formed by alternating units of deoxyribose sugar and phosphate, while the rungs are composed of pairs of nitrogenous bases. One end of each nitrogenous base is attached to a sugar-phosphate unit, and the other end is linked to its partner on the opposite side of the ladder to complete the rung. These nitrogen compounds are only four in number: adenine, thymine, guanine and cytosine or, as they are referred to in scientific shorthand: A, T, G, and C. However, the pairing of these bases is highly specific, as A is so constructed that it will fit precisely only with T, and G only with C. Thus the sequence of bases along one side of the ladder must necessarily determine the sequence along the other. This fact is of fundamental importance in understanding the ability of DNA to duplicate itself prior to cell division. Figures 11-3 and 11-4 illustrate the basic structure of DNA.

Although the sides of the ladder are an important part of the DNA molecule, it is the order or sequence of bases in the rungs of the ladder that constitutes the so-called "genetic code." In other words, the order in which A, T, G, and C appear apparently "spells out" the genetic instructions that control the activities of the cell, in general, and the construction of complex protein molecules in particular. Because most of the molecules in every cell are proteins, their production is the key to life itself. For example, enzymes (the essential organic catalysts of the body) are proteins, and every one of the *thousands* of different chemical reactions that take place in the body is expedited by a specific enzyme. Thus DNA has the monumental task of directing the formation of thousands of different proteins just to meet the enzyme requirements of the body. Added to this task is the formation of many other proteins that serve as the major structural components of skin, muscle, blood vessels, and all internal organs.

How does DNA accomplish this task? First let us think of a protein molecule as resembling a line of alphabet blocks, each lettered block representing one of 20 amino acids; the sequence of these amino acid blocks determines the protein "word" that will be spelled out. Inasmuch as the fact that DNA carries the genetic code letters A, T, G, and C has already been established, it now remains to see how this chemical alphabet of only 4 letters can be used to write "protein words" that may contain anywhere from a mere 50 letters to tens of thousands of letters. The secret lies in the fact that this 4-letter alphabet is used to write only *3-letter code words.* Because a total of only 20 code words (one for each of the amino acids) is needed to construct any one of the thousands of body proteins, the 4 letters are more than adequate. For example, when one does not have to worry about pronouncing the words, any 4 letters can be so arranged as to form 64 different 3-letter combinations or code words. Then, if one thinks of the 20 amino acid code words as being analogous to 20 letters of the English alphabet, it does not require too much imagination to visualize the almost infinite number of protein words of varying lengths that could be constructed. As a matter of fact, it has been estimated that if all of the coded DNA instructions found in one single cell were translated into English they would more than fill 1000 volumes of an encyclopedia. Figure 11-4 illustrates the spiral ladder appearance of only a small fraction of a DNA molecule because if all of the DNA in a single human cell nucleus were stretched out in a thin thread it would be about 3 feet long!

In addition to the chromosomes, the nucleus also contains one or more small rounded bodies known as nucleoli (sing. nucleolus). The function of a nucleolus is still shrouded in mystery, but it may be the place where another nucleic acid, known as ribonucleic acid (RNA), is stored until needed. RNA is formed from DNA and is part of an elaborate "messenger system" that enables DNA to control the manufacture of protein. The nucleolus also may be the place where the actual "protein factories" (ribosomes) are assembled, and from whence they migrate into the cytoplasm where the bulk of protein synthesis occurs.*

## Body Fluids

The cell membrane plays an important role in regulating cell activities, since it controls what passes into and out of the cytoplasm. It contains tiny openings (pores) which act more or less like filters, allowing the passage of some molecules and rejecting others. Because of this characteristic, the cell membrane, or cell wall, is described as *semipermeable.* There are many factors influencing this mechanism, but before discussing them, it is necessary to understand something about the water (body fluids) in which all cells are bathed.

There is a large amount of water in all living material. Life cannot exist for long without it, since it is the medium which holds the various components of protoplasm (both solids and gases) in solution and is necessary for all of the chemical reactions which occur in the cell. Water comprises about 60 per cent of our body weight. About three fourths of this water is found within the cells, and is called *intracellular fluid* ("intra" means "within"). The remainder is found outside of the cells and is called *extracellular fluid* ("extra" means "outside"). About one fourth of the extracellular fluid is found in the blood vessels as plasma—the liquid portion of the blood—and the remaining three fourths is in the spaces between the blood vessels and the cells. The latter is known as *intercellular fluid* ("inter" means "between"), *tissue fluid* or *interstitial fluid.* It acts as a vehicle for the exchange of substances between the blood stream and the cells—a process known as osmosis. For example, oxygen is carried by the blood and eventually passes through the walls of the capillaries (the smallest of the blood vessel network) into the intercellular fluid. It then circulates in this fluid and is ready to enter the cells for use in metabolism. The waste materials of metabolism pass through the cell membranes in the opposite direction, circulating through the intercellular fluid into the

---

* Chaffee, E. E., and Greisheimer, E. M.: *Basic Physiology and Anatomy,* 2nd Edition. Philadelphia, J. B. Lippincott Co., 1969.

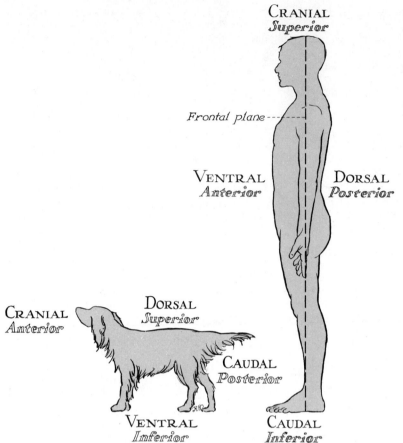

Figure 11-5. Comparative terminology in quadruped and man, for location or position; frontal plane is indicated by broken line. (Greisheimer, E. M., and Wiedeman, M. P.: Physiology and Anatomy, ed. 9. Philadelphia, Lippincott, 1972)

blood or lymph vessels, which transport them to the systems of excretion. This is illustrated diagrammatically on page 122.

Many elements such as sodium, potassium, magnesium, and calcium *ionize* when they are dissolved in water; that is, they acquire electrical charges. Hence, we have given them the name *electrolytes*. Electrolytes may take the form of acids, alkalies (bases), or salts. In order for the body to function normally, electrolytes must be present in precisely the right quantities in both the intracellular and the extracellular fluids. Electrolyte balance is extremely critical; if the fluid is too acid or too alkaline, it may have highly destructive effects on the cells. Normally, this balance is maintained automatically by various mechanisms, chiefly by the action of the kidneys. Many illnesses and surgical procedures disturb this balance, but fortunately we can usually control it by injecting solutions containing electrolytes into the body. Maintenance of

fluid and electrolyte balance is discussed in greater detail in Chapter 32.

## Tissues

We have said that the body is organized in a definite pattern. Cells of the same type and structure join together to form tissues, each of which has a special function. The list below identifies the types of tissue and tells what they do and where they are located:

*Epithelial:* Covers body surfaces, lines cavities (skin, nails, hair, lining of parts of the body such as the nose and the throat) and forms glands

*Connective:* Anchors and holds other tissues together

*Muscular:* Contracts and stretches, causing motion

  A. *Skeletal (striated)*—attached to bones

  B. *Smooth (visceral)*—found in the walls of blood vessels and internal organs such as the stomach

  C. *Cardiac*—found in the walls of the heart

*Nervous:* Receives stimuli and conducts impulses to and from all parts of the body

*Blood:* Carries food and oxygen to the cells, removes wastes and fights infection and poisons. (NOTE: The presence of cells places this liquid in the category of a tissue. Blood is really a form of connective tissue, but it has so many special characteristics that we study it separately.)

## Membranes

Certain kinds of epithelial and connective tissues act together, serving a special function as membranes. We have already spoken of the cell and nuclear membranes which really are considered parts of a single cell. However, "tissue" membranes are made up of many cells. Both tissues and membranes will be discussed in the next chapter.

**Tumors.** In discussing cells and tissues we have considered normal structure and growth. Occasionally, a cell or group of cells will grow into an abnormal mass of tissue called a *tumor,* which has no function whatever.

## Organs and Systems

Different kinds of tissues form organs. For example, the heart is a combination of muscle, nerve, blood, and epithelial tissue. An *organ* is defined as a part of the body which performs a definite function. It does not work independently but is associated with other organs and may have many functions. These group associations are called *systems*—groups of organs in which each contributes its share to the function of the whole. Systems do specialized work in the body, but all body systems are dependent on each other. Your understanding of the structure and the functions of the systems is the basis for your own health habits and your care of patients. Here is a bird's-eye view of the systems, showing how organs are grouped together for specific purposes:

*Skeletal:* Bones, which are the body framework

*Muscular:* Muscles, attached to bones, which make the body movements possible

*Circulatory:* Heart, blood and blood vessels, lymph and lymph vessels. These organs carry food, water, oxygen, and wastes in the body.

*Digestive:* Mouth, salivary glands, pharynx, esophagus, stomach, intestines, liver, and pan-

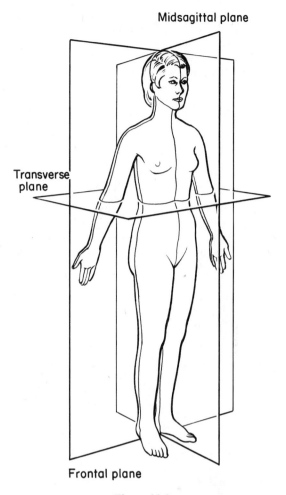

Figure 11-6

creas. These organs take in food and convert it into substances the cells can use.

*Respiratory:* Nose, pharynx, larynx, trachea, bronchi, and lungs. This system supplies the body with oxygen and eliminates carbon dioxide as waste.

*Urinary:* Kidneys, ureters, urinary bladder, and urethra. They eliminate waste products from the body. Sometimes this system is discussed under the classification of the *excretory system,* which includes the respiratory and digestive systems and the skin as well.

*Reproductive:* Ovaries, fallopian (uterine) tubes, uterus, vagina, and mammary glands (breasts) in the woman; testes, accessory glands, and penis in the man. This system makes possible the perpetuation of the species.

*Endocrine:* Ductless glands (pituitary, thyroid, parathyroids, adrenals, testes, ovaries, thymus, pineal, and islands of Langerhans in the pancreas). These glands secrete hormones that regulate various body processes, such as growth, cell metabolism, etc.

*Nervous:* Brain, spinal cord, and nerves, which control and coordinate the activities of the body.

*Sensory:* Eyes, ears, taste buds, organs of smell, touch, pain, etc. These organs operate in special ways to bring stimuli from the outside to the brain.

The next 10 chapters will be devoted to a description of each of these systems.

## BODY DIRECTIONS

A number of terms are used to designate certain areas and directions of the body. They help to specify the location of an organ or system in studying anatomy and physiology and also give the doctor and the nurse a guide in noting and recording signs and symptoms. As we discuss some of these terms, it is important to remember that they refer to the body in the "anatomic position" (i.e., the body is erect with arms at the sides and palms turned forward). (See Fig. 11-5.)

*Superior:* "Above" or in a higher position
*Inferior:* "Below" or in a lower position
 *Examples:* The head is superior to the neck.
  The chest is inferior to the neck.
*Cranial:* Near the head
*Caudal:* Near the lower end of the body (i.e., near the end of the spine)
 *Examples:* The brain is in the cranial cavity.
  The buttocks, the muscles upon which we sit, are located at the caudal end of the body.

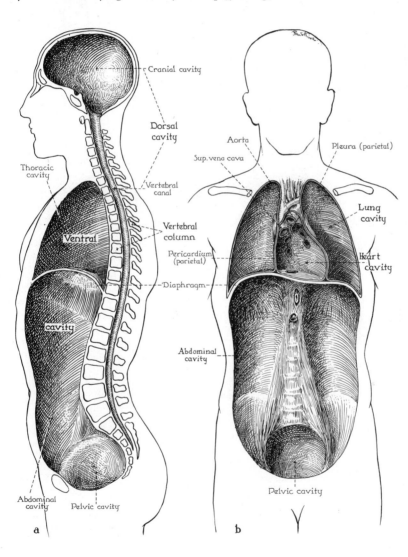

Figure 11-7. Diagram of body cavities. (a) The vertebral column, the dorsal cavity, and the ventral cavity are shown. The diaphragm separates the abdominal from the thoracic portion; the lower portion of the abdominal cavity is called the pelvic cavity. (b) The divisions of the ventral cavity are shown. The thoracic division of the ventral cavity is subdivided into the pleural and the pericardial cavities. (Greisheimer, E. M.: Physiology and Anatomy, ed. 8. Philadelphia, Lippincott)

*Anterior or ventral:* Toward the front or "belly" surface of the body

*Posterior or dorsal:* Toward the back of the body

    *Examples:* The nose is on the anterior, or ventral, surface of the head.

    The calf is on the posterior, or dorsal surface of the leg.

*Medial:* Nearer the midline

*Lateral:* Farther from the midline, toward the side

    *Examples:* The nose is medial to the eyes.

    The ears are lateral to the nose.

*Internal:* Deeper within the body

*External:* Toward the outer surface of the body

    *Examples:* The stomach is an internal body organ.

    The skin covers the external surface of the body.

*Proximal:* Nearest the origin of a part

*Distal:* Farthest from the origin of a part

    *Examples:* In the upper extremity (arm), the upper arm above the elbow is proximal to the lower arm below.

    In the lower extremity (leg), the lower leg below the knee is distal to the thigh.

*Central:* Situated at or pertaining to the center

*Peripheral:* Situated at or pertaining to the outward part of surface

    *Examples:* The brain and the spinal cord are part of the central nervous system.

    The peripheral nerves go out to the body parts and return to the central nervous system.

*Parietal:* Pertaining to the sides or the walls of a cavity

*Visceral:* Pertaining to the organs within a cavity

    *Examples:* The abdominal cavity is lined with a membrane called the parietal peritoneum.

    The stomach and the intestines are visceral organs in the abdominal cavity.

In order to show a better relation of the position of the body structures to each other, the following imaginary planes are used to divide the body into sections (also see Fig. 11-6).

*The Midsagittal Plane:* Divides the body into right and left halves by passing through the midline from top to bottom.

*The Frontal (Coronal) Plane:* Divides the body into front and back parts by passing through the body longitudinally from head to toes.

*The Transverse (Horizontal) Plane:* Divides the body into upper (superior) and lower (inferior) parts by passing through the body horizontally. Various levels of the transverse plane are possible.

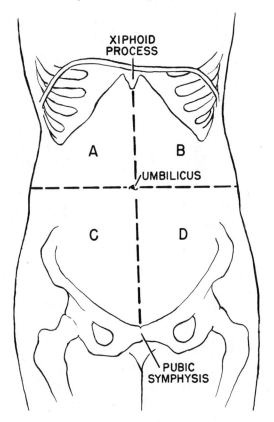

Figure 11-8. Quadrants of the abdomen: (A) The right upper quadrant—RUQ; (B) The left upper quadrant—LUQ; (C) The right lower quadrant—RLQ; (D) The left lower quadrant—LLQ. (Fuerst, E. V., and Wolff, L.: Fundamentals of Nursing, ed. 4. Philadelphia, Lippincott, 1969)

## BODY CAVITIES

Within the body are 2 groups of spaces (or cavities) which contain various organs. They are the *dorsal* and the *ventral cavities.*

The dorsal cavity consists of the cranial portion, which houses the brain, and the vertebral portion, which houses the spinal cord.

The ventral cavity consists of the thoracic and abdominal (or abdominopelvic) portions which are separated by a large muscle called the diaphragm. (The diaphragm will be discussed in Chapter 13.) The thoracic cavity comprises the pericardial cavity, which contains the heart, and 2 pleural cavities, each of which contains a lung. In addition to the heart, the space between the lungs (called the

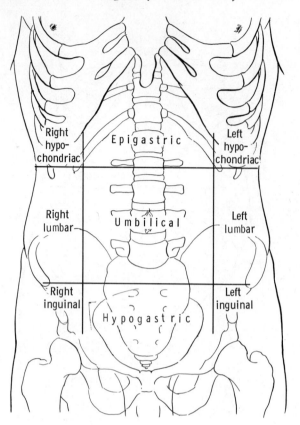

Figure 11-9. Regions of the abdomen. (Greisheimer, E. M.: Physiology and Anatomy, ed. 8. Philadelphia, Lippincott)

mediastinum) also contains structures such as the large blood vessels, the trachea, the esophagus, and the thymus gland.

The upper part of the abdominal cavity contains the stomach, most of the intestines, the liver, the gallbladder, the pancreas, the spleen, the kidneys, the adrenal glands, and the ureters. The lower portion, called the pelvic cavity, contains the urinary bladder, the remaining part of the intestines, the rectum, and the internal reproductive organs.

The body cavities are lined by serous membranes, which protect the internal organs and contain them within the appropriate space. These will be discussed further in Chapter 12.

## Regions in the Abdominal Cavity

The abdominal cavity has been divided into quadrants to help in describing signs and symptoms and locating the viscera from the surface. These are the right upper, the left upper, the right lower, and the left lower quadrants as shown in Figure 11-8. There is another division which divides the abdominal cavity into 9 regions. These are illustrated in Figure 11-9.

# The Body's Cell Pattern: Tissues and Membranes

---

### BEHAVIORAL OBJECTIVES

*The student successfully attaining the goals of this chapter will be able to:*

- *list the 4 major types of tissues in the body.*
- *differentiate between types of epithelial tissues and describe each type.*
- *name the types of connective tissue and describe the function of each type.*
- *name and describe the types of muscle tissue.*
- *define the term membrane; list the types of membranes; describe the function of each type.*
- *identify the layers of skin, as well as its "appendages"; locate all of these on a chart; list the functions of each.*

---

## TISSUES

Cells which are grouped together according to their functions are called tissues. The following give further descriptions of the kinds of tissues within the body and their functions.

### Epithelial Tissues

Epithelial tissues are those which cover the body surfaces or line the cavities of the body. An important characteristic of epithelial tissue (also called *epithelium*) is that its cells are packed closely together with very little intercellular material between them. This arrangement enables them to protect other parts of the body.

Some epithelial cells have fine hairlike processes on them called *cilia,* which move in waves and carry or transport materials, such as mucus. Other epithelial cells are heavily supplied with nerve endings, such as those found in the fingertips.

Groups of epithelial cells shaped like tiny goblets have the ability to form secretions; these are called *glands.* They release their secretions either into a duct or directly into the bloodstream. Another kind of epithelium is especially adapted to the function of absorption, such as that found in the intestines.

The epithelium may be described according to its various characteristics. Its cells may be 1 layer in thickness (simple epithelium), may be 2 or more layers (stratified epithelium), or, as was already mentioned, may be grouped together in glands (glandular epithelium). The cells, in turn, have their own designation. According to their shape, the cells are called *cuboidal* (cube-shaped), *squamous* (flat or like a plate), or *columnar* (tall and thin). The epithelial tissues found in glands may be in the shape of a tube (*tubular*) or a flask (*alveolar*) and may be branched or unbranched.

Because the outer layers of the epithelial cells are constantly being worn off at the surface, the bottom layers of epithelium are continually producing new cells. Thus the epithelium is in a continuous state of regeneration.

## Connective Tissues

Connective tissues are found everywhere in the body. They do what their name suggests—bind or tie together other cells, tissues, or organs of the body and anchor organs in place. One type of connective tissue, the blood, is active in protecting the body from infection by producing antibodies to immunize against reactions to disease. This will be discussed in Chapter 15.

Connective tissue, unlike epithelium, has few cells for a given amount of tissue. The material between cells is a nonliving substance called *intercellular substance*. It varies in nature from the liquid found in the blood to the hard compound of bone. The intercellular substance in connective tissue is abundant, whereas the cells are few. The situation is opposite in the case of the blood.

There are several different kinds of connective tissue. *Adipose* tissue is fatty in substance; *cartilage* tissue serves as a shock absorber between bones; and *elastic* tissue which is found in the walls of the various tubes of the body and is more flexible due to the presence of a network of elastic fibers in its intercellular substance.

Connective tissue may also be described as *hard* or *soft*. Bone and cartilage are examples of hard connective tissue which is also considered osseous tissue in this case. Adipose tissue is an example of soft connective tissue. Soft connective tissue has the ability to repair itself as does muscle and nerve tissue. The formation of a scar is the result of this function.

## Muscle Tissue

Muscle tissue contracts or extends to provide motion. Skeletal (striated) muscle looks like the meat we eat—red and soft, sometimes stringy, and usually held in large bundles and shaped into muscle masses. This is the muscle tissue that is attached to bone to provide body movements. It is called *voluntary muscle* because its movements originate in an act of will. Smooth (visceral) muscle tissue makes up the walls of the intestines and the blood vessels. This is known as *involuntary muscle* because it acts independently of the will; that is, we cannot voluntarily control the action of smooth muscle tissue. A third kind of muscle tissue is cardiac, the muscle of the heart. This is also an involuntary muscle.

## Nerve Tissue

Nerve tissue will be discussed in Chapter 14 on The Nervous System.

# MEMBRANES

Membranes are thin soft sheets of tissue which cover surfaces, line body cavities, or divide organs. All have protective and secretory functions. Some membranes absorb or excrete as well.

There are 2 basic types of membranes: *epithelial membranes* (the outer surface is covered with epithelial tissue), which secrete lubricants and protect the body against infection, and *connective tissue membranes* (composed of connective tissue), which anchor and support the organs and cover bone and cartilage. Both types of membranes are divided into 2 further categories. The 2 types of epithelial membranes are the mucous membranes and the serous membranes. The 2 types of connective tissue membranes are the synovial membranes and the fascial membranes.

*Mucous membranes* line cavities of the body which open to the exterior, such as the mouth, the nose, and the intestinal or urinary tracts. They secrete a substance called mucus and form a protection against bacterial invasion as well as other foreign particles. They may be ciliated.

*Serous membranes* line the cavities that do not open to the exterior; they cover organs such as the lungs, the stomach, and the heart. The pleurae (singular, pleura) enclose the lungs, the pericardium covers the heart, and the peritoneum lines the abdominal cavity. These membranes secrete a thin fluid which prevents friction when organs are in contact with one another.

*Synovial* or *skeletal membranes* line joint cavities between bones and cover tendons and bursal sacs. They provide for smooth motion without friction.

*Fascial* or *fibrous membranes* underlie the skin and attach it to underlying structures. Deep fascia surrounds the muscles and supports the internal organs.

## THE SKIN

The skin, known as the integumentary system and sometimes classified as a membrane, is one of the largest and most important tissues of the body. It is generally soft and elastic with a resistive outer layer that serves as a protection.

Its function as a protection serves the body in several ways. It prevents the entrance of microorganisms or other foreign substances; it also prevents injury to more fragile organs within the body and usually keeps the body from suffering from too great a loss of water.

The skin contains many nerve endings or receptors for the nervous system and, therefore, serves as an organ of sensation. Along with our sense of touch, we can perceive warmth, cold, pain, etc.

One of the important duties of the skin is to help regulate body temperature. In hot weather, the blood vessels dilate, bringing the blood to the surface of the skin for cooling. If the blood vessels constrict (that is, become smaller), the amount of heat lost through the skin is reduced. The evaporation of water through the sweat glands also cools the body.

The skin has the powers of absorption and excretion. Some medications are applied to be absorbed through the skin. Because the sweat glands excrete excess water and salts, some authorities classify the skin as part of the excretory system.

The skin is composed of 2 layers: the dermis and the epidermis. Directly under the dermis, but not part of the skin, is the subcutaneous tissue. The *epidermis* (outer layer) protects the layer beneath. It is thicker over the soles of the feet and palms of the hands—places that undergo considerable wear and tear. The cells on the outside or the top layer are constantly being rubbed off by the friction of movement, bathing, etc. (*desquamation*). The live inner cells continually replace these cells by mitosis; these live cells push up to the surface to replace the dead cells. The living cells contain pigment, the coloring matter of the skin. The amount of pigment varies in races and individuals—the Nordic peoples and other blondes have less pigment than the Asiatic people and other brunettes, and both have less pigment than the African races. Although skin color is inherited, exposure to the sun increases the amount of pigment in the skin. There are no blood vessels in the epidermis.

The *dermis* (inner layer), usually called the "true skin," is composed entirely of live cells enclosed in a network of lymph vessels, capillaries, and nerves projecting out to form ridges (papillae) in the epidermis. These ridges make the individual pattern of fingerprints and footprints that are used for identification. The nerve endings provide us with a sense of touch. The cells in this layer give the skin elasticity, allowing it to stretch. There are also fat cells in this layer which give the skin a smooth appearance. As aging occurs, the loss of subcutaneous fat and elastic tissues causes wrinkles to appear.

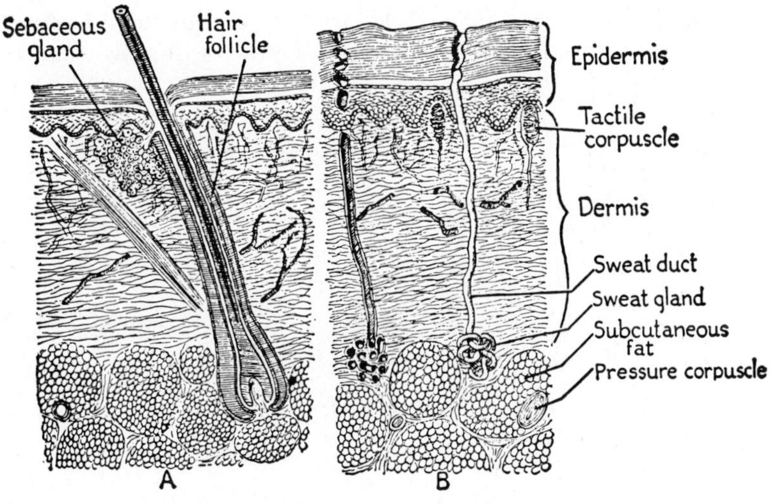

Figure 12-1. Section through skin: (A) with hair follicle; (B) with sweat glands and nerve endings. (Baillif and Kimmel: Structure and Function of the Human Body. Philadelphia, Lippincott)

The hair, the nails, the sebaceous (oil) glands and the sweat glands are called the "appendages" of the skin.

**Hair.** The skin is covered with hairs except in a few areas such as the palms of the hands and the soles of the feet. Hair serves to protect the head from sunburn and to protect the nose and the eyes from foreign objects. The part of the hair seen above the skin is the shaft; the part lying below is the root. The shaft runs slantwise from the body. The organs of touch lie in the true skin, close to the hair follicle, so that only a slight movement of the hair will cause the sensation of touch. The skin hairs have their roots in tiny sacs, called the hair *follicles.* Each follicle contains a single hair root, which, as long as it is alive, will continue to grow a hair that projects above the skin. (Two gray hairs cannot come in for every one that is pulled out!) Diseased or injured follicles destroy hair roots.

The hair obtains its nourishment entirely from the blood stream serving living cells at its roots. Since hair growth takes place here, cutting or trimming the ends will not stimulate growth. However, brushing the hair or massaging the scalp may be effective. The color of the hair is due to pigment that is deposited in a layer of the hair; when hair turns gray, there is a reduction of pigment and an increase in the light-reflecting air spaces between the cells. Baldness may be associated with the endocrine system, or it may be due to a factor of heredity. Constriction of the scalp by tight hat bands may contribute to baldness.

Surrounding each hair follicle are small muscles called the *arrectores pilorum.* If you become cold and the body wants to generate heat rapidly by widespread muscle action, these small muscles contract and the hairs stand erect. This is commonly called "goose flesh."

**Sebaceous Glands.** The sebaceous or oil glands lie close to the hair follicles into which they empty oil (sebum). The oil travels from there to the surface of the skin. These glands provide a natural oil to keep the skin soft and make the hair glossy. Overactive oil glands make your skin and hair unattractive. Pimples are caused by inflamed or infected oil glands.

**Sweat Glands.** The sweat glands (*sudoriparous glands*) remove waste from the body in the form of perspiration. They extract water and salt wastes from the blood and discharge them through the tiny outlets on the skin surface called the *pores.* These openings are countless—there are millions in the skin of an adult—especially in the hands, the feet, the forehead, and the axillae (armpits). Perspiration also helps to control the temperature of the body. If the body becomes too warm, the dermal capillaries expand and more blood flows to the surface. The sweat glands then have more blood from which to take water and other materials; therefore, they pour out more perspiration. Greater evaporation increases the cooling effects on the body, just as wetting the porch roof or the sidewalks makes the surrounding air cooler on a hot summer day.

**Nails.** The nails are tightly packed cells of the epidermis that protect the tips of the fingers and the toes and help in handling and picking up objects. Their roots are live cells, but the outer ends are dead. An injured nail will grow again if the root cells are still alive. After middle age, the nails usually become thicker and more brittle.

# 13

# The Musculoskeletal System

---

## BEHAVIORAL OBJECTIVES

*The student successfully attaining the goals of this chapter will be able to:*

- *discuss the interrelationships of all the systems of the body in the maintenance of life, movement of the body, and other body processes.*
- *compare the interrelationship of the muscular and skeletal systems; relate these functions to the external movements of the human body.*
- *list at least 4 functions of the skeletal system.*
- *differentiate between the axial and appendicular skeleton and give at least 2 examples of the groups of bones located in each.*
- *list the 4 general types of bones and give an example of each.*
- *diagram a long bone and label the diaphysis, epiphysis, red marrow, yellow marrow, periosteum, and endosteum.*
- *name the 3 major kinds of joints and give an example of each; further differentiate between the 4 types of synovial joints and give an example of each.*
- *define facet, tuberosity, process, spine, ridge, foramen, meatus, sinus, fossa, and suture in relationship to bone markings.*
- *discuss the interrelationships between ligaments, cartilage, and the bones as they all affect the movements of the body.*
- *define flexion, extension, abduction, adduction, circumduction, rotation, supination, pronation, protraction, retraction, inversion, and eversion; demonstrate each movement with his or her own body.*
- *list the 3 major divisions of the skeletal system and give examples of each; locate these on a skeleton or chart.*
- *locate and name the major bones of the body and describe their function.*
- *discuss the structure and function of the muscles; identify the general characteristics of all muscles.*
- *define insertion, origin, prime mover, antagonist, and synergist, in relationship to movement of the body.*
- *locate and name on a chart, the major muscle groups in the human body; indicate the actions of each group.*
- *classify the major muscles of the body as abductors, adductors, levators, depressors, flexors, extensors, rotators, or sphincters.*
- *relate the concept of metabolism to the ability of the muscles to move.*

---

## THE BODY'S FRAMEWORK

The skeleton is the living bony framework for the rest of the body. It supports and gives shape to the body and protects vital organs and delicate soft tissues. It serves also as an anchor for the skeletal muscles by providing attachments for tendons and parts of the muscles thereby allowing motion. Some of the individual bones of the skeleton serve as levers to assist in movement. In addition to these functions of the skeletal system, the bones store calcium, and the bone marrow manufactures red blood cells, some white blood cells, and the platelets—the solid elements of the blood tissue.

For study purposes, the human skeleton is divided into two main parts—the axial skeleton and the appendicular skeleton. The axial skeleton is composed of the bones of the skull, the thorax, and the vertebral column. These bones, 80 in number, form the *axis* of the body. The *appendicular* skeleton consists of the bones of the shoulder, the upper extremities, the hips, and the lower extremities. These bones, 126 in number, are attached to the axial skeleton as *appendages*.

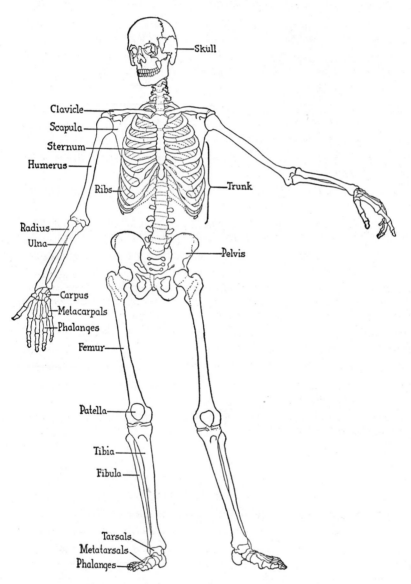

Figure 13-1. The skeleton, front view.

## Structure of Bones

There are more than 200 bones in the body which can be classified as *long bones,* some of which provide support (such as the tibia); *short bones* (such as the carpals) which facilitate greater motion within parts; *flat bones* (such as the scapula) which give protection, and *irregular bones* (such as the vertebrae) which vary in size and shape to accommodate other structures. Included in this last category are the *sesamoid bones,* which are small rounded bones that develop in the capsules of joints or in tendons (the only exception is the patella, or kneecap).

Although bone tissue is hardened by deposits of calcium and phosphorus, bones are made up of living cells. The *periosteum,* a membrane that covers every bone, contains the blood vessels that supply the oxygen and the nutrition to the bone cells to keep them alive. The blood vessels also bring the bone building materials and minerals that harden the bone by filling the intercellular spaces.

Bones are living active organs that change greatly in the lifetime of an individual. The small, partially cartilaginous bones of the baby grow in diameter and length and continue to harden until the individual's growth

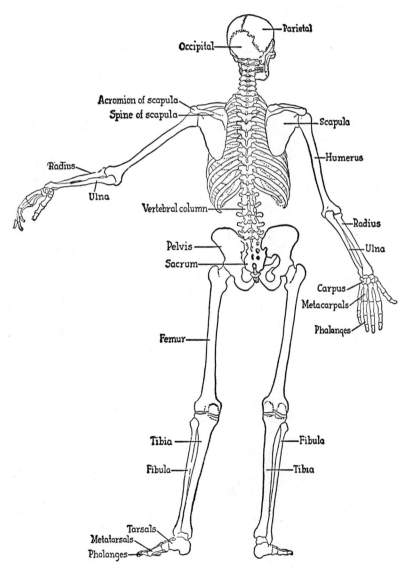

Figure 13-2. The skeleton, back view.

is complete, which usually occurs between the ages of 18 and 21. The ossification process which hardens the bones through an increase in calcified tissue, progresses from the middle of the shaft outward. Although the bone structure and size are altered primarily to accommodate growth, change continues into later life when most growth has stopped. Bone cells multiply rapidly in the growing years, but thereafter new cells are formed only to replace dead or injured ones and to repair breaks. Bones become harder and more brittle, breaking more easily with age.

Two types of osseous (bone) tissue enter into the construction of the long bones of the extremities. The shaft, or *diaphysis,* is hard and compact, while the end, or *epiphysis,* is spongelike and covered by a shell of harder bone (see Fig. 13-3). The diaphysis and the

epiphysis do not fuse until full growth is reached.

The outside surface of the bones is hard; the hollow inner part is filled with a soft substance called marrow. (The prefix referring to bone marrow is *myelo-.*) There are 2 kinds of marrow: yellow and red. The yellow kind, which we have seen in "soup bones," is found in the central cavities of the long bones. The red marrow, which is found in the ends of long bones as well as in the bodies of the vertebrae and the flat bones, is responsible for the manufacture of red blood cells, white blood cells, and probably also blood platelets.

The lining of the hollow marrow cavity is called the *endosteum.* The covering or outside layer of the bone is called the *periosteum* and has the ability to form new bone tissue.

## Joints

The points at which the bones are attached to each other are called joints or articulations. Because of the way the bones are attached, the body position can be changed, and hundreds of motions are possible. (The prefix *arthro-* refers to a joint.)

**Kinds of Joints.** There are primarily 3 different kinds of joints. The first is the type in which there is no motion at all, as in the bones of the skull which are fitted together with interlocking notches. These are referred to as immovable or *fibrous joints.* Within the second kind, known as slightly movable or *cartilaginous joints,* there is a slight degree of motion or flexibility, as is found in the vertebral column. The third type of joint is classified as "freely movables" or *synovial* or *diarthrodial joints* and can be found in many parts of the body, such as the shoulder.

There are several kinds of freely movable joints. Your finger and knee joints move like a door on its hinges and are appropriately called hinge joints. In the shoulders and the hips, ball-and-socket joints allow rotating motions—the rounded end of one bone (the ball) fits into the hollowed-out end of the other (the socket). The elbow is an example of a pivot joint, which makes it possible to turn the forearm as in turning a doorknob (see Fig. 13-4). The wrist is an example of a gliding joint.

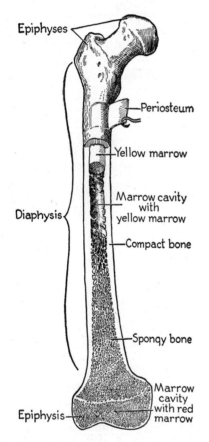

Epiphyses

Periosteum

Yellow marrow

Marrow cavity with yellow marrow

Diaphysis

Compact bone

Spongy bone

Marrow cavity with red marrow

Epiphysis

Figure 13-3. Bone as an organ. (Baillif and Kimmel: Structure and Function of the Human Body. Philadelphia, Lippincott)

## Bone Markings

The contour of bones resembles the configuration of an interesting landscape with its hills and valleys; there are hundreds of these bone markings or landscapes, each type identified by special characteristics. A *facet* is a small plane or smooth area. A *tuberosity* is a projection. Any bony prominence is called a bony *process*; a *spine* is a sharp process; a *ridge* or *crest* is thin or narrow. A hole through which blood vessels, ligaments, and nerves pass is called a *foramen*; a long tube-like hole is called a *canal* or a *meatus*. A *sinus* is a spongelike air space inside a bone. A dent or depression is usually called a *fossa*. The enlargement at the end of the long bone is called the *head* of the bone. A *suture* (or suture line) is the line where skull bones have joined.

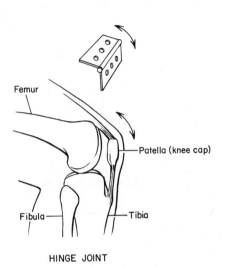

HINGE JOINT

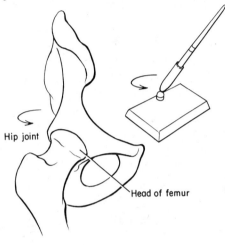

BALL-AND-SOCKET JOINT

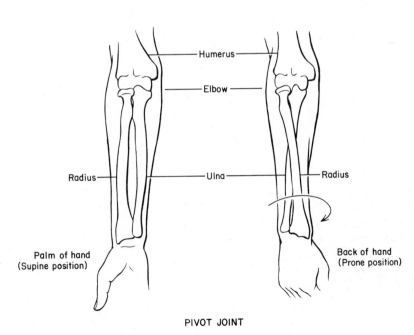

PIVOT JOINT

Figure 13-4. Some freely movable joints.

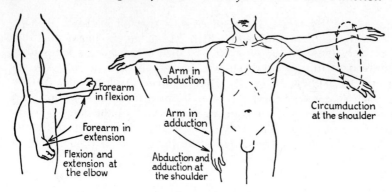

Figure 13-5. Movement types. (Baillif and Kimmel: Structure and Function of the Human Body. Philadelphia, Lippincott)

## Ligaments and Cartilage

Strong, fibrous bands, called ligaments, hold bones together. Cartilage plates on the ends of bones make a slick surface for rotation, and absorb shocks and jars. (The prefix which refers to cartilage is *chondro-*.) The moving joints are lined with a membrane that secretes a fluid called *synovial fluid,* which keeps them lubricated and working smoothly.

## Bursae

The body contains sacs called *bursae,* which are also lined with synovial membrane. These act as cushions between the ends of the bones and also are found between muscles and bones or between tendons, wherever motion is likely to produce friction.

## Movements

Some of the many different motions that the body can perform have definite names so far as function is concerned. *Flexion* decreases the angle between 2 bones or bends a part on itself, as in bending the elbow; *extension,* or straightening, is the opposite. *Abduction* is movement away from the midplane of the body; *adduction,* the opposite, is movement toward the midplane. If you hold your arm out straight and then move it around in a circle, all these movements are combined; the resulting motion is *circumduction.* A different kind of motion is *rotation,* which is twisting one part with respect to that which joins it, but without changing the angle between the two. An example of rotation is twisting the head in the familiar gesture of saying "No."

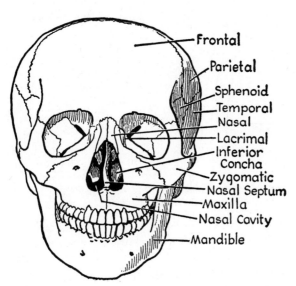

Figure 13-6. Anterior view of the skull. (Baillif and Kimmel: Structure and Function of the Human Body. Philadelphia, Lippincott)

Some joined structures have special movements. If you stand with your arms hanging down and your palms facing forward, the movement that brings the forearm into this position is *supination*. Now, if you reverse your hands so that the backs of them face forward, the movement is called *pronation*. These movements are special because, as you reverse your hands, the 2 bones in the forearm actually cross one another (see Fig. 13-4).

The ankle joint also has special movements. If you bend your ankle so that the sole of the foot faces the opposite foot, the motion is called *inversion*. If you bend your ankle the opposite way, with the sole facing outward, the movement is known as *eversion*.

The lower jaw can move forward (*protraction*) and backward (*retraction*).

## THE SKULL

The 3 main parts of the skeleton are the skull, the trunk, and the extremities. The skull has 2 parts: (1) the thin, flat bones of the *cranium*, which protect the brain, and (2) the facial bones, which are light, irregularly shaped, and generally small. The lower jaw bone, the mandible, is the only movable facial bone. The cranial and the facial bones give the face its individual shape.

Figures 13-6 and 13-7 show the bones of the skull. The following list is the simplest way of describing their arrangement.

### BONES OF THE CRANIUM

2 parietal
top and sides of head

1 occipital
back of head

1 frontal
forehead

2 temporal
contain ear cavities, mastoid cells in tip

1 sphenoid
center of base of skull

1 ethmoid
roof of nasal cavity

### BONES OF THE FACE

2 nasal
bridge of nose

1 vomer
divides nasal cavity (as part of nasal septum)

2 inferior turbinates (conchae) in the nostrils

2 lacrimal (orbitals)
front part of eye sockets

2 zygomatic
prominent part of cheeks
base of eye sockets

2 palate (palatines)
roof of mouth

2 maxillae
upper jaw

1 mandible
lower jaw

A small horseshoe-shaped bone, the *hyoid*, lies just behind and below the mandible; the tongue muscles are attached to it.

Four pairs of cavities in the cranial bones make your skull lighter and give back the sound of your voice. They are the *sinuses* and are named for the bones in which they lie: the frontal, the ethmoid, the sphenoid, and the maxillary. These sinuses are lined with mucous membrane continuous with the nasal mucosa and drain into the nasal cavity.

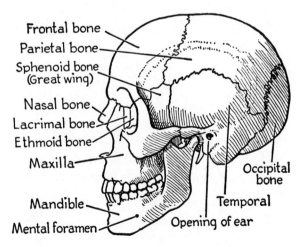

Figure 13-7. Lateral view of the skull. (Baillif and Kimmel: Structure and Function of the Human Body. Philadelphia, Lippincott)

## THE TRUNK

### The Vertebral Column

The vertebral column, or spine, holds the head, stiffens and supports the midportion of the body, and provides attachments for the ribs and the pelvic bones. It also protects the spinal cord, which passes from the brain down through the bony rings which make up the spinal canal. The vertebrae are constructed on a common plan; there are slight variations in their structure, but each one is made to adjust to the one beneath. They are separated from each other by plates of cartilage called *intervertebral disks,* which act as shock absorbers when you walk, jump, or fall. On the inner side of the vertebra is a bony structure called the *arch,* which forms an opening or spinal foramen through which the spinal cord passes. Jutting from the arch are several fingerlike extensions, or *processes,* on which ligaments and tendons of the muscles of the back are anchored (see Figs. 13-8 and 13-9). The muscles, the ligaments, and the cartilage disks help to make the vertebral column strong yet flexible: we can bend forward, backward, and to either side and can accomplish a considerable rotation of the central portion of our body as well.

The spine has 4 normal curves that help to balance the body. Disease or injury and poor posture distort these curves. Increased abnormal thoracic curvature of the lumbar spine is called *lordosis* or *swayback.* An increased lateral curvature is called *scoliosis.* An increased curvature of the thoracic spine is called *kyphosis* (hunchback).

### Division of the Vertebrae

The 26 vertebrae are divided into groups. The top 7, or cervical vertebrae, are located in the neck; the first (the *atlas*) supports the skull, and the second (the *axis*) has an especially wide surface so that the head can be turned freely. The next 12 are the thoracic vertebrae, to which the ribs are attached. The next 5, the lumbar vertebrae, are in the small of the back. The 5 sacral vertebrae form 1 solid bone, the *sacrum,* which anchors the

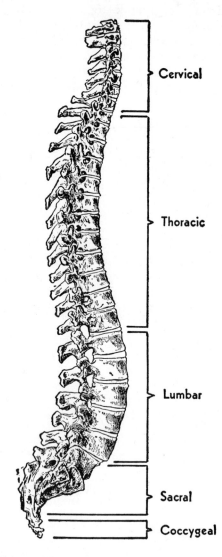

Figure 13-9. Lateral view of an adult vertebral column, showing the curves and the divisions of the columns with reference to the spaces from which the spinal nerves emerge. Note the cartilage disks in the spaces between the bodies of the vertebrae.

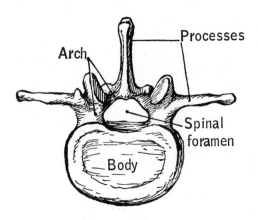

Figure 13-8. Transverse section of a vertebra.

pelvis. The last 4 vertebrae, small and incomplete, form the *coccyx*. These two sections (sacrum and coccyx) are commonly called the tailbone (see Fig. 13-9).

### The Thorax

The *thorax* is a cavity formed by the ribs (costae), attached anteriorly to the sternum and posteriorly to the thoracic vertebrae. The thorax protects the heart, the lungs, and the great thoracic blood vessels. It is also a supportive structure for the bones of the shoulder girdle. The floor of the thorax is the diaphragm.

The front boundary of the upper part of the thorax is the *sternum* (or breast bone), a flat, sword-shaped bone in the middle of the chest opposite the thoracic vertebrae in the back.

The ribs make the cage that supports the chest and protects the heart and the lungs. These flat, narrow bowed bones are arranged in pairs, 12 on each side. From their attachment to the spine at the back, the ribs curve out and to the front like barrel hoops. The upper 7 pairs are attached to the sternum in front, the next 3 pairs are attached to each other and indirectly to the sternum, and the last 2 pairs are free in front. These "floating ribs" are shorter than the rest. The relatively elastic cartilage on the ends of the ribs allows leeway for the chest and the abdomen to expand.

## THE EXTREMITIES

### The Pelvis

Although it is not considered a part of the extremities, the pelvic girdle is discussed here because it anchors the legs to the central part of the body. It is formed by the 2 large, irregularly shaped *innominate* (hip bones or os coxae) attached posteriorly to the sacrum. These bones spread outward at the top and become narrow at their front lower edges. In fetal development, these bones develop as 3 separate bones known as the *ilium,* the *ischium,* and the *pubis,* which usually fuse by the time growth is completed. The ilium is the upper flaring portion that one usually identifies as the hip bone. The ischium is the lower, stronger portion, which you may be

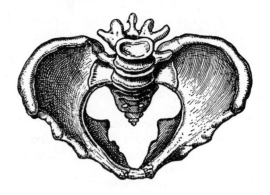

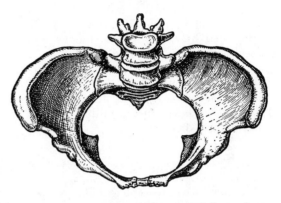

Figure 13-10. Pelvic girdles viewed from above. (*Top*) Male pelvis. (*Bottom*) Female pelvis. (Baillif and Kimmel: Structure and Function of the Human Body. Philadelphia, Lippincott)

conscious of only after horseback riding. The pubic bones meet in front and are joined by a pad of cartilage. This juncture is called the *symphysis pubis.* Connected to the sacrum and the coccyx posteriorly, these bones form your pelvic cavity, which houses the urinary bladder, the rectum, and, in a woman, the reproductive organs. A woman's pelvis is larger and wider than a man's, which is Nature's way of providing room for the development and birth of a baby (see Fig. 13-10). A hollow on the outer side of each innominate bone makes a socket for the upper end of the femur and provides attachments for thigh and abdominal muscles.

### The Leg (Lower Extremity)

The *femur* (thigh bone), the upper bone of the leg, supports the weight of the trunk and is the longest and strongest bone of the body. Its upper end is attached to the pelvic bone in a ball-and-socket joint, where its rounded end (the head) fits into the depression on the outside of the innominate bone; the other end is attached to the tibia in the lower leg. The head of the femur joins the shaft (the cylindrical long portion) by a short length of bone called the neck. (This area is a common site of fractures in the elderly.) Elevation on either side of the junction of the shaft and the neck are called the *trochanters,* which serve as points of attachment.

There are 2 bones in the lower leg; the *tibia,* or "shin bone" and the *fibula.* The upper end of the tibia is attached to the lower end of the femur in the knee joint. The front of this joint is protected by a small bone, the *patella,* or "knee cap," which is buried in a tendon that passes over the joint. The other bone in the lower leg, the fibula, is smaller than the tibia and is attached to it at the upper end. The lower ends of these bones meet the bones of the ankle to form the ankle joint.

### The Foot

The foot is constructed to hold the weight of the entire body and, at the same time, give flexibility and resilience to our motions. The 7 *tarsal* bones of the ankle are compact and shaped irregularly; the largest of these bones is in the heel. They join the 5 *metatarsal,* or "instep bones," to form 2 arches: the longi-

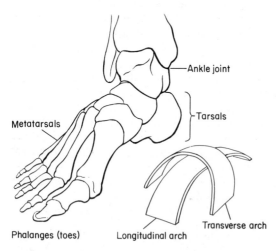

Figure 13-11. Bones of the right foot and ankle. The longitudinal and the transverse arches are illustrated diagrammatically.

tudinal arch, which extends from the heel to the toe; and the transverse or metatarsal arch, which extends across the foot. The weight of the body falls on these arches, and the many joints spring and give when you walk. Weak muscles lessen this "spring," and high, spiky heels and poor posture upset the body balance, flattening the arches. The 14 bones of the toes, the *phalanges,* are attached to the metatarsal bones. The great toe has 2 phalanges; each of the other toes has 3.

In general, the hands and the feet are built alike, but in the hands, the bones are finer and the joints more numerous (there are 29 in the wrist and the hand). The hands are designed for fine and flexible movements; the feet, for support. Together these bones number about half of those in the body.

### The Shoulders and the Arms (Upper Extremity)

The shoulder girdle, which anchors the arms, is formed by 4 bones. Two long, thin bones, the *clavicles,* or "collar bones," are attached to the sternum and extend outward at right angles to it on either side. Opposite the clavicles at the back are the *scapulae,* the "shoulder blades." They are flat, triangular bones attached to the outer ends of the clavicles and to the humerus in the upper arm. Look at these bones on the skeleton. You can see that they are attached to the trunk of the body at only one place—the sternum. This is why you can move your shoulders and arms so freely. But because the shoulder is not securely anchored, it can be easily dislocated.

The *humerus* is the single long bone in the upper arm; the upper end is attached to the scapula, and the lower end meets the larger of the 2 forearm bones, the ulna, to form the elbow joint.

There are 2 bones in the forearm. The larger, the *ulna,* has 2 hollows in its upper end; the lower end of the humerus fits into one of these depressions, and the upper end of the second forearm bone, the *radius,* fits into the other. The radius lies beside the ulna and is attached to it at the upper end; both the radius and the ulna are attached to the wrist bones to form the wrist joint. The arrangement of these bones lets you turn your palm forward (supine position) or backward (prone position), and the radius and the ulna move so freely with the wrist bones and each other that, when you turn your palm down, the radius crosses the ulna. The relationship of these bones in movement is shown in the illustration of a pivot joint in Figure 13-4.

## The Hand

The bones of the hands and the feet are especially structured for their unique functions. One of the differences between man and the other animals is his ability to use his hands.

More than one fourth of the total number of bones in the human body are found in the hands and the wrists. Because of the many small bones which allow for a great range of motions—twisting, bending, grasping, squeezing—you can do such things as play a violin, write your name, and pick up minute objects with your thumb and forefinger.

The 8 *carpal,* or wrist, bones are small, irregular bones that support the base of the palm and are attached to the radius, to the ulna, and to the 5 long, slender, and slightly curved *metacarpal* bones that form the palm of the hand. The other ends of the metacarpal bones are attached to the *phalanges,* or finger bones. There are 3 phalanges in each finger and 2 in the thumb.

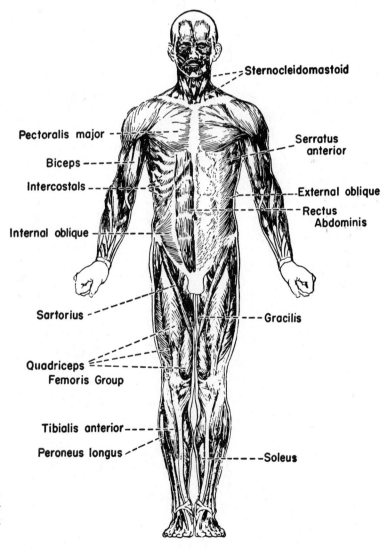

Figure 13-12. Muscles of the body, front view. The deeper muscles are shown on the right side of the abdomen.

## MUSCLES

Although the functions of the skeleton include giving shape to the body and providing joints for the purpose of allowing body motion, neither of these functions is carried out without the aid of other body systems, including the muscles. Muscles lie in sheets and cords beneath the skin and cover the bones. The skeleton determines the size of the framework, but the muscles (plus fat!) determine the body shape. The prefix which denotes muscle is myo.

Muscles and tendons move the bones; muscle cells are like millions of little motors moving your body, just as a motor moves an automobile. Without muscles your body would be as stationary as the classroom skeleton.

The muscles are arranged in fine elastic threads, or *fibers*. Each fiber is comparable in size with a human hair and will hold about 1,000 times its own weight. The fibers are wrapped together in *bundles*, with several bundles forming a muscle.

Each muscle is covered by a sheath of connective tissue called *fascia*, the ends of which lengthen into tough cords called *tendons*.

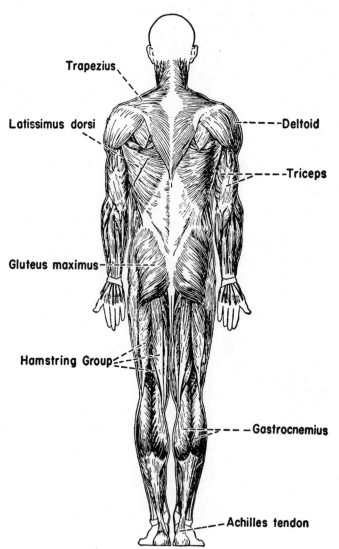

Figure 13-13. Muscles of the body, back view.

The muscles are attached to bones by means of these tendons. The tendons have sheaths lined with a synovial membrane which permits a smooth gliding movement. The thick meaty portion of the muscle is called the body or the *belly* of the muscle.

To understand the anatomy of a muscle and its tendon, place your hand on the thick muscle at the calf of your leg. Here are located some of the strongest muscles in the body. Move your hand toward your ankle and you will find that as both the leg and the muscles become narrower, the tissues become tough, fibrous, and ropelike. (Flex and extend your foot to emphasize this.) This occurs because approximately halfway to the ankle the muscle is attached to a tendon, the tendon of Achilles, which extends down to the heel and attaches to the calcaneus (the large bone of the heel).

All living cells have certain characteristics. Specialized cells exhibit special characteristics. The specialized muscle cells have the characteristic of *contractility*—the ability to shorten and become thicker—which is how the muscles accomplish their work. Muscle tissue is also said to have the property of *extensibility*, or the ability to stretch. Because it possesses *elasticity*, the muscle tissue returns to its normal length after it has been used. Some of the characteristics of muscle tissue can be observed by stretching a heavy rubber band, which exhibits many similar traits.

Muscles are attached to bones at points which will bring about the most effective motions. Since muscles work by contracting or shortening (and thereby pulling), most muscles attach one bone to another or extend from one part to another. One end of the muscle, the *origin*, is attached to the nonmoving or less movable bone or part, while the other end, the *insertion*, is attached to the part or bone being moved.

Muscles are elastic and work in pairs having opposite actions—when one muscle contracts, the other relaxes. A movement is initiated by a single muscle or a set of muscles called the *prime mover*. When an opposite movement is to be made, another set of muscles called the *antagonist* takes over. Muscles that assist one another in the movement are called *synergic* or *synergistic* muscles. When you bend your elbow (flexion), you can feel the muscle in your upper arm contract, grow hard, and thicken as the muscle fibers shorten to raise the forearm. At the same time, the muscles on the back of your upper arm relax, lengthen, and pull against the front muscles. If you permit, they will pull your forearm straight (extension) (see Fig. 13-14).

Muscles may be classified by their actions. The muscles that move the body part away from the trunk are called *abductors*; those that move the part toward the body are called *adductors*. *Levators* raise the part; *depressors* lower the part. *Flexors* bend joints; *extensors* extend the joints. *Rotators* rotate the joint around the axis; and *sphincters*, which are circular muscles, serve to close off body openings.

Figure 13-14. Diagram of co-ordinated movement. (*Left*) In flexion of the forearm the biceps brachii is contracted (note the bulging), and the triceps is relaxed. (*Right*) In extension, the reverse condition holds. (Redrawn from Keith; Greisheimer, E. M., and Wiedeman, M. P.: Physiology and Anatomy, ed. 9. Philadelphia, Lippincott, 1972)

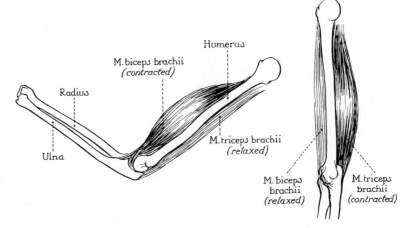

Radius

M. biceps brachii
*(contracted)*

Humerus

Ulna

M. triceps brachii
*(relaxed)*

M. biceps brachii
*(relaxed)*

M. triceps brachii
*(contracted)*

## Types of Muscles

Three different kinds of muscle tissue can be identified through a microscope (see Fig. 13-15). Those which you can control consciously are called *voluntary muscles.* They are made of special types of cells that are long and give the appearance of being striped; therefore, they are also known as *striated* muscles. Since it is the voluntary striated muscles which control the skeletal movements (they are attached to the bones), they are also called *skeletal* muscles.

The second kind are not striped like the voluntary muscle but are smooth and thus are called *smooth muscle.* They are also called *involuntary* because these muscles work automatically; you do not control their actions. The involuntary muscles control motion inside body organs (the viscera). For example, they move food along the digestive tract, make eye adjustments, and dilate and contract the blood vessels to assist the circulation of the blood.

The third type of muscle tissue is found in the heart and is called *cardiac muscle.* It works automatically but looks somewhat like the striped or striated muscle. However, these fibers are formed in a continuous network rather than being wrapped in sheaths. Since you do not control cardiac muscle, it is referred to as involuntary muscle.

## Power Source

Muscles need energy to move any part of the body. The foods we eat furnish carbon, hydrogen, and oxygen from which the body makes glycogen, a special form of carbohydrate used by the body for fuel. (It is also called animal starch.) Oxygen and glycogen (sugar), brought to the muscle cells by the blood, react with each other, and the result of this oxidation or burning process is energy and heat. In fact, most of the heat that is produced in the body originates from muscle activity. When muscles are very active they draw on the reserve glycogen stored in their cells. The body makes use of our muscles' ability to produce heat rapidly by the automatic device of general muscle action or shivering when we are cold. To produce a great amount of necessary heat in an emergency, the body produces the more violent exercise of chilling.

**Waste Products.** Carbon dioxide and lactic acid are waste products produced in the process of oxidation. The blood carries carbon dioxide to the lungs, where it is removed in breathing; lactic acid is removed through the urinary system and the sweat glands. Vigorous or prolonged muscle action produces such a quantity of waste products, especially lactic acid, that the blood cannot carry it away fast enough, and some of it accumulates in the muscle cells. This is why your muscles are fatigued, ache, or feel sore after violent exercise or prolonged use. A simple formula might help you to summarize the action of muscles:

Muscle Cell + Food and Oxygen

↓

Heat and Energy

↓

By-Products: Lactic Acid and Carbon Dioxide

## Muscle Tone

Because man stands erect against the constant pull of gravity, many of his muscles are constantly in a mild state of contraction to help him to maintain his balance. Even relaxed muscles are always ready to go into action if they are in good condition. This state of slight contraction and this ability to spring into action is called *muscle tone* (*tonus*). When muscle tone is good you feel springy and alive: your walk is firm, your head is erect, and your eyes are wide open and alert. Poor muscle tone makes you feel dragged out: your head droops, your body sags. Physical exercise improves the tone of the muscles and builds them up. An idle muscle loses its tone and wastes away. This is why it is important for children who sit in school all day to have an opportunity for vigorous play after school; their muscles need such stimulation. If a patient does not use certain muscles or uses them very little, they become flabby and weak (*atonic*).

Pressure on the nerves in muscles makes

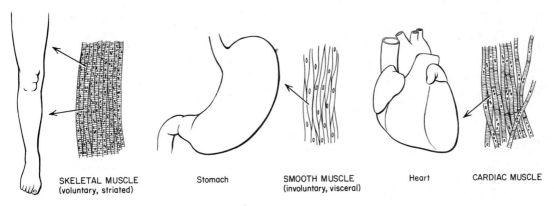

SKELETAL MUSCLE
(voluntary, striated)

Stomach

SMOOTH MUSCLE
(involuntary, visceral)

Heart

CARDIAC MUSCLE

Figure 13-15. The 3 types of muscles in the human body.

them sore; patients who must lie on their backs most of the time complain of aches and pains in these muscles. Strains or inactivity also affect them. For these reasons, a back rub can be comforting. It is also advisable to adjust the patient's body to positions that do not cause strain, to change his position frequently, and to support him the first time he stands on his feet.

**Rehabilitation.** An injured or inactive muscle can be retrained to do its work. Retraining usually requires working with more than one muscle because, as previously stated, muscles work in groups, except for the simplest movements. Fine work is being done today in helping people to recover the use of injured or inactive muscles. Rehabilitation activities are prescribed by physicians, and trained physiotherapists and occupational therapists carry them out. Nurses work under the direction of these specialists to help the patient with selected exercises. Reeducating muscles is sometimes a long process; improvement is likely to be so gradual that it is hardly noticeable from day to day, and the patient often needs encouragement to persevere. The general principles of rehabilitation will be considered in more detail in Chapter 34.

## Important Muscles

**Neck and Shoulders.** The *sternocleidomastoid* is the strong muscle on the side of the neck which helps to hold the head erect. When it becomes diseased or injured, the head is permanently drawn to one side, a condition known as torticollis or wry neck.

From the nurse's standpoint, the most important muscle of the shoulder is the *deltoid*. Aside from moving the upper arm outward from the body, it is used as a site for intramuscular injections.

**Arm and Anterior Chest.** The *triceps* and the *biceps* are used to extend and flex the forearm. The biceps is located on the front of the upper arms; the triceps, posteriorly to it. The *pectoralis major* and *minor* and the *serratus anterior* are large anterior chest muscles. The pectoralis helps to bring the arm across the chest.

**Respiration.** One group of muscles assists in the process of breathing. A large, flat dome-shaped muscle, the *diaphragm,* lies between the abdominal and the thoracic cavities. When the diaphragm contracts, it moves downward, making the chest cavity larger and forming a partial vacuum about the lungs, which causes air to rush into the lungs. As the diaphragm relaxes, it pushes up and the air is forced out of the lungs. An easy way to check this change in the size and the shape of the rib cavity is to place a tape measure around the chest and inhale and exhale. Notice the difference in your chest measurements. The intercostal muscles located between the ribs also aid in respiration by helping to enlarge the chest cavity.

**Abdomen.** The abdominal muscles are the flat bands that stretch from the ribs to the pelvis and support the abdominal organs. The main muscles found here are the *internal* and the *external oblique,* the *transversus abdom-*

*inis* and the *rectus abdominis.* These are arranged to give support by overlapping in layers from various angles. Any opening in a muscle creates an area of weakness within it because the opening may stretch or enlarge. There are weak places within the abdominal muscles where a hernia (rupture) may occur with pressure from or protrusion of part of the intestine. These weak places are areas where blood vessels, nerves, ligaments, and cords extend through the muscles. The inguinal rings, the femoral rings, and the umbilicus are common sites for hernias.

Healthy abdominal muscles "give" just enough to permit the organs to move when you breathe; when they lose some of their contracting power, the abdominal organs drop out of place or bulge outward against the muscles.

**Back and Posterior Chest.** Large muscles lie across the back and the posterior chest.

Two of these are the *trapezius* and the *latissimus dorsi.* The trapezius is also called the "swimming muscle" and helps to lift the shoulder area. The latissimus dorsi and other muscles of the back often work in groups to help you to stand erect, balance when you carry heavy objects, and turn or bend your body.

**Gluteal Muscles.** The large muscles forming the buttocks are called *gluteal muscles* (gluteus maximus, medius, and minimus). You use these muscles in changing from sitting to standing positions, as well as in walking. These muscles are frequently used as a site for intramuscular injections.

**Thigh and Lower Leg.** A large group of muscles on the front of the thigh is called the *quadriceps femoris* group. On the posterior surface, another group called the *hamstring* group flexes and extends the leg and the thigh. The *gracilis* and the *sartorius* are

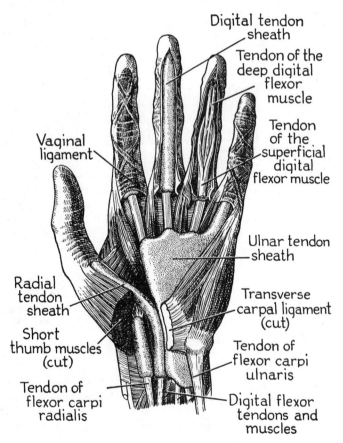

Digital tendon sheath

Tendon of the deep digital flexor muscle

Tendon of the superficial digital flexor muscle

Vaginal ligament

Ulnar tendon sheath

Radial tendon sheath

Transverse carpal ligament (cut)

Short thumb muscles (cut)

Tendon of flexor carpi ulnaris

Tendon of flexor carpi radialis

Digital flexor tendons and muscles

Figure 13-16. Deep structures in palm and wrist. (Baillif and Kimmel: Structures and Function of the Human Body. Philadelphia, Lippincott)

thigh muscles. The latter is called the "tailor's muscle," since it allows a person to sit crosslegged.

The *tibialis anterior* is located in the front of the lower leg. The *gastrocnemius,* the *soleus,* and the *peroneus longus* give the rounded appearance to the calf of the leg. The *Achilles tendon* is a name taken from Greek mythology to designate the tendon which attaches the calf muscle to the heel bone. The calf muscles allow you to extend your foot to give you the "spring in your step" when walking or running.

**Hands and the Feet.** The muscles and the tendons of the hands and the feet are planned in a slightly different manner from those of the rest of the body. There are many bones in the hands and the feet to permit their more intricate functions, and many muscles and tendons are necessary to move them. However, bulky muscles would make clumsy motions, so the larger muscles that move the hands and the feet are located in the forearm and the lower leg. When you flex your fingers to clench your first, you can feel the muscles move and tighten in your forearm. Some muscles begin from the wrist. These muscles extend into long thin tendons that attach to the bones of the fingers, permitting accuracy as well as a wide range of motion (see Fig. 13-16).

You can stand on your toes, your heels, and the ball of your foot. Consider the many motions of the dancer, and you will understand that to accomplish such fine movements, the structure of the foot is similar to that of the hand. Their variance in design allows a difference in function.

# 14

# The Nervous System

## BEHAVIORAL OBJECTIVES

*The student successfully attaining the goals of this chapter will be able to:*

- *diagram 2 nerve cells, indicating each cell body, nucleus, cytoplasm, neurilemma, nerve fiber group, dendrite, axon, synapse, and myelin sheath (when present); indicate the direction of the impulse through these neurons.*
- *differentiate between nerve tract and ganglion.*
- *identify the functions of sensory, motor, and connecting neurons.*
- *define the term receptor; differentiate between exteroceptor, proprioceptor, and interoceptor.*
- *define the term effector; differentiate between somatic-voluntary and visceral-involuntary.*
- *discuss the actions and the interrelationships between the sympathetic and the parasympathetic divisions of the autonomic nervous systems.*
- *diagram the human brain, showing the hemispheres of the cerebrum and indicating the frontal, parietal, temporal and occipital areas; indicate the thalamus, the hypothalamus, and the cerebellum; and indicate the pons and the medulla in the midbrain; discuss the major functions of each of these.*
- *list the functions of the spinal cord.*
- *diagram the location of the meninges, the dura mater, the pia mater, and the arachnoid; describe each; locate the cerebrospinal fluid and describe its functions.*
- *briefly describe the peripheral nervous system.*
- *compare and contrast the actions of the autonomic nervous system and the portion of the central nervous system which is under conscious control.*
- *relate the functions of the nervous system to those of the musculoskeletal system.*

Our bodies are made up of billions of cells, divided into systems according to either their structure or the functions they perform. None of these systems functions alone; their activities are interrelated, integrated, and coordinated by messages carried from one system to another. The hormones and the enzymes of the body act as chemical messengers, but our major system of *communication* from both within and without is the nervous system.

The nervous system brings us all the im-

pressions and the information that we have from the world outside us (*external stimuli*), and it stores this information (*memory*) for future reference and application. It serves as the center that coordinates the messages from the internal body systems (*internal stimuli*), and it makes it possible for us to readjust constantly to both our internal and our external environment. Thus the nervous system is the director of all body activities.

The nervous system is often likened to the

operations of a telephone exchange. Through a network of wires, messages come into the central switchboard, where the necessary connections are made to direct them to the right places. Your nervous system is organized to bring messages into a center which relays them to certain parts of the body. The brain and the spinal cord are the switchboard. Anatomically, this functions as the *central nervous system*. The nerves are the wires that carry incoming and outgoing messages and make up what is called the *peripheral nervous system*.

## THE NERVE CELL

The nervous tissue is made up of special cells called *neurons*. The neuron consists of a cell body containing a nucleus, granular cytoplasm, and threadlike projections of the cytoplasm called nerve fibers. Scattered throughout the cytoplasm are Nissl bodies which are concerned with the nutrition of the cell. The fibers which bring the impulses to the cell are called *dendrites*; those which carry the impulses away are called *axons*. Each neuron has one axon and several dendrites (see Fig. 14-2). Within the central nervous system, a bundle of nerve fibers is called a *nerve tract*; outside the central nervous system, it is called a *ganglion*.

There are 3 types of neurons: *sensory, motor,* and *connecting*. Sensory neurons receive messages from all parts of the body and transmit them to the central nervous system. Motor neurons transmit messages from the central nervous system to all parts of the body, either to alter muscle activity or to cause glands to secrete. The impulse is carried through pathways between the sensory and the motor neurons by the connecting neurons.

Because of their fibers or processes, the neurons are able to carry out their unique activity of transmitting signals from one neuron to the next. The nerve fiber is an axon or a dendrite that extends from the central nervous system out into the body. Some of these fibers are several feet in length.

When one neuron receives a signal, it sends it on to the next neuron across a small space or junction between the axon and the den-

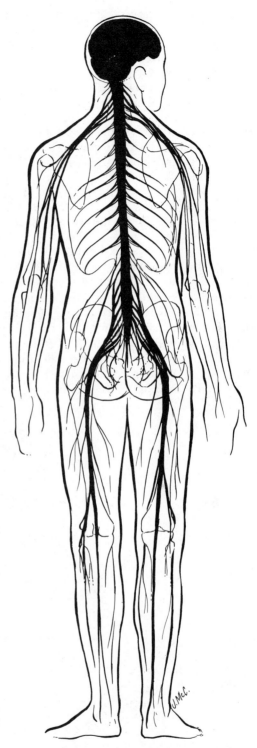

Figure 14-1. Diagram illustrating the brain, the spinal cord and the spinal nerves.

drite called a *synapse*. Impulses pass only from axon to dendrite or to cell body across the synapse. Hence, if a nerve impulse is blocked, the blocking takes place at the synapse. The sensory neurons begin to bring information to the brain by means of *receptors* (end organs which are the initial receivers of sensations from outside the body). The receptors are usually classified as follows: the *exteroceptors*, which are concerned with touch, cutaneous pain, heat, cold, smell, vision, and hearing; the *proprioceptors* which carry sensations of position and balance and of muscle sense; and the *interoceptors* which respond to changes in the viscera, such as visceral pain, hunger, and thirst.

Once the receptors have picked up the impulse the sensation is carried to the central nervous system via the fibers of the sensory neurons; it is sent through the connecting neurons through complex pathways for interpretation and decision for action. If a corresponding action is required, further impulse is sent via the fibers of the motor neurons to bring about the proper response. (The structures which carry out the activity are called

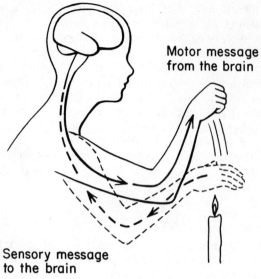

**Motor message from the brain**

**Sensory message to the brain**

Figure 14-3. Sensory and motor processes involved when the hand is held over a flame.

effectors, either somatic-voluntary or visceral-involuntary.) For example, the initial sting of a mosquito bite is made known to the brain by a sensory neuron; the brain interprets the sensation for what it is; the con-

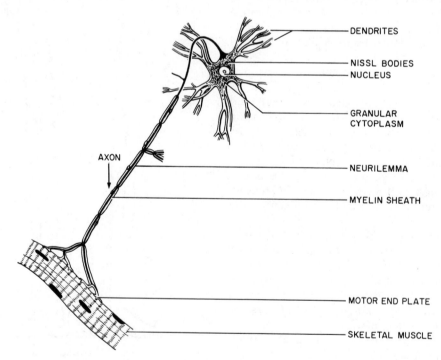

DENDRITES

NISSL BODIES
NUCLEUS

GRANULAR CYTOPLASM

AXON

NEURILEMMA

MYELIN SHEATH

MOTOR END PLATE

SKELETAL MUSCLE

Figure 14-2. Diagram of a typical neuron showing the motor end plate, the point of contact between the axon and the skeletal muscle.

necting neurons carry the message via the proper paths to the motor neuron; the brain sends the order to slap the insect away, by means of a motor neuron to the appropriate muscles. (A similar illustration is shown in Fig. 14-3.)

The nerve fibers dispatch messages to the brain by electricity manufactured by and in the neurons. Recordings of the impulses have been made, and the electrical impulses, no matter what the sensation or its source, all sound the same. However, the various areas of the brain decipher the signals and relay them to the proper channels.

The axons of the nerve fibers in the peripheral nervous system are covered by a thin, protective sheath called the *neurilemma.* Its most important function is to aid in the regeneration of nerve fibers. Regeneration of nerve fibers is very slow, so the symptoms of nerve injury may persist for a long time. Certain nerve fibers are also covered by the *myelin sheath,* which is under the neurilemma when both are present. Those fibers which are covered with myelin conduct impulses faster than others; thus, myelin is thought to have an effect upon the speed of impulse transmission.

Nerve tissue is very fragile and easily subject to injury. For this reason, the central nervous system has top priority on the oxygen supply from the circulatory system. It is also well protected by the skull bones and by the surrounding structures of the vertebral column. If the nerve fiber is injured, eventually it may repair itself. If the neuron itself is destroyed, it will never be replaced. When the nucleus of a neuron is destroyed, it is lost forever.

There are many possible pathways that messages can take. It is amazing that they take the quickest route (the body is very thrifty in its use of body products and its automatic activities) and that the same kind of messages tend to follow the same paths every time. Motions that you repeat become more or less automatic habits, which are patterns that you have built up by using the same nerve pathways over and over.

There are some actions which are considered *reflex acts.* For example, you close or blink your eyes to protect them from danger. You do this before any conscious stimulus

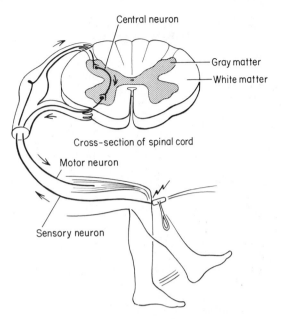

Figure 14-4. Diagrammatic section of the lower part of the spinal cord to illustrate a simple reflex arc as elicited by the knee jerk. When the tendon of the patella (knee cap) is tapped, the receptors in the tendon are stimulated. The impulses pass over the sensory neurons to the spinal cord where they are transmitted over the central neurons to the motor neurons leaving the cord. The effectors of the motor neurons are in the anterior thigh muscles which, when stimulated, contract and extend the leg.

reaches the brain; the stimulus enters and leaves at the level of the spinal cord. It is a simple entrance of the stimulus through the sensory nerve, across the connecting neurons in the spinal cord and out via the motor neuron. The simplest "reflex arc" in man is the knee jerk triggered by a light blow below the knee (see Fig. 14-4).

Although the nervous system is complicated, you are relieved of some of the responsibility in the operations of your body. You choose and direct the actions that make life pleasant; you can protect yourself from dangers; you can think and feel. However, one part of your nervous system works on its own and requires no planning from you. It directs such things as the digestion of food and circulation of the blood.

Thus, the nervous system has 2 sections— one you control, and the other, though closely related, is automatic and is called the *autonomic* nervous system.

## AUTONOMIC NERVOUS SYSTEM (INVOLUNTARY)

The autonomic nervous system has 2 divisions: the *sympathetic* and the *parasympathetic* which regulate the action of the glands, the smooth muscles, and the heart. These structures receive their stimuli from both divisions; however, their effects are opposite. For example, the sympathetic nerves speed up the heart rate, constrict the blood vessels, and dilate the pupil of the eye; the parasympathetic nerves constrict the pupil of the eye, dilate the blood vessels, and slow the heart rate.

Knowledge of the actions of the autonomic nervous system is important in giving medications which affect one or the other division.

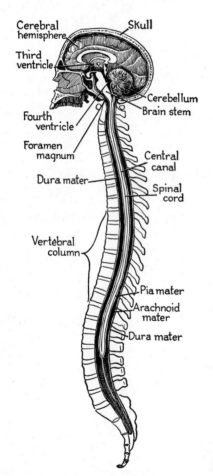

Figure 14-5. The central nervous system. (Baillif and Kimmel: Structure and Function of the Human Body. Philadelphia, Lippincott)

To illustrate, atropine, a drug used in examining the eye, inhibits (slows down) the action of the parasympathetic division and thus causes a dilation of the pupil of the eye. On the other hand, pilocarpine, which is used in certain disease conditions, stimulates the parasympathetic division and causes the pupil to become more constricted.

The close relationship between the two parts of the nervous system (that controlled consciously and the autonomic system) can be illustrated if you visualize a large, juicy, sizzling steak. If it is an idea which stimulates your appetite, your mouth will water—saliva and other digestive juices will flow. The flow of digestive juices is a function controlled by the autonomic nervous system, which works automatically. However, you know that control of the appetite by the individual is a conscious function, and you can decide not to supply food for the juices to digest, if you so wish.

## THE CENTRAL NERVOUS SYSTEM

### The Brain

As stated previously, the central nervous system is made up of the brain and the spinal cord (*neuraxis*). The human brain is the center for thought. It weighs about 3 pounds, has 3 divisions, and is located within the skull. The largest division of the brain is the *cerebrum*, which fills the upper part of the cranium. The cerebrum is divided into halves (*hemispheres*), one on either side of the cranium. The outside of the cerebrum (the *cerebral cortex*) is made of soft grayish matter that is mostly nerve cells. Underneath this is the white matter, which contains the nerve fibers that connect with the cells. (The myelin sheaths which cover the nerve fibers give the white appearance.) The cerebral cortex is wrinkled and folded upon itself many times. This gives a greater surface in a small area. It is divided into 4 *lobes* which are named from the overlying cranial bones—frontal, parietal, temporal, and occipital. A number of special centers in the cerebrum enable it to carry out the work of associating impressions and information, which becomes our knowledge. After comparing and combining knowledge, we think and arrive at judgments, the highest function of the human mind. While it has been suggested that our mental faculties of memory, reasoning, and intelligence involve the cerebral cortex, exactly where or how these processes are performed is not known.

Other centers in the cerebrum are related to hearing, seeing, moving, speaking, and other activities. There are duplicate motor control centers in the right hemisphere and the left hemisphere of the brain. The right center controls the muscles on the left side of the body, and the left center controls the muscles on the right side of the body. This is a result of *decussation* (crossing) of the nerve tracts within the brain. Some of the functional areas of the cerebrum are shown in Figure 14-6.

Directly beneath the cerebral hemispheres and covered by them are 2 centers called the *thalamus* and the *hypothalamus*. The thalamus is a relay station for nerve stimuli. It receives impulses from every part of the body and relays them to appropriate parts of the cortex. Investigations indicate that the thalamus may contain a center for interpreting whether or not actions or sensations give us pleasure.

The hypothalamus contains centers that control many of the autonomic functions, as well as heat regulation and food and water metabolism. Some authorities think that the center for appetite control as well as our "waking center" is located here. The hypothalamus also is involved in the expression of certain emotions and is closely associated with pituitary activities.

The *cerebellum* is the second largest part of the brain and is concerned with muscle tone, coordination, and equilibrium; it coordinates the action of voluntary muscles. It helps keep you balanced when you walk, makes your movements graceful, and affects your skill in sports and other muscle activities.

The brain stem includes the *midbrain,* the *pons,* and the *medulla.* The midbrain is located at the very top of the brain stem and functions as an important reflex center. It is believed that the center for mood and behavior control is located in the midbrain. The word "pons" means "bridge," and reflects the fact that the pons has nerve tracts within it which carry messages between the cerebrum and the medulla.

The medulla lies just below the pons and

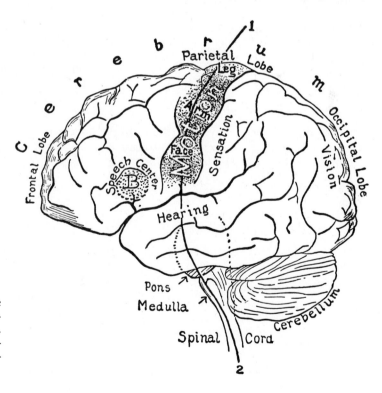

Figure 14-6. Side view of the brain, showing some of the functional areas of the cerebrum. (Emerson and Bragdon: Essentials of Medicine, ed. 17. Philadelphia, Lippincott)

rests on the floor of the skull. It is continuous with, but not a part of, the spinal cord. Messages go to and from the cerebrum through the medulla. It also contains centers for many vital body functions: the rate of the heart beat, the constriction of blood vessels, control of respiration, and control of swallowing are all part of its activities. Other activities are concerned with such reflexes as coughing, sneezing, and laughing.

## The Spinal Cord

The *spinal cord* is a long mass of nerve cells and fibers extending through a central canal from the medulla to the approximate level of the first or the second lumbar vertebra. It is well protected from shocks and injuries by its position within the vertebral column. The spinal cord has 2 main purposes: it acts as a conductor of impulses to and from the brain and is a reflex center. The reflex centers in the cord receive and send out messages through the nerve fibers. They act as substations for messages and relieve the brain of routine work. Some nerve fibers in the cord are sensory, that is, they carry messages to the brain, while other nerve tracts are motor— they carry messages away from the brain. The nerve fibers of the spinal cord do not regenerate after an injury. The peripheral spinal nerve fibers originate within the brain and spinal cord.

## The Meninges

The brain and the spinal cord (the central nervous system) are covered with 3 protective membranes called the *meninges*. The outer one (*dura mater*) is a tough, fibrous covering which adheres to the bones of the skull. The inner layer (*pia mater*) lies closely over the brain and the spinal cord. It is a thin vascular layer containing many blood vessels which bring oxygen to nourish the nervous tissue. The middle layer is a delicate weblike tissue called the *arachnoid*. The space between the middle layer and the inner layer (*subarachnoid space*) is filled with *cerebrospinal fluid*. Cerebrospinal fluid is produced constantly, mainly by filtration from the blood in the capillaries of the brain, but it is also produced in the brain in spaces called ventricles. This liquid circulates around the brain and the spinal cord, maintaining an even pressure and acting as a cushion or shock absorber for these delicate structures. In order for the amount to remain constant it is continuously absorbed into the blood vessels in the brain.

## THE PERIPHERAL NERVOUS SYSTEM

The peripheral nervous system is made up of 2 nerve groups: the cranial nerves and the spinal nerves. There are 12 pairs of cranial nerves which attach directly to the brain. Most of them carry impulses to and from the brain and various structures about the head (the sensory organs, the organs of swallowing and speech, the facial muscles, etc.). However, other cranial nerves act on the organs of the thorax and the abdomen.

The spinal nerves attach to the spinal cord. They carry such impulses as temperature, touch, pain, muscle tone, and balance. They also transport motor impulses to the skeletal muscles.

# 15

# The Circulatory System

---

## BEHAVIORAL OBJECTIVES

*The student successfully attaining the goals of this chapter will be able to:*

- *list the functions of the circulatory system and discuss how this system is related to the activities of all other systems in the body.*
- *identify the components of plasma and list the functions of each component.*
- *describe the red blood cell and its functions.*
- *list the characteristics common to all white blood cells; identify the types of white blood cells and describe the functions of each.*
- *state the most important function of platelets.*
- *define blood pressure; locate several pressure points in the body.*
- *identify the 4 blood groups and state which is the universal donor.*
- *discuss the mechanism of blood clotting; identify a situation in which clotting is helpful and one in which clotting is dangerous.*
- *diagram the heart, showing the 4 chambers and the valves, and identify the pericardium, endocardium, and myocardium.*
- *trace the circulation of blood through the heart and lungs; identify at which points the blood is oxygenated; discuss the oxygen supply to the heart muscle itself.*
- *on a chart, trace the route of circulation of blood throughout the body, indicating by name the major blood vessels.*
- *compare pulmonary circulation to general circulation; identify the phase during which the blood is oxygenated.*
- *differentiate between arteries, arterioles, veins, venules, and capillaries, with regard to the structure and function of each.*
- *discuss the portal circulation and its role in digestion and elimination, as well as its value in maintaining the general well-being of the body.*
- *describe the lymphatic circulation and state its chief function.*
- *name at least 3 functions of the spleen.*

---

The circulatory system is a meticulously organized plan for communication of each of the cells with various other parts of the body. Even though a cell may be located in the tip of your toe or at the end of your fingers, it gets oxygen from the lungs and food from the intestines and sends its wastes back to the kidneys. The circulatory system is composed of the blood, the heart, and the tubes or vessels (arteries, veins, capillaries) which are the routes over which the blood travels. The blood carries the necessary products to the cells and carries away wastes; the heart provides the force to pump the blood through the body; and the arteries, veins, and capillaries contain and transport the blood.

## FUNCTIONS

The circulatory system has many functions, some of which you already know. The following is a list of its more important duties:

It carries oxygen from the lungs to the cells.

It carries carbon dioxide from the cells to the lungs.

Food is picked up (absorbed) from the small intestine and brought to the cells by the blood.

Certain waste products of the work of the cells are transported by the blood to the kidneys to be eliminated from the body.

The products of the endocrine glands, the hormones, are carried to their destinations by the blood.

The blood and the blood vessels contribute to the regulation of body temperature. If the body needs to become cooler, surface blood vessels dilate, giving off heat. For example, the flushed face which occurs after strenuous exercises is a result of the dilation of the facial blood vessels. If the body needs to conserve heat or energy, the surface blood vessels constrict, thereby reducing heat loss. Heat from muscle activity is also transported in the blood.

The blood assists in maintaining the acid-base balance of the body. There are alkaline products in the blood which constantly work against (buffer) the acids formed by metabolism within the body; the acids also guard against excessive alkalinity by buffering the alkaline (base) substances in the blood.

The circulatory system helps to maintain the fluid balance of the body. As was stated in Chapter 11, within and surrounding all cells is body fluid. In a healthy person this fluid remains fairly constant in amount. Although we take in extra liquid every day, the body eliminates an approximately equal quantity through the evaporation of perspiration and through the kidneys. The circulatory system serves as a transport medium for this fluid.

The circulatory system defends the body against disease by means of its white cells. It also produces antibodies and antitoxins, important in immunity and disease control.

## THE BLOOD

If you wish to consider the marvels of your body, the blood alone can be a source of wonder. The blood is a liquid within the body, yet it can coagulate quickly to form a solid clot, although under normal conditions coagulation does not take place within the body.

It is a *liquid tissue,* because the fluid portion, called plasma, contains many cells and other substances. Within this watery intercellular substance are the formed elements, consisting of white blood cells, red blood cells, and platelets. The average adult body contains about 12 pints of blood.

### Blood Plasma

Plasma is the liquid portion of the circulating blood. It is composed of 90 per cent water, a combination of various salts, and numerous other substances associated with the body processes.

It is interesting to note that scientists speculate that the concentration of salts in the blood is similar to the salt content of the sea when life on earth first began. This is one of the theories which led them to believe that life originally arose in the warm currents of the sea.

The salts contained in the plasma are sodium, calcium, potassium, and magnesium, as well as the ions of other elements in the forms of bicarbonates, sulfates, chlorides, and phosphates. These salts are absorbed by the plasma from the foods we eat and are used by the cells. The maintenance of these salts within the plasma (in special quantities to act as neutralizers or buffers to each other) controls the chemical and acid-base balance of the blood, as well as contributing to the chemical and fluid balance of the entire body.

The plasma also contains antibodies, food elements (carbohydrates, fats, proteins), nitrogenous waste products such as urea and ammonium salts, and small amounts of gases such as oxygen, carbon dioxide, and nitrogen. Hormones are carried in the plasma, as are the chemicals involved in the process of the clotting of blood. Some of the plasma proteins are albumin, a main constituent of cells, serum globulins, which are related to disease protection, and fibrinogen, one of the clotting substances.

### Red Blood Cells

Although the red blood cells (*erythrocytes*) give blood its red color, they appear under the microscope as faintly pink disks, thinner in the center than at the edges. These cells are different from other cells of the body in that they have no nucleus when they are mature. There are so many red blood cells that the blood appears to be packed solid with them, but they are so tiny that approximately 3,000 of them could be placed side by side within the distance of 1 inch. There are about 25 trillion red blood cells in the whole body. They are the most numerous of the blood cells.

The erythrocytes get their color from an iron compound which they contain called *hemoglobin* (heme: iron; globin: protein). As the blood passes through the lungs, the iron in the hemoglobin picks up oxygen in a loose chemical combination and carries it to the body cells. When hemoglobin is saturated with oxygen, it is bright red. As the erythrocytes circulate through the capillaries in the tissues, the hemoglobin gives its oxygen to the cells and picks up their carbon dioxide. Carbon dioxide makes the blood darker red.

Often a count of the blood cells is made to determine if the body is producing the normal amount. The average number of the red blood cells (R.B.C.) is 4½ to 5 million per cubic millimeter, the amount of blood in a tiny drop. An abnormally high red cell count is called *polycythemia*; an abnormally low count (or low hemoglobin content) is called *anemia*. It is believed that erythrocytes survive for about 3 to 4 months. They are made in the red marrow of the bones at the rate of about 1 million per second. They wear out and are destroyed at the same rate in the liver and the spleen, an organ of the lymphatic system sometimes referred to as the "graveyard of the red blood cells" (see p. 124).

## White Blood Cells

White blood cells (*leukocytes*) are colorless cells that defend the body against disease organisms, toxins, or irritants. They have a nucleus and are larger and far fewer in number than the red cells. The normal white blood count (W.B.C.) is 5,000 to 10,000 per cubic millimeter of blood.

There are 2 subgroups of white cells: the granular and the nongranular leukocytes. The 3 types of granular leukocytes—baso-

phils, eosinophils, and neutrophils—are characterized by a speckled or grainy cytoplasm. They are produced in the bone marrow and function by surrounding and dissolving the body's invaders. The nongranular leukocytes, classified as lymphocytes and monocytes, are produced in lymphatic tissue, such as lymph nodes and the spleen, and have relatively clear cytoplasm. Their exact function is unknown, but some believe that they have a relationship to antibody formation in producing immunity to certain diseases.

Unlike the red blood cells which remain inside the blood vessels to do their work, the leukocytes leave the blood stream to travel to the affected site. They can move by changing shape, a process known as *ameboid* movement. They push or squeeze themselves through the capillary wall and rush to the threatened spot. They increase in number, engulf and devour the invaders (*phagocytosis*), and assist in repairing the damaged tissues. Sometimes they die in this activity and collect with bacteria to form *pus*. The average life of a white blood cell is 9 days.

Since in some diseases the white blood cells increase in number (*leukocytosis*) or decrease in number (*leukopenia*), a white cell count is a valuable aid to diagnosis. A drop of blood is viewed under the microscope, and the number of white cells is estimated. The normal white count of 5,000 to 10,000 may increase to 25,000 or higher when infection is present. In some diseases, the relative proportion of the kinds of white blood cells may vary, and therefore a differential count is made, in which the number of granular leukocytes is compared with the number of nongranular leukocytes. This count gives further diagnostic clues to the doctor. The presence of immature white blood cells may indicate *leukemia*.

## Platelets

The blood platelets, sometimes called *thrombocytes*, are smaller than erythrocytes and leukocytes, with a life span of about 4 days. They are thought to be manufactured in the red bone marrow, as are the other formed elements of the blood. There is a wide variance in the normal count, but 250,000 to 500,000 per cubic millimeter of blood could be considered as being normal. They are essential in the clotting of blood. Figure 15-1 diagrammatically illustrates the red and the white blood cells and the platelets.

## Blood Pressure

The blood in the arteries always exerts some pressure against their walls, as water does when running through a garden hose. When the heart muscle contracts to pump the blood during the *active phase* (also known as *systole*), the force increases the pressure against the blood vessel walls, as it would against the garden hose if you had the water pressure up to full. When the heart relaxes during the *resting phase* (also known as *diastole*), the pressure decreases as it would if the water pressure were turned down; then the water would trickle through the hose. When you take a person's blood pressure, both pressures are recorded with the figure of the higher or systolic pressure reading written over the lower or diastolic pressure reading. For example, a nor-mal blood pressure (B.P.) reading for some individuals might be $\frac{120}{80}$.

Children normally have lower blood pressures than adults. Some people have lower than average blood pressure (*hypotension*), but unless this is caused by disease, their prospects for a long life are good. The statement that your blood pressure should be "your age plus 100" is not true.

Blood pressure varies from time to time, depending on activity, emotion, and strain. Such changes are normal and are only temporary.

There are many factors other than the force of the pumping of the heart which are related to the control of blood pressure, such as the muscles in the capillary walls, kidney function, and hormones. The arteries naturally become less elastic with age, but this condition begins much earlier in some people than in others. The reasons for this are not known completely, but scientists believe that diet, physical and emotional stress, and heredity are responsible. (Blood pressure and the method of measuring it will be described in more detail in Chapter 27.)

## The Clotting of Blood (Coagulation)

The blood protects the body from losing vital plasma fluid and blood cells by sealing off broken blood vessels through a process of clotting called *coagulation*. Otherwise, we would not survive minor cuts and wounds. The process in clot formation is not a simple one but is the result of a number of activities within the blood, some of which are not totally understood. Calcium must be present for clotting to occur. When the tissue is injured, the platelets break down and cause the release of a chemical, *thromboplastin*. This interacts with *prothrombin*, a protein substance in the blood, which further reacts with *fibrinogen* in the blood to form threads of fibrin. The threads of *fibrin* form a net which entraps the cells which build up to form the clot. The clot acts like a plug in a hole and tends to draw the injured edges together. As the clot shrinks, a clear yellow liquid called *serum* is squeezed out. Serum is much like plasma except that fibrinogen and other clotting elements needed in the coagulation process are

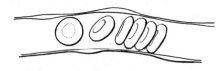

RED BLOOD CELLS (in capillary)

Basophil    Eosinophil    Neutrophil

GRANULAR LEUKOCYTES

NONGRANULAR LEUKOCYTES

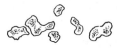

BLOOD PLATELETS

Figure 15-1.

no longer present. Coagulation is a complicated mechanism and will not take place if any of the necessary elements are missing.

A clot that forms within a blood vessel and remains at the formation site is called a *thrombus*. One that moves from its original site is called an *embolus*.

## Hemorrhage and Blood Types

Literally, the definition of hemorrhage is the escape of blood from blood vessels, but we usually think of a hemorrhage as the loss of a considerable amount of blood. A cut or torn blood vessel allows blood to escape. As soon as a clot forms, the bleeding stops. Therefore, once a blood vessel is broken, the clotting of the blood becomes very important. Severe hemorrhage is serious because the body loses so much fluid and oxygen-carrying red blood cells that death can result. The strength of the force behind the flow of blood (as in an injured artery), the size of the wound, the volume of the blood lost, or a deficiency in any of the coagulant substances can prevent clotting.

Severe hemorrhage is treated by replacing the blood lost with blood from another person. This replacement of blood is called *transfusion* (see Chapter 47). Blood usually falls into 1 of 4 main groups: A, B, AB, and O. Blood group O can be given safely to any other group and is known as the *universal donor*. About 40 per cent of all people have Type O blood. Likewise, group AB can receive the blood of any other group and is known as the *universal recipient*. Plasma transfusion is almost always safe and is quicker than a transfusion of whole blood; but blood plasma does not contain red and white blood cells, so a doctor may prefer that whole blood be used. Blood may also be given in the form of packed cells. This is a blood transfusion in which much of the plasma has been removed, so the patient receives more blood cells with less volume. Packed cells are less likely to overload the circulation or to overhydrate the patient. In this way a larger amount of blood can be given in a shorter time.

There are other ways that plasma and its elements can be used to help patients. Plasma is sometimes used in a paste form to treat external injuries, such as burns. In addition gamma globulin or serum globulin can be injected to treat an infection.

Some people have mistaken notions about blood and blood transfusions. It is important to remember that, except for the usual blood type variations, there is no difference in the blood of healthy persons of different races. Blood does not carry or transmit mental, emotional, or racial characteristics. However, some diseases, such as serum hepatitis, can be transmitted by transfusion.

Since the value of transfusions has proved itself beyond doubt, almost every community has established blood banks to cover emergency needs. The American National Red Cross Blood Donor Service is known all over the world and serves all communities.

## The Rh Factor

The Rh factor is another red-cell protein which is inherited just as blood type is inherited. About 85 per cent of white Americans have this factor in their blood and are said to be Rh positive (expressed Rh+). Those who do not have this factor in their blood are said to be Rh negative (Rh−). The percentage of Rh-negative people is lower in some races than in others. For instance, only 7 per cent of the Negro race and 1 per cent of Oriental peoples are found to be Rh negative. The Rh factor and its effects upon pregnancy are discussed in Chapter 36.

## THE HEART

### The Heart Chambers

The heart is a strong muscular pump, about the size of a doubled-up fist, which lies in the lower left central part of the chest cavity. Its shape is that of an irregular and slightly flattened cone. The base of the cone is directed upward and to the right. The apex (the pointed part) is directed downward, anteriorly and to the left. It is hollow and made of thick strong muscles that contract to force the blood into the arteries. The heart is covered by a thin sac, the *pericardium*. The membrane that lines the heart and the substance of the valves is called the *endocardium*. Its cells resemble squamous epithelium. The muscular part (thickest layer) of the heart is known as the *myocardium*. The heart itself is supplied by the coronary arteries. A blockage of these arteries causes myocardial insufficiency or infarction.

The heart is divided into 4 chambers. The 2 upper chambers, the *atria* (auricles), receive the blood; and the 2 lower chambers, the *ventricles,* pump the blood out. Between the atria and the ventricles are "one-way" flaps of tissue (valves), whose purpose is to prevent the backflow of the blood. The valve between the right atria and the right ventricle is called the *tricuspid* valve, because it is formed of 3 flaps of tissue. The valve between the left auricle and the left ventricle is called the *mitral* or bicuspid valve, since it has only 2 flaps of tissue.

The heart does its work by opening and closing the hollows within it at an average rate of 72 times per minute, or 100,000 times a day. The blood is literally squeezed out of the heart's chambers. This squeezing or pumping drives 5 to 6 quarts of blood per minute through thousands of feet of blood vessels in the body. Each pumping is called the heart beat.

The heart is divided into a right and a left half by a complete muscular wall, the *septum*. The 2 sides are completely separated with no communication from the right to the left side. Each side is a separate pump.

When the heart is resting between beats, the atria fill. When the heart contracts, the atria squeeze down to force the blood through the mitral and the tricuspid valves into the ventricles below. The wave of contraction continues to the ventricles and forces the blood from the left ventricle through the aortic valve into the *aorta* (the large artery leading to all body parts) and from the right ventricle through the pulmonary semilunar valve into the pulmonary artery leading to the lungs. After blood is squeezed from the atria into the ventricles, the mitral and tricuspid valves close to prevent the blood from flowing back into the atria when the ventricles contract. The semilunar valves close after the blood has been forced into the aorta and pulmonary artery. Because the left ventricle must contract with sufficient force to send the blood to the entire body, its muscle walls are thicker than the other chambers of the heart. The contraction which pumps the blood from the heart is called the systole, and the period when the heart is relaxed or at rest is called the diastole.

Blood that has delivered its food materials and oxygen to the cells and has accumulated waste products from the body flows into the right atrium, goes down into the right ventricle, and is pumped through the pulmonary artery to the lungs to get rid of the carbon dioxide and to pick up a supply of oxygen. This phase is designated as *pulmonary circulation*. The blood has now exchanged its carbon dioxide waste for oxygen; it returns to the heart at the left atrium, enters the left ventricle, and is pumped into the aorta, carrying the precious oxygen supply to all the body cells. The circulation of oxygenated blood from the left ventricle to the body cells and back again to the right atrium is designated as *general circulation*. The oxygenated blood

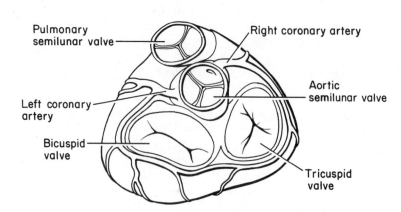

Pulmonary semilunar valve

Right coronary artery

Aortic semilunar valve

Left coronary artery

Bicuspid valve

Tricuspid valve

Figure 15-2. Valves of the heart, viewed from above toward the ventricles. The atria and the greater part of the aorta and the pulmonary artery have been removed. Note the flaps of tissue which form the tricuspid and the bicuspid valves. Each semilunar valve is formed by a set of 3 pocketlike flaps. The right and the left coronary arteries which branch from the aorta to supply the heart muscle with oxygen and nourishment are also shown.

on the left is separated from that carrying carbon dioxide on the right by the solid wall of the septum.

## The Nerve Supply of the Heart

The nerve supply of the heart is a part of the autonomic nervous system. It is a complex distribution possessing both accelerating and braking devices. This results in an accurate and delicate control of the rate. The vagus nerve fibers are the "brakes." They serve to slow the heart and reduce the force of its beats. The fibers of the accelerator nerve have the opposite action to that of the vagus; they increase the rate and the force of the heart beat. The result of both actions is a delicate balance. If the action of the vagus is reduced and the accelerator action is increased, then faster than normal acceleration of the heart is brought about.

There are special bundles of unique tissue in the heart—a combination of muscle and nerve tissue. The first of these bundles is embedded in the wall of the right atrium at the junction of the superior and the inferior venae cavae. It is called the *sinoatrial node* or the S.A. node and is the "pacemaker" of the heart. The other bundle is found in the lower part of the septum between the atria. This bundle is the *atrioventricular* or A.V. node. Originating from this area is a bundle of fibers, the *bundle of His.* It is called the coordinator.

It is in the S.A. node that the heart beat originates. It sets the pace, and the rest of the heart follows its bidding. The swift message is sent out through the muscular tissue of the atrium, which contracts; then the A.V. node picks up the message like a receiving station and relays the message on to the muscle fibers of the ventricle which contracts in turn. The heart then rests for a short period between beats. Failure of this electrical impulse results in *heart block.*

## THE BLOOD VESSELS

### The Arteries

The blood is carried through the body in a set of tubes or blood vessels: *arteries, capillaries,* and *veins.* The arteries carry blood

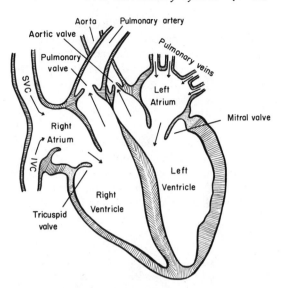

Figure 15-3. These points will help in remembering how the heart and the circulation operate: (1) The auricles (atria) are receiving stations only. (2) The ventricles are dispensing stations only. (3) The right side of the heart contains only "blue" (deoxygenated) blood. (4) The left side of the heart contains only "red" (oxygenated) blood. (5) all arteries carry blood **away from** the heart. (6) All veins carry blood **to** the heart. (7) All arteries carry red blood (**except the pulmonary artery**). (8) All veins carry "blue" (deoxygenated) blood (**except the 4 pulmonary veins**). (After Kimber, Gray, Stackpole and Leavell: Anatomy and Physiology, New York, Macmillan)

away from the heart, the capillaries serve as "in-between" channels, and the veins carry blood to the heart. As the blood leaves the left ventricle of the heart, it surges into the largest artery of the body, the aorta, which is divided into the ascending aorta, the aortic arch, the thoracic aorta, and the abdominal aorta. The arteries have in their walls smooth muscle cells, one layer of which runs lengthwise and another layer of which is circular. The circular band of muscle tends to protect a person when an artery is severed. If the artery is just nicked so that the circular band cannot contract, hemorrhage is much more likely to occur. As in all muscle cells of the body, the contraction of these cells (and therefore the size of the opening in the arteries) is controlled by the nervous system. The arterial walls are strong and elastic and expand as the heart pumps the blood out to be carried *away* to the cells of the body. (This is the *pulse*.) The pulse can be felt at places where the arteries are close to the surface; the wrist (radial), the neck (carotid), the back of the knee (popliteal), the groin (femoral), the ankle (tibial), and the temple. *Blood pressure* is usually taken over the brachial artery in the arm.

From the aorta the arteries branch into smaller and smaller vessels, just as do the branches from the central trunk of a tree (see Fig. 15-4). The smallest of the arteries are called arterioles. From the arterioles the blood flows into the smallest blood vessels of all, the capillaries.

## The Capillaries

The *capillaries* are so small that the minute red blood cells must pass through them in single file. Their walls are 1-cell layer thick. The capillaries must be plentiful, since it is through their walls that the oxygen and the food finally are supplied to the individual cells. (One estimate of the total length of the blood vessels of the body is 70,000 miles, most

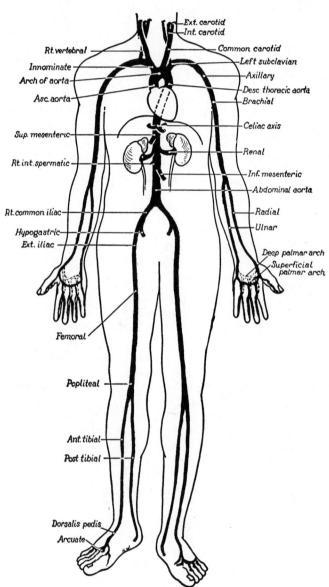

Figure 15-4. The main arteries of the body. (Anthony, C. P.: Textbook of Anatomy and Physiology, St. Louis, Mosby)

of which is made up of capillaries.) The blood flow into each capillary from the arteriole is guarded by a sphincter muscle. This slow single file passage of the blood through the capillaries allows time for the oxygen, the food, and the white blood cells to leave the blood vessels and enter the tissues. Part of the plasma of the blood, the lymph, which is the intercellular fluid that surrounds all body cells, also seeps through the capillary walls, as do the salts and other materials necessary for the health of the tissues. It is ruptured capillaries which result in the bruise ("black-and-blue" mark).

## The Veins

At the same time that materials are being delivered to the cells, waste products are being picked up from the cells by the capillaries. The blood starts traveling back to the heart through the venules, the smallest veins. The branches of the veins grow larger and fewer as they near the heart (see Fig. 15-5), until

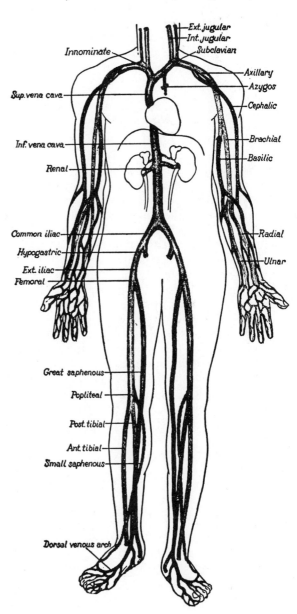

Figure 15-5. The main veins of the body. (Anthony, C. P.: Textbook of Anatomy and Physiology, St. Louis, Mosby)

finally the blood reaches the superior and the inferior venae cavae, the 2 large veins that deliver the blood to the right atrium. (This blood is dark red because the oxygen has been replaced with carbon dioxide waste.)

The blood in the veins has lost the force from the contractions of the heart during the slow journey through the capillaries, therefore, veins do not pulsate. Our bodies provide an extra push for venous blood because the veins are located between skeletal muscles. The contractions of the skeletal muscle squeeze the blood forward. In addition to this help, a backflow of blood in the veins is prevented by a system of valves that permits the blood to flow in one direction only. These valves contribute to the efficient venous flow from the extremities.

## The Circulatory Route

The route of the blood through the entire system is as follows: The blood leaves the left ventricle of the heart through the largest artery, the aorta. It travels through smaller and smaller arterial branches to all parts of the body. From the smallest arteries, the arterioles, the blood enters the capillaries where the oxygen and the food is exchanged for waste products. The blood then begins its journey back to the heart from the capillaries to the venules, the larger veins, and then the inferior and the superior venae cavae to the right atrium (see Fig. 15-6). The route thus far is the general (*systemic*) circulation. The blood now begins the pulmonary circulation to the lungs to rid itself of the carbon dioxide.

From the right atrium the blood flows into the right ventricle; from the right ventricle the blood is pumped into the pulmonary artery, the only artery in the body which car-

ries unoxygenated blood. The blood goes to the capillaries in the lungs where the carbon dioxide, carried in the hemoglobin, is exchanged for the oxygen. The blood in the lung capillaries is collected by small veins that combine eventually into the 4 pulmonary veins, which pour the oxygenated blood into the left atrium. From here the blood is pumped into the left ventricle, which contracts, forcing the oxygenated blood into the aorta and back into the general circulation again.

## The Coronary Arteries

The heart muscle itself must have its own supply of blood, since none of the blood which flows through the heart chambers is absorbed for use by heart tissue itself. The first branches from the aorta are those which return to supply the heart tissue with oxygen and nourishment. They are called the *coronary* arteries because they fit over the heart like a crown (corona). A narrowing of these arteries or an obstruction from a blood clot interferes with the heart's own blood supply, resulting in coronary artery disease (see Fig. 15-2).

## The Portal System

Another area of the circulatory system is called the portal system. The veins from the stomach, the intestine, the spleen, and the pancreas all empty into a common vessel, the *portal vein,* which leads to the liver. The liver extracts food materials from this blood for storage and chemical modification (including removal of toxins). Then the blood leaves the liver by way of the *hepatic veins* and empties into the inferior vena cava. It is through

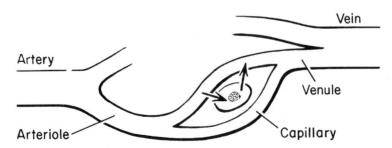

Figure 15-6. Diagrammatic view of an artery, arteriole, capillary, venule and vein. The arrows indicate the passage of oxygen and food from the capillary through the tissue fluid, into the body cell, and in reverse, from the body cell through the tissue fluid, into the capillary.

the portal system that the digested foods from the intestine reach the general circulation for distribution to the tissues.

## THE LYMPHATIC SYSTEM

The body cells normally are bathed in tissue fluid. Some of this fluid drains into the blood capillaries which go directly to the veins. However, there is another group of vessels called the *lymphatic system* which also drains this fluid. The first group of these vessels is a network of tiny lymph capillaries in which excess fluid and certain other waste products collect to form the thin watery liquid known as *lymph*.

Since lymph originally is derived from plasma, its composition is much the same, except that it is lower in protein content. Lymph that is drained from the intestinal area may contain large amounts of fats after a fatty meal, which gives this lymph a milky

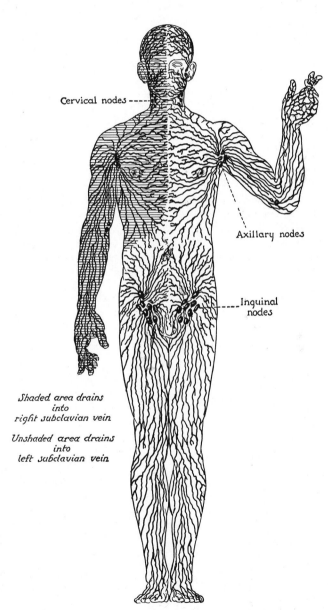

Cervical nodes

Axillary nodes

Inguinal nodes

*Shaded area drains into right subclavian vein*

*Unshaded area drains into left subclavian vein*

Figure 15-7. Diagram of the superficial lymphatic vessels and the cervical, axillary and inguinal nodes. (Greisheimer, E. M., and Wiedeman, M. P.: Physiology and Anatomy, ed. 9. Philadelphia, Lippincott, 1972)

white appearance. The lymph capillaries empty into progressively larger vessels that finally end in 2 main channels: the thoracic duct and the right lymphatic duct. These 2 ducts enter the veins at the base of the neck where the lymph mixes with the blood plasma and becomes part of the general circulation. It is through these 2 vessels that the digested fats from the small intestine finally reach the bloodstream. The lacteals in the villi (the small projections in the lining of the intestine) are small lymphatic capillaries which absorb digested fats and eventually empty into the thoracic and the right lymphatic ducts.

Lymph flows very slowly in the lymphatic system of channels. As in the venous system, it is aided by pressure from the contractions of muscles which keep the lymph moving, as well as by valves which prevent the backward flow.

Small bundles of special lymphoid tissue called *lymph nodes,* or lymph glands, are situated at various points in the lymphatic system. Many of these nodes appear in the neck, the groin and the armpits (see Fig. 15-7). Before the lymph reaches the veins, it passes through the nodes traveling through passages lined with cells, which devour bacteria, and filters waste products and other foreign sub-stances. The chief function of the lymphatic system is filtration. Another function of the nodes is to manufacture lymphocytes and monocytes and add them to the lymph for transportation to the blood.

Lymphoid tissue also forms a few body organs, such as the tonsils, the adenoids, and the spleen.

## THE SPLEEN

The *spleen,* another mass of lymphoid tissue, is often classified as part of the lymphatic system. It is a somewhat flattened dark-purple organ about 6 inches long and 3 inches wide located directly below the diaphragm, above the left kidney and behind the stomach. Its functions are somewhat of a mystery, but it is known to act as a blood storage reservoir and to destroy red blood cells, filter out dead blood cells and cancer cells, destroy bacteria, and manufacture one type of white blood cells, the lymphocytes. (In the fetus, it produces red blood cells.) It also produces antibodies which give us an immunity to certain diseases. Although the functions of the spleen are very important, it can be removed without ill effects.

# 16

# The Respiratory System

## BEHAVIORAL OBJECTIVES

*The student successfully attaining the goals of this chapter will be able to:*

- *differentiate between internal and external respiration.*
- *discuss the relationship between the respiratory and the circulatory systems.*
- *define ventilation, inspiration, and expiration.*
- *diagram the upper and lower respiratory tract and trace the pathway of oxygen as it enters the body; describe how oxygen is carried to the cells; describe the removal of carbon dioxide.*
- *discuss the protective mechanisms within the nose, the pharynx, and the larynx.*
- *locate and identify by name the major structures of the respiratory system.*

Your body cells must have oxygen in order to survive. If you are without oxygen for more than a few minutes, the brain cells are injured and the rest of the body slowly begins to fail. The air you take in through your respiratory system (ventilation), is about 20 per cent oxygen and provides a more than ample supply for your needs.

Respiration consists of taking oxygen into the body through the lungs and eliminating the waste product, carbon dioxide, and water. Breathing the air in is called *inspiration* (inhaling), and breathing it out is called *expiration* (exhaling).

There are 2 kinds of respirations: external and internal. The exchange of oxygen for carbon dioxide within the alveoli of the lungs is called external respiration (lung breathing). The trade of oxygen for carbon dioxide within the cells is called internal respiration (cell breathing).

## THE UPPER RESPIRATORY TRACT

### The Nose

The air begins its journey into the body through the nose, which is divided into 2 sides or cavities by the *nasal septum,* a structure consisting of bone and cartilage. The nerve endings in the septum and the nasal passages are responsible for the sense of smell. The nasal cavities are lined with mucous membrane richly supplied with blood vessels which aid in warming and moistening the air before it reaches the lungs. The mucus is sticky and traps within itself dust particles, dirt, and microorganisms from the air. The hairs at the entrance of the nostrils and the tiny hairlike projections (cilia) on the membrane serve as filters to remove some foreign particles which otherwise might be carried to the lungs.

Three small bones, the *turbinates (conchae),* project into the nasal cavity to increase the surface lining of the nose. The *nasolacrimal (tear) ducts* open into the upper nasal cavities, which explains the "runny nose" that occurs when crying. Also communicating with these cavities are the sinuses in the frontal, maxillary, ethmoid, and sphenoid bones. (These were described in Chapter 13.) The lining of the sinuses is continuous with the mucous membrane of the nose and therefore is subject to infection from the nasal cavity.

## The Pharynx (Throat)

Air travels from the nose to the *pharynx* (pronounced *fair' inks*), a tube-shaped passage for both air and food. The section of the pharynx which lies behind the nose is called the *nasopharynx* and contains a mass of lymphoid tissue called the adenoids. The part behind the mouth is the *oropharynx,* commonly called the throat. The tonsils, also masses of lymphoid tissue, are in the back of the oropharynx. Both the tonsils and the adenoids serve as filters for microorganisms and other foreign substances. The *eustachian tubes,* which open into the pharynx, are passageways which connect the middle ear with the pharynx in order to equalize the pressure in the middle ear.

## The Larynx (Voice Box)

From the pharynx, the air passes into the *larynx* (*lair' inks*), a boxlike structure made of cartilages held together by ligaments. It is located in the midline of the neck. (The largest and most prominent cartilage is the thyroid cartilage, commonly known as the "Adam's Apple.")

The pharynx is a dual passageway for air and food, but only air is allowed to pass into the larynx. The entrance to the larynx is guarded by a lid or cover called the *epiglottis.* This cover to the larynx automatically closes when you swallow and therefore prevents food from entering the lower respiratory passages. If, by accident, a portion of food becomes lodged in the larynx, usually it can be dislodged by coughing. If not, the air passage may be blocked and prove to be fatal unless proper emergency treatment is rendered.

Within the larynx are the *vocal cords,* 2 triangular-shaped membranous folds which extend from front to back. As air leaves the lungs and passes over the vocal cords, the cords vibrate and produce sounds. The size of the vocal cords and the size of the larynx vary in different individuals, which causes the difference in voices. A man has a larger larynx and therefore a deeper voice than a woman. Your voice becomes louder and stronger when you rapidly force out a large amount of air.

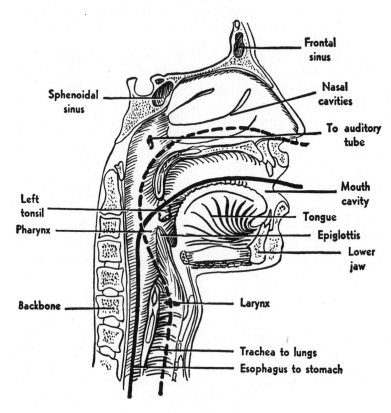

Figure 16-1. Section through the middle plane of head, neck and thorax. The air path is indicated by the dotted line, the food path by the solid line. The 2 paths cross in the lower pharynx.

## The Trachea (Wind Pipe)

The air passes from the larynx into the *trachea*—a tube made of horseshoe-shaped rings of cartilage (which keep it open) and connective tissue—which extends from the lower end of the voice box into the chest cavity behind the heart. Immediately posterior to the larynx and the trachea is the tube called the esophagus which transports the food from the pharynx to the stomach. The cartilaginous rings of the trachea provide sufficient rigidity to keep it open at all times for the air to pass through; yet they are flexible enough to permit bending the neck. The trachea is lined with ciliated mucous membrane. As in the nose, the mucus in the trachea traps inhaled foreign particles, which the waves of cilia carry out of the respiratory tract through the pharynx.

## THE LOWER RESPIRATORY TRACT

### The Bronchi

As the trachea enters the chest cavity, it divides into 2 smaller tubes called the *bronchi*. The bronchi enter the lungs and divide into smaller and smaller branches to form what is commonly called the "bronchial tree" which is spread throughout the lung tissue. As the bronchi become smaller and smaller their walls become thinner, and they become known as *bronchioles*. The bronchi and the bronchioles continue to be lined with ciliated mucous membrane. The bronchioles termi-

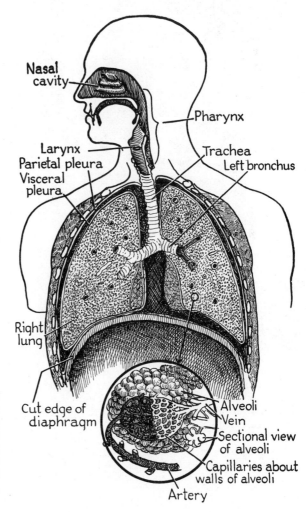

Figure 16-2. The respiratory system showing nasal cavity, pharynx, larynx, trachea, lungs, bronchi and alveoli. Note the enlarged diagram of the alveoli with surrounding blood capillaries through which the exchange of gases takes place between the inspired air and the blood. (Baillif and Kimmel: Structure and Function of the Human Body. Philadelphia, Lippincott)

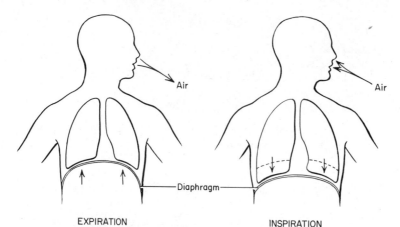

Figure 16-3. The mechanics of breathing. (*Left*) Chest space and lung size when air is exhaled and the muscles of respiration are relaxed. (*Right*) Expansion of the lungs in the vacuum created by an increase in the size of the chest upon inhalation. The ribs are lifted and the diaphragm contracts.

EXPIRATION

INSPIRATION

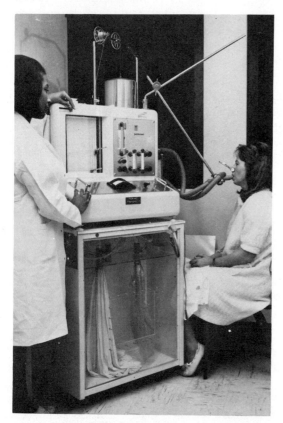

Figure 16-4. Pulmonary function testing is done to determine the ability of the lungs to handle the oxygenation of the blood. In many disorders, the ability of the lungs or the capacity of the lungs is decreased. (See Chapters 48 and 31.) The normal breath is called the *tidal volume*; the amount the lungs can hold at maximum is called the *vital capacity*. (University of Minnesota Health Sciences Center)

nate in microscopic balloonlike structures or air sacs called *alveoli,* which somewhat resemble a bunch of grapes. These microscopic "balloons" give the lungs their spongy appearance.

It is through the alveoli that the exchange of gases (oxygen and carbon dioxide) takes place. The walls of the alveoli are 1-cell layer thick. They are surrounded by the equally thin blood capillaries. When oxygen enters the lungs it travels through the walls of the alveoli into the capillaries, where it combines with hemoglobin, the main chemical component of the red blood cells. In this manner the oxygen is distributed to the body cells by the bloodstream. After it gives up its oxygen, hemoglobin combines with carbon dioxide, a waste product of cells. This carbon dioxide is released into the lungs for removal by exhalation in exchange for oxygen. An enlargement of the alveoli is shown in Figure 16-2.

## The Lungs

The *lungs* are the stations where the blood picks up oxygen and drops off its load of carbon dioxide. The lungs are 2 cone-shaped organs which fill the chest cavity. The term *apex* is given to the top of the triangular cone. The lower wide portion which fits over the diaphragm is called the *base.* The lungs are spongy tissue, filled with alveoli, nerves, and blood and lymph vessels. They are separated by the heart, the large blood vessels, the esophagus, and other contents of the *medias-*

*tinum,* the area which lies between the lungs in the thorax.

The lungs are divided into sections called lobes. The right lung has 3 lobes; the left has 2. On the inner surface of the lungs is an indented area called the *hilum.* The arteries, the veins, the bronchi, and the nerves enter the lungs at the hilum.

The lungs are covered with a smooth double-layered sac called the *pleura.* One layer covers the lungs, while the outer layer lines the chest cavity. Their surfaces are in constant contact and are moist, allowing the lungs to move without pain or friction against the chest wall.

## THE MECHANICS OF BREATHING

As mentioned previously in Chapter 13, the lungs do not move by themselves during the process of breathing—they are inflated and deflated by the muscles which surround them. The intercostal muscles contract to lift the ribs when you inhale, and they relax when you exhale. The diaphragm, the dome-shaped muscle which separates the thorax and the abdominal cavities, contracts and flattens to increase the chest space. The resulting partial vacuum inflates the lungs as the air rushes in. When the diaphragm relaxes, it curves upward into the thorax, presses against the lower surface of the lungs and pushes the air out of them (see Fig. 16-3).

The respiratory center which controls breathing is in the medulla in the brain. Breathing is also affected by the amount of carbon dioxide in the blood. Therefore, if you take deep breaths and breathe in a large amount of oxygen, you do not need to breathe as often. When you exercise strenuously, your muscles need more energy for power, and you breathe more rapidly to supply more oxygen.

Even when you have exhaled all the air you can from your lungs, there is still slightly more than a quart (1,100 ml.) of residual air remaining constantly in the alveoli. If filled to capacity, the lungs will hold approximately 1 gallon (4,000 + ml.), but the intake and the output with every normal breath is about 500 ml. or 1 pint. Adults usually average between 14 to 20 respirations per minute. The rate is much higher for children. Normal respiration is called *eupnea;* difficult breathing is known as *dyspnea.*

# 17

# The Digestive System

---

BEHAVIORAL OBJECTIVES

*The student successfully attaining the goals of this chapter will be able to:*

- *discuss the relationship of the digestive system to the other systems of the body.*
- *trace the digestive pathway, indicating the physical and chemical alterations which food undergoes at each stage of the digestive process.*
- *describe the term enzyme and discuss the general functions of enzymes in digestion; list the major enzymes, state where they enter the digestive tract, and indicate the action of each.*
- *diagram a tooth, showing the crown, neck, root, enamel, cement, dentin, and the pulp cavity; identify the chief function of the teeth.*
- *diagram the stomach, indicating the fundus, body, pyloric portion, and cardiac and pyloric sphincters; describe what digestive processes occur in the stomach.*
- *define and state the function of bolus, peristalsis, chyme, rugae, gastrin, mastication, digestion, absorption, villi, feces, peritoneum, and mesentery.*
- *outline the contributions of the accessory organs of digestion (the liver, gall bladder, and pancreas) to the digestive process; describe the functions of the liver which are not directly related to the digestive process.*
- *locate on a chart or model the small intestine, indicating the duodenum, jejunum, and ileum, and state the colloquial name for each; discuss the digestive activities which occur in the small intestine.*
- *locate the large intestine, indicating the ileocecal valve, the cecum, and the vermiform appendix; the ascending, transverse, and descending colon; the sigmoid colon, the rectum and anal sphincter; describe the functions of the large intestine.*

---

## FOOD MATERIALS AND ENZYMES

Because the body must have energy to perform its many tasks, it has to have a supply of fuel and water. You are able to breathe, your heart beats, you talk and laugh and move because your digestive system supplies you with food which gives you the fuel for your energy demands. The digestive system changes the food we eat into a usable form.

The foods that provide fuel for the body are carbohydrates (starches and sugars), proteins, and fats. Some of their main sources are listed on page 163. These organic food materials are made up of carbon, hydrogen, and oxygen. The proteins also contain nitrogen. The function of the organs of the digestive system is to break down the food into its most simple forms—small units or molecules —that can be carried by the circulatory vessels and can pass through cell membranes to be used by the cells. The cells use the simple forms of food molecules for energy, as well as to build, maintain, and repair body tissues.

This wonderfully efficient machinery which your body uses for processing food to be supplied to body cells is called the digestive tract (see Fig. 17-1). It is also called the alimentary canal, the GI tract, and the gastrointestinal system. This tract or canal is like a tube, about 30 feet long, which runs through your body and is open to the outside at both ends. Because of this last feature, it is not sterile. Actual absorption of nutrients occurs outside the alimentary canal.

The conversion of the mass of food to the basic food materials is called digestion. The chemicals that accomplish most of the digestive processes are called *enzymes*. An enzyme is a substance produced by the body to aid or speed a chemical reaction. Enzymes act only on specific substances; for instance, some act only on proteins, others on fats, and still others on carbohydrates.

# THE ORGANS OF DIGESTION
## (The Alimentary Canal)

### The Mouth (Oral Cavity or Buccal Cavity)

Food is taken into the body through the mouth, where digestion begins. The teeth cut, chop, and grind the food so that the particles become smaller and more food surface is exposed to the actions of the digestive juices and enzymes.

### The Teeth

The teeth are set in spaces or sockets in the upper and lower jaw bones—the *maxilla* and the *mandible*. Humans have 2 sets of teeth: the deciduous or baby teeth and a permanent

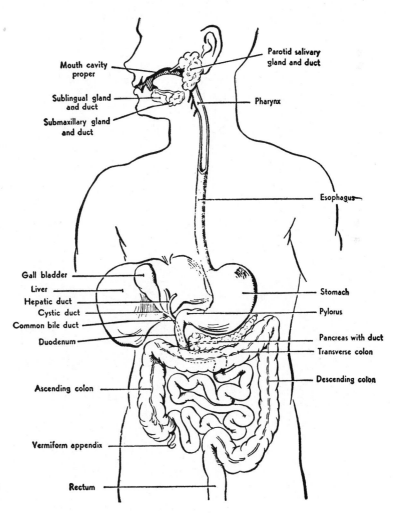

Figure 17-1. Diagram of the digestive system.

or adult set (see Fig. 17-2). A baby's deciduous teeth usually begin to erupt when he is from 6 to 8 months old, and the total of 20 is usually complete by the time he is 2½ years old. When the child is about 6, the permanent teeth begin to appear. As they grow in, they push out the deciduous teeth, replace them, and fill in the spaces in the jaw. There are 32 teeth in the permanent set. The front and the side teeth are biters and cutters; the back teeth, or molars, are grinders. The last permanent teeth, the *wisdom teeth,* sometimes do not appear before adulthood. If the jaw is small and the jaw space limited, they may not have room to erupt and may have to be removed surgically.

A tooth has 3 parts: the exposed part or *crown,* the narrowed *neck* at the gumline, and the *root* in the bony socket. The crown is covered by enamel, which is the hardest structure in the body. Covering the root is another substance called *cement.* Beneath the enamel and the cement is a hard bonelike substance called *dentin,* which is the bulk of the material of the tooth. The center of the tooth is the pulp cavity. The pulp contains many nerves and blood vessels which enter from a canal through the roots from the sockets. The teeth are imbedded in and nourished by bone.

As previously stated, the chief function of the teeth is to break the food into small particles. This is accomplished through the act of chewing or *mastication.*

## The Tongue

The tongue is muscular and flexible and has many functions. (The prefix referring to the tongue is *glosso-* or *lingua-.*) The rough upper surface is sprinkled with taste buds—small organs containing nerve endings that distinguish between salty, bitter (back of tongue), sweet (front of tongue), and sour tastes. The taste of food is also dependent upon the sense of smell. The tongue also helps us to know whether food is hot or cold, and whether it is smooth, lumpy, or stringy. It mixes food with saliva and moves the food beneath the teeth to be chewed. It begins the swallowing process (*deglutition*), by pushing the food into the pharynx, the next portion of the digestive tube.

Three pairs of salivary glands from the mouth (sublingual), the cheek (parotid), and the jaw (submaxillary) pour saliva into the mouth. Saliva is a thin watery fluid that contains *ptyalin.* Ptyalin is also called *salivary amylase* (*amyl:* starch; *ase:* pertaining to enzymes). Saliva moistens the food particles, (which stimulates the taste buds), makes the food easier to swallow, and, through the action of the enzyme, begins the breakdown of starch into smaller sugar molecules. The salivary glands also excrete other substances.

## The Pharynx and the Esophagus

The tongue lifts the ball of food (called a *bolus*) which it has mixed with saliva into the

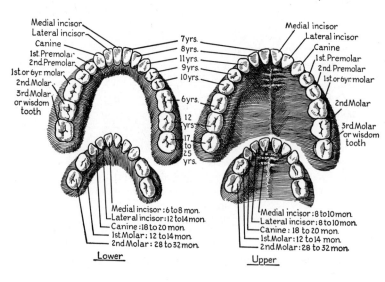

Medial incisor
Lateral incisor
Canine
1st. Premolar
2nd. Premolar
1st. or 6 yr. molar
2nd. Molar
3rd. Molar or wisdom tooth

7 yrs.
8 yrs.
11 yrs.
9 yrs.
10 yrs.

6 yrs.

12 yrs.

17 to 25 yrs.

Medial incisor
Lateral incisor
Canine
1st. Premolar
2nd. Premolar
1st. or 6 yr. molar
2nd. Molar
3rd. Molar or wisdom tooth

Medial incisor : 6 to 8 mon.
Lateral incisor : 12 to 14 mon.
Canine : 18 to 20 mon.
1st. Molar : 12 to 14 mon.
2nd. Molar : 28 to 32 mon.
Lower

Medial incisor : 8 to 10 mon.
Lateral incisor : 8 to 10 mon.
Canine : 18 to 20 mon.
1st. Molar : 12 to 14 mon.
2nd. Molar : 28 to 32 mon.
Upper

Figure 17-2. Permanent and deciduous teeth. (Baillif and Kimmel: Structure and Function of the Human Body. Philadelphia, Lippincott)

muscular tube behind the mouth, the *pharynx*. After the food is swallowed, the movement of food becomes *involuntary*. Contractions of the pharynx continue the act of swallowing and push the food into the esophagus. The *epiglottis* covers the larynx and prevents the food from entering the respiratory tract. The contractions in the pharynx begin the automatic journey of the food through the digestive tract. The smooth or involuntary muscles pass the food along by waves of contractions called *peristalsis*. Peristalsis is the alternate relaxation and contraction of the muscles to push the food through the digestive tube.

From the pharynx, the food passes down the muscular *esophagus* (or gullet). The esophagus averages about 10 inches in length and extends from the pharynx into the neck and the thorax and, through an opening in the diaphragm, to the stomach. Its role in digestion is merely to serve as a passageway. The stomach opening, the *cardiac orifice*, is guarded by a muscle called the *cardiac sphincter*. As the waves of peristalsis push the food through the lower esophagus, the cardiac sphincter opens and allows the food to enter, and closes to prevent food from regurgitating.

## The Stomach

The *stomach* is a muscular, collapsible pouchlike sac which is capable of great distention. It is located in the upper left side of the abdominal cavity and receives its blood supply from the ciliac artery. The rounded portion at the top of the stomach is called the *fundus*. The central portion is called the *body*; the lower portion, which attaches to the small intestine, is called the *pyloric portion* (see Fig. 17-3). (The prefix referring to the stomach is *gastro-*.)

The strong walls of the stomach consist of 3 layers of smooth muscle: a circular layer, a longitudinal layer, and an oblique layer. This spread of the muscles in all directions allows great motion in stirring and churning the food and breaking it up into small particles.

The stomach is lined with mucous membrane. In addition to the glands that secrete mucus, the gastric lining also secretes gastric juice, which consists mostly of water, enzymes,

and hydrochloric acid. The hydrochloric acid activates some enzymes and also destroys organisms. Too much of this acid can cause an ulcer or upset the action of the enzymes. The enzymes in the stomach are mostly concerned with the digestion of protein. The enzyme *pepsin* begins the breakdown of proteins; *rennin* curdles the protein in milk, making it more easily digestible. Some authorities state that *lipase,* another enzyme present in small quantities, acts on emulsified fats (those which have already been broken down into tiny droplets). However, most of the fat digestion takes place later in the small intestine.

In the stomach, all foods are mixed with the gastric juices and churned until they are in a semiliquid form called *chyme*. This process usually takes from 3 to 5 hours. Peristalsis in the smooth muscles of the stomach normally moves the food toward the pyloric outlet. The pyloric sphincter at the lower opening contracts to keep the food in the stomach until it is thoroughly mixed. It then relaxes to let the peristaltic waves push the food in small amounts into the small intestine. If the stomach is irritated or overfull, sometimes the direction of the waves of peristalsis reverses and forces the material back into the lower end of the esophagus. Reverse peristalsis

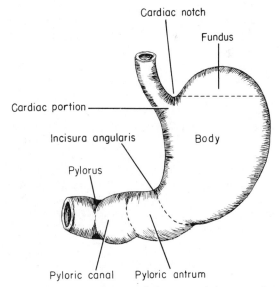

Figure 17-3. Diagram of the parts of the stomach. (From Grant, J. C. B.: A Method of Anatomy, ed. 5, Baltimore, Williams & Wilkins)

## TABLE 17–1.   ENZYMES AND THEIR ACTIONS

| Area of Digestive System | Secretion | Enzyme | Action |
|---|---|---|---|
| Mouth | Saliva from the salivary glands | Amylase (also called ptyalin) | Begins digestion of starches |
| Stomach | Gastric juice from the stomach lining (includes hydrochloric acid—HCl) | Pepsin | Begins digestion of proteins |
| | | Lipase | Acts on emulsified fats |
| | | Rennin | Acts on casein in milk (a protein) |
| Small intestine | Bile from the liver | No enzyme | Emulsifies fats |
| | Pancreatic juice from the pancreas | Trypsin (Protease) | Digests proteins to amino acids |
| | | Amylopsin (Amylase) | Digests starches to sugars |
| | | Steapsin (Lipase) | Digests fats to simplest forms— fatty acids and glycerol |
| | Intestinal juice from the intestinal lining | Erepsin (Proteases) | Digests proteins to amino acids |
| | | Lactase Maltase Sucrase | Digests sugars to simplest forms—glucose, fructose and galactose |
| | | Enterokinase | Activates trypsin to act on proteins |

within the stomach plus contractions of the abdominal muscles and the diaphragm force the food back through the esophagus and out through the mouth, causing vomiting.

When the stomach is empty, it collapses and lies in folds called rugae.

The actions of the digestive system are subject to the control of the nervous system. It is known that there are also hormones (chemical messengers carried in the bloodstream) which control certain actions. For instance, *gastrin* is a hormone of the stomach which appears to be related to the control of gastric secretions. There are many other known hormones of the digestive system and others which are being investigated.

## The Small Intestine

The small intestine is about 20 feet long and 1½ inches in diameter and lies coiled upon itself in the abdominal cavity. It is about 18 feet longer than the large intestine which follows it. The first portion is the 10 to 12 inch "C"-shaped *duodenum*. (The prefix referring to the intestines is *entero-*.)

As the chyme enters the duodenum, more digestive juices are added. *Bile,* a greenish-brown liquid which is manufactured by the *liver* and stored in the *gallbladder,* pours in through the *common bile duct* to emulsify fats in preparation for further digestive action. The *pancreas* is a glandular organ behind the stomach which adds 3 enzymes in the secretions it sends through the *pancreatic duct: protease* or *trypsin* for proteins, *amylase* or *amylopsin* for carbohydrates, and *lipase* for fat digestion. Pancreatic juice is vital for life. The common bile duct and the pancreatic duct enter the duodenum a short distance beyond the pyloric sphincter of the stomach. The small intestine itself secretes enzymes for the digestion of all foodstuffs. Together these juices break up the fats, the carbohydrates, and the proteins into materials that the cells can use.

In order to be absorbed by the blood and the lymph capillaries, the carbohydrates must be in the form of the simple sugars: glucose, fructose, and galactose. The proteins must also be digested to their simplest state, amino acids, and the fats must be converted to fatty acids and glycerol. Table 17-1 summarizes the action of the enzymes in preparing food for absorption. Most *digestion* (conversion of foods into simpler compounds) takes place in the stomach and duodenum. Most *absorption* (passage of food into the bloodstream for use by the body) takes place in the remainder of the small intestine.

The chyme travels on through the remaining portions of the small intestine, the *jejunum* and the *ileum*. (The jejunum is called "the empty intestine" because it always empties after death. The ileum is called "the twisted intestine" because of its many coils and twists.) Like the rest of the alimentary canal, the entire intestinal tract is lined with mucous membrane. Throughout the whole length of the small intestine are tiny finger-like projections called *villi*. These villi projecting from the walls add a tremendous amount of absorption area to the intestines, just as deep pleats in a skirt add to the amount of material needed to make it. They wave to and fro to keep the food molecules thoroughly mixed with digestive juices. It is through the villi that about 85 per cent of the food is absorbed as it flows over their surfaces.

Since the villi play such an important part in absorption, they are heavily supplied with blood capillaries. In the center of each villus there is also a lymph capillary called a *lacteal*. The digested carbohydrates and proteins pass into the villi and are absorbed by the blood capillaries, while most of the digested fat is absorbed into the lacteals and is carried in the lymph. The fats eventually reach the bloodstream by way of the thoracic and right lymphatic ducts in the region of the neck. The completely digested foods are then ready for distribution to the various body tissues. We have already mentioned the processes by which the food needed by cells passes through the capillary walls into the surrounding tissue

fluid and then through the cell membrane into the body of the cell.

After the food has been in the small intestine for about 4 to 6 hours, it passes on into the large intestine; all that remains of it are water and waste products. A sphincter muscle, located where the large and the small intestine meet, acts as a valve to prevent the backflow of material to the small intestine and also regulates the forward flow. It is called the *ileocecal valve* from the names of the 2 joining parts, the ileum (small intestine) and the cecum (large intestine).

## The Large Intestine

The large intestine (sometimes called the *large bowel* or *colon*), is much wider than the small intestine (diameter about 2½ inches) but is only about 6 feet long. It has no villi, does not coil or lie in folds, and is divided into different areas by name.

The first portion is the *cecum,* a blind pouch about 2 to 3 inches long. A small fingerlike projection of the cecum is the *vermiform appendix,* which has no known function. It has some of the same lymphoid tissue as the tonsils and, like the tonsils, frequently becomes infected, a condition called *appendicitis.* It is prone to infection because fecal material enters and cannot always drain out. The cecum and the appendix are located in the right lower quadrant of the abdominal cavity.

The next and longest portion of the large intestine is the *colon,* a continuous tube divided into 3 parts, taking their names from the course they follow: the *ascending colon* travels up the right side of the abdominal cavity; the *transverse colon* crosses to the left side in the upper part of the cavity; the *descending colon* goes down the left side into the pelvis. The next and last portion, which is called the *sigmoid* (sigma: Greek letter for S) ends at the *rectum*. The rectum is about 5 inches in length and terminates at the *anal canal*. This is the terminal portion of the large intestine. It is about 1 to 1½ inches long, and its opening to the outside, the *anus,* is guarded by internal and external sphincter muscles. The external sphincter is under the control of the will and can be consciously contracted and relaxed.

Since most of the valuable food products are absorbed in the small intestine, the main function of the large bowel is the absorption of water. There are no enzymes in the large intestine. It is lined with mucous membrane. As the contents move along, most of the water is absorbed through the walls of the large intestine into the circulation to assist in maintaining the body's fluid balance. As the water leaves, the cellulose, left from food, masses together and passes into the rectum. This solid waste, the *feces,* also contains bacteria, mucus, and a small amount of water. As the feces enter the rectum they stimulate sensory nerve endings, causing the sensation of accumulating bulk. The peristaltic waves push the contents against the anal muscles as a signal to empty the rectum. Relaxation of the external sphincter muscle (the anus) and the pressure from peristalsis plus that consciously exerted by the diaphragm and the abdominal muscles brings about defecation, the emptying of the rectum. If the sensation for defecation is ignored, the impulse dies.

## THE ACCESSORY ORGANS OF DIGESTION

### The Liver

The digested food which has reached the blood through the villi in the small intestine passes through the *liver* and undergoes vital changes. The liver is the largest glandular organ in the body and lies just below the diaphragm in the upper right quadrant of the abdominal cavity. It receives its blood supply from the hepatic artery. (The prefix referring to the liver is *hepato.*) In man, the liver weighs about 3 pounds and resembles in color and texture the calf liver that we eat. The liver plays such an important part in overall bodily functions that a person cannot live long if it is severely diseased or injured. It can be likened to:

*A filtration plant.* The phagocytic cells lining the sinusoids of the liver engulf bacteria and other particles. It filters and detoxifies the blood.
*A chemical laboratory.* It breaks down digested fats and proteins into substances which can be

used or stored by the liver or elsewhere in the body. It prepares products from the breakdown of red blood cells for further use by the body and detoxicates bacterial and other poisons such as alcohol and drugs that have gained entrance into the blood stream.
*A manufacturing plant.* The liver produces bile, glycogen (a form of stored sugar) and a substance called heparin which prevents the clotting of blood in the blood vessels. It also produces most of the blood proteins, such as albumin, prothrombin, and fibrinogen (which is needed for blood clotting).
*A warehouse.* It stores carbohydrates, fats and proteins as well as vitamins and minerals, changes their form and releases them to the body as needed. It stores iron and copper.
*A waste disposal plant.* It prepares many substances for excretion, including urea, the chief waste product from the utilization of amino acids.
*A regulation plant.* It regulates the concentration of each amino acid in the body (its most important function) and helps to regulate the *blood volume* of the body, thereby influencing blood pressure.
*Vitamin control.* It forms vitamin A from carotene, as well as storing vitamins A, D, and B complex.
*A heating plant.* The burning of the simple sugars, the amino acids and the fatty acids in the liver produces body heat second only to the amount produced by the skeletal muscles.

### The Gallbladder

The *gallbladder* is a muscular sac resembling a small pear and is located on the undersurface of the liver. Some authorities regard it as an enlargement of the cystic duct through which it drains. Its main function is to store and release bile as it is needed in the small intestines to emulsify fats.

Cells within the liver manufacture bile. Small ducts from these cells emerge and join to form the hepatic duct, which then joins the cystic duct coming from the gallbladder. At this point it is called the *common bile duct* which, with the pancreatic duct, empties into the duodenum at the major duodenal papilla, an opening a small distance beyond the pyloric portion of the stomach. This was mentioned earlier in this chapter in discussing digestion in the small intestine. As bile is produced, it flows down the hepatic duct and up into the cystic duct for storage in the gallbladder. With the appearance of fats in the intestines, the hormone *cholecystokinin* activates the gallbladder to release the bile; then it flows through the cystic duct into the common bile duct for deposit in the duodenum. This system of passageways for the transport of bile from the liver to the gallbladder to the intestines is known as the *biliary apparatus* and is shown diagrammatically in Figure 17-4.

Obstruction of the biliary apparatus can cause cholelithiasis (gallstones) or cholecystitis (inflammation of the gallbladder).

## The Pancreas

The *pancreas,* a long fish-shaped gland behind the stomach, has tissues for 2 distinct functions. Certain cells secrete pancreatic juice for food digestion. These enzymes, which were discussed previously, are carried to the small intestine by way of the pancreatic duct. Cells of other tissues, called the *islets of Langerhans,* secrete *insulin* which the body cells must have to utilize sugar. Without adequate insulin, the blood sugar (the blood glucose) level rises to abnormal levels.

## The Peritoneum

Lining the walls of the abdominal cavity is a large sheet of serous membrane called the *peritoneum* which reflects itself (turns itself back) to cover all of the abdominal organs. The peritoneal cavity is the very small space between the layer covering the organs and the layer lining the walls. It contains a small amount of fluid which permits the organs to glide freely against each other and against the wall without friction. Because of the continuity of this membrane, an infection which reaches it from a diseased organ can spread very rapidly and be very serious. Such an infection is known as *peritonitis*; fortunately, it

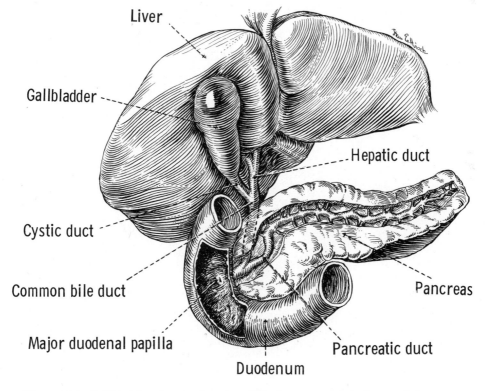

Figure 17-4. Gallbladder, showing location. Bile ducts, pancreatic ducts and the entrance of the ducts into the duodenum are shown. (Greisheimer, E. M., and Wiedeman, M. P.: Physiology and Anatomy, ed. 9. Philadelphia, Lippincott, 1972)

can usually be controlled by the use of anti-biotic drugs.

Folds of the peritoneum which support the intestines are called the *mesentery*. Between the folds are the blood and the lymph vessels and the nerves which supply the intestines. Another large fold of peritoneum, the *greater omentum*, lies anteriorly over the abdominal cavity like an apron, serving as an insulator and a protective covering. The *lesser omentum* extends from the stomach to the liver. Some structures, such as the pancreas, duodenum, and kidneys lie behind the peritoneum, and are said to be *retroperitoneal*.

## METABOLISM

The term *metabolism* is applied to the sum total of all those body functions which serve to convert simpler compounds into the living tissue of the body. These changes involve *physical changes* (chewing—breaking down food into smaller particles) and *chemical changes* (the action of enzymes upon food to change the food into chemically smaller substances). The conversion of foods into the living body is called constructive metabolism or *anabolism*. The reconversion of these materials into simpler compounds with the resulting release of heat and energy is called destructive metabolism or *catabolism*.

The term *basal metabolism* refers to the amount of energy (calories) used by the body while it is at rest. This is measured by the amount of oxygen used or by the amount of energy released. The basal metabolism is the amount of energy needed to sustain life.

# 18

# The Urinary System

## BEHAVIORAL OBJECTIVES

*The student successfully attaining the goals of this chapter will be able to:*

- *discuss the principles of homeostasis, in relationship to all the systems of the body and as it relates specifically to the urinary system.*

- *diagram a kidney, showing its location in the body along with the renal fascia, hilum, ureter, cortex, and medulla; describe the functions of each structure.*

- *identify the functions of the nephron, pyramids, renal pelvis, papillae, calices, glomerulus, Bowman's capsule, the proximal and distal convoluted tubules, the loop of Henle, the connecting tubule, renal arteries, renal veins, ureters, urinary bladder, and urethra; locate each of these structures on a chart.*

- *recognize the amount of urine normally contained in the bladder before distention occurs.*

- *list the characteristics of normal urine and identify abnormal components of urine.*

- *discuss the blood pressure within the kidneys and the influence of the kidneys upon the systemic blood pressure.*

## FUNCTIONS

As the body builds and repairs tissues and produces energy for the life processes, the food supplied by the digestive system is burned into waste in the cells. The respiratory system and the skin remove some of the water, the carbon dioxide, and the nitrogenous wastes in breathing and perspiration, while the digestive system removes the bulk wastes of food in the feces. However, the urinary system, also called the excretory system (see Fig. 18-1), is vital in eliminating other wastes of metabolism. Since these wastes are carried by the circulating blood from the cells to the kidneys for elimination in the urine, the urinary system has been called the body's filtration and removal plant.

In addition to being the primary source for eliminating protein wastes and other toxic material from the body, the urinary system provides the life-saving process of maintaining the steady composition of the blood (homeostasis):

The degree of acidity and alkalinity of the blood and the fluid in the tissues must be balanced. The kidneys aid in this control by eliminating excess acid or alkaline substances from the blood.

The amount of water in the body must remain at a fairly constant level. The kidneys maintain this water balance by excreting excess water or by conserving it according to body needs.

The salts in the body fluids are present in specific amounts. The kidneys balance the body salts by regulating their excretion from the body. (An accumulation of water in the tissues is known as *edema*; an abnormal decrease is known as *dehydration*.)

## STRUCTURES OF THE URINARY SYSTEM

### The Kidneys

The *kidneys* are 2 reddish brown bean-shaped organs located in the small of the back at the lower edge of the ribs on either side of the vertebral column. They are about 4 inches long, 2 inches wide, and 1 inch thick; they are very vascular (heavily supplied with blood vessels). Each kidney is embedded in fatty tissue and is surrounded by a fibrous tissue covering called the *renal fascia*. (The word renal relates to the kidneys; the prefix *nephro* is also used to designate kidney.) The fatty pads plus the renal fascia, which is anchored to surrounding tissues, help to hold the kidneys in place. On the medial surface of each kidney is an indented area called the *hilum*, through which the blood vessels and the nerves, plus the structure known as the ureter, enter.

If the kidney is cut in half longitudinally, you can see that it is divided into 2 parts: the outside, the *cortex*, and the inner portion, the *medulla*.

**The Cortex.** The cortex is smooth and solid in appearance. The greater portion of the nephron, the unit of function of the kid-

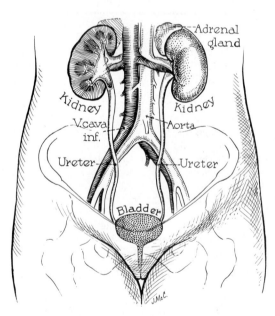

Figure 18-1. The urinary system.

ney which filters the waste products from the blood, is located in the cortex.

**The Medulla.** The medulla consists of 12 *pyramids*, cone-shaped structures, which drain the wastes and the excess water into the basin of the kidney. This receiving space is called the *renal pelvis*. (The word pelvis means *basin*, the prefix which refers to the pelvis of the kidney is *pyelo-*.) The pyramids are composed of tiny collecting tubules which give the kidneys a striped appearance. At the tip or apex of the pyramids are the *papillae*, with openings through which the urine passes into the *calyces*, which are bell-shaped cups continuous with the renal pelvis.

**The Nephron.** There are over 1,000,000 functional units, or *nephrons*, in each kidney. These microscopic structures are composed of a cluster of capillaries, the *glomerulus*, partially enclosed in a funnel-shaped structure called *Bowman's capsule*. The blood with its filterable products enters the glomerulus through the afferent arteriole which divides to form the capillary loop. Water, wastes, glucose, and salts filter through the thin walls of the capillaries and into the Bowman's capsule in a very dilute solution. The capillaries unite to form the efferent arteriole through which the remaining blood leaves the glomerulus.

Extending from Bowman's capsule is a long twisted tube called the *convoluted tubule*. The first portion is called the *proximal convoluted tubule*; the next, the *loop of Henle*, and the final portion, which is the end of the nephron unit, the *distal convoluted tubule*. The water with its dissolved contents travels the length of this tubule. It is surrounded by capillaries whose job it is to reabsorb the water and the salts needed by the body, as well as all of the glucose. (There is normally no sugar in the urine.) The remaining concentrated mixture of waste products and water is *urine*. The end of the distal convoluted tubule is attached to a *collecting tubule*. These collecting tubules join in the renal pyramids and dump their contents, the urine, into the renal pelvis (see Fig. 18-2).

The kidneys receive their generous blood supply from the renal arteries. Since these are one of the early branches from the aorta, the blood enters at high pressure and thus can be spread throughout the glomeruli. It circulates at much lower pressure after it leaves the glomeruli and travels around the tubules for reabsorption of the necessary products. It leaves the kidneys through the renal veins which enter the inferior vena cava. The kidneys have a definite influence on blood pressure.

### The Ureters

Urine travels from the pelvis of the kidneys into the *ureters*. The ureters are narrow tubes about one fifth inch in diameter and about 10 to 12 inches long. They are attached to the kidney at the renal pelvis and carry the urine from the kidneys down to the urinary bladder. In the walls of the ureters are smooth muscles which contract in peristaltic waves (similar to the peristalsis in the intestines) to carry the urine, drop by drop, to the bladder.

### The Bladder

The *bladder* is a hollow muscular sac which when empty lies behind the symphysis pubis. When full, it may extend well up into the abdominal cavity. It is lined with mucous membrane, as is the entire urinary tract. The capacity of the bladder varies, but usually the desire to empty the bladder (void) is present when it fills to about 200 to 300 cc. Since the bladder is the reservoir where urine is stored, the muscles in its walls distend as it fills with urine and contract as it empties itself. A moderately full bladder holds about 500 cc. of urine.

### The Urethra

The bladder wall contains 3 openings: 2 from the ureters and 1 from the *urethra,* the tube through which the urine passes to the outside. In the male, the urethra is about 8 inches long. It passes through the prostate gland where 2 ducts from the male sex glands join it and then through the length of the penis, the male organ of copulation (Fig. 19-1). The female urethra is short, about 1½ inches long, and opens to the outside at the urinary meatus. In both male and female, the meatus is controlled by a voluntary sphincter. The female urethra is a passageway for urine only. In the male, the urethra serves the reproductive system as well and is the passageway for both urine and sperm, the male sex cells.

## OTHER CONSIDERATIONS

### Voiding

The release of urine from the body is called *voiding* or *micturition*. (Involuntary voiding is called *urinary incontinence*.) The urine flows from the collecting tubules into the

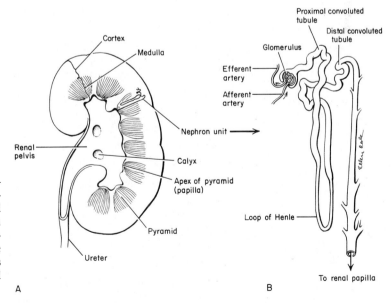

Figure 18-2. (A) Longitudinal section of the kidney showing portion of an enlarged nephron. (B) Diagram of an enlarged nephron. The horseshoe-shaped Bowman's capsule surrounding the glomerulus connects with the convoluted tubule.

renal pelvis, down the ureters and slowly enters the bladder. This sac, which is flat when empty, slowly fills. As the urine distends the bladder, it stimulates the nerve endings in the bladder walls. The brain interprets the message that soon the bladder will have to be emptied. The internal and the external sphincter muscles which control the opening to the urethra are stimulated by the nervous system to relax. However, the external sphincter can be controlled voluntarily. Therefore, when the person wills, the external muscular ring relaxes, the muscles in the bladder wall contract, and the urine which has accumulated within the bladder is forced out.

## The Urine

About 1,000 to 1,500 cc. (2 to 3 pints) of urine are excreted from the body daily. However, the quantity is influenced by many things: the amount of fluid taken into the body, perspiration, hemorrhage, blood pressure, external temperature, drugs, fever, various diseases and many other factors.

Urine is initially a clear amber liquid, with a very characteristic odor. (It may become cloudy when exposed to air.) It is acid in reaction but upon standing may become alkaline as certain substances within it break down into ammonia bodies. Normal urine is only slightly concentrated, with a specific gravity of about 1.010 to 1.025. A higher specific gravity can indicate dehydration or urinary retention.

Certain wastes are always present in urine, but careful analysis will show whether substances which are not normally found in urine are present. The composition of normal urine is:

*Water,* about 95 per cent. The water serves as the solvent.

*Nitrogenous waste products* from the breakdown of proteins. Common protein wastes are urea, uric acid, and creatinine. (A condition in which waste products accumulate because of defective function is called uremia and is often fatal.)

*Excess minerals* from the diet such as sodium, potassium, chlorides, calcium, sulfates, and phosphates.

*Toxins*

*Hormones* (especially those related to the sex of the person).

*Yellow pigment* from certain bile compounds.

Abnormal products such as blood, glucose, pus, casts, and albumin may be present and indicate disease or malfunction. Urine is normally sterile; nonsterile urine implies disease or infection. If a catheter is being used in the treatment of a patient, it might very well be the source through which infection is introduced into the urinary system. Thus the nurse must be extremely careful when inserting a catheter and in seeing that it is kept sterile.

# 19

# How Life Begins:
# The Reproductive System

## BEHAVIORAL OBJECTIVES

*The student successfully attaining the goals of this chapter will be able to:*

- *describe the secondary sex characteristics which are present in the adult male and the adult female.*
- *describe the production of sperm and the seminal fluid; trace the route of these through the reproductive organs of the male; identify the role of sperm in human reproduction.*
- *identify on a chart the structures involved in the manufacture of sperm and semen, the penis, Cowper's glands, urethra, prostate gland, seminal vesicles, and ejaculatory ducts; describe the functions of each.*
- *diagram the ovaries, the fallopian tubes, the uterus (noting the cervix, the body, fundus, myometrium, and endometrium) and vagina; outline the functions of each structure in human reproduction.*
- *describe the phases of the menstrual cycle if the ovum is not fertilized; if the ovum is fertilized.*
- *define menarche, menopause, and climacteric.*
- *locate on a chart, the structures which are considered the external genitalia of the female, the mons pubis, labia majora, labia minora, clitoris, vestibule, Bartholin's glands, and perineum; describe the functions of these structures as a unit.*
- *describe the function of the breasts during and immediately after pregnancy.*
- *discuss the concept of fertility and be able to name factors which could render the male or female infertile; identify the conditions necessary for pregnancy to occur.*

You know that cells within the body wear out and that these cells are constantly replacing themselves by a process of cell division. That the millions of body cells can accomplish this feat in such a systematized and routine manner is wonderful enough—but the function of the reproductive system in man is the most awesome and impressive of all. From the union of 2 small cells (*gametes*), the total being of another person develops, whose millions of body cells perform their individual and intricate functions; a being who can think, reason, and plan—an entire human organism.

The general body structures of boys and girls are similar until they reach the stage of *puberty,* which occurs around 12 years of age in girls and 14 years in boys. At this time the sex glands become active, the organs of the reproductive systems begin to function, and *secondary sex characteristics* appear.

The boy develops the hard musculature of

the adult male. His glands of perspiration become more active. He develops a beard, and pubic and axillary hair, and there is a general increase in hair growth all over his body. His body outline changes to the broader shoulders and the narrow hips, and a change in voice to the deeper tones is marked. The development of these secondary sex characteristics in the male is dependent upon the hormone testosterone, which is secreted by the testes, the male sex glands.

The girl at puberty exhibits many changes as well. The curved feminine contour appears; breast tissue develops; and fat deposits accumulate which alter the angular shape of childhood to a more rounded appearance. The glands of perspiration become active, and hair appears in the pubic and the axillary areas. Although voice changes are not as marked as those in the male, there is a deepening and maturing in voice tone and quality. As the glands of reproduction become active, menstruation appears. All secondary sex characteristics in the female are dependent upon the secretions of the hormones, estrogen and progesterone, which are produced in the ovaries, the female sex glands.

## THE MALE REPRODUCTIVE SYSTEM

### The Testes

The gonads or sex glands in the male are called the *testes* (singular = *testis*). (The prefix relating to testis is orchi.) These are 2 almond-shaped glands which are composed

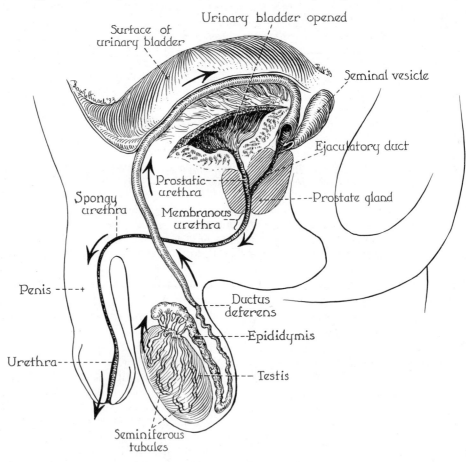

Figure 19-1. Male reproductive system. The various organs of the male reproductive system are shown. The path of the spermatozoa from the time they leave the testis until they leave the body is indicated. (Greisheimer, E. M., and Wiedeman, M. P.: Physiology and Anatomy, ed. 9. Philadelphia, Lippincott, 1972)

of long lengths of convoluted (*seminiferous*) tubules whose function is to produce the male reproductive cells called *spermatozoa*, commonly known as sperm. The testes also secrete the main part of the *semen* or seminal fluid in which the sperm are carried. The sperm are very small cells which look like tadpoles when viewed by microscope; they have a "head" and a whiplike "tail" which provides them with motility—they swim very rapidly in the semen. Sperm are produced in very large numbers: millions of sperm can be found in 1 drop of seminal fluid. Between the seminiferous tubules are small groups of cells which secrete the male hormones.

The testes develop before birth in the abdominal cavity. Usually by the time a male infant is born, the testes have descended into a sac called the *scrotum,* which is composed of skin and muscle and is suspended below the groin between the thighs. Occasionally, the testes remain inside the abdominal cavity; undescended testes do not usually produce sperm, although they do manufacture male hormones. It is believed that the testes lie outside the body cavity because they are very sensitive to heat, and the higher temperature within the body is unfavorable to the production of sperm. The descent of the testes from the abdominal cavity makes a weak spot in the muscle wall of the abdomen. This is thought to account for the frequent number of inguinal hernias which occur in males.

## The Epididymis

The sperm travel from the testis to a tightly coiled tube called the *epididymis.* This tube is approximately 20 feet long but is so tiny that it can barely be seen with the naked eye. It lies along the top and the posterior surface of each testis. The sperm mature here and some sperm are stored here. Some semen is also secreted here.

**The Ductus Deferens.** The sperm continue their journey through a tube called the *ductus deferens* (vas deferens) which is actually an enlarged continuation of the epididymis. The ductus deferens passes through the inguinal canal in the muscles of the abdominal wall into the abdominal cavity and continues over the top and down the posterior surface of the bladder, into the pelvic cavity. Each joins a

duct from the seminal vesicles, and together with blood vessels, lymphatic vessels, nerves, and covering, makes up a *spermatic cord.*

**The Seminal Vesicles.** The 2 *seminal vesicles* are pouches which store sperm and secrete a fluid which adds to the semen. Each vesicle has an excretory duct, which joins with 1 of the 2 ductus deferens to form the *ejaculatory duct.*

## The Prostate Gland

The *prostate gland* is a doughnut-shaped gland lying just below the bladder, surrounding the neck of the bladder and the urethra. It adds an alkaline secretion to the semen, which is thought to increase the motility of the sperm. The urethra runs through the prostate gland and joins the 2 ejaculatory ducts. This passageway continues through the length of the penis and serves as the outlet tube for both urine and semen. Any swelling or growth in the prostate gland causes pressure on the urethra and can easily stop the flow of urine, which is a fairly common condition in elderly men.

At the base of the penis and emptying into the urethra are 2 small glands called the *bulbourethral glands (Cowper's glands).* Their function is to secrete an alkaline substance into the urethra. Since the urine is usually acid in its reaction, this alkaline secretion tends to neutralize the urethral environment. Sperm survive better in an alkaline than in an acid medium.

## The Penis

The penis is a cylinder-shaped organ located externally immediately above the scrotum. It is made up of *erectile tissue* with cavernlike spaces in it. At the time of sexual excitement, blood fills these spaces, changing the soft, limp penis to an enlarged rigid erect organ. The smooth cap of the penis is called the *glans penis* and is covered by a fold of loose skin which forms the hoodlike *foreskin* or prepuce. Removal of this foreskin (circumcision) is a frequently performed operation. The penis and the scrotum are referred to as the external genitalia in the male. The penis also serves as part of the urinary tract in the male.

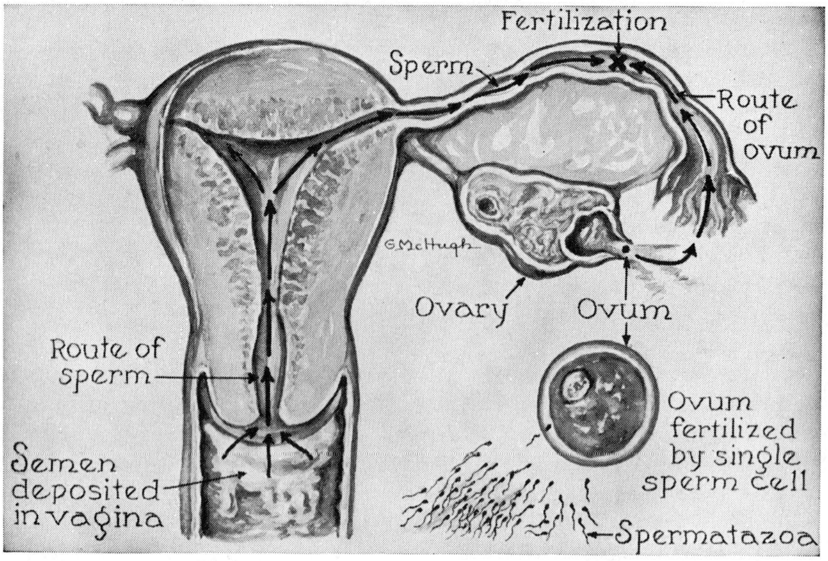

Figure 19-2. The process of fertilization. Note the ovum leaving the ovarian follicle and its subsequent course into the tube. Sperm deposited in the vagina travel upward through the cervix and the uterus into the outer end of the tube, where fertilization takes place. The insert shows the relative sizes of the sperm and the ovum. (DeLee, S. T.: Safeguarding Motherhood. ed. 6. Philadelphia, Lippincott, 1969)

## Copulation

Sexual intercourse or sexual union between the male and the female is also called copulation or coitus. The erect penis is inserted within the vaginal canal, and sperm are deposited or ejaculated within the vagina by means of waves of contractions of the ducts through which the semen travels. The amount of semen in each ejaculation is about 3 to 5 milliliters. There are about 120,000,000 to 300,000,000 sperm per milliliter. If the sperm count falls below 60,000,000 per milliliter, the individual is considered to be infertile. The sperm cell determines the sex of the unborn child.

## THE FEMALE REPRODUCTIVE SYSTEM

The female reproductive system includes the paired *ovaries,* the paired *fallopian (uterine) tubes,* and the single *uterus* and *vagina,* with their associated structures, the *external genitalia* and the *mammary glands (breasts).*

### The Ovaries

The ovaries are 2 almond-shaped glands about 1½ inches in length located within the brim of the pelvis, one on either side of the uterus, the hollow organ in the center of the pelvic cavity where the unborn infant grows.

The prefix which refers to the ovaries is oophoro-.

The ovaries are composed of connective tissue and are covered with a special epithelium in which are imbedded thousands of microscopic structures called *graafian follicles.* Ova (egg cells) develop and mature within the follicles. From the time of puberty until menstruation ceases, at approximate monthly intervals, a follicle ripens and pushes its way to the surface of the ovary. It is during the ripening of the follicle that the hormone, estrogen is released. The mature ovum then ruptures the surface of the follicle and is discharged into the pelvic cavity. This release of the ovum is called *ovulation.* Ovulation usually occurs about halfway between the average 28-day menstrual cycle, or about 14 days before the onset of the next menstrual period. Usually only one ovum at a time is released. However, it is believed that some females ovulate more than once during their menstrual cycle.

After ovulation, the follicle is replaced by a yellowish substance called the corpus luteum. The corpus luteum then secretes the hormone, progesterone, to thicken and enrich the uterine lining in preparation for pregnancy. If the ovum is not penetrated (fertilized) by the sperm, the corpus luteum degenerates after approximately 2 weeks and forms scar tissue. If the ovum is fertilized, it remains for about 3 months and aids in the development of the fertilized egg cell.

## The Fallopian Tubes

As the mature ovum bursts from the ovary into the pelvic cavity, it is picked up by the open fringed ends of the uterine (fallopian) tubes. There are 2 of these tubes, one attached to either side of the uterus. They are lined with cilia which help guide the ovum to the uterus, which takes about 5 days. (The prefix salpingo- refers to the uterine tubes.)

Fertilization of the ovum (i.e., the meeting of the sperm and the ovum) usually takes place about midway in the fallopian tube. (If the fertilized ovum stays there, an ectopic or tubal pregnancy results.) From here the fertilized ovum travels to the uterus where it becomes embedded in the uterine lining in preparation for growth.

## The Uterus

The uterus is a hollow, muscular, pear-shaped organ in the center of the pelvic cavity, immediately posterior to the bladder. It is about 3 inches long and usually lies tipped slightly forward over the bladder. The broader section above is called the *body,* and the narrower section below is called the *cervix.* The round surface which bridges the level where the tubes enter is the *fundus.* The myometrium is the thick smooth muscle layer of the uterine wall; it can expel the baby at delivery as well as the menstrual flow in the nonpregnant woman. The inside of the uterus is lined with a tissue called the *endometrium,* a mucous membrane containing many blood vessels. The uterus in general is very vascular. Although it is very movable, the uterus is held in position by strong structures called the broad and the round ligaments.

The function of the uterus is to receive the fertilized ovum and to provide housing and nourishment for the developing baby (fetus). The uterus must be capable of great expansion, since it is the organ in which the baby develops. The prefix for uterus is hystero.

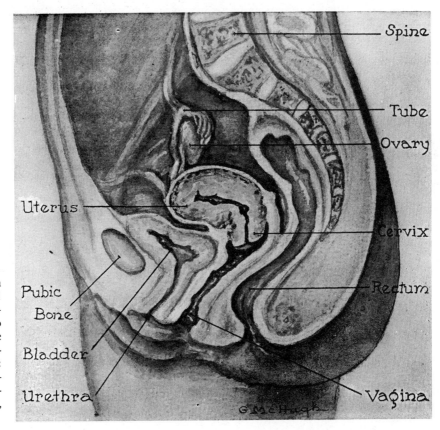

Figure 19-3. Mid line section through the pelvis viewed from the side, showing the relationship of the uterus to the bladder and the rectum. (DeLee, S. T.: Safeguarding Motherhood, ed. 6. Philadelphia, Lippincott, 1969)

## The Vagina

The neck of the uterus projects into a 3-inch muscular canal, the vagina, which extends from the cervix and opens to the outside of the body. It is located behind the urethra. The vagina is the female organ of intercourse and forms part of the birth canal. Its inner surface is moistened by the secretions of many glands from the mucous membrane lining its walls. It lies in folds, called rugae, which are expandable to permit passage of the fetus. A fold of membrane, the *hymen,* is sometimes found closing the external opening of the vagina, but since it can be injured in various ways, it is not considered a sign of virginity.

## The External Genitalia

The external genitalia (vulva) of the female consists of the *mons pubis (veneris),* the *labia majora,* the *labia minora,* the *clitoris,* and the *vestibule* (see Fig. 19-4). The mons pubis is a fatty pad over the symphysis pubis which is covered with pubic hair after the age of puberty. Posterior to the mons pubis are the

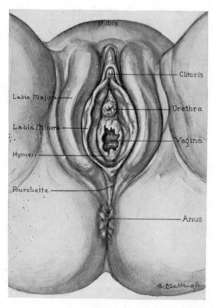

Figure 19-4. External genitalia viewed from below. (DeLee, S. T.: Safeguarding Motherhood, ed. 6. Philadelphia, Lippincott, 1969)

other external organs. The labia majora are 2 large outer folds of fat and skin which extend backward almost to the anus. Under and between the labia majora are the labia minora which do not have pubic hair but contain many glands. At the anterior junction of the labia is the clitoris, a very small structure comparable with the penis in the male. It is composed of erectile tissue which is stimulated by sexual sensations. Posterior to the clitoris and between the labia minora is the space called the vestibule. Within the vestibule is found the urinary meatus and the vaginal opening, referred to as the vaginal orifice. The vestibule also contains the *Bartholin's glands,* which are considered to be glands of lubrication. If the openings to these glands become obstructed, Bartholin cysts result.

The space between the vaginal orifice and the rectum is called the *perineum.* It is made up of strong muscles which act as slinglike supports for the pelvic organs. These are the muscles that are sometimes torn or incised (episiotomy), during childbirth.

## The Mammary Glands (The Breasts)

The mammary glands (breasts) are usually classified as organs of the reproductive system because they are stimulated by hormones to secrete milk after childbirth (lactation). These 2 glands, on the outside of the chest wall, are composed of glandular tissues and varying amounts of fat covered by rather thin skin. Each breast is divided into 16 to 20 separate lobes that secrete milk. The duct from each lobe converges toward the nipple, like the spokes of a wheel, and terminates in small openings through the nipple. The breasts enlarge during pregnancy due to the stimulation of estrogen and progesterone, and skin around the nipples, the *areola,* becomes more heavily pigmented. The raised areas on the areola are called the *glands of Montgomery;* they are sebaceous glands which keep the nipples from drying out. After the termination of pregnancy, the production of milk by the mammary glands is stimulated by a hormone of the anterior pituitary gland. The size of the breasts has no relationship to success in nursing a baby.

## Menstruation

Throughout the universe we find many examples of Nature's "rhythms" or cycles. The phases of the moon change regularly; the ocean tides have a rhythm of their own. The human body also has several of these built-in clocks; for instance, you sleep and eat in fairly regular cycles. Another of these cyclic activities is menstruation in the female. This rhythmic series of changes which occurs about every 28 days is called the *menstrual cycle*. Menstruation, which is the flow of blood and other substances from the vagina caused by the shedding of the lining of the uterus, usually begins between the ages of 10 and 14. The first menstrual period is called the *menarche*. The various changes that occur are brought about through the action of several hormones.

The onset of menstruation is the beginning of the cycle, i.e., the first day of menstruation is the first day of the cycle. The menstrual flow usually lasts from 3 to 5 days. During the next phase of the cycle, the graafian follicle in the ovary ripens, and the ovum within begins to mature. It finally ruptures about the fourteenth day, and the ovum is released, a process called ovulation, which was discussed earlier in this chapter. The anterior pituitary gland in the brain secretes the hormones which stimulate this action in the ovary.

The level of the ovarian hormones (estrogen and progesterone) is now high, and their action has caused the endometrium to become greatly thickened and vascular, preparing it for possible pregnancy. Toward the end of the menstrual cycle, if the enriched uterine lining is not needed, the action of the hormones decreases. This affects the blood supply of the endometrium so that it begins to degenerate. The capillaries within the uterine wall begin to bleed, and the endometrium is sloughed off. The menstrual flow, consisting of blood, mucus, and cells then occurs.

Authorities differ in their ideas of the time during which the ovum can be fertilized following ovulation, opinions varying from 15 minutes to 72 hours. The length of time that sperm survive after intercourse is also debated. However, for fertilization to occur, the sperm must meet and penetrate the ovum in the fallopian tube. Their 2 nuclei then join to form the 23 pairs of chromosomes, the beginning of a new individual. The average time for ovulation to occur is 14 days before the next menstrual period, regardless of the length of the cycle. For example, in a 28-day cycle, the 14th day is the probable time of ovulation. This can be calculated if the menstrual periods occur at regular intervals. This method of computation is called the rhythm method and is used both for planning and for preventing pregnancy. If intercourse is avoided for 5 days before and 5 days following ovulation, fertilization of the egg cell is not likely to occur. If pregnancy is desired, sexual relations at the probable time of ovulation will enhance such a possibility. It is obvious that this method of calculating the time of ovulation is not suitable if menstrual periods are irregular.

## The Menopause

Menstrual cycles continue as long as ovarian hormones stimulate the uterine lining. Normally, when a woman is between 40 and 50, her ovaries become less active and cease producing both ova and hormones. Menstruation may terminate abruptly, but it is usually a gradual process. The cessation of the menstrual cycles is called the *menopause,* and the period during which the ovaries are undergoing these changes is called the *climacteric*.

The menopause is a normal process and may be so gradual that the body adjusts to it without difficulty. However, since many hormonal changes are involved, some unpleasant symptoms such as headaches and sensations of heat (*hot flashes*) may occur. If too severe, usually these can be treated satisfactorily with temporary hormonal therapy. Men may experience a similar phase, but it is a much slower process, and usually there is no sharp demarcation of beginning or end as there is in the female. However, some authorities refer to it as the *male climacteric*.

# 20

# The Endocrine System

## BEHAVIORAL OBJECTIVES

*The student successfully attaining the goals of this chapter will be able to:*

- *differentiate between exocrine and endocrine glands.*
- *define a hormone and discuss the actions of the major hormones of the body.*
- *relate the activities of the endocrine system to those of the other systems in the body.*
- *locate on a chart, the major endocrine glands, state what hormone(s) they secrete, and list the chief actions of each hormone.*

## FUNCTIONS

The endocrine system comprises a group of glands located in various parts of the body (see Fig. 20-1). Because they do not send their secretions through pipes or ducts but pour them directly into the blood stream instead, endocrine glands are also called the *ductless glands* or the glands of internal secretion. The chemical substances which they manufacture are called *hormones*.

The hormones are chemical regulators, which integrate and coordinate the activities of the body. They not only speed up or slow down the activities of entire body organs, but some affect the rate of various activities of individual cells of the body. Hormones also affect each other: too much or too little of a particular hormone interferes with the actions of other hormones. There is a fine balance within the endocrine system that promotes normal body functions (see Fig. 20-2). Most hormones are either steroids (derived from fats) or proteins. Their production may be brought about by nervous stimulation, by the level of some substance in the blood, or by another hormone.

Some authorities feel that there is a close relationship between the endocrine system and the nervous system, since both have the function of stimulating as well as controlling actions of the body. However, the effect of nerve stimuli is immediate and lasts only as long as the stimulation is present; the action of an endocrine gland is slower and is a more prolonged stimulation and regulation.

There is also a close relationship or dependency between the endocrine glands and the circulatory system, because the hormones travel via the blood stream.

Little was known about the endocrines before 1900. Research is still being conducted to learn more about their function.

### The Pituitary Gland (The Hypophysis)

The *pituitary* gland is a small gland about the size of a pea, located in a saddlelike hollow (the sella turcica), in the phenoid bone at the base of the brain. It is made up of 2 parts: the *anterior lobe* and the *posterior lobe;* for this reason sometimes it is classified as 2 separate glands.

The anterior lobe secretes a large number of hormones. Five of these control the action of other endocrine glands; therefore, the pituitary is often referred to as the "master gland." One of these hormones, ACTH, stimulates the adrenal cortex; another regulates the thyroid hormone. Three other hormones stimulate the testes and the ovaries, as well as the mammary glands following pregnancy.

The sixth hormone secreted by the anterior pituitary is called the *growth hormone* (somatotropic hormone or STH); it controls protein anabolism and the release of glucose from the liver, as well as influencing growth. If the pituitary secretes too much growth hormone in childhood, it causes gigantism. The bones in the face, the hands, and feet enlarge to abnormal size, a condition called acromegaly. Too little of this hormone in childhood results in dwarfism.

The posterior lobe secretes 2 different hormones: oxytoxin and vasopressin. Oxytoxin stimulates contractions of the uterine muscles and the formation of milk. Vasopressin stimulates smooth muscles in the walls of blood vessels and in the gastrointestinal tract. Thus, it increases blood pressure and influences re-

absorption of water by the tubules of the kidney.

One of the most important portions of vasopressin is ADH (antidiuretic hormone). A lack of this hormone results in diabetes insipidus.

## The Thyroid Gland

The *thyroid* gland, the largest of the endocrine glands, lies in front of the neck just below the larynx, with a wing (lobe) on either side of the trachea. The thyroid secretes the hormone *thyroxin,* which it manufactures from iodine absorbed from the blood. Thyroxin regulates the metabolism of the body; that is, it controls the rate at which each of the individual cells carries on its work, building and repairing itself, producing energy, etc. Thus it regulates the rate at which the cells burn food. If the thyroid does not secrete

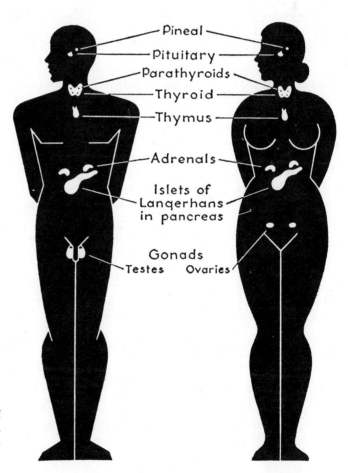

Figure 20-1. The endocrine glands. (Hirsch, J.: Minnesota Department of Health; Todd and Freeman: Health Care for the Family, Philadelphia, Saunders)

enough thyroxin (hypothyroidism), the cells oxidize food too slowly. This interferes with the cells' activities and slows down body functions. If the hypothyroidism is severe, the person may be retarded physically and mentally, a condition known as cretinism. Hypothyroidism can also cause abnormally slow sexual development. If the thyroid secretes too much thyroxin, all body functions are speeded up. The cells burn food too rapidly and produce more energy than is needed. This is termed hyperthyroidism, or Graves disease and causes such symptoms as nervousness, hy-peractivity, irritability, and protrusion of the eyeballs (exophthalmia).

The thyroid removes iodine from the blood to make thyroxin. This iodine must be supplied through the diet. If the diet lacks iodine, the thyroid grows larger in overworking to make more thyroxin. An enlarged thyroid gland is called a goiter. In areas of the country where the soil lacks iodine, sufficient quantity in the diet is assured by the use of iodized salt.

The proper functioning of the thyroid gland is measured by a basal metabolism test,

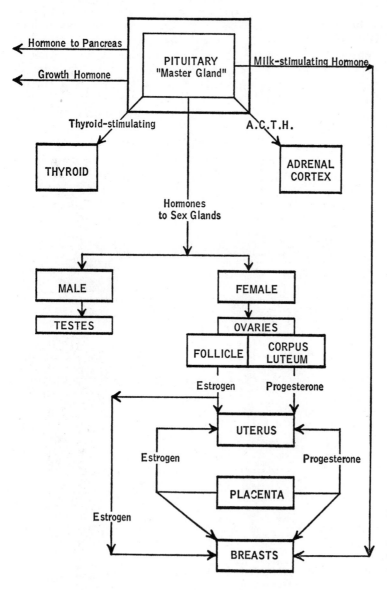

Figure 20-2. Endocrine relationships (simplified) in the human body. Note the many functions of the pituitary gland and its effect upon both the male and the female reproductive systems. (After Cole and Elman: Textbook of General Surgery, ed. 6, New York, Appleton-Century-Crofts, 1952)

which measures the amount of oxygen needed to carry out basic body functions. Another test called a PBI (protein-bound iodine) measures the amount of iodine in the blood and is considered to be more accurate.

## The Parathyroid Glands

The *parathyroids* are small glands, each about the size of a pea, which lie on either side of the under part of the thyroid gland. They are 4, 6, or 8 in number; despite their size, they are essential to health and to life itself. The parathyroids secrete a hormone parathormone, which regulates the amount of calcium and phosphorus in the blood, which in turn affects nerve and muscle irritability. Too little calcium causes tetany, a condition marked by muscle spasms, convulsions, and possible death (not to be confused with the infection called tetanus or lockjaw). If the parathyroids secrete too much of the hormone, the diet cannot supply enough calcium, and the calcium salts are drawn from the bones, making them soft and unable to support weight.

## The Adrenal Glands

The 2 *adrenal* glands (also known as the suprarenal glands) sit like hats on top of each kidney. Like the pituitary gland, the adrenal glands have 2 parts which produce different hormones. (In some animals other than man, they occur as 2 separate glands.) The central portion, called the *medulla,* secretes the hormone epinephrine (adrenalin) which brings many body processes into action quickly. Epinephrine makes the heart beat faster, contracts blood vessels, raises blood pressure, and increases muscle power by causing the liver to release glucose for energy.

The medulla also secretes the hormone norepinephrine which has some but not all of the actions of epinephrine. The hormones from the medulla "mimic" the action of the sympathetic nervous system. However, the medulla is not necessary for life because its activities can be taken over or assumed by the sympathetic nervous system. The adrenals are active in emergencies: emotions of fright, anger, love, or grief stimulate them. They are said to

prepare us for "flight or fight." The functions of the medulla are important in that they apparently help us adapt to stress.

The outer part of the adrenals, the *cortex,* is now known to secrete many compounds, and probably more will be discovered. Their actions are so widespread and so complex that they are difficult to enumerate. The hormones of the adrenal cortex are called steroids. Some of the functions of adrenocortical secretions are to sustain the ability of the individual to withstand stress and infections, to stimulate repair of injured tissue, to regulate the behavior of salts in the body, to control water retention, and to control carbohydrate, protein, and fat metabolism and storage. Male and female hormones are also secreted by the adrenal cortex. Hyperactivity can hasten sexual development in boys or cause masculine sex characteristics (such as facial hair and deeper voice, lack of menstruation) to appear in girls.

The hormones of the adrenal cortex are necessary for life. Many, such as cortisone, are available commercially, and prospects are good for others to be available in the future.

## The Pancreas

The pancreas is located behind the stomach between the duodenum and the spleen. Within its tissue are cells called the *islets of Langerhans,* consisting of alpha cells and beta cells. Beta cells secrete the hormone *insulin.* Without insulin, cells are unable to utilize glucose, a condition called diabetes mellitus. The alpha cells produce *glucagon,* which causes an increase in blood sugar level by breaking down liver glycogen into glucose (glycogenesis).

## The Gonads

The *gonads* are the glands of reproduction: the testes of the male and the ovaries of the female.

In addition to producing sperm, the *testes* produce testosterone, the male sex hormone. Testosterone controls the development of the sex organs of the male as well as influencing such characteristics as male body form, hair distribution, and voice. There are also other steroid hormones which produce masculinizing effects. As a group they are called *androgens.*

The ovaries produce estrogen and progesterone, hormones which stimulate maturing of the female sex organs. These hormones also influence development of secondary sex characteristics such as breast development, voice quality, and the broader pelvis of the female body form. Menstruation occurs because of the hormone production of the ovaries. Estrogen is responsible for most of these changes. Progesterone apparently is concerned primarily with body changes that favor the implantation of the fertilized ovum and continuation of pregnancy. Both hormones seem to influence the mood changes and the emotional climate of the female.

## The Thymus and Pineal Gland

The *thymus* gland lies behind the sternum (breastbone). Efforts to discover any definite contribution of the thymus to the endocrine system have not yet been successful. It is made up of lymphoid tissue and is known to produce lymphocytes. Recent studies indicate that the thymus, which is comparatively large in infants, has an important role in establishing antibody formation in the newborn. It supposedly continues its functions related to immunity reactions through puberty but atrophies by the time of adulthood.

The *pineal* gland, another endocrine puzzle, is attached to the brain. No secretion has been discovered, and its function is unknown.

## Other Hormones

There are other hormones which are known and others which are being investigated and discovered. The stomach wall secretes a hormone, *gastrin,* which stimulates the secretions of the gastric glands. The lining of the upper part of the small intestine secretes the hormone, *secretin,* which stimulates the pancreatic juices, and also another hormone which causes the gallbladder to contract.

The placenta is also a temporary endocrine gland that secretes hormones that help to maintain pregnancy. The presence of high levels of these hormones in the body provides the basis for the commonly used tests to determine pregnancy.

# 21

# The Sensory System

BEHAVIORAL OBJECTIVES

*The student successfully attaining the goals of this chapter will be able to:*

- *identify the sensory receptors of the body in terms of location and function; identify the areas of the brain which interpret the sensations from each.*
- *discuss the concept of pain and its transmission to the brain.*
- *locate on a chart, the major structures of the ear, including the auricle, auditory canal, tympanic membrane, malleus, incus, stapes, eustachian tube, cochlea, oval window, organ of Corti, acoustic nerve, and semicircular canals; discuss the function of each; identify the boundaries of the outer, middle, and inner ear.*
- *define cerumen, eye-blink reflex, accommodation, rods and cones, and optic chiasm.*
- *locate on a chart, the major structures of the eye, including the conjunctiva, eyelid, lacrimal gland, nasolacrimal duct, sclera, cornea, choroid, ciliary body, iris, pupil, lens, retina, aqueous humor, vitreous humor, and optic nerve; discuss the function of each structure; differentiate between the 3 layers of the eye; describe how the eyeball itself is moved.*
- *discuss awareness of hunger, thirst, taste, and smell; list the sensations which are transmitted by the organs of taste; state how the sense of taste is related to the sense of smell.*
- *discuss the concept of balance or equilibrium and how it is maintained.*

An often-repeated statement is that "all knowledge comes to us through our senses." The obvious sensory perceptions you think of are those of seeing, hearing, smelling, tasting, and feeling. There are many more. You can also receive impressions of warmth, pressure, softness, and pain. A very important impression is your sense of equilibrium: you know whether or not you are moving and the posture and the position of your body.

From your study of the nervous system, you know that to be aware of information from the world around you, you must have receptors which receive the stimuli, nerve routes which carry the sensation or stimuli to the brain, and centers in the brain to interpret the stimuli, such as "red," "sweet," or "loud."

## THE EAR

The ear is the special sense organ for hearing. It is an especially adapted apparatus for bringing the vibrations in the air to your nervous system for interpretation as sound. For instance, a piano being played produces vibrations or sound waves in the air which cause thousands of hairlike cells in the ear to carry a pattern to the brain which you translate as music. The prefix referring to ear is oto-.

The ear has 3 parts: the *external (outer)*, the *middle,* and the *inner* ear. These lead to the acoustic nerve and then to the center for hearing which is located in the temporal lobe of the cerebrum.

The external ear, called the *pinna* or *auricle,* is the only readily visible part. It is composed mostly of cartilage and is shaped like a funnel to gather and guide sound waves into its small opening, which extends into a tube called the *auditory canal.* The lining of the auditory canal is covered with tiny hairs and secretes a waxy substance called *cerumen;* both the hairs and the wax aid in protecting the ear from foreign objects. The auditory canal is very short, about 1 inch in length, and extends to the ear drum, a thin membrane called the *tympanum.* This tympanic membrane separates the external and the middle ear.

On the other side of the tympanum is the middle ear, a small cavity in the temporal bone. Within this cavity, between the ear drum and the inner ear, are 3 small bones called the *malleus* (hammer), the *incus* (anvil), and the *stapes* (stirrup). These 3 bones are called *ossicles* and are so small that sound waves can set them in motion. The sound waves start vibrations of the ear drum and the malleus or hammer which is attached to it. The malleus stimulates vibrations in the incus, which in turn moves the stapes. As the vibrations pass through the middle ear, the effect of the vibrations is magnified.

Extending from the middle ear are 2 openings: 1 leads into the mastoid cells behind it, and the other into the eustachian tube which communicates with the nasopharynx. The eustachian tube opens during swallowing or yawning. Its function is to equalize the pressure in the middle ear with atmospheric pressure. By this means, the pressure on both sides of the drum membrane is equalized, and the drum can vibrate freely. The middle ear, the eustachian tube, and the passage to the mastoid cells are lined with a continuous coat of mucous membrane.

The inner ear (labyrinth) has 2 parts. One is the *cochlea,* which is shaped like a hollow snail shell and is filled with fluid. Along the cochlea are hairlike processes which are thought to be the receptors for the *organ of Corti.* The organ of Corti is said to be the true organ of hearing, because this is where the transmission of nerve stimuli begins.

The base of the stapes fits into an opening between the middle and the inner ear. This opening is covered by a thin membrane and is called the *oval window.* The stapes vibrates against the membrane, setting the fluid in the cochlea in motion. The fluid in motion passes the vibrations on to the tiny hairlike nerve endings or receptors in the organ of Corti which transmits the impulses to the *acoustic nerve.* The acoustic nerve sends them to the center for hearing in the brain, which then interprets these impulses as sounds (see Fig. 21-1).

Another section of the inner ear is the *semi-circular canals.* Shaped like horseshoes, they lie behind the cochlea. They too contain hairlike nerve endings which are set in motion by fluid within the canals. Motion in the

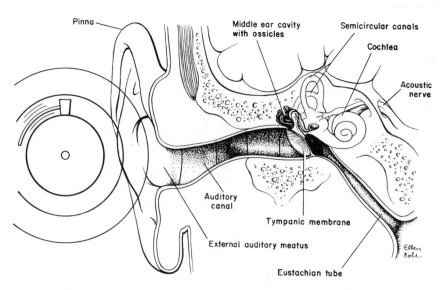

Figure 21-1. How we hear.

fluid is caused by head or body movements. The receptors lead to the acoustic nerve, but the pathway of this section of the acoustic nerve goes to the cerebellum and is concerned with balance and coordination. A defect of the inner ear usually causes dizziness.

## THE EYE

The eye is constantly compared with a camera, and although this analogy is not totally correct, there are many parts to each apparatus which have corresponding functions. One marked difference is that the camera shows 1 image, but the eye registers 2, which the brain then combines into a single image. This *binocular vision* is possible because coordinated muscles move the eyeballs. The eye also automatically perceives depth, whereas in photography, this is an illusion.

The eye lies in a protective bony orbit in the skull. Between the eye itself and its bony surroundings is a cushion of fat. The eyelids, the brows, and the lashes serve as further protection for the eye. The eyelid is the cover for the anterior surface of the eye which is deprived of the protection of the skull. A reflex, the eye blink, protects the eye from foreign objects or blows. Also covering the anterior eye, beneath and lining the eyelids, is a thin transparent mucous membrane called the *conjunctiva* which is well supplied with blood vessels and nerve endings.

In order to keep the surface of the eye moist, it is supplied with the *lacrimal glands* which produce tears. The lacrimal glands are located at the outer edge of the corner of the eye. Tears drain through a small opening in the inner canthus or corner of the eye, the nasolacrimal duct, into the nose. The tears are slightly antiseptic in their effect.

The eyeball is a hollow sphere made up of 3 layers of tissue. The tough protective outer layer is the *sclera* or white of the eye. In order to allow light rays to enter the front of the eye, the sclera has a transparent section over the front of the eyeball; this transparent section is called the *cornea* which does about two-thirds of the focusing of the eye. The middle layer, or the *choroid,* is a vascular layer which brings oxygen and nutrients to the eye. The choroid extends to the ciliary body which helps to control the shape of the lens. Over the front of the eyeball, the choroid develops into a pigmented section, the *iris,* which gives the eye its individual color. Within the iris are muscles which control the size of the opening within its center, the *pupil.* The pupil regulates the amount of light traveling through the eye. It always appears black because it looks into the dark inner chambers of the eye.

The *lens* is a structure immediately behind the iris and does about one-third of the focusing of the eye. It is a transparent body whose function is to bring the light rays into focus to allow a clear image. Then the image is reflected on the *retina,* which is the nerve center of the eye. Parallel rays of light, passing through the lens, are refracted or bent so

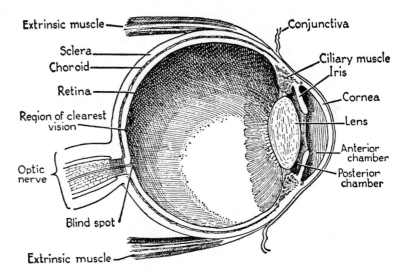

Figure 21-2. Section through the eyeball. (Baillif and Kimmel: Structure and Function of the Human Body, p. 281, Philadelphia, Lippincott)

Extrinsic muscle

Conjunctiva

Sclera

Choroid

Ciliary muscle
Iris

Retina

Cornea

Region of clearest vision

Lens

Anterior chamber

Optic nerve

Posterior chamber

Blind spot

Extrinsic muscle

that they focus on the retina. This adjustment by the lens to make a sharp clear image is called *accommodation* and is controlled by the autonomic nervous system. If the eyeball is too short, the light rays are focused behind the retina instead of on it. This causes *farsightedness (hyperopia)*. In *nearsightedness (myopia)*, the eyeball is too long or the lens too strong, and the light rays are focused in front of the retina.

The space between the cornea and the lens is filled with a liquid called the *aqueous humor*; the space behind the lens is filled with a gelatinlike material called the *vitreous humor*. It is these fluids which give shape to the eyeball.

The inner layer of the eyeball is the *retina,* which contains the receptors of the optic nerve. Some of the neurons of the retina cells are shaped as rods and cones. The cones permit perception of color; the rods are concerned with the perception of light and shade.

Light must pass through the cornea, the aqueous humor, the lens, and the vitreous humor before coming into focus on the retina. The receptors in the retina send the nerve impulses through the nerve fibers to the nerve of sight, the *optic nerve.* The optic nerve carries the stimuli to the occipital area of the brain where visual images are interpreted. The optic nerves cross before entering the brain (*optic chiasm*). The *ophthalmic nerve* carries sensations of pain and temperature to the brain. If a foreign object is in the eye, this nerve carries that sensation. (The prefix ophthalmo- relates to the eye.)

Smooth muscles (extraocular muscles) in the eye control the size of the pupil and the action of the lens in accommodation. Three pairs of muscles, attached to its outer coat, move the eyeball. Another muscle attached to the upper eyelid holds the eye open; when the eyelids shut, this muscle is relaxed.

## OTHER SPECIAL SENSES

**Taste.** The nerves of taste provide you with 4 taste sensations: sweet, salty, bitter, and sour. The receptors for taste, located on the tongue, are what we commonly call the taste buds. Many foods are combinations of more than one taste sensation.

**Smell.** The nerve of smell is the *olfactory nerve,* and the receptors for the sense of smell are located in the upper third of the nasal cavities. The sense of taste and the sense of smell work very closely together. Many times it is the odor of a food that makes it pleasant to eat. Think how tasteless your food is when you have a head cold. Smell and taste combine to give foods flavor.

**Touch.** Your touch receptors, mostly in the skin, are constantly receiving nerve impulses, allowing you to feel pain, as well as the pleasures of softness and warmth, and the dangers of too much heat or cold. There are many more touch receptors in some areas, such as the fingertips and around the lips, than are found in other areas.

These special senses are as interesting and as useful as your eyes and ears, but because they are not so often involved in illness or disease, they are not studied in such detail.

# Unit 5:
# Meeting the Nutritional Needs of People

22. *Food for Growth and Energy*
23. *From Market to Meals*
24. *Special Diets to Meet Patients' Needs*

# Food for Growth and Energy

## BEHAVIORAL OBJECTIVES

*The student successfully attaining the goals of this chapter will be able to:*

- *discuss some of the factors which can contribute to an inadequate diet.*

- *identify the major cause of obesity, list at least two adverse physical conditions which are attributed to obesity.* *heart disease & diabetes*

- *exemplify a knowledge of proper nutrition by practicing good dietary habits.*

- *describe the science of nutrition; discuss the value of nutrition information in nursing practice.*

- *list the 6 classes of nutrients; identify the function of each, and give an example of each.*

- *define nutrient, protective foods, obesity, and Basic 4.*

- *describe the nutritional value of the carbohydrates; list several good sources; identify several sugars and describe them; identify which form of sugar can be directly used by the body without alteration; and describe the functions of starch and cellulose.*

- *describe the storage of carbohydrates in the body.*

- *describe what is meant by a fat; list at least 5 functions of fats in the body; list good food sources; and differentiate between saturated and unsaturated fats.*

- *describe the nutritional values of protein; identify good sources; describe protein digestion; and differentiate between complete, partially complete, and incomplete proteins.* *C – PC – IC*

- *define calorie; state the number of calories yielded upon burning 1 gram of protein, fat, and carbohydrate.*

- *plan a daily diet for a family or for any age group, utilizing the Basic 4.*

- *describe the function of minerals in the body; identify good sources of each major mineral; identify deficiency conditions caused by lack of calcium, phosphorus, iron, magnesium, and iodine; list 4 considerations in diet planning which will ensure an adequate mineral supply.*

- *define vitamin; list several general characteristics of vitamins; classify vitamins as fat-soluble or water-soluble; identify the major vitamins, food sources, and specific function in the body.*

- *discuss the importance of a well-distributed diet, with special emphasis upon an adequate breakfast.*

*Table 22-1*

## FOOD AND HEALTH

Food plays a vital part in our lives. Although it is natural to eat because we enjoy food, it is also necessary to eat to live and be healthy. People today are healthier than people were in previous times; this is partly due to increased knowledge about food and to the greater availability of foodstuffs. In America food is plentiful. Although poverty and lack of food still haunt many, most people in the United States are probably better fed than any

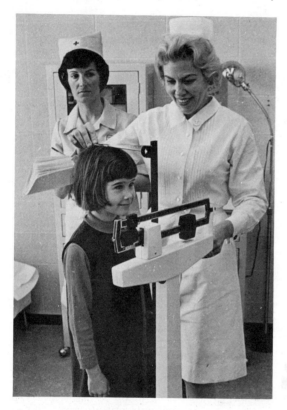

Figure 22-1. Although there are differences between individuals, there are general weight and height averages which are considered within normal limits. Most schools have a program of regular weight and height measurement in order to determine great deviations from normal. Often, if a great deviation can be detected in childhood, the causative factor can be identified and corrected. Many deficiencies or problems of overweight are due to faulty eating patterns, and the family can be educated to prevent further difficulties. The practical nurse, as a mother, may be asked to assist in the screening of students in the local schools. (American Red Cross Photo for the St. Louis Globe-Democrat by Paul Ockrassa.

other people in the world. Yet we are told that half of our population do not eat enough of the essential foods, such as milk, vegetables, meats, and fruit. It has been estimated that 20 per cent of school-age young people suffer from malnutrition, which may be defined as a lack of necessary nutrients in the body. While malnutrition may be due to some physical dysfunction, it often can be traced to poor eating habits.

Perhaps subnutrition is a better word to use to describe the problem in America. Most persons have sufficient food available and eat an adequate quantity, but they may not eat wisely.

### Excessive Weight

Because of poor eating habits, many people in this country are overweight. This condition is very rarely due to a physical disorder; it is almost always the result of overeating. Unfortunately, people who are chronically overweight are prone to develop many other physical disorders, including heart disease and diabetes. Therefore, it is to their benefit to take off the extra weight. How effectively or safely they accomplish this feat depends on the method they use. Many physicians and psychologists specialize in helping people to lose weight.

### Normal Nutrition

Normal nutrition is the science concerned with the use of food by the body to (1) provide energy, (2) build and repair tissues, and (3) regulate body processes. Good nutrition contributes to health, happiness, enjoyable, productive work and play, and a long life relatively free from illness.

What can be done to improve nutrition? Teach people the facts about nutrition! This kind of education is going on constantly in our schools, the logical place to begin it. It is also carried on in homes, industries, clubs, and agencies associated with clinics and hospitals.

### Essential Nutrients

You think of food as cereals, vegetables, meat, fish, eggs, milk, cheese, and desserts from which you choose your 3 meals a day and the snacks in between. However, the body cells are interested only in extracting from food the materials which they can use. These materials are called *nutrients,* from the word *nutrire* meaning to *nourish* or to *feed.* We list them here, with their uses in the body:

1. Carbohydrates (starches and sugars): provide heat and energy.
2. Fats: provide heat and energy; build fatty tissue.
3. Proteins: build and repair tissues; provide heat and energy.
4. Minerals: build and repair tissues; regulate body processes.
5. Vitamins: regulate body processes.
6. Water and cellulose: regulate body processes.

The amounts of these nutrient materials present in individual foods vary considerably. Some foods contain large amounts of one nutrient and small amounts of others; other foods contain small amounts of several nutrients. The purpose in planning meals is to provide the essential nutrients in the amounts necessary to keep the body healthy. These food combinations make up an adequate diet. But you also want meals to be appetizing and attractive; so, to make the plan complete, you need to know which foods provide which nutrients (see Table 22-1). The foods which provide for the needs of the body in the greatest measure are called "protective foods."

## The Basic 4

A good daily food guide should include the protective foods, in 4 groups which are essential for good nutrition and should be included in the daily food plan. Each group contributes to the essential nutrients—no one group will provide all of them.

1. *Milk group:* includes some milk every day in the following amounts:

| | |
|---|---|
| Children | 3 to 4 cups |
| Teen-agers | 4 or more cups |
| Adults | 2 or more cups |
| Pregnant women | 4 or more cups |
| Nursing mothers | 6 or more cups |

Part of the milk can be replaced by cheese, ice cream, or other milk products.

2. *Meat group:* 2 or more servings of beef, pork, veal, lamb, fish, poultry, or eggs. Alter-

## TABLE 22–1. GENERAL CLASSIFICATIONS OF THE SOURCES OF NUTRIENTS

| Carbo-hydrates *sugars starch* | Proteins | Fats |
|---|---|---|
| Provide fuel for energy and heat | Build and maintain body tissues | Provide fuel for energy and heat |
| Flour | Lean meats | Cooking fats |
| Breads | Fish | Salad oils |
| Cereals | Poultry | (mayonnaise, |
| Sugar | Eggs | French dressing) |
| Sweets (honey, jelly, syrups, candy) | Milk | Butter |
| | Cheese | Margarine |
| Vegetables (potato) | Legumes (dried peas, beans) | Animal fats (bacon, lard, salt pork, suet) |
| Fruits (dates) | Nuts (particularly peanuts) | Bitter chocolate |
| Carbonated beverages | | |

nates can be dry beans, peas, lentils, or nuts.

3. *Vegetable-fruit group:* 4 or more servings to include:

A. A dark-green or deep-yellow vegetable at least every other day. *Vit A stored*

B. A citrus fruit or other fruit or vegetable (tomatoes) every day. *Vit C not stored*

C. Other fruits and vegetables—including potatoes.

4. *Bread-cereals group:* whole-grain, enriched or restored: 4 or more servings daily.

This gives you the foundation of a good diet. Other foods not mentioned in these groups will be used to make meals more appetizing, such as butter, margarine, oils, and sugars—especially when combined with baked dishes and desserts and as flavoring for vegetables. Some people will also use more of the basic foods to satisfy their individual requirements.

## Carbohydrates

The carbohydrates are the most economical and available sources of energy. The body uses carbohydrates more completely and readily than any of the other nutrients (see Chapter 17), and they are widely distributed in nature. Next to water, they make up the greatest amount of bulk in plants. Carbohydrates are valuable because they supply quick energy and provide roughage and give satisfaction in the diet; they are low in cost and can be stored easily without spoiling.

The important sources of carbohydrates are the sugars and the starches in our diets. In relation to sugars, it may surprise you to learn that there is more than one kind of sugar. Starches are the more complex forms of sugars. Some forms are found in the foods we eat; others are made in the body in the process of digestion. Sugar is of no use to the tissues of the body until it is in the form which the body can use readily. This means that some sugars must be changed within the body into this usable form called *glucose*.

**Sugars.** *Glucose* is the only form of sugar which can be absorbed and carried in the blood stream ready for use by the body tissues. All the other forms of sugar must be changed into glucose, the sources of which are natural glucose, which is found in honey, fruits, and most vegetables, and other sugars and starches which are changed into glucose within the body.

2. *Sucrose* is the form of sugar that probably is the most familiar to you. It tastes sweet; as crystallized sugar, it is used on the table and in cooking. The sources of sucrose are sugar beets, sugar cane, and the sap of the maple tree.

3. *Fructose* is another form of sugar which is found mostly in honey and fruits and in some plants. It tastes almost twice as sweet as sucrose.

4. *Lactose* is the sugar which is found in milk. It is neither as soluble nor as sweet as sucrose. It encourages the growth in the intestine of certain bacteria which aid in the use of vitamin K and niacin.

5. *Galactose* is not found naturally but is a product of the digestion of milk.

6. *Maltose* is the product of sprouting grain and of the digestion of starch within the body. It is readily soluble and easily changed into glucose, so it is often used in infant formulas, in preference to other sugars.

**Starch.** Starch is the form of carbohydrate which is found in plants; the main sources are grain, roots, bulbs, tubers, and seeds. The starch grains are encased in a tough covering which is broken down in the process of digestion. The cooking of foods containing starch speeds up digestion. Enzymes in the saliva can act upon cooked starch but have no effect on raw starch. Starch must be changed into carbohydrate in order to be utilized by the body.

**Cellulose.** Cellulose is classified as a carbohydrate, but it has no actual food value; it consists of the fibers of plant framework, which are insoluble and indigestible. However, it does have a definite use in providing bulk which helps in the elimination of food residue from the intestine. Bran, whole-grain cereals, fibrous vegetables, and fruits are the main sources of this roughage.

**Absorption and Digestion.** Simple sugars are ready to pass into the blood stream without any digestive change. The more complex sugars have to be carried through several stages of digestion before they are ready for use. We have already mentioned the various enzymes in the saliva and the intestinal tract which carry out this breakdown.

Too much sugar in the diet takes away the appetite for other essential foods; also, it may ferment in the digestive tract and irritate it. The waste products from the use of carbohydrates by the body are carbon dioxide and water.

**Glycogen.** The body can store a reserve of carbohydrate in the liver in the form of glycogen; it can be changed into glucose and released into the blood stream as it is needed.

Carbohydrates taken into the body in excess of its immediate needs for heat and energy will be changed into fatty tissue. This can serve as a source of fuel stored for future use. If the intake of food is lowered, the body can call upon stored carbohydrates for energy. Carbohydrates also aid in the consumption of fats to keep them from burning up too rapidly. The presence of too much fatty tissue is called *obesity*.

## Fats

Fats furnish a concentrated form of energy. Deposits of fat in the body guarantee a large and lasting supply of fuel. Certain fats are important in the function and the structure of body tissues, especially nerve tissue. Fat also serves as protection from mechanical injury and as a padding around vital organs; a layer of fat underneath the skin conserves body heat. Like carbohydrates, fat also can be used by the body for energy when the protein intake is low. It also lubricates the intestinal tract to help in elimination. Fat makes the diet more attractive and tasty and prevents hunger, since it remains in the stomach longer than other nutrients. Another important function of fats is to aid in the utilization of vitamins A, D, E, and K.

The sources of fats are plants or animals. Fats are composed of carbon, hydrogen, and oxygen and vary in consistency. They are classified as *saturated* or *unsaturated* fats. The saturated or solid fats (animal fats, butter, lard, hydrogenated shortenings) already contain their full complement of hydrogen, in their natural form or because hydrogen has been added by hydrogenation.

The unsaturated fats (soft or liquid fats or oils) are capable of taking on more hydrogen. (Manufacturers add hydrogen to the oily fats to make them solid.) The relatively inexpensive vegetable oils, such as corn, cottonseed, soybean, and coconut oils, are used for this purpose. Margarine, which is also made in this way, is processed with cultured milk to give it a butter flavor, with vitamins A and D added. Fortified margarine has approximately the same nutritional and caloric values as butter.

Fats are insoluble in water. There is no digestion of fats in the mouth and very little in the stomach. When fats reach the small intestine, bile secreted by the liver breaks them up into tiny droplets (emulsifies them). Then the intestinal and pancreatic juices can break up these droplets into fatty acids and glycerol —simple forms which the body cells can use. Three of the fatty acids essential for the body (linoleic, linolenic, and arachidonic) come from fats which are found only in butter, meats, egg yolks, soybean, cottonseed, corn, and olive oils. Therefore, some of these fat sources must be included in the daily food supply.

As the body uses fatty acids, it breaks them down into other substances called acetone or ketone bodies. These substances are further broken down into carbon dioxide and water and are excreted as waste products.

Cholesterol, a combination of fatty acids and alcohols, is found in all body tissues, especially in the liver, the blood, the brain, and the nerve tissue. Studies have shown that a high intake of certain fats may produce an abnormal storage of cholesterol in the blood, possibly causing fat deposits in the lining of the blood vessels and leading to atherosclerosis and heart disease. There is as yet no absolute proof that this is true, but much research is being done in this field. Among the foods which contain substantial amounts of cholesterol are butter, meat fats, poultry, shellfish, and egg yolks.

Fats vary in digestibility. Foods fried in fat, especially at high temperatures, are digested more slowly than foods boiled or baked. Although fats will produce about twice as much energy as equal amounts of carbohydrate, they are much more expensive as energy sources.

The average person in this country consumes more fat than the necessary amount, which should be about 20 to 25 per cent of his diet. His diet consists of about 33 per cent fat, which may have some bearing on the prevalence in the United States of heart and blood vessel difficulties, as well as problems related to excess weight.

## Proteins

Every animal, man included, must have protein to remain alive and to grow. Protein is the foundation element of every body cell. It is the only nutrient which will build tissue; it is the chief substance of muscles and glands, internal organs, brain, nerves, skin, hair, and nails and of essential enzymes and hormones. *"Protein"* comes from the Greek word which means "to take first place" and seems to be unquestionably the most important of all food substances.

Proteins come from both animal and plant food sources. Like carbohydrates, they contain carbon, hydrogen, and oxygen, but, in addition, they contain nitrogen; some proteins also contain phosphorus, sulfur, and iron.

Protein digestion starts in the stomach where an enzyme (pepsin) breaks down the proteins, to be further acted upon in the intestines by another enzyme (erepsin) and the pancreatic juice. The end products of these processes of digestion are chemical compounds called *amino acids.* Twenty-two amino acids are known at present—10 of them are essential for growth and body maintenance. Many years ago experiments to determine the value of proteins in the body showed that rats would not grow properly, or even stay alive, if some of the amino acids were omitted from their diet.

The number of amino acids and the amounts of each in individual proteins vary widely. Accordingly, proteins are classified as *complete, partially complete,* and *incomplete.* The complete proteins contain the essential amino acids in sufficient quantities for maintenance and normal growth; milk, meat, fish, poultry, eggs, and cheese are complete proteins. Partially complete proteins will maintain life but will not promote normal growth; they are found in cereals and vegetables and are important in the diet to supplement the complete proteins. Incomplete proteins alone will neither maintain life nor promote growth; the proteins in corn and gelatin are in this group. Because we usually combine a variety of foods in every meal, we obtain a combination of proteins that supplement each other. However, every meal should provide some form of complete protein.

Your daily selection of protein foods should allow an intake well above your needs to ensure an adequate supply of the essential amino acids. The daily requirement for good nutrition for a healthy person varies with age and body weight. The Food and Nutrition Board recommends protein as about 10 to 15 per cent of the total daily calories for men and women, estimated as 1 gm. per Kilogram of body weight; growing children need more per unit of weight. Pregnant women and nursing mothers need a higher percentage because they are supplying 2 people. In body conditions involving tissue damage or loss, the protein allowance is increased to help in tissue repair.

The blood stream carries the unneeded amino acids to the liver where they are changed into urea which is excreted by the kidneys and into sugarlike compounds which are used to provide energy. One of these compounds, glycogen, is stored in the liver; the others are changed into fatty tissue.

## Energy

Although science does not know exactly what energy is, it has been defined as the ability to do work. We can understand and measure several of the forms that energy assumes, such as light, heat, motion, sounds, and electricity.

The human body uses these different forms of energy in its many activities: for breathing, for circulating the blood or transmitting nerve stimuli; for moving the body or any part of it; and for the processing involved in digestion, absorption, and the utilization of food.

The process of using food to produce energy for the total activities of the body is called metabolism (mentioned already in previous chapters). Even an inactive person continually uses some energy for the work of the heart, the lungs, and all the tiny muscles in the body systems. The rate of this burning or oxidation process in the tissues producing the energy required just to keep him alive, to sustain only those activities fundamental or basic to living, is called the "basal metabolic rate" (BMR). In diagnosing certain illness conditions, it is sometimes necessary to determine the patient's BMR.

The amount of energy (measured in calories) which a normal individual needs depends on age, sex, weight, and the make-up of his body. It also is influenced by the kind of work he does. Children need a great deal of energy for growing and because they are very active. Older people use less energy. People at desk jobs need less than laborers, who are using their muscles a great deal. Men need more energy than women; large people use more than small people. Some people use a great deal of energy in the things they do for fun, such as walking or taking part in sports and games. Some household jobs take more energy than others—for example, sweeping takes more energy than mending. Certain body disturbances, such as fever or exophthalmic goiter, increase the amount of energy the body uses. Other disorders can prevent the proper utilization of food. It all amounts to this: the energy requirements of an individual are the sum of the amounts necessary to keep his body processes going and to carry on his activities. He provides this energy by the food he eats. Additional food intake or calories are stored as fat.

## What is a Calorie?

The unit of measurement for food energy is called a *calorie,* and the caloric value of foods can be determined in the laboratory. In this process an apparatus is used which measures the increased temperature of water as heat

## TABLE 22–2. RECOMMENDED DAILY DIETARY ALLOWANCES*

Designed for the Maintenance of Good Nutrition of Practically All Healthy People in the U.S.A.

| | Age | Average Weight | Average Height in Inches | Daily Caloric Need (calories per kilogram of weight) |
|---|---|---|---|---|
| Infants | to 1 year | 7–27 lb. | 18–31 | 100–120 |
| Children | 1–4 years | 26–35 lb. | 28–43 | 1100–1400 |
| | 4–6 years | 42 lb. | 38–49 | 1600 |
| | 6–8 years | 51 lb. | 42–54 | 2000 |
| | 8–10 years | 62 lb. | 46–59 | 2200 |
| Males | 10–puberty | 75–130 lb. | 55–67 | 2500–3000 |
| | puberty–22 years | 147 lb. | 69 | 2800 |
| | 22–35 years | 154 lb. | 69 | 2800 |
| | 35–55 years | 154 lb. | 68 | 2600 |
| | 55–75+ years | 154 lb. | 67 | 2400 |
| Females | 10–12 years | 77 lb. | 56 | 2250 |
| | 12–18 years | 97–119 lb. | 61–63 | 2300–2400 |
| | 18–22 years | 128 lb. | 64 | 2000 |
| | 22–35 years | 128 lb. | 64 | 2000 |
| | 35–55 years | 128 lb. | 63 | 1850 |
| | 55–75+ years | 128 lb. | 62 | 1700 |

(Pregnancy: add 200 calories)
(Lactation: add 1000 calories)

* Adapted from *Eat to Live*. Wheat Flour Institute, Chicago, 1969, p. 26.

given off by the burning of test food passes into it. Consequently, the definition of calorie is "the amount of heat required to raise the temperature of 1 kilogram of water 1° centigrade." A calorie is sometimes designated by a large "C" and is also called a *Kilocalorie*. The caloric values of the energy-producing foods have been determined as follows:

1 gram of protein will yield 4 calories
1 gram of fat will yield 9 calories
1 gram of carbohydrate will yield 4 calories

Table 22-2 lists the calorie allowances for individuals of various body weights and ages. Remember that this chart is based upon desirable weight, not upon actual weight. Remember also that each pound of excess weight represents 3500 extra calories.

Guides have been worked out naming the foods and estimating the amounts of each that a normal individual needs for light, moderate, or heavy work.

Calorie charts, giving the number of calories in a serving of the foods we use, are available without cost from a number of sources. The National Dairy Council puts out many excellent booklets which you can get from your local dairy council.

## Minerals

Minerals are vital to the body for building bones and teeth; they help to maintain muscle tone, to regulate body processes, and to maintain the acid-base balance in the body. Some minerals are used more readily by the body than others, and foods vary considerably in the amount of minerals they contain. Some minerals are lost in cooking, and some are lost in body wastes.

**Calcium.** Calcium, the mineral which the body needs the most, is the one most likely to be left out of the ordinary diet. Most of the calcium in the body is in the bones and the teeth. It has other important uses in keeping the body fluids balanced, helping with the clotting of the blood, and regulating heart and muscle and nerve responses. Calcium deficiencies cause poor teeth, rickets, damage

## TABLE 22–3. CALCIUM AND IRON IN PATTERN DIETARY FOR 1 DAY

| Food Group | Amount in Gm. | Household Measure | Calories | Calcium Mg. | Iron Mg. |
|---|---|---|---|---|---|
| Milk or equivalent......... | 488 | 2 cups | 332 | 570 | .4 |
| Egg ................. | 50 | 1 medium | 81 | 27 | 1.1 |
| Meat, fish, poultry ........ | 90 | 3 ozs. cooked | 256 | 11 | 3.2 |
| Vegetables: | | | | | |
| Potato, cooked ......... | 100 | 1 medium | 65 | 6 | .5 |
| Green, leafy, and yellow .. | 75 | 1 serving | 18 | 36 | .6 |
| Other ............... | 75 | 1 serving | 37 | 13 | .6 |
| Fruits: | | | | | |
| Citrus ............... | 100 | 1 serving | 43 | 19 | .3 |
| Other ............... | 100 | 1 serving | 85 | 11 | .8 |
| Bread, white, enriched ..... | 70 | 3 slices | 189 | 67 | 1.8 |
| Cereal, whole grain or | | | | | |
| enriched .............. | 30 | 1 oz. dry or | | | |
| | | 2/3 c. cooked | 86 | 13 | .9 |
| Butter or margarine ....... | 14 | 1 tbsp. | 100 | 3 | .. |
| | | | 1,292 | 776 | 10.2 |

Mitchell, H. S., Rynbergen, H. J., Anderson, L., and Dibble, M. V.: Cooper's Nutrition in Health and Disease, 15th Edition. Philadelphia, Lippincott, 1968.

to a mother's teeth and bones both before and after a baby is born, slow clotting of the blood, and disabilities of the muscles and nerves.

Milk contains more calcium than any other food. A quart of milk for a child and a pint for an adult will supply the body with its daily calcium requirement. Milk products are also high in calcium. Vegetables contain varying amounts of calcium, but some of them in a form which the body cannot use readily. The richest vegetable sources are broccoli, kale, turnip, and collard greens; other good sources are cheese and molasses. See Table 22-3 for the amount of calcium found in foods composing a satisfactory daily diet.

**Phosphorus.** Phosphorus is a constituent of every body cell, but most of it is in the bones and the teeth. It helps the cells to use proteins, fats, carbohydrates, and vitamins and regulates the acid-base balance in the blood. So many ordinary foods contain phosphorus that the body is almost certain to get enough of it. The best food sources are milk, fish, poultry, cereals, cheese, nuts, dried beans, and peas.

**Iron.** The body needs a relatively small amount of iron, but this amount is vitally important because it is an essential part of every body cell and a constituent of hemoglobin (which carries oxygen) in the red blood cells. The body is very thrifty with its supply of iron and uses it over and over by salvaging the iron from worn-out red blood cells. The best sources of iron are liver, meat, legumes, whole or enriched grains, green leafy vegetables, and dried fruits (see Table 22-3). Molasses and raisins are rich in iron, but are used in the diet in such small quantities that they are not practical sources.

**Sodium, Potassium, Magnesium, and Chlorides.** These minerals work together in a very close relationship and have many similar functions. They are essential for maintaining the osmotic pressure balance between the cells and the surrounding cell fluids; they also help to maintain the normal acid-base balance in the body. *Sodium chloride* is readily available in common table salt; sea food is another good source. Cereals, legumes, meats, and vegetables provide *potassium*. Since the amount required daily is relatively small and this mineral is found in so many foods, the ordinary diet provides adequate amounts.

*Magnesium* serves as a regulator of the action of other minerals and lack of it increases muscular irritability. It is present in large amounts in many foods, particularly in green vegetables; therefore, the ordinary diet provides an adequate amount.

**Sulfur.** Sulfur is a necessary constituent of the amino acids and is most highly concentrated in the bones, the hair, and the nails, although it is present in all body cells. Good food sources are liver, chicken, bluefish, dried beans, and peanuts, but it is widely available in protein foods.

**Iodine.** Although the amount of iodine in the body is small, the thyroid gland cannot function properly without it. The sources of iodine are sea water and sea salt and water in localities where the soil contains iodine. Some sea foods also contain iodine. Some parts of the United States have almost no iodine in the soil, especially near the Great Lakes and in parts of the Rocky Mountain regions. Since food products from these areas also lack iodine, goiter is common. This deficiency can be remedied by using *iodized salt*—a recommended practice in parts of the country where iodine is lacking.

**Trace Elements.** Some minerals are present in the body in very small amounts but are important in body processes. These elements are arsenic, aluminum, bromine, cobalt, copper, fluorine, manganese, nickel, silicon, selenium, and zinc. The ordinary diet provides an adequate supply.

*Copper* is an essential agent in the process of changing iron into hemoglobin.

*Cobalt* and *manganese* play a part in blood formation.

*Fluorine* is essential in forming tooth enamel.

*Zinc* is associated with enzyme activity.

No functions are known for the other trace elements although they are present in plant and animal tissues.

**Diet Planning.** The problem is to plan for an adequate mineral supply and yet keep the diet interesting. For example, the body needs a considerable amount of calcium. Turnips contain calcium, but the amount is so small that you would have to eat a great many turnips to supply your body needs for only 1 day. However, there is more calcium in milk than in other foods, and milk is easy to incorporate

into the diet, because you can use it in so many ways.

In choosing foods to supply minerals, select: (1) foods with the greatest amount of the minerals, (2) foods with the mineral in the form which the body can use readily, (3) foods with minerals which will remain in the body, and (4) foods high in minerals which can be appetizing in quantity.

## Water

Except for oxygen, nothing is more essential to life than water. Man can survive for weeks without food, but not without water.

We noted in Chapter 11 that about 60 per cent of the body's weight is water. Ordinarily the body excretes about 2½ quarts per day—in perspiration, in urine, and in the breath. In order to maintain the fluid balance in the cells of the body, the amount lost must be replaced. Food provides us with some fluid intake, but we must supplement this amount by drinking water and other liquids. Most authorities say the average adult needs 6 to 8 glasses of fluid every day.

The importance of water in the diet is evident. In studying the cells of the body, we learned that water was part of their major make-up. The nutrients are distributed to the body cells by the blood, of which water is one of the essential components. The presence of water within the body allows vital chemical changes to take place and is necessary in the control of body temperature. No organ of the body can function without water. Water is so necessary to life that Nature has provided man with an inborn safety device: thirst is his strongest appetite.

## The Vitamins

The word *vitamin* is a key to the importance of these substances in foods—*vita* is the Latin word for life. Vitamins have been recognized since 1911; they were discovered one after another, and new information is continually appearing. The body, with a few exceptions, cannot produce vitamins, nor can it store most vitamins; therefore an adequate daily supply is essential for health and growth.

Foods are the natural sources of vitamins and should supply our vitamin needs. (Vitamins are available in concentrated form, and physicians prescribe them for marked deficiencies.) Because some of the vitamins are not stored in the body, it is doubly important to ensure a daily supply; an all-around vitamin deficiency may not be the cause of a specific disease, but it does impair general health and efficiency.

Foods differ greatly in the amount and the number of vitamins they contain. Vitamins vary as to their solubility in fat (fat-soluble) or in water (water-soluble) and also in the degree to which they are affected by cooking temperatures. The following information applies to vitamins in general:

Some vitamins are lost by exposure to the air. They also may be lost in the storage of food. Frozen foods are second to fresh foods for retaining vitamins; canned foods retain a higher vitamin value if they are canned carefully and are not stored too long.

Some vitamins are soluble in fats and are stored in the body in this form. This means that the diet must include a sufficient amount of fat to provide an adequate supply of these vitamins.

Some vitamins are soluble in water. Therefore, foods should be cooked in a small amount of water and the cooking water should be used, if possible, in gravies and sauces.

High temperatures destroy vitamins; food should not be overcooked and should be served at once, in order to preserve vitamin content.

In some foods, the vitamin content is in the portion that is likely to be thrown away, such as the outer leaves of lettuce and the peelings of vegetables.

## Fat-Soluble Vitamins

VITAMIN A. Vitamin A (carotene) promotes growth, sustains normal vision, supports normal reproduction, and maintains healthy skin and mucous membrane, promoting resistance to infection.

The best sources of vitamin A are liver, spinach, and green and yellow vegetables. A bright yellow color identifies fruits and vegetables as being good sources. It is found also in cream, butter, and egg yolk, in highly concentrated amounts.

Surplus amounts are stored in the body; it is not destroyed by cooking.

VITAMIN D. Vitamin D (calciferol) is essential in regulating the use of calcium and phosphorus in the body. A marked deficiency in vitamin D hampers growth and affects the hardness of bones. This deficiency, plus an inadequate supply of calcium and phosphorus, causes rickets—a condition in which the bones do not harden as they should and bend into deformed positions, such as bowlegs. Before and after a baby is born, a mother must provide herself with enough vitamin D to prevent rickets from developing in the baby and to preserve her own bones and teeth. However, studies have shown that an overdose of vitamin D can have toxic effects, such as abnormal calcification of growing bones and the hardening of soft tissues, and may develop other serious complications. Therefore, large supplemental dosages should be given only under the guidance of a physician, especially when the pregnant mother and the growing child are concerned.

The best sources of vitamin D are the fish-liver oils. Vitamin D is formed in the body by the action of sunlight on the cholesterol products in the skin. Milk is not high in vitamin D, but the content is increased by irradiation and by adding vitamin D concentrate. Infants and children need supplemental amounts, but under normal conditions it is not usually considered necessary to provide supplemental vitamin D for adults. It can be stored in the body to some extent, primarily in the liver.

VITAMIN E. Vitamin E is called the reproductive or the antisterility vitamin. So far, there is no proof that vitamin E is necessary for human beings, but it has been proved that some animals definitely require this vitamin to reproduce successfully. It is found in many foods, especially in wheat-germ oils and green, leafy vegetables; it is also present in egg yolks and margarine. Heat seems to have little effect on it.

VITAMIN K. The body extracts vitamin K from its food sources via the same route that it absorbs fats from the small intestine. Any interference with fat absorption may result in a poor supply of any of the fat soluble vitamins, including vitamin K.

Vitamin K is essential in the formation of prothrombin, a substance necessary for the clotting of blood.

The average diet supplies an adequate amount of vitamin K, as it is found in a variety of foods. Good sources are liver, cauliflower, cabbage, spinach, and other green leafy vegetables. Margarine, soybean, and other vegetable oils are also sources. The limited amount stored in the body is found in the liver.

Deficiencies of vitamin K produce hemorrhagic symptoms. Intramuscular administration of vitamin K is often used to overcome hemorrhagic tendencies in the newborn.

### Water-Soluble Vitamins

VITAMIN C. Vitamin C is probably equally well known by its other chemical name, *ascorbic acid*. Its function has been recognized for many years, but further uses are still being discovered.

One of the contributions of vitamin C to our vital processes is the maintenance of the intercellular substances of the body. Since these are everywhere in our bodies, vitamin C contributes to healthy tissues and proper functioning of the blood vessels, skin, gums, bones, joints, and muscles—indeed, all tissues and organs of the body. Maintenance of these healthy organs helps to provide us with additional resistance to disease.

At present it is thought that vitamin C is related to both the formation and the hemoglobin content of the blood cells. Patients treated by surgery are frequently given large doses of ascorbic acid, since it is essential to and promotes healing of wounds.

The century-old classic disease of vitamin C deficiency is scurvy, a disease marked by bleeding gums, loose teeth, sore stiff joints, tiny hemorrhages, and great loss of weight. Lesser deficiencies affect health by causing listlessness, irritability, and lowered resistance to disease.

Vitamin C is probably the most unstable of the vitamins. It is destroyed by exposure to the air, drying, heating, and storing. Because vitamin C survives longer in acid surroundings, baking soda should not be added to foods in cooking, since it counteracts acids. Tomatoes retain vitamin C better than other vegetables because they contain acid. Freezing fruits and vegetables helps to preserve their vitamin C content, but they should be used immediately after thawing. Fruits and vegetables canned commercially retain this vitamin because the air is excluded during the canning process.

Since vitamin C is destroyed by heat as well as being water-soluble, cooking should be done in as little water as possible (the cooking water or juices should be used for other preparations). Overcooking should be avoided also.

VITAMIN B COMPLEX. At first, the group of vitamins presently known as the vitamin B complex was thought to be a single entity and was named vitamin B. Further research with the so-called vitamin B led to the discovery of several vitamins within the one, and each was given a name.

The B complex vitamins share the characteristics of being widely distributed in foods and soluble in water, but each of the members is chemically distinct. Each has functions which can be isolated, and each produces its own deficiency symptoms.

*Thiamine (B₁).* Thiamine promotes general body efficiency. It is necessary for growth, stimulates the appetite, aids the digestion, regulates the nervous system, and aids reproduction and lactation. Signs of a deficiency of thiamine are poor appetite, fatigue, irritability, listlessness, loss of weight and strength, depression, and poor intestinal tone. A very great deficiency causes beriberi, a disease of the nervous system which leads to paralysis and then to death from heart failure.

The best food sources of thiamine are the whole grain and enriched products: peas, beans and soybeans, pork, liver, meats from the glandular organs, and dried yeast. Some of the thiamine in milk is lost in pasteurization.

Thiamine is not stored in the body to any extent; it is soluble in water and is destroyed by heat.

*Riboflavin (B₂).* Riboflavin is essential for growth and plays a part in protein metabolism. A deficiency leads to skin and eye irritations. Riboflavin is not stored in the body to any extent; therefore, a steady supply must be provided.

Riboflavin is available in a wide variety of foods but only in small quantities. The best sources are liver, meats, milk and milk products, eggs, green leafy vegetables, whole grain or enriched bread, and cereals. If it is exposed to light while in solution, it disintegrates.

*Niacin.* Niacin (nicotinic acid) is essential to metabolism. A marked niacin deficiency in the body leads to the disease *pellagra*. The mucous membranes of the mouth and of the

## TABLE 22–4.  SUMMARY OF NUTRIENTS AND FUNCTIONS*

| | Key Nutrients | Important Functions | Important Sources |
|---|---|---|---|
| | **Protein** | Builds and repairs all tissues<br>Helps build blood and form antibodies to fight infection<br>Supplies energy | Meat, fish, poultry, eggs<br>Milk and all kinds of cheese<br>Dried beans and peas<br>Peanut butter, nuts<br>Bread and cereals |
| Water is also an essential, although people do not usually think of it as a food. Water helps in carrying nutrients to cells and waste products away, in building tissue, regulating temperature, aiding digestion, replacing daily water loss. | **Fat** | Supplies large amount of energy in a small amount of food<br>Helps keep infant's skin healthy by supplying essential fatty acids<br>Carries vitamins A, D, E and K | Butter and cream<br>Salad oils and dressings<br>Cooking and table fats<br>Fat in meat |
| Other B-vitamins are essential human nutrients: vitamin $B_6$, $B_{12}$ and folacin. Folacin and vitamin $B_{12}$ have antianemic properties, while vitamin $B_6$ helps enzyme and other biochemical systems to function normally. The three vitamins are widely distributed in foods—from meat, fish, poultry, whole grain and enriched bread and cereals, dark green and leafy vegetables. Milk provides vitamin $B_{12}$ and folacin. | **Carbohydrate** (Sugars and Starch) | Supplies energy | Bread and cereals<br>Potatoes, lima beans, corn<br>Dried beans and peas<br>Dried fruits, sweetened fruits; smaller amounts in fresh fruits<br>Sugar, sirup, jelly, jam, honey |
| | **Minerals**<br>Calcium | Helps build bones and teeth<br>Helps blood clot<br>Helps muscles and nerves to work<br>Helps regulate the use of other minerals in the body | Milk<br>Cheese, but less in cottage cheese, ice cream<br>Sardines, other whole canned fish<br>Turnip and mustard greens<br>Collards, kale, broccoli |
| Although the exact biochemical mechanism whereby vitamin E functions in the body is still unknown, it plays an important role as an intracellular antioxidant thus inhibiting the oxidation of unsaturated fatty acids and vitamin A. It is found in a variety of foods such as wheat germ oil, vegetable oil, egg yolk, milk fat, meats, butter, cereal germs and leafy vegetables. | Iron | Combines with protein to make hemoglobin, the red substance in the blood that carries oxygen to the cells | Liver, other meat and eggs<br>Dried beans and peas<br>Green leafy vegetables<br>Prunes, raisins, dried apricots<br>Enriched or whole grain bread and cereals |
| | Iodine | A constituent of thyroxine, a hormone that controls metabolic rate | Seafoods, iodized salt |
| | **Vitamins**<br>Vitamin A | Helps keep skin clear and smooth<br>Helps keep mucous membranes firm and resistant to infection<br>Helps prevent night blindness and promote healthy eyes<br>Helps control bone growth | Liver, eggs<br>Dark green and deep yellow vegetables<br>Deep yellow fruits, such as peaches or cantaloupe<br>Butter, whole milk, fortified skim milk, cream<br>Cheddar-type cheese, ice cream |

* Reprinted by permission of the National Dairy Council from *Nutrition Source Book*, page 5, 1971.

TABLE 22–4.   SUMMARY OF NUTRIENTS AND FUNCTIONS (*Con't.*)

| Key Nutrients | Important Functions | Important Sources |
|---|---|---|
| Thiamin or Vitamin B₁ | Helps promote normal appetite and digestion<br>Helps keep nervous system healthy and prevent irritability<br>Helps body release energy from food | Meat, fish, poultry—pork supplies about 3 times as much as other meats<br>Eggs<br>Enriched or whole grain bread and cereals<br>Dried beans and peas<br>Potatoes, broccoli, collards |
| Riboflavin | Helps cells use oxygen<br>Helps keep eyes, skin, tongue and lips healthy<br>Helps prevent scaly, greasy skin around mouth and nose | Milk<br>All kinds of cheese, ice cream<br>Enriched or whole grain bread and cereals<br>Meat, especially liver<br>Fish, poultry, eggs |
| Niacin or its Equivalent | Helps keep nervous system healthy<br>Helps keep skin, mouth, tongue, digestive tract in healthy condition<br>Helps cells use other nutrients | Peanut butter<br>Meat, fish, poultry<br>Milk (high in tryptophan)<br>Enriched or whole grain bread and cereals |
| Ascorbic Acid or Vitamin C | Helps make cementing materials that hold body cells together<br>Helps make walls of blood vessels firm<br>Helps in healing wounds and broken bones<br>Helps resist infection | Citrus fruits—orange, grapefruit, lemon, lime<br>Strawberries and cantaloupe<br>Tomatoes<br>Green peppers, broccoli<br>Raw or lightly cooked greens, cabbage<br>White potatoes |
| Vitamin D, The Sunshine Vitamin | Helps absorb calcium from the digestive tract and build calcium and phosphorus into bones | Vitamin D milk<br>Fish liver oils<br>Sunshine on skin (not a food) |

digestive tract become red and inflamed; lesions appear on the skin. The victims lose their appetite and lose weight; they experience vomiting and diarrhea and become weak and irritable; they also may become mentally disturbed. A lesser deficiency brings on these same symptoms in a milder form.

The best sources of niacin are lean meat, liver, whole grain and enriched products, and fresh and dried peas, and beans.

Niacin is a water soluble vitamin, not readily destroyed by heat and is stored in the body to a limited extent.

*Biotin.* Biotin is thought to be involved in the metabolism of amino acids. Although its exact function has not yet been established definitely, it is often included in multiple vitamin preparations. Food sources are liver, organ meats, whole grain cereals, and leafy vegetables.

*Folacin (Folic Acid).* Folic acid is an essential component of tissues and seems to be necessary in the formation of red blood cells. A deficiency causes certain types of anemia (a decrease in the number of red blood cells). It is a recent addition to the B complex group, and its use in the body has not been fully determined. Good sources of folic acid

*folic acid*

are liver, meat, eggs, fish, and green leafy vegetables.

✓ *also*

*$B_{12}$*. Vitamin $B_{12}$ is related to folic acid but is far more potent. It also is involved in the formation of red blood cells. A deficiency leads to anemia and to retarded growth in children. Food sources are the same as for folacin.

*Inositol*. The function of this vitamin is not known for human beings, although it seems to be necessary for animals. It is abundant in the average diet.

*Choline*. Choline is associated with the metabolism of fat and its storage in the liver. It is manufactured in the body, and since it is widely available in animals and plants, the average diet supplies it also.

*$B_6$ (Pyridoxine)*. Vitamin $B_6$ is one of 3 closely related chemical compounds which function in the cellular metabolism of amino acids. A deficiency causes retarded growth and nervous irritability. Although the exact requirement is not yet known, a sufficient quantity is assured in the average diet.

*Pantothenic Acid*. Pantothenic acid is involved in a number of metabolic processes in animals—especially in the metabolism of carbohydrates and of fats. Its importance in human nutrition has not been established yet, and although the requirement has not been determined, it is thought that the average diet supplies a sufficient amount.

*Para-Aminobenzoic Acid (PABA)*. There is no evidence of deficiency of this vitamin in man. Its functions are not yet verified, but it has been shown to be necessary for growth and for prevention of the graying of hair in certain experimental animals. Food sources are yeast, liver, whole grains, and molasses.

## A Daily Menu for Normal Healthy Persons

Eat at regular intervals, and remember that *breakfast* is the most important meal, because it follows a long period of fasting and sets the pattern for the day. Eating a nutritious breakfast will help keep you alert until lunch time. If you skip breakfast, you will be hungry and sleepy in the middle of the morning and unable to concentrate. To avoid feeling hungry by mid-morning, include some protein in your breakfast.

The largest meal should be eaten at noon, since afternoon activity will deplete the body's store of food. If the largest meal is eaten in the evening, the food may not be completely "used up," and the extra calories will be stored in the body as fat. As a nurse, of course, you may need to alter your meal plans to fit your working hours.

# 23

# From Market to Meals

---

### BEHAVIORAL OBJECTIVES

*The student successfully attaining the goals of this chapter will be able to:*

- *describe at least 6 factors to consider in planning meals.*
- *consider the attractiveness and palatability of foods when preparing or serving food trays.*
- *serve the correct tray to the correct patient at the correct time, always considering the desires, individual needs, and safety of the patient.*
- *report pertinent information regarding the patient's diet, accurately and appropriately.*

---

Food goes with friendliness and hospitality, especially on such occasions as morning coffee and afternoon tea, a picnic on the shore, or dinner by candlelight. To break bread with a man means to entertain him and honor him as a friend. The Bible speaks of manna in the wilderness and the miracle of the loaves and the fishes. Modern poets write about the delicious smell of new-baked bread and the spicy fragrance of pickles cooking.

## PLANNING AND PREPARING MEALS

You need up-to-date information about nutrition and preparing food (1) for your own health and (2) for the health of your patient. Diet is an important part of nursing care. Even if you do not always prepare your patient's food yourself, you are responsible for carrying out the doctor's orders. Sometimes it is necessary to consider racial and religious food customs in serving and preparing meals and diets. You cannot guide someone else in planning and preparing your patient's meals unless you yourself know how. Sometimes you may need to use tact in explaining changes in family meal plans and cooking methods; you can manage this if you stress the needs of the patient. Every-

body in the family is interested in your patient's recovery.

## Meal Patterns

Meals follow a pattern in any household or hospital. The same basic pattern can be used to meet the nutritional needs of everyone. You must think of:

1. The cost of meals
2. The types of meals
3. The attractiveness of meals
4. Foods that go together in flavor
5. Variety in texture of foods
6. Individual preferences or individual requirements (activity, age, illness, or body disturbances)
7. Safety of storage and preparation techniques

Most people are used to the pattern of 3 meals a day; the hours for serving these meals may vary to fit into family schedules for school, work, or leisure time. These meals are usually breakfast, lunch, and dinner. If dinner is served at noon, supper is the evening meal, with much the same kind of food as would be served for a noon lunch. It is possible to keep to a familiar pattern, to include the essential foods, and to provide variety through their preparation. Below are examples of adequate meals:

### BREAKFAST

| | |
|---|---|
| Fruit or fruit juice | Eggs or bacon |
| Cereal or bread and butter | A beverage—coffee, tea, milk, or cocoa |
| Cream, sugar | |

### LUNCH (OR SUPPER)

| | |
|---|---|
| Soup and/or salad | Fruit or other dessert |
| Sandwich or roll or bread and butter | Beverage |

### DINNER

| | |
|---|---|
| Meat, fish, cheese, or eggs | Vegetable and/or salad |
| | Dessert |
| Potatoes or rice or macaroni | Bread and butter |
| | Beverage |

## ATTRACTIVE SERVICE

Eye appeal is the first appeal to anyone's appetite. Can you think of a more appetizing sight than a golden-brown Thanksgiving turkey on a silver or china platter? Attractive service makes the most of food by giving it the best possible setting. Modern equipment for the table is so varied and colorful that you can make any table or any patient's tray alluring without using expensive linen, china, or silver; there are many attractive and inexpensive substitutes in cotton, paper, and plastics.

### Serving Food

Follow these simple rules when you serve food:

Keep the servings small. The sight of quantities of food may take away the appetite.

Serve hot foods hot and cold foods cold. Cover hot dishes.

Avoid dribbles of food on the edges of dishes.

Fill cups and glasses about three quarters full to avoid spilling the contents.

## PREPARING THE PATIENT

A tired patient, or one in pain, will neither take nor digest food well. Plan to carry out a lengthy or an uncomfortable procedure well before or after mealtimes. Emotional upsets affect the appetite and the digestion. Patients get the best effects from food when they are comfortable, happy, and relaxed. As far as possible, have your patient ready for a meal before you bring the tray. Wash his hands, and make him comfortable by giving him the bedpan, if necessary. Adjust his pillows and backrest if he is allowed to sit up; a patient with a poor appetite sometimes eats more if you can plan to give him a meal at the times when he is allowed to sit up in bed or in a chair. Do not let him get overtired before the tray arrives.

**Factors Influencing the Patient's Eating Pattern.** Pain and nervousness have already been mentioned as factors interfering with a person's appetite. Aside from these factors, the patient may not like the food served him, he may resent having to follow a particular diet, or the food served may not be in keeping with his religious or cultural customs. He may also find the diet too bland; medication can affect the taste of food. By explaining to the patient that the diet offered him has been "tailored" to his needs and by visiting him during mealtime, you can make mealtimes more pleasant.

## HOSPITAL FOOD SERVICE

The regular meals and the special diets for the patients in a hospital are planned and prepared by the dietary department headed by the chief dietitian. Hot food may be served from heated carts brought into the wards or the floor diet kitchens, where the trays are set up. Each tray is labeled with the patient's name and the appropriate type of diet. Nonetheless, it should be checked with the posted diet list or the Kardex. Every hospital has its own system of food service.

Train yourself to check each tray with the diet ordered. Learn to notice whether a napkin, a spoon, or a glass is missing before you carry the tray to the patient. See that bedside tables or overbed tables are ready; see that the patients are prepared for their meals. If you have a patient who must be fed, serve the trays to the other patients first. You are responsible for recording the necessary observations on the patients' charts and also for calling the attention of the head nurse to any unusual occurrence—from a poor appetite or the refusal of food to nausea or vomiting. This is important for the patient because you will need direction about what to do next to provide him with the food which is so essential for his recovery.

# 24

# Special Diets to Meet Patients' Needs

## BEHAVIORAL OBJECTIVES

*The student successfully attaining the goals of this chapter will be able to:*

- *demonstrate an understanding of the importance of the diet as an integral part of the patient's treatment by encouraging him to follow his diet and by providing meaningful patient teaching.*
- *briefly describe the full or general diet; identify some common modified diets, list foods included, and state an example of a physical disorder in which each might be prescribed.*
- *identify the consistency modifications in the diet as the patient progresses toward a full diet immediately after a major surgical procedure; give examples of other situations in which this progression might be used.*
- *demonstrate an understanding of the bland, high or low residue, high or low calorie, high iron, controlled carbohydrate, low sodium, and low purine diets by being able to recognize whether or not an individual patient's food tray has been correctly prepared and by identifying incorrect foods on the tray in an effort to protect the patient.*
- *effectively teach the person who is allergic to foods, so that the patient will have the most desirable diet which is possible for him.*

It will be easier to satisfy a finicky patient if he has a considerable margin of choice in the diet he is allowed, but many patients are on a diet prescribed as a part of the treatment of more than one body disturbance. For example, a patient with a heart condition also may be underweight; a convalescent surgical patient also may be a diabetic.

You can help a patient to like his diet by using color, variety, and camouflage. Many a milk hater has had his daily allowance of milk in soup, ice cream, or pudding, without being any the wiser. Attitudes about food are hard to change, especially if nutrition is a completely new idea to your patient, who may believe firmly that his stomach will tell him what is good for him. People also have many other false ideas about food, such as the acid in tomatoes sears the stomach, or a sick person will "lose his strength" if he does not have solid food. Sometimes it is difficult to make people see that the intestinal tract welcomes a rest after it has been upset. So you must persevere with a diet until the improved condition of the patient speaks for itself.

## KINDS OF DIETS

You will find that the patient is far more amenable to diet restrictions if he is not constantly reminded of his particular disease or condition by having diets classified according to the name of a disease. For instance, referring to the diabetic patient's diet as "controlled carbohydrate" deemphasizes diabetes and concentrates attention on dietary habits you want him to develop. The following classifications tell how diets are modified in the treatment of patients:

Diets with modification according to consistency

Liquid, soft, light, full, bland, high residue, low residue

Diets with modification according to energy value

High calorie, low calorie

Diets with modification of 1 or more of the nutrients

High iron (anemia), controlled carbohydrate (diabetic), controlled fat (cardiac), high protein (liver), low sodium (cardiovascular), acid-alkaline (kidney), low purine (gout), high vitamin (arthritis)

These titles show the kind of diet prescribed, although the amounts or the specific nutrients may be varied for an individual patient according to the doctor's orders. If there are no restrictions or special requirements, the patient may have any of the foods listed on his type of diet; you will be expected to know, generally, the kinds of food which will be allowed. Although the individual trays are checked carefully in a hospital, mistakes can happen. You should be able to recognize each type of diet and examine each tray with the patient in mind.

## Consistency Modifications

**Liquid Diets.** These diets consist of liquids only. They are given as a patient's first steps toward taking solid foods after an operation; they are given during an acute illness, or they may be the sole diet in specific body disturbances, such as irritation of the intestinal tract. According to the individual patient's needs, they may be *full* or *limited* liquid diets and are often used progressively. Feedings may be given every 2, 3, or 4 hours, as prescribed.

CLEAR LIQUID DIET

Fat free meat broth
Tea, coffee (without milk or cream)
Gelatin or Jello
Carbonated beverages
Sherbet

FULL LIQUID DIET

Soup—clear, strained or milk
Milk, cream
Milk sherbet
Plain ice cream
Well-beaten eggs in beverages
Cereal gruels
Strained vegetable or fruit juices
Tea, coffee

A full liquid diet can be used for long periods to supply adequate amounts of protein, fat, and carbohydrate if the patient is confined to bed. A limited or clear liquid diet is sufficient to replace body fluids but does not meet other nutrient requirements. For this reason, the patient progresses to a full liquid diet as soon as possible.

**Soft Diet.** A soft diet includes semisolid foods and is often supplemented with between-meal feedings; usually it is high in calories and is easily digested. The foods included are:

Soups—clear, strained vegetable, cream
Eggs—except fried
Milk, cream, butter, cottage cheese, cream cheese, mild cheddar cheese
Baked or mashed potato, milk flavored or sieved vegetables
Cooked or refined ready-to-eat cereals, refined rice, macaroni
Refined bread, crackers
Ground meats, white meat of poultry, fish
Milk puddings, plain ice cream, custards, gelatin desserts, sherbets, sponge or angel food cake
Sugar—a small amount
Tea, coffee

The doctor may order a modification of this diet that does not allow all of the foods listed above.

**Light Diet.** The light diet is sometimes called the *convalescent diet* and is the diet for preoperative and postoperative patients. It is more varied than the soft diet and precedes the full-diet stage. Usually it includes a liberal amount of calories, and the foods allowed are easily digested. The foods which are permitted are:

Soft diet foods
Broiled lamb chops, ground beef, liver, bacon
All but strongly flavored vegetables, dried beans, or gas-forming vegetables
All fruits
Salads and salad dressings
Macaroni, spaghetti, noodles; all cereals but bran products
Any kind of bread but bran
All desserts except rich pastries
Small amounts of concentrated sweets, such as jam, jelly, honey
Butter, cream
Tea, coffee

**Full Diet.** The full diet is really a normal diet; sometimes it has to be modified to meet individual needs, but it allows a wide choice of foods and includes everything but rich pastries and foods likely to cause digestive disturbances. Since all patients are comparatively inactive, the number of calories should be kept within the requirements for an inactive person.

The full diet is the most frequently used of all hospital diets. It is given to all ambulatory and bed patients whose condition does not require a special diet. It may also be called a general diet, a house diet, or a regular diet.

## DIETS AS TREATMENT

Diet plays an important part in the treatment of many diseases and in the correction of nutrition disorders. These special (therapeutic) diets will be discussed as a part of the treatment in the various conditions of illness. Some of the purposes of therapeutic diets are:

To regulate the amount of certain food constituents in disorders of metabolism (diabetes).

To increase or decrease body weight by adding or limiting calories (overweight or underweight).

To reduce or prevent edema (an accumulation of fluid in the tissues) by restricting salt (cardiac conditions).

To aid digestion by avoiding foods which irritate the alimentary tract or interfere with stomach action (ulcer).

To help an overburdened organ to regain its normal function (nephritis).

### Bland Diet

Diarrhea is a symptom of such intestinal disturbances as food poisoning, colitis, or typhoid fever, or it may be the result of improper eating or of taking laxatives. The diet prescribed depends on the cause of the diarrhea, but usually it is limited at first to clear broth and weak tea, then increased gradually. It is safer to give too little food rather than too much until the symptoms disappear.

This diet is designed to prevent stimulation of peristalsis and the flow of gastric secretions caused by chemical or mechanical irritation and also to reduce inflammation. It is employed in the treatment of ulcers, diarrhea, and colitis (inflammation of the colon).

In spastic constipation, the nerve endings in the intestines become oversensitive and irritated; this causes spasms and pain. Smooth, nonirritating food is given to soothe and rest the intestine until the spasms are relieved.

The diet of the patient with a severe ulcer may consist at first of one half milk and one

half cream (*Sippy diet*). Later, this is increased by adding puréed vegetables and fruits, strained cereals, eggs, and tender meats. Spiced or salty foods, tea, coffee, gravies, or broths are not allowed. The feedings are small and given frequently to keep the gastric juice in the stomach diluted and so reduce irritation of the ulcer. The temperature of the food served should not be extremely hot or extremely cold. This type of diet is called a *bland* diet.

### High Fiber Diet

A poorly balanced diet may be one of the causes of *atonic* constipation. The intestines need bulky waste to stimulate movement, so the diet for constipation, caused by a lack of bulk, includes plenty of the vegetables high in cellulose, fruits except blackberries, whole-grain cereals, and plenty of water, milk, cream, and butter. Fats in the diet serve to oil and soften the contents of the intestines.

### Low Residue or Residue-Free Diet

This diet is made up of foods which can be absorbed completely so that there is no residue left for the formation of feces. It may be used in cases of severe diarrhea and colitis, before and after surgery on the lower intestine and the rectum, and in partial obstruction. Suitable foods include tender meat, fish and poultry, fruit juices, gelatin desserts, rice, clear soups, and hard-cooked eggs. Coarse breads, cheese, milk, fried foods, fruits and vegetables and tough meats are to be avoided. Since this diet is deficient in both vitamins and minerals, it should be used for as short a time as is possible.

### High Calorie Diet

Science has changed the old saying: "Feed a cold and starve a fever." Studies have proven that the body cells burn food rapidly in fevers; therefore, the body needs *more* instead of *less* food in the case of a fever. The prescribed diet (high calorie) for a fever is usually high in fats, carbohydrates, and proteins. A fever interferes with the appetite, so you may need to give smaller and more frequent feedings. Unless there is a definite reason for excluding it, the patient is usually allowed solid food if he can chew and digest it easily. The high calorie diet also may be used whenever it is necessary to replace lost weight, as in cases of hyperthyroidism. It is used for weight-gaining in general undernutrition.

## Low Calorie Diet

When the body weight is more than 10 per cent above the average weight for height and age, this type of diet can be used.

The standard tables for *normal weight* according to height and age will not apply to everyone because some people have larger bones and are more active than others. This is why a reducing or a weight-increasing diet should be prescribed by a physician; he allows for these differences and for body disturbances.

*Overweight* comes from an oversupply of fat in the body tissues when a person takes in more food than he uses for energy. A safe reducing diet provides the necessary amounts of proteins, vitamins, and minerals and cuts down on the fat-making foods. Extreme diets followed by faddists are dangerous because these diets are usually completely unbalanced.

A diet of from 1,200 to 1,800 calories per day brings a weight loss of from 1 to 3 pounds a week—gradual enough to be safe. Here are some important points about this diet:

1. The normal amount of protein is allowed; 1 pint of milk, 1 egg, 2 servings of lean meat, poultry, fish, or cottage cheese will supply it.

2. The rest of the calorie allowance is divided between fruits, vegetables, butter, and whole grain cereals to supply minerals and vitamins. Liberal servings of low calorie vegetables and fruits help also to allay feelings of hunger.

3. Cream and sugar are not allowed, and the amount of butter is limited to 1 teaspoon per meal.

4. Water and salt are not restricted unless there is a special reason for cutting down the amounts.

5. If the diet is cut to 1,000 calories or less, the vitamin content becomes dangerously low, and concentrates should be prescribed and taken.

## High Iron Diet ANEMIA

The high iron diet is prescribed for patients with *anemia,* a condition in which either there is not enough blood (as a result of hemorrhage) or the red cells are deficient in quantity or quality. Iron is a necessary element in normal red cells. If it is deficient in the body, it can be supplied in the diet.

The diet given in anemia will depend on the type of anemia that the patient has. Before liver extract was developed, the diet for anemia included substantial amounts of liver. Today, doctors prescribe liver extract, to be given intramuscularly; the patient still may have some liver in his diet, but the amount required is less. The advantage of natural liver is that it contains iron, which liver extract does not. The diet for anemia also includes large amounts of red meat (kidneys, gizzards, sweetbreads, and brains) and green vegetables and fruits (peaches, apricots, prunes, raisins, apples, and grapes). It cuts down the amount of fats, sweets, and salt.

## Low Carbohydrate Diet

The low carbohydrate diet is used mainly by the diabetic patient in controlling his disease. Diabetes mellitus is a disease of metabolism in which the body is either partially or completely unable to utilize sugar (glucose), owing to the failure of the pancreas to produce enough of the hormone *insulin,* which regulates the amount of sugar used by the tissues. There are 2 main aspects of the treatment of diabetes. One is by giving doses of insulin. The other is to modify the diet so that no more carbohydrates are given than are necessary for the patient to maintain health and carry on normal activities.

## Low Sodium Diet

The low sodium diet is one which, while otherwise normal, has a decreased sodium content. This diet is given to patients with cardiovascular diseases, as well as certain kidney diseases such as nephritis and nephrosis, among others.

These patients sometimes are unable to excrete normal amounts of water and salts, with the result that these accumulate in the tissues and cause swelling (particularly in the extremities). This swelling is called *edema*.

If the sodium intake is reduced, the sodium and the water already in the tissues tend to flow back into the blood, where they are excreted. At the same time, the edema is relieved.

The diet for chronic heart disease is usually given in 5 or 6 small meals and omits gasforming or bulky foods. Bland, easily digested foods are given. Carbohydrates and protein are given in sufficient amounts; but such foods as milk, meat, eggs, fish, and fowl, all of which are high in sodium content, are limited. There is no restriction on whole-grain cereals, bread, fruits, vegetables, and unsalted butter. In this diet, no salt is added to foods, and foods preserved with salt are not allowed.

The overweight cardiac patient is usually on a reducing diet as well, since weight adds to the work of the heart. In arteriosclerosis and hypertension, the diet regimen is one that prohibits excessive amounts of fluid, alcoholic beverages, carbohydrate, protein, and fat.

### Acid-Alkaline Diet

If this diet is planned carefully, it can meet the requirements for normal nutrition. It is used in such conditions as kidney stones and edema to adjust the reaction of urine so that salts will be held in solution. Neutral foods such as butter, sugar, oils, and fat can be included. If an *alkaline urinary reaction* is desired, fruits, milk, and vegetables are emphasized. If an *acid reaction* is desired, flesh meats, eggs, cereals, breads, plums, prunes, and cranberries are served in large quantities. Supplementary vitamin A is usually given to reinforce the deficiency in this diet.

### Low Purine Diet

This diet is usually a normal diet with restriction of foods containing purine and is usually given in cases of gout. (Purine, one of the products of protein metabolism, further breaks down into simpler products, one of which is uric acid.) Since there is a disturbance of purine metabolism in gout, foods such as meats—especially organs—fish, gravies, whole grain cereals, breads, and such vegetables as spinach, cabbage, onions, and asparagus are restricted. Excessive seasonings, relishes, and alcoholic beverages are also eliminated. Obesity is frequently present; therefore, the patient may be placed on a low calorie diet as well (see Low Calorie Diet).

### High Vitamin Diet

A well-balanced diet, plus food high in vitamins, is indicated in arthritis, pernicious anemia, hyperthyroidism, malnutrition, pregnancy, and lactation. Foods to be included are: liberal amounts of eggs, milk, butter, liver, pork, whole grain cereals, citrus and other fruits, and green and yellow vegetables. If the deficiency is severe, vitamins should be given in concentrated amounts.

## DIET IN FOOD SENSITIVENESS OR ALLERGY

"It must have been something I ate!" It probably was. People who complain of indigestion usually find that it can be traced to food. Other signs of food sensitiveness are hives, hay fever, or asthma. Allergy specialists have found that milk, eggs, and chocolate seem to be the great offenders—cabbage, onions, tomatoes, pork, and strawberries are also high on the list. Some people are sensitive to wheat in any form, to potatoes, and to seafoods. The doctor finds the troublesome food by starting with a diet of foods that seldom cause trouble, such as lamb, rice, butter, sugar, and canned pears. If the symptoms disappear, other foods are added, one at a time, until the harmful food is found.

It takes skill to feed people who are highly sensitive to common foods. Substitutes containing the same food elements must be found. However, large amounts of these, given every day, may make the person sensitive to the substitutes. Avoid this problem by rotating these foods and giving small amounts at a time. Be careful, too, about giving dishes that are prepared from the offending foods, such as cakes made with wheat flour if the person is sensitive to wheat. A person who is only moderately sensitive to a particular food may eat it occasionally—for instance, if he is sensitive to eggs, an egg twice a week will not make him uncomfortable, but he cannot eat one every day.

# Unit 6:
# Deviations from Normal

25.  *The Signs and the Symptoms of Illness*

# 25

# The Signs and the Symptoms of Illness

## BEHAVIORAL OBJECTIVES

*The student successfully attaining the goals of this chapter will be able to:*

- *demonstrate an understanding of normal body structure and function by recognizing, reporting, and appropriately dealing with deviations from that condition recognized as normal.*
- *differentiate between a functional and an organic disorder; discuss how the 2 can become interrelated.*
- *define and give an example of each of the following classifications of physical disorders—hereditary, congenital, infectious, deficiency, metabolic, neoplastic, traumatic, and occupational.*
- *differentiate between subjective and objective symptoms and give an example of each; differentiate between acute and chronic conditions.*
- *observe the patient effectively, so that no pertinent symptom goes unnoticed; demonstrate an awareness of the meaning of these symptoms by reporting them at an appropriate time and in an effective manner.*
- *describe and report signs and symptoms of the patient in a consistent manner, avoiding ambiguous medical terminology, so that other members of the health care team will interpret the student's description accurately.*
- *describe edema and list at least 4 precipitating possible causes.*
- *list and define several objective words which could be written in the patient's chart to describe a cough, breathing, skin color or condition, emesis, hemorrhage, stool, body temperature, or pain.*
- *discuss the importance of good patient observation and list and describe 12 specific areas toward which the nurse's observational skills should be systematically directed.*

*Illness* and *disease* are the opposites of health and normality. Illness is a disturbance of the normal functions of the body and the mind as a result of a condition that is not normal. Disease is a change in the tissues of the body, in the operation of body systems, or in mental adjustments. *Infection* is a form of change in body tissues brought about by disease organisms. It is not to be confused with pathology, which is the study of *disease processes* in the body.

## Organic and Functional Diseases

You often hear a disease described as *organic* or *functional*. Organic disease means that some change has occurred in one or more organs, preventing them from carrying on their activities normally; functional disease means that no observable change has occurred in any organ, yet the patient feels sick and is sick. You can understand that the person with a functional disease can suffer just as much as the person with an organic disease. In many instances organic disease and functional disease seem to overlap. A peptic ulcer is considered by many physicians to be such a disease: at first the person experiences severe psychological stress (functional); eventually, if the cause of the stress is not corrected, physical changes occur which prevent normal function (organic).

## Categories of Deviation from Normal

There are various classifications of disease, or deviations from normal, none of which is really satisfactory because categories continually overlap. For example, diseases may be classified: (1) according to their cause; (2) according to the system of the body that is affected; and (3) according to the way in which they are acquired. Classifying disease according to cause is not always satisfactory because the ultimate cause of many diseases is still unknown.

Some common classifications of disease and causes of illnesses are:

*Hereditary Diseases:* If one or both parents pass on to the embryo a trait through genes that impairs some body function, the resulting disease is called hereditary. Hemophilia (prolonged blood-coagulation time) is inherited. Hemophilia is transmitted by the female but appears only in the male. The mother is the "carrier" and is free of symptoms.

*Congenital Diseases:* Congenital diseases are also present at birth, but unlike hereditary diseases, they are not transmitted through the genes. They are due to the effects on the fetus of some unfavorable condition which interferes with its normal development. Syphilis in the mother can be transmitted through the placenta; German measles, contracted by the mother during pregnancy, or drugs (thalidomide is an example) may cause body abnormalities or defects. Examples of abnormal fetal development are cleft palate, congenital heart disease, and clubbed feet (deformities of the bones in the feet).

*Infectious Diseases:* The most common of all causes of disease is invasion of the body by microorganisms, such as bacteria, viruses, and animal parasites.

*Deficiency Diseases:* These are disorders of nutrition as a result of deficiency of one or more vitamins in the diet. For example, lack of vitamin C causes scurvy. Deficiency in several vitamins, or general malnutrition, is more common in this country than a single vitamin deficiency.

*Metabolic Diseases:* These disorders are caused by a disturbance of one or more of the glands of internal secretion. These glands, known as endocrine glands, secrete hormones, which regulate body processes.

*Neoplastic Diseases:* This term is used to describe new growth of abnormal tissue, or tumors, which may be benign or malignant. A benign tumor is a growth of cells similar to the tissue in which it appears and is surrounded by a capsule. Once removed, it usually does not recur. It may be disfiguring, but it is not dangerous unless it crowds other structures or robs surrounding tissues of their blood supply. A malignant tumor (any form of cancer) is a wild and disorderly growth of cells that are unlike the tissues where they are located. This cell growth weakens bones, causes breaks in blood vessels, and robs normal tissues of nutrients; the cells also tend to spread to other parts of the body—this process is called metastasis.

*Traumatic Injuries:* This type of illness is the result of physical or mental injuries or shocks. It includes physical injuries, such as those incurred in automobile accidents or falls, or mental suffering, as from a personal loss.

*Occupational Diseases:* Certain occupational groups suffer from conditions peculiar to their jobs.

## The Course of Disease

Diseases progress in short or more lengthy stages. An *acute* disease comes on suddenly and runs its course in days. A *subacute* condition may go on for weeks or even months. The course of a *chronic* disease may be prolonged for years or for a lifetime. Complications involving other parts of the body may occur at any stage.

## Symptoms

Symptoms are the *signs* of disease. *Subjective symptoms* are sensations that only the patient knows about and can report—pain, itching, nausea, fear, worry. *Objective symptoms* are those signs that can be noted by an observer, such as a doctor or a nurse—a rash, swelling, pallor, pulse and temperature changes, hysteria, or weeping. Symptoms may be *local*, that is, limited to the affected part (swelling), or *general*, affecting most or all of the body (fever). In any case, it is clear that a nurse must first know what is normal, before she can recognize the deviations that she should record and report.

Some symptoms that are commonly associated with specific diseases will be fully discussed under the disease itself. Because they may also occur in other illnesses we mention them briefly here.

*Cough* usually indicates irritation somewhere along the respiratory tract. It is present in most respiratory diseases and in some heart conditions. A cough may be helpful or harmful. In some diseases it aids greatly in draining an infected area. In the absence of pulmonary secretions it serves no useful purpose and may even be harmful.

*Dyspnea* (difficult breathing) and *orthopnea* (inability to breathe except when upright) usually indicate some difficulty in obtaining or utilizing oxygen. These symptoms are frequently seen in cardiac and respiratory conditions.

*Cyanosis* (blueness of the skin due to a lack of oxygen in the blood) often occurs in the 2 conditions mentioned above. With diminishing bright red color in the blood, the patient's skin assumes a bluish pallor especially noticeable in the lips or the fingernails. This is true for Caucasian or Oriental patients.

*Jaundice* is another change in the color of the patient's skin. The patient generally develops a yellowish color, first noticeable in the whites of the eyes.

*Edema* (swelling) is the result of an abnormal amount of water in the tissues; there are several reasons for it. (1) If the return flow to the veins is obstructed in some way the pressure on the capillaries increases, forcing more fluid into the tissues. (2) Normally, the plasma proteins are retained in the blood vessels and help to maintain the osmotic pressure which keeps fluid in the blood vessels. If these proteins are reduced by disease, the fluid escapes into the tissues. (3) A high intake of salt tends to keep water in the tissues because the body attempts to retain fluid to dilute the salt. (4) Obstruction of the lymph vessels prevents them from carrying off tissue fluid. (5) Injury to blood vessels, causing them to lose plasma proteins, will cause edema.

Edema frequently occurs in loose tissues, such as the eyelids and the genitalia, while tightly constructed tissues resist edema formation. Edema is also more likely to occur in areas where the return flow of blood is slowest —in the fingers and the ankles, for example. Since edema fluid is toxic, the patient's fluid intake is not always radically restricted because fluids are needed to dilute these toxins.

*Emesis* (vomiting) has many causes. Sometimes it follows mental or emotional disturbance and has no physical cause. It may be due to disturbance or obstruction of the alimentary tract, varying in form according to the location of the difficulty; the vomited material also tells much about this. Fermented, undigested food indicates it has been returned from the stomach; bile-stained fluid is returned from the upper small intestine; fecal vomitus is returned from the colon. Blood in the vomitus indicates hemorrhage and is always regarded as a serious symptom.

*Hemorrhage,* or abnormal loss of blood into the tissues, may also indicate certain conditions. In the emesis or the sputum, blood may be a sign of disease of the digestive or the respiratory systems. Bright red or blackish, tarlike blood in the stool indicates digestive tract disturbance. Hemorrhage from accidental or surgical wounds can be fatal in a short space of time if it is not controlled. Bleeding into the tissues in varying amounts may be associated with diseases of the digestive and the urinary systems.

*Diarrhea,* or the passage of liquid, unformed, watery stools, may be caused by physical or emotional difficulties. It is sometimes a protective mechanism that the body uses to get rid of irritating or toxic materials. If diarrhea is the result of a deep-seated emotional problem, a nurse can help the psychiatrist or the physician in guiding the patient to a better understanding of and an adjustment to the problems of daily living.

*Fever* is an elevation of body temperature above normal and is another sign of the body's attempt to fight disease. It may develop suddenly or gradually. Associated with rise in temperature are 2 other symptoms of body changes: *increase in pulse and in respiratory rates,* which rise proportionately as the body temperature goes up.

*Fatigue,* as a symptom of disease, is extreme

tiredness for which no reasons can be found; sometimes it is due to the toxic effects of the disease.

*Loss of appetite or general weakness* may also be a symptom of illness.

A *sharp increase or decrease in blood pressure* may indicate signs of illness.

*Inflammation* is the body's attempt to fight infection or to cope with damage to body cells as the result of an injury which has caused a break in the skin (a wound). The following symptoms usually are found in some degree where there is injury or infection: (1) pain, (2) redness, (3) swelling, (4) heat, (5) loss of function, and eventually (6) the formation of pus.

| Symptom | Cause |
|---|---|
| Redness | Increase in circulation to the part |
| Swelling | Fluid and leukocytes leave blood stream to enter tissues |
| Pain | Pressure of fluid on nerve endings |
| Heat | Increased circulation |
| Loss of function | The body's attempt to keep injured area at rest |

Inflammation may be subacute or chronic. In acute inflammation an excess of fluid and cells is usually present in or issuing from the tissues (*exudate*). Exudates may be *clear* (serum) such as the discharge from a nasal cold; *fibrinous,* which causes adhesions to form as the tissues are repaired; *bloody,* as a result of small hemorrhages in the area; and *purulent,* due to bacteria. The formation of pus is called *suppuration.* In this process, the poisons of the bacteria kill off white blood cells and destroy tissue. The death of tissue is called *necrosis.*

The destroyed tissue may be cast off (*slough*), leaving behind it an area which needs to be filled in with new tissue. Sometimes there is a local unhealed area (of epithelial tissue), called an *ulcer.* A blind channel from a twisting wound which does not heal is called a *sinus;* a wound which has a small persistent opening that does not heal and connects with an internal hollow organ is called a *fistula.*

A *chronic* inflammation is one that persists over a long period of time and does not follow the usual process of healing.

## OBSERVING THE PATIENT

Because the nurse is with the patient for extended periods, her observations are invaluable as a guide to the doctor in determining the patient's treatment and in judging its effects. The doctor depends on you to include everything that is important. Your notes about every patient should create a picture of the person as an individual during his illness.

### What to Look For

The patient is able to give only part of the information about himself because he reports only the things that seem important to *him.* The nurse must be aware of signs she can see, hear, smell, and feel which are her responsibility to observe and report. It is the doctor's responsibility to decide what the symptoms mean and to prescribe the necessary treatment, but he depends on the nurse to observe them accurately. The nurse, in turn, must understand the significance of certain symptoms in order to give intelligent nursing care. Before taking up these observations in detail, it will help to consider the general categories to be included in observations of patients, such as:

1. Pain or discomfort
2. The food he eats
3. The amount and type of rest he gets
4. His body processes, including elimination
5. His behavior and body positions
6. His activities and interactions with others
7. His emotional and mental reactions
8. Treatments and their effects
9. Effects and side effects of medications
10. Observations of blood, urine, and other output
11. What the patient says about his condition
12. Objective symptoms which you can observe

1. *Pain or Discomfort:* Pain has been defined as a disagreeable sensation elicited by a potentially harmful stimulus. Its purpose is mainly protective.

MEASUREMENT OF PAIN:

Nature: Is it sharp, dull, burning, aching, squeezing, deep, pulsating?
Intensity: Is it mild, moderate, severe?
Location: Where did the pain start?
Duration: Is it intermittent or persistent? When did it begin?
Localization: Is it confined to one area or does it radiate to other parts?

Relation to circumstance: Is it associated with certain events?

How is it controlled? Is it relieved by medication, backrub, or other measures?

Pain is so much a part of illness and is so often misunderstood that we need to discuss it more fully than other symptoms. Pain may cause both physical and emotional discomfort, which varies greatly in intensity among individuals. The sensitivity of various parts of the body also differs. Some patients will try to conceal pain; others will exaggerate their symptoms. Still others complain of pain when no cause for it can be found. Thus, personality has a bearing on reactions.

Pain may be *local*, that is, affecting one part of the body, or it may be *general*, affecting more than one part. Pain is sometimes felt in one part of the body while the cause of it is located in another—this is *referred* pain.

2. *The Food He Eats:* Does the patient appear to be overweight or underweight? Does he exhibit any obvious signs of malnutrition? Is he eating the food served him? What does he say about the food? Is he nauseated? Does he vomit? Is he unusually hungry or thirsty? What is the condition of his mouth and teeth? Can he chew and swallow?

3. *The Amount and Type of Rest He Gets:* Does the patient complain of not being able to sleep? Does he seem tired, relaxed, restless?

4. *His Body Processes, Including Elimination:* Can the patient control his voiding and bowel movements? Are his elimination habits regular? Does he complain about elimination? Is his skin clammy, hot, moist; does he perspire profusely? Does he complain about being cold or too warm? Are his reflexes appropriate; do his eyes react to light? Does he have a cough, watering eyes, or runny nose?

5. *His Behavior and Body Positions:* Can he walk, sit, stand without assistance? Does his position seem to indicate that he is comfortable? Does he look worried or anxious? Is he expressionless? Is his face puffy? Is he pale or flushed? Are his movements jerky? Does he have tremors or muscle spasms?

6. *His Activities and Interactions With Others:* Does he visit with his roommate? Does he have visitors? Does he have some sort of diversional activity to keep him occupied?

7. *His Emotional and Mental Reactions:* Is he alert, disoriented, or unresponsive? Is there a language difficulty? Can he hear and see well? Is he oriented to time, place, and person?

8. *Treatments and Their Effects:* How does the patient react to nursing treatments? What do you observe about the positive or negative effects of treatments?

9. *Effects and Side Effects of Medications:* Are you aware of the expected effect and the possible side effects of the medications which you are giving?

10. *Observations of Blood, Urine, and Other Output:* The blood and the urine help to indicate the condition of the internal environment of the body. Is the urine clear or cloudy; does it contain sediment, blood, pus? What is the color of the urine; the amount? How would you describe the emesis; bowel movements; drainage? What do the laboratory reports state about the patient's blood and other output?

11. *What the Patient Says About His Condition:* The patient can often tell you how he feels. His own description is often a valuable guide and should be incorporated into his chart when possible.

12. *Objective Symptoms Which You Can Observe:* Does the patient have bruises, cuts, bedsores? Does his skin color provide any information about his condition? What information can be gained from his vital signs?

## Attitudes

You learn how a patient feels *about* himself and his treatment by observing his actions and listening to what he says. Is he cooperative, unreasonable, fearful, worried, cheerful? Does he talk about his problems? What clues does he give to his physical and mental condition? Again, you can report what you see him do, but he is the only one who can give you his reason for doing it. He may not give the real reason, but the reason that he gives may be a clue to his behavior and is valuable information for the doctor. This is why it is important to report this kind of information in the patient's own words. Be sure to include this information within quotation marks, so the doctor will know that it is a direct quote in the patient's exact words.

# Unit 7:

# Fundamental Nursing Skills

26. *The Patient in His Surroundings*
27. *Introducing the Patient to the Hospital*
28. *Assisting the Physician*
29. *Assisting the Patient to Meet Daily Needs*
30. *Nursing Treatment to Meet Special Patient Needs*
31. *The Patient With Special Oxygen Needs*
32. *Nursing Intervention for Patients Having Surgery*
33. *Administering Selected Medications to the Patient*
34. *Rehabilitation*
35. *First Aid and Care in Emergencies*

# 26

# The Patient in His Surroundings

---

BEHAVIORAL OBJECTIVES

*The student successfully attaining the goals of this chapter will be able to:*

- *integrate all of the concepts in this chapter into nursing practice, so that a safe and comfortable patient environment is maintained at all times.*
- *demonstrate a knowledge of cleaning methods used for various materials, such as glassware, metalware, instruments, and rubber or plastic items, as well as the items of furniture within the patient unit.*
- *safely clean a patient unit after discharge or death of the patient, taking into consideration the reason for the patient's hospitalization.*
- *inspect a patient unit and determine whether or not it is properly arranged and completely equipped; replace missing items.*
- *operate all equipment within the patient unit, including the bed and its attachments, the intercom, and the emergency call system.*
- *make an unoccupied bed, practicing protective body mechanics.*
- *make an occupied bed, providing safety, privacy, and comfort for the patient, while conserving the nurse's energy and while practicing efficient body mechanics, still protecting the nurse, as well as other patients from cross-contamination.*
- *allow for individual patient needs or desires in bedmaking; adjust bedmaking technics to attachments or appliances within the bed itself.*

---

## THE CARE OF A PATIENT AT HOME

Many practical nurses are employed in hospitals today, but there is also a great need for practical nurses to take care of patients who are sick in their own homes. Modern medicine encourages home care for patients who do not need the special services of a hospital during a long-term illness. With a shortage of hospital beds, home care makes more beds available for acutely ill patients. Also many patients are happier in a home environment.

Although your first experience with patients will be in a hospital, directions for their care also apply to the care of the patient who is sick at home or who needs additional nursing care after discharge from the hospital. The hospital has all the necessary nursing equipment, but in the home, the patient must provide it. The local visiting nurse service and the local Red Cross chapter frequently lend equipment for home use. In addition some types of equipment can be rented from a surgical supply house.

## THE HOSPITAL

In the hospital the patient is the center of nursing care; all hospital functions revolve around him. The nurse, as a member of the hospital team, assists by teaching the patient self-care and by doing for or with the patient those things which he cannot do by himself.

In the hospital, you will have more than one patient to take care of and you will need to consider hospital routines. Meal hours, doctors' rounds, patients' appointments for the operating room or the x-ray room and for laboratory procedures must also be considered when you make your work plan. You may be asked temporarily to assist with the emergencies that come up on a busy service. In any situation, remember that your patients are your first responsibility.

In a hospital, much of the housekeeping may be taken care of by other workers; but you are responsible for keeping your patient's immediate surroundings neat and clean, and the head nurse expects you to cooperate with other workers who may help with this part of your work.

Hospitals today give a great deal of thought to providing patients with surroundings that are pleasant as well as practical. Walls that once were a muddy beige may now be a restful pale green or blue; draperies adorn bare windows; attractive furniture has replaced those dull brown or glaring white pieces. The patient has a light that he can control and adjust, and he may have a telephone, a radio with earphones, and a television. In a ward or semiprivate room, cubicle curtains give him privacy. In addition, air-conditioning equipment regulates temperature and ventilation.

## Ventilation

Ventilation means providing a supply of clean air, with the proper amount of moisture, at a comfortable temperature. The problems of ventilation vary with the climate, the season, the living quarters, and individual preferences. In any case, some way must be found to keep the air moving because the comforting and healthful effects of good ventilation are produced by the movement of the air currents against the skin.

**Air.** Pure air is composed of gases in approximately these percentages: oxygen, 20 per cent; carbon dioxide, 0.04 per cent; and nitrogen, 78 per cent. Of course, we never breathe absolutely pure air because air always contains organisms and particles of dust; however, we do want clean air, which is air that contains a minimum amount of dust and other particles and is free from unpleasant odors.

**How to Ventilate a Room.** Warm air is lighter than cold air, and outside air is often colder than inside air; if you open a window from the top and from the bottom, the warmed used air escapes and the cooler fresh air comes in. An electric fan will keep the air moving in a room.

**Precautions in Ventilation.** Always protect your patient's body from contact with strong air currents or drafts, to prevent chilling. Open a window that is not parallel with his bed; if his bed and the door are parallel, use a doorstop to prop the door part way open. If there is no choice of windows, put a screen between the window and the bed.

When a patient is out of bed, you can protect his body from chilling by using extra clothing and blankets and by placing his chair out of the way of drafts.

Air-conditioning equipment now washes and strains fresh air, heats or cools it to a comfortable temperature, brings it to the proper degree of humidity, and circulates it.

It is the temperature of the air around you that affects your comfort. The balance between the heat you lose and the heat you produce must be right. The room temperature that keeps this balance is between 68° and 74° F.

## Using Electrical Equipment

Remember that water conducts electricity, so be sure that your hands are dry before you insert a plug in an electric outlet; never turn a light off or on or touch a radio when you are in the bathtub or standing on a wet floor. Always disconnect equipment by grasping the plug—pulling on the cord loosens it from its plug connection. Always have frayed or worn cords repaired to prevent short circuits and blown fuses. Disconnect equipment or turn off motors as soon as you have finished using electrical apparatus. Motors are lubricated with grease packed inside; some equipment is lubricated with light oil. Motors should not be overheated or allowed to run dry; excess heat or burning odors from a running motor indicate that something is wrong.

## Intercommunication System ("Intercom")

If the hospital has an "intercom" system, you will learn how it works, so that you can teach the patient. Since it is bewildering to a patient to be faced with unfamiliar equipment, you will want him to know how to use it so that he will not be frightened by it and will not hesitate to use it if he needs assistance.

**The Nurse's Call Light.** The signal cord or call light must always be within reach of the patient. Remind him to use it whenever he needs assistance.

## Ward Order

The patient's unit should be kept neat and orderly at all times. Good housekeeping helps to prevent accidents and helps the nurse to carry out her duties efficiently. Everything should be so arranged that it can be located by all personnel. These measures help the patient to feel secure and make it less likely that the staff or the patient will fall or trip.

## HOW TO CLEAN EQUIPMENT

Wash glassware in soap or detergent solutions. When washing glass syringes, use the special small brushes which are available for cleaning the inside of the syringe. To prevent material from drying on the surface soak the items before washing.

Clean monelmetal and enamelware with soap or detergent solution and remove stubborn spots with an abrasive. Sterilize under steam pressure if possible. Pay special attention to cleaning bedpans and urinals. Equipment for flushing bedpans after use is provided in many hospitals. Bedpans should be handled in the same manner as other similar ware.

Instruments are made of stainless steel, nickel-plated steel, or chromium. Scrub instruments with a brush and soap or detergent solution to remove material from grooves and crevices. Dry them well to prevent rust. Instruments should be sterilized under steam pressure except for those with a cutting edge, which are sterilized with dry heat or sometimes with a chemical disinfectant.

Wash rubber items with soap or detergent solution, forcing the solution through catheters or tubing to clean the inside. They should be rinsed as soon as possible after being used. Rubber goods are best sterilized under steam pressure although dry heat or boiling may be used. Almost all rubber or plastic goods are discarded after use.

Rubber gloves are powdered before they are sterilized so that they will slip on easily; a packet of sterile powder is provided to powder the hands. In some hospitals plastic disposable gloves are used. Gloves may be sterile or unsterile, depending upon the purpose for which they are used. In any case, they should be airtight (unperforated).

Normal laundry processes are usually considered adequate for cleaning linens. In hospitals, linen from patients with infectious diseases is placed in specially marked bags to be washed with special precautions.

Many items used in the modern hospital are disposable; that is, they are used one time or for only one patient and are then discarded. This is a much safer method because it prevents the spread of disease from one person to another via equipment.

Once you know how to take care of wood surfaces, enamelware, glass, rubber goods, and linens, you can apply what you have learned to either housekeeping or nursing equipment. Oil will have the same effect on an enema tube as grease will on a rubber-covered dish drainer. Boiling water poured over a glass measuring graduate will behave like boiling water poured on a drinking glass at the kitchen sink. The scouring powder used on enamel saucepans will be equally effective on enamel bath basins.

## THE PATIENT UNIT

We call the place where the patient's bed is located *the patient unit*. It includes the bed and the other furniture and most of the equipment used in his care. This unit may be in a private or a semiprivate room or in a ward.

The basic equipment for a patient unit includes:

*Furniture:* Bed, bedside table and chair, lamp, overbed table

*Linen:* Sheets, drawsheet, pillow cases, blankets,

spread, bath blanket, face towel, bath towel, wash-cloth, bedpan cover, gown

*Toilet equipment:* Wash basin, soapdish, tooth-brush container, kidney basin (emesis basin), tumbler, comb and brush, toothbrush, nail brush, bedpan (and urinal for male patient)

*Other equipment:* Moisture-proof drawsheet, water pitcher and drinking glass, thermometer in container, call bell or button, screen or curtain

Equipment for nursing treatments is kept outside the unit, in the treatment, tray, or utility room. The unit should always be complete and ready to use. This saves steps and time, as well as delay which is wearing for the patient.

## Restocking the Unit

Check and replace used supplies; check the equipment and inspect it for breaks, cracks, or rough places that might injure patient or nurse. Replace broken or damaged equipment and report the damage to the head nurse so that the equipment can be replaced or re-paired. It is customary in many hospitals to keep an inventory of the equipment on each floor as a basis for ordering new articles or replacing damaged ones.

## Cleaning the Patient Unit After Use

For years, cleaning the unit had been the nurse's responsibility. In many hospitals to-day, auxiliary personnel attached to the nurs-ing or the housekeeping departments are responsible for this procedure, thus giving nurses more time for the care of patients. However, every nurse should know how to clean a unit according to the policy of the hospital and the principles of asepsis. In some situations, this procedure is still the nurse's responsibility.

Everything in the unit is considered soiled and must be cleaned before it can be used by another patient. This prevents the possibility of transferring infection from one person to another, and it is esthetically satisfying to the patient to know that he is not using someone else's things.

You clean the unit after a patient has been discharged from the hospital or transferred to another room or ward, or after a patient dies. It is important to handle pieces of bed linen separately, making certain none of the pa-

tient's possessions are discarded with the soiled bedclothes. Remember that the hospital is responsible if a patient's personal possessions are lost.

KEY POINTS IN THE PROCEDURE

Avoid touching your uniform with soiled linen or equipment.

*Principle: Microorganisms are transmitted by contact.*

Use a dampened brush to remove dust or lint, thus avoiding the scattering of micro-organisms.

*Principle: Microorganisms are found on dust particles.*

Wash furniture with soap and water or spe-cific detergent and rinse in clear water and dry.

*Principle: Cleansing removes organisms and foreign material.*

Clean the least soiled areas first.

*Principle: Moving from a soiled area to a cleaner area spreads organisms.*

Wash all equipment used by the patient with soap and water or detergent before steril-izing it.

*Principle: Cleansing helps to make steriliza-tion more effective.*

# BEDS AND BEDMAKING

## Types of Beds

Rest in bed is usually a part of the patient's treatment—sometimes the all-important part, as it is for patients with heart conditions or tuberculosis. Therefore, the bed must be right for comfort and for good posture. A good bed is made of metal or wood and is durable, light-weight, easy to move, and easy to clean. These are the measurements that meet the require-ments for comfort: 6 feet 6 inches long; 3 feet wide; and 26 inches from the floor to the springs. Most hospital beds today are the Gatch type, equipped with a spring frame and a crank or electric motor so that they can be adjusted to different positions.

Hospital beds (Hi-Lo) are now available and are equipped with an electrical mecha-nism to lower and raise the bed so that the patient can get in and out of it easily. The patient who is being encouraged to help himself can operate this mechanism. The CircOlectric bed makes it possible to put the quadriplegic patient in an upright position or to turn a patient more easily.

## Purpose in Bedmaking

The main objective in bedmaking is to add to the comfort of the patient. This means clean linen—a tight lower sheet to prevent wrinkles which might irritate the skin; and upper bedclothing which does not weigh on the patient's body or restrict his movements, but still covers his shoulders. Adjustments in the procedure may be necessary for the comfort and the convenience of individual patients and to suit temperature conditions and the patient's condition.

Making the bed every day is a routine procedure in patient care which is carried out after breakfast or following the patient's bath or morning care. Exceptions to this rule are made when changing the bed may prove harmful to the patient. For example, a patient may be bleeding, may be having a special treatment, or may be too weak or exhausted to move.

Keep the patient's body in as good alignment as possible while making his bed. At the same time, be certain *you* are practicing good body alignment.

## Making a Bed

Each hospital has its own method for making different types of beds, and you will learn the procedure followed by the hospital in which you are working. The details may vary, but the principles to follow are the same. Since you will make a great many beds while you are a student nurse and many more as a graduate, it is important to know how to make them correctly and with the least amount of effort. Good body mechanics are essential.

BODY MECHANICS IN BEDMAKING

Face in the direction of your work and move along with the work as you place bedclothing on the bed to avoid twisting and over-reaching.

*Principle: Muscles work in groups. Twisting distorts their position and causes strain.*

Separate your feet slightly and flex your knees when tucking bedding under the mattress.

*Principle: The longest and the strongest*

*muscles are made to do the work when the knees are flexed and the back is in good alignment.*

Open and spread bed linen on the edge of the bed. Lifting it to shoulder level puts strain on the back.

*Principle: Lifting uses more energy to overcome the pull of gravity.*

Work with your hands palms downward when pulling sheets tight, using arm and shoulder muscles. Advance one foot and rock back.

*Principle: The longest and the strongest muscles are the most efficient. Firm support and rocking backward and forward add the power of body weight and reduce the effort required of the muscles.*

## Making a Closed Bed or an Unoccupied Bed

You usually make a closed bed when preparing the unit for a new patient, or when your patient is able to get up in the chair or walk. Follow the same procedure as in making an occupied bed with these exceptions:

Start with an empty bed.
Stay on one side of the bed until it is finished completely.
Fold the top sheet back over the blanket before putting on the spread.
The top of the spread is even with the top edge of the mattress.
The pillows are placed one above the other with the open edges facing away from the door.

## Making an Occupied Bed

The method used to make an occupied bed should be one that disturbs the patient the least and requires minimum exertion for patient and nurse. Opinions vary as to the most efficient ways of reducing efforts, but with any method, you will need to make necessary adjustments for the individual patient. For example, bed cradles and other appliances require special arrangements of the bedclothing. Some patients need extra blankets for additional warmth, and some may have fractures or injuries that necessitate their being turned or moved in a special way.

**Equipment.** The amount of linen listed here is what you would use to change a bed completely or to make up a bed after cleaning

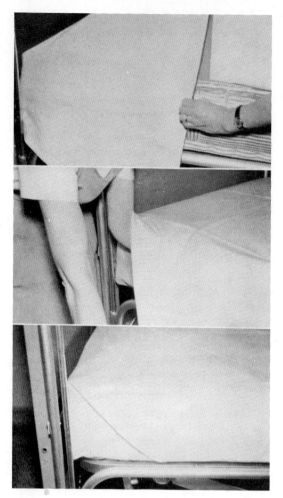

Figure 26-1. (*Top*) The first step in making a diagonal corner. (*Center*) The second step in making a diagonal corner. (*Bottom*) The completed corner.

a unit. Hospitals do not usually allow this much clean linen every day; adjustments in using the necessary minimum amount are explained:

| | |
|---|---|
| 1 bed pad | May not be used in some hospitals or may not need to be changed daily. |
| 2 large sheets | One clean sheet may be allowed if the used top sheet is to replace the bottom sheet on the bed or if you have a cotton drawsheet. |
| 1 cotton drawsheet (optional) | If a folded top sheet is used for this, you will need 2 large sheets. |
| 2 pillowcases | You may use only 1 and change the pillowcase on alternate pillows every day. |
| 2 blankets | The number of blankets depends on the weather, the patient's condition, and his preference. |
| 1 bedspread | |

### SUGGESTED PROCEDURE

Bring clean linen to bedside table or chair.

*Guide: The linen should be placed on a clean, clear space and arranged in the order in which it is to be used.*

Loosen the linen all around the bed.

*Guide: Place one hand under the mattress to prevent tearing the linen.*

Pull mattress up to the head of the bed.

*Guide: Ask the patient to help or get assistance, if necessary.*

Fold back and remove the spread, placing it over the back of the chair.

*Guide: Fold the top down to the bottom and pick it up in the center. If the spread is to be discarded, put it in a laundry bag or a hamper for soiled linen. Never put soiled linen on the floor (which is always contaminated) or allow it to touch your uniform. Do not shake linen—this spreads organisms.*

Fold the blanket, remove it, and place it over the back of the chair.

Place the bath blanket over the top sheet.

*Guide: If the patient's condition warrants it, ask him to hold the top of the blanket in preparation for the next step; if not, tuck it under his shoulders.*

Remove the top sheet.

*Guide: Fold from head to foot and place it on the back of the chair if it is to be used in remaking the bed.*

Remove pillows and one or both cases.

*Guide: Leave 1 pillow if the patient is uncomfortable without it; put the soiled case or cases with the soiled linen.*

Turn patient toward the other side of the bed.

Roll soiled drawsheet toward the patient—repeat with the protective sheet and bottom sheet.

*Guide: Gather together in folds and push close to patient.*

Pull mattress pad smooth if it is not being changed.

*Guide: Patients with excessive drainages may have to have the pad changed daily. It is rolled toward the patient in the same manner as above.*

Place a clean large sheet or used top sheet on the bed.

*Guide: Center it lengthwise, lower edge even with the mattress surface. If it is long enough after allowing 18 inches at the top, the sheet will also tuck under the bottom.*

Gather the farther half of the sheet into a roll and push it against the patient and under the soiled bottom sheet.

Tuck a clean sheet under the mattress at the top.

*Guide: Pull it under and toward the foot as far as you can reach easily.*

Make the corner: Pick up the selvage edge; lay a triangle back on the bed; tuck the hanging part under the mattress; drop the triangle over the side of the bed; and tuck the hanging edge under the mattress (see Fig. 26-1).

*Guide: The selvage is straight up and down against the side of the mattress—the palm of one hand is next to the springs.*

Tuck the sheet under, all along the side of the bed.

*Guide: If the sheet covers the lower end of the mattress, make a corner. Fitted sheets are often used and are much more convenient.*

Tuck the nearer half of the drawsheet under the mattress, if a drawsheet is used.

Turn the patient back toward you—lift his feet over all sheets.

*Guide: Lift the edge of the blanket slightly so that he will not lie on it. Be sure that he cannot roll out of the bed.*

Push the rolled sheets out.

Go to the other side of the bed and pull the sheets through.

Roll and remove the soiled bottom sheet—straighten the rubber sheet—remove the soiled drawsheet.

*Guide: Bunch each soiled sheet as you remove it and put it with the soiled linen.*

Turn the patient on his back.

*Guide: Do not turn him if you want him to lie on his side or if he is unable to lie on his back.*

Adjust the bottom sheet.

*Guide: Tuck it under at the top, make a corner, tuck in the sides—pull all the way down to the side, a diagonal pull—tight and*

smooth; brace your thigh against the bed and keep your back straight for good posture and efficient body mechanics.

Pull the rubber sheet tight and tuck it under the mattress—repeat for the drawsheet.

Put the clean pillowcases on one pillow or both.

*Guide: Do this with the pillow resting on a flat surface. Open the case down into corners and grasp it at the outside at the center of the end seam. Turn the case back over your hand and grasp the pillow from the outside and adjust the corners into the case. Turn the case up over the pillow and adjust it evenly; the pillow should not touch your clothing.*

Place and adjust the pillow or pillows under the patient's head.

Place the top sheet over the bath blanket.

*Guide: Place it wrong side out. This will be right side out when turned back over the blanket. Allow sufficient length to turn it back.*

Remove the bath blanket. Put the blanket over the sheet.

*Guide: The patient can hold the sheet at the top if he is able; pull the bath blanket out. Place the wool blanket shoulder high.*

Make a box pleat in the blanket and the sheet together at the center of the lower end of the bed.

*Guide: This allows for toe room.*

Tuck together under the mattress—make a corner.

Put on the spread; turn the top edge back under the top edge of the blanket.

*Guide: The upper edge extends beyond and above the end of the blanket. The turn-under holds the top covers and protects the blanket.*

Turn the top sheet down over the spread.

*Guide: This protects the spread, and the hem is now right side out.*

## Opening a Bed for a Patient

A bed is opened for a new patient, or it may be left this way when the patient is out of bed for a short time.

### SUGGESTED PROCEDURE

Turn the spread down from the top and fold it under the top edge of the blanket. Turn the top sheet back over the spread.

*Guide: This protects the blanket, keeps the rough blanket away from the patient's skin,*

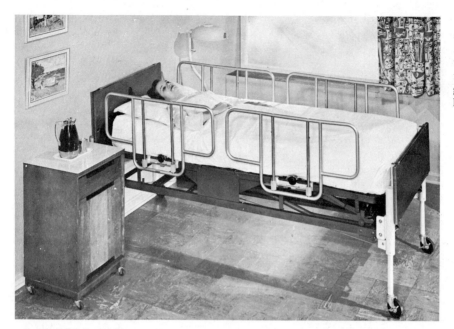

Figure 26-2. Metal side attachments for hospital beds used when patients are restless and likely to get out of bed. (Hill-Rom Co. Inc., Batesville, Ind.)

*and makes it easier for the patient to handle the bedclothes.*

Turn the top bedding down to the foot of the mattress and fold it back on itself.

*Guide: This shows the patient that his bed is ready for him. It is also easier to help him back into the bed when it is open.*

*Always* leave the bed in low position to prevent falls.

## Using a Bed Cradle

A bed cradle is a frame used to keep the bedclothes from touching all or part of the patient's body. A wide cradle fits across the bed; a narrow one fits along the bed lengthwise—it can be used over one arm or leg. Bed cradles usually are made of metal.

A cradle is used for fractures, extensive burns, and wounds. Some cradles are equipped with light bulbs fastened under the top of the frame; they are used to supply heat or for special treatments. If you are using an electric heat cradle, make sure that the temperature of the patient's skin is checked frequently to prevent burns. With impeded circulation, the patient may not be aware of excessive heat. Be careful not to get water on the connections when you clean this kind of a cradle; be sure that your hands are dry if you handle it when the current is on. Clean a

cradle as you would any metal or enamelware.

A patient using a cradle may feel chilly with so much air space around him. You will make the foot end of his bed first, using extra linen if the cradle is over his feet and legs. This provides covering long enough to protect his shoulders and to tuck in snugly over the cradle.

## Adjusting Bedsides

Bedsides, also called side rails or safety sides, are used to prevent restless patients from getting out of bed and to protect others from falling out of bed (see Fig. 26-2). Metal bedsides with self-adjusting hooks covered with rubber to protect the bed are easy to handle. Most hospital beds are now equipped with side rails.

Bedsides are used for restless or irrational patients or those who are unable to control their movements. If a patient resents bedsides, remember that this is natural. Most people have a fear of being shut in or of being treated as if they were irresponsible. Try to make a patient understand that the bedsides are used to protect him. Explain this to the family, too. Failure to provide for the safety of the patient until the need arises may result in injury to the patient. Because courts have held the nurse liable in similar situations, it is always wise to know the policy of the institution in which you are employed.

Usually the patient shows signs of confusion and loss of muscle control before actually needing the bedsides. Report such signs. If you have any reason to think that it is dangerous, never leave a patient alone. Sometimes the patient's condition changes so rapidly that you need to provide this protection for him suddenly. Let the head nurse know immediately if this happens. Never put on the sides or remove them without permission. You can remove one side when you are bathing a patient or giving him other care. Be sure that help is near if the patient is likely to try to get out of bed. If it is necessary to protect the patient from pressure or injury, pad the bedsides. Restless patients may press or throw themselves against the hard metal.

## Other Bed Parts and Equipment

*The Footboard:* A footboard may be attached to the foot of the bed to prevent the deformity called footdrop. This device is discussed in greater detail in Chapter 45.

*The Bed Board:* A board may be placed under the mattress to provide greater back support.

*Traction Equipment:* The patient may be placed in traction; or a trapeze may be necessary so that he can pull himself up to a sitting position. These devices are usually attached to a large frame, which is attached to the bed.

*The I.V. Stand:* Most hospital beds are equipped with a means for attaching a standard that holds bottles for intravenous or blood therapy.

*The Emergency Headboard:* Most hospital beds are equipped with a detachable headboard that may be placed under the patient in the event that emergency cardiopulmonary resuscitation is needed. (See Chapters 35, 47, and 48.)

*The Overbed Table:* The patient unit also includes a table that fits over the bed. It is useful when the patient is eating, reading, or grooming himself. The table can be opened; usually there is a mirror inside and a place to keep small toilet articles. The top is adjustable to permit the patient to place the book at a comfortable angle so that he can read without becoming overtired.

## The Bedside Stand

In the hospital, the bedside table is made of metal or plastic, which makes it durable and easy to keep clean because it can be washed with soap and water. The legs are rubber tipped or have casters so that it can be moved easily and quietly. The top is covered with a composition material that prevents noise when you place things on it. Bedside tables come with a drawer and an enclosed storage space below, with shelves. Some of them have a ring attached to hold the wash basin.

The drawer provides a place for personal belongings—comb and brush and toothbrush. Basins and bath blankets are stored on the top shelf of the table; if the patient's bedpan and urinal are kept at the bedside, this equipment and the toilet tissue go on the bottom shelf. In any storage arrangement, always keep the bedpan and the urinal apart from other personal things.

# HOSPITAL PERSONNEL AND SERVICES

## Diagnosis and Treatment Departments

In the *clinical diagnostic laboratory* numerous tests are done to assist the doctor in diagnosing the patient's disorder.

The pathologist and his associates in the *pathology laboratory* have considerable responsibility for determining the underlying nature of the patient's disease through their examination and study of specimens of tissue. Autopsies are also performed here.

Some large teaching hospitals also include a *research laboratory,* where studies and experiments on animals are carried out in efforts to cure or to prevent human disease.

In the *radiology department,* diagnostic x-ray studies are done to aid the physician in determining the exact location and nature of the patient's disorder, and radiation therapy is given in the treatment of certain diseases.

The *dietary department* is responsible for the preparation of all meals for patients in accordance with the diet instructions given by the physician.

The *pharmacy* is responsible for dispensing medications ordered by the physician.

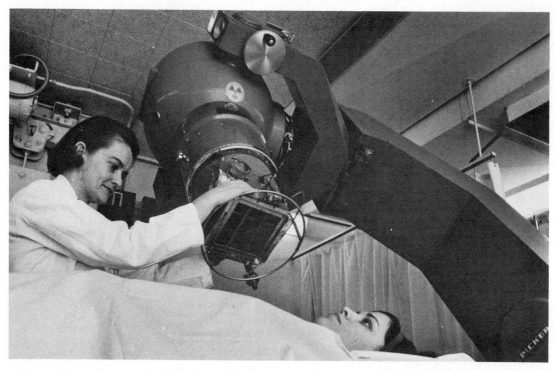

Figure 26-3. The equipment in the x-ray department can be very frightening to the patient. It is up to the nurse to provide explanations and reassurance to the patient, so that he will receive the greatest possible benefit from either diagnostic x-ray or x-ray therapy. (University of Minnesota Health Sciences Center)

## Direct Patient Care Departments

The *physical therapy department* (PT) directs its efforts toward preventing physical disability. Here the staff assists the patient in regaining the best possible function of affected parts through an individually planned program of exercise and activity.

Through the use of diversional or craft activities in the *occupational therapy department* (OT), the patient is helped toward rehabilitation. The occupational therapist may assist in job retraining as well.

Some hospitals contain facilities for *music therapy, recreational therapy,* and *play therapy.*

The staff in the *operating room* (OR) and the *postanesthesia recovery room* (PAR) are, of course, concerned with the care of the surgical patient during surgery and in the hours immediately after surgery.

## Specialized Units

Various other specialized units may be found in large hospitals.

The *emergency room* (ER) is where accident victims or other persons requiring immediate attention are taken. The hospital ambulance service and the cardiopulmonary resuscitation service are components of emergency room functions.

The *intensive care unit* (ICU) provides for the care of critically ill patients.

In the *coronary care unit* (CCU or ACU) patients with serious heart disorders are attended by a specially trained nursing staff.

Patients who need chronic renal dialysis are treated in the *dialysis unit.*

The *inhalation therapy* (or *respiratory therapy*) *department* is responsible for carrying out measures prescribed by the physician to assist the patient suffering from certain cardiac or respiratory diseases.

# 27

# Introducing the Patient to the Hospital

---

## BEHAVIORAL OBJECTIVES

*The student successfully attaining the goals of this chapter will be able to:*
- always *treat each patient as an individual, as a unique person.*
- *recognize that a patient comes to the hospital with concerns and fears and that the procedures and equipment used are often unknown to him.*
- *carry out all necessary admission procedures with consideration and tact.*
- *list information which should be included in admission charting for all patients.*
- *demonstrate orientation of a newly admitted patient to his unit, including explanations regarding equipment in the room and usual hospital routines.*
- *review orally the anatomical concepts relating to pulse and blood pressure which were presented in Chapter 15; define pulse and relate this definition to at least 5 possible patient disorders; define blood pressure and relate this to at least 5 possible patient disorders.*
- *demonstrate accurate measurement of the pulse in at least 3 points in the body; list and define 10 descriptive terms relating to pulse.*
- *with another student, correctly measure apical-radial pulse; discuss the meaning of apical-radial pulse and implications of a pulse deficit.*
- *obtain an accurate brachial blood pressure measurement in 5 patients of varying ages and of varying states of illness, as verified by instructor.*
- *review orally the anatomical concepts relating to respiration as presented in Chapter 16; define respiration; demonstrate ability to count patient's respiration; identify conditions in which the respiration might be altered; list and define 5 descriptive terms relating to respiration.*
- *identify some of the conditions which may cause a rise or fall in body temperature; describe and demonstrate 3 methods of measuring body temperature and state situations in which each method could or could not be used; state the usual normal reading for each method.*
- *demonstrate ability to chart temperature, pulse, respiration, and blood pressure.*
- *discuss importance of urinalysis; discuss some of the information which can be gained through the urinalysis.*
- *demonstrate ability to collect various types of urine samples.*
- *discuss importance of blood analysis in treatment of the patient.*
- *discuss the interrelationships of all vital signs and laboratory tests in the evaluation of the patient's health status.*
- *safely and tactfully transfer a patient to another unit within the hospital.*
- *assist in the predischarge teaching and in the safe discharge of a patient from the hospital; chart the discharge; and discuss the types of nursing and medical services available to the patient after discharge.*
- *discuss the legal and ethical considerations concerned with the patient's discharge release, if the patient signs himself out of the hospital against medical advice, and if the patient offers a student a tip or a gift.*

---

## ADMITTING THE PATIENT

### The Patient's Feelings

Any person who is hospitalized is bound to feel anxious and nervous about what is going to happen to him or his family while he is in the hospital. This stress can cause physical and emotional tension and might even contribute to the disease process itself. Of course, people react differently to stress; what might be upsetting to one person may have no effect on another. In the case of illness, the degree of anxiety may vary with the degree of severity of the illness. The nurse can help by recognizing the patient's anxiety and allowing him to verbalize his feelings. She should also be aware of any nonverbal means by which a patient may express anxiety; he may look upset, may talk incessantly or refuse to talk, may have his call light on all the time, or may assume an unnatural or uncomfortable position in bed. If you are perceptive, you will notice these signs of apprehension.

There are many reasons why a patient experiences such apprehension. Perhaps the most intense fear comes from fear of the unknown—of not knowing what is going to happen. The patient may be afraid of death or serious illness, or he may feel that the doctor is not telling him the truth and that his disease is really more serious than it actually is.

Patients also react intensely to any threat to their body images. Everyone has an image of himself as a "total" human being. Many people find it difficult to face an illness, especially if it involves surgery. This can happen even when the surgery will not cause disfigurement. However, should the surgery involve amputation of a limb or removal of a breast, the possibility of disfigurement is far more real. Such a possibility can create disturbing fears about what the spouse may think or about the possible loss of a job or friends. In these instances, the nurse who helps the patient work through these feelings will help him to face the realities of life in the future.

Another fear which haunts many patients is the fear of financial burden. Many patients cannot afford the expense of hospitalization and are concerned about how the family will manage while they are in the hospital. Since such preoccupation with financial problems can affect the patient's reaction to his illness, the nurse should try to be as reassuring as possible.

Even if a patient has none of these fears, he may still feel uneasy. If this is his first hospital experience, he may be embarrassed because personal services have to be performed for him. Added difficulties may arise from superstitions and ignorance about the body or from a limited understanding of the English language.

### The Nurse's Reaction

**Be Friendly.** Wherever you meet the patient, the most important thing is to be friendly. The patient must feel at ease with you and trust you if you are going to gain his cooperation and confidence. You will not know very much about his background at this first meeting, but you do not need this information to be courteous and friendly. Introduce yourself at once; learn the patient's name and use it. It makes a patient feel that he is more than a body in a room or a bed number.

**Explain.** You can sense when a person is worried, frightened, or confused. Put the new patient at ease by explaining the arrangement of his room, by making comments on everyday things, by letting him know that you were expecting him. You need to be sensitive to his mood at the time—do not begin by trying to be funny with a frightened person. Feel your way. Explain hospital procedures if this is his first experience; if he has been in a hospital before, let him see that you understand that he is familiar with one. Don't forget that the nurse who is in the hospital, as a patient, also has questions.

These guides apply to the family, too. They will feel more confident if they know that you are kind and that they can trust you. Tell them the hours for visiting and the general rules of the hospital (such as bringing food for the patient). Explain that the patient will have 24-hour care and that the hospital will contact them immediately if an emergency should arise. Let them see that you understand their anxiety, and that you see them as individuals whom you are happy to know. Treat them as welcome guests and try to make them comfortable while they are visiting the patient.

## The Admitting Department

Certain general routines are necessary for the admission of the patient and are usually carried out in a separate department. A member of the clerical staff records such information as age, sex, and marital status and whether or not the patient has hospital insurance. An identification band also is applied at this time. During these preliminary procedures, every effort is made to make the patient feel at home and to alleviate any feeling of tenseness he may be experiencing.

Someone from the department or a member of the auxiliary personnel then brings the patient to his unit. Every hospital has its own admitting procedures, but most follow the general pattern described here.

## The Patient Arrives

Before the patient arrives, check the unit to be sure that it is equipped completely and in order, and open the bed. The patient may walk in or may arrive in a wheelchair or on a stretcher. Unless there are orders to the contrary, the patient undresses, puts on a hospital gown, and goes to bed in preparation for an examination by a physician—a routine procedure in most hospitals.

**Removing the Patient's Clothes.** Give the patient whatever assistance he may need in undressing; sometimes a member of the family can be of assistance, particularly when the patient is a child, for he may resist being undressed by a stranger or may not understand the need for going to bed during the day.

**Undressing the Helpless Patient.** If the patient is a female, push a garment off one shoulder. Push the sleeve down in a roll to the wrist, then slip it off. Unfasten the waistband; push all the lower garments down as far as you can around the hips—then ask the patient to raise her hips (if she is lying down) while you pull the clothes down. Take the upper garments off over the head in the same manner. If the garments must come off over the head, slip the arms from the sleeves, push the clothing up to the hips, and ask the patient to raise her hips. Pull the garments up to the shoulders—you can turn the patient's shoulders first to one side and then to the other—and slip the garments off over the face.

Raise the head and remove the clothes, gathering them together into a roll as much as possible to keep them from dragging over the patient's face. When putting the gown on the patient, cover her with a bath blanket and work under it as much as possible to avoid exposing or embarrassing her. If you remove the garments above the waist first and put on her gown, she will not be exposed while you take off her lower garments.

**Placing the Patient in Bed.** If a patient is weak or tired, remove his shoes and outdoor clothing and put him on the bed immediately; then cover him with a bath blanket or with the bedclothes. This prevents more fatigue. He already has exerted an extra effort in making the trip to the hospital.

Find out from the head nurse or team leader what the patient is allowed to do for himself; if he is allowed bathroom privileges, show him the bathroom and put his bathrobe and slippers where he can reach them. Since in most instances a urine specimen is to be saved, give him instructions about using the urinal instead of the toilet. Arrange his things and tell him where they are; put special items on his bedside table where he can reach them. Show him how the communication system works and put a signal cord where he can reach it. Be sure that the shades are adjusted; regulate the ventilation and adjust the bed for his comfort. If the patient will be getting in and out of bed without assistance, adjust the bedside footstool for his convenience or put the bed in low position.

Explain how the bed works as you adjust it—tell him that if it is not comfortable, you can change it. Inform him of the hours for meals and that you will find out what he may have to eat and when. Sometimes a patient goes without a meal because he does not know what to expect, and the nurses have overlooked him. If he is in semiprivate accommodations, introduce him to the other patients.

**Toilet Equipment.** Every hospital has its own system for supplying such essential toilet articles as toothbrushes, toothpaste, combs, and toilet soap. Usually the supplies are available for purchase in the hospital pharmacy or gift shop if the hospital does not supply them. Many patients have personal preferences and like to provide these articles themselves. Disposable tissues are provided, either at the hospital's or the patient's expense.

Patients usually bring their own bathrobes and slippers with them. However, most hospitals provide these articles if the patients are unable to supply them. For bed patients it is customary to use the gowns provided by the hospital. They can be sent to the hospital laundry and are easy to put on and remove. Explain to the patient that the hospital gown is used for its convenience, comfort, and economy. During convalescence or as patients become ambulatory, they may wear their own nightgowns, pajamas, or bed jackets, provided they are able to make arrangement for the laundering of these articles outside of the hospital.

Private and ward patients alike should learn as soon as possible that individual equipment is set aside for them during their stay in the hospital—these are *their* things and no one else uses them. Any one of us ought to be able to feel confident that a ward is as safe and clean a place as a private room. The luxuries are lacking in a ward, but the necessities are provided, and no patient should have any reason to feel that equipment used for him is also used indiscriminately for someone else. This is especially important in an open ward where the patients have an opportunity to see so much of what goes on with all kinds of illnesses.

**Identification.** Be sure that the patient receives and wears an identification band. Then check the information on the band. Also check the tag on the bed and make sure the patient is properly identified. The tag should also indicate whether the patient is allowed to be up, what his diet is to be, and other pertinent information. This information can be checked with the doctor's order sheet.

## Essential Information

The following information is essential for the doctor and for the patient's record: Be sure to check and sign the chart. Chart accurately and completely.

1. Note the date and hour of admission and his name—his ward number or section.
2. Indicate how he was admitted—walking,

in a wheelchair, on a stretcher. Who was with him?
3. Note temperature, pulse, respiration, and blood pressure. Note also if blood was drawn.
4. Record the amount of urine voided for specimen—unusual appearance, if any—note that it was sent to the laboratory or that the patient was unable to void.
5. Record any symptoms that the patient tells you—headache, nausea. Ask him why he came to the hospital.
6. Indicate what you notice about him—flushed face, swelling, discomfort, fear, irritability, difficulty in moving.
7. Record weight and height.
8. Note the state of consciousness and level of orientation to his surroundings. (See Chapter 46.)
9. Ask the patient if he has any allergies. If he does, this must be noted on the front of the chart and on the kardex.
10. Ask the patient if he is regularly taking any medications and be sure to note this in the chart. It is important to continue anticoagulants, birth control pills, insulin, and other medications.
11. Note if the patient wears a prosthesis, dentures, contact lenses.
12. Indicate what was done with his valuables.
13. Note any special procedures done, such as x-rays, an EKG, or a catheterization.

## Care of the Patient's Clothing

A private-room patient has more leeway with his belongings than other patients. Clothing can be hung in the closet of his room; he has a place for his bathrobe and slippers; and dresser drawers provide space for personal things.

Ward patients' clothing may be sent to a special room for storage. No matter what the condition of the clothes, they should be placed on hangers and protected from dust. Many hospitals provide garment bags for this purpose. The ward patient has little space for personal belongings at his bedside. If he is using a robe and slippers provided by the hospital, they should be set aside for him and not serve as common property in the department. List every item of clothing for every patient. It is important to follow the system that the hospital has established; it protects the patient, the hospital, and you.

## Care of the Patient's Valuables

Valuables, such as a watch, jewelry, and money, must be put in a safe place. Usually the items are listed and kept in the hospital safe. When the patient learns that he will not be able to keep these things at his bedside or wear them, he may prefer to send them home with his family. Again, it is important to list them carefully for everyone's protection. The fact that the patient or a member of the family signs the slip verifies the list.

## Reporting

Report to the head nurse when you have completed the admission procedures. She is a busy person and does not always know exactly when a new patient reaches her department. She is the one who is responsible for seeing that there are instructions about the patient. She relays the order for his diet to the dietary department and notifies the physician of the patient's arrival. Report everything you can about the patient; you have been making notes on paper and in your head all the time you were with him. Anything that you can tell her is important for the patient's care.

## Checking the Doctor's Orders

When a patient is admitted, the admitting nurse checks the doctor's order sheet for any *stat* orders, such as medications to be given or tests to be done at once. Any special orders must also be noted and carried out. If you do not know how to do a certain procedure, be sure to ask.

## THE VITAL SIGNS

Body temperature, the pulse, the respiration (TPR), and the blood pressure often show changes which are going on in the body and affecting a patient's condition. They have long been called the vital signs or *cardinal symptoms*. Although modern medicine now has many other methods for detecting body changes, these signs are still important. If you

are uncertain whether you have observed them correctly, ask your supervisor to check your observations. Unusual changes should also be called to her attention—for example, a marked increase in the pulse rate or a sudden rise in temperature.

The temperature, the pulse, and the respiration are usually observed together. It has been the practice in hospitals to require this observation morning and evening as a routine procedure for every patient. In some hospitals today, these routine observations are omitted for certain patients, such as those in self-care units, long-term patients, or those under psychiatric observation, unless the doctor asks that they be made. In some illnesses it is important to make frequent observations of these symptoms, such as every 4 hours in the postoperative period; observations may be made more often if the nature of an illness makes it necessary. In some illnesses it may be necessary to check the pulse frequently; in others the respiration is the most significant symptom. Changes in one of these symptoms may affect the others, which is one of the reasons for observing them at the same time.

## THE PULSE

Every beat of the heart produces a wave of blood which causes pulsations through the arteries. Just as you can hear the slap of waves against the side of a boat, you can *feel* the vibrations of a wave of blood in the arteries. This vibration is the *pulse*. You can feel it through the nerves in your fingertips if you place your fingers over one of the large arteries that lie close to the skin, especially if the artery runs across a bone and has very little soft tissue around it. You can feel the pulse most plainly over these arteries:

> Temporal—just in front of the ear
> Mandibular—on the lower jawbone
> Carotid—on each side of the front of the neck
> Femoral—in the groin
> Radial—in the wrist at the base of the thumb

The radial artery is the one most commonly used to count the pulse, because of its convenient location. In taking a pulse, use your first 3 fingers—your thumb has a strong pulse of its own which may be stronger than the patient's pulse.

## The Rate

The pulse tells how often the heart beats; the pulse rate varies with the age and size and weight of an individual. The normal rate for an adult man is from 60 to 65 beats per minute; it is slightly faster in a woman. The pulse of a newborn infant varies from 120 to 140 beats per minute. Rates for children are between the adult and the infant rates, according to the size and the age of the child.

Activity affects the pulse rate; the heart does not work as hard when a person is sleeping as when he is sitting or standing; if he runs or takes violent exercise or does heavy physical work, the heart beats faster and the pulse rate increases. Excitement, anger, and fear increase the rate; some drugs increase it—caffeine, for example. The pulse rate is more rapid in fever and when the thyroid gland is overactive. It increases in proportion to the temperature— the pulse rate goes up about 10 beats for every 1° rise in body temperature. Many of these conditions cause a rapid rate *temporarily,* but an abnormally rapid rate may be a sign of heart disease, heart failure, hemorrhage, or other serious disturbance. If the pulse rate is consistently above normal, the condition is called *tachycardia;* the first treatment is rest. The doctor may also order that certain drugs be given to decrease the heart rate.

Sometimes the pulse rate is continuously slow—below 60 beats per minute. This condition is called *bradycardia;* it may occur in convalescence from a long, feverish illness. It is a serious sign in cerebral hemorrhage because it shows increased pressure on the brain. It is also a sign of complete heart block.

## The Volume

The volume of the pulse varies with the volume of blood in the arteries, the strength of the heart contractions, and the elasticity of the blood vessels. In hemorrhage, when a considerable amount of blood has been lost, every pulse beat may be *weak* or *thready.* When every beat is strong, we describe the pulse as *strong.* A normal pulse can be felt with a moderate pressure of the finger—a stronger pressure obliterates the beats. If a pulse is difficult to obliterate it is called *full* or *bounding.* The pulse may have both strong and weak beats within the minute—then the force is *irregular.*

## The Rhythm

The rhythm of the pulse is the spacing of the beats. With normal or *regular* rhythm the intervals between the beats are the same. When the pulse occasionally skips a beat, this irregularity is described as an *intermittent* or irregular pulse. A pulse may be regular in rhythm but irregular in force; that is, every other beat is weak. In fact, these beats may be so weak that they are not felt in the pulse at all. This is very serious because the heart is actually beating twice as fast as the pulse rate indicates. If a patient is having treatment with digitalis—which decreases an overrapid heart rate—it may seem that the treatment is satisfactory, when the real truth is that the patient is having too much digitalis, which is actually increasing the heart rate alarmingly and harming the heart itself.

The pulse may be irregular in both force and rhythm—a sign of some forms of heart disease or an overactive thyroid gland.

## Radial Pulse

### KEY POINTS IN THE PROCEDURE

When taking a radial pulse rest the patient's arm and hand at his side, palm upward.

*Reason: An uncomfortable position can increase the pulse rate.*

The radial artery is on the inside of the wrist.

Press the 1st, the 2nd, and the 3rd fingers gently on the artery and against the radius until you feel the contraction and expansion of the artery with each heartbeat.

*Reason: The radial artery lies along the radius close to the skin surface. Excessive pressure will obliterate the pulse. You may be counting your own pulse if you use your thumb, which has a strong pulse of its own.*

Using a watch with a second hand, count the pulse beats for a half-minute and multiply by 2. Count for a full minute if the pulse is abnormal in any way. Repeat if necessary.

*Reason: Irregularities can be detected in a half-minute—counting for a full minute makes allowance for irregular spacing between beats and is more accurate.*

Record the pulse rate, noting irregularities that have been observed.

*Reason: Pulse irregularities are significant symptoms. Take an apical pulse if there is any question.*

## Apical Pulse

The doctor may order that the apical pulse be taken. In this procedure, the nurse listens at the apex (the pointed end) of the heart with a stethoscope and counts the beats she hears. This procedure should be done for 1 full minute. Generally, the apical pulse can be heard best in the left center of the chest, just below the level of the nipples. The apical pulse should aways be taken if there is any question about the rhythm or rate of the heart or if it appears that the heart has stopped.

## Apical-Radial Pulse

If the apical-radial pulse is ordered, 2 nurses carry out the procedure at the same time. Using the same watch, 1 nurse counts the apical pulse for 1 minute, while the other nurse counts the radial pulse. One gives the signal to start counting and both start at the same time. The 2 numbers are charted and identified. For example: A-R pulse 76/72. If there is a difference and the apical pulse is higher, this means that some beats are not strong enough to reach the wrist. If there is a difference between the 2 readings, it is called the *pulse deficit*. The existence of a pulse deficit is important to the doctor. Normally, these 2 readings should be the same.

## TAKING THE RESPIRATION

*Respiration* is the process that brings oxygen into the body and removes carbon dioxide wastes. This exchange takes place in the lungs.

Oxygen keeps body cells alive; accumulated carbon dioxide wastes kill them. Therefore, it is vitally important to observe respirations closely in order to detect signs of interference with the breathing process.

## Respiration Control

Respiration is controlled and regulated by the respiratory center in the brain and by the proportion of carbon dioxide in the blood. Injury to the respiratory center or to the nerves which connect it with the lungs will affect respiration; too little or too much carbon dioxide in the blood affects it. The body apparatus which accomplishes breathing include the chest muscles and the diaphragm; injuries to these parts of the body will affect breathing.

Normally, respiration is automatic; you breathe without thinking about it. You can control the action of your breathing apparatus to some extent, by taking deeper or shallower breaths or even by holding your breath for a limited time; when the limit is reached, the automatic control takes over, and your chest muscles relax in spite of your efforts.

## Rate and Depth of Respiration

The rate of respiration for a normal adult is from 14 to 18 per minute, with women having a more rapid rate than men. For the newborn infant, the rate is about 40; for children, it varies from 25 to 30 per minute. Excitement, exercise, pain, and fever increase the rate. Rapid respiration is also characteristic in the diseases which affect the lungs, such as pneumonia. Heart disease, hemorrhage, and nephritis also increase the rate, as well as some drugs. Rapid respirations indicate that the body is making an increased effort to maintain the right balance of oxygen and carbon dioxide. The body also tries to adjust the balance by taking deeper breaths.

If a patient takes in and breathes out small amounts of air, the respirations are described as *shallow*. Pressure on the respiratory center in the brain decreases the rate of respirations; cerebral hemorrhage has this effect. Some drugs, such as opium preparations, depress the respiratory center, and poisons that accumulate in the body in uremia and diabetic coma also slow the respirations. Respirations *below* 8 or *above* 40 per minute are serious symptoms.

## Sounds of Respiration

Snoring or *stertorous* breathing occurs when the air is passing through the secretions in the air passages. These bubbling noises or rattles are characteristic before death when the air passages fill with mucus. Obstructions near the glottis cause a hissing, crowing sound.

## Difficult Breathing (Dyspnea)

When a person is making a definite effort to get more oxygen and get rid of carbon dioxide, his breathing is *difficult*: the term for difficult breathing is *dyspnea*. This may be a temporary condition, such as when a runner breathes in gasps at the end of a race or when you run upstairs and pant "to get your breath" at the top. Normal exertion may make breathing difficult for fat people. In some diseases, breathing difficulty is more or less constant, as in the acute stage of pneumonia, in emphysema, or some types of heart disease. When the difficulty is so marked that the patient can breathe only when he is in an upright position, it is called *orthopnea*.

Obstructions of the air passages, either by secretions (croup) or by a foreign object, interfere with breathing. Asthma causes difficult breathing because the bronchial tube muscles contract; fluid in the abdomen also interferes with the action of the diaphragm. Normally, the proportion of respirations to the heartbeats is 1 to 4. Respirations usually increase if the pulse rate increases, but not always in a definite proportion; usually the pulse rate goes up faster than the respiration rate. However, the respiration rate goes up faster in respiratory diseases.

**Signs of Breathing Difficulties.** The characteristic signs of breathing difficulties are heaving of the chest and the abdomen, a distressed expression, and cyanosis (bluish tinge) in the skin—especially in the lips. In severe conditions, cyanosis spreads to the nails and the extremities and eventually is apparent over the entire body. It is much more evident in Caucasians.

## Cheyne-Stokes Respirations

Cheyne-Stokes respirations are periodic, that is, the patient breathes deeply and rapidly for about 30 seconds, stops breathing for from 10 to 30 seconds, then repeats the cycle. The respirations are slow and shallow at first and gradually grow faster and deeper, then taper off until they stop entirely. Cheyne-Stokes respirations constitute a serious symptom and usually precede death in cerebral hemorrhage, uremia, or heart disease.

KEY POINTS IN THE PROCEDURE

Count the respirations with your fingertips on the patient's pulse.
*Reason: The patient thinks you are count-*

*ing his pulse—if he knows you are counting his respirations, he may not breathe naturally.*

Count the respirations by watching the rise and fall of the patient's chest. You can also place his arm on his chest and feel the rise and fall without looking at his chest.
*Reason: Taking in and expelling air constitute 1 respiration.*

Count for a half-minute and multiply by 2 to get the rate per minute. Count for a full minute if the respirations are abnormal.
*Reason: The timing between abnormal respirations may be uneven.*

Record the procedure on the patient's chart, noting the respiration rate and anything that is unusual, such as noisy or Cheyne-Stokes breathing or cyanosis.

## BODY TEMPERATURE

*Body temperature* is the measure of the heat in the body—the balance between heat produced and heat lost. The body generates heat when it burns food. It loses heat through the skin, the lungs, and the body discharges. When heat is produced and lost in the proper balance, the body temperature is normal—98.6° F. If the temperature goes much higher or lower, it means that the balance is upset. The signs of an elevated temperature are easy to recognize: a flushed, hot skin, unusually bright eyes, restlessness and thirst. A lifeless manner and pale, cold, and clammy skin are signs of a subnormal temperature.

## Body Temperature Regulation

The heat-regulating centers in the brain control body temperature through the temperature of the blood when it reaches the brain. Heat is a product of metabolism. Muscle and gland activities generate most of the heat in the body. When you are cold, exercising your muscles warms you; if you get angry or excited, the adrenal glands become very active and you feel warm—probably this is the reason for using the expression "hot under the collar." The process of digestion increases the body temperature. Drugs, cold, and shock depress the nervous system and decrease heat production.

## Normal Body Temperature

Temperature is measured on the Fahrenheit (F.) or on the centigrade (C.) scale. If you have been using a Fahrenheit thermometer and are asked to use one with centigrade markings it is easy to convert the reading to Fahrenheit. To change centigrade to Fahrenheit, multiply by 9/5 and add 32. To change Fahrenheit to centigrade, subtract 32 and multiply by 5/9.

Average normal temperatures for adults are:

| | | |
|---|---|---|
| Mouth (oral) | 98.6° F. | (37° C.) |
| Rectal | 99.6° F. | (37.5° C.) |
| Axillary | 97.6° F. to 98° F. | (36.7° C.) |

*Normal* temperature varies. A difference of 0.5 to 1 degree either way is within normal limits. Body temperature is usually lowest in the morning and highest in the late afternoon and evening. The normal temperature for newborn infants and children is usually higher than the normal adult temperature. Other influences on body temperature have already been mentioned.

**Elevated Body Temperature.** An elevation above normal body temperature is called *pyrexia* (fever). It often accompanies illness and may be a sign that the body is fighting infection and attempting to destroy bacteria.

The body temperature rises when heat production increases in the body or when heat loss is decreased. Both of these processes may be going on at the same time. Extremely high temperatures can have fatal effects; patients with a temperature of 108° F. seldom survive. Fever temperatures range from low fever of 100° F., to 103° F. to 105° F., which is high fever. A frequent complication of a high fever is convulsions. A temperature that alternates between fever and normal, or subnormal, is called an *intermittent* or *undulating* fever. A temperature that rises to several degrees above normal, then drops a little but never reaches normal is a *remittent* fever. A *continued* fever stays elevated. A sudden drop from fever temperature to normal is called a *crisis*. If a fever temperature gradually returns to normal it is called *lysis*.

**Lowered Body Temperature.** A temperature below normal is called *hypothermia*. Such temperatures usually precede death. Survival is rare when it falls below approximately 93.2° F. (34° C.). In some instances, body temperature slightly below normal is helpful because it slows body metabolism and decreases the body's need for oxygen.

## The Clinical Thermometer

Body temperature is measured by a *clinical thermometer,* marked in Fahrenheit or centigrade measurements (more commonly in Fahrenheit). The clinical thermometer is a hollow glass tube, or stem, with a bulb filled with mercury on one end of it; the other end is sealed. Heat expands mercury, which makes it rise into the stem which is marked in degrees and two-tenths degrees. The markings range from 93° F. (33.9° C.) or 94° F. (34.4° C.) to about 108° F. (42.2° C.), which cover the average range of temperatures possible for a living person.

The thermometer tip is placed where it will be completely surrounded by body tissues. The usual places are the mouth, the rectum and the axilla. Every hospital establishes its own routine about taking temperatures and the method to be used; for instance, a hospital may require temperatures to be taken by rectum whenever possible. The main thing is to use the method that will give the most accurate reading in the light of the patient's condition.

There are 2 types of thermometer tips: thin and slender, or rounded and bulb-shaped (see Fig. 27-1). The bulb-tipped thermometer is used for taking rectal temperatures because it is safer for insertion; the slender-tipped or mouth thermometer is used in taking oral temperatures. Some mouth thermometers also have a bulb tip. Thermometers used for taking the temperature by mouth should not be used interchangeably with thermometers used for taking rectal temperatures and vice versa.

## The Oral or Mouth Temperature

The oral method is never used if a patient is unconscious, delirious, or otherwise irresponsible. Nor is this method used with an infant, because of the danger of injury from a broken thermometer. This method is also contraindicated in surgery or injury of the

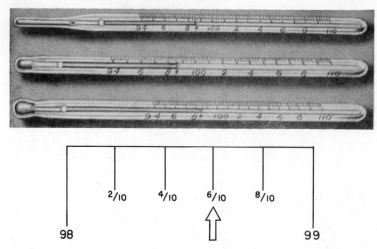

Figure 27-1. (*Top*) Clinical thermometer used for measuring body temperature. The 2 upper thermometers are used to record mouth temperatures. The thermometer at the bottom is used for rectal temperatures. Note that the column of mercury is at 98.6° F. in all 3 thermometers. (Becton, Dickinson & Co., Rutherford, N. J.) (*Bottom*) Sketch of 1 degree magnified.

nose or mouth or in conditions where the patient must breathe through his mouth. If a patient has had a hot or a cold drink, wait 15 minutes before taking a mouth temperature; the temporary effects of heat or cold will have disappeared from the tissues in that time. Chewing gum and tobacco smoking can also affect the patient's temperature.

## The Rectal Temperature

The rectal temperature is the most accurate, since the thermometer is placed in an enclosed cavity and is not affected by the temperature of the patient's environment. If there is any question about the accuracy of an oral temperature, it can be checked rectally. Some hospitals make it a policy to check oral temperatures by the rectal method when they are above a certain level. This method is used for unconscious or irrational patients and for infants and young children. To prevent injury, the nurse holds the thermometer in place. The method is contraindicated in such conditions as diarrhea, rectal disease, or rectal surgery.

## The Axillary Temperature

Taking the temperature by axilla is the method of last resort when conditions make it impossible to use any other method. The axillary temperature is the least accurate because the skin surfaces in the axillary space may not come together to form a closed cavity around the thermometer tip. It is necessary for the nurse to hold the thermometer in place while the temperature registers. An axillary temperature should never be taken immediately after washing the axilla because the temperature of the water and the friction used in washing and drying the skin alter skin temperature.

## Taking the Temperature

A patient who is ill at home must have his own thermometer; hospitals either provide individual thermometers for the patients or supply a number of thermometers in each nursing division. Individual thermometers usually are kept in the patient's unit and are cleansed after use, wiped dry, and kept in a safe container. If a common supply is used, provision must also be made for disinfecting each thermometer after use, before it is used for another patient. This means that each thermometer must be cleansed after it is used, then placed in a disinfectant solution long enough to destroy harmful organisms. Every hospital has its own method for thermometer care, but the principles are the same no matter what solution is used; it is most important to follow the directions for the time that the thermometers must remain in the solution, because the time varies according to the effectiveness of the solution.

### EQUIPMENT

| | |
|---|---|
| Thermometer | Jar of tissue wipes |
| Thermometer container | Waste container |
| Container with soap or detergent solution (cleansing solution) | Lubricant for rectal temperature |

**The Oral Method.** If the thermometer is kept in a chemical solution, dry it with a wipe. Wipe up from the bulb with a twisting motion. You may need to rinse in *cold* water.

*Principle: Chemicals irritate mucous membranes and may have an unpleasant taste. Twisting ensures contact with all of the surface. Wiping from the cleaner to the less clean area prevents spread of organisms.*

Hold the thermometer firmly by the thumb and forefinger. With quick snaps of the wrist, shake the mercury down to the lowest marking on the thermometer. Be careful not to hit the thermometer against your uniform or anything else—the thermometer may break.

*Principle: The constriction above the mercury tip keeps the mercury column at the previous reading until it is shaken down.*

Check the drop in the mercury column by holding the thermometer at eye level, turning it slowly until you can see where the mercury stops.

*Principle: Holding at eye level gives the true level of the mercury column. Moving an object brings it in focus.*

Place the mercury tip under the patient's tongue, telling him to close his lips but not to bite down.

*Principle: Enclosing the tip on the superficial blood vessels under the tongue ensures a reliable temperature registration.*

Leave the thermometer in place for 3 to 4 minutes (unless otherwise drected).

*Principle: It takes a certain amount of time for the mercury to register the temperature of the tissues.*

Remove the thermometer and wipe it toward the bulb.

*Principle: Mucus on the thermometer obscures the column of mercury and the markings. Movement is from the cleaner to the less clean surface. Friction loosens materials.*

Read the thermometer and shake it down as before.

Follow the hospital procedure for disinfecting and storing the thermometer.

*Principle: Disinfection of contaminated articles keeps organisms from spreading.*

Record the temperature on the patient's chart. Always record to the even two-tenths of a degree.

**The Rectal Method.** Wipe and shake down the thermometer as in taking an oral temperature.

Lubricate the bulb and the area up to 1 inch above it with lubricant placed on a wipe.

*Principle: Lubrication reduces friction and makes it easier to insert the thermometer without injuring the tissues. Applying the lubricant with a wipe prevents contamination of the supply of lubrication.*

Turn the patient on his side. Fold back the bed clothes and separate the buttocks so that the anal opening is easily seen. Insert the thermometer about 1½ inches. Hold it in place. Keep the patient covered.

Leave the thermometer in the rectum for 2 minutes.

*Principle: It takes a definite amount of time to register the temperature of the tissues.*

Remove and wipe the thermometer as with the mouth thermometer.

*Principle: Fecal matter on the thermometer obscures the mercury and the markings. Friction is an aid in cleansing.*

Read the thermometer. Shake it down.

Follow the hospital procedure for disinfecting and storing the thermometer.

Record the temperature on the patient's chart. Indicate that the temperature was taken rectally.

**The Axillary Method.** Wipe and shake down the thermometer as in taking an oral temperature.

Place the thermometer in the axilla and point the bulb toward the patient's head. Bring his arm down against his body as tightly as possible, with the forearm resting across his chest.

*Principle: Close contact of the thermometer with the superficial blood vessels in the axilla ensures a more accurate registration of temperature.*

Keep the thermometer in place for 10 minutes.

*Principle: It takes longer to get an accurate temperature reading when the thermometer is less tightly enclosed.*

Remove, read, and shake down the thermometer. Disinfect and store it according to the hospital procedure.

Record the temperature on the patient's chart.

## Cleansing and Disinfecting Clinical Thermometers

It is impossible to use heat as a thermometer disinfectant because heat expands mercury; a temperature high enough to destroy organisms will expand the mercury out of the thermometer tube. Many sad stories are told of the student nurse who boiled the thermometers or rinsed them in hot water; therefore, clinical thermometers must be disinfected by a chemical solution. The procedure is the same for each type of thermometer, with one exception—attention must be given to removing the lubricant from a rectal thermometer. Lubricants form a film on the thermometer which prevents the disinfectant from reaching organisms on the surface. Detergents are more effective than soap and water in removing oily substances.

KEY POINTS IN THE PROCEDURE

Wipe the thermometer with a soft tissue, using a clean tissue each time.

*Principle: Body material on a surface prevents a disinfectant from reaching organisms. Soft tissues contact a surface more closely than harsh ones.*

Wipe from the top downward, with a twisting motion.

*Principle: Spreading organisms from the more contaminated area to a cleaner area is poor practice.*

Using a wipe and friction, cleanse the thermometer with soap or detergent solution.

*Principle: Soap or detergent solutions help to loosen material from a surface.*

Rinse the thermometer under *cold* running water.

*Principle: Rinsing removes organisms, loosened material and soap solution. Soap interferes with the disinfectant action of some chemicals (Zephiran is one of them). Cold water must be used to avoid breaking the thermometer.*

Dry the thermometer.

*Principle: Water left on the thermometer reduces the strength of the disinfectant solution.*

Place the thermometer in the disinfectant called for in hospital procedure for the designated time.

*Principle: To be effective, chemical solutions must be used at a definite strength and for a definite length of time.*

After disinfection, rinse the thermometer with water.

*Principle: Traces of chemical solutions can irritate mucous membranes (the mouth and rectum) and may have an unpleasant taste.*

Store the thermometer according to hospital procedure.

*Principle: A thermometer is used in unsterile body cavities—it is not necessary to keep it sterile after disinfection.*

## The Graphic Chart

The temperature, the pulse, and the respiration are recorded on the graphic chart; this chart shows the relationship between these 3 symptoms. The readings throughout the patient's illness are recorded in continuous lines which show the peaks and the levels of each—one below the other across a page. Each reading is recorded as a dot in the proper space, with lines connecting the dots. Every hospital has its own printed graphic form and method for recording the temperature, the pulse, and the respiration, with space for recording other information, such as the blood pressure, the total intake and output of fluids, and weight.

## TAKING THE BLOOD PRESSURE

Measuring blood pressure is important for patients who have unusually high or unusually low blood pressure, for postoperative patients after anesthesia, or for patients who have sustained serious injury or shock. The blood pressure gives significant information about changes that may be taking place in the patient's body in certain types of illness. In most routine care of patients, blood pressure is measured once daily.

Because the heart *forces* the blood into the circulation, there is a certain amount of pressure in the arteries. Two things determine the degree of pressure: the rate of the heartbeats and the ease with which the blood flows into the smallest branches of the arteries. If the normal elasticity of the arteries and the

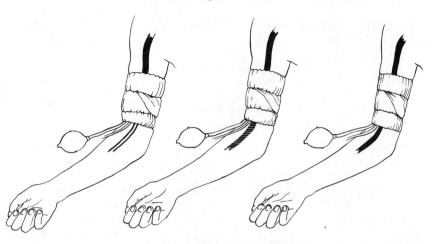

Figure 27-2. When the cuff has been inflated sufficiently, it will occlude the flow of blood into the forearm (*left*). No sound will be heard through the stethoscope at this time. When pressure in the cuff is released sufficiently for blood to begin flowing through the brachial artery (*center*) the first sound is recorded as the *systolic* pressure. As the pressure in the cuff continues to be released, the last distinct sound heard through the stethoscope is the *diastolic* pressure. At this time, blood flows through the brachial artery freely (*right*).

arterioles is maintained and the heart contraction exerts normal force, the blood pressure will be within the normal limits. However, if the heart rate or force is increased due to exertion or illness, the blood pressure will increase. If the quantity of blood within the circulatory system is reduced (as in hemorrhage) with the other factors remaining normal, the blood pressure will fall. By contrast, if the blood volume is normal and the rate and the force of the heartbeat are normal, but the elasticity of the arteries is reduced, the blood pressure will rise (typical of aging).

Measuring the level of the pressure is called taking the blood pressure. The pressure is at its height with each heartbeat when the heart is contracted—this is called the *systolic* pressure or systole. The pressure diminishes as the heart relaxes and is at its lowest when the heart is relaxed before it begins to contract again—this is the *diastolic* pressure. The difference between the two readings is called the *pulse pressure*. The average of the two is called the *mean arterial pressure*.

## Normal Blood Pressure

Normally, the difference between these 2 pressures is a number which is a third of the highest, or systolic, pressure. Both pressure readings give information; for example, a wide difference between the 2 pressures is a symptom of some kinds of heart disease. Normal systolic pressure for a man at the age of 20 is

about 120, diastolic pressure about 80. Blood pressure increases gradually with age; at 60, the systolic pressure can be expected to reach 140, as a result of the effects of aging on the heart and the arteries. This pressure might be alarming in a person of 20. Any pressure that is very much higher than the normal for the person's age is a sign of difficulty in the circulatory system (hypertension). If the blood pressure is very low (hypotension), it may indicate hemorrhage or shock.

## Measuring Blood Pressure

Blood pressure is measured with an instrument called the *sphygmomanometer* (usually called the blood pressure apparatus). The apparatus includes a cloth-covered broad rubber bag, or cuff, with 2 rubber tubes extending from it. One tube is connected to a rubber bulb air pump; this bulb has a valve which can be opened and closed. The other tube is connected to a glass tube of mercury, the manometer, which is closed at the top and marked for the blood pressure readings. It may also be connected to an aneroid dial. The manometer is fastened firmly to a standard or to a case. You obtain the blood pressure reading by listening to the heartbeats with a stethoscope, which you place over the artery on the inside bend of the elbow (over the branchial artery). The stethoscope magnifies sounds in the arteries. With another type of apparatus, a dial is attached to the arm

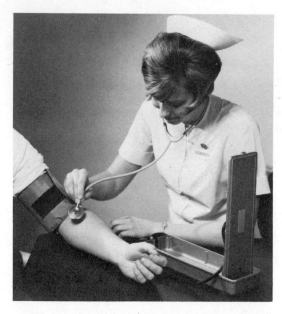

Figure 27-3. During the measurement of the blood pressure, the patient may be sitting or lying down, as long as he is resting and not bearing weight on the arm. The manometer is placed at the level of the arm and read at eye level. The bell or diaphragm of the stethoscope is placed on the brachial artery on the inside of the bend of the elbow. (Medical Products Division, 3M Company)

wrap instead of the mercury manometer. This method is considered less accurate, but it is more convenient for use. This is called the *aneroid manometer.*

When you take a blood pressure, you must do 2 things at the same time: *listen* to the heartbeat through the stethoscope and *watch* the manometer. You listen for the first sound to appear and listen for its disappearance or a distinct change in the sound. You note the manometer figures at these points—they are the 2 pressure readings.

Take the blood pressure when the patient is resting and quiet; physical exertion or emotional distress will affect the level of blood pressure. Prepare the patient by explaining that the cuff on the arm may feel tight for a second or two—otherwise the procedure will not bother him, and he only needs to keep his arm quiet for a few minutes. Tell him that taking the blood pressure is one method of obtaining information about any adult patient. Be sure that there are no leaks in the rubber bag or the valve.

KEY POINTS IN THE PROCEDURE

Cleanse the stethoscope and earpieces before and after the procedure.

Make the patient comfortable; he should be lying down or resting comfortably in a chair with his arm supported and his palm turned upward to expose the brachial artery on the inside of the elbow. Remove any constricting clothing.

*Principle: A more normal reading is obtained when a person is lying down (at rest). The stethoscope is placed over the brachial artery (Fig. 27-3).*

Sit to take blood pressure, so you can read the height of the mercury column on the manometer at eye level. It must be level with the patient.

*Principle: An accurate reading is ensured at eye level.*

Let the air out of the cuff. Apply the cuff just far enough above the elbow to leave the space over the brachial artery free—wrap it firmly around the arm and tuck in the end under the last turn of the cuff, or fasten the clip or Velcro closure.

*Principle: Smooth and even wrapping ensures even pressure on the arm to obtain an accurate reading. Accuracy is ensured by using the correct size cuff.*

Find the pulse in the artery and place the stethoscope over the spot where you can feel the strongest pulsations.

*Principle: The beat is easier to hear with the stethoscope directly over the artery.*

Pump the manometer bulb until the mercury rises to about 20 mm. above a possible systolic pressure—this allows leeway in releasing air.

*Principle: As pressure on the cuff increases, it shuts off the flow of blood in the brachial artery.*

Manipulate the valve on the manometer bulb to gradually release air from the cuff—note the level on the mercury column at which you first hear a heartbeat. This is the systolic pressure.

*Principle: As pressure in the cuff is reduced, the heart is able to force blood into the brachial artery. The point at which the heartbeat can be heard measures that force.*

Continue releasing small amounts of air from the cuff—the point on the column of mercury when the heartbeat cannot be heard is the diastolic pressure reading.

*Principle: Diastolic pressure is the point at which the only pressure on the blood is exerted by the walls of the arteries, with the heart at rest.*

Release the remaining air from the cuff.

Record the blood pressure reading on the patient's chart by writing the systolic pressure above the diastolic pressure (use only even numbers). For example:

$$\text{B.P.} \frac{\text{(systolic)}}{\text{(diastolic)}}$$

You may also chart the blood pressure on a graph with dots or check marks.

When blood pressure is taken in the leg, the popliteal space is used (popliteal artery) and the cuff is applied above the knee. You should indicate when you take a blood pressure reading at any place other than the arm.

## WEIGHING THE PATIENT

The patient is weighed on admission, at which time his height may also be recorded. These measurements indicate whether the patient is retaining fluids and whether he is overweight or underweight; they also establish a baseline for further observations. The patient may stand on the balance scales (use a transfer paper for cleanliness), or he may be weighed on a litter scale or other special scale. The weight is charted on the graphic sheet and also in the nurse's admission notes.

## OBSERVATION OF THE URINE

### Urinalysis

Urinalysis is included in a health examination and is a part of the examination of every patient at the beginning of an illness. One of the first things done for a patient on admission is to collect a specimen of urine and to send it to the laboratory. Except for simple tests, it takes special knowledge to analyze a specimen of urine. In the hospital, trained technicians do the urine examinations.

The urine may be examined from time to time during an illness; in some illnesses it is examined every day. About four fifths of the excess water, some carbon dioxide, most of the solid wastes of the body, and poisons that appear in the blood are removed from the body in the urine. In disturbances of the urinary system, the urine tells a great deal about the condition of the kidneys and the bladder.

**Amount.** Urine is secreted by the kidneys and carried through the ureters to the bladder reservoir, which expels it from the body through the urethra. The amount voided in 24 hours averages from 500 to 3,000 cc.; the total output is influenced by the amount of fluid taken into the body and the amount removed by the lungs, the skin, and the intestinal tract. In hot weather, or when a patient perspires freely, the amount is less than in cold weather; it is less in illnesses when perspiration is present or fluid is retained in the body tissues. To keep a normal balance of fluid in the body, from 6 to 8 glassfuls of fluids are required every day. If this amount is supplied and other conditions are normal, between 1,000 and 1,500 cc. would be a normal output of urine. The normal output for an adult naturally will be more than for a child.

A great increase in the amount of urine is called *polyuria*—an output of over 3,000 cc. a day. It may be the result of drinking a large amount of water, diabetes mellitus, diabetes insipidus, and nephritis (at some stages). A marked decrease in the amount is called *oliguria*. It may be due to the amount of fluid taken into the body or to other causes that will be discussed shortly. *Anuria* is the total absence of urinary output.

**Color.** Freshly voided normal urine is transparent and light amber in color. The kinds and the amounts of wastes in the urine make it lighter or darker. Blood in the urine colors it. If the amount of blood is large, the urine will be red. Practically always, some red blood cells are present in the urine during a flare-up of chronic nephritis and give the urine a smoky appearance. Some medications will discolor the urine, each of these medicines having a distinctive coloring effect; for example, Pyridium gives a bright orange-red urine, which may frighten a patient not forewarned of this effect.

**Odor.** Normal freshly voided urine has a characteristic aromatic odor. When the urine stands, certain changes take place which give it an ammonia odor. These changes affect the urine so that some tests will not be reliable indications of urine conditions. Sometimes preservatives are added to a urine specimen to keep it in good condition for examination. If this is necessary, the doctor will tell you what preservatives to use. Ideally, a urine specimen that is not examined at once should be kept in a refrigerator.

**Retention.** Usually, when the bladder contains about 200 to 250 cc. of urine, a person feels the distention and has a desire to void. Failure of the bladder to expel the urine is called *retention*. If the amount of urine increases, the bladder muscles stretch, with the danger of weakening them or making them less sensitive. One cause of retention is an obstruction of the bladder outlet or of the urethra. This may be due to swelling in the tissues or to masses of fecal material in the rectum pressing on the urethra. Fear or pain may cause tension in the muscles which control the urethral opening so that they will not relax to expel the urine. Another common cause of retention is the position of the bladder when the patient is lying down.

A number of things may help to relieve retention. The sound of running water, putting the patient's hands in warm water, or pouring warm water over the genitalia of the female patient often help to stimulate the muscles to function. If the doctor can allow the patient to sit up, either in bed, on the edge of the bed, or on a commode, she may be able to void.

**Incontinence.** Incontinence is the opposite of retention. Loss of muscle tone, injuries, or paralysis destroy the ability of the urethral muscles to constrict and so to keep the urine outlet closed; thus the urine dribbles constantly. If the nerve pathways to the control center in the brain are injured, the patient either does not feel the impulse to urinate or is unable to control the outlet muscles and voids involuntarily.

**Suppression.** In some illness conditions, the kidneys fail to secrete urine. This brings about suppression of urine or the condition called *anuria*. This condition occurs if both kidneys are injured or destroyed by disease, if a poison stops their work, or if the ureters are blocked. Remarkably enough, when one kidney is destroyed or removed, if the other is normal, it is able to take over the work of both. Other signs of suppression which may appear with the failure to void urine are headache, dizziness, puffiness beneath the eyes, spots before the eyes, nausea, and dim vision. Suppression is dangerous because poisonous wastes accumulate in the body.

The treatment for suppression is to stimulate the skin and the bowels to eliminate wastes more freely, to rest and to relieve the kidneys by diet (low salt), to force fluids in order to dilute the wastes, and to give medications that stimulate the kidneys to be more active.

## The Urine Specimen

You know now what to observe about urine and why observations about the amount, the color, and the odor of urine are important. You also know what normal conditions are. Nursing procedures in relation to urine include observing, measuring and recording the amount and collecting urine specimens. The contents of every bedpan and every urinal are important for giving information which will help the doctor in treating the patient. This means that you must know when the urine is to be measured and when a specimen is required, so that you do not dispose of the urine until it has been measured. Prevent the patient from unknowingly destroying a specimen and encourage him to void by explaining that the doctor needs the information that a urine test will give. Tell the patient who has bathroom privileges to use the bedpan or the urinal instead of the toilet. Always save an unusual specimen and show it to the doctor or the head nurse.

Measure the urine in a graduated container marked in *ounces* or *cc's*. Note the number of ounces or cubic centimeters voided each time and record your observations on the patient's chart. The doctor may or may not want you to measure the urine as the patient convalesces. Always measure the urine until the doctor says that it is no longer necessary.

## Collecting a Single Specimen of Urine

The amount and the content of a urine specimen vary with the time of day, the food taken in, and the amount of rest. The doctor may ask for specimens at different times in the day. Usually, it is customary to collect a routine specimen when the patient wakes up in the morning. A specimen of urine is usually collected as soon as the patient is admitted to the hospital. It may be a hospital rule to collect a specimen of urine from every patient on a specified day of the week. It is important to note on the specimen label if the patient is menstruating at that time. Because of the bacteria normally present on the labia, the perineum, and around the anus of the female patient, it is easier to contaminate a voided urine specimen. To avoid this possibility, and the necessity of collecting another specimen (with the extra cost to the patient), soap and water cleansing of the genitals immediately preceding the collection of the specimen is advocated.

### EQUIPMENT

Covered 6-ounce specimen bottle (wide-mouthed bottle is best)
Label
Bedpan or urinal

#### SUGGESTED PROCEDURE

Instruct the patient to void. Remove the bedpan or urinal after the patient has voided.

*Guide: If the patient feels that his bowels may move, ask him to urinate first. Remove the bedpan with the specimen and if the patient is a woman give her another bedpan.*

Pour about 120 cc. of the urine into the specimen bottle and cover the bottle.

*Guide: It is important to have enough urine to do the required tests.*

Label the bottle with the date, the patient's name, room, and department identification, and the doctor's name. A tag should be fastened on with a rubber band. Take or send the specimen to the laboratory.

*Guide: Note on the label whether other than routine tests are to be done.*

## Midstream Urine Collection

This is the most common way of obtaining a specimen from an adult patient. The patient is instructed to thoroughly cleanse the urethral area. Kits, which contain all the necessary equipment, or cotton balls and Zephiran may be used. The female patient must be sure to cleanse from front to back and to cleanse each side with a separate cotton ball, saving the last cotton ball for the urethral area itself. The male specimen is almost always obtained in this way. The last of the male stream is considered prostate washings.

The patient is instructed to void a small amount into the toilet to rinse out the urethra, then to catch the middle of the stream, and to discard the last of the stream. The midstream is considered bladder and kidney washings. The patient then gives the specimen to the nurse. Be sure to properly label it and take it to the laboratory without delay.

Catheterization is avoided, if possible, because of the danger of infection.

Note on the chart that this procedure was done, since it is routine for all patients admitted. Also note if the patient is unable to void, if he has any difficulty, or if the urine has an abnormal appearance.

## Collecting an Accumulated Specimen of Urine

An accumulated specimen of urine gives more detailed information than a single specimen because it shows what wastes the kidneys are eliminating and the amount of each. The urine may be collected for 24 hours or for some part of that period; this depends on the specific information desired. The fractional specimen is often collected from a patient with diabetes mellitus because it helps to determine the diet and the amount of insulin needed. You can start to collect the specimen at any time, but you begin by asking the patient to void and discard that single specimen. However, you note the *time,* as the beginning of the 24-hour period. This may be done by catheter or by voiding.

### EQUIPMENT

Large, clean bottle with cover or stopper
Measuring graduate
Bedpan or urinal
Ice

#### SUGGESTED PROCEDURE

Give the bedpan or urinal to the patient and ask him or her to void. Discard the urine and record the time on the patient's chart.

*Guide: Collection begins with an empty bladder.*

Measure each specimen of urine voided and pour into the bottle; record each amount on the chart.

*Guide: Continue for 24 hours from the time the urine was discarded. Caution the patient as before in relation to bowel movements.*

At the exact hour, 24 hours after beginning the collection, ask the patient to void. Pour the specimen into the bottle. A 24-hour specimen is kept on ice.

*Guide: The last voiding completes the 24-hour total; collection ends with an empty bladder.*

Label the bottle as for a single specimen and add the *time* collection began and ended, along with the *total amount* of urine. Cork the bottle and take it to the laboratory.

You will need more bottles if the urine is to be collected for separate parts of the 24-hour period. You begin the collection at the time that you discard the first specimen. If the periods run from 6 A.M. to 12 NOON, 12 to 6 P.M., 6 P.M. to MIDNIGHT, 12 to 6 A.M., you ask the patient to void and discard the specimen at 6 A.M.; at noon you complete that fraction of the 24-hour period by asking the patient to void and by saving the specimen. The next period then begins properly with the bladder empty.

The common tests made on a single specimen are for: acid or alkaline reaction, specific gravity, sugar and albumin. Some tests are done to find out how efficiently the kidneys are working.

Means for assisting patients who cannot void are discussed in Chapter 29.

## BLOOD SPECIMENS

It often happens that a blood specimen is taken when the patient is admitted. This is done to obtain information about the different kinds of cells and to look for disease organisms. In some body disturbances, one or another of the different kinds of blood cells will increase in number or change in shape. Thus, the number and the shape of the red cells give information about anemia; the number of the leukocytes tells about infection. The organism that causes syphilis is found in the blood; this is also true of malaria.

A specimen of the patient's blood is obtained by inserting a needle into a vein and drawing out the required amount of blood with a syringe. If only a few drops are needed, they are obtained by puncturing the patient's finger and smearing the blood directly on a glass slide. Blood usually is taken from a vein on the inside surface of the forearm, near the elbow. The veins are near the surface and easy to see or feel, although other areas where the veins stand out prominently may be chosen. The patient lies on his back with his arm resting comfortably on the bed. The tourniquet is applied around the upper arm, tightened, and secured by a slip knot. The tourniquet prevents the blood from flowing back, and the vein enlarges and stands out. The patient can also force more blood into the vein by opening and closing his fist several times. The area over the vein is cleansed before the needle is inserted in order to remove infectious organisms from the skin. The protective sheet is placed under the arm to prevent soiling the bed; when the required amount of blood has been collected the tourniquet is released. A sponge is laid over the needle where it enters the skin, the needle is withdrawn, and the patient bends his elbow to put pressure on the vein and check bleeding.

A blood specimen is obtained from an infant or a young child by puncturing the jugular vein in the neck. In this case, the mummy type of restraint is used. The nurse holds the child with his head over the edge of the treatment table and steadies his head.

The doctor or the laboratory technician usually collects a blood specimen, although the professional nurse may sometimes do this procedure. The equipment is provided by the laboratory. You will often be asked to assemble the equipment.

The specimen is labeled and taken to the laboratory. In caring for the equipment after use, it is important to rinse the syringe with cold water and to force cold water through the needles. Then the needles and the syringe must be sterilized. If scratches or cuts are present on your hands and are not covered with a dressing, use especial care in handling this equipment. Remember that harmful organisms enter the body through cuts and scratches.

## THE ROUTINE CHEST X-RAY EXAMINATION

Most patients are given a routine chest x-ray examination, unless they have had one within the previous 6 months. This is done to rule out tuberculosis or tumors of the lungs and to help determine whether the heart is enlarged or other lung disease is present.

## TRANSFERRING A PATIENT TO ANOTHER UNIT

There are a number of logical reasons for transferring a patient to another unit: the assignment to a certain unit is only temporary; a change in condition necessitates placing the patient in another department; he requires a quieter environment, he may be disturbing others; he needs a less expensive room because his stay is unexpectedly prolonged; or his condition becomes serious and alarms the other patients.

To transfer a patient, place him in the wheelchair or on the stretcher together with his belongings and chart. Be sure that he is protected from drafts in the halls as he travels from one unit to another. As a friendly gesture, see that he is comfortably established in his new unit. Don't forget to transfer his rented television, his mail, and his telephone, and be sure to take all of his belongings with him. Report to the nurse who is receiving the patient and give her the patient's chart.

## WHEN THE PATIENT IS DISCHARGED

In the hospital, the head nurse is responsible for seeing that the patient or the family has the necessary instruction. She begins to make a plan as soon as she knows that the patient is about to be discharged. You may be asked to assist with some part of it. You should know what such a plan includes so that you can give her any information that you have about the patient's problems.

The patient, at discharge, must know:

*The day and the date* for the next visit to or by the doctor or to the clinic for a checkup. Remind him to get advice from the doctor when he needs it.

*How and when to give medications.* Explain the need for care, caution and accuracy. Teach him to do it exactly as you do.

*How to change dressings.* Show how and explain why. Tell him where to get the dressings.

*The amount of rest* that the patient must have and the amount of activity that he is allowed.

*The diet.* Describe it as simply as possible. Name the foods that are not allowed, the foods that are "musts" every day, and the amounts allowed. The patient might make out a day's menu and discuss it with you. In the hospital the dietitian usually gives instructions about a special diet.

*For a bed patient,* give instructions about making the bed, giving the bath, moving and turning the patient, giving the bedpan, adjusting the pillows, and keeping good body alignment.

*Equipment needed.* Find out what equipment he already has at home. Tell the family what they must buy and discuss substitutes which can be used for some equipment. Discuss the need for a hospital bed or the way to use blocks or other means to make a home bed higher and the need for a wheelchair and the possibility of renting equipment from a medical supply house.

*Danger signs to watch for.* These will vary with the individual and may include an abnormal reaction to insulin or other medications, excessive drainage or bleeding on the dressings, or pressure areas from casts, splints, or prolonged bed rest.

*Ways that you have learned to get the patient to cooperate with you;* the patient's own preferences; things to be firm about and those you can be lenient about without doing harm.

*Things the patient can do for himself.* He should be encouraged to continue doing them. If the family knows that this is a part of getting well, they are less likely to coddle the patient unnecessarily.

*Services offered by the visiting nurse association.* Sometimes a visit once or twice a week is enough to take care of special treatments or essential nursing.

As you take care of a patient, you have an opportunity to learn a great deal about his habits, his problems, his interests, and his family. This is what helps you to plan his future care.

### The Day He Leaves

Before the day comes for the patient to go home, discuss the best time to leave. The family is instructed to bring clothing, pillows, or blankets, if they are needed. If he is anxious to go home, as most patients are, he probably can hardly wait to get dressed when the day arrives. If he seems to be eager to be ready, and his condition permits it, he can get dressed and rest on his bed until it is time to leave. These are the things to be done before the patient leaves:

The discharge order must be signed by the doctor. This prevents misunderstandings and protects the patient and the hospital.

The medications he is to take with him are ready. The patient knows the date of his next visit to the doctor.

A wheelchair is ready to take him to the hospital exit. He may walk if he has been an uppatient and his condition warrants it. Otherwise, use a wheelchair to prevent fatigue. Some hospitals require all patients to be discharged on a wheelchair.

His clothes and valuables are returned to him; he checks the list with the nurse and signs it. As was previously stated, this list, signed when he came in and before he goes home, is a safety measure.

The nurse takes him to the business office where he pays his bill, or a member of the family may attend to this detail. If the patient or a member of the family says the bill is paid, check with the business office before you take the patient to the waiting car or taxi. You tactfully can say that every nurse must report when she brings down a patient for discharge. Accompany the patient to the car and help him to get in; this gives him a feeling of security.

## The Release

The nurse who assists with discharging the patient brings the chart up to date, records the hour of discharge, and how the patient left—walking, in a wheelchair, or by ambulance. This rounds out the record of his stay in the hospital.

**Tips or Gifts.** If a patient offers you money or a personal gift, the situation must be handled with tact, since he usually means well. Generally, the nurse should not accept gifts from patients. However, it is usually permissible to accept a box of candy or a bouquet of flowers, which can be shared by all the nurses. Personal gifts should not be accepted.

**Leaving the Hospital Against Advice.** At times a patient may leave the hospital without the doctor's permission. In this case, he must sign a release slip which releases the doctor and hospital from all responsibility in the event he suffers complications. The practical nurse should report to the team leader if any patient says that he is leaving the hospital against advice.

# 28

# Assisting the Physician

## BEHAVIORAL OBJECTIVES

*The student successfully attaining the goals of this chapter will be able to:*

- *discuss the legal aspects of the medical record and demonstrate an awareness of the importance of this record by always charting accurately, completely, and carefully.*
- *keep in confidence all information about the patient which he or she may learn while in the medical facility or when reading a chart.*
- *discuss the function of the Kardex and the nursing care plan and demonstrate their correct use in the clinical area.*
- *assist with physical examinations in such a way as to be of the greatest assistance to both the doctor and the patient.*
- *place a patient in horizontal recumbent, dorsal recumbent, prone, Sims's, Fowler's, knee-chest, and dorsal lithotomy positions, demonstrating a thorough knowledge of the procedure to be done and consideration for the patient's physical comfort by utilizing the correct position; and consider the patient's emotional comfort by utilizing proper draping technic and by giving emotional support to the patient.*
- *assemble the correct equipment and effectively assist with a gynecological, rectal, or other examinations.*
- *practice proper restraint and reassurance procedures to effectively assist with the examination of a child.*
- *correctly and helpfully assist in making rounds with a doctor.*
- *demonstrate a knowledge of the valuable communication functions of the telephone by tactfully, efficiently, and accurately handling all calls.*

Judgment is needed when taking care of patients to decide what procedures can be done safely without an order and what procedures require definite orders from the doctor or the head nurse. Sometimes a professional nurse must perform even the simplest procedures for a patient, such as when he is critically ill or requires special treatments or close scientific observation. You learn that certain symptoms are serious and that others are only signs of discomfort.

In a hospital, the professional nurse interprets the doctor's orders to you; someone is always there to turn to if advice or help is needed. Everything about your patient is reported to your team leader or to the professional nurse to whom you are responsible. You record information of this type on each patient's chart.

For the practical nurse who works in a doctor's office or clinic and helps in examining and treating patients, specific training is provided by the physician concerning the various procedures used in the office or clinic.

## THE DOCTOR'S ORDERS

You rely on the doctor's orders, and in turn, the doctor will depend on you to interpret his orders correctly, to make accurate observations about the patient, and to record them. The doctor's orders tell you what to do, and nursing procedures show you how to do it. In their orders, doctors use abbreviations and symbols that all nurses learn. Many of them are abbreviations of Latin words, some of which are also used in prescriptions, and are translated by the druggist into the language that the patient can understand. It is important for the druggist to see what the doctor has written; this prevents mistakes that might be made in copying or in reading a prescription over the telephone.

The doctor may give verbal directions to explain the written ones. However, read his orders before he leaves to be sure that you understand them. Some orders are absolute and positive; others may require judgment on your part. For example, you must be sure you know what the doctor means when he writes "S.S. enema (soapsuds), if necessary." Does he mean that you will give an enema as soon as the patient says he is uncomfortable or has not moved his bowels or should you wait to see if perhaps the patient will have a bowel movement later on?

## THE PATIENT'S CHART

The standard hospital chart includes forms for recording the temperature, pulse, and respiration, the fluid intake and output, the laboratory and x-ray reports, the doctor's orders, the patient's history, and the bedside notes. The charting system used will be explained to you in the individual hospital.

### How to Chart

Because most of the observations recorded on the patient's chart are made by the nurses, it is important to know how to chart plainly and accurately; you must also know what is important to record. You learn the customary expressions to use, but you must say what you mean, and people must be able to read and understand it. Nurses' notes are always printed because individual handwriting is often difficult to read.

You record what you learn about the patient and what is done for him and what he tells you about himself. Record favorable changes in the patient's condition—they are as important as the unfavorable ones. There are standard expressions to use; perhaps soon some of them will be improved to give a better picture of the patient as a person. It was a shock to one patient, a nurse who had the doctor's permission to see her chart, to find herself described as a "middle-aged female lying quietly in bed!"

Avoid using too many abbreviations; some are permitted because they save time and space—for example, *lab.* for laboratory, *T.P.R.* for temperature, pulse and respiration and $\bar{c}$ for with. A list of the abbreviations commonly used with medications is included in Chapter 33.

### The Kardex and the Nursing Care Plan

Many hospitals record the patient's treatment plan on a card called the "Kardex." A separate card is drawn up for each patient and is usually kept in the nurses' station.

The Kardex is your guide to nursing care; on it are specified the treatments and medications which have been ordered by the doctor. It is your responsibility to check the Kardex frequently to make sure that you are doing what is ordered. If the orders are changed during your shift of duty, the charge nurse or team leader should tell you about the changes, but you should check occasionally, just to make sure.

The nursing care plan is the plan concerning the nursing approach for each patient. The entire nursing team plans the care in a team conference. (The team conference will be discussed later in this book, but you should know that the nursing student is very much a part of the nursing team and has a great deal to contribute to the nursing care plan.) The plan defines specific nursing problems and suggested approaches for solving these problems. An individual nursing care plan should be set up for each patient and should be kept up-to-date by the team leader and other members of the nursing team. If you notice something which is out of date on the care plan, you should point this out to the team leader.

Figure 28-1. Body Positions. (A) The horizontal recumbent position. (B) The dorsal recumbent position. (C) The prone position. (D) Sims's position.

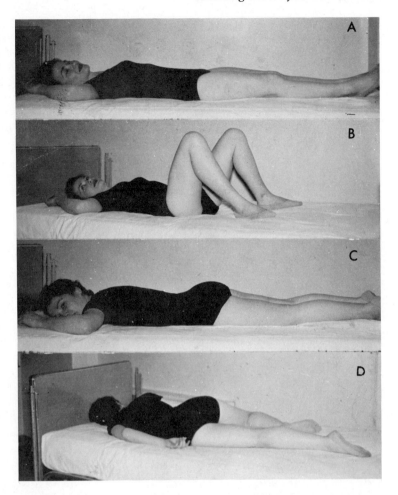

## THE PHYSICAL EXAMINATION

The doctor relies on the physical examination and the patient's history for much of his information about the patient. The history tells the doctor about the patient's parents, his past illnesses, his habits, and his present complaints. From the physical examination he learns the patient's height and weight and makes general observations. He examines the body from head to toe including the eyes, ears, nose, mouth, throat, neck, chest, breasts, abdomen, and extremities. He listens to the heart and lung sounds. A vaginal, rectal, or other such internal examinations are performed as indicated. (A vaginal examination is considered essential for women over 20 because of the possibility of cancer.)

Certain laboratory tests, such as urine and blood examinations and a chest x-ray, are included routinely as part of the physical examination.

## Assisting With the Physical Examination of an Adult

The doctor usually questions the patient first and writes down what is said. In a hospital, an intern may take this history. You should already have told the patient that he is to have an examination and explained the reason for it. When assisting in a physical examination, remember your own health examination and do everything you can to make the patient feel comfortable and unembarrassed. You come in when the doctor is ready and arrange the covering sheets, hand equipment to the doctor, and put the specimens in a safe place. If the patient's temperature has not been taken, you do that also. The patient will lie flat on his back with 1 pillow under his head for most of the examination; he sits up while the doctor examines his chest. The doctor may also want the patient to stand so that he can check his posture and examine

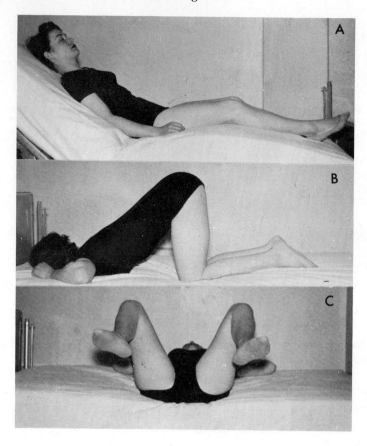

Figure 28-2. Body Positions. (A) Fowler's position. (B) The knee-chest position. (C) The dorsal lithotomy position.

his spine. Spread paper towels on the floor for him to stand on.

A physical examination is most satisfactory if the patient is relaxed and cooperative. Explaining the procedure beforehand and assuring privacy for him will contribute to his mental comfort and make him less tense and apprehensive. Since the patient wears a hospital gown, which is easy to adjust and affords movement without exertion, the doctor can examine him without exposing him unduly. Equipment should be assembled beforehand:

| | |
|---|---|
| Hospital gown or pajamas | Tape measure |
| | Tongue depressors |
| Sheet or bath blanket | Ophthalmoscope |
| A tray with: | Otoscope |
| Flashlight | Blood pressure apparatus |
| Rubber gloves | |
| Lubricant | Percussion hammer |
| Basin for soiled instruments | Red and blue pencils |

You may also need slides, blood tubes, or other equipment, depending upon what tests are to be done. Add a rectal and a vaginal speculum if the doctor wants to examine the rectum or the vagina.

When the examination is over, have the patient put on his gown. Draw up the bedclothes, remove the bath blanket, and make the patient comfortable. He may want another pillow under his head or the back rest raised and his bed adjusted. If specimens were sent to the laboratory, make a note on the chart of the time and the kind of specimen sent.

## Putting a Patient in Different Body Positions

Patients are sometimes put in special positions as a part of their treatment or examination; a number of different positions are used for a physical examination, for nursing treatments and for tests and to obtain specimens. Since you will put patients in some of these positions and will see other positions used, you should know how to assist the patient and adjust the necessary drapes.

**Horizontal Recumbent Position.** (Fig.

28-1A.) Put the patient on his back, with 1 pillow under his head and with his legs extended and his arms above his head, folded on his chest, or lying along his body. This is his position during most of a physical examination. Cover him with a bath blanket.

**Dorsal Recumbent Position.** (Fig. 28-1B.) Put the patient on his back with the knees flexed and the soles of his feet flat on the bed. Put a sheet or a bath blanket folded once across his chest; put a second sheet crosswise over his thighs and legs; wrap the lower ends of the sheet around the legs and the feet and expose the genital region.

**Prone Position.** (Fig. 28-1C.) Put the patient on his abdomen—turn his head sidewise for comfort; put his arms above his head or along his body; cover him with a bath blanket. This position is used to examine a patient's spine and back or when a patient has had a back injury or an operation. If a patient has an abdominal incision, is unconscious, or has difficulty in breathing, he cannot lie in this position.

**Sims's Position.** (Fig. 28-1D.) Put the patient on his left side with a pillow under his head; flex his right knee against his abdomen; flex his left knee but not as much; put his left arm behind his body—his right arm in the position most comfortable for him. Cover him with a bath blanket. This is the position for a rectal examination. A patient with leg injuries or arthritis cannot assume this position.

**Fowler's Position.** (Fig. 28-2A.) Adjust a back rest to the desired height; raise the bed section under the patient's knees slightly. As a brace against his feet and to keep him from sliding down, a rolled pillow can be placed between the patient's feet and the foot of the bed. This position is used for most patients to help drainage or to make breathing easier. Watch the patient for dizziness or faintness.

**Knee-Chest Position.** (Fig. 28-2B.) Put the patient on his knees, with the chest resting on the bed; rest the elbows on the bed or put the arms above the head. The thighs should be straight up and down and the legs flat on the bed. This position is used for rectal and vaginal examinations and as a treatment to bring the uterus into a normal position. A patient in this position might become dizzy or faint and fall out of bed so do not leave him alone.

**Dorsal Lithotomy Position.** (Fig. 28-2C.) The patient is placed in the same position as dorsal recumbent except that the legs are well separated and the thighs and the legs are more acutely flexed. This position is used for examinations of the urinary bladder, vagina, cervix, rectum, and perineum.

## The Gynecologic Examination

Some women are likely to look upon a vaginal or gynecologic examination with mixed feelings—partly dread and partly embarrassment. A woman may fear the examination because she thinks that it may be painful or that it may show that something is wrong. She also may be embarrassed by a dread of physical exposure or of questions which the doctor may ask. This is when the nurse's matter-of-fact, friendly attitude is very comforting, as is her assurance that she will stay with the patient throughout the examination. An informed patient is a more relaxed one, and relaxation is an aid to the doctor in obtaining the information he wants.

**Assisting With a Vaginal Examination.** The purpose of a vaginal or pelvic examination is to examine the external genitals and the pelvic organs for signs of irritation, growths, displacement, or other abnormal conditions and to take vaginal smears.

The patient is given a gown to protect the upper part of her body during the examination. Be sure that she empties her bladder prior to being examined. You assist the doctor by putting the patient in the lithotomy position (see Fig. 28-2C), adjusting the drape and placing the examining tray conveniently near.

The doctor palpates the pelvic organs by inserting 2 fingers in the vagina, at the same time placing his other hand on the patient's lower abdomen. He inspects the vagina and cervix after inserting the lubricated speculum. If he wants to take smears of vaginal or cervical secretions, he uses applicators and glass slides.

Stay by the patient, helping her to relax. After the examination is over, wipe traces of the lubricating jelly from the perineum and adjust her position; provide her with a sanitary pad if necessary. Label the specimens if any have been taken and send or take them to the laboratory. Make a note of this on the

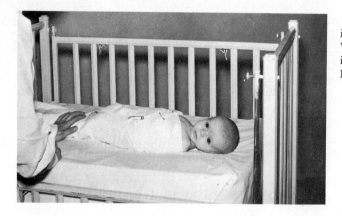

Figure 28-3. Method of restraining an infant with a blanket. (From Blake, F. G., Wright, F. H., and Waechter, R. N.: Nursing Care of Children, ed. 8, Philadelphia, Lippincott)

patient's chart, with the time and the kind of specimen. Care for the equipment as indicated on your procedure sheet.

These are the guides to remember in carrying out this procedure:

The lithotomy position, with the knees drawn up, relaxes abdominal muscles.

Mental reassurance also promotes relaxation.

Lubrication of the speculum reduces discomfort during the insertion.

Proper aftercare of the equipment prevents infection.

This procedure is discussed further in Chapter 51.

## The Rectal Examination

The purpose of the rectal examination is to inspect the rectum for signs of hemorrhoids, fissures, growths, or irritations, or for examination after surgery on the rectum. Rectal examinations are made also periodically during labor.

A rectal examination is usually included in the physical examination of a man over 40 years of age because digital examination of the rectum is an aid in discovering cancer of the prostate gland while it is still in an early stage.

The patient is placed in either the dorsal recumbent position with the knees flexed or in the Sims's position (see Fig. 28-1D). However, if the patient has a rectal condition which requires examination with special instruments (proctoscopy) the patient is placed in the knee-chest position (see Fig. 28-2B). This procedure is usually carried out in the operating room or treatment room. An enema, to empty the lower bowel, precedes a proctoscopic examination. The nurse explains the procedure beforehand, shows the patient how to assume the knee-chest position, and encourages him to have patience with its awkwardness.

## Assisting With a Physical Examination of an Infant or a Child

The equipment is the same as for an adult. One of the most important aids in this examination is the child's cooperation; if he is too young or too ill to understand how to cooperate, you will have to restrain him for parts of the examination. Figure 28-3 shows how to restrain an infant or a small child with a blanket; Figure 28-4 shows how to restrain an infant or a child while the doctor examines the front chest and the abdomen. For exam-

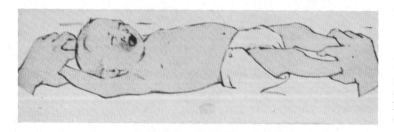

Figure 28-4. Method of restraining an infant for an examination of his head, anterior chest and abdomen. (Wolf, L.: Nursing, New York, Appleton-Century)

ination of the spine and the chest, hold him upright, with 1 of your arms around his legs, the other supporting the lower end of his spine, and his head against your shoulder. Restraint frightens the child more than the examination—no one likes interference with his body movements. So do your best to get a child to cooperate without restraint.

## MAKING ROUNDS WITH THE DOCTOR

The nurse will often be asked to accompany the physician as he makes his rounds. Generally, the practical nursing student will not be asked to make rounds with the physician by herself, but the Licensed Practical Nurse may be asked to do so. If you have a chance to accompany the doctor on his rounds, be sure to take advantage of this valuable learning experience. When a nurse is assigned this duty, she must be ready to assist the doctor with procedures and to follow up on orders. (Specific procedures will be discussed later in this unit.)

## TELEPHONE ETHICS

The nurse, whether working in the hospital or the doctor's office, will often be asked to answer the phone. When doing so, be sure to give the name of the department and your name and position so the caller knows to whom he is speaking. For example, you might answer the phone as follows: "Station Main 2 West, Miss Adams, practical nursing student, speaking." The caller then knows if you can help him or if he needs to ask for someone else.

It is important to answer the phone as promptly as possible. It may be an emergency and the caller may become very excited while waiting for the answer. Be sure to take messages correctly and to deliver them promptly. This is especially vital in the case of laboratory reports, especially if the doctor needs to be notified immediately of a certain labora-

tory finding. You should know when to pass on information, but if you have any questions about this, you should be sure to ask.

The practical nursing student should *never* take doctors' orders over the phone. This is a legal responsibility which you are not prepared to assume. If the doctor wishes to leave phone orders, you must find someone who is qualified to take them.

Many types of information should not be given over the phone; therefore if you are unsure on these matters, be sure to ask the team leader. For example, if someone calls to ask a patient's condition, generally only the nurse will be allowed to state the condition listed on the Kardex. If someone wants more information than this, you should turn the call politely over to the team leader.

It is very impolite to cover the receiver and continue a conversation with someone else. Since the caller can usually hear what was said, it is advisable to finish the call and then carry on your conversation.

It goes without saying that the nurse does not chew gum while on duty, but this is especially true when she is conducting hospital or office business by phone; it is particularly annoying to talk on the phone with someone who is chewing gum or candy.

There are times when you will have to make an emergency call, such as in the case of a patient who has suffered cardiac arrest. Be sure to give all the necessary information and not to panic. Your prime responsibility in an emergency situation is to get assistance, but you will not be able to do so effectively, unless you are calm and give all the necessary information.

Whenever you call someone else, be sure to state who you are and to whom you wish to talk. If you are calling a doctor, you may need to explain to his nurse what you want and whether or not it is an emergency. If you become frustrated with this procedure, remember that you may be an office nurse some day and may need to screen calls to conserve the doctor's time.

# 29

# Assisting the Patient to Meet Daily Needs

---

## BEHAVIORAL OBJECTIVES

*The student successfully attaining the goals of this chapter will be able to:*

- *explain the relationships between the basic needs of all people and the special needs of people who are ill.*
- *demonstrate in clinical area a thorough knowledge and understanding of the basic principles which guide all nursing care; discuss these.*
- *identify the nursing procedures which generally comprise early morning care, morning care, and evening care in the hospital.*
- *identify at least 3 components of a safe patient environment; demonstrate a knowledge of the hospital's fire procedure and emergency plan; demonstrate emergency evacuation of a helpless patient; demonstrate emergency resuscitation procedures and methods for summoning the rescue team.*
- *demonstrate ability to correctly place a helpless patient into at least 3 comfortable and safe positions and describe the reasons for using various devices to maintain positioning.*
- *list the basic principles of good body mechanics; personally maintain good body alignment and practice good body mechanics.*
- *correctly carry out passive or active range of motion exercises, so that all of the patient's joints and muscles will be maintained in as well-functioning a state as possible, so that deformities will be prevented.*
- *safely assist patients in varying stages of recovery to dangle, get out of bed, walk, or sit in the chair; safely transfer a helpless patient to and from litter, commode, or wheelchair.*
- *demonstrate safety and tactfulness in serving a food tray or in assisting to feed patients; correctly chart and report patient's intake and output.*
- *tactfully and correctly assist a patient to the bathroom, or to use the urinal, bedpan, or commode; correctly insert a rectal tube or suppository and record the results; demonstrate the ability to manually remove feces; and kindly and effectively assist the patient who is vomiting.*
- *describe and demonstrate basic principles of using a retention catheter by caring for catheterized patient and accurately recording urine output.*
- *demonstrate ability in the clinical area of giving cleansing, retention, and Fleet's enemas to persons in all age groups and with various illnesses.*
- *effectively observe and report signs of possible skin or muscle breakdown, as well as carry out preventive measures in this regard; define decubitus ulcer and list several predisposing possible causes.*

---

## THE PATIENT'S NEEDS

Many of the needs of patients are the normal needs of every human being, plus the special needs connected with illness. Patients have essential needs for:

| | |
|---|---|
| Cleanliness and comfort | Pleasant and safe surroundings |
| Proper food | |
| Sleep and rest | Correct body position and exercise |
| Elimination of body wastes | Essential medical treatment |
| Emotional and spiritual support | Restorative encouragement |
| | Diversional interests |

As you can see, the above needs are physical, mental, and emotional. The patient's progress toward recovery, his comfort, and his happiness depend upon the extent to which these needs are satisfied. Meeting them involves teamwork between the doctor, the professional nurse, the practical nurse, the aide, the social worker, and the technicians—in fact, by anyone who comes in contact with the patient, including the patient's family. If any one team member fails to do his or her part, the patient suffers.

## NURSING PROCEDURES

Practical nursing students usually learn nursing procedures as practiced in the hospital where they are receiving their nursing training. However, there may be minor differences in procedures among different hospitals. For instance, the policy in one institution may be to make square corners on the beds, while in another, the corners may be diagonal. Disposable equipment may be widely used or utensils may be made of different materials. Such differences do not matter. There are reasons why certain steps in every nursing procedure must be followed to achieve the desired results. These reasons are the *principles,* or known facts, which guide you in making a procedure effective. The steps tell you what to do, and the principles tell you why. It is important to know the guiding principles for the key points in every procedure.

Individual procedures vary, but the general directions given here must be followed for each one. To avoid tiresome repetition, they are not listed with the individual procedures, but they must be included as an important part of each.

### GENERAL DIRECTIONS

Wash your hands before carrying out a procedure and after it is completed.

Assemble all the necessary equipment so that the procedure can be carried out as expeditiously and effectively as possible.

Explain the procedure to the patient to allay his fears of pain or discomfort. Patients are likely to be apprehensive about apparatus or machines, especially if appliances have electrical connections. They also may fear sharp instruments or needles, applications of heat or cold, or any apparatus which covers the face. Avoid using the words "hurt" or "painful." Instead, say "you will feel a pin prick" or "you will have to lie in one position, but we will help to make you comfortable." Emphasize the positive aspects—"it won't take long" or "it will make you feel better." A patient will be more cooperative if he knows what to expect. Never tell a patient "there is nothing to it" when you know a procedure has some painful or uncomfortable aspects. Make him as comfortable as possible before beginning the procedure.

Assure the patient of privacy by closing the door or using cubicle curtains or screens.

Care for the equipment and store it as indicated by hospital policies and by the procedure itself (wash, sterilize, store, or return to surgical supply department).

Record the treatment, the time it was given, and the results, including any unusual patient reactions.

## Grouping Nursing Procedures

You carry out many nursing procedures for the patient's health and grooming and for his comfort. You often do several procedures in connection with each other, but each procedure is complete in itself. Some procedures are grouped together because they are associated with a time of day or a special kind of treatment—these blocks of nursing care are known to nurses by group names. Here are some examples:

EARLY MORNING CARE—given before breakfast for health and comfort:

| | |
|---|---|
| Washing face and hands | Taking temperature, |
| Brushing teeth | pulse, respiration and |
| Giving bedpan or urinal | blood pressure |

Adjusting bed and bed-
clothes

Changing patient's po-
sition

Adjusting table for the
tray

LATER MORNING CARE—given after breakfast
for health and comfort:

Giving bath
Making bed with clean
linen
Changing patient's po-
sition—ambulation
Giving back rub

Combing hair
Caring for nails
Tidying and dusting
unit
Caring for flowers

EVENING CARE—given for health and comfort
—prepares the patient for the night:

Washing face and hands
Brushing teeth
Giving back rub
Combing and tidying
hair

Giving bedpan or urinal
Changing patient's po-
sition
Adjusting bed and bed-
clothes

## Progressive Patient Care

Progressive patient care is organized to give
patients the amount of medical and nursing
care needed for different degrees of illness. It is
set up this way to provide:

*Intensive care*—for the critically ill patient.

*Specialized care*—for a certain patient problem
(coronary, dialysis).

*Intermediate care*—a moderate amount of care.

*Self-care*—for the patient who is physically able
to take care of himself but needs restorative care,
such as teaching and rehabilitative activities, or
for the patient who is having diagnostic tests.

*Long-term rehabilitative care*—requires hospital
services.

*Home care*—the patient is at home, but the hospital plans and helps with his care. The Public
Health Nurse is often involved in this kind of
care.

# 1. Providing a Safe Environment

The patient has a right to expect that the
environment of the hospital will be safe
enough to protect him from the danger of
contracting another disease or suffering injury
while in the hospital. Safety measures in the
hospital include such obvious things as fire
safety, disaster plans, and emergency evacuation plans. Other safety measures include
provisions for emergency resuscitation, the
prevention of the spread of infection from
patient to patient, and the administration of
correct medications and treatments. A more
subtle aspect in hospital safety is proper waste
disposal to prevent environmental contamination. Obviously, *everybody* in the hospital is
involved in the patient's safety.

## Fire Emergency

As a nurse, you must know where the emergency equipment is kept in the hospital. You
are responsible for locating the fire extinguisher and fire call on each station to which
you are assigned. You must know how to use
the fire extinguisher and what type of extin-

guisher to use on each type of fire. You must
know the routine for calling in a fire alarm
and the procedures for the immediate safety of
the patients in the area of the fire.

## Disaster Emergency

In the case of disaster, a specific plan goes
into effect for each hospital. You are responsible for knowing the disaster plan for your
hospital and for carrying it out calmly in the
event of an emergency. Many hospitals have
fire and disaster drills to allow their staffs to
practice emergency skills. If you have an opportunity to participate in a drill, you will
probably be calmer if an emergency arises.

## Resuscitation

The nurse must know where the emergency
resuscitation equipment is kept. Each station
generally has an Ambu bag available; you
should learn where this is and how to use it.
You should also know the procedure for calling the cardiopulmonary resuscitation team.

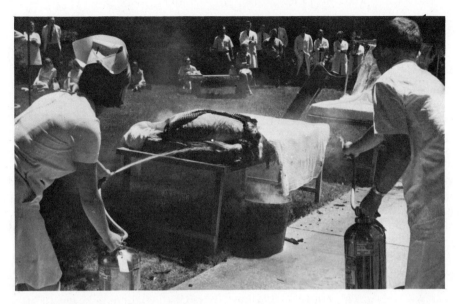

Figure 29-1. The nursing student should have an opportunity to practice with fire extinguishing equipment, in order to know how to use it in the event of a fire. Most hospitals have a fire safety program, which allows hospital staff to practice with equipment in a safe environment. It is important to remember that water cannot be used on an oil or electrical fire. Many fires can be put out by suffocating the flames, that is, by removing the oxygen supply to the fire. (University of Minnesota Health Sciences Center)

## Other Protections

Many other hospital safety measures are designed to prevent accidents, deformities, and infection. These will be discussed throughout this book. Such appliances as side rails, wheelchair restraints, and handrails next to the bathtub serve as safety devices. Footboards, splints, and trocanter rolls are examples of devices which prevent deformity.

## Handwashing Technics

The most important safety measure and the basis of many nursing technics is proper handwashing. The nurse *must* wash her hands properly before and after caring for each patient in order to prevent the spread of disease from one patient to another.

PROCEDURE

1. Turn on water without contaminating the faucets. This is easier to do if there are knee or foot controls. If these devices are not present, you must use a paper towel to turn on the water, discarding the towel afterward.
2. Wet hands and forearms with water and apply an antibacterial soap, such as pHisoHex.
3. Lather well with soap and additional water as needed. Be sure to scrub all areas of your hands and forearms thoroughly. Use a brush, if necessary. Be sure to clean under your fingernails. (Keep your fingernails short, to lessen the chance of spreading infection.)
4. Rinse thoroughly, allowing the water to drip off your fingertips. (This keeps contamination from spreading to your upper arms.)
5. To ensure thorough cleaning, repeat the procedure again.
6. Dry hands thoroughly with paper towel and discard the towel. Reusable towels are discarded and laundered after each use. Under no circumstances, is a towel hung at the sink and reused.
7. Use a clean paper towel to turn off the faucets, so that you do not contaminate the faucets or contaminate your hands in the event that the faucet is already contaminated.

# 2. *Assisting the Patient to be Comfortable*

## CHANGING BODY POSITIONS

You change the position of a patient's body for several reasons: to restore body functions, to prevent deformities, to relieve pressures and strains, to stimulate circulation, and to give treatments. If the doctor specifies a certain position or forbids another, you follow his order exactly. You never let a patient sit up or get out of bed until the doctor has left an order permitting the change from one of these positions to the other. You never use fracture boards, splints, body frames, or other appliances, unless the doctor orders them. You may use comfort devices, such as pillows, rolls, pads, and bed cradles, except in certain conditions. You will learn what these conditions are, and the doctor will point them out to you. You must use these devices in such a way as to promote good body alignment and comfort, not to interfere with it.

The points to remember in changing the patient's position are: good body alignment; the safety of the patient; the need to reassure the patient; proper handling of the patient's body to prevent pain or injury; your posture in order to do the procedure effectively without strains on your own body; and assistance, if you need it, for heavy or helpless patients.

### EQUIPMENT

| | |
|---|---|
| Pillows—large and small | Pads—folded towels and |
| Bed boards for a sag-ging mattress | sponge rubber |
| | Sandbags |
| Rolls for support—cot-ton blankets | Bed cradles |
| | Footboards |

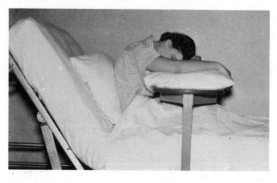

Figure 29-2. This is a restful position for a patient who is unable to lie down in bed.

## Turning a Patient and Maintaining a Side-Lying Position

Sometimes turning the patient is such an important part of his treatment that the doctor specifies how often to do it. This is especially important for elderly patients to prevent lung congestion. In other conditions, it may be impossible to turn the patient (as in the case of fractures with traction appliances), or it may be harmful (with spinal injuries). You may want to turn a patient only to wash or rub his back or change his bed. Many patients are able to help themselves; others need some assistance; you will have to turn the helpless patients—*you* may even need assistance, if the patient is heavy, to keep him from falling out of bed and to prevent pain. When turning a patient on his side, you put him in the *side-lying* position. You proceed in the same way to turn him temporarily on his side (to rub his back, for instance) or to leave him in that position. You may not need pillows for support in the temporary position unless he is very uncomfortable without them (see Fig. 29-3). The following key points will guide you in placing a patient in the side-lying position:

### KEY POINTS

Stand on the side of the bed opposite the side which the patient will be facing when he is turned.

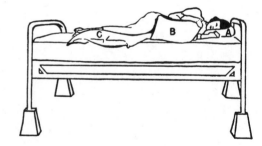

Figure 29-3. Side-lying position to add to the patient's comfort. Small pillow (A) supports head and neck in the midline position. A folded pillow (B) provides support for the upper arm, so that it does not fall forward across the chest. The underneath hip and knee are in very slight flexion, and the upper leg is brought forward to rest on pillow (C) to avoid pressure on the leg underneath.

Slip one arm under the patient's shoulders, the other under his hips.

Advance one foot, bend forward from your hips, and move the patient toward you without lifting. However, do not drag the patient over the sheets so that his skin is damaged.

Roll the patient over on his side, supporting his back and his hips.

Flex the underneath knee and hip slightly to prevent strain on the hip joint.

Bring the upper leg forward to rest on a pillow, thus preventing pressure on the underneath leg.

Put a folded pillow in front of the chest to keep the upper arm from falling across the chest and to keep the shoulders in line.

Put a folded pillow against the back if it makes the patient feel more secure.

## Adjusting the Back Rest and Pillows

If your patient is in a Gatch bed (one that can be adjusted to different positions), it is no problem to raise or lower the back rest. However, to adjust the pillows, his shoulders and back must be lifted. The following are the key points:

### PROCEDURE

Stand facing the patient with one foot forward and the body bent forward from the hips.

Put one arm under the patient's shoulders—put his nearest arm over *your* shoulder—put your other arm under his and across his back.

Tighten your thigh and hip muscles and bring your body and the patient's body upright together.

Continue supporting the patient while you adjust the pillows or back rest with the hand under his back.

## Putting a Patient on a Back Rest (Sitting Position)

A patient may be sitting up for a short time to eat his meals, to work on a table or to change his position. Or he may need to be in this position continuously to make breathing easier (as in cardiac conditions). Support is needed when the body is resting in a sitting position. Pillows support the back, the neck, and the head to keep the spine in its normal curves. Folded pillows support the arms and keep the shoulders up. Pads in the hands

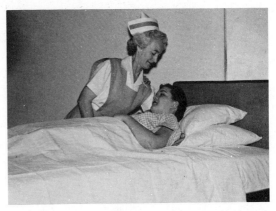

Figure 29-4. Helping the patient to sit up.

support the wrist and keep the fingers bent a little and the thumb out—the position for grasping things. The knees are supported in a comfortable position—the slanting footrest is comfortable for the feet and prevents footdrop.

Figure 29-5 shows a Gatch bed, but you can use any back rest so long as you keep the body alignment the same.

There is more of a tendency for the mattress to slip to the foot of the bed when a back rest is used. This makes it difficult to keep the body in good alignment. To avoid this, a pillow or rolled blanket is sometimes placed in the space between the edge of the mattress and the lower end of the bed.

The bed must be flat to move the mattress

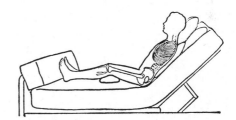

Figure 29-5. Patient in a Gatch bed, backrest position, with 3 pillows arranged to support the normal spinal curves. This drawing pictures the body and the skeletal landmarks with a small pillow under the slightly flexed knees and the feet against the slanting footrest, which enables the patient to relax in a position to preserve function. In addition, pillows, not shown in the drawing, are placed one under each arm from elbow to fingertips, and in each hand are small pads to support the wrists. The fingers and the thumb are in moderate flexion.

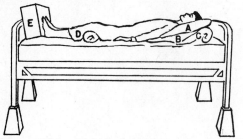

Figure 29-6. This bed is elevated on blocks (head and foot) to place the patient on a more convenient level to save the nurse from unnecessary backstrain. Note the position of the patient on the bed and the arrangement of the 3 pillows (A, B, C) where the middle pillow (B) supports the lumbar spine and pillows A and C the head and the shoulders. Cotton-roll pillow (D) is placed under the knees, and the feet are kept against the pad (E) to maintain their position at right angles.

to the top of the bed in its proper position. If the patient can help, he grasps the bars at the head of the bed, while you grasp the mattress at the top and the side. Then pull together. It is easier if someone pulls with you on the opposite side of the mattress.

You put a patient in the sitting position for the first time during an illness only on the doctor's order. He should be observed closely for signs of fatigue and faintness until his body has adjusted to the change.

## Good Body Alignment With the Patient on His Back

Many patients must lie on their back for a good part of the time; in fact, some patients may stay in this position through a long illness. It is important to make such a patient as comfortable as possible and to prevent body deformities. Figure 29-6 shows how to preserve good body alignment when a patient is lying on his back. Look at the 3 pillows—the middle one supports the lumbar part of the spine, the other 2 support the shoulders and the head. This position gives the breathing and the digestive organs room to work normally. The small knee roll supports the knee at a normal angle; the covered box or footboard is slanted to support the feet at right angles to the legs—a normal angle—and prevents footdrop.

If the patient's body trunk must lie flatter, he will have only 1 pillow to support his head

and neck, the knee roll will be lowered; he will have a pad under his ankles to prevent pressure on his heels; the box at the foot will be more nearly upright.

Remember that the patient's body alignment when he is lying down should be approximately the same as if he were standing.

## Moving Specific Parts of the Body

Parts of the body may be elevated to improve the circulation, to relieve congestion or pain, or to check hemorrhage. Pillows are used to elevate a leg or an arm; protect a pillow with a rubber pillowcase if necessary. Sandbags also may be used to keep the part in position. You would not elevate any part of the body without an order from the doctor—but if you do it in an emergency, such as a hemorrhage, then call the doctor and report what you have done and why.

Always support an arm or a leg along its entire length when you move it. Move it gently and slowly.

## Instructing the Patient

Explain to the patient why you are changing his position and how you will do it. Tell him that you will not hurt yourself because you know how to lift him. If a patient can help, tell him what to do. Your own posture is an important part of the know-how in lifting or moving the patient. You advance one foot—this gives you a wider base to balance your body. You keep your back straight and bend forward from your hips, so that you use your strong thigh and hip muscles.

## Giving a Body Rub

You will not be expected to give massage, since this is the job for an expert with special training. However, the doctor may want a patient to have *light massage* which you can give; find out specifically just what he wants you to do.

Massage is applying pressure and friction to the body with your hands; it may be given for a stimulating or for a soothing effect. Light pressure is soothing; heavier pressure is stimulating. These are the movements used in light massage:

*Stroking (effleurage):* Stroke the large surfaces of the body with the palms of your hands; stroke in the direction of the venous circulation *toward* the heart. You can use your thumb and fingers for the smaller surfaces; keep the strokes and the pressure even. You begin and end light massage with *stroking*.

*Kneading (Pétrissage):* Press on muscle groups or single muscles, picking them up and squeezing them gently. Use the palms of your hands for the large muscles; use your fingers and thumbs for the single muscles. Use this movement for the extremities, the abdomen, and the back.

*Friction:* This is rubbing around the bony prominences of the body, such as the end of the spine and the shoulder blades.

These are the simplest and most effective movements for the kind of light massage that you can give to stimulate circulation and relax contracted muscles. You would give this kind of body rub only after the doctor orders it. Do not give a rub of this kind if the patient is bleeding or shows signs of phlebitis (inflammation of a vein).

## Giving a Back Rub

A back rub is refreshing and relieves tired muscles; it stimulates the circulation, so it is especially helpful over pressure areas to prevent pressure sores. Alcohol hardens and dries the skin—pressure sores are more likely to develop if the skin is moist. Skin lotions containing oil are widely used because of their soothing and softening effect on overly dry skin. You rub the back when you give the morning bath and as a part of the evening care of the patient; you will do it at other times during the day and the night when it is necessary in the patient's treatment or for his comfort. Warm your hands and the skin lotion or alcohol before you begin, to prevent chilling the patient. Be sure that your nails are short enough to rub the back effectively without scratching it. Make sure you are not wearing any jewelry, since jewelry can also scratch the patient. Use long, firm strokes and give extra attention to pressure areas.

### EQUIPMENT

Skin lotion or 50 to 70 per cent rubbing alcohol
Bath powder

The following detailed procedure may sound complicated, but with practice, it can be done easily and quickly. Patients find it very comforting.

### PROCEDURE

Place the patient comfortably on the side or prone, with the entire back exposed. Apply lotion or alcohol to the entire area of the back, rub dry, and dust powder on the hands and apply it to the back if alcohol has been used. Then proceed with the following steps; in each step, repeat the motion 3 times.

Using the first 3 fingers of both hands, rub under the hairline with a circular motion.

Using the first 3 fingers of one hand, rub in the hollow at the back of the neck with a circular motion.

Separating the thumb and the finger of 1 hand, place on either side of the neck and beginning at the hairline, rub the length of the neck with a circular motion.

Using the first 3 fingers of both hands, continue the circular motion down each side of the spine to the coccyx.

Using the heel of the hand, make a firm, circular motion over the coccyx.

Using the flat of both hands, with the fingers extending toward the front, rub the shoulders with a circular motion.

Continue the circular motion with the flat of the hands down the entire surface of the back and the buttocks.

Separating the first and the second fingers of one hand, place the hands on either side of the spine and run them lightly up from the coccyx to the hairline and firmly down.

Remember to use long, firm strokes combined with circular strokes and massage. You may also gently tap the buttocks with the sides of your hands.

Finish with a dusting of powder.

**Your Posture.** Pay attention to your posture when you are giving a back rub. This will sound familiar—stand with one foot slightly forward and your knees bent slightly, with the patient as near your side of the bed as possible. This enables your strong arm and shoulder muscles to do the work and prevents back strain.

# 3. Assisting the Patient to Move

## BED EXERCISES

Bed exercises are sometimes necessary to prepare the patient for getting out of bed and for such activities as walking, getting into a wheelchair, or crutch-walking. These exercises strengthen those muscles in the arms, shoulders, legs, and thighs which have become weakened from lack of use.

It is vital that all patients have some exercise and regular change in body position. When a patient is helpless, a *turning schedule* must be set up and followed whereby the patient is turned at regular intervals to prevent deformities and complications. The patient is also assisted by the nursing staff in other exercise activities called Passive Range of Motion. If the patient can do his own exercises, it is called Active Range of Motion, but nursing supervision may still be necessary to assure that the patient is really moving all of his joints and using all of his muscles.

In other activities, the patient sits up in bed and lifts his hips by pushing his hands down into the mattress. For push-up exercises, he lies face downward and extends his elbows stiffly to raise his head and chest up off the bed. The thigh and leg muscles can be strengthened by asking the patient to contract the *quadriceps femoris,* the large muscle on the anterior thigh. This gives him the feeling that he is pushing the popliteal space behind the knee downward into the mattress and pulling the foot forward.

Some of the daily activities of a patient can be turned into useful exercise. These include such things as reaching for objects on the bedside table, pulling the overbed table forward and pushing it away, and brushing the hair. Muscles are strengthened by using them, and the patient will many times create his own exercises when he understands their purpose.

The physical therapist sometimes introduces the exercises to the patient, but since they are often repeated several times a day, the nurse must be able to supervise them.

## GETTING A PATIENT OUT OF BED

Some patients are allowed out of bed for the entire day. Others are up for a certain length of time each day as their condition improves or permits. This helps to change position, to strengthen muscles, and to prevent deformities.

The patient usually views being up and dressed as a hopeful sign. He is encouraged to wear his own clothes if they are available and if his condition warrants it. However, some patients show little interest in being dressed. They may dread the fatigue of putting on clothes or the pain of moving. Others know that dressing means getting well and resuming problems that they do not want to face. Look for the reason when a patient does not want to be up and dressed.

The doctor will tell you when a patient may be up for the first time and for how long. Remember that merely being up is tiring after an illness.

Decide on the best time to get the patient up. He should be rested, and the room should be warm enough. Most patients enjoy having a meal out of bed or talking to visitors at that time. Be careful about tiring the patient the first time he gets up. If you need assistance in helping the patient to get up, choose a time when the assistance is available.

### Reassurance and Protection

Reassure the patient by explaining how he will be protected—patients worry about falling or getting tired. Tell him not to worry if he is not as strong as he expected to be. Even 1 day in bed can cause wobbly legs and a feeling of needles in the feet. Tell him that as he uses his muscles again, his strength will come back. Protect him in the following way:

Keep him out of drafts and protect him with clothing and blankets.

Spare him extra exertion by using fewer clothes and more blankets; lift or support him as he moves. You will need help in moving the more helpless or the weak or the unusually heavy patient.

Choose a chair that will not slide; keep a footstool steady; use extra care if the floor is slippery.

Check the pulse rate before and after putting the patient into a chair. The change in position affects the circulation and the supply of blood to the brain. He may feel faint and you must watch for signs of fatigue.

Place the signal cord within easy reach of the patient.

A comfortable chair with arms, or a wheelchair
Pillows, blankets, footstool—as necessary
Dressing gown, stockings, and slippers or shoes
Moisture-proof pillowcase, if necessary

## Preparation

Move the chair close to the bed; put a pillow in the seat and cover it with a moisture-proof pillowcase if the patient is likely to soil it; put a pillow lengthwise against the back. Spread a blanket across the seat and leave enough at the lower end to spread beneath the patient's feet if he needs extra warmth.

## Dangling

Dangling the legs over the bed (sometimes called pedangling) is the transitional procedure used before the patient is ready to get up in the chair. Sometimes, the patient is only strong enough to dangle and then lie down again. Sometimes, the patient will need to dangle his legs over the side of the bed for a few minutes before being assisted into the chair. If the patient is to be dangled, he must have something upon which to rest his feet; If the bed is low enough, his feet will touch the floor. But if not, he should be given a footstool or a chair upon which to put his feet. Be sure the patient is covered, so he does not become chilled.

## Getting a Patient Into a Wheelchair

A wheelchair is used to move patients who cannot walk or who should be spared fatigue as much as possible.

**Precautions.** The first thing you do is check the wheelchair you are going to use.

Look at the tires; they should be intact—broken tires cause bumps and jars as the wheels move. The footrest should stay in position when you adjust it, and the rods that hold the back up should stay adjusted at any angle. If everything is in good working order, the wheelchair is safe and comfortable. Hospitals are liable for accidents that harm a patient; thus it is dangerous to take chances by using a wheelchair that is broken or out of order.

Ease the patient's fears of falling by explaining how you will protect him. These are the precautions you take when putting a patient into a wheelchair:

Get someone to help you if the patient is helpless, heavy, or unusually nervous.
Bring the chair against the bed and steady it.
Fold back the footrest so that the patient will not step on it and tip the chair.
Lock the wheels to keep the chair from moving.

**The Procedure.** First, put the bed in low position. Lock the wheels of the wheelchair and place it by the side of the bed, facing the head. If the wheels cannot be locked, an assistant must steady the chair. Prepare the chair with a blanket and pillows as described above. Bring the patient to the side of the bed and assist him to sit up. Proceed slowly: a change in his position may make him feel faint.

Supporting the patient's shoulders and legs, swing him around with his legs over the side of the bed until his feet rest on a chair. This prevents him from sliding off the bed and is more comfortable than if his feet are allowed to hang.

At this point, it is easy to put on the patient's robe, stockings, and slippers or shoes. Facing the patient, with his hands on your shoulders, put your hands, thumbs up, under the axillary region. In this position you are able to support him if he falters or falls forward, as he steps onto the footstool (if one is needed), and to the floor. Let him rest for a few seconds between steps. Then, turning him with his back to the chair, lower him to the edge of the chair and assist him to move back on the chair seat. Practice good body mechanics—stand with one foot slightly forward and your knees flexed. Prevent strain on your back

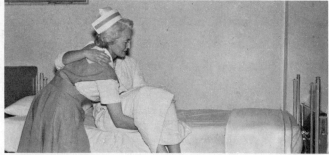

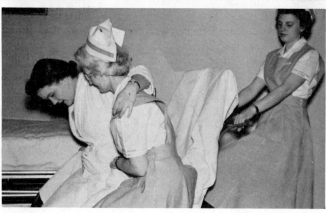

Figure 29-7. (*Top*) While an assistant brings a wheelchair forward, the nurse swings the patient's legs over the edge of the bed. (*Bottom*) The nurse helps the patient to lower herself into the wheelchair. Her assistant steadies the chair.

by using your arm and leg muscles as a lift and lower the patient (see Fig. 29-7).

Adjust the wheelchair footrests, the pillows, and blanket. If the patient is left alone, be sure that the signal cord is within easy reach and is secured so that it cannot be displaced. You may need to restrain the patient in the wheelchair for safety.

### Putting a Patient on a Stretcher (Litter)

A stretcher is a 4-wheeled, rubber-tired cart with a moisture-proof mattress. It is used for the following purposes:

1. To move patients who cannot sit up.
2. To move patients with appliances or casts which would not fit into a wheelchair or would be disarranged.
3. To move patients to the operating room or the x-ray department or to rooms for special tests, treatments, or examinations.
4. To transfer patients from one unit to another.

The tires should be intact so the patient will not be jarred. The stretcher covering should be clean, and enough blankets should be provided to keep the patient warm. You

protect the patient from injury by lifting him correctly and putting him down carefully, by having enough people to lift him, and by never leaving him alone when he is on the stretcher unless he is restrained.

If the patient is able to help himself, place the stretcher parallel to the bed. Be sure the wheels of the bed and the stretcher are locked. Cover the patient with a blanket and turn back the bedclothes; steady the stretcher and assist the patient to move onto it from the bed. It takes 3 people to move a helpless or unconscious patient to a stretcher (see Fig. 29-8). An extra person may also be needed in handling a patient with an injured arm or leg. A strap fastened across the patient's body prevents the patient from falling.

## MOVING AND LIFTING HELPLESS PATIENTS

Some patients can help to get themselves in and out of bed; others are partially helpless; still others, such as paralyzed or unconscious patients, are completely helpless and unable to move their bodies or stand on their feet. A change in position helps the patient's muscles as well as his morale.

Figure 29-8. (*Top*) The 3-man lift. The patient has been brought to the edge of the bed, the stretcher is at a right angle to the foot of the bed and the 3 persons preparing to lift the patient have their arms well under the patient with the greatest support being given to the heaviest part of the patient. Each has a wide base of support and each is leaning over close to the patient in preparation for the lift.

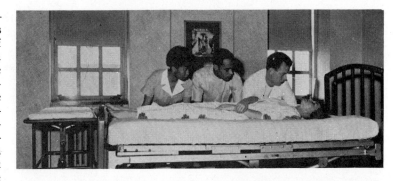

(*Bottom*). On a given signal, the 3 persons rock back and simultaneously lift the patient and logroll her onto their chests. They then pivot and place the patient on the stretcher. As the patient is being lowered onto the stretcher, all 3 carriers maintain a wide base of support and flex their knees.

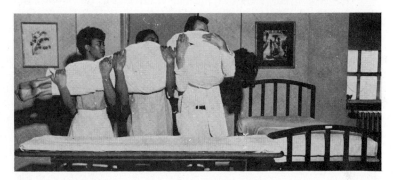

## Body Mechanics

The secret in lifting and moving any weight lies in using good body mechanics. By following these principles, a nurse can move and lift helpless patients with the least amount of strain on the patient or herself.

## Moving a Helpless Patient Up in Bed

It is usually quite easy to slide children or lightweight adults up in bed by yourself, but with heavier adults, you need another person to help you. After locking the bed wheels, 1 person stands on each side of the bed, facing the head. Ask the patient to flex his knees. Each of you puts your nearest arm under the patient's axilla—1 person will be responsible for moving the pillow up against the head of the bed as the other supports the patient's head. Advance 1 foot and flex your knees; on signal, the patient pushes with his feet as you rock forward, sliding the patient toward the head. The pillow keeps the patient's head from hitting the bed frame as he is moved.

If the patient is unable to push with his feet, you flex his knees, holding them in place if necessary. The pillow is placed against the head of the bed. You stand facing each other on opposite sides of the bed at the patient's hips. Flexing your knees and leaning close to the patient, join hands under his hips and shoulders and on signal rock toward the head of the bed, sliding the patient up. Care must be taken to avoid twisting the patient's head and neck.

When absolutely necessary, you can move a patient by yourself by standing at the head of the bed and pulling him up in bed. Stand on the bed frame or a footstool. Put 1 hand under each of the patient's armpits. Rock backward, pulling the patient up in bed. This is a 2-person method which is easier for all concerned. Lock the bed wheels and slip a wide draw sheet or folded large sheet under the patient, from his head to below the buttocks. Roll the sides of the sheet close to his body— this gives you a firm hold. Stand opposite each other, near the patient's shoulders and chest; face toward the foot of the bed, with the leg nearest the bed behind the other leg. Grasp the sheet near the neck and near the lumbar region, lean forward, and rock backward together. Your combined weight slides the draw sheet and patient up toward the head of the bed.

## The 3-Man Lift

This method is used to move a helpless patient, while maintaining his horizontal position. The procedure described here is for moving a patient from his bed to a stretcher (see Fig. 29-8).

Lock the bed wheels.

Place the stretcher at a right angle to the foot of the bed.

Carrier No. 1, the tallest, stands at the patient's head; next tallest is No. 2; the shortest is No. 3.

*Related body mechanic: The tallest people have the longest arms making it easier to support the patient's head and shoulders.*

No. 2 slides both arms under the patient's buttocks.

*Related body mechanic: The heaviest part needs the strongest support.*

No. 1 puts one arm under the patient's neck and shoulders with the other arm against the arm of No. 2.

*Related body mechanic: The touching arms add support.*

No. 3 puts one arm against the arm of No. 2, with the other arm under the patient's ankles.

All 3 lean over the patient and moving on signal, together they rock the patient back and slide him to the edge of the bed.

*Related body mechanic: The lifters' weight and arm-and-knee power combine to move the patient.*

The lifters slide their arms farther under the patient, advance one foot, flex their knees, and logroll the patient onto their chests, then pivot around to the stretcher and lower the patient onto it, bringing their bodies down with him.

*Related body mechanic: Logrolling brings the centers of gravity closer together to stabilize lifting power and reduce strain. The large leg and arm muscles are stronger than the back muscles.*

## Moving a Helpless Patient From the Bed to a Chair

This is a useful technic, especially when a helpless patient is too heavy for 1 person to lift alone and no other help is available. It also can be used to slide a patient onto a commode.

Place the chair facing and against the bed and opposite the patient's buttocks.

Slide your arms under the patient's head and shoulders and advance one foot. Rock backward drawing the upper part of the patient's body to the edge of the bed.

From behind, put your arms well under the patient's axillae, resting his head and shoulders against you.

*Related body mechanic: Distributing the weight makes lifting easier.*

Move around to the back of the chair, drawing the patient into it as you move. Rock back, pulling the patient into the chair.

*Related body mechanic: Brace yourself and the chair by leaning against the chair back.*

Grasping it at the seat, slowly pull the chair back until only his feet and ankles are resting on the bed.

Flex the patient's knees and legs as you lower his feet to the floor, keeping your knees flexed.

*Related body mechanic: Leg and thigh muscles are stronger than back muscles.*

## Moving a Helpless Patient From a Chair to a Hospital Bed

This procedure is slightly different from the one you follow when the bed and the chair levels are the same. In this instance the hospital bed is higher than the chair.

Bring the chair to the side of the bed, with the patient facing the center.

*Related body mechanic: If the chair does not roll, slide it to the bed rather than lifting it. This conserves energy.*

Stand behind the patient, to one side of the chair and place your arms under the patient's axillae drawing him close against you.

*Related body mechanic: Arm and shoulder muscles are long and strong for lifting. Supporting the upper portion of the patient's body on your body reduces the weight to be moved.*

Standing with the foot nearest the chair drawn back and the other foot forward, rock the patient's trunk strongly upward, lifting the entire body and the buttocks onto the bed.

*Related body mechanic: Rocking adds the weight of the body to muscle power.*

Supporting the thighs by resting against them, slide the chair away with your foot.

Lift the patient's legs onto the bed and roll and slide him into position.

*Related body mechanic: It takes less energy to move an object by rolling or sliding it than by lifting it.*

### Assisting the Patient to Move to the Side of the Bed

One nurse, using proper body mechanics, can move a small or large patient. Place your arm and hand under the patient's body, supporting his head and shoulders with one arm and his upper back with the other arm. Lift and move him gently, so that you do not irritate his skin. Bend at the knees and move from front foot to back foot to prevent injury to yourself. After you have moved the pa-

tient's shoulders, repeat the same procedure with his hips and legs. When it comes to moving a very large patient, 2 nurses are better than 1.

### Other Devices for Assisting the Patient to Move

There are many mechanical devices which assist the patient to move. For example, the paralyzed patient may be placed in a CircO-Lectric bed or a Stryker frame, while the patient-lift may be used to conserve the nurse's strength. Many slings and braces are available to help the patient move his fingers or hands, while crutches and walkers give the patient some assistance in getting about. You will learn to use these devices during your practical nursing program. Many of them are discussed in Chapter 46.

## 4. Assisting the Patient with Food and Fluids

### Serving a Food Tray

Most likely, the first contact you will have concerning the nutrition of the patient, will be serving the patient his dinner tray. You must remember that eating is one of the events of the hospitalized patient's day.

Be sure that you are serving the tray to the correct patient. Check his name band with the name on the food tray before giving the tray to him.

### Feeding the Patient

Even patients who can feed themselves may need some assistance in spreading butter on bread, cutting meat, or pouring tea. Always warn a patient about extremely hot foods to prevent him from burning his mouth, especially if he is using a drinking tube. Encourage him to help himself—it develops his self-confidence and his sense of progress toward getting well.

You will have to feed very young or helpless or irrational patients to make sure that they take the necessary food and to protect them from possible injuries or accidents. Use your

judgment about how much the patient can help—sometimes he can hold a piece of bread although he cannot manage other food.

### Encouraging Fluid Intake

Often, the doctor orders "force fluids," which means that the patient is to be encouraged to take as much fluid as possible. The patient will find it much more interesting if fluids are varied and are given in small amounts. Depending upon the patient's diet, offer him some ice cream, jello, coffee, or other fluid occasionally, rather than just water. Whenever you go into his room offer him some fluids in small amounts.

### Intravenous Feeding

A later chapter will discuss the methods and principles related to intravenous therapy; however, in the context of feeding the patient, you must realize that intravenous therapy is another means of giving food and fluids to the patient, as well as medications and blood. Do not forget that this total must be included in the total intake of fluid for the day.

Your responsibility related to intravenous therapy, at this point in your practical nursing education, is to observe to make sure that the fluid is dripping properly and that there is no abnormal swelling in the patient's arm at the site of the needle insertion. You will need to take the presence of the needle and tubing into consideration when you are giving care to the patient. Don't forget to report any abnormalities to the charge nurse or team leader.

## COMMON DIGESTIVE COMPLAINTS

Part of the nurse's responsibility in observing the nutritional status of the patient is to note any discomfort or digestive complaints expressed by the patient.

### Heartburn and Belching

Sometimes the stomach regurgitates part of its contents into the esophagus, where it burns and stings the linings. Although this is called *heartburn,* the heart has nothing to do with causing it. It usually happens after hearty eating or in connection with emotional stress. Another annoyance is *belching,* which is the result of swallowing great gulps of air while eating—a habit some people unwittingly fall into when they are upset. Making people aware of this practice will often help them to overcome it.

### Overeating

The opposite extreme from refusing to eat is eating too much, a habit which is easy to acquire and to find excuses for. Obesity, aside from being a health problem (as in diabetes and heart disease), is also a social liability. It may be the result of lack of exercise, an unbalanced diet, or emotional tensions. If weight reduction is a major problem, it should be carried out under the direction of a physician.

### Vomiting (Emesis)

Vomiting is the result of expelling partially digested food from the stomach. *Regurgitation* is sometimes used to define spitting-up small amounts of food. Persistent vomiting is serious because the body is deprived of essential foods and fluids. Rectal and intravenous feedings are sometimes needed to replace these losses.

Observe and report any of these symptoms carefully—they give the doctor important information. Vomiting may be due to various causes. Always remember that the patient who vomits should not have anything by mouth until the doctor has given instructions.

Note the type of vomiting. For example, in brain disturbances and in some obstructions of the intestines, vomited material is ejected with great force—this is called *projectile vomiting.*

**Vomitus.** Vomiting is not an illness in itself but is a symptom of illness. Vomitus is stomach contents; its appearance and odor tell something about the cause of the vomiting. Notice whether it is undigested food, is odorless or has a sour smell, or is liquid. Does it contain mucus or pus? Vomitus containing bile is a yellowish or greenish color. If it is material which has been forced back into the stomach from the intestine, it has a fecal odor. It may also have a *coffee-ground* appearance, which is evidence of bleeding.

**Specimens.** Always save for inspection any unusual vomitus. Note the amount of vomitus, if possible; it can be measured. The doctor may want the entire specimen sent to the laboratory for examination or may send only a portion of the vomited material. As with other specimens, a single specimen should be in a moisture-proof, covered container and properly labeled.

**Care of the Patient.** If the patient is lying down when he starts to vomit, lift his head slightly and place a curved basin under his chin. Always turn his head to the side to aid in draining material from the mouth and to prevent it from entering the air passages (*aspiration*). If the patient is sitting up, hold the basin for him and support his head with your other hand on his forehead. A towel under the basin protects the bed. If vomiting is frequent, protect the pillow with a moisture-proof covering under the pillow case. Remove soiled linen and wash the face and the hands, if necessary, to remove all traces of offensive and nauseating odors. Rinsing the patient's mouth helps to eliminate a disagreeable aftertaste. Once the patient is comfortable, you can empty the emesis basin and wash it.

## 5. *Assisting the Patient with Elimination*

### NUTRITION AND ELIMINATION

You have previously studied the anatomy and physiology of digestion and elimination. It is important for you to realize that these two processes are interdependent. If nutrition or digestion fails, elimination suffers also. If the patient is unable to eliminate his wastes, these build up in his body and cause disease or a worsening of the existing disease condition.

Next to oxygen, the basic needs of digestion and elimination are perhaps the 2 most important basic needs for maintenance of life. Remember that elimination involves not only the elimination of urine and feces, but also elimination of sweat via the sweat glands and other body fluids via emesis and wound drainage.

### OBSERVATION OF THE FECES

The feces are mostly refuse left from the food we eat. The amount of the feces expelled at any one time is called the *stool*—commonly known as a *bowel movement*. The process of expelling the feces is called *defecation*; the common expression is to say that the *bowels move*. This term is used because *bowels* is another word for *intestines*.

The feces are an important source of information about conditions of the digestive system. They tell about digestion, inflammation or obstruction of the intestinal tract, and the presence of parasites or blood. The appearance of the feces tells much about the way it has moved through the digestive tract. Because the food mass loses water as it moves along, liquid feces indicate a rapid movement; while hard feces indicate that a slower rate has taken place or that the feces have been in the rectum for some time. Observation of the feces includes a number of things, such as consistency, color, and odor.

**Consistency.** Normal feces are soft, formed stools. Liquid feces show irritation of the intestinal tract which may be due to a chronic inflammation or to a temporary irritation.

Hard, dry-looking stools indicate constipation. The size of the mass shows the amount of roughage or waste material in the diet and the time that it has accumulated. The feces are always considered in relation to the diet.

**Color.** Normal feces are a greenish brown; this color comes from bile. Clay-colored stools show that the normal amount of bile is lacking—a mark of gallbladder disturbances. Light-colored stools are sometimes due to undigested fat. A dark, tarlike stool is a sign of hemorrhage, either in the stomach or high up in the intestines. Bright red blood in the stool indicates hemorrhage lower down in the intestinal tract—perhaps in the rectum—with the blood free and not mixed with the stool. The digestive system tries to digest everything that appears in the food passage, including blood. Digested blood is dark and makes the stool tarry. Some foods and medications also affect the color of the stool.

*Pus* in the stool may be due to intestinal infection or the rupture of an abscess into the intestinal tract. *Mucus* indicates irritation of the lining of the intestinal tract. *Blood,* of course, indicates hemorrhage and is always a danger signal which should be reported at once.

**Odor.** The odor of the feces is characteristic, but unusual odors should be noted. Some medications affect the odor; protein decay in accumulated feces also affects it.

**Foreign Objects.** There may be times when a patient will be admitted to the hospital with a history of having swallowed a foreign object. This is especially true in the pediatric department where we find children who have swallowed buttons, safety pins, marbles, or other objects. You will be expected to save each fecal specimen, break it down from the solid mass, and examine it carefully to see if the object has been passed. If you place a small amount of warm water in the bedpan and use wooden tongue blades to stir the mass, it will facilitate the examination of the stool. Any stool that is unusual should be reported to the head nurse or to the doctor. If there is any question in your mind, save the bedpan for inspection by your superior.

## Collecting a Specimen of Feces

### EQUIPMENT

Clean bedpan and cover—2, if the patient wishes
  to void
Paper container and cover
Wooden tongue blades
Paper bag for used tongue blades

### SUGGESTED PROCEDURE

Give the bedpan to the patient and ask
him to defecate. Use a *clean* bedpan.

*Guide: Give another bedpan or urinal first
if patient wishes to urinate.*

Remove the bedpan. Put a portion of the
feces in the container and cover it.

*Guide: Use the tongue blade to transfer the
specimen.*

Label the container in the same manner as
for a urine specimen.

*Guide: Note any special examination re-
quested.*

Take the container immediately to the laboratory. Sometimes the bedpan and the entire
contents are taken to the laboratory.

*Guide: Stools should be examined when
fresh. Examinations for parasites, eggs (ova),
and organisms must be made when the stool
is warm.*

When an infant's stool specimen is to be
examined, take the diaper to the laboratory
wrapped in a paper towel or bag and label it.

## INTAKE AND OUTPUT RECORDS

In many cases, it is vital for the doctor to
know exactly how much fluid (and sometimes
solid food) the patient consumes in one day
and how much he eliminates. This is referred
to as Intake and Output.

*Intake* includes all fluid taken by mouth
and by other means, such as intravenous
therapy or proctoclysis. *Output* includes all
urine and other output, such as wound drainage, emesis, and bleeding. As part of the
record, it is usually noted if the patient ate
all of his food or a portion of it and if he had
a bowel movement or not. In some cases,
every bite of food is weighed and recorded;
and sometimes, all stools are weighed, so the
doctor knows exactly what the total intake
and output was.

Generally, when a patient is on intake and
output all fluid intake and output must be
measured. Don't forget that such things as
jello, ice cream, and thin cereal are considered liquid intake. Each hospital has a listing
of the amounts of liquid contained in various
containers and in different foods and you
should follow this in your recording. Generally, the Intake and Output sheet is kept at
the patient's bedside, and each nurse is responsible for recording the intake and output
which she observes. Be sure to find out the
policy of the hospital for recording water-
pitcher intake. Sometimes, it is recorded
when it is filled and sometimes when it is
empty. Do not fill a pitcher or empty one
unless you are sure of the procedure because
you may cause an error in the recording for
that day. Do not dump a bedpan or urinal
without first finding out if the patient is on
Intake and Output.

**Urine Specific Gravity.** Often, when a
urine output recording is ordered, a specific
gravity measurement is also ordered. This
determines the concentration of the urine.
Generally, the order calls for urine volume
and specific gravity at specified intervals. To
obtain this information, first measure the
urine. Then fill the specific gravity beaker
and gently drop in the measuring instrument,
the hydrometer (also called the *urinometer*).
When the hydrometer stops bouncing up and
down, read the specific gravity. Be sure to
have the instrument at eye level, so that you
get an accurate reading. And be sure to read
at the bottom of the meniscus of the fluid.
The reading is measured in fractions above
1.000 (which would be the reading for pure
water). The normal range for specific gravity
is about 1.003 (very dilute) to 1.025 (quite
concentrated).

*Cautions:* The urinometer must not be
touching the side of the tube or beaker, or
the reading will be incorrect. Also, the urine
must be within a normal range of temperature, or the reading will be incorrect. Finally,
if you read at the top of the meniscus, the
reading will be incorrect.

After the volume and specific gravity (vol.
and spec.) have been recorded, discard the
urine and rinse out the equipment in cool
water (warm water coagulates the proteins in
urine and will cause the equipment to be
unclean). Be sure to wash your hands thoroughly before touching anything else, including your pencil and paper.

## ASSISTING THE PATIENT TO THE BATHROOM

Probably the first duty which you will be asked to perform in this regard is that of assisting the patient to the bathroom. First, be sure to check that he has permission to be up. Then check to find out if the patient is on *Intake and Output* before assisting him to the bathroom. If he is on recorded Output, you may place the bedpan on the chair and then measure the urine, or you may place the bedpan under the toilet seat in the bathroom, so that the patient can collect the specimen himself. Find out how strong the patient is, so that you may obtain additional assistance, if needed. You can walk with the patient just to make sure that he does not fall, or you may need to actually physically assist him to walk. Some patients are taken to the bathroom in the wheelchair or by litter. Other patients use the bedside commode.

Stay with the patient if he is weak, or stay outside the door so that he can call you if he feels faint. Be sure to explain to the patient that there is a nurse's call button in the bathroom which he can use if he needs help. (Usually, the call button in the bathroom activates an alarm, so that the nurse may use it if she needs immediate assistance, such as when a patient falls or suffers cardiac arrest.)

## GIVING AND REMOVING A BEDPAN AND A URINAL

The patient eliminates urine and feces as waste products from the body by voiding and defecating. The utensils used for this purpose if the patient is confined to bed are the *bedpan* and the *urinal*. Females use the bedpan for both; males use the bedpan for defecating and the urinal for voiding. A female urinal may be used for a female patient in certain conditions, such as when she is in a body cast or in some other constricting appliance.

Bedpans are usually made of metal, enamelware, or plastic. They may feel cold on the skin and should be warmed before being placed under the patient. Some of the newer bedpans are made of nylon resin which feel warmer to the touch, are less noisy to handle, and can be cleaned and sterilized by conventional methods (or are disposable).

The position of the body which the patient must assume often makes it difficult to get on and off the bedpan, so that many need assistance. Male nursing personnel usually help male patients who cannot manage by themselves. In any case, it is essential to provide privacy for the patient.

A full bladder makes a patient uncomfortable; in a hospital it is customary to *pass bedpans* to the patients before meals, before visiting hours, and when they settle down for the night.

It is harmful to keep a patient waiting for a bedpan; it weakens the tone of the sphincter muscles in the urethra and the rectum and distresses the patient physically and emotionally. Most patients feel embarrassed about having anyone do such a personal service for them; explain to a patient that there is no need to feel self-conscious about the natural functions of the body; assure him that he will have privacy and that you can place the bedpan to avoid soiling the bed. If a patient is restless or unable to follow directions, protect the bed with a pad.

## The Bedpan Procedure

There is less strain on the patient's back if the head of the bed is elevated slightly before he is placed on the bedpan. Folding back one corner only of the upper bedclothing makes it possible to slip the bedpan under him without exposure. If he needs some assistance, you can help him to raise himself by putting your hand under his buttocks and lifting. If he is unable to help himself, turn him on his side and hold the bedpan against his buttocks as he is rolled back onto it. It is sometimes difficult to do this by yourself.

After giving a patient the bedpan, be sure that the signal bell is within reach and that toilet tissue is conveniently placed. Soap and water for washing his hands should also be available. Always cover a bedpan when taking it to the patient and immediately after it is used.

If a patient is forced to wait when he needs a bedpan or he does not have prompt attention after using it, he may try to walk to the bathroom on his own and fall and injure himself, or he may upset the bedpan and soil the bed. Many patients become emotionally upset in such situations which, of course, is detrimental to their condition.

A child's bedpan is smaller than the standard size; you may be able to use a small bedpan for an adult who is helpless or unable to lie on the larger pan. A fracture pan, which is small and flat, is also available.

A female patient may be allowed to sit up on the bedpan or even to dangle her legs over the edge of the bed if she is having difficulty in voiding. However, she must have whatever back support is necessary and should not be left alone.

## Observation and Recording

The urine and the feces tell many things about the patient's condition, especially in disturbances of the digestive and the urinary systems. You always observe the contents of a bedpan or urinal carefully and note unusual conditions. Be alert about orders to save specimens of urine or feces; save the entire content if you note unusual conditions and show it to the doctor or head nurse. Record difficulties in voiding or in eliminating feces.

## The Urinal Procedure

The urinal is used for a male patient for voiding. Cover the urinal when you bring it to the patient and when you remove it. Help the patient to place the urinal if necessary; provide for washing his hands. After urination, measure urine, and rinse the urinal first with cold water, then with hot. If the urinals are kept in the utility room for general use, sterilize each one in the same way as the bedpan is sterilized every time it is used.

## Using a Commode

Some people have great difficulty with urination and bowel movements when using a bedpan. If such a patient is unable to go to the bathroom, the doctor may permit him to get out of bed in order to use a commode at the bedside. A commode is a straight-back chair or wheelchair, with an open seat and a place beneath to hold a bedpan or other receptacle. Stay with the patient if he is weak and likely to become faint. The directions for using a bedpan also apply to using a commode—wash the patient's hands, note the contents of the commode, and clean the com-

mode after use. It is better to keep the commode out of sight, but it may be covered and kept at the bedside.

## Care of a Patient Who Has a Retention Catheter

Undoubtedly you will be taking care of patients who have retention catheters inserted to care for urine drainage. It is your responsibility to care for the equipment that is used and to see that the drainage apparatus is working properly. The equipment consists of the drainage tubing attached to the catheter and the container for the urine. You never remove the catheter without a doctor's order. If it should come out report the incident to the head nurse.

In observing this type of drainage apparatus, check the following points:

The catheter should be in place.

The tubing should be long enough to allow the patient to turn freely without displacing it from the drainage container.

The tubing should reach well into the container, but the end of it should be above the level of the urine.

Note whether or not urine drainage is taking place by looking at the glass or plastic connecting tube and the level of drainage in the container.

The tubing should pass over the patient's thigh. If it passes under the thigh and buttocks, pressure may interfere with drainage. The adhesive tab around the tubing should be pinned to the sheet, allowing enough leeway for the patient to turn without pulling on the catheter but not so much that the tubing will become tangled. Catheter or tubing should never be bent as this shuts off the flow of urine.

The catheter, tubing, and drainage bag are considered a closed, sterile system and are *not* disconnected unless this is specifically ordered.

Measure all urine that is collected. If you are to irrigate the catheter, you will be shown the method to use.

## Inserting a Rectal Tube To Relieve Flatus

Sometimes a rectal tube is used to aid the patient in expelling flatus (gas) from the intestines. Inserted in the rectum, the tube provides an outlet for accumulated gas and relieves the discomfort of intestinal distention. Insert the tube as for an enema and place the outer end in a urinal, a small basin, or a cardboard sputum or specimen container. A piece of tubing can be attached to the rectal tube and the end placed in a container with sufficient water to cover it; air bubbles in the water will show whether or not gas is being expelled. From 20 to 30 minutes is long enough to leave the tube in the rectum; after that time the sphincter muscles become numbed and the tube ceases to stimulate peristalsis. Note the result on the patient's chart—the length of the insertion, the amount of gas and feces expelled, if any, and whether or not the patient felt relief.

### Inserting a Suppository

A suppository is a small solid substance which melts at body temperature, such as cocoa butter, or glycerin, and is inserted into the rectum to stimulate peristalsis and defecation. Some suppositories contain medication to relieve pain and irritation. Since a small amount of absorption takes place in the large colon, some medications for systemic effect can be given by a suppository.

The intake of food and fluids usually stimulates peristalsis; therefore, a suppository is likely to be more effective if it is inserted half an hour before a meal. This allows time for it to soften feces in the rectum and makes defecation easier.

Insert the suppository past the internal anal sphincter (2 inches). Lubricate it to make insertion easier and protect your finger with a rubber glove or finger cot. Explain the purpose of the procedure and tell the patient it may be half an hour or more before it is effective. If the patient is tense, instruct him to breathe through his mouth to help relax the internal sphincter. Some patients may be able to learn how to insert a suppository for themselves.

## ENEMAS

An enema is the injection of fluid into the large intestine (the colon) through the rectum.

To understand the uses of enemas we begin with the digestive system. The digestion of food results in certain waste materials which normally are moved along the intestinal tract by peristaltic waves until they reach the lower colon and are expelled through the rectum

(see Chapter 17). In supposedly healthy people, poor health habits, such as failure to eat the right foods or to drink enough fluids or to get sufficient exercise, may interfere with this process. Also certain types of illnesses interfere with bowel elimination, especially those which require a restricted diet, prolonged bed rest, or immobilization of the body in one position for a long period of time. Enemas may then be necessary. Enemas are also essential to empty the intestinal tract before a surgical operation or before x-ray or rectal examinations. They are useful in giving certain types of medicines and in relieving distention caused by gas (flatus) in the intestines.

### The Methods and Equipment

In addition to the commercially prepared, disposable enema unit, an enema may be given by 2 other methods: the can and tubing method and the funnel method. With the *can and tubing method,* the solution flows from a can or bag through a length of tubing which is attached to the rectal tube by a connecting tip. With the *funnel method,* the solution is poured from a pitcher into a funnel attached to the rectal tube.

The height at which the solution is poured affects the force and speed of its flow—the higher the can is held, the greater the force. The can is *never* held more than 18 inches above the mattress. With the funnel method, the height is limited to the length of the rectal tube; this makes it impossible to introduce the fluid at a pressure which might harm the colon or distend it so rapidly that it would be impossible to give enough to make an enema effective. Therefore, the funnel method is safer.

**The Rectal Tube.** All enemas are given with a rubber or plastic rectal tube, which is smooth and flexible so that it will not irritate the rectum if it is inserted carefully. A rectal tube may also come with a disposable kit, such as a Fleet enema. Rectal tubes come in different sizes—the larger the size, the more it stimulates the anal sphincter muscles to expel the rectal contents. The sizes used for a cleansing enema range from No. 26, Fr. to No. 32, Fr.; for an enema to be retained, No. 14, Fr. to No. 20, Fr. are used. A retention enema is given when results are not expected immediately. Smaller amounts of solution are given (150 to 200 cc.) so that the patient is able to retain the amount. The size of the rectal tube also affects the rate of the flow of fluid; it will flow faster and with more force through a larger tube.

**The Solution.** The temperature of the solution should be only slightly higher than body temperature to avoid injuring the lining of the intestine. From 105° to 115° F. is usually considered a safe range. This refers to the temperature when the solution is prepared —if it is to be given with a can and tubing, naturally it will be cooler when it reaches the patient. Disposable enema units are usually stored at room temperature. Patients sometimes complain of chilliness with disposable enemas, so these units should never be stored in a cool place.

It is difficult to determine the amount of solution which is necessary for a cleansing enema, because so much depends on the individual patient's ability to retain fluid and on how easily the impulse to empty the rectum is stimulated. Usually, the amount needed for an adult ranges from 750 to 1,000 cc. It is needlessly distressing for the patient if the nurse insists on giving the maximum amount, if satisfactory results can be accomplished with less. On the other hand, larger amounts may be needed and sometimes a patient needs a great deal of encouragement to retain fluid at all—this is especially true of patients who are tense and fearful.

**Effective Enemas.** Certain factors, such as the size of the rectal tube, the method of giving the enema, and the amount and temperature of the solution have a great deal to do with making an enema effective. Never underestimate the importance of giving an enema correctly.

## Kinds of Enema

Enemas are classified according to their purpose:

Purgative or cleansing—to aid in expelling feces
Carminative—to stimulate peristalsis as an aid in expelling gas
Anthelmintic—to destroy intestinal parasites
Emollient—to soothe or protect the mucous membrane

Medicated—to administer medication
Nutritive—to supply food materials

**The Cleansing Enema.** The purpose of the cleasing enema is to inject enough fluid into the colon to soften the feces, stimulate the peristaltic waves, and produce a bowel movement that empties the rectum and the colon. This procedure often is a necessary part of the treatment in illness when body functions are disturbed. Otherwise, a proper diet, sufficient fluids, and a certain amount of exercise, together with regular elimination habits should make the need for enemas unnecessary.

Usually, after breakfast, a peristaltic wave is set up which moves the feces from the colon into the rectum: the fecal mass stimulates the nerve endings in the rectum and brings the desire to empty it. If this impulse is ignored, it disappears, the feces become dry and hard, and defecation is difficult. The colon and the rectum become distended and lose muscle tone as the feces accumulate. An enema provides an artificial stimulus and helps to remove the feces, but, unless normal stimulation and regular defecation are established, taking an enema can become a habit.

A variety of fluids may be used for a cleansing enema such as soap solution, hypertonic solution, normal saline solution, tap water or cottonseed, mineral, or olive oil. Oil is given when it is necessary to soften and to lubricate the feces. It is given in small amounts because it must be retained for a time to be effective. Sometimes, if an oil solution has not been effective after several hours, it is necessary to follow with an enema of soap or saline solution.

Soap solution, saline, or tap water enemas are prepared in larger amounts (500 to 1,500 cc.), enough to stimulate peristalsis and expel the feces. Action may result immediately or it may take longer—usually it occurs in less than 15 minutes.

Soap solution is easily made by dissolving a bland white soap in the water if prepared soap solution is not available. Adding prepackaged soap concentrate to water is a more accurate method. Soap is added because it irritates the mucous membrane of the colon and stimulates peristalsis. Mild soap is used to avoid excessive irritation. Some *proctologists* (rectal disease specialists) forbid the use of soap in enemas before rectal examinations or for patients known to have rectal disease. Tap water is the most common solution for enemas.

The commercially prepared, disposable enema unit contains a hypertonic solution in small amounts—usually 4 ounces (120 cc.). Acting on the principle of osmosis, it draws fluid from the body to create fluid bulk in the colon. The solution is not irritating; it is easily given and usually brings good results in less than 10 minutes. It is especially useful for patients who are unable to retain larger quantities of fluid or have anal incontinence. It helps to prevent anal impaction in patients who must lie in one position or who are unable to sit up. The disposable enema is also widely used in preparing a patient for x-ray or rectal examinations. It comes ready for use and the equipment can be discarded afterwards.

**The Carminative Enema.** The carminative enema is given to stimulate peristalsis to expel gas from the intestine. The solutions used are milk and molasses, turpentine, and mixtures of magnesium sulfate, glycerin, and water. These, however, are rarely required.

The combination of magnesium sulfate, glycerin, and water is known as the 1-2-3 enema because it contains 30 cc. of magnesium sulfate solution, 60 cc. of glycerin, and 90 cc. of water. Together, these ingredients irritate the mucous membrane and distend the colon to stimulate peristalsis and expel the accumulated gas.

**The Anthelmintic Enema.** Anthelmintic drugs help to destroy intestinal parasites and usually are given orally. Because they are toxic drugs, they must be given carefully and are unsafe for some patients, such as those with liver damage. In such instances, a solution of an anthelmintic drug may be instilled into the rectum to be retained.

**The Emollient Enema.** An emollient enema consists of a small amount of olive or cottonseed oil, given to protect or soothe the mucous membrane of the colon. This enema is to be retained.

**The Medicated Enema.** The medicated enema, which involves inserting a drug into the rectum, sometimes is the only way to give a patient a drug. It also may be the best way to make a drug effective quickly—some drugs are absorbed by the mucous membrane very rapidly. This is true of some anesthetics, such as Avertin, and of sedative drugs, such as paraldehyde and chloral hydrate. It is almost impossible to take paraldehyde by mouth because of its offensive taste. The drug is combined with a small amount of oil or saline to reduce its irritating effect on the mucous membrane and to lessen the desire to expel it, since it is given to be retained.

**The Nutritive Enema.** This method of supplying nutritive materials has been replaced largely by intravenous feeding, which is more efficient. It is impossible to maintain adequate nourishment by rectal feeding since the colon is very selective in what it will absorb. A solution of dextrose is used most often.

## Emergency Measures

Occasionally, fluids are given by rectum to tide the patient over an emergency until more effective methods are available.

A quantity of fluid can be given by rectum over a long period of time by a drip method known as *proctoclysis*. Equipment similar to that included in the can method of giving an enema is used and the rate of flow is controlled by a clamp. This procedure is less common since other methods of administering fluids have been perfected.

## Explaining the Procedure

Many patients are familiar with the cleansing enema, which is given to produce a bowel movement, but do not understand the purpose of an enema to be retained. In any case, the procedure and the reason for it should be explained as simply as possible. A nurse may have an opportunity to relate the patient's diet and fluids to their effects in preventing constipation. The patient who is having an enema for the first time may be fearful of pain or of soiling the bed. The patient's cooperation has much to do with making an enema effective.

## The Patient's Position

The descending colon lies on the left side of the abdomen so it has always been assumed that an enema would be more effective if it were given with the patient lying on his left side. Today, it is thought that it is relatively unimportant, as the fluid runs into the colon as easily from one side as the other. In fact, if the patient is in traction, an enema can be given while he is lying on his back. So there is no need to be unduly concerned if the patient is unable to lie on his left side. However, an enema should never be given with the patient sitting up because without the help of gravity, it takes a great deal of pressure to force the fluid into the colon; also the patient may be unable to retain it long enough to make the procedure effective.

## Inserting the Rectal Tube

The anus has an inside and an outside sphincter muscle which control the opening (see p. 135). The tube should be inserted past both of these muscles—3 or 4 inches would be more than sufficient, since the anal canal is only 1 to 1½ inches long. Attempts to force the tube into the rectum against resistance may harm the tissues. If the tube does not go in easily, let a small amount of solution enter and withdraw the tube slightly, then reinsert it. Resistance may be caused by a kink in the tube, by a spasm of the colon, or by feces impacted in the rectum. Running a small amount of the fluid through the tubing warms it so that the fluid reaches the patient at the proper temperature from the beginning of administration.

## Giving a Cleansing Enema (Can and Tubing Method)

### EQUIPMENT

| | |
|---|---|
| Irrigating can and tubing, glass connecting tip, clamp | Solution as prescribed |
| | Lubricant |
| Rectal tube No. 26 to No. 32, Fr. (Use a catheter for an infant or a child) | Protective sheet and cover |
| | Standard toilet tissue |
| | Bedpan and cover |
| | Bath blanket |

### KEY POINTS IN THE PROCEDURE

Prepare the solution as ordered, 750 to 1,500 cc. for an adult at a temperature of 105° to 110° F.

*Principle: The adult colon holds 750 to 2,000 cc. The solution should be approximately at body temperature when it reaches the colon. It loses heat as it travels through the tubing. Heat stimulates the mucous membrane.*

Lubricate the tip of the rectal tube for 2 to 3 inches.

*Principle: Lubrication prevents friction when the tube is inserted.*

Put the patient on his left or right side. If this is impossible, he can lie on his back.

*Principle: Gravity aids the flow of fluid.*

Let some fluid run out of the tube.

*Principle: You must determine that the tube is patent (open) and you do not wish to introduce air into the colon from the tubing.*

Slowly insert the rectal tube for 4 to 5 inches.

*Principle: The anal canal is 1 to 1½ inches long, and 4 to 5 inches ensures entering of the colon. Slow insertion is less likely to cause spasms of the intestinal wall.*

Raise the can (or funnel) high enough to allow the fluid to flow into the rectum slowly—let the patient indicate when the flow may be too rapid. You may stop the flow for a few seconds and then resume.

*Principle: Gravity aids the flow of fluid. The higher the container is held, the more rapid the flow and the greater the pressure on the colon and the desire to expel the fluid.*

When the patient feels a strong desire to empty the rectum, discontinue the flow of fluid and withdraw the rectal tube gently.

*Principle: Distention of the colon stimulates peristalsis and a desire to expel the rectal contents.*

Put the patient on the bedpan (sitting up, if possible) or assist him to the commode or bathroom toilet.

*Principle: Contracting the abdominal and perineal muscles helps to empty the colon. This is easier in a sitting position.*

Encourage the patient to retain the fluid for a short time.

*Principle: Most patients think the enema should be expelled immediately. Fluid helps to soften the feces and makes expelling it easier.*

Record the treatment on the chart, noting any unusual conditions, characteristics of feces, flatus expelled, and the patient's reactions.

## Care of Enema Equipment

Autoclaving is considered the safest way to care for enema equipment, unless disposable equipment is used, in which case it is simply discarded. Sterile equipment is not necessary in giving an enema, but it is important to sterilize enema equipment *after* it has been used, to prevent carrying infection to others. In many hospitals this is taken care of by preparing enema sets in the surgical supply room.

## When the Patient Is Unable To Retain an Enema

If the patient is unable to contract the anal sphincter muscles or if the muscles have lost their power to contract, it will be necessary to give the cleansing enema with the patient on the bedpan. Elevating the head of the bed slightly and placing a pillow in the lumbar region help to prevent back strain. The advantage of using a disposable enema unit for this type of patient is that it is given in a small amount.

## When the Patient Is Unable To Expel an Enema

When the muscles do not respond to stimulation and the patient is unable to expel an enema, the solution must be withdrawn. The bedpan is placed on a chair at the bedside, beneath the level of the rectum. When the rectal tube is directed into the pan the force of gravity helps to drain off the fluid. If this is not effective the fluid is siphoned off.

## Giving an Enema to a Child

An infant or a small child will not be able to retain an enema, so you must provide a pad and a basin or a small bedpan to catch the solution, which is almost sure to be expelled as you give the enema. It may be necessary to restrain the child or to ask someone to assist you.

It is difficult to state the specific amount of solution that should be given because this depends on the age and size of the child. For an infant, the amount of solution should not exceed 300 cc. and might be less. The amount increases with the age of the child but usually is no more than 500 cc. up to the age of 14.

The irrigating can or the funnel should not be more than 18 inches above the mattress; use a No. 10, Fr. to 14, Fr. catheter for an infant; a No. 14, Fr. to 16, Fr. rectal tube for a child.

A rubber-tipped bulb syringe (100 cc.) is easy to manage with infants or small children. The fluid should be injected with the least possible amount of pressure.

## The Doctor's Orders

An enema is never given without a doctor's order. The order may be for an enema every day, or it may state "when necessary," which leaves the decision up to the nurse. She is guided somewhat by the patient's feelings—some people are distressed if they do no have a bowel movement every day. In the hospital, the practical nurse consults her supervisor about carrying out a "when necessary" (p.r.n.) order.

## COLONIC IRRIGATION

A colonic irrigation is a prolonged washing-out of the large intestine. It bathes the intestine with a considerable amount of fluid, some of which the intestine absorbs. Occasionally, colonic irrigation is given to cleanse the colon and as a treatment for such conditions as colitis and uremic poisoning; it is also given to supply heat and fluid to the body.

Obviously, no one should have a colonic irrigation unless his doctor prescribes it. In the past, this treatment led to a widespread form of quackery—the colonic irrigation operators. When the doctor prescribes a colonic irrigation, he is also concerned about other aspects of the patient's treatment, as for example, the diet. Self-prescribed colonic irrigations may actually do harm by delaying proper treatment.

A colonic irrigation consists of introducing water into the colon and siphoning it off. The kind, the amount, and the temperature of the solution are determined by the reason for giving the irrigation. This treatment is rarely prescribed today. If you are asked to do a colonic irrigation, consult the hospital's procedure manual and your supervisor.

## COLOSTOMY IRRIGATION

The method of removing fecal material from the bowel after a colostomy has been performed is known as colostomy irrigation. This procedure is described in Chapter 49.

## DIGITAL REMOVAL OF FECES

Sometimes, the feces becomes so impacted and hard, that the patient cannot expel it. In this case, and with a doctor's order only, the nurse may be instructed to manually remove the feces. Put on an unsterile rubber glove and lubricate one finger well. Insert the finger carefully into the rectum and break up the stool. Do this procedure very gently, since it may be very uncomfortable for the patient. Usually, after the stool is broken into pieces, the patient will be able to expel it. He may also be given an enema to assist in expelling the feces. In some cases, the nurse is instructed to remove the particles of feces after breaking the stool. Be sure to obtain instruction in this procedure the first time you do it.

If the patient is a woman, a sterile glove may be applied to the other hand, lubricated, and inserted into the vagina. The 2 gloved fingers can then break up the stool at the same time. This method is often more effective than just the rectal method.

## DISORDERS OF ELIMINATION

### Diarrhea

People sometimes have a wrong conception of true diarrhea—doctors define it as frequent, loose watery stools and consider the *consistency* of the stools more important than their frequency.

### Constipation

Conversely, constipation is characterized by hard, dry, and infrequent stools. It may be the result of a lack of roughage in the diet or of ignoring the impulse to empty the rectum, thereby allowing the feces to become dry and hard. Some medicines, such as barium have a constipating effect.

# 6. *Assisting the Patient with Personal Cleanliness*

## WASHING THE PATIENT'S FACE AND HANDS

Wash the patient's face and hands before breakfast, during a bath, and before dinner. You may also do it at other times for comfort and you always see that his hands are washed after he has had a bedpan or a urinal.

If he is able, the patient who can sit up should be encouraged to wash his face and hands himself. Arrange the equipment conveniently on the overbed table, so that he will have no difficulty. This is a step in rehabilitation.

#### GENERAL DIRECTIONS

Protect the bedclothing with a towel placed under the patient's chin.

Wring the washcloth sufficiently to prevent dripping.

Do not use soap on the face unless the patient wants it. Never use soap on the eyes, and if soap is used on the face, remove it thoroughly by rinsing.

Wash each eye from the nose outward.

Put the patient's hands in the basin of water to wash them and use soap. Use a hand brush if necessary for grimy nails.

## GENERAL MOUTH CARE

Many disease organisms enter the body by the mouth, and food particles in the crevices between the teeth cause decay and breath odor. Some illnesses cause irritation or dryness or brownish deposits on the tongue and the mucous membranes. Some infections of the gums are communicable. Any mouth condition which interferes with taking food or causes infection in the mouth or another part of the body harms the patient's health. Breath odors or decayed teeth make sensitive people self-conscious.

People who have not learned good health habits need to be taught why good mouth care helps them to keep well. Poor teeth and other mouth conditions prevent people from eating necessary foods and interfere with the appetite. When you tell a patient why you are doing any nursing procedure, two things happen: (1) you reassure him, and (2) he learns something. Patients do learn to improve their health habits if a tactful nurse is really interested in helping them. If you want a patient to go on brushing his teeth after he leaves the hospital, you might comment on such things as the improved appearance of his teeth and how much better his appetite is. Be sure to offer the patient the opportunity to brush his teeth after each meal.

## Observations

Observe the condition of a patient's mouth and teeth and record the effect of brushing. Note such factors as bleeding, swelling, or unusual mouth odor, on the chart. If the gums or teeth are unusually sensitive, it may be necessary to use applicators or a tongue depressor wrapped in gauze, rather than a toothbrush.

### EQUIPMENT

| | |
|---|---|
| Toothbrush | Small curved basin |
| Toothpaste, powder, or mouthwash | Container, if mouthwash is used |
| Glass of cool water | Towel |

If the patient is able to brush his teeth himself, see that he is sitting up comfortably and that the equipment is placed conveniently.

### PROCEDURE

Protect the patient's gown and the bedclothing.

Turn the patient's head to one side if he is lying down.

Caution the patient about swallowing the mouthwash.

Provide sufficient water for rinsing and rinse freely.

See that he brushes his teeth effectively—show him the correct method, if it is necessary to do so.

Wipe his mouth and chin and rinse the toothbrush well.

## Caring for the Mouth When a Patient Wears Dentures

People may be sensitive about wearing dentures, so be careful about privacy for these patients when you give them the toothbrushing equipment. If the dentures are left out of the mouth, put them in an opaque container —preferably covered—out of sight. Keep them in water. Handle the dentures carefully to avoid breaking them; they are expensive, and the patient is handicapped without them. Be sure to label them and be very careful not to lose them.

Frequently you find a patient who is constantly removing his dentures; you may find them under the pillow or on the bedside table. In these instances, look for irritated areas in the mouth; many dentures fit poorly. Poorly fitting dentures are often the reason for poor eating habits and poor nutrition; the afflicted person neither chews his food well nor eats the proper foods. This is one of the reasons for older people's dietary problems.

The mouth needs the same care when dentures are worn as it does with one's own teeth. Mouths and dentures that are not clean cause breath odor—toothpaste advertising makes a great point of "denture breath." Specially designed brushes and preparations for soaking dentures to remove deposits are available. Always hold dentures over a basin of water when cleansing them, if they should be dropped on a hard surface they are likely to break.

Most dentists encourage their patients to wear their dentures all the time. If dentures are removed for long periods, the gum line changes and the dentures do not fit. If they must be removed, they should never be stored in cups or glasses which are used for drinking.

Always remove dentures if a patient is unconscious or irrational or having convulsions; remove them if a patient is going to the operating room. The danger is not that the patient may swallow them, although removable bridges have been swallowed, but that they may obstruct the trachea and cut off the patient's air supply.

## Special Mouth Care

If a patient is helpless, you will have to care for his teeth; you may have to give special mouth care in some illnesses if brownish material (*sordes*) collects on the tongue and teeth, or if the patient breathes through his mouth. If the patient cannot take fluids by mouth or if fluids are restricted, it may be necessary to give special mouth care as often as every hour. If a patient needs to be encouraged to take food, cleansing the mouth before eating helps to make food more palatable.

Some patients like the aromatic taste of a medicated mouthwash, but water or salt water is just as effective. Hydrogen peroxide may also be used.

If the patient is unable to cooperate by opening his mouth, a tongue blade can be used to hold it open. Sometimes it is necessary to use a mouth gag. Never try to hold open a patient's mouth with your fingers—you may be bitten.

### PROCEDURE

Turn the patient's head to one side to keep the patient from aspirating the slightest amount of fluid.

Cotton applicators of a suitable size and gauze wrapped around a tongue blade are effective cleansing tools, for all surfaces (mouth and tongue).

Moisten the mucous membrane with water after cleansing.

Apply an emollient cream to the lips to prevent drying and cracking—moisture evaporates rapidly from the thin skin of the lips.

If the patient has an infectious mouth condition, use the same precautions in the care of his equipment, wastes, linen, and dishes as for any communicable disease. Explain to the family why you use these precautions and caution them about touching things which the patient handles. People put their hands to their mouths more often than they realize.

## BATHING THE PATIENT

A complete daily bath is not necessarily essential or even advisable for every patient.

In many instances, the patient's condition, or the weather, may determine how often a bath is necessary; personal bathing habits have an influence on the frequency of bathing. Until comparatively recently, it was almost universal hospital practice to expect nurses to have all the patients bathed by the middle of the morning at the latest, or by the time the doctors began to make their rounds. Today, we try to be more considerate of the patient's comfort and not so concerned with a deadline for having everything tidy. If a patient has had an uncomfortable sleepless night, a rest after breakfast may be much more appealing than a bath. In some cases, a bath may do the patient more harm than good.

Another long-standing (and disturbing) custom was the practice of washing the patient's hands and face hours before his breakfast was served. This often necessitated waking the patient at a very early hour, rousing him so thoroughly that he was unable to go back to sleep. In some cases, having a good night's sleep may be much more important to the patient than being bathed. Many hospitals have adjusted their routines with the patient's comfort in mind. Modern equipment includes showers and bathtubs equipped with self-help devices for patients who are able to bathe themselves. Daily baths now are considered less of a sacred ritual "to be observed at any cost."

A bath helps the process of elimination by removing the waste products of perspiration from the skin; it also stimulates circulation and is refreshing. The main purpose of a bath is to keep the body clean. The 3 kinds of cleansing baths are the shower, the tub, and the sponge bath given in bed. The patient's condition determines which kind of bath is the safest and the best for him. A sponge bath involves the least exertion for the patient and is the safest if he has any difficulty in moving or is irresponsible.

## Giving a Tub Bath

Some patients can safely have a shower or a tub bath on admission to the hospital. Convalescent patients progress to the point where a tub bath is another step toward their normal habits. A patient gains independence and is encouraged by this evidence that he is getting well. Always get permission to give the first tub bath when you have been giving bed baths to a patient. It is better not to give a bath immediately after a meal because a bath draws the blood to the skin and takes it away from the digestive organs.

You must be the judge of how much assistance the patient will need. Some patients may prefer to wait until they are able to carry on alone; others will not feel embarrassed by assistance. In any event, you can do much to spare the patient exertion; you are also responsible for his comfort and safety.

### EQUIPMENT

| | |
|---|---|
| Blanket | Bath powder |
| Bath mat | Clean gown or pajamas |
| Bath towels | Clean bed linen as in |
| Face towel | "Making an Occupied |
| Washcloth | Bed" (Chap. 26) |
| Soap | Bath thermometer |

**Preparation.** Check the temperature of the bathroom. If you use an electric heater, put it at a safe distance from the tub; caution the patient about touching it with wet towels or hands. Place a chair near the tub with a bath blanket opened over it. This is convenient for the patient to sit on while he dries himself or while you dry him; it prevents fatigue and allows him to keep part of his body covered as he dries himself, to prevent chilling and exposure. Place towels, washcloth and soap where he can reach them easily. Fill the tub about half full of water—less for a child. The temperature varies anywhere from warm to very warm—never hot or over 100° to 110° F. Test the water with a bath thermometer. Elderly and thin people usually find a warmer temperature more comfortable.

Place the bath mat in front of the tub. Bring the patient to the bathroom. Help him to remove his dressing gown, gown, and slippers and help him into the bathtub, if he needs assistance—otherwise you may leave him.

**Safety Precautions.** Devices attached to the tub or a rail on the wall make it easier to get in and out of a tub without assistance. A rubber mat in the bottom of the tub prevents slipping. By sitting on a chair beside the tub, the patient can ease over onto the tub's edge and then swing his feet into the tub; by steadying himself on the opposite edge he can gradually lower himself into a sitting position. This procedure is good muscle exercise. Remind the patient that there is a nurse's call light in the bathroom which he can use if he needs help.

Ask him not to lock the door—tell him that you will see that no one comes in and that you will be near if he needs help. Come back in a few minutes and call through the door to find out whether he is all right or if he wants anything. Do this often enough to be sure that he is safe. Never leave a child or a depressed person alone in a tub or a person who is unsure or unsteady in his movements—poor eyesight and stiff joints cause accidents—many home accidents happen in the bathroom. If the patient's condition allows it, he may luxuriate in his bath for 10 or 15 minutes; you will need to check with him frequently to see that he does not go to sleep or become faint and slip under the water.

Help him out of the tub and dry him, if he needs assistance. Put on his gown, dressing gown and slippers and assist him back to bed.

## The Shower Bath

A guide rail on both the inside and the outside of a shower stall is essential. Two rails are better than one—one rail at a level the patient can reach for support when he is sitting down on a stool and the other higher up for support when he is standing. When the shower is attached to the bathtub rather than being in a separate stall, the suggestion of using a stool in the tub is often welcomed by some apprehensive patients. It is safer for most patients to sit down while taking a shower, especially if they are elderly or weak. In fact, any patient who is very weak or unsteady should not be permitted to take a shower unattended. The patient should have the necessary assistance, and the same precautions should be taken for his safety as for a tub bath. Regulate the temperature of the water first and protect the hair of a woman patient with a waterproof covering. Caution the patient about standing on one leg, as the stool is there to sit on while he washes his feet and legs.

## Giving a Bed Bath

The bath is given in such a way as to get the desired effect with the least exertion for the patient and without chilling him. Patients do not always look forward to having a bath—

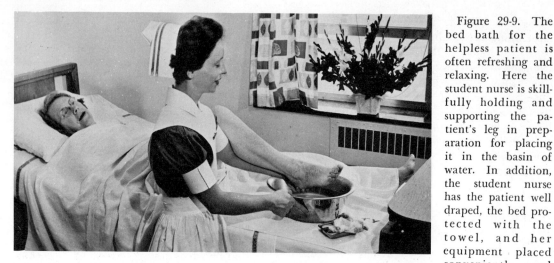

Figure 29-9. The bed bath for the helpless patient is often refreshing and relaxing. Here the student nurse is skillfully holding and supporting the patient's leg in preparation for placing it in the basin of water. In addition, the student nurse has the patient well draped, the bed protected with the towel, and her equipment placed conveniently and ready for use. (Fuerst, E. V., and Wolff, L.: Fundamentals of Nursing, p. 237, ed. 4. Philadelphia, Lippincott, 1969)

some people are shy and embarrassed; others are afraid of being chilled; another may dread a bath because it hurts to move or because he feels too tired to make an effort. You can reassure a patient by explaining that the door will be closed or the cubicle curtains drawn, that he will be covered with a blanket to keep him from "catching cold," and that you will close the window and use comfortably warm water.

In some instances a sponge bath is harmful for a patient, such as those who have considerable pain, are bleeding, or are weak. You will have to decide when a patient can be allowed to help with his bath and when you must spare him every bit of exertion you can. For instance, some patients can turn and move themselves—others must not be allowed to make the slightest effort. It is also important to consider the patient's feelings—if he is uncomfortable unless he has 2 pillows under his head, if he wants another blanket over him, if he says the water feels cold—try to make him comfortable while he is having his bath.

The time when a bath is most refreshing is in the morning or at night before he goes to sleep. A bath during the day may also prove comforting to the patient. If a patient perspires a great deal or feels hot and uncomfortable, a bath at night may help him to sleep. However, an hour or so after breakfast is the usual time for bathing a patient.

In the hospital, the time for the bath is governed by a patient's condition and the number of patients for whom you are responsible. You have less leeway in choosing the time for a bath but you can plan to bathe the most uncomfortable patients first or to leave to the last any patient who has been vomiting or has just had a painful treatment or dressing. You also must take into consideration appointments with P.T., x-ray, or other departments.

You will be able to give the bath itself in about 20 minutes when you become skillful; however, you have to allow extra time for the other procedures which go with the bath—getting ready for it, making the bed, and caring for the equipment, the soiled linen, and the unit afterward. Sometimes other workers, such as ward aides, tidy and dust the unit. It is not always possible to give every patient a bath every day in a public hospital ward. A common procedure is to give 2 complete baths a week and partial baths on the other days. The very sick patients may have a complete bath every day. You make a plan every day according to the number of patients you are assigned and the number of complete or partial baths you are giving. The head nurse or your team leader helps you with this plan; it changes every day because the doctors' orders change or because the patient may go to the operating room or the x-ray department or have special tests or treatments.

| | |
|---|---|
| Check the patient unit for: | Clean bedspread, if necessary |
| Bath basin | Clean linen, as allowed and necessary |
| Bath blanket | |
| Bath towel | Washcloth |
| Face towel | Patient's gown or pajamas |
| Rubbing alcohol or lotion | Extra bath towel |
| Bath powder | Soap |
| | Laundry bag or hamper |

## Preparation

The preparation for the bath is especially important because you should be able to complete the procedure without leaving the unit for forgotten equipment. When the bath is interrupted, the patient may become chilled and uneasy and the bath water becomes cold. The following key points can be used when preparing for a bed bath:

Tell the patient about the bath.

Check the temperature of the room; protect the patient from drafts and close the window if necessary.

Close the door or draw the cubicle curtains and place a straight chair beside the bed at the foot.

Clear the bedside table for bath equipment.

Fill the bath basin ⅔ full with quite warm water—it can be about 120° F. because it will cool slightly while you are getting the patient ready.

Remove the bedspread, fold it, and hang it over the back of the chair. If you are discarding the spread, put it in the receptacle for soiled linen.

Place the bath blanket on the bed and draw it down, remove and fold the bed blanket, and hang it over the back of the chair.

Remove and fold the top sheet and place it over the back of the chair.

Remove all but 1 pillow. Remove the patient's gown and place it with the soiled linen.

The suggested procedure described assumes that the patient is unable to move without assistance.

Bring the patient to the side of the bed nearest you by segmentally moving his head and shoulders, hips, thighs, and lower legs.

*Guide: Stand facing the bed, opposite the part to be moved each time, with one leg forward and the knees flexed. Slide your forearms under the part, lean forward and rock back, making effective use of the longest and strongest muscles.*

Spread a bath towel under the patient's chin and wash the face.

*Guide: See "Washing the Patient's Face and Hands," p. 254.*

Use soap to wash the ears and the front of the neck. Rinse and dry.

*Guide: Have the washcloth wet enough to rinse well without dripping. Make a mitt over your hand by folding and tucking in the washcloth ends.*

Put the towel over the chest and fold the blanket back. Wash, rinse, and dry the chest.

*Guide: Expose the areas under the breasts and observe for irritation.*

Allow the towel to remain on the chest and turn the bath blanket back. Wash, rinse, and dry the abdomen.

*Guide: Wash well around to the back, over the pubic area and the upper thighs. If necessary, use a cotton-tipped orangewood stick moistened with oil to cleanse a dirty umbilicus.*

Remove the towel and replace the blanket. Uncover the arm nearest you and place a towel under it. Wash, rinse, and dry the arm.

*Guide: Support the arm—lift it and wash the axilla.*

*Guide: Always protect the bottom bedding with a towel while washing any part of the body to prevent the linen from becoming wet and chilling the patient.*

Wash the hands and care for the nails. Replace the bath blanket.

*Guide: See "Caring for the Fingernails" p. 260.*

Repeat for the other arm and hand from the same side of the bed.

Wash, rinse, and dry the thigh and the leg nearest you.

*Guide: Flex the patient's knee and drape the bath blanket around the thigh to prevent the exposure of the genital area.*

Place the soapdish and the basin of water at the foot. Support the leg on your arm and carefully place the foot in the basin. Wash, rinse, dry, and clean the toenails.

*Guide: See "Caring for the Toenails" p. 261.*

Repeat for the other thigh, leg, and foot from the same side of the bed. You may wish to soak the patient's feet. This is very comforting to the patient.

Change the bath water.

*Guide: Always change the water at this point, but change it more often if it becomes excessively soapy or soiled. Carry the basin close to the body to reduce strain on the arm muscles.*

Turn the patient on his side and bring him close to the edge of the bed.

*Guide: While the patient is on his back, cross his nearest leg over the opposite one— place the arm he will be lying on away from his body with the elbow bent and the hand pointed toward the head of the bed. Go to the opposite side and put one hand on the patient's shoulder, the other on his buttocks. Standing with one leg forward and braced against the bed with your knees flexed, rock back, bringing the patient over on his side.*

Go to the other side of the bed and slip your hands under the hips and draw them to the edge of the bed.

Place the towel along the back. Turn the bath blanket back and wash, rinse, and dry the back of the neck, the shoulders, the back, the buttocks, and the posterior upper thighs.

*Guide: Stand with one foot forward and rock slightly forward with the upward strokes and backward with the downward strokes. Rocking helps to make strokes even and smooth.*

Rub the back with alcohol or lotion and powder the back following an alcohol rub.

*Guide: Do not use powder with the lotion. It will cake and cause irritation of the skin.*

Roll the patient back to the back-lying position.

*Guide: Put one hand on the patient's shoulder and one on his hip. Place one foot forward and pull him over by rocking back. Go to the other side of the bed. Put your hands under his buttocks. Separate your feet and rock back to bring the patient's body in good alignment.*

Wash the genital area if the patient is unable to do so. Otherwise place the necessary equipment within easy reach and leave the unit. Ask the patient to "finish his bath."

Put a clean gown on the patient, and make the bed and comb his hair.

*Guide: A towel can be used to protect the bed from combings.*

If a male patient is unable to finish his bath unaided, a member of the male nursing personnel can perform this service for him with the least embarrassment. However, if a male nurse or attendant is not available and the nurse neglects this necessary procedure, she is guilty of poor nursing. No patient should be penalized because of his sex.

The sponge bath provides an opportunity for the nurse to give close scrutiny to the condition of the patient's body. She should record the type of bath given and any significant observations such as skin eruptions or reddened pressure areas.

## Giving a Partial Bed Bath

The patient should have a partial bath on the days when he does not have a complete one. It consists of bathing the face and the hands, the axillae, the back, the buttocks, and the genital area. Some patients are able to do this for themselves. You draw the cubicle curtains, regulate the room temperature, prevent drafts and prepare the equipment. After the bath, remove the equipment and make the bed. A patient may need some assistance, especially in washing the back area. Every patient should be encouraged to accomplish as much of the procedure as possible because it is good muscle exercise and helps to make him self-sufficient.

## Caring for the Fingernails

The patient's general condition and his health habits affect his nails. Brittle, broken nails may be the result of improper diet or fever. Emotional tensions cause nail-biting. Some types of work make the nails stained and broken, while water, strong soaps, and washing powders make the nails and the cuticle dry. Well-cared-for nails are pleasing to look at and are a health protection; conditions like torn cuticle are an invitation to infection. Thus reddened areas or breaks in the cuticle should be reported. Dirty nails can carry infection through handling food or scratching the skin. It is better to file the nails than to cut them since filing prevents rough edges that catch on the clothing and cause the nail to break.

Essential daily care is cleaning beneath the nails and pushing back the cuticle. The best time to do this is after the patient's hands have been in water. Soap and water loosen dirt and soften the cuticle temporarily. Oil on the nails and the cuticle softens dry, tight cuticle and dry nails. Use an orangewood stick to clean the nails and to push back the cuticle. The stick is blunt and smooth and less likely to injure the nails than the tip of a metal nail file. Cut off hangnails with manicure scissors to keep them from tearing still more.

The convalescent patient may be able to care for her own nails. Arrange the necessary equipment on the overbed or bedside table. You will need:

| | |
|---|---|
| A basin ⅓ full of warm water | Orangewood stick |
| Soap | She may have other things she wants to use such as nail polish, cuticle oil, nail file |
| Towel | |
| Nail brush | |

Never give sharp-pointed or cutting equipment to a patient who has unsteady hands or is depressed—he may injure himself.

## Caring for the Toenails

In caring for the toenails, you follow the same procedure as for the fingernails, with some exceptions. If the toenails are thick and hard, you may have to cut them first, then smooth them with a file or emery board. Cut them straight across; if you cut the corners down, you may encourage ingrown nails. If the nails tend to grow inward at the corners, a wisp of cotton tucked under the nail prevents pressure on the toe. Toenails need the same care as fingernails. Long toenails may scratch the skin and may catch on the bedclothes and break. Dirty toenails may cause infection by scratching the skin. Do not cut toenails of patients with diabetes or the nails of newborn babies. Cutting toenails is not a nursing measure unless specifically ordered. Sometimes, very thick, hard toenails must be surgically removed.

While caring for the toenails, notice any corns and calluses; you may apply oil to soften them but nothing else. If the patient is distressed by corns, calluses, ingrown nails, or bunions, report these conditions. People sometimes have infected corns or calluses as a result of cutting them with razor blades or using corn removers that contain salicylic acid. You may cover an infected area with a sterile dressing, but the doctor prescribes any other treatment.

## Caring for the Patient's Hair

Brushing and dressing the patient's hair is part of daily care. It keeps the hair in condition and makes the patient feel better; it also gives the nurse an opportunity to note scalp disorders or pediculi. Brushing stimulates the scalp circulation and distributes the oil over the hair to give it sheen. Short hair should have the same care as long hair. When a patient is ill for some time, he or she may need the services of a barber to cut the hair. In some hospitals, beauty parlor and barber services are available for patients who need them. Although you will not have time to do elaborate hair arrangements for patients try to arrange a patient's hair as becomingly as you can in the time you have—it gives any woman a bit of an uplift to feel that her hair looks well. Using ribbons may also help to raise the spirits of both adults and children. Encourage patients to comb their own hair— it is good exercise for the shoulder joints.

Comb one strand at a time, beginning at the end; wrap the strand firmly around your forefinger, leaving it slack between your hand and the patient's head so as to avoid pulling. Braid long hair to prevent tangles and avoid using hairpins or bobby pins that might be uncomfortable or might injure the patient's head. Start the braids toward the front so the patient does not have to lie on them, and fasten them at the end with rubber bands or ribbons. This is the easiest and least disturbing way of caring for the hair if a patient is very ill or unable to move her head.

Wash the brush and the comb frequently; this helps to keep the hair clean and prevents reinfection of the scalp in infectious conditions. Report such conditions as excess dandruff, falling hair, or crusts or sores on the scalp.

**Giving a Shampoo.** The purpose of a shampoo is to cleanse the hair and the head; it may be necessary after ointments or other medications have been applied to the scalp, following an EEG during which paste is used, or as a part of the treatment for pediculosis, or for cleanliness during a long-term illness. A shampoo is never given without the doctor's permission nor should it be given if the patient is weak or exhausted, has a respiratory infection or fever, or is not allowed to exert herself. Sometimes a patient is admitted to the hospital with really dirty hair and should have a shampoo, but usually shampooing is not necessary during a short stay in the hospital.

The procedure for giving a shampoo is determined by the equipment available in the individual hospital. Some of the larger institutions have beautician services available for patients, or equipment similar to that used in beauty parlors may be provided. However, it is often necessary to give a shampoo without these aids, using ordinary equipment and methods which are simple and effective.

Precautions to observe in giving a shampoo:

Protect the patient from drafts and be sure that the room is warm enough.
Use warm water (105° to 110° F.).
Protect the patient's eyes and ears.
Use enough solution to make a thick lather.
Rinse and dry the hair thoroughly.
Protect the bed and the floor.
Assure continuous drainage for the shampoo water.

Usually a solution of a mild soap is used. Find out about the patient's preferences. She may want to provide a soapless shampoo or a special soap preparation for you to use. Soap and water and soapless shampoos remove the oil from the hair. However, if used too frequently or too lavishly, they may remove too much. Oily hair, on the other hand, is not affected by them as easily as dry hair.

**Giving a Shampoo to an Ambulatory Patient.** The patient who is up can have her shampoo in the bathroom, using the lavatory bowl. Choose a chair low enough to let the patient's head rest comfortably on the edge of the bowl. She may prefer to sit facing the bowl, resting her forehead on the edge and holding a folded towel over her eyes. If a spray is used, adjust the temperature of the water before you begin. If the patient feels faint, stop the procedure, wrap her head in a bath towel, and get her back to bed at once.

The patient who can be moved on a stretcher can be wheeled to a convenient sink for a shampoo while she is lying on the stretcher.

**Giving a Shampoo to a Bed Patient.** The most difficult part of this procedure is providing continuous drainage of the shampoo to prevent wetting the patient and the bed.

EQUIPMENT

| | |
|---|---|
| 2 Bath towels | Safety pins |
| 1 Large pitcher of water 105° to 110° F. | Nonabsorbent cotton Moisture-proof sheet |
| 1 Small pitcher for pouring | 1 Pail Newspapers to protect the chair or the floor |
| Small container for shampoo solution | Moisture-proof pillowcase |
| 1 Hand towel | |

SUGGESTED PROCEDURE

Cover the patient with a bath blanket and turn back the bedclothing.

Cover the pillow with a moisture-proof case and a cotton case and place it under the patient's head.

Move the patient's head and shoulders to the edge of the bed.

*Reason: It is easier to use the strongest muscles efficiently when working close to the body.*

If it is necessary to improvise a trough, roll the sides of a good-sized moisture-proof sheet over towels toward the center or use a Kelly pad.

*Reason: The flow of water is directed by a confining trough.*

Pin a folded towel around the patient's neck to absorb dripping and keep water from running down the patient's back. Cover her eyes with a folded towel and put cotton in her ears.

*Reason: Wet clothing causes chilling. Soap and detergents may injure delicate structures.*

Put one end of the trough (or Kelly pad) under the patient's head; direct the other end into the pail at the side of the bed—protect the floor with newspaper.

*Reason: The pull of gravity aids in the flow of fluids.*

Wet the hair thoroughly, apply the shampoo and rub it into a good lather and rinse well.

*Reason: Friction loosens particles; soap (or detergents) and water wash away loosened particles.*

Apply shampoo, rub, and rinse again. Rinse until the hair squeaks.

Wrap a towel around the patient's head and slip the trough into the pail. Rub the hair dry with a bath towel.

*Reason: Moisture absorbs heat and causes chilling.*

## Treating Pediculosis

*Pediculi* are lice; these tiny insects live on blood of the person they infest and are found on the hairy parts of the body. There are over 50 kinds of pediculi, but the ones found on the body are head and body lice.

*Body lice* are found on the clothing and *crab* lice on the hairy parts of the body, especially the pubes. They cause itching on the back, the neck, the abdomen, and the pubic area; be suspicious of scratches on the body in these areas.

*Head lice* are found on the hair and the scalp. They are tiny, oval-shaped, grayish insects. The eggs—*nits*—look like dandruff but are solid specks, not flakes; they stick tightly to the hair and are hard to destroy.

Pediculi spread disease and harm the body in many ways; they cause itching and scratching, and the scratches sometimes become infected. They spread from person to person on clothing, bedding, and combs and brushes.

Part of your observation of a patient on admission to the hospital is to notice signs of skin irritation and pediculi. Pediculi are not always a sign of unhygienic living and indifference to cleanliness.

If you find pediculi on a patient's head or body, treatment will kill the live ones and destroy the nits. Be tactful and matter-of-fact when you tell the patient what you are going to do—it can always be assumed that the pediculi came from someone else's clothing that the patient had touched.

If you find pediculi, report your discovery to the head nurse or the doctor; either one will tell you what treatment to use. Every hospital usually has its own method of treating pediculosis. A number of effective preparations are available, some of which will destroy both lice and nits.

It is usually necessary to repeat treatments of pediculosis several times, after which a bath is given. Treatment may also include shaving the pubes and axillae.

Sometimes the patient's clothing is infested with body lice. If badly infested, it may have to be burned; otherwise, it can be disinfected.

## Shaving a Male Patient

Most men feel and look untidy if they are unable to shave every day. A barber is usually available to shave male patients in the hospital, but it is often necessary for you to shave a patient or for a patient to shave himself. However, caution must be taken with certain patients. A patient with unsteady hands and poor eyesight should not be allowed to shave himself, nor should a patient who is mentally depressed or upset. If it is safe, allow a patient to shave himself because it encourages him to do one more thing for himself as a part of his recovery. You can get the equipment ready for him, make him comfortable, and provide a mirror and a good light.

It is possible that you may have to shave a patient if no one else is available to do it. Be sure the razor is sharp—dull blades make shaving a painful process. Always use plenty of lather and shave in the direction of the hairs, holding the skin taut. Be careful not to nick the skin—broken skin provides an avenue for infection.

The procedure described here applies to the use of a straight or safety razor. If an electric razor is used, study the directions carefully and follow them. Generally, an electric razor is easier and safer to use.

### EQUIPMENT

| | |
|---|---|
| Basin of hot water | Powder |
| Shaving brush | Shaving soap or cream |
| After-shave lotion | Razor, straight or safety |
| Tissues | Mirror |
| | Light |

### SUGGESTED PROCEDURE

Place a light so no shadows fall on the face.

Put a safety razor together tightly—use a sharp blade.

Use plenty of lather to soften hairs.

Shave with the direction of the hairs; hold the razor at an angle of about 250°; use short firm strokes; hold the skin taut.

Wipe the hairs and lather from the razor frequently.

Shave carefully around the nose and lips— these areas are especially sensitive; wash the face to remove soap.

Lotion and powder are soothing, however, some men may not like to use them.

If the skin is nicked, apply an antiseptic and cover with a sterile dressing.

# 7. *Preventing Deformities and Disease*

## DECUBITUS ULCERS

### Observing Pressures on the Body

Continuous pressure on any part of the body makes a patient uncomfortable, hampers the circulation, and may cause pressure sores (also called bedsores or decubitus ulcers— Fig. 29-10). Thin people who must lie in bed for some time, especially suffer from pressures on the bony parts of the body not protected by fat pads. The main pressure areas include: the shoulder blades, the elbows, the buttocks, the end of the spine, the heels, and the back of the head. Tight bedclothes also press on the legs and the feet.

You always should be on the alert for signs of pressure on the body especially when you bathe a patient or rub his back. The condition of an individual patient and the probable length of his illness tell you when you should be using aids to prevent pressure sores. The patient also tells you about painful spots. Report signs of pressure and be suspicious of reddened areas that stay red after being rubbed.

### Preventing and Taking Care of a Bedsore

The preventive treatment for bedsores is most important. Bedsores are caused by pressure on the parts of the body that are not covered by pads of fat or other tissues, thereby causing a break in the skin and destruction of the tissues beneath it. The skin is more likely to break down if the area is continually moist or is not clean. In addition, rest in bed affects the circulation and increases the pressure on the bony prominences of the body, such as the spine, the shoulder blades, and the elbows. The dangers are increased if a patient must lie in one position or if he has a cast or splints or a disease condition that affects the circulation. As soon as a break in the skin occurs, the way is open to infection.

Gently rubbing reddened areas, keeping the skin dry, removing wastes from the skin when caring for incontinent patients, and changing the patient's position to relieve pressures are good preventive treatment.

If a bedsore does develop, 2 points in the treatment are most important: (1) protecting the broken area by sterile dressings and (2) relieving the pressure on the area as much as possible. The doctor will prescribe the treatment to be used for the ulcer. He may order application of such ointments as zinc stearate, Peruvian balsam, or scarlet-red ointment or

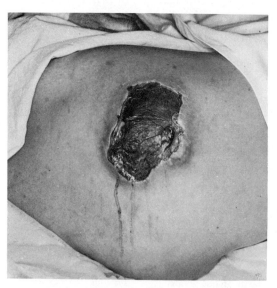

Figure 29-10. There is absolutely *no excuse* for allowing a severe decubitus ulcer (bedsore) to occur in the modern hospital or nursing home. Good nursing care can prevent this deformity. Once a patient has a bedsore, it is very difficult to cure. The best cure is *prevention*. There are commercial products on the market which toughen the skin and help to prevent bedsores or cure bedsores, but the best cure is ambitious, constant *excellence in nursing care*. (Medical Products Division, 3M Company)

exposure to light rays or to heat from electric light bulbs. It is essential to keep the area *clean* and *dry*. When a patient lies on a sheet over a rubber or synthetic protective material for a long period of time, moisture from perspiration does not evaporate. The moisture, combined with continuous pressure, predisposes to bedsores. While the skin can cope with its own flora of microorganisms, the presence of microorganisms from an infected wound or feces can be dangerous, particularly if there is a break in the skin.

An airfoam mattress aids in distributing pressure evenly on every part of the body; smooth, tight undersheets also eliminate skin irritation. At the first signs of redness, the best treatment is washing with soap and water and rubbing with skin lotion. The area should be covered with large cotton pads which are changed frequently: airfoam or lamb's wool pads are excellent because air spaces in the wool permit the skin to dry.

**The Alternating Pressure Mattress Pad.** If a firm mattress places constant pressure on one or more parts of the body, causing a bedsore, an alternating pressure mattress pad may be used. This pad is constructed in such a way that sections of it are distended with air or fluid, while other sections stay flat: then the flat sections fill and the distended sections flatten out. This alternating process is continuous and prevents steady pressure on any one point. Patients seem to have little diffi-culty in adjusting to this mattress. However, be very careful not to use pins with this mattress—you may puncture the mattress.

**The Floatation Pad.** This is a heavy semiliquid pad which is placed under the patient to prevent pressure areas. These pads are available in all sizes, although the pad about 2-feet square is the most commonly used. This can be placed into the bed or a larger pad can be placed in the wheelchair under the paraplegic patient, to prevent pressure areas.

**Foam Pads.** Various forms of foam rubber pads are available which can be applied to specific areas of the body to prevent pressure areas. If the patient already has a pressure area, a hole is cut in the pad and the pad is placed around the pressure area. Heels and elbows are often padded to prevent skin breakdown, as is the stump of an amputation to prevent irritation from the prosthesis.

Authorities no longer recommend the use of doughnuts, air cushions, or air rings for most patients; instead of relieving pressure, these devices create a circle of pressure and constrict the circulation. Instead, large soft pads placed next to the pressure point to provide a smooth distribution of pressure are recommended. However, an air ring (covered by a pillow case to absorb perspiration) is acceptable as a temporary aid for a short time after rectal or perineal surgery.

These methods are all fully discussed in Chapter 45.

## 8. Meeting Emotional Needs

The basic need of communicating one's feelings has been discussed elsewhere in this book, but you should be reminded that the patient needs to communicate, perhaps more so than other people, because he is more likely to be anxious. Do not forget that we communicate in nonverbal ways, as well as in verbal ways.

## 9. Providing Diversion for the Patient

Another way of increasing the self-esteem of the patient is by allowing him to spend some time in a diversional activity which he considers worthwhile. It becomes very boring for the patient if he has nothing to do to divert his attention from himself and his illness. A contact with the Occupational Therapy Department often provides an appropriate activity which the patient can enjoy. Frequently a patient becomes so engrossed in making gifts for his family and friends or small items to sell to others that he forgets about his illness.

# 10. *The Spiritual Needs of The Patient*

Since you will take care of people of different faiths and creeds it is important to realize that religion is a vital part of people's lives. Thus you often find the Bible and a prayer book on many bedside tables. Since people need reassurance when they are sick, they may sometimes talk to you about their illness and their beliefs. Remember to respect these confidences as professional secrets. You should also be sensitive to the clues which indicate that a patient would like to talk to a clergyman or a priest or a rabbi. A patient may think that you have no time for his spiritual needs, so let him feel that you are sympathetic to this part of his life, too.

## Religious Faiths and Rituals

Every nurse should be familiar with the customs of the 3 most common religious faiths—Protestant, Catholic, and Jewish—and should understand their significance.

**The Protestant Faith.** There are many denominations in the Protestant faith. They agree on some things and disagree on others. While their forms of worship are different, most of them recognize 2 ceremonies—baptism and communion. Therefore members of the different denominations would be expected to consider these ceremonies important. Individual needs differ. A person who has found strength and comfort in talking with his minister is more likely to want to see him when he is ill. Yet you must never upset a patient by ushering in a minister without first finding out whether or not he wants to see him.

**The Jewish Faith.** The Orthodox Jew follows many ancient and honorable religious customs which are sacred to him. The custom that perhaps matters most and is most difficult to follow when he is sick is related to his food. It is impossible to serve kosher meat in a non-Jewish hospital, but you can be sure not to serve meat and dairy foods together or pork of any kind to an Orthodox Jewish patient. You can let the head nurse know that the pa-

tient is an Orthodox Jew so that she can tell the dietary department. In this way you can assure the patient that his religious beliefs will be respected. Even though the Jewish patient is not required to observe these dietary regulations when he is ill, he is very reluctant to disobey a sacred religious law.

**The Catholic Faith.** The Roman Catholic Church considers Baptism, Confession, Holy Communion and Extreme Unction as basic sacraments of the Church. These ceremonies are a vital part of a sincere Catholic's faith.

During a long illness a Catholic patient usually wants a priest to hear his confession and to give him communion. Some Protestant patients also may wish to observe Holy Communion. You should provide as much privacy for the patient and the clergyman as possible.

Extreme Unction is a sacrament of comfort and consolation; it is not offered solely to prepare a Catholic patient for death. Many Catholics look upon Extreme Unction as a positive sign that death is imminent. Because they are unable to face that knowledge, they may delay in receiving the sacrament.

If a Catholic patient has been ill for some time, his family will be aware of his spiritual needs. However, you may be responsible for telling them of sudden serious changes in his condition which may indicate that death is near. Many patients are brought into hospitals unconscious or in a serious condition. Always look for indications that such a patient is a Catholic, if he is unable to tell you. You may find a rosary or a medal on his person or information on an identification card. Always call a priest so that the patient may have Extreme Unction; if the patient is conscious, he also should have an opportunity to confess and receive communion. To prepare the patient for Extreme Unction, loosen the covers at the foot of the bed.

The last rites of the Church are a vital part of the Catholic faith and comfort both the patient and the members of his family. If a patient dies suddenly, the priest can administer them conditionally within 2 hours after death.

# 30

# Nursing Treatments to Meet Special Patient Needs

---

## BEHAVIORAL OBJECTIVES

*The student successfully attaining the goals of this chapter will be able to:*

- *discuss the effects of heat application to the body and describe the dangers involved in the use of external heat; demonstrate skill in the various methods of applying external heat in the clinical area, including the warm-water bottle, the electric pad, immersion of a body part, or warm packs.*
- *discuss the effects of application of cold to the body and describe the dangers involved; demonstrate skill in administering external cold to the body in the clinical area, including the ice pack, cold moist-compresses, the alcohol or cold sponge bath.*
- *utilize various bandages and binders effectively; demonstrate the proper application of the roller bandage and the elastic stocking; state at least 3 reasons for using these; identify the type of patient who will be most likely to need these.*
- *differentiate between medical and surgical asepsis.*
- *discuss ways in which diseases are transmitted and give examples as to how the spread of disease can be blocked; discuss maintenance of medical asepsis within hospital situations.*
- *discuss the major considerations in isolation technic; demonstrate safety and skill in the isolation room, including proper use of gowns, masks, gloves, and the double-bagging procedure; discuss reverse isolation technic and demonstrate skill in this procedure.*
- *discuss the concept of surgical asepsis and identify situations in which it is used; utilize the principles of surgical asepsis, gown and glove without contamination, demonstrate the opening of a sterile pack, and assist with procedures which involve sterile technic.*
- *discuss the reasons for a douche; demonstrate the ability to perform this procedure and discuss precautions to be observed.*
- *list possible reasons for catheterization; list the types of catheters; demonstrate ability to safely perform·this procedure on patients of varying ages of the same sex as the nurse; describe the procedure for a patient of the opposite sex.*
- *discuss the general concept of death, including the emotional stages through which the patient and his family resolve their feelings and the physical changes which take place within the patient's body.*
- *describe the procedure for caring for the body after death.*

---

# 1. *The Application of Heat and Cold for Therapeutic Purposes*

## APPLYING HEAT TO THE BODY

Applications of heat are used widely to treat disease and to relieve pain. Heat may also be used to make the chilly patient more comfortable or to raise the temperature of the body. Since heat must be fairly intensive to produce the desired effect, there is one great danger in using it—the danger of *burns*.

### Sensitivity to Heat

Precautions to prevent injury from burns are necessary for these reasons:

The nerves in the skin are numbed easily, and the patient may not feel the pain of a burn, especially if he has had repeated heat applications.

Some parts of the body are especially sensitive to heat—such as the eyelids, the neck, and the inside surface of the arm.

Large applications provide more heat to the skin than small ones.

Infants, older people, and people with fair, thin skin have less resistance to heat. Lowered body resistance also makes the body tissues less resistant to heat.

Patients who are unconscious or under anesthesia, or some patients suffering from cerebral hemorrhage cannot tell when heat is intense.

Impaired circulation and some metabolic diseases make people more susceptible to burns. This is true of the patient who is in shock or has diabetes.

Heat is applied only when ordered by a doctor. This is true regardless of the form of application.

### Dry Heat

Heat, either dry or moist, is usually applied for its local effects. The common methods for applying dry heat are exposure to the sun, a warm-water bag, an electric pad, a heat lamp, or an electric cradle.

When you apply heat to any patient, think of the reasons why this particular individual may be sensitive to heat. It helps you to determine what degree of heat is safe for him and how long you can safely leave any heat application on the skin. The application must be hot enough to accomplish its purpose but must be kept within the safety range. For example: the doctor leaves orders to apply an electric pad to the patient's back continuously; if you find that the skin is becoming red and sensitive, you report this condition and decide whether you should keep the pad at a lower temperature or leave it off altogether for a time.

### Preparing and Applying a Warm-Water Bag

A warm-water bag is applied to relieve aches and pains, to increase the circulation, or to warm a patient. It must be leakproof to prevent burning the patient and wetting his clothing or his bed. The temperature of the water in a warm-water bag may be anywhere up to 125°F., depending on the area to which it is applied and the age and condition of the patient. Tell the patient that you have tested the temperature of the water but that some people are more sensitive to heat than others, so he must tell you how it feels to him. The bag always is placed in a cover which can be previously warmed or moistened to hasten the transmission of heat.

Never place a warm-water bag directly against the skin of an unconscious patient or a patient in shock. Never allow a patient to lie on a warm-water bag or a heating pad. If possible, place the heating unit on the top of the area to be warmed. When the heat is confined in a small place, the possibilities of burning are increased. If you are going to treat a patient by applying heat to the back, turn the patient onto his side or abdomen. Regulate the temperature of the water in a warm-water bag so that it will be safe for a patient who may shift it to a sensitive area in an effort to obtain relief from pain. Never make it hotter than 125°F. A safe temperature range is:

Infants under 2 years of age: 105° to 115° F.
Children over 2 years of age and adults: 115° to 125° F.

Refill the bag often enough to maintain the desired temperature. Inspect the skin regularly to see whether or not it looks red. When the bag is no longer needed, empty it and hang it upside down to drain and dry. Prevent losing the stopper by putting it in a safe place or tying it to the bag. When the bag is dry, screw in the stopper, leaving the bag inflated to keep the sides from sticking together. Store the bag in its accustomed place.

### EQUIPMENT

Warm-water bag and cover (cotton flannel or a bath towel makes an excellent cover)
Pitcher of hot water
Bath thermometer

### SUGGESTED PROCEDURE

Inspect the stopper to make sure the bag will not leak.
*Reason: Leakage wets clothing and the bed and may burn the patient.*
Test the temperature of the water with a thermometer. Bring it to the temperature desired, not over 125°F.
*Reason: A thermometer is accurate. Hand testing is unreliable.*
Pour the water into the bag, filling it about ½ to ⅔ full.
*Reason: The heavier the bag, the more uncomfortable it is on the patient and the more difficult it is to adjust.*
Expel the air: place the bag flat on the table—when the water is seen in the neck, screw in the stopper.
*Reason: Air distends the bag and makes it hard and unadjustable.*
Test for leaks by holding the bag upside down.
*Reason: A missing washer or a loosely screwed-in stopper causes leaks.*
Dry the bag and apply the warmed cover.
*Reason: A warm cover helps the heat to reach the body more quickly.*
Apply as ordered and record the treatment on the patient's chart.

## Applying an Electric Pad

An electric pad is a covered network of wires which give off heat when an electrical current passes through them. Pads with a waterproof covering are best and the only kind safe to use in moist conditions. Never put pins through a heating pad—if a pin touches the electric wires it may cause an electric shock. If the wires are crushed or bent

the pad may overheat and cause burns or even a fire. And always remember that the pad may get too hot—the temperature of the water in a hot water bag goes down, but in the heating pad the temperature is constant. This means that there is a greater danger of burning the patient.

Special precautions are necessary when electric pads are used for children, for very old people, or for irrational or unconscious patients.

Before you apply the pad, connect it with an electric outlet, turn the heating switch to "high" to see whether the pad heats promptly, and then turn it off and disconnect from the outlet. Cover it with its washable case or a towel, connect to the outlet at the bedside, adjust to the proper temperature, and apply. Inspect frequently to prevent the patient from being burned.

In addition to the regular electric pad, there is a special pad called the Aquamatic-K Pad (Aqua-K), which contains tubes which are filled with water heated by an electric current. This pad is much more reliable and easier to use. For example, the temperature is set by a key and can only be regulated with a key. Thus the patient is unable to change the temperature, whereas with an ordinary pad, a patient may accidently turn up the temperature. Aside from this advantage, the Aqua-K pad can be used in combination with warm moist packs, making them more effective.

## Giving Lamp Treatments

Lamp treatments usually are given by trained personnel because exposure to light rays must be regulated carefully to prevent injury to the patient. Information about light rays is included here to explain why lamp treatments may be dangerous unless they are given properly.

*Infrared* rays are used to relax muscles, stimulate the circulation, and relieve pain; they have the same effect on the body as other forms of dry heat. *Ultraviolet* rays are not so penetrating as infrared rays—sunlight provides mild ultraviolet light rays. However, prolonged exposure to the sun will burn a sensitive skin. Utraviolet rays are used to treat skin infections and wounds.

## Moist Heat

Water is a better heat conductor than air; therefore, moist hot applications heat the skin more quickly than applications of dry heat. This is why you wring warm wet compresses or packs as dry as possible—excess water may burn the skin. Prolonged applications of moist heat also soften and weaken the skin. Moist heat is more penetrating than dry heat and is more effective for relieving pain in the deeper tissues. Gauze compresses, woolen or flannel packs (stupes), baths, and inhalations are used to apply moist heat.

## Applying Warm-Moist Compresses and Packs

Warm moist compresses and packs are used to apply heat to an area to stimulate circulation and to promote drainage in infections. Packs are made of wool, flannel or cotton and are used on larger body areas than are gauze compresses. (Terrycloth toweling may be substituted for packs if wool or flannel material is not available.) The applications need not be sterile unless there is a break in the skin. Water or a mild antiseptic solution such as 2 per cent boric acid or normal saline may be used.

The doctor prescribes the kind of application and how it is to be used; it may be applied for long or short periods at a time, or it may be changed more frequently to keep it warm. The length of time varies from 10 to 30 minutes, with changes of application every 2 to 5 minutes. Thick compresses or packs, covered to keep the heat in, will stay hot longer than thin ones. They are applied as hot as the patient can comfortably tolerate them. During the procedure he may feel chilly, so take precautions to keep him warm and protected from drafts.

The preparation of the patient is especially important because the sight of hot steaming water is rather frightening; explain that you wring the material very dry so that there is no danger of dropping hot water on his skin and that the compress loses heat quickly and will not be nearly as hot as the water by the time it reaches his skin. Apply it gradually so that he can tell you how hot it feels—only the patient knows when an application is too hot for comfort.

### EQUIPMENT

| | |
|---|---|
| Basin containing the prescribed solution | Oiled silk, plastic or aluminum foil |
| Hot pack machine | Dry pack |
| Compresses or packs of suitable size | Applicators |
| | Petroleum jelly |
| 2 Forceps or wringer | Waste container |

### KEY POINTS IN THE PROCEDURE

Heat the solution until it steams, or use hot tap water (a hot-packer, which heats the packs to the correct temperature, may also be available).

Immerse the compresses or packs in the hot solution.

*Principle: Woolen material absorbs water slowly but holds moisture. Gauze absorbs moisture quickly and dries out quickly.*

Arrange the waterproof cover and the dry pack to place over the moist compress or pack after it is applied.

*Principle: Covering the moist pack or compress keeps air out. Contact with the air cools the pack.*

Apply petroleum jelly to the area with an applicator.

*Principle: Coating on the skin allows heat to penetrate gradually.*

Wring the compress or the pack with forceps or wringer, removing as much of the water as is possible.

*Principle: Hot water burns the skin.*

Shake the packs lightly.

*Principle: Slight heat loss from contact with the air reduces the possibility of burning.*

Apply to the area lightly at first, gradually pressing against the skin. In a few seconds lift the pack slightly to inspect the degree of redness of the skin.

*Principle: Air is a poor heat conductor. Eliminating air spaces between the compress or the pack and the skin makes it more effective. The degree of redness of the skin shows whether or not the pack is too hot.*

Cover the moist compress or pack with the dry pack and moisture-proof cover.

*Principle: Covering provides insulation against heat loss and evaporation of moisture.*

Change the compress or pack often enough to keep the area heated.

*Principle: Small applications cool more quickly than large ones.*

Continue the treatment for the prescribed

time, then remove the dry and moist applications. Dry the skin and cover it.

*Principle: Moisture softens the skin and makes it susceptible to chilling.*

Make the patient comfortable and care for the equipment.

Record the treatment on the patient's chart, noting the patient's reactions.

## Applying Warm-Moist Compresses to the Eye

The eyelid and the skin around the eye are thin and delicate structures; therefore precautions to prevent burning of these tissues are especially important. If the eye is discharging, discard each compress when you remove it. Remember also that all equipment is sterilized after the treatment. If compresses are applied to both eyes, use separate equipment for each to prevent spreading the infection. Eyesight is very precious, and eye treatments must be given carefully, since they may be the deciding factor between preserving and losing sight.

## Soaks (Immersion)

Moist heat also can be applied to the extremities or to an area of the torso by immersing the part in warm water or a solution, for a prescribed time. This procedure is called a soak. The purpose in giving a soak may be to improve circulation, to increase the blood supply in an infected area, to aid in breaking down infected tissues (*suppuration*), to apply medication, or to cleanse discharging or encrusted wounds. This treatment requires a basin or receptacle large enough to hold sufficient water to cover the part and to accommodate it comfortably. A tub shaped for giving arm or leg soaks is available in most hospitals.

Usually, it is not considered necessary to sterilize the tub, but it should be cleaned thoroughly with soap, a disinfectant, such as O-syl, and water. Tap water is used for soaks unless otherwise specified since it is generally recognized as being free from harmful bacteria.

The temperature of the water usually ranges from 105° to 110° F., although the doctor may prescribe a definite temperature. The usual length of a soak is 15 to 20 minutes. The temperature of the water should be tested frequently and hot water added as needed. When adding hotter water, pour it in near the edge with your hand between the stream and the patient's body, stirring the water as you add it to distribute the heat evenly.

If a soak is given with the patient in bed, protect the bed with a waterproof covering beneath the tub. Place the basin or tub so that the patient's body is in good alignment and in a comfortable position, avoiding pressure on the arm or leg. If necessary, place a folded bath towel over the edge of the tub beneath the body part and a folded pillow beneath the knee or elbow. Depending on the patient's condition, a soak may be given with the patient in bed or sitting in a chair.

The procedure described here applies to an arm or leg soak.

### EQUIPMENT

| | |
|---|---|
| Arm or foot tub | Bath towels |
| Bath thermometer | Bath blanket |
| Pitcher of hot water or solution | Sterile dressings, if necessary |
| Protective sheet and cover | |

A whirlpool circulator may be placed in the tub or the physical therapy department may give this treatment in a regular whirlpool or Hubbard tank.

### KEY POINTS IN THE PROCEDURE

Adjust the protective sheet and cover it with a bath towel. Prepare the water in the tub (105° to 110° F. unless otherwise specified).

When the tub is removed at the end of the bath, the arm or leg can rest on the towel.

Remove the dressings, if there is a wound, and lower the part into the water gradually.

Adjust the pad on the edge of the tub and support the knees or elbow with a folded pillow if necessary.

*Principle: Pressure on the blood vessels on the backs of the legs or the arms interferes with the circulation. Unsupported parts cause fatigue and poor alignment.*

Test the temperature at intervals.

*Principle: The proper degree of heat is necessary to make the treatment effective.*

Add hot water as needed to maintain the required temperature, stirring the tub water as it is poured.

*Principle: Stirring the water hastens the diffusion of the hot water in the cooler water and distributes the heat evenly.*

Remove the part from the bath in 15 or 20 minutes (or as ordered). If there is a wound, apply a sterile dressing. Dry the other areas.

In the case of a discharging wound, sterilize the equipment.

*Principle: Contact with infected material spreads infection to others.*

Record the treatment on the chart, noting the patient's reactions.

## Hip or Sitz Bath

The purpose of a sitz bath may be to apply heat to the pelvic area, to cleanse a wound or to relieve pain. It is also known as a hip bath and consists of placing the patient in a tub containing enough water to reach the umbilicus. A regular bathtub can be used, but a special sitz tub or seat built to accommodate the patient's hips and buttocks may be provided if the baths are ordered frequently. The advantage of a sitz tub is that the patient's legs and feet do not have to be in the water and heat is concentrated on the pelvic area. If the aim of the bath is to apply heat, the temperature of the water should be 110° to 115° F. If it is given for cleansing purposes and to promote healing, the bath temperature should be from 94° to 98° F. The doctor will prescribe the length of the treatment according to its aim. It is usually 15 to 20 minutes.

The effect of heat on a relatively large area of the body may make the patient weak or faint. He should be observed closely and protected from drafts and chilling by covering the upper part of his body with a blanket. The same precautions should be taken after the bath. Usually the patient goes to bed for a time until the circulation has returned to normal.

Since the height of a sitz tub cannot be adjusted, a short patient may need a stool under his feet to prevent pressure on the blood vessels in his legs. A folded towel in the lumbar area will help to support his back and keep his body in good alignment during the treatment.

KEY POINTS IN THE PROCEDURE

Fill the tub to the required depth with water of the specified temperature. Put a large bath towel in the bottom of the tub, for patient comfort.

*Principle: Higher temperatures produce relaxation of the body parts to relieve pain. Moderate temperatures relieve congestion and aid in cleansing.*

When the patient is in the bath, cover the upper part of his body with a blanket.

*Principle: Exposure to cold and drafts causes chilling.*

Test the temperature of the water often and add hot water as needed to maintain the required temperature. You may be able to adjust the tub water supply and drain so that a constant circulation of water can be maintained.

*Principle: A constant degree of heat is necessary to make the procedure effective.*

Watch for signs of fainting or weakness. Make sure the patient has a call light.

*Principle: The supply of blood to the brain is reduced as heat stimulates the circulation in the pelvic area.*

Assist the patient in getting out of the bath after the specified time.

*Principle: The success of the treatment depends on sufficient exposure to heat.*

Protect the patient from drafts and chilling by covering him adequately in bed. Request ambulatory patients to remain in bed for a short time.

*Principle: It takes a little time for the pelvic circulation to return to normal.*

Record the treatment on the chart, noting the patient's reactions.

## Giving a Steam Inhalation

A steam inhalation is a method of administering soothing drugs and warm moist heat to irritated and congested mucous membranes in the nose and throat. The drug is added to heated water which vaporizes and carries the drug to the affected part as the patient breathes in the vapor. Moist heat alone is effective in relieving inflammation and congestion. *Compound benzoin tincture* and *oil of eucalyptus* are drugs that are often used in inhalations for their soothing effects.

Most hospitals are equipped with electrically heated apparatus for giving steam inhalations.

Continuous inhalations sometimes are given following operations on the larynx or trachea. Some kind of an enclosure may be necessary to confine the steam to the patient's breathing area. The front of the tent should be open so that the patient's face can be seen.

A tent over the crib is the best method of ensuring a high humidity in the air when giving a steam inhalation to an infant or a child; this is a common treatment for croup. The tent is called a croupette and is discussed in Chapter 39. A child should have particularly close attention during an inhalation.

### EQUIPMENT

Inhaler or croup tent      Towel
Solution ordered

#### KEY POINTS IN THE PROCEDURE

Prepare the solution as it was ordered.

Attach the inhaler to an electric outlet.

*Principle: Heating a liquid produces steam.*

Move the apparatus to the bedside when the steam rises, and place it on a chair or stool near the head of the bed.

Protect the patient's eyes with a folded towel.

*Principle: Concentrated heat may irritate the eyes and forehead.*

Direct the spout toward the patient's nose and mouth.

*Principle: Moist heat soothes irritated mucous membranes and relieves congestion.*

Replenish the solution in the inhaler if necessary.

*Principle: Steam is produced by the evaporation of water. Constant heat causes evaporation.*

At the end of the prescribed period, discontinue the treatment. Dry the patient's face and neck and protect him from the cold air or drafts.

*Principle: Moist heat dilates surface blood vessels. Heat loss from the skin causes chilling. Exposing the patient to a change in the temperature of the room can counteract the beneficial effects of an inhalation.*

Record the treatment on the chart, noting the patient's reactions.

## APPLYING COLD TO THE BODY

The first effect of cold on the body is to contract the surface blood vessels. This prevents the escape of heat from the body and also controls hemorrhage. Cold affects the skin like a local anesthetic because it numbs the nerve endings. Prolonged applications of cold can be as damaging to the tissues as prolonged heat. If the patient complains of numbness in the area and the skin looks white or spotty, the applications should be discontinued. Cold applications as a continuing treatment may be discontinued at intervals to prevent tissue injury.

Cold is applied to sprains or bruises to prevent swelling (edema). However, it will not reduce edema which is already present in the tissues. As cold decreases the flow of blood in one area of the body, it increases the flow to other areas. This explains why cold or chilling drafts striking the body often cause congestion in the nasal passages. Continued applications or prolonged exposure to cold affects the deeper tissues (frostbite).

Cold applications relieve pain, such as a headache, and make the patient with a fever more comfortable. They slow up bacterial activity in infections and relieve congestion in the parts where they are applied. They may also be used to slow down or stop bleeding. Cold is applied to the body by using icecaps, ice collars, compresses, or cool sponge baths.

### Filling and Applying an Icecap or an Ice Collar

The doctor prescribes the application of an icecap to specific parts of the body. However, you may apply an icecap for headache or in an emergency, such as a nosebleed, without an order from the doctor. Always remember that cold has harmful effects on a weakened or an undernourished person although it may be stimulating to a healthy person.

An icecap is a flat, oval rubber bag with a leakproof, screw-in top. The opening in an icecap is wide so that it can be filled easily. An ice collar is a narrow rubber bag curved to fit the neck. These bags are used for headache and after throat operations or tooth extractions to check and prevent bleeding. They are also used to prevent intestinal movement in abdominal inflammation, such as appendicitis, to relieve pain in engorged breasts, and to prevent painful swelling in injured tissues. The procedure described here applies to either an icecap or an ice collar.

EQUIPMENT

Icecap or ice collar
Icecap cover—cotton flannel or a towel
Basin of ice
Safety pins for towel

KEY POINTS IN THE PROCEDURE

Inspect the stopper of the bag and test the bag for leakage.

*Reason: Leaking water will wet the bed-clothes and chill the patient.*

Fill an icecap about ¾ full, using small pieces of ice.

*Reason: It is easier to fit it closely to the body if the ice is in small pieces.*

Flatten the icecap on a hard surface, and press on it to expel the air.

*Reason: Air is a poor conductor of heat and interferes with the removal of heat from the body.*

Screw in the top, making sure that the stopper is in place.

*Reason: The properly inserted stopper prevents leakage.*

Dry and cover the icecap with an absorbent cover or towel. Be very careful not to puncture the bag with a pin. Masking tape may also be used.

*Reason: Moisture condenses on the outside which is uncomfortable for the patient if the icecap is uncovered.*

Adjust the icecap on the part of the body to be treated.

Apply the icecap for ½ to 1 hour as directed. Leave it off for 1 hour before reapplying unless directed otherwise.

*Reason: Prolonged applications of cold slow up circulation which may cause tissue damage.*

Record the treatment on the patient's chart, noting "on" and "off" periods.

Many hospitals provide icecaps which are filled with a solution and are kept frozen in a refrigerator ready for use. This does away with refilling, since the used icecap can be disinfected and returned to the refrigerator for refreezing.

An ice pack is also available for 1-time emergency use. By breaking a capsule, a chemical is released, which causes the bag to freeze. Once it thaws out, it cannot be refrozen.

## Applying Cold Moist Compresses

One method of applying moist cold to a part of the body is by means of cold compresses. Cold compresses are often applied to relieve pain and inflammation in eye injuries or after a tooth extraction. Sometimes they are applied to hemorrhoids. They may be made of gauze or of thin pads of cotton covered with gauze, depending on the thickness which is most suitable for the condition to be treated. A folded washcloth can be used as a compress for the forehead, cheek, or jaw. Cold compresses are not sterile.

The patient needs to know that the treatment is given to relieve his discomfort and that it will not do him any harm—some patients live in fear of "catching cold."

THE PROCEDURE

Put the compresses in a basin containing pieces of ice and a small amount of water.

*Principle: The amount of water increases as the ice melts. Water also increases the cooling effects of the ice.*

Wring the compress thoroughly to prevent dripping; apply the compress to the part to be treated. Change it frequently.

*Principle: The compress absorbs heat from the body. A warm compress will not accomplish the purpose of the treatment.*

Continue the treatment as ordered, usually for 15 to 20 minutes, to be repeated every 2 to 3 hours.

If the patient is able, he can be allowed to apply the compresses himself.

*Principle: Encouraging a patient to help himself is a rehabilitative measure and helps a patient to become more self-reliant.*

Record the treatment on the patient's chart, noting the duration and patient's reaction.

## Giving an Alcohol or Cold Sponge Bath

An alcohol or cold sponge bath is ordered occasionally to reduce elevated temperature.

Usually, this bath is given with tepid rather than cold water (then called a tepid sponge bath), with alcohol sometimes added to the water. The first effect of cold water on the skin is the constriction of the blood vessels and the reduction of heat elimination. Alcohol evaporates rapidly from the skin and aids in eliminating heat.

The patient's first reaction to a cold or cool sponge bath is chilliness, which disappears as the body adjusts to the cold temperature. Therefore, the bath must be continued long enough to allow for this adjustment—at least 25 to 30 minutes. Each extremity is sponged for 5 minutes, the back and the buttocks for 5 to 10 minutes more. Moist cloths placed in the axillae and the groin reduce temperature in the large blood vessels which lie close to the surface in these areas. A warm-water bag (about 100° F.) at the patient's feet reduces chilliness; an icecap applied to his head helps to prevent congestion and headache. The patient's body temperature shortly after the bath has been completed (½ hour) shows the effect of the treatment. A cold sponge bath is often given for its temporarily soothing effect and may not produce a marked temperature drop. In conditions which cause a dangerously high temperature, such as neurosurgery, an ice mattress (hypothermia blanket)—a plastic mattress pad through which ice water flows continuously—can be used.

**Contraindications.** Some patients react unfavorably to cold baths; others are unable to tolerate them. Cold baths are not advisable for older people with inelastic arteries, arthritic patients, patients with lowered resistance, or very young children. The first effect of cold on the body is depressing and may produce undesirable reactions. If the patient has a weak, rapid pulse, bluish lips and nails, and chills, the bath should be discontinued and moderate heat applied.

**Reassurance.** Explain the procedure to the patient. Point out that the room is warm to keep him from catching cold; explain that he will be covered as in any bath. If the patient is nervous and fearful, the bath is not likely to be effective. Explain the procedure to the family, who probably realize that the patient has an elevated temperature and are apprehensive. Give the patient a urinal or a bedpan before the bath.

## EQUIPMENT

| | |
|---|---|
| Basin of water (70° to 85° F.) | Face towel |
| | 2 Washcloths |
| Basin of chipped ice | Hot-water bag and |
| Bath thermometer | cover |
| Bath blanket | Icecap and cover |
| Bath towel | |

### KEY POINTS IN THE PROCEDURE

Take the patient's rectal temperature before beginning the procedure.

*Principle: You must have a base-line temperature upon which to guide your treatment. Be sure to note if the patient has had aspirin or another antipyretic, since this may influence the effects of the sponge bath.*

Add ice to the water to bring it to the required temperature (65° F. to 80° F.).

*Principle: Cool water brings blood to the surface of the skin.*

Add alcohol if prescribed.

*Principle: Alcohol evaporates rapidly from the skin and removes heat.*

Apply a warm hot-water bag to the patient's feet and an icecap to his head.

*Principle: Warmth reduces chilliness, and cold prevents congestion and headache.*

Place moist, cool cloths in the axillae and groin. Wring the cloths just enough to prevent dripping.

*Principle: Large blood vessels are close to the skin in the groin and the axilla. Temperature reduction takes place through the evaporation of water.*

Sponge each limb for at least 5 minutes. Sponge the back and the buttocks for 5 or 10 minutes more.

*Principle: It takes about 25 to 30 minutes for the body to respond to cold applications.*

Take the patient's rectal temperature ½ hour after the procedure is completed. If the treatment is continued for more than ½ hour, the temperature must be taken and recorded at least every ½ hour. Rectal temperature is more accurate.

Record the treatment on the patient's chart, noting his reactions. Be sure to note the patient's various rectal temperatures.

## THE USE OF IRRITANTS AND COUNTERIRRITANTS

Irritants are chemicals used on the skin to produce a process similar to inflammation, causing dilation of blood vessels and increased circulation. The skin reacts much the same as it does from the local application of heat. When a chemical is used for other than local effects (as in the deep underlying tissues), it is called a counterirritant.

Less use is being made of irritants and counterirritants today because antibiotics and pain relievers are more effective. However, many people, especially older persons, still cling to a faith in proprietary remedies to be rubbed on the skin as a cure for colds or bronchitis.

# 2. Applying Binders and Bandages

### Binders

**Straight Binder.** Straight binders are made of 2 thicknesses of muslin stitched together on the edges. A straight binder can be used to keep dressings in place on the wider areas, such as the abdomen or the back; it should be at least 12 inches wide and 36 inches long, or even larger for some people. To apply a straight binder, follow this procedure: gather half the length of the binder into folds and slip it under the patient; pull it through and adjust it evenly. Lap one end over the other (fold the upper lap under, if necessary); pin with safety pins from the bottom upward, spacing the pins about 2 inches apart, keeping the end of the binder in a vertical straight line. Adjust fullness at the sides by pinning in pleats from the top downward until the binder fits. Put the fingers of one hand between the patient and the binder as you insert the pins to prevent pricking the patient's skin.

Perineal straps can be attached to a straight binder by pinning 1 or 2 strips, 2 inches wide, to the bottom of the binder at the back; the other ends of the straps are drawn between the legs and pinned to the bottom of the binder in the front. You can attach shoulder straps to a chest or a breast binder in a similar manner.

**T Binder.** A T binder gets its name from its shape—it is made of 2 strips of muslin, 3 or 4 inches wide, which are fastened together. This binder is used to hold rectal or perineal dressings in place. The perineal strap is split through the middle to make a T binder for a male patient. Put the band around the patient's waist, bring the perineal strap through between the legs and pin through the band and the strap at the midline.

**Many-Tailed Binder.** The many-tailed, or *scultetus,* binder is made by sewing 3- or 4-inch overlapping strips of cloth together. The 48-inch long strips overlap each other by half their width and are stitched together for about 10 inches, leaving strips about 19 inches long hanging loose at each end of the binder. To apply the binder, begin with the bottom strips, slanting one strip across the abdomen and pinning it to its opposite. Continue alternating opposite strips until you reach the last one—bring this around the waist and fasten. You can pin the strips at the crossing point before you fasten the final strip, to make the binder firm for support. This binder can be used to exert pressure on the upper abdomen by applying it from the top downward.

**Adhesive Tape Straps.** Strips of adhesive or hypoallergenic tape of various widths are often used in place of bandages and binders to hold dressings in place or to give support. Tape is also commonly used for a sprained ankle or fractured ribs. The skin should be shaved before applying massive dressings of adhesive tape, because hairs stick to the tape and make its removal a painful process. Ether or benzine, applied to the skin at the edge of the applied strip, helps to remove adhesive tape painlessly. Keep moistening the skin close to the adhesive as you peel the tape off gently. These substances can also be used to remove tape marks. Never use these liquids near an open flame, because they are highly flammable.

## The Elastic Roller Bandage

The stretchable roller bandage is often used to apply gentle pressure to a part of the body, to provide support, or to hold a dressing in place. This could be to give support to the legs, to encourage circulation after surgery, or to arrest bleeding by direct pressure. It is important to apply the bandage (sometimes called the ACE bandage, although newer forms are available) correctly.

Application of the roller bandage to the leg or arm is done from the toes or the fingers up toward the hip or shoulder. It is important to wrap the bandage firmly, but not too tightly. You must remember that the bandage may tighten as you wrap, so be sure to check the circulation of the toes after the bandage is in place.

**Procedure.** The doctor will order the specific part to be wrapped. For example, the order might say, "ACE bandages, both legs, foot to above knee." The order will also include how often this is to be done or if the bandages are to remain in place continuously. If the latter is the case, elastic stockings may be ordered instead.

The bandage must be rolled when you begin. If you are rewrapping a bandage, roll it up as you take it off. Be sure to explain to the patient what you plan to do. The part to be wrapped should be elevated or at least be level with the body when it is wrapped. This will help to drain some of the excess blood out of the leg, so the wrapping will be more effective.

Wrap around about 2 times, overlapping the strips, to anchor the bandage. Then proceed to wrap around the foot and on up the leg. It is often helpful to wrap around the foot, then the ankle, then the foot again. This alternation helps to keep the bandage from slipping down.

Continue wrapping, moving up the leg and keeping steady pressure on the bandage to assure even tension. Overlap each succeeding layer about half the width of the bandage. Anchor the top with clips, pins, or tape.

Points to remember:

1. Be sure to check the foot after the bandage is applied to make sure it is not too tight.
2. Be sure to use enough bandages to completely wrap the leg to the height ordered.

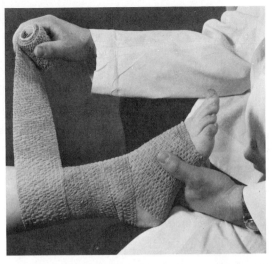

Figure 30-1. Roller bandages must be rewrapped at intervals to ensure their effectiveness. They must be rewrapped at least once every 8 hours, and more often, if needed. During the wrapping procedure, the foot is elevated to the level of the body or higher. Firm, even pressure is applied on the bandage as it is applied. Each successive wrap covers about half of the previous part of the bandage. The particular type of bandage pictured stays in place much better and gives more air circulation to the leg than the older type of elastic bandage. (Medical Products Division, 3M Company)

3. Protect the patient if you use clips or pins to secure the bandage.
4. The bandage must be released at least once every 8 hours and rewrapped. The leg should be exercised at this time and some soothing lotion applied.
5. If the patient complains of pain or itching, check it immediately.
6. The width of the bandage is determined by the part to be wrapped. Generally, however, a bandage wider than 3 inches is difficult to keep in place on the leg or arm. Wider bandages may be used to hold dressings in place on the chest or abdomen.

Figure 30-1 illustrates the correct way to wrap the foot and leg.

**Elastic Stockings.** Many doctors order elastic stockings routinely for all postoperative patients. These are firm stockings which cover the foot (except the toes) and leg up to the knee. They give support to the blood vessels in the leg, thus helping to maintain an adequate blood pressure and prevent emboli from forming.

The stocking should be applied slowly from toes up, with even pressure applied the length of the stocking. Before the stocking is applied, it should be gathered up, since it is not possible to adequately and evenly pull the entire length of the stocking over the foot, without gathering it.

## Slings

Sometimes, the nurse is called upon to put a sling on a patient's arm in order to hold the arm in place. The sling is often used when there is a cast on the arm, since the cast is heavy and will make it difficult for the patient to hold his arm up without assistance. The application of the sling is covered in Chapter 35.

# 3. Medical Asepsis

## ASEPTIC PROCEDURES IN COMMUNICABLE DISEASE

Certain diseases are easily communicated from one person to another through direct contact with the organisms of the disease which are present in body discharges or in droplets in the air from coughs and sneezes.

### Transmission of Disease

There are various means by which communicable diseases spread. The route of spread depends upon the specific disease and sometimes upon the particular patient. If the cause of disease is unknown, strict isolation must be maintained, so that all routes of spread are stopped or blocked.

Diseases may be spread by contact, by vehicle, by air, and by a vector.

*Contact* spread involves either direct contact, which means that the disease is spread by actually touching the infected patient, or indirect contact, which means that infected articles which the patient has infected serve as the route of spread. Included in the latter category are linens, dishes, or bedding from the patient's room. Contact spread of infection is also possible through droplets from the patient's mouth and nose. This requires close proximity to the patient, because droplets usually cannot travel further than 3 feet.

The *vehicle* route concerns the spread of diseases by contaminated food, water, or drugs, or by direct transfer of blood from an infected patient to another person.

*Airborne* transmission of disease occurs via dust particles in the air or from droplets particles which are able to survive longer than ordinary droplets.

A *vector* is an insect, such as the mosquito or the tick, which spreads disease from one person to another.

You, as a nurse, can think of many ways in which to stop the spread of infection, by remembering how infections are spread.

The purpose of the procedures discussed here is to prevent the spread of communicable disease organisms. This can be done: (1) by keeping the patient and everything that is in direct or indirect contact with him away from other people; (2) by destroying the organisms that leave his body; and (3) by taking protective measures for the person who is taking care of him.

### Concurrent Disinfection

The practice of disinfecting all contaminated articles and body discharges and disposing of contaminated materials during the daily care of the patient is called *concurrent disinfection*. It is very important in controlling the spread of communicable disease because it reduces the number of organisms in the patient's surroundings; this protects the patient from reinfection and leaves fewer organisms to spread to others.

### Isolation Technic

The patient may be isolated in his own unit or in a special hospital unit; the actual facilities for carrying out isolation technics may not be the same in every hospital, but the guiding principles in carrying out the

Figure 30-2. Most often, the isolation unit is set up in the patient's room or in a special isolation area of the hospital. In this illustration, a special isolation environment is set up. The climate and everything in it is controlled. This type of unit may be used for either protective isolation or for isolating a patient with a communicable disease. The nurse must wear special clothing to protect the patient and to prevent the spread of infection. The isolation unit may also

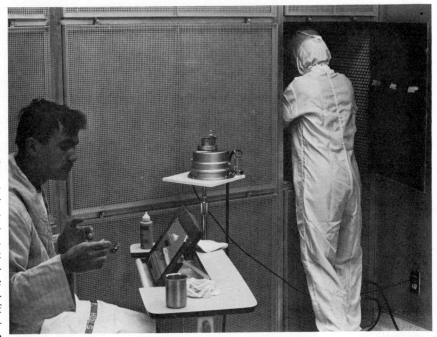

be set up to involve only the patient's bed; the unit looks like a large oxygen tent. This isolates the patient without making him feel so alone, since he can see through the tent. (University of Minnesota Health Sciences Center)

procedures are the same, whatever the method.

The first thing a nurse does in setting up isolation procedures is to explain them to the patient and to the patient's family. You explain how easily disease germs can be spread unless certain precautions are used and why visitors are not allowed to touch the patient or anything around him. Explain that children are not allowed to visit a patient with a communicable disease because they are extremely susceptible to these diseases. Explain the reason for wearing a gown and the care of the dishes and linen, so that the members of the family will co-operate with you intelligently when you need assistance.

It is important to remember that isolation can be frightening for the patient alone in a unit, sometimes with strange and frightening equipment. He may fear that he has some dreaded disease and that people are afraid to come near him. He may be lonely in a room by himself, missing the companionship of other patients and the normal contacts with hospital personnel, such as the maid who sweeps the floor and the aides who bring his tray. Therefore, it is important that the nurs-

ing staff not avoid this patient, even though it takes more effort to go into his room. Try to plan your work so that you can stay in the room as long as possible at one time. Even when you are not going into the room, stop by the door and say hello.

## Specific Diseases and How They Are Spread

Certain contagious diseases are spread via the following routes.

1. *Respiratory:* The disease is spread by sneezing, coughing, or talking. Included in this category are upper respiratory infections, pneumonia, tuberculosis, measles, mumps, and the common cold.

2. *Gastrointestinal:* The disease is spread by contact with contaminated excreta. These diseases are the dysenteries, infectious hepatitis, and contagious diarrhea in children.

3. *Blood and Serum:* The disease is spread by transfer of blood from one person to another. This may be done by a contaminated needle, by an insect, or by a blood transfusion from an infected person. The diseases spread

this way are malaria, syphilis, and serum hepatitis.

4. *Skin and Mucous Membranes:* Some diseases may be spread by mere contact with the skin of the infected person, others must involve contact with the mucous membrane or with an open wound in the mucous membrane. These diseases include syphilis, gonorrhea, impetigo, scabies, staphylococcal infections, and the gas gangrenes.

### Preventive Measures

The first step to be taken in the control of communicable disease is to break the chain of infection or set up barriers to any further spread. The route of spread will influence the control technics used.

1. In the diseases spread by respiratory secretions, handwashing and the wearing of masks and gowns are imperative. In addition, oral and nasal discharges, and sometimes excreta, must be specially disposed of.

2. Diseases spread through the gastrointestinal system: Again handwashing and gowns are necessary. Concurrent disinfection of all items taken out of the room must be done and the excreta must be specially cared for. Adequate screening is important, since flies and other insects can carry the disease.

3. Diseases spread by serum: The nurse should always use disposable syringes and needles. Care should be taken when obtaining blood for transfusion to make sure the donor is well.

4. Diseases spread by contact with skin or mucous membranes require full isolation technic. This includes gown, mask, and gloves, as well as concurrent disinfection. All disposable items must be removed from the room and burned. All nondisposables must be disinfected.

## PROTECTIVE TECHNICS IN CARING FOR PATIENTS IN ISOLATION

### Handwashing

Handwashing is a basic technic in all nursing procedures. The nurse must always wash her hands thoroughly between patients to prevent cross-contamination. Isolation handwashing involves a complete scrub, such as is done before surgery. However, in isolation technic, the hands are pointed downward to prevent the spread of infection to the upper arms. The sink should have foot or knee controls, as well as a soap dispenser, and paper towels should be used. The hands are thoroughly scrubbed at least twice, with special attention given to the nails. The nurse should not touch any part of the sink nor should she wear rings, which might harbor disease, when caring for the isolation patient. (Handwashing technic was discussed previously in this unit.)

### "Scrubbing-Out" of a Room

Whenever you leave the room of an isolation patient, you must take care to disinfect yourself, so that you do not spread the infection to other patients. The procedure of discarding your gown and mask without contaminating yourself and scrubbing your hands without contaminating your upper arms, is known as "scrubbing-out" of the room. It is vital to follow correct procedure, since all the isolation technics are useless unless you get out of the room without carrying contamination to the outside.

### Putting On and Removing the Gown

You wear a gown to keep your clothing clean while you are caring for the patient. Here are certain points to keep in mind when putting on or removing the gown. The *inside* of the gown is clean; the outside is contaminated. The gown must be long enough to cover your uniform completely; it must open down the back and must be full enough to overlap at the back; a tie around the waist keeps the gown in place. The neck of the gown is clean because you never touch that part of the gown with contaminated hands. If you have a long-sleeved uniform, roll your sleeves above your elbows before you put the gown on.

Everyone coming into close contact with an isolated patient must wear a gown. Two technics, the re-use technic or the throw-away technic, are used when donning a gown. With the re-use technic, the nurse's gown hangs in the unit with the *contaminated side out*. With the throw-away technic, the gown is discarded after it is used by folding it *inside out* and

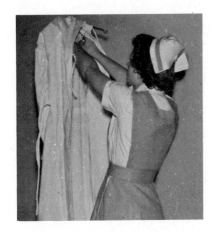

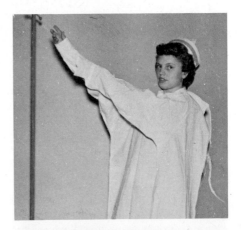

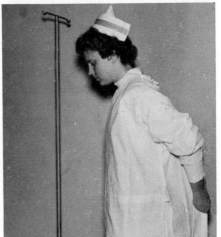

Figure 30-3. (*Top, left*) Removing the gown from the hook. The nurse grasps the gown at the inside of the neckband.

(*Top, right*) The nurse keeps 1 hand *inside* 1 sleeve as she adjusts the other.

(*Bottom*) The nurse draws the back edges together and away from her body before folding the back over and fastening the ties.

placing it in the receptacle provided for contaminated linen. A supply of clean gowns is ready outside to put on before entering the unit. After removing the gown, the wearer washes her hands.

The following procedure describes the re-use technic:

### SUGGESTED PROCEDURE

Slip your hands inside the shoulders of the gown and lift it from the hook.

*Principle: Clean hands touch the clean inside of the gown.*

Slip your arms into the sleeves and keep one hand inside on the sleeve as you adjust the other.

*Principle: A clean hand touches the clean inside of one sleeve.*

Without touching the front of the gown, fasten it at the neck, keeping the sleeves away from your hair.

*Principle: Clean hands touch the clean neck.*

Bring the back edges of the gown together at the waistline, drawing them away from your body and folding them over. Tie the belt.

*Principle: Clean hands are now contaminated by touching the contaminated part of the gown.*

### REMOVING THE GOWN

Untie the strings at the waistline.

*Principle: Contaminated hands touch the contaminated strings.*

Wash your hands—unfasten the neck strings.

*Principle: Clean hands touch the clean neck.*

Wriggle your arms and shoulders out of the gown, drawing hands up through the sleeves.

*Principle: Clean hands touch the clean inside of the gown.*

With hands inside the shoulder of the gown, bring the shoulder seams together and grasp the gown and hang it on the hook. Wash your hands.

*Principle: Clean hands are contaminated by touching the contaminated outside of the gown.*

## Masks

Since some communicable diseases are transmitted through the respiratory tract, it becomes necessary to wear a mask. The individual hospital establishes a policy about wearing masks. In some hospitals, everyone in contact with the patient, including visitors, wears a mask; in others, the patient also wears one. In other situations, only the patient wears a mask.

The principal reason for wearing a mask is to keep organisms from entering and leaving the respiratory tract. When a patient with a severe upper respiratory infection is being cared for, the masks protect those who are attending the patient. In the operating room or in the nursery, masks protect the patient from possible infection by the nursing staff or other personnel. It is generally agreed that the best mask is the disposable type.

Once a mask is removed from the nose and mouth, and once it becomes wet, it should be discarded. The mask which dangles like a necklace beneath the nurse's chin, when not in use, is a menace rather than a protection. Generally to be effective, masks should be changed often. Be sure to wash your hands after removing the mask and to touch the mask only by the strings.

## "Double-Bagging"

The double-bag procedure is carried out by 2 nurses. The nurse on the inside of the room is considered contaminated and the nurse on the outside is considered clean. The contaminated nurse places items from the room into bags held by the clean nurse. The clean nurse folds all bags over to protect the top of the bag and her hands from contamination. The bags are sealed carefully and labeled with isolation tags, indicating the contents of the bags. This procedure is done for paper and other burnable items, as well as for linens or dishes. Instruments must also be double-bagged, but they must be labeled if they will be ruined by autoclave sterilization.

## Specific Isolation Procedures

**Disposing of Excreta.** In some communities, sewage disposal technics destroy organisms. In diseases where the organisms are excreted in the urine or feces, special precautions are needed to destroy these organisms if the sewage disposal system is inadequate. One technic for disposing of hospital waste is to burn as much of it as possible.

**Disposing of Other Body Discharges.** Discharges from the patient's eyes, nose, and mouth require the use of paper wipes that are disposed of immediately by being dropped into a paper bag pinned to the patient's bed. The closed bag can then be "double-bagged" out of the room and burned.

**Care of Linen.** Modern processes in a hospital laundry are generally effective for destroying most communicable disease organisms. However, linens contaminated by spore-forming organisms, such as those causing tetanus or anthrax, are an exception and should be sterilized first by steam pressure before they are handled by laundry workers. If disposable linen is not used in the care of a patient with a communicable disease, then the linen must be placed in a double bag before it is removed from the room.

**Care of Dishes.** Mechanical dishwashers are an ideal solution to the problem of disinfecting dishes used by a patient with a communicable disease. However, disposable dishes and tray-setting materials may be used which leaves only the silverware to be disinfected. By far the best method is the use of disposable dishes and "barrier" trays. It is safe, saves time, and disposes of the unappetizing sight of a used tray lying around.

**Administering Medications.** If you are giving medicine by mouth, use disposable medication cups. If you are not going to touch the patient, you may just wear a mask, if required. Be sure you do not touch the patient or anything in the room, and be sure to wash your hands after leaving.

If you are giving an injection, you must wear gown and gloves if required. Dispose of all needles and syringes in the room, and be sure to break needles off disposable syringes and label them, to protect the housekeeping personnel. Any I.V. bottles which are taken from the room must be labeled as "glass."

**Sending a Specimen to the Laboratory.** If you are sending a blood, urine, or other specimen to the laboratory, you must double-bag it out of the room and label it. Then, a clean nurse takes it to the laboratory immediately. You can do this yourself, after you have given yourself a thorough scrubbing.

**Taking Vital Signs.** When taking vital signs for a person in isolation, be sure to leave the various items used, such as thermometer, blood pressure cuff, and stethoscope in the patient's room, and disinfect them when the patient is removed from isolation. Since you use your watch in some of these procedures, place it on a clean paper towel and do not touch it for other reasons while in the room.

**Transporting the Patient to X-ray or Other Areas of the Hospital.** In very rare cases, it is necessary to transport the patient, who is in isolation, to another part of the hospital. The patient is given a clean gown and mask to wear. The wheelchair or litter is draped with a clean bath blanket, which is then wrapped around the patient, so that only his face is exposed. In this way, the outside of the blanket is still clean, and the person transporting the patient will touch only the outside of the blanket. Be sure that the x-ray department or other department knows that this patient is contaminated, so that they can take the proper disinfection precautions. They must know why the patient is isolated, so they will know what precautions to take.

**Care of the Body after Death.** When a patient dies while in isolation, you must take precautions to prevent the spread of infection. The body should be wrapped while in the room and then transferred to a cart which has been draped with a clean bath blanket or shroud. This is then wrapped around the body by a "clean" person outside the room. If you are the person who has touched the body inside the room, you are considered contaminated and must scrub before leaving the room. Thereafter, you may touch only the outside of the wrapping. Be sure to label the body, so the pathologist knows that this patient was in isolation.

**Terminal Disinfection.** Terminal disinfection means the care of a patient's unit and belongings after the infectious period has terminated. The process is the same whether the patient remains in the hospital, has been discharged, or has expired. Sometimes the sanitary code of the city or community prescribes the methods to be used. The methods should be sufficiently thorough to destroy the particular organisms causing the disease. Medical science has given us so much information about organisms that cause disease that it should be possible to select the best and most appropriate methods of disinfection in each instance. Some organisms are harder to destroy than others and ordinary methods are not effective.

*A reminder:* The nurse must remember that anything which touches the isolation patient is contaminated and must be sterilized before it can touch the nurse or another patient. *Stop and think* before you do anything for the patient in isolation or else you might become contaminated and spread the disease. *Only one break in technic is all it takes to spread infection.* Good handwashing is vital in the isolation technic. If in doubt, wash your hands.

## Reverse Isolation (Protective Isolation)

Sometimes, it is the patient who must be protected from the environment. In this case, modified surgical asepsis is used, whereby the patient is placed in a special room and everything which comes in contact with him is sterile. The type of patient who might be placed into protective isolation is the burn patient who is not receiving open treatment, the patient with a blood defect which renders him unable to fight off infection, the patient with very low resistance from some other cause, or the patient with a large, open wound.

Just remember that you are trying to protect the patient from contamination. Therefore, use only sterile equipment and linens when caring for him, and wear sterile gown, gloves, and mask, as well as a cap which covers all your hair. This technic is very similar to surgical asepsis, which is used in the operating room or in other sterile procedures.

# 4. *Surgical Asepsis (Sterile Technic)*

Surgical asepsis is accomplished by making and keeping objects sterile—first, by sterilizing them to destroy all bacteria and secondly, by avoiding any contact with unsterile objects. When a sterile object is touched by an unsterile object it becomes contaminated and is no longer sterile. Surgical asepsis is essential in surgical operations and in deliveries and in many nursing procedures, such as giving hypodermic injections and catheterizations. We call this method *surgical aseptic technic.*

Surgical asepsis or sterile technic differs from medical asepsis in that *all* microorganisms are destroyed. This technic implies that no organisms will be carried to the patient. Therefore, anything which comes in contact with the patient is sterile. You must remember that if you are wearing sterile gloves, you *cannot* touch anything which is unsterile or you will be contaminated. On the other hand, if you are unsterile, you cannot touch anything which is sterile, or you will contaminate it. Try to think of unsterile things as having insects on them. Then, think before you touch anything, so that you do not carry the contamination to something which is sterile.

You must understand the difference between clean and sterile. *Clean* applies to medical asepsis and implies that all gross contamination is removed and that many microorganisms have been removed. Clean can be accomplished by mechanical cleansing. *Sterile* means that the item is free of all microorganisms, dangerous or not, and all spores. Sterile to sterile remains sterile. Sterile to clean becomes contaminated.

## GENERAL PRINCIPLES

Once you have on sterile gloves and/or a gown, you cannot touch anything which is not sterile.

Reaching over a sterile field, while the clothes you wear are not sterile, contaminates the area.

If a sterile wrapper becomes wet, it is no longer sterile.

Skin cannot be sterilized; it can only be cleaned.

The parts of the body which are not exposed to the outside are considered sterile. This includes the abdominal cavity, the urinary bladder, and usually the uterus. The gastrointestinal tract is not sterile, because it is actually a tube within the body which opens on both ends to the outside. In addition, unsterile items (food) are introduced into the GI tract daily.

## Sterilization and Disinfection

Sterilization and disinfection are necessary in carrying out surgical asepsis, but they are also necessary in preventing spread of harmful bacteria from one patient to another. Sometimes we know that a patient harbors specific organisms, but we know that others may be present also—others about which we know nothing. Therefore, we sterilize equipment used for a patient before we use it for another. For instance, when a patient is discharged, we sterilize the wash basin, mouth care utensils, and the bedpan he used while in the hospital. Thus we know that any remaining organisms have been destroyed, and the next patient can safely use the equipment.

## Methods of Sterilization

Sterilization is exposing articles to heat or to chemical disinfectants long enough to kill all microorganisms and spores. Some germs are harder to destroy than others. However, boiling for 10 minutes destroys most organisms; exposure for 15 minutes to steam under 18 pounds of pressure at a temperature of 257° F. will kill even the toughest ones. (Pressure steam sterilizers are known as *autoclaves.*) Chemical disinfectants powerful enough to destroy germs cannot be used for some articles; for example, phenol (carbolic acid) would destroy organisms on a rectal tube but would also destroy the tube. Moist heat destroys the sharp cutting edges of some instruments; therefore, they are better sterilized by dry heat or chemicals. Another method is dry heat (hot-air sterilization or gas sterilization), which involves the use of equipment similar to the ordinary baking oven.

Equipment for nursing treatments is sterilized in various ways. In some hospitals, the treatment trays are prepared and sterilized in a central supply room. Many sterile items are used one time and then discarded, to prevent cross-contamination.

## Sterile Supplies

The supplies used for surgical and other sterile procedures must be free of all organisms, both pathogenic and nonpathogenic. Anything which comes into contact with an open wound or break in the skin, or is introduced into a sterile body cavity, or punctures the skin must be *sterile*. In most hospitals today, sterile supplies are prepared in a central supply unit or are packaged in a sterile condition and disposed of after being used. Gauze sponges and compresses, pads, cotton balls, applicators, and towels are sterilized, are packaged in cloth, paper or plastic wraps, are secured with masking tape, and are labeled. Some institutions prepare certain types of supplies in covered glass enamel or metal containers. It is more difficult to keep supplies sterile in containers because once the container is opened, the contents are exposed to air contamination. Packaged supplies can be put up in "one use" amounts. If many people are using supplies from a container, the chances for contamination are increased.

## HANDLING STERILE SUPPLIES AND EQUIPMENT

Remember these 2 points in handling sterile equipment: (1) never touch sterile articles with unsterile ones and (2) discard an article if you should happen to contaminate it or if you are not sure if it is contaminated. It is better to discard an item than to take a chance on using a contaminated item. Every movement in aseptic procedures is a link in the chain of asepsis—if you break one link by contaminating something, the chain is broken, and you open the door to infection.

## The Transfer Forceps

You can handle sterile equipment with a forceps which is sterile on the end which touches the sterile articles. A long forceps with a flat broad tip—a sponge forceps—is often used to handle sterile materials, or in removing sterile dressings from containers, or sterile instruments and basins from the sterilizer, or to set up trays. (The transfer forceps is used less frequently than in the past, because prepackaged items are now available.) The forceps is kept in a tall wide-mouthed jar of antiseptic solution, such as alcohol, which is a sterilizing agent and keeps the forceps sterile. The container and the forceps are sterilized; the container is filled with enough solution to cover at least two-thirds of the forceps; and the forceps is placed in the solution, ready for use.

Follow these directions in using transfer forceps:

Never put more than one forceps in a container because it is difficult to remove one of them without touching the sterile part against the unsterile handle of the remaining forceps.

Keep the prongs of the forceps together and avoid touching the rim of the container.

*Always* keep the tip of the forceps pointed downward to prevent the solution from flowing down over the unsterile handle and then back onto the sterile part.

Avoid touching the rim or outside of a container with a sterile article when removing it.

Discard the forceps if you think you may have contaminated it.

## The Sterile Tray

A sterile tray can be prepared by covering a tray with a sterile towel and placing the sterile equipment on it with the sterile handling forceps. In removing supplies from sterile jars, put the covers down *inside up,* to keep them sterile, and avoid touching the outside unsterile part of the jar with the sterile forceps or with the sterile article you are removing. If you spill liquid on the sterile towel covering the tray, it is no longer sterile because the wet spot furnishes a point for organisms to penetrate from the unsterile tray beneath.

## The Surgical Mask

The newer type of disposable masks are much more effective in preventing the spread of germs through droplets in the air. Place the mask over your mouth and nose. If you wear glasses, be sure to bend the metal strip

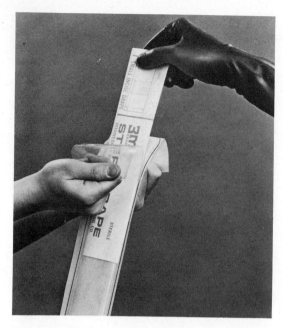

Figure 30-4. The proper method of opening a sterile package. The nurse on the left (the unsterile hands) opens the package, touching only the flaps and the outside of the package. The nurse on the right (with sterile gloves) touches only the inside of the package. The contents of a sterile package may be dropped onto a sterile field without becoming contaminated. (Medical Products Division, 3M Company)

on top of the mask to fit your nose, otherwise your glasses will steam up. You may tie the two strings of the mask behind your head or you may loop the top string around your ears and tie it under your chin, with the bottom string tied behind the head at neck level. This position is often more comfortable and makes it easier to take off the mask; just unloop the strings around your ears and the mask will fall away from your mouth and nose.

Remember that the mask must be put on before your gloves, that it is not effective if it becomes wet, and that once used, it is considered contaminated and must be discarded.

## The Surgical Hood

In the case of a male nurse with a beard, a hood is often worn to cover the entire face, except the eyes.

**The Hair Covering.** In some cases, especially in the operating room, you will be asked to wear a cap or hood which will cover all of your hair. Remember that none of your hair can be showing. If you have long hair, you will need to wear a special type of hood. If your hair is short, you can wear a surgical cap.

## The Sterile Gown

Remember that you can only touch with your hands the parts of the gown which will touch your body after the gown is in place. Therefore, touch only the inside of the gown. Someone will tie the strings for you; the back of your gown is considered contaminated, even though it was sterile when you put it on. Any part of the gown below the level of your hips is also considered contaminated. Be careful when you are wearing a sterile gown not to touch anything which is not sterile. If, for example, you are observing in the operating room, remember not to touch anything without thinking first.

Your instructors will give you specific instructions in how to put on a gown and gloves without contaminating yourself or anything else in the sterile area.

## Sterile Gloves

For some procedures, you will be expected to put on sterile gloves. Remember that once you have the gloves on, you cannot touch anything which is not sterile without contaminating your gloves. Therefore, you must make all your preparations before you put on your gloves. Open the glove package, using sterile technic. Do not touch the inside of the wrapper with your hands. Remember that your hands can touch only those parts of the gloves which they will touch when the gloves are on. With the first hand, hold one glove by the inside. Pull it on and leave the cuff in place. With the other hand (the one with the sterile glove on) pick up the other glove, now touching only the sterile side. Keep your fingers inside the cuff and snap the glove in place. You can now adjust your gloves touching only the sterile surfaces.

Once you have your gloves on, you must remember that you cannot touch anything which is not sterile.

## The Sterile Package

When you are asked to open a sterile package, the most important thing to remember is which part of the package is contaminated and which part is sterile. If you are opening the package, you can touch only the outside of the package, since your hands are not sterile. If you are receiving the contents of the package, you will have sterile gloves on and can touch only the inside of the package, because this is sterile.

Figure 30-4 shows the correct way to hand a sterile item to a doctor or another nurse.

## The Dressing Change

When you make rounds with the doctor, you may be asked to assist with a dressing change. At a later time, you may be permitted to change a dressing on a small wound by yourself. The principles of aseptic or sterile technic apply here as usual. The doctor may ask for ABD (abdominal) pads, sterile 4-by-4 inch pads, kerlix, tape, or other types of pads and dressings. You can take your cue from the dressing which is taken off the patient; chances are, the doctor will put on much the same type of dressing.

If irrigation of the wound is done at the same time, you will need a basin to catch the drainage, sterile solution, a syringe (perhaps an Asepto), and other equipment specified by the doctor.

Your most important role is to anticipate the needs of the doctor and to have the necessary items ready. Remember not to contaminate any sterile items and to use good technic when handing things to the doctor. You will become more proficient as you practice.

When giving injection drugs to a doctor who has sterile gloves on, you must show him the label and then hold the bottle while he draws the drug up into the syringe. The syringe which he is using is sterile, but the bottle is not. Don't forget that the bottle must be tipped upside-down while the drug is drawn up. Again after the drug is drawn up show the doctor the label and mention the name of the drug. It is also your responsibility to keep track of drugs used and to chart this information, noting the dose and the time of administration.

## Removal of Stitches or Skin Clamps

Sutures (stitches) and skin clamps are often removed at the time of the dressing change. Frequently, a suture removal kit is used and discarded after use. If this is not available, you will need a sterile tweezers and a very small sterile scissors, as well as a few sterile 2-by-2 inch gauze pads. If you are asked to remove stitches, you must have instruction, but remember to cut the suture and to pull on the side of the knot to remove the stitch. Use sterile technic in doing the procedure.

# 5. *Assisting the Female Patient*

## VAGINAL TREATMENTS

### Vaginal Irrigation (Douche)

This consists of directing a flow of fluid into the vaginal canal and allowing it to flow out by gravity. The purposes of a vaginal irrigation are to cleanse the vaginal canal of discharge and to apply heat or medications to relieve pain and inflammation.

The vaginal canal is a passage about 3 inches long, which is lined with mucous membrane and extends from the uterus to the vulva. The inner labia enclose the vaginal opening and the secretions of the mucous

membrane protect it from infection. Therefore, it is not desirable to wash away these secretions by douches unless such treatment is necessary. Nor is it wise to use strong irritating solutions which may also set up inflammation in the vaginal canal. Mild antiseptic solutions, such as boric acid or normal saline, are suitable and safe for vaginal irrigations. Sodium bicarbonate solution is sometimes used for an overacid condition, while a solution of potassium permanganate may be used for an odorous discharge. Vinegar solution (2 tablespoons to a pint of water) may be used because it resembles normal vaginal secretions.

The doctor will specify the kind of solution to be used.

The temperature of the solution for a cleansing vaginal irrigation should be about 105°F. If the doctor prescribes a hotter douche, it may be given at a temperature of from 110° to 115°F. The inside of the vagina can safely stand a considerable degree of heat, but the hotter fluid may burn the more sensitive vulva and the perineum. These parts should be protected with an application of oil if the temperature of the solution is as high as 110°F.

A vaginal irrigation is given with an irrigating can and tubing attached to a douche tip, which is inserted into the vaginal canal. Douche tips are made of glass, hard rubber, or plastic. (Plastic douche tips cannot be sterilized by steam or boiling; a disinfectant must be used. This is an argument in favor of using disposable tips.) The douche tips must be inspected before they are used to be sure that they are in good condition; a cracked, rough, or broken tip would injure the vaginal tissues.

The vaginal canal curves up and back when the patient is lying down; the tip is inserted to follow this direction. The flow of the fluid into the vagina should be gentle, to prevent forcing infection into the uterus. The cervix projects down into the vagina in such a way that a pocket is formed between the cervix and the rear wall of the vaginal canal. The douche tip is rotated during the irrigation to be sure that the solution washes out discharge collected in this pocket and reaches every part of the vagina.

**Infectious Conditions.** If the patient has a gonorrheal or a syphilitic infection, special precautions are necessary, to protect both the patient and the nurse. The patient should be instructed to keep her hands away from the perineal area in order to prevent carrying infection to her eyes. The nurse wears gloves and may also wear goggles to prevent possible splashing of infected material into her eyes. A thorough hand-washing is vital, and the equipment must be sterilized after use.

The can, the tubing, and the douche pan for an unsterile vaginal irrigation are *clean,* while the douche tip is *sterile.* In some hospitals, the complete equipment for a vaginal irrigation is done up as a sterile package in the central supply room.

## EQUIPMENT

| | |
|---|---|
| Irrigating can or bag tubing, and clamp | Standard (short I.V. stand) |
| Douche tip and container | Bath thermometer |
| Douche pan and cover | Protective pad and cover |
| Solution as prescribed | Perineal pad |
| | Tissues |

### KEY POINTS IN THE PROCEDURE

Have the patient void before beginning the treatment.

*Reason: A full bladder interferes with the insertion of the douche nozzle.*

Prepare the prescribed solution (about 1,500 cc.) at the required temperature (100° to 110° F.) according to the purpose of the treatment.

*Reason: Heat relieves inflammation but solution at high temperatures will burn the mucous membranes and the skin around the meatus when flowing back.*

Put the patient on her back with only one pillow under her head and place her on the douche pan. This procedure may also be done while the patient is sitting on the toilet.

*Reason: Gravity aids the flow of solution to reach the farthest part of the vagina.*

Place the irrigating can slightly above the level of the patient's hips to insure a continuous but gentle flow of the solution. (*Never more than 18 inches higher than the hips!*)

*Reason: The higher the can, the more forceful the flow. Force can drive infectious material into the cervical opening.*

Release the clamp to let the air out of the tubing before you begin. Separate the labia and insert the nozzle, directing it downward and backward.

*Reason: In the dorsal recumbent position, the direction of the vaginal canal is down and back.*

Rotate the nozzle gently during the treatment.

*Reason: Rotation of the nozzle directs the fluid over all parts of the vagina.*

Clamp the tubing and withdraw the tip from the vagina. Detach the tip from the tubing and place it in the waste basin.

*Reason:* Microorganisms cause infection. Harmful organisms are transferred to individuals and to clean objects by contact.

If the patient is able, have her sit up on the pan for a few minutes, to drain the fluid from the vagina. Then place a pad over the vulva.

*Reason:* Draining fluid soils the bed and makes the patient uncomfortable.

Disinfect the douche tip and the waste basin before returning the equipment to the surgical room.

*Reason:* Disinfection kills harmful microorganisms and prevents the spread of infection.

Record the treatment on the patient's chart.

## Inserting A Vaginal Suppository

Vaginal suppositories are used to apply medication to the vaginal canal. The medication is incorporated in a round cocoa butter base. Like the rectal suppository, it melts after it has been inserted. The suppository can be inserted with the patient lying on her back or on her side. Use a water-soluble lubricant for the suppository and insert it full length into the vagina; wear a rubber glove or finger cots on the right-hand thumb and finger. Record the kind of suppository used and the patient's reaction.

## CATHETERIZATION

Catheterization is the procedure of inserting a catheter through the urethra into the bladder to remove urine.

The bladder is the reservoir for the urine secreted by the kidneys (see Chap. 18). Usually, when 200 to 250 cc. accumulate, the urge to void occurs. If the bladder cannot be emptied normally, urine accumulates, distending the bladder, or it dribbles continually from the urethral opening.

### Reasons for Catheterization

The urethra and the bladder are delicate structures; injury to the mucous membrane or infection in these organs can have serious effects on the patient. On the other hand, if the bladder becomes overdistended or retains urine for a long period, these conditions may also be harmful. Some of the reasons for catheterizing a patient are:

To relieve the retention of urine when the patient is temporarily unable to void.

To remove the urine remaining in the bladder when voiding only partly empties it (residual urine).

To empty the bladder of an incontinent patient at regular intervals—to keep the patient dry and to prevent bedsores.

To obtain a sterile specimen of urine.

To prevent urine from touching stitches in the perineum.

**Modern Practices.** The need for catheterization following a surgical operation has diminished, as the practice of early ambulation for surgical patients has increased. *Position* is a very important aid in emptying the bladder. Women who cannot void lying down often are able to void if they are allowed to sit up. Men find it easier to void when standing. With support in these positions, many patients are able to void normally.

Formerly, catheterization was considered necessary to obtain an uncontaminated specimen of urine. Normally, the inside of the bladder is considered sterile. Many doctors now feel that catheterization may carry infectious material from the urethra into the bladder to contaminate the urine specimen. They recommend a method instead which is called "clean catch." This procedure is discussed in Chapter 27.

In any catheterization procedure it is not considered safe to remove more than 750 to 1,000 cc. of urine from the bladder at any one time. If the flow of urine seems undiminished after this amount is withdrawn, report it to the head nurse so the doctor can be notified and determine further action. If a patient is admitted to the hospital with a greatly distended bladder, it is usually considered safer to relieve the distention gradually to prevent bladder damage and possible shock.

### Types of Catheters

The catheters most commonly used are made of rubber or plastic, although glass or metal catheters are used occasionally. Catheters should be discarded after removal. It is very difficult to adequately sterilize a catheter. Every type of catheter has a rounded tip, to prevent injury to the meatus or the urethra. Catheters are graded in the same way as rectal tubes. Sizes No. 14, Fr. and No. 16, Fr. are suitable for the female patient. For the male patient, sizes No. 20, Fr. and No. 22, Fr. are usually used. Sizes No. 8, Fr. and No. 10, Fr. are appropriate for children.

**The Retention (In-dwelling) Catheter.** The retention catheter provides temporary or permanent drainage of urine. This may be necessary for incontinence in an unconscious patient, for bladder injury or surgery, or in other bladder conditions, such as cancer or infection.

The Foley catheter is a commonly used retention catheter. It has a small tube within it that opens into a small balloon below the opening in the tip which provides an outlet for the urine. After the catheter is inserted, the balloon is inflated with sterile water or saline through a small projecting tube near the outer end of the catheter, and the tube is clamped off. The inflated balloon keeps the catheter from slipping out. There are other varieties of the retention catheter which may be used, such as the so-called mushroom type. This is discussed in Chapter 50.

## Preparing the Female Patient

Explain to the patient that you are going to drain urine from the bladder to make her more comfortable and that you will use a small tube that slips in easily because it is lubricated. Explain how she can help by relaxing—that she will barely notice when you slip in the tube if she is not tense. Be sure that the room and the patient are warm enough. Chilliness makes people tense. Ask her to breathe through her mouth to assist relaxation.

## Essential Precautions

Catheterization is an aseptic procedure which requires sterile equipment. In the hospital sterile catheterization sets are prepared in the surgical supply room, or sterile disposable equipment may be provided. These sets are so wrapped that the catheters lie straight and are easy to handle.

The position of the female patient is the same as for a vaginal examination.

EQUIPMENT

| Sterile | Unsterile |
|---|---|
| Rubber catheters No. 14, Fr. and No. 16, F. (2). If one catheter becomes contaminated, another one is available. | Protective sheet and cover |
| | Towel |
| | Extra bath blanket |
| | Waste container |
| 1 Small basin | Accessory lamp |
| 2 Large basins | |
| Sponges or cotton balls | |
| Solution | |
| Lubricant | |
| Specimen bottle and cover, if required or disposable catheterization tray. | |
| Forceps | |
| (or disposable catheterization tray) | |

KEY POINTS IN THE PROCEDURE
(FEMALE PATIENT, USING DISPOSABLE TRAY)

Place the patient on her back.
*Principle: Gravity aids the flow of urine.*
Adjust the drapes and cover the patient's chest as conditions indicate.
*Principle: Embarrassment and chilliness increase tension. Tension interferes with the insertion of the catheter.*
Open the package, using sterile precautions. Prepare the cleansing solution and squeeze the sterile lubricant onto the catheter.
*Principle: Thorough preparation aids speed and efficiency.*
Arrange the equipment for convenience and to prevent contaminating the catheters.
*Principle: Reaching across sterile equipment may contaminate it.*
Put on gloves; separate and press upward on the inner labia. Touch the patient with your left hand only. Keep your right hand sterile.
Cleanse the area according to the prescribed procedure, using and discarding cotton balls until the area is clean.
*Principle: Microorganisms introduced into the bladder will cause infection.*
*Principle: Lubrication reduces friction.*
Pick up the catheter 3 inches from the tip.
*Principle: The sterile tip prevents bladder contamination.*
Insert the catheter for 2 to 3 inches or until

urine begins to flow. You may hold it with your left hand.

*Principle: The female urethra is about 1½ inches long.*

To collect a specimen, pinch off the catheter. Place the end of it in the sterile specimen container and let the urine flow. Place your hand on the pubis to help to keep the catheter in place.

*Principle: Moving the catheter back and forth increases the possibility of contamination.*

When the urine flow begins to diminish, withdraw the catheter slowly by half-inches until only a drip of urine appears. If the catheter is to remain in place do not withdraw it. Inject solution to blow up the balloon as instructed. Keep the drainage set intact—breaking the seal can lead to contamination.

*Principle: The catheter continues to remove urine as it is withdrawn.*

Make the patient comfortable and clean all the equipment immediately or dispose of it.

*Principle: Secretions and other substances are more easily removed when not coagulated.*

Record the amount of urine obtained, noting its appearance (clear or cloudy), evidences of blood or pus, and the patient's reactions.

## The Lateral Position for Catheterization

In many cases, a side-lying position for catheterization of the female is preferable to the back-lying position. It allows less exposure of the patient, is more comfortable because the legs can be relaxed and is the only position possible for the patient who has had back surgery or who has contractures of the legs. This position also makes it easier to maintain sterile technic because only one labia must be held into position, while gravity maintains the other. And since the nurse does not need to reach over the patient's leg she is less likely to contaminate the catheter. The patient cannot see the equipment, so she is not as apprehensive. The patient is more relaxed, making the insertion of the catheter easier.

The patient lies on her side with her knees drawn up on her chest. If the nurse is right-handed, the patient should lie on her left side. The patient's buttocks should be close to the side of the bed where the nurse is standing and the patient's shoulders should be close to the other side of the bed.

## Catheterization of the Male Patient

It is more difficult to catheterize a male patient because the urethra in the male is longer and has more curves than that of the female. In addition, an enlarged prostate gland constricts or obstructs the male urethra. Previous infection in the urethra also causes strictures. Usually the doctor or a male nurse is the one who catheterizes a male patient, but any nurse should be prepared to do it, if necessary. It may seem embarrassing to a male patient, but a matter-of-fact, assured attitude helps to put the patient at ease and to prevent body tensions that might interfere with the procedure.

The main difference between catheterizing a female and a male patient lies with the insertion of the catheter because of the differences in shape between the female and male urethra. The male urethra is longer with 2 curves in its passage to the bladder, which makes inserting a catheter more difficult. One of these curves can be straightened out by lifting the penis; the other one is fixed. For this reason, the penis is held upright, at right angles to the patient's body when the catheter is inserted.

The patient lies on his back with his legs spread apart and his knees flexed slightly. The receptacle for the urine is placed between his thighs. With the end of the penis held between the thumb and the forefinger, the nurse cleans the meatus as in the female patient. Holding the penis upright, exert slight pressure on the organ to widen the opening for the insertion of the catheter, which has been lubricated for 1½ inches. A drop of sterile lubricant on the meatus also aids in the insertion of the catheter.

If slight resistance is felt, usually it can be overcome by twisting the catheter a little. With more pronounced resistance, the pull on the penis can be increased as the catheter is withdrawn slightly, then pushed ahead, with a series of short shoves, until the urine begins to flow.

Instructing the patient to breathe deeply helps to relax the perineal muscles and to overcome resistance to the entry of the catheter.

# 6. *Assisting the Dying Patient and His Family*

## THE FINAL HOURS

Despite the great advances in technology, medical science cannot cure every illness. Thus you may find yourself nursing a patient with a terminal illness, who, to the best medical knowledge, has no chance of recovering from a fatal process.

As a nurse, you may well be the person to give the last comforting services to the patient and provide a source of comfort to his family as well. The last days in a patient's life offer you one of the greatest challenges in your nursing career.

All too often, nursing texts deal with the physical aspects of death and ignore its emotional impact. Death is, no doubt, one of the most profound emotional experiences which you will encounter as a nurse and as a family member. It is very definitely the most meaningful and moving emotional experience which you will encounter as a person.

It is difficult for the nurse to resolve herself to the fact of death. Somehow, it seems like a failure on the part of the medical staff and the nurse. Because we are constantly preoccupied with preserving life at all costs, it is difficult to admit that the patient cannot be cured.

Before the nurse can be helpful to the dying patient and his family, she must effectively work out her own feelings about death as it relates to her personally, and she should be able to consider the assistance she gives a dying patient and his family as a nursing opportunity and not as a failure.

Dr. Kübler-Ross, in discussing the increasing loneliness of death, notes that in the past, people were allowed to die at home with their friends and family in attendance. Today, the patient is rushed into the emergency room with equipment surrounding him, with ambulance sirens screaming, and with all the people busy attending to the machines. With everything becoming more mechanical and dehumanized, it is difficult to determine exactly when death occurs. "He may cry for rest, peace, and dignity, but he will get infusions, transfusions, a heart machine, or tracheostomy if necessary. He may want one single person to stop for a single minute so that he can ask one single question—but he will get a dozen people around the clock, all busily preoccupied with his heart rate, pulse, electrocardiogram or pulmonary functions, his secretions or excretions, but not with him as a human being . . . all this is done in the fight for his life, and if they can save his life they can consider the person afterwards."*

## The Psychology of Death

Dr. Elisabeth Kübler-Ross in her book, *On Death and Dying*, has so impressively discussed many psychological aspects of death that every nursing student should read this book. Many of her ideas have been incorporated into this discussion of death.

Death should be considered as a part of life, as an extension of birth and a natural part of living. Unfortunately, all too often we do not share such a healthy view. We often do not allow children to be exposed to death, and thus, we do not prepare them to deal with death, when it does occur. As a result many people develop an unnatural fear of dying, a fear which is intensified in some cases by guilt feelings or anger or by fear of the unknown, or by fear of pain or anguish in the actual act of dying.

Our attitudes are further shaped by the fact that each one of us considers himself immortal, in a way. While each of us can imagine other people dying, we cannot imagine our own death. Nor can we conceive of our death as occurring from within; rather it must be caused by something from outside our body. Thus when a patient is faced with the prospect of death, he may not actually believe that he is going to die.

## The Stages of Coping with a Terminal Illness

Dr. Kübler-Ross, as well as other authors, have described certain phases through which a patient passes in his attempt to cope with the fact that he is going to die. All patients pass through some, and hopefully all, of these

---

* Kübler-Ross, E.: *On Death and Dying*. Macmillan, 1969.

stages before death, except when death is instantaneous or when the patient is unable to resolve his conflicts.

**Denial and Isolation.** In this stage the patient does not believe that the diagnosis is correct—"This can't be happening to me!" This is the stage during which the patient may seek the advice of several doctors, hoping that one of them will offer a more hopeful prognosis. Quacks capitalize on this patient and take advantage of his desperate feelings.

**Anger and Rage.** Next, the patient asks "Why did this happen to me? Why now?" Often, he envies the person who is young and healthy, and may strike out at the nursing staff and be difficult to relate to. The nurse must understand that this is a phase of the patient's illness and that the anger being expressed is being directed at the situation and not at the nurse as a person. What the patient is rebelling against is the feeling of sudden helplessness. You can imagine how you would feel if you had always been in control of your life and suddenly met a situation which you could not control.

**Bargaining—Developing Awareness.** During this stage, which may be very short or entirely absent, the patient makes "deals" with God or with himself. "If I can just live 2 more weeks, I can see my boy get married." When the time has passed, the patient often feels like making another bargain, postponing death indefinitely. You may meet many patients who seem to make up their mind to live until a certain event and then die quickly after that time.

**Depression.** The patient suddenly realizes that he is going to die and there is absolutely nothing which can be done to stop it. He may feel a severe sense of loss concerning his job, the money spent on medical bills, his children and loved ones, and, of course, the greatest loss of all—life itself.

The depression often passes through two phases: the verbal and the nonverbal stages. During the verbal stage, also called *reactive depression,* the patient concentrates on past losses. He can be reassured and encouraged to smile and to cheer up because things could be worse. Later, during the nonverbal stage, also called *preparatory depression,* the patient realizes the impact of his future loss. During this phase encouragement is not meaningful be-cause the patient realizes that he will be leaving everything he has known behind. He may wish to pray and to plan for life after death, if this is his belief, or he may daydream or sleep a great deal, in an effort to escape reality. The nurse can be most helpful by being present and by not trying to "cheer him up" with empty talking. Just a touch of the hand or a kind word will be more helpful than a great deal of meaningless chatter. Let the patient know that you care and that you are available, but do not push yourself on him.

**Acceptance and Peace.** As the patient resolves his emotional conflicts about death, he enters the stage where he realizes and accepts the inevitability of his fate. To reach this point, the patient must have had time and assistance in working through the previous stages. While he may sleep a great deal, it is no longer a means of escape, but is necessary because of weakness and fatigue. As the patient resigns himself to the fact that he is going to die, he seems to be devoid of all feeling. This is a particularly difficult time for the family, because they interpret the patient's acceptance of death as a rejection of life and of them. They must be assisted to understand that the patient will not be able to die until he has been helped to give up everything associated with life, and that while the patient is often unable or unwilling to communicate at this time, he usually will appreciate short visits or the presence of a family member who is just there but who does not attempt to hold a conversation with him.

**Decathexis.** The final stage is called *decathexis,* during which time the patient gradually separates himself from the world so that there is no longer a 2-way communication between himself and those around him. Since the patient may be apparently unconscious during this time, nursing care can now be primarily directed toward the physical needs of the patient. However, the nurse must remember that the patient often can hear what is being said even though he may not answer or respond.

**The Role of Hope.** Through most of the stages preceding death, the patient clings to hope and usually does not give up until the very end, when he finally accepts his fate. Until then he should be allowed to maintain hope. While the nurse should not discourage hope, she should not give any false hope of a miracle. Dr. Kübler-Ross states that a good nursing or medical response would be "To my knowledge I have done everything I can to help you. I will continue, however, to keep you as comfortable as possible."

## THE PATIENT'S FAMILY

Often the patient's family feels this trying period more keenly than the patient; they already feel the sense of loss that death will bring and yet they feel they must try to appear as usual. If the patient is suffering, you can explain how the family can make death easier by avoiding emotional behavior and by taking turns in staying with the patient. Too many people in the room may upset the patient.

Encourage the members of the family to keep the family life on as even a keel as possible. Explain the need for rest and food. In the hospital, it is a great kindness to a patient's family to offer them a cup of tea or coffee when the waiting period has been long and exhausting. If possible, the family should have a place where they can be alone when they are not with the patient. If the waiting period is likely to be long, encourage the family to go out for meals and rest, assuring them that they will be called if any change occurs in the patient's condition.

You may need to prepare the family for changes in the patient's appearance. You can explain that even though the patient seems distressed, decreasing sensibility reduces pain.

When it comes to the everyday problems which confront a family at this time the nurse, social workers, chaplain, and other members of the medical team can assist in such matters as financial difficulties, arranging for baby sitting and for transportation to and from the hospital, and indicating where to find temporary housing for out-of-town families, and who to consult on religious questions and other such matters.

Since the dying person can offer comfort to his family by sharing his feelings and thoughts, the nurse can encourage such communication. The sooner the patient shares the prognosis with his family, the longer the time they will have to work out the situation together. After all it *is* a sad situation and the family can feel free to share this time and feeling with the patient; the family who hides all their feelings may give the patient the impression that they do not care about him or about the fact that he is dying.

After death has occurred, do not forget about the family. They may wish to see the body or to be alone to talk for a while. While you would be kind to offer them a cup of coffee and any other assistance, do not hover in the background.

## PHYSICAL ASPECTS OF NURSING CARE

Once the actual physical process of dying has begun, the nurse's main job is to assist in the supportive and symptomatic care of the patient, rather than to engage in any heroic measures. Alfred Worcester in his book, *The Care of the Aged, the Dying and the Dead,* states that "The history of the patient as well as the nature of his disease may help in differentiating the approach of death from similar states of collapse where restoration is possible. . . . Old age is the only natural cause of death, and natural death is merely falling asleep."

As with all nursing care, it is important to allow the patient to maintain his self-esteem and personal dignity. Therefore while the nurse can assist the patient with those things which he cannot do, she should never do things which he can do for himself.

**Changes Before Death.** The unmistakable signs of death appear as gradual physical changes. Usually movement and feeling in the lower limbs are lost before the arms are affected. Action ceases in the stomach and the intestines, even though the patient can still swallow; therefore, it is useless to give the patient nourishment, which may cause distress by distending the stomach and impairing respiration, which already may be difficult. When the patient's mouth becomes dry and parched, a few sips of water or weak tea with lemon will help relieve the discomfort. If the patient is unconscious or chokes on fluids, the lips and the tongue can be moistened or a gauze-wrapped piece of ice can be placed between the tongue and the cheek. As death approaches, the face may become pinched and drawn, the eyes sunken, and the mouth open (called the *facies Hippocratiea*). When the actual process of dying has begun, resuscitation measures may be more harmful than helpful.

The changes which take place can be placed into 5 general categories:

1. Loss of muscle tone (from the feet up).
2. Cessation of peristalsis.
3. Slowing of circulation (pulse is often rapid and irregular; blood pressure loss).
4. Labored respirations (fast or shallow; irregular).
5. Loss of senses. (Hearing is the last sense to be lost.)

The loss of the sense of touch is called *the anesthesia of the dying,* and the unconsciousness which often occurs is called *in extremis.*

**Care of Mouth, Nose, and Eyes.** The mouth needs regular care—it should be swabbed with mouthwash as often as is necessary to keep it clean; mineral oil and lemon juice should be applied to the tongue and inside the cheeks. If there is an excess of secretion in the mouth, as happens sometimes, turn the patient on his side to make drainage easier. The nostrils should be freed of crust and moistened and soothed with applications of mineral oil. The eyes may be kept clean by wiping them with wipes or cotton balls moistened in normal saline. The tongue may become dry and should be moistened with a water-soluble lubricant, so that it does not stick to the roof of the mouth. Be sure the airway is kept open.

**Change of Position.** Turn the patient frequently, if possible, to make him more comfortable. He may not be able to tell you that he would like a change of position. Support him with pillows when he is on his side. *Do not* leave him on his back.

**Breathing Difficulties.** Cheyne-Stokes respirations are common in the dying patient. They are less distressing if the patient can be turned on his side or propped up in a partly sitting position. Always preserve good posture and provide enough support. Make certain that the tongue does not drop back and obstruct the air passageway. If it should, pull it forward with a gauze and turn the patient on his side with his head elevated to prevent a recurrence. The collection of mucus and secretions causes a sound called the "death rattle." Gentle suctioning or a change in position may relieve this as will a dose of atropine.

**Incontinence.** The patient may be incontinent, or the bladder may become distended. Keep the patient dry and clean. Notify the doctor if the patient does not void.

**Relief of Pain.** Medication is often given to relieve pain. Some authorities say that a dying patient, even though not actually in pain, should have some drugs for distress and exhaustion to make him comfortable and to make death easier. During the early stages of the death process, there may be some pain. Medications, such as the opiates should be given to relieve as much pain as possible. Large doses may be given because as the circulation fails the drug will have more difficulty in reaching the brain and because the doctor is no longer worried about the possibility of addiction. The opiate may also be given directly into the heart.

Just before death, pain usually disappears, as the result of failing sensation. The sudden disappearance of pain in a dying person is usually a sign of impending death. The patient who has been confused or unconscious up to now may suddenly be very lucid and alert. This may be due to the sudden drop in blood pressure which relieves the congestion in the brain.

**Failing Circulation.** As the circulation fails, the body becomes cold and frequently is covered with perspiration. In spite of this, the patient usually does not feel the cold, and heavy coverings make him restless. Provide light covering and keep it loose over the feet—use a bed cradle, if necessary. The room should be well ventilated and well lighted. The dying patient is likely to feel a sense of increasing darkness as his vision begins to fail and often turns toward a window or other source of light.

**Ventilation and Air.** The room should be kept well ventilated. Although air should be allowed to circulate, be sure that it is not blowing across the patient's face. Oxygen is usually not helpful at this stage, although it may make breathing slightly easier.

**Failing Senses.** It is important to remember that the patient usually can hear until death comes. Speak distinctly to him and do not whisper or talk about him, even though he cannot answer. Many patients enjoy soft music.

## Determining When Death Occurs

Death occurs when respiration and heartbeat have stopped for several minutes. (Assuming, of course, that the patient is not being maintained on a respirator or cardiac pacemaker.) The nurse must be sure to note the exact time when the respirations stop (usually before the heartbeat stops) and when the heart stops beating. The doctor, of course, will have been notified prior to this.

## Helping the Family After Death

The family must be supported and given assistance to work out their grief. Since the doctor may ask to perform an autopsy (postmortem examination), the family may have questions to ask about this. You should prepare the body so that they can see the patient if they wish. Be sure that all tubes are disconnected, all tape marks removed, and all blood or body discharges removed from the body. You will wish to place a clean sheet over the patient, not covering his face. He should be placed as comfortably as possible. The family should be allowed to be alone in the room, knowing that the nurse is available, if needed. Muted lighting is usually most comforting.

After the family leaves, the nurse is responsible for preparing the body for autopsy or for the transportation to the funeral director.

## CARE OF THE BODY AFTER DEATH

The doctor pronounces the patient dead and signs the death certificate. After the family has left the room, you straighten the body and place a pillow beneath the head. Remove jewelry if the patient is wearing any.

Sometimes the patient before death or the family requests that a wedding band remain on the finger. If so, it must be taped in place, and a notation made on the chart. All other personal belongings should be listed and signed for when given to relatives. Close the mouth by placing a rolled towel as a support under the chin. Close the eyes; you may need to tape them lightly with hypoallergenic tape. Remove all extra equipment, such as cradle or hot-water bags, from the bed; remove all top bed linen but the sheet that covers the patient.

Bathe any part of the body that has been soiled with discharges; it is usually not necessary to give a complete bath, but the body should be clean. Remove soiled dressings and replace them with clean ones. Pack the rectum and the vagina with absorbent gauze to absorb discharges. Comb and arrange the hair as the patient usually wore it. The wrists and the ankles are padded and tied loosely together to make handling the body easier. Most morticians prefer placing dentures in the mouth themselves.

Every hospital has its own procedure for the care of the body after death. Usually a shroud is provided to wrap the body before it is taken to the hospital morgue. Before the body is removed to the morgue, two tags are attached to the body—one tied to the foot or wrist, the other to the covering sheet; these tags are marked with the patient's name, ward or room number, and the diagnosis.

The patient's chart is completed with a notation of the exact time of death; the unit is cleaned as after the discharge of a patient. If the patient had an infectious disease, special precautions must be taken with the body and in cleaning the room.

# 31

# The Patient With Special Oxygen Needs

## BEHAVIORAL OBJECTIVES

*The student successfully attaining the goals of this chapter will be able to:*

- *list the chief circulatory and respiratory disorders which cause the patient to have a special need for oxygen.*
- *list several descriptive terms related to breathing and define each.*
- *discuss the concept of shock and list at least 5 signs of shock; state the first supportive nursing measure in the event of shock.*
- *discuss the physical and emotional aspects of the administration of oxygen to the patient; list the methods of administration; list at least 5 general precautions which must be observed; demonstrate ability to carry out these procedures in the clinical area, considering the physical and emotional support of the patient and his family.*
- *describe the opening of an oxygen cylinder and demonstrate skill in this procedure, if appropriate; describe the wall outlet for piped-in oxygen and demonstrate skill in using this apparatus; demonstrate ability to connect the oxygen tubing to the source, attach the humidifier and heater, and attach the device to be used to deliver the oxygen to the patient.*
- *demonstrate ability to administer oxygen by various means, such as the nasal catheter, the face mask, the IPPB apparatus, and the oxygen tent or croupette; identify advantages and disadvantages of each method; list the steps to take in installing the equipment in the patient's room and bringing the oxygen to the patient; and discuss the emotional support required for the patient receiving oxygen.*
- *discuss the administration of oxygen in an emergency situation; demonstrate skill in mouth-to-mouth or mouth-to-nose resuscitation; demonstrate skill in the use of the Ambu bag.*
- *briefly discuss the 2 general types of external respirators and identify how each is used; discuss the difference between the patient-cycled respirator and the controlled respirator.*
- *describe a tracheostomy, list the situations in which the procedure might be done, and describe the role of the nurse in assisting with the surgical procedure; discuss the care of the patient with a temporary tracheostomy and demonstrate skill in this care; discuss the nursing care involved in caring for the patient with a permanent tracheostomy and demonstrate skill in the care of this patient; demonstrate effective patient and family teaching.*
- *discuss the administration of oxygen to a child; to a person for the purpose of administering a drug; demonstrate skill in the clinical area in these procedures.*

You will recall from previous discussions that oxygen is one of the basic needs of all people and animals. Without oxygen, the brain begins to die within 2 or 3 minutes, with death occurring within 4 to 6 minutes.

The tissue cells must have a constant supply of oxygen to live, but since oxygen is not stored in the body, the body's supply of oxygen normally is obtained from the air (air is approximately 20 per cent oxygen). In some types of illness, the body is unable to take in enough oxygen or cannot use it effectively.

## REASONS FOR OXYGEN NEEDS

### Circulatory Disorders

As you know, the oxygen is carried to the body tissues by hemoglobin in the blood. If, for one reason or another, the blood cannot get to the tissues, the oxygen supply is cut off. There are 3 chief circulatory disorders which may account for a decrease in oxygen supply: lack of hemoglobin in the blood, failure of the heart to pump, and blockage or rupture of a blood vessel.

A lack of hemoglobin in the blood is called *anemia* and indicates that the body will not get enough oxygen because there is not enough hemoglobin to carry the oxygen.

Failure of the heart to pump may be caused by a lack of blood supply to the heart itself (myocardial infarction) or by the stoppage (cardiac arrest) or improper beating (fibrillation) of the heart, which is the pump for the blood.

If the blood cannot get through a blood vessel because of a clot or a stricture or because of gradual atherosclerosis, the blood supply is reduced or stopped completely. This happens in a cerebral vascular accident when a blood vessel which supplies the brain is blocked, in a thrombosis (clot) when a blood vessel is plugged or partially plugged or in a ruptured aneurysm when the aneurysm (outpouching of a blood vessel) breaks.

### Respiratory Disorders

There are many instances when the body does not get enough oxygen because of a disorder in the respiratory system: the airway may be blocked, in which case, respiration will cease; the lungs may be congested, in which case respiration will be difficult and may gradually become worse; an injury to the chest or lungs may cause difficulty in breathing; or chronic or acute infections in the lungs may interfere with breathing.

In these instances, the decrease in oxygen may be sudden or gradual. For example, if the person chokes on a piece of meat, the supply of air or oxygen is suddenly cut off and the person will die if his airway is not restored within a matter of minutes. On the other hand, in many infectious or chronic conditions of the lungs, breathing is impaired but not stopped completely. In these instances, most of which are not emergencies, the nurse can help to maintain life by assisting the patient to breathe or to obtain oxygen.

## SYMPTOMS

The nurse must learn to recognize the symptoms of respiratory or circulatory complications in order to assist the patient to meet the need for oxygen.

**Difficult Breathing.** One of the most obvious signs of a respiratory problem is difficulty in breathing, or *dyspnea,* which may be categorized into several classifications. Cardiac dyspnea is a result of heart disease; renal dyspnea is a result of kidney disease. Expirational dyspnea refers to the blockage of air removal from the lungs while inspirational dyspnea indicates that air is blocked from being drawn into the lungs. When there is difficulty in expanding the chest and drawing air into the lungs, the term expansional dyspnea is used. Paroxysmal dyspnea indicates that the breathing difficulty comes and goes. *Orthopnea* denotes that the patient is only able to breathe while sitting up. *Cheyne-Stokes respiration* is a type of breathing characterized by periods when breathing stops and then resumes.

**Apnea.** Absence of breathing (*apnea*) indicates a cessation of breathing. Other terms for such an emergency are *respiratory arrest* or *asphyxia.*

**Hyperventilation.** Hyperventilation denotes a period of rapid breathing, which may be a dangerous sign.

**Cardiac Signs.** The basic disorder involves

a failure of the heart to provide blood and, thus, oxygen to the tissues. The symptoms include arrhythmias, fibrillation, and cardiac standstill (*cardiac arrest*).

## Shock

Shock is the way in which the body reacts to lack of oxygen. It is associated with a general depression of all body functions and may be caused by lowered blood volume (as in hemorrhage), by lack of circulation (as in cardiac arrest), or by lack of respiration (as in blockage of the airway and respiratory arrest). It may also be caused by allergy, (anaphylactic shock), by a severe trauma (such as an electrical shock), or by other factors, such as an overdose of a drug or an extreme psychological shock.

### Recognizing Shock

Since shock is a complication which may follow any surgery, illness, or trauma, the nurse must be aware of its symptoms and should be on the alert for them at all times.

1. *Drop in Blood Pressure.* In every case of shock, the blood pressure, as measured by the sphygmomanometer, drops. If the systolic reading falls below 90, generally this is considered a sign of possible shock. A systolic reading below 80 is considered to be a symptom of actual shock. Of course, this varies with the individual, so that the nurse must know what each patient's usual reading is. The central venous pressure will either go up or down greatly, depending upon the cause of the shock.

2. *Increase in Pulse Rate.* In an attempt to offset the lowered blood volume or blood pressure, the heart beats faster, thereby causing an increased pulse rate. It often does not beat as hard as before, so that the pulse will be *thready* as well as rapid.

3. *Narrowing of Pulse Pressure.* The difference between systolic and diastolic blood pressure readings is known as the pulse pressure. When the heart begins to beat faster and less effectively, the difference between these two readings becomes smaller.

4. *Air Hunger.* The patient becomes dyspneic; he has difficulty in breathing and actually gasps for air.

5. *Skin Color.* Change in skin color is easier to recognize in the Caucasian or Oriental patient, since the nail beds and lips take on a bluish color (*cyanosis*). The Black patient will also show a darkening of the lips and nail beds.

6. *Other Signs.* The patient often is restless and anxious, complains of thirst, and has cold, moist, and pale skin. His temperature may drop, and he may complain of ringing in his ears or spots before his eyes.

### Treatment of Shock

While treatment of shock is discussed in Chapter 32, a brief summary will be presented here. The patient is positioned with his head lower than his feet (Trendelenburg position) and is kept from losing body heat. Hemorrhage is controlled, blood replacement is given, and oxygen and vasopressor drugs are administered.

## OXYGEN THERAPY

Oxygen is used to reinforce the oxygen supply in the blood in such conditions as (1) pneumonia, (2) carbon monoxide gas poisoning, (3) severe asthma, (4) heart failure, (5) respiratory failure in nervous system injuries, and (6) severe abdominal distention caused by bowel paralysis.

In these instances, oxygen makes the patient more comfortable; he breathes easier, his pulse rate drops, and he takes food more readily. The cooperation of the patient is highly important in oxygen therapy. He is likely to be apprehensive and worried about the treatment and especially fearful of apparatus. Therefore, the nurse must reassure the patient and provide emotional support so that he will cooperate. Since the patient needs to feel secure about the procedures being done, the nurse should be calm and confident.

### The Airway

The most important consideration in the administration of oxygen is the presence of a *patent* (open) *airway*. It does *no good* to administer oxygen or artificial respiration if the airway is blocked. The nurse can check the airway in an unconscious person by breathing

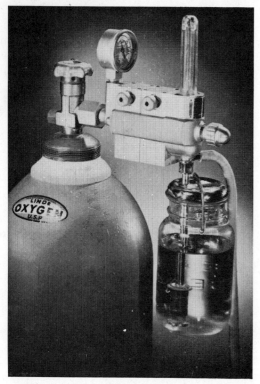

Figure 31-1. The regulation apparatus which is attached to the top of the oxygen supply tank gives an easily readable record of both the amount of oxygen in the tank and the rate at which it is being dispensed. By passing the oxygen through the humidifier, patient discomfort is alleviated. Many hospitals use the humidifier as a routine measure. (Linde Company, Division of Union Carbide Corporation)

into his nose or mouth and watching a rise and fall of the chest and listening to hear if air is being exchanged.

The airway is best opened by flexing the patient's head as far backward as possible. (The head is hyperextended with the mouth open.) The lower jaw is then pulled forward and down. This may be done, in an unconscious person, by grasping the jaw with your thumb in his mouth, holding his tongue down.

Sometimes, an endotracheal tube or a tracheotomy tube must be put in place to open the airway, or suctioning may be done or drugs administered to remove or loosen secretions which are blocking the airway. At times,

a patient who cannot cough may need assistance in opening his airway.

At this point, mouth-to-mouth resuscitation or Ambu bag resuscitation may be given to the person in respiratory arrest.

## Methods of Administration

Oxygen can be administered by face mask, nasal catheter, cannula, oxygen tent or respirator either with or without a tracheostomy. The method chosen depends on the patient's condition, the facilities available for giving oxygen, the concentration of oxygen needed, and the method preferred by the patient and the doctor. Any method requires an oxygen-supply and a reducing gauge. Oxygen is given in different concentrations, which are measured by the flow of liters per minute and which may vary from 20 to 100 per cent.

### EQUIPMENT

Oxygen cylinder or piping system

Regulator—reduces high pressure of oxygen coming from cylinder and controls oxygen flow

Gauges (2)—Oxygen contents gauge (attached to regulator) shows how much oxygen is in cylinder. Liter-flow gauge (attached to regulator) shows flow of liters per minute. (Wall oxygen has only the liter-flow gauge.)

## GENERAL RULES FOR ADMINISTERING OXYGEN

### Precautions

Everyone, including the patient, his visitors, and other patients in the same unit, should know the precautions that must be taken when oxygen is used. Oxygen *by itself* cannot burn; but if oxygen comes in contact with anything that is burning, even so small as a spark, the result is a fire of almost explosive violence. The following precautionary measures should be taken when oxygen is being administered:

1. Explain the dangers of lighting matches or smoking cigarettes or pipes. Be sure the patient has no matches or cigarettes in his bedside table.

2. Warning signs should be posted on the patient's door or bed: (OXYGEN—NO SMOKING).

3. Electrical devices, such as heating pads,

electric blankets, or the ordinary signal light must not be used. Some hospitals provide a special kind of signal light, which has a grounding device, or a tap-bell.

4. Oil must not be used on the oxygen regulator because oil can ignite by itself if it is exposed to oxygen. The nurse should be sure there are no traces of oil on her hands before she adjusts oxygen apparatus.

5. Woolen blankets should never be used; and nylon or rayon clothing are never permitted. Static electricity from these materials may cause a fire. For this reason many hospitals require nurses to wear cotton uniforms when working with oxygen in high concentrations.

## Oxygen Cylinders

Oxygen is stored in tanks or cylinders. In some hospitals, an oxygen therapy technician is responsible for oxygen apparatus; he sets it up, keeps it in working order, inspects it while it is in use, and cleans and stores it. Otherwise, the nurse is responsible. Since oxygen equipment is available for use in private homes, the nurse should be aware of how to use it.

### PROCEDURE FOR PREPARING CYLINDER FOR USE

Remove the protective cap from cylinder.

With the outlet pointing away from you, open the cylinder valve a *very little* and close it *quickly*. This blows away any dust that may be in the valve opening.

Insert the regulator inlet into the valve opening and tighten the nut with the wrench.

Loosen the flow-adjusting handle on the regulator. This must be done before opening the valve on top of the cylinder.

Open the cylinder valve very slowly until the neede on the nearest gauge stops moving.

Tighten the flow-adjusting handle (turn to right, clockwise) until prescribed flow of liters per minute is registered on the liter-flow gauge.

Loosen the flow-adjusting handle (turn left, counterclockwise) until needle on the liter-flow gauge returns to zero. Now you are ready to connect the oxygen equipment to the face mask, catheter, or oxygen tent.

The wrench *must* stay with the cylinder.

When the oxygen is to be discontinued for 30 minutes or more, or an empty cylinder must be replaced with a full one, follow this procedure:

Close the cylinder valve.

When needles on both gauges have returned to zero, loosen the flow-adjusting handle until it moves freely.

Disconnect the regulator from the cylinder by unscrewing inlet nut with the wrench.

## The Oxygen Wall Outlet

The nurse should practice this procedure, so that in an emergency she will be able to act without difficulty. The connecting apparatus must be put into the 2 holes right-side up or it will not fit; since the prongs match the holes in the wall outlet, the nurse can check to see how they should fit. A strong push will be required to insert the apparatus into the wall socket, and a pop will occur when the equipment is in place. After the regulator is inserted into the wall, no oxygen should escape around the apparatus. If oxygen is escaping, reinsert the socket. To remove this apparatus from the wall, push in all the way and then pull it out fast.

Be sure that this connection is made before attaching the tubing to the patient, and be sure that the liter-flow regulator is working correctly.

## Regulation

In oxygen therapy, it is important to maintain the prescribed liter flow and to understand how to operate the regulator and keep the patient as comfortable as possible. When oxygen therapy is discontinued, it should be done gradually, allowing the patient to be without it for short periods at a time (weaning). He should be watched closely. If he shows signs of difficulty with breathing and becomes pale or cyanotic, if his pulse rate goes up or he complains of pain in his chest or of fatigue, oxygen should be resumed at once.

Explaining the treatment and reassuring the patient about his breathing and the relief that oxygen will give him are essential in oxygen therapy.

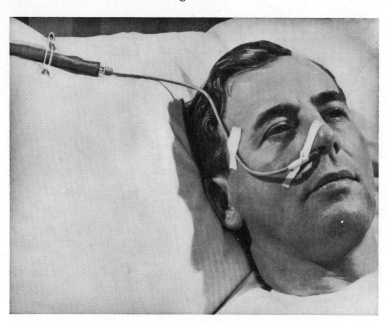

Figure 31-2. Oxygen administration via nasal catheter. Note the placement of the adhesive tape to maintain the position of the catheter. The large safety pin is placed through a small amount of the material of the pillowcase on either side of the rubber tubing. Care should be taken to prevent puncturing the tubing. (Linde Company, Division of Union Carbide Corporation)

## ADMINISTERING OXYGEN TO THE PATIENT WHO CAN BREATHE

### Nasal Catheter

The nasal catheter, which is green to help distinguish it from any other type of catheter, has the advantage of allowing the patient more freedom of movement. However, it may become irritating to the nose and cause the nostrils to become dry. It is not possible to determine the concentration of oxygen as easily when a catheter is used. Another disadvantage is the possibility that an irrational patient may easily dislodge or pull the catheter out.

The catheter should be changed at least every 8 to 12 hours and more often if necessary. If possible, it should be alternated from one nostril to the other. Another device, the nasal cannula, has 2 short tubes, one for each nostril, instead of the single catheter (see Fig. 47-2). The catheter should be disposed of or washed and sterilized before it is reinserted. If a nasal catheter is washed and reinserted, be sure that all the water is out of the tube, to prevent any chance of the patient aspirating water.

#### EQUIPMENT

Rubber catheter (size No. 8, Fr. to 10, Fr. for children, No. 12, Fr. to 14, Fr. for adults)
Rubber tubing (5 feet)
Connector to attach catheter to tubing
Lubricant (water soluble)
Humidifier and, maybe, a heater
Adapter
Source of oxygen
Distilled water for humidifier.

#### PROCEDURE

Attach catheter to one end of the rubber tubing with the adapter. Attach the other end of the tubing to the humidifier.

Attach the humidifier to the oxygen regulator.

Measure on the catheter the distance from the tip of the nose to the lobe of the ear and mark it with tape.

At the taped mark, hold the catheter between the thumb and the forefinger to determine natural "droop" of the catheter.

Adjust the flow of oxygen to about 3 liters per minute.

Lubricate the catheter lightly while oxygen is flowing; hold the tip in a glass of water to be sure that the holes are open.

Grasp the catheter at the taped mark between the thumb and the forefinger and slowly rotate it until the tip hangs at its lowest level.

With the oxygen flowing, elevate the tip of the nose and insert the catheter slowly in the nostril to the mark.

To make sure that the catheter is placed correctly, insert it slightly beyond the mark until the patient has swallowed a gulp of oxygen; then draw it back until he no longer swallows (about 1/4 inch).

Tape the catheter over the end of the nose and on the forehead. It may be taped to the cheek and brought over toward the ear and taped to the side of the face if the patient prefers. Use hypoallergenic tape as much as possible, to avoid irritation.

Increase the oxygen flow up to 4 to 6 liters per minute, or as the doctor orders.

Pin the tubing to the pillow or back of the mattress, leaving enough slack so that the patient can move his head without displacing the catheter.

Be sure that the patient is comfortable and his call bell is within reach before you leave him.

Check the humidifier at regular intervals and add water when necessary. Turn off the oxygen before adding water and fill the humidifier quickly so that the patient will be without oxygen for the least possible time.

## Face Mask

The advantages of using a face mask are several; it is not irritating, it provides the best concentration of oxygen, it does not interfere

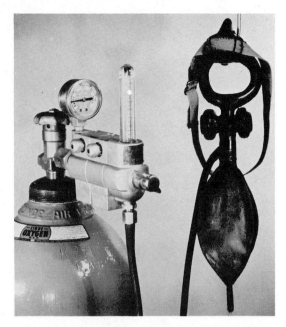

Figure 31-4. Open-type face mask for the administration of oxygen. Linde Company, Division of Union Carbide Corporation)

with nursing care, and it does not give the patient a feeling of being "shut in" as a tent may do. The main disadvantage is that oxygen must be discontinued when the patient eats or drinks if the mask covers both the mouth and the nose.

The mask should fit properly to prevent loss of oxygen; pressure on the face should be relieved by thin pads if necessary. The mask should be removed at regular intervals and washed and dried. The patient's face should also receive this attention.

### EQUIPMENT

Face mask—There are 2 kinds, one which covers the nose and one which covers both mouth and nose. The mask may be attached to a breathing bag and tubing; in this case, part of the exhaled air stays in the breathing bag and is rebreathed.

Disposable face mask—These do not have the rebreathing bag.

Humidifier, gauge, and oxygen source.

### PROCEDURE

Attach the end of the rubber tubing to the outlet of the regulator (below the liter-flow gauge).

Turn the regulator handle until the needle

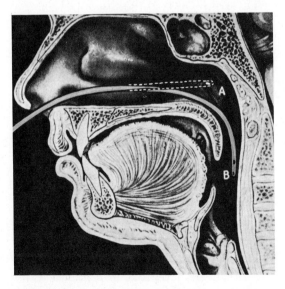

Figure 31-3. Position of catheter in: (A) nasopharynx, (B) oropharynx. (Barach, A. L.: Physiologic Therapy in Respiratory Diseases. Philadelphia, Lippincott)

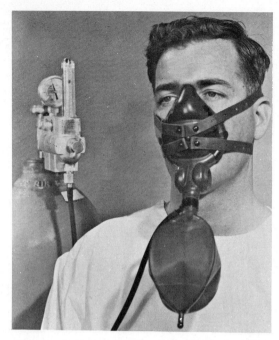

Figure 31-5. Closed type face mask, including the rebreathing bag, for the administration of oxygen. (Linde Company, Division of Union Carbide Corporation)

on the liter-flow gauge registers a flow of 10 to 12 liters per minute.

Apply the mask to the patient's face, asking him to exhale as it is applied.

When first deep and rapid breathing subsides, adjust the oxygen flow so that the breathing bag almost, but not quite, collapses when the patient inhales. This allows a flow of from 6 to 8 liters per minute.

With the disposable mask, the liter flow is simply adjusted to the doctor's order and applied.

## Oxygen Tent

The oxygen tent is made from a transparent plastic material and provides a cool, humidified atmosphere. Some types cover the entire bed. However, the one most frequently used covers only the upper third of the bed. The patient's movements are restricted to the extent that he must not be allowed to displace the tucked-in edges of the tent. These edges must be tucked in closely to preserve oxygen

concentration. The tent is the most expensive method of giving oxygen. It is also the most dangerous, since it provides the greatest concentration of oxygen. The tent is explosive when filled with oxygen, so the nurse must be alert to prevent fire, which would most likely kill the patient should it occur. Perhaps for these reasons, the oxygen tent is the least frequently used means of administering oxygen today.

### EQUIPMENT

Motor-driven or motorless tent
Canopy to cover the patient (rubberized fabric or plastic film)
Cabinet connected to a supply of oxygen
Rubber or plastic cover for the mattress and pillow

### PROCEDURE

Check the tent outside of the patient's room to make sure that the unit is complete; fill the cabinet with chunks of ice. The newer models have a self-contained refrigeration unit. No ice is necessary.

Bring the tent to the bedside and explain what you do as you go along (you have already talked to the patient about the treatment). Put a bath blanket around the patient's shoulders.

Turn on the flow of oxygen; adjust the canopy over the patient, keeping it from touching his face. Tuck the canopy in as far as possible under the mattress at the head and the sides of the bed. Make a wide double cuff with a bath blanket and tuck the remaining edge of the canopy into it, then tuck the ends of the bath blanket under the mattress.

Raise the oxygen flow to 15 liters per minute and keep it there for about 15 minutes. Then analyze the atmosphere within the tent to be sure that the patient is getting the right concentration of oxygen. Usually 50 per cent is prescribed.

Put a drain bucket in place and open the water drain, if necessary.

Check the thermometer in the tent to be sure that the temperature is not too cold for the patient. If he is cold, give him an extra blanket and turn the temperature control to medium or warm.

After analyzing the oxygen content in the

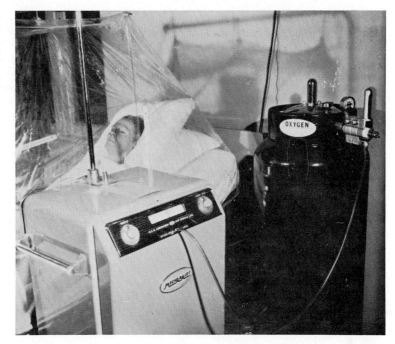

Figure 31-6. Use of the oxygen tent with the automatic humidification and refrigeration apparatus in the care of the bedfast patient. The clear plastic canopy enables the nurse to make frequent visual checks of the patient and also helps to prevent the "closed-in" feeling of which the patient sometimes complains. (Linde Company, Division of Union Carbide Corporation)

tent, if the concentration of oxygen is as prescribed, reduce the liter flow to between 6 to 10 liters per minute.

Be sure the patient has his call bell before you leave him.

The air within the tent should be analyzed regularly (every 3 or 4 hours) and after the canopy has been opened for treatments or examinations. When the tent is no longer needed, it should be washed with soap and water and aired before being stored. Handle the canopy carefully—do not fold it. Tears in plastic material can be mended with cellophane tape.

Don't forget that the patient in the oxygen tent needs to be turned frequently and encouraged to cough. He may be afraid to do this because of the apparatus.

### Patient-Tripped Respirator

If the patient is breathing on his own, but needs some assistance, the doctor may put him on a respirator which is *patient-cycled*. This means that the patient breathes on his own, but the respirator assists him by giving an extra boost. Thus the patient obtains more oxygen than he would on his own. If a speci-

fied amount of time elapses and the patient has not taken a breath, the machine will initiate a breath for the patient. The most commonly used respirators are the Bird and the Bennett.

These machines may be used to assist the patient, to maintain the patient who is in respiratory arrest, or to administer selected medications in aerosol form. Generally, when these respirators are used to assist the patient to breathe, a tracheostomy tube is in place. If not, they are used with an endotracheal tube, which passes through the patient's mouth.

As the patient begins to breathe more normally on his own, the assistance of the respirator is removed, since the patient may begin to fight the respirator, and cause it to do more harm than good.

### ADMINISTERING OXYGEN IN EMERGENCY SITUATIONS

In instances of acute respiratory failure, "sudden death" may occur, which means that the patient has stopped breathing and his heart has stopped beating. In such an emergency, resuscitation must be initiated or brain death will occur in about 6 minutes. The first thing the nurse should do when she notices that a patient is not breathing is to initiate respiration and maintain heartbeat (see Chapter 47 for discussion of external cardiac massage).

## Mouth-to-Mouth and Mouth-to-Nose Resuscitation

One way of establishing the exchange of air into and out of the patient's lungs is by using mouth-to-mouth resuscitation. This is the method to use until help arrives and an Ambu bag is made available. (See page 582 for discussion on when to use the Ambu bag.)

### PROCEDURE

1. Make sure that the airway is open. Clear the mouth of mucus and foreign objects. Tilt the patient's head as far back as it will go.

2. With one hand pull the lower jaw upward and hold the jaw forward so that it "juts out." This pulls the tongue forward and opens the air passage and permits inflation of the lungs.

3. Pinch the nose closed with the thumb and forefinger of the other hand.

4. Take a deep breath, exhale this air into the victim's mouth. Remove your mouth from the mouth of the victim and allow this air to be expired. Repeat about 18 to 20 times per minute. You must be sure that the airway is open. If the victim shows any resistance to the passage of air, clear the mouth with your finger or by turning the head so that fluid or other material may drain clear. The victim's chest should rise and fall with each breath. Make sure the patient has a pulse during this procedure.

5. A mouth-to-nose method may also be used. The victim's mouth is held closed and his chin up while you place your mouth over his nose and blow in. This inflates the lungs if there is no obstruction. When your mouth is withdrawn, the victim should expel air through the nose.

Remember that when the patient is small, as with a child, there is an added danger of overinflating the lungs. Use just enough breath until you feel the resistance of the victim's lungs.

## The Ambu Bag

This is a much more sanitary method of resuscitation than the mouth-to-mouth method. The face mask of the Ambu bag is placed over the mouth and nose of the patient. Room air may be used or the bag may be hooked up to oxygen for more oxygenation. The important thing is to start treatment immediately and to make sure the airway is open.

## Surgical Bag Breathing With Intubation

An endotracheal tube, either cuffed or non-cuffed, is placed into the patient's throat and trachea to establish an emergency source of oxygen until a tracheostomy can be performed. During surgery, this is done routinely once the patient is anesthetized, after which the patient is maintained by use of a face mask or oxygen supply connected directly to the endotracheal tube and controlled by the anesthetist. The bag is squeezed, forcing air and oxygen or other gasses into the lungs. This is sometimes done at the nursing station by the Anesthesia or Inhalation Therapy Departments while a tracheostomy is being performed. It is important for the nurse to know that the patient often has a sore, irritated throat following removal of the endotracheal tube (*extubation*).

## External Respirators

If the patient is in a state of *respiratory arrest,* which means he cannot breathe by himself, he will need to be maintained by means of an external respirator. There are 2 basic types of respirators; the *negative-pressure* respirator which encloses all or part of the body and operates by forming a vacuum which causes the chest to expand, and the *positive-pressure* respirator, which operates by forcing oxygen into the lungs from outside. Respirators can also be pressure-cycled (also designated pressure-limited) whereby a preselected pressure is reached, the inspiration cycle is shut off and expiration is passive, or they may be volume-limited (also designated volume-cycled) whereby a preset volume is delivered, regardless of resistance, although there is a

Figure 31-7. Gauze squares, slit half-way down, are placed around the tube to catch secretions. These dressings are changed by the nurse as often as it is necessary. Note the tapes that hold the outer tube in place. The tapes are tied in a knot at the back of the patient's neck. (Smith, D. W., Germain, C. P., and Gips, C. D.: Care of the Adult Patient. ed. 3. Philadelphia, Lippincott, 1971)

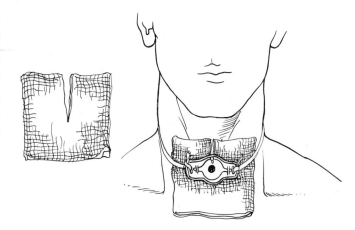

safety valve. The doctor chooses the type of respirator, the settings, and the cycle which best fit the individual patient.

The nurse must be aware that this machine is maintaining the patient's life. If it is disconnected or malfunctioning, the patient will die quickly. Thus the electric plug must be taped in place, so that it cannot be pulled out accidently. Usually, a special type of plug which cannot be pulled out is used. When a patient is being kept alive by means of a respirator, emergency resuscitation equipment (such as an Ambu bag) must be kept at his bedside at all times.

## THE PATIENT WHO HAS A TRACHEOSTOMY

A tracheostomy tube may be inserted into the trachea for several reasons. It may be an emergency life-saving device in a situation of sudden blockage of the mouth or throat; or it may be a permanent breathing orifice for the person who has had mouth or throat surgery, such as a laryngectomy.

### Assisting With a Tracheostomy

The nurse in the Intensive Care Unit or Emergency Room may be asked to assist the doctor while he does a tracheostomy (or *"trach"*). The nurse is responsible for assembling the equipment, which usually comes set up on a "trach" tray. She must know what is on the tray and what else will be needed for the proce-

dure. Usually, in addition to the tray, she will need a local anesthetic, such as novocaine, gloves for the doctor, a strong light, and an emergency breathing apparatus, such as the Ambu bag. A source of suction must also be available, and a source of oxygen is desirable. If there is time, the doctor will want to "gown and glove" sterilly.

The nurse may be asked to hold the patient's head during the procedure. A folded towel should be placed behind the neck to hyperextend the neck, exposing the trachea to the best advantage. It is important that the patient lie very still during the procedure. Thus the nurse will need to provide emotional support to the patient during this frightening procedure.

The nurse also assists by recording pertinent information about what was done and by whom. She may also be asked to provide oxygen through an endotracheal tube while the tracheostomy is being done. This procedure is most often done with an Ambu bag.

If a respirator is to be used with the "trach" tube, the cuffed variety of "trach" tube will be used. This tube has a small bag around it, which is inflated to prevent leakage of air from the tube while the respirator is in operation. It is important for the nurse to find out whether the "trach" tube is cuffed or not, because usually this cuff will need to be released at intervals to prevent damage to the trachea and throat. The nurse must also be aware of the possibility of swelling and may need to release the cuff to allow the patient to breathe through the "trach" tube.

### Care of the Tube

The tracheostomy tube has 3 parts: an outer tube, an inner tube, and an obdurator. The obdurator is inserted in the outer tube, with its lower end protruding from the tube, which is then inserted into the tracheal opening. When the outer tube is in place, the obdurator is withdrawn and replaced by the inner tube, which is locked in position. Tapes are attached to each side of the outer tube and tied behind the neck to hold it firmly in position. A gauze sponge that has been split halfway is placed under the tube to catch the leakage from secretions (Fig. 31-7).

The inner tube is removed and cleaned at intervals under cold running water. Sometimes, a stronger solution, such as peroxide, is used. If this is not sufficient to remove the secretions, a pipe cleaner or a small test tube brush might be helpful. At first, the doctor removes the entire tube when it needs to be changed; later, the patient may be allowed to do this himself. By the time the patient with a permanent "trach" is ready to go home, suctioning usually is no longer necessary, but if it is he must have a suction machine at home. At this point he is bathing and dressing himself and is taking care of the tracheostomy tube.

### Nursing the Patient With a Tracheostomy

The following steps are part of the nurse's responsibility in caring for a tracheostomy patient:

1. The outer tube is held in place by a woven cotton tape which encircles the neck and ties at the back. This tape should never be untied, cut, or changed by the practical nurse because of the danger of the patient coughing out the cannula.

2. An extra tracheostomy set should be kept in the patient's room at all times.

3. All equipment for cleaning and caring for the "trach" should be kept at the bedside.

4. In normal breathing, the air is warmed and cleansed by the action of the nose and throat. In the person with a "trach", this must be done artificially by means of a humidifier, a room air purifier, or an air condi-

tioner which warms and cleans the air. Sometimes, a small humidifier is placed directly over the "trach" tube.

5. Secretions must be removed as soon as they appear, so that they will not be aspirated back into the "trach" tube. Frequent suctioning is *vital*.

6. Gauze dressings around the tube must be bound with tape so that the loose strings will not be aspirated. Cotton filled gauze should not be used.

7. The inner cannula and the outer cannula are usually made of very soft metal and can be bent or damaged by careless handling. Some of the newer tubes are of a plastic or teflon material.

8. Until he becomes accustomed to breathing through the tube the patient may be very apprehensive and easily upset by coughing. He will need continued reassurance and competent, well-informed nurses in attendance.

9. Never suction beyond the length of the laryngeal tube and do not suction while inserting the suction tube. Use intermittent suctioning (maximum 10 seconds), withdraw the tube, and rotate it on the way out. Stop suctioning if the patient coughs very hard, but suction as much as you can to remove the mucus.

## ADMINISTERING OXYGEN IN SPECIAL SITUATIONS

### For a Child

There are 3 chief ways in which the child will receive oxygen: in the newborn *isolette,* in the *incubator,* and in the *croupette.* The newborn *isolette,* into which almost every newborn is placed, provides some oxygen and warmth for the new baby. The premature baby who needs a larger amount of oxygen is placed into an *incubator.* (The care of the baby in the incubator is discussed more fully in Chapter 38.) The child who has a respiratory condition is often placed in a *croupette,* which provides oxygen and humidity to liquify secretions and to assist in breathing. (This will be discussed more fully in Chapter 39.)

It is difficult to administer oxygen to the small child by nasal catheter or by face mask, because it is difficult for him to understand or to cooperate. Therefore, the equipment used generally covers the child's entire body.

## For Drug Therapy

IPPB treatments (intermittent positive pressure breathing apparatus) are often ordered for patients who have undergone surgery or who have a chronic condition of the lungs. This method of therapy utilizes a respirator, such as the Bennett or Bird and is administered by the nurse or by the inhalation therapist.

The drug ordered, sometimes saline or a solution to loosen secretions, such as Isuprel, Alevaire, or a bronchodilator, is given to the patient in a mist or aerosol form. The medication ordered, usually mixed with water or saline, is put into the nebulizer, and the rate of oxygen flow is set. The patient is then instructed to plug his nose and to breathe through his mouth, inhaling the medication and oxygen as deeply as possible. In addition to this treatment the patient should be encouraged to move about, to breath deeply, and to cough. He should also be encouraged to cough out as much mucus as possible. If necessary, this treatment may be combined with postural drainage to remove more secretions.

By this method, the patient receives medication and oxygen together. In addition, he is forced to breathe more deeply by the action of the machine and is forced to cough out secretions by the action of the medication.

# 32

# Nursing Care for Patients Having Surgery

---

## BEHAVIORAL OBJECTIVES

*The student successfully attaining the goals of this chapter will be able to:*

- *prepare patients of all age groups and with various illnesses for surgical intervention, in such a way that the patient's physical and emotional needs are met.*

- *explain the reasons for and skillfully carry out specific procedures related to surgery, such as skin preparation, intestinal preparation, and administration of preoperative medications.*

- *assist the patient's family so that they will be as informed and comfortable as possible during the patient's hospitalization; teach the patient so that he is as comfortable as possible about his operation.*

- *identify the 2 chief classifications of anesthetics and describe the major effects of each.*

- *describe the 4 stages of general anesthesia.*

- *list the equipment necessary for immediate postoperative care, whether in the recovery room or the patient's unit; demonstrate skill in using this equipment in various situations; demonstrate ability to care for an immediate postoperative patient, and to make a surgical bed.*

- *list 11 procedures to be performed as soon as the patient arrives from the recovery room.*

- *identify and describe the symptoms of the 3 most common immediate postoperative complications and the nursing management of each.*

- *list 7 common postoperative discomforts and the supportive nursing measures which may be employed for each; demonstrate skill in these nursing measures in the clinical area.*

- *discuss later postoperative complications and their treatment, as well as preventive measures.*

- *effectively assist the patient to meet his basic needs after surgery, as well as to meet special needs which are a result of the surgery.*

- *discuss the theory of parenteral replacement therapy and recognize the signs of difficulty in a patient receiving an I.V.*

---

One of the common treatments of disease or body disorders is that of surgery or surgical intervention. It is called intervention, because the surgeon actually intervenes in the disease process by operating on the patient's body in order to repair, remove, or replace body tissues or organs.

## PREOPERATIVE NURSING CARE

In the beginning of her experience with patients, it is impossible for the student to have detailed information about each disease and the specific nursing care entailed. However, it is reassuring if she has a good basic knowledge of how certain types of patients may look and behave, what their common problems may be, and how she can best take care of them. More information about the surgical patient and the nursing care needed in specific illnesses will be given in the chapters which are devoted to such illnesses.

### Preparing a Patient for a Surgical Operation

In the hospital, you will be asked to assist the professional nurse in the care of preoperative patients. It is very important to carry out preoperative orders exactly—they affect the success of the operation. These orders concern the physical preparation of the patient, but, as you carry them out, remember the patient's feelings and his need for reassurance.

No patient looks forward to an operation. In fact, he is more likely to dread or fear the ordeal. Therefore, it is up to the nurse to explain what is about to happen and to provide an opportunity for the patient's questions, to let him express his doubts and fears without losing face. Agreeing with him that it is natural to feel apprehensive is vastly more reassuring than saying there is nothing to worry about, no matter how true that may be. Remember that even the simplest operation can present some danger to an individual patient.

**The Patient's Feelings.** If you ever have had an operation, you should be able to put yourself in the patient's place and sense his feelings. To begin with, his previous experiences will affect him now: if he has had an operation before, he is thinking of all the things that happened then—perhaps he had nausea, pain, a draining wound, a long illness. If this is his first experience, he may have all sorts of vague fears. People are likely to imagine large sharp knives and torturing instruments as being a part of an operation. Some people dread losing consciousness or being "sick from the anesthetic." Most people fear pain after the operation. Others are afraid that they will die. Some are fearful of having cancer or of being disabled. The mother worries about her children's care while she is in the hospital; the father, about his family's support.

Explain the preparations for the operation to the patient as you go along—how each step helps him and the doctor. Observe and report to the team leader anything unusual that happens.

### Skin Preparation

One of the most important procedures in the preparation of the patient for a surgical procedure is the cleansing of the skin. Because the skin is normally oily and contains a large quantity of bacteria, care must be taken to cleanse it properly and to remove as much of this material as possible to prevent contamination of the wound.

Preparation will begin on the evening before the scheduled day of operation, except in the case of emergency. Cleansing agents, either soap and water solution or one of the many proprietary skin detergents such as pHisoHex, will be used. As you have been shown previously, mild friction in washing is one of the most efficient ways to remove foreign material. Once the skin is cleansed the area is carefully shaved, because microorganisms stick to hair. The hair growth on many parts of the body is very fine and can be seen only in a brightly illuminated room. Therefore, make sure that your lighting facilities are adequate.

Be careful not to cut the skin with the razor and thereby open up a potential source of infection.

Prepare an area in excess of the actual operation field. This allows for the proper draping of the patient without contamination caused by touching an unprepared area.

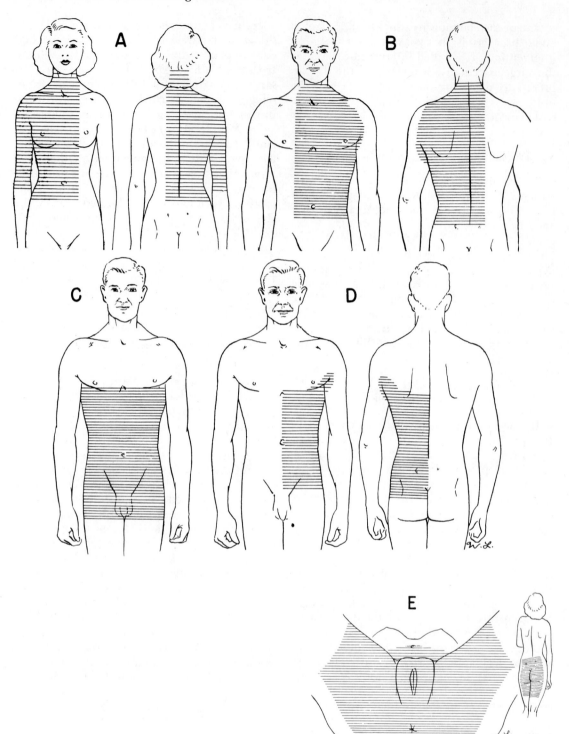

Figure 32-1. (*Caption on facing page.*)

Unless you have been expressly directed as to the area to be prepared, follow the diagram in Figure 32-1.

## Intestinal Preparation

The preparation of the patient will be in keeping with the orders of the doctor, the kind of operation to be performed, the type of anesthetic to be used, and the patient's condition. Since the intestinal tract should be as empty of feces as possible, the patient is usually given an enema to empty the colon; this makes the operation easier for the surgeon and prevents distress. Be sure that the patient has expelled all of the enema, because when he is relaxed under an anesthetic, he may expel the remainder on the operating table.

Usually no food is given on the morning of the operation and probably a very small amount the night before. Again, this depends on the type of operation and the time of day that the patient goes to the operating room. A patient is less likely to be nauseated or to vomit if his stomach is empty; a general anesthetic tends to aggravate nausea, and vomiting interferes with the anesthetic. An empty stomach also helps to prevent aspiration.

## Preoperative Medication

Before giving the preoperative medication, you should explain to the patient the purpose of the drug and what effects it might have— it might make him drowsy; it might make his mouth dry, or it might affect him in some other ways. Explain to the patient that this drug is preparation for the anesthetic and not the anesthetic itself. He needs to understand that he will still be awake when he goes to the operating room. You should also explain that for the patient's own safety, the side rails will be put up on his bed and that he should ask for assistance if he needs to get up to go to the bathroom.

The nurse should also explain to the patient's family that the patient has been partially sedated. They may stay with him but should not expect him to carry on a conversation. He will be less anxious if his family can stay until he goes to the operating room.

## Organization of Preoperative Care

**The preceding afternoon:**

1. Check the chart and note the doctor's preoperative orders (enema, catheterization, medication.)
2. See that the operation permit is signed. This must be witnessed. Student nurses should not witness legal papers of any type.
3. Prepare the operative area (if ordered).
4. See that all specimens and blood samples have been collected and sent to the laboratory.
5. Note and attend to change in diet (as ordered).
6. In the evening, give the sedative if ordered.
7. Withhold fluids and foods as directed.

**The morning of the operation:**

1. Record T.P.R. and B.P. Report immediately any marked deviation from normal to the nurse in charge, so that she can report it to the doctor.
2. Help the patient with bath and cleanliness measures. Be sure the patient has a

---

Figure 32-1. (*Facing page.*) Common areas to be prepared for operation. The shaded areas are those to be shaved. (A) Preparation for amputation of breast. Note that the area to be prepared includes the front and the back of the trunk and extends from the neck to the umbilicus. The axilla and the upper portion of the arm also are included. (B) Area of preparation for operation on the thorax. (C) Area of preparation for operation upon the abdomen (laparotomy) and for hernia. The preparation should extend from the nipple line to well below the crest of the ilium. For herniorrhaphy the upper limit of preparation may be the area of the umbilicus. (D) Area to be prepared for nephrectomy. Note that the preparation should be on both the anterior and the posterior sides of the trunk. (E) Area to be prepared for operations on the perineum. These areas should be shaved completely for all gynecologic operations, operations around the anus and for such combined operations as an abdominoperineal resection of the rectum. Other areas may be prepared for other procedures. The preparation is often done by the operating room staff.

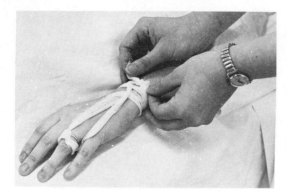

Figure 32-2. To prevent loss during surgery, the nurse has secured this patient's wedding band to her hand by slipping the gauze under the band and looping it around the finger and ring as shown. It is important not to tie it so tightly as to impair circulation.

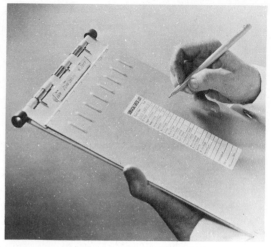

Figure 32-3. The nurse checks off the items on the preoperative check list immediately before the patient goes to the operating room. The items included on the list are: ID band; permit; "prep" and shave; blood work done; urinalysis; TPR (temperature, pulse, respiration) and BP (blood pressure); dentures removed, contact lenses or glasses removed; jewelry removed or secured; the patient voided or catheterized; hair pins, makeup, and nail polish removed; NPO after midnight. In this way, everyone is sure that all things are done. The nurse who checks the patient out and sends him to surgery, signs the check list. (Professional Tape Company, Inc., Hinsdale, Illinois)

bath and clean gown before going to surgery.

3. Remove prostheses if present. Also remove wigs, contact lenses, false eyelashes, and glasses.

4. Remove jewelry and valuables and put them in a safe or give them to the family. Be sure that the wedding band is included with these, unless the patient does not wish to remove it and it is securely bound to the hand. (See Fig. 32-2).

5. Help the patient put on elastic stockings if ordered.

6. Have the patient void immediately before going to the O.R. (if the patient is unable to void, tell the charge nurse and report this fact on the chart).

7. Remove any hair pins which the patient may have.

8. Remove dentures, complete or partial, and put them into a denture cup with clear water. Label carefully and put into a safe place such as the drawer of the bedside table.

9. Remove any make-up or nail polish. The anesthetist watches the nail beds and lips for signs of cyanosis (lack of oxygen).

10. Be sure that all the items on the preparation check-list have been carried out and signed and attached to the chart (see Fig. 32-3). The chart will be taken to the operating room with the patient.

## Transporting the Patient

The patient is transported to the operating room on a stretcher. It is important that the nurse prepare the room so that the operating room staff can conveniently move the patient. Furniture should be moved so that the operating room cart can be put next to the bed, and all items should be taken off the bedside stand so they will not be knocked off. During the moving procedure the patient should be made as comfortable as possible. Since his chart will accompany him, make sure the check list is complete and signed. You should also send a clean bath blanket with him.

The chart is given to the anesthetist or operating room nurse by the person who takes the patient to the operating room. It is never left with the patient or in his room. Another reminder—Be sure to note on the front of the chart if the patient has any drug allergies or is taking cortisone, insulin, an anticonvulsant, or anticoagulants.

Always be certain that the patient is properly identified before taking him to the operating room. Identification bracelets help to prevent errors.

Explain to the patient and to his family that he will be going to the recovery room for a period of time immediately following the surgery. There he will be observed by specially trained personnel and will be returned to his room upon recovery from the anesthetic.

## Considering the Patient's Family

The thoughful nurse will explain to the patient's family that the patient will be taken to surgery ½ to 1 hour before he actually goes into the operating room and will be going to the recovery room for several hours after the surgery, so they should not become alarmed at the length of time he is gone.

The nurse will also explain to the patient's family where they may wait for the patient. Many hospitals have a special room for this purpose. Often the family is notified when the patient leaves the operating room and goes into the recovery room. Since the doctor often talks to the family after the surgery, the nurse should tell them where to wait for him.

## ANESTHESIA

It is most helpful if the patient can meet the anesthetist before the surgery and have a short visit with him. Some anesthetists make it a point to visit a patient the day before the operation. This gives the patient an opportunity to ask questions and to receive explanations which will do away with many of his anxieties. It is also pleasant for the patient to recognize someone when he comes to the operating room.

**Anesthesia Personnel.** A physician trained in anesthesiology is called an anesthesiologist and a registered nurse trained in anesthesiology is called an anesthetist. Many hospitals have both persons on their staff.

## Anesthetics

Anesthetics have been divided into 2 main classes: (1) general anesthetics which suspend the sensations of the whole body and (2) local, regional, or spinal anesthetics which bring about the insensitivity of parts of the body without general unconsciousness. General anesthetics can be administered intravenously or rectally or by inhalation. The most common anesthetics given by inhalation are halothane, nitrous oxide, and cyclopropane. The patient is most often prepared for inhalation anesthesia by the intravenous injection of sodium pentothal. This injection puts the patient to sleep, after which he is intubated and maintained on an inhalation anesthetic. Pentothal is sometimes given alone for minor procedures or may be used in combination with inhalation anesthesia for longer or more complex procedures.

## Stages of Inhalation Anesthesia

General anesthesia is described as having 4 stages:

1. *Stage of Beginning Anesthesia.* First, the patient feels drowsy and warm, with a heavy "drugged" sensation. He is still conscious but cannot lift his arms or his legs. He can still hear, even to an exaggerated point, but he cannot speak. At this time most patients remember a feeling of anxiety lest the operation begin before they have completely lost consciousness.

2. *Stage of Excitement.* Many times the patient will begin to struggle (possibly because he wants to show that he is not yet unconscious). There should be no preparatory work on the operative site at this time, since it only aggravates the patient's excitement. The pupils become dilated but will still contract with light. The pulse rate becomes rapid, the respirations irregular.

3. *Stage of Surgical Anesthesia.* The patient becomes totally unconscious. The pupils are small but will respond to light. Respiration is regular, and the pulse is normal and of good volume. The skin is warm and pink. This stage may be continued for hours if the proper administration of anesthesia is main-

tained and the patient's condition remains good.

4. *Stage of Danger.* The patient may react to the anesthetic in an adverse way and thus become too deeply anesthetized, so that all body functions are slowed too much. At this time, the surgery is discontinued until his vital signs become normal again. Fortunately, this is a rare occurrence.

## THE PRACTICAL NURSE IN THE OPERATING ROOM

Often, the practical nursing student will observe in the operating room as a part of her student experience. This will not only give her a better idea of operating procedures, but will also help her to understand the patient's feelings and apprehensions. Sometimes, graduate practical nurses are specially trained to work in the operating room or postanesthesia recovery room.

## POSTOPERATIVE NURSING CARE

### The Recovery Room

Nearly all hospitals now have a room, or a suite of rooms, set aside for the care of patients immediately after surgery. This *recovery room,* as it is called, ideally should be on the same floor as the operating rooms so that doctors and nurses are quickly available if a postoperative patient needs emergency attention. Concentrating postoperative patients in a limited area makes it possible for one nurse to give close attention to 2 or 3 patients at the same time. She would not be able to do this if they were scattered throughout a ward or were in separate private or semiprivate rooms.

**Equipment.** Another advantage of the recovery room is that it has every type of equipment at hand ready for use. This includes:

1. Breathing aids: oxygen, tracheostomy sets, laryngoscopes, suction equipment, emergency airways, and an Ambu bag or other resuscitation equipment.

2. Circulatory aids: blood pressure apparatus (sphygmomanometer), stethoscope, intravenous and cut-down trays, universal donor blood, plasma, intravenous solutions, cardiac arrest equipment, tourniquets, syringes, and needles, cardiac drugs and respiratory stimulants as well as heat monitors.

3. Narcotics, sedatives, emergency drugs, and surgical dressings.

Each patient unit has a recovery bed, equipped with side rails for the patient's protection, intravenous poles, wheel brakes, and a chart rack. The bed can be moved easily and can be adjusted to elevate the head or the foot. The unit has a bedside stand which holds tissue, emesis basin, tongue depressors, face cloth, and towel. Each unit has its own outlet for piped-in oxygen and for suction.

**The Trip to the Recovery Room.** When moving patients every effort is made to avoid unnecessary strain or possible injury and to accomplish the transfer as quickly as possible with the least amount of exposure.

The anesthesiologist goes to the recovery room with the patient to make certain that the patient's condition is satisfactory before leaving his care. The doctor reports the patient's condition to the nurse in charge and leaves postoperative orders and any special directions about what to watch for.

No patient should be left alone until he has fully regained consciousness. Check the doctor's orders and carry them out immediately—such as giving oxygen, connecting drainage tubes, giving special medications, and using suction.

Occasionally, the nurse will find herself caring for the immediate postoperative patient in the patient unit. Before the patient arrives she should be prepared with the same equipment as would be found in the recovery room.

### Receiving the Patient from the Recovery Room

The recovery room staff should call the nursing station and give a report on the patient's condition and indicate what special equipment will be needed for the patient when he returns to the station. The nurse will then have time to prepare any special equipment which will be needed before the patient arrives.

The preparation of a room for any surgical patient includes making the surgical bed and arranging the furniture so the patient can be easily transferred from the recovery room cart to the bed. The nurse should also have on hand tissues, an emesis basin, the blood pressure cuff and stethoscope, a rectal thermometer, a vital signs chart, and suction and oxygen equipment if required.

When the patient arrives from the recovery room, the nurse should immediately take the blood pressure to make sure it compares favorably with the readings obtained by the recovery room staff. She should receive a report from the person who brings the patient. She may also assist in the transfer of the new surgical patient from the cart to his bed.

When the patient is settled in his bed and his vital signs have been taken, and all immediate orders are carried out, the nurse should see that the patient's family is notified that the patient is back in his room. Although the family should not visit for long periods of time, they can help reassure the patient if they can stop in to see him.

### Procedures to be Performed Immediately

1. Carry out any orders which call for the immediate administration of drugs or oxygen.
2. Attach drainage apparatus as ordered for bottle drainage from cholecystostomy, catheters, chest tubes.
3. Attach gastric or other tubes to the appropriate suction device.
4. Take vital signs as ordered. Blood pressure is usually taken often for the first hour and gradually less often if it is stable.
5. Inspect dressings and note signs of hemorrhage and any unusual amount of drainage. If necessary, reinforce but *do not change* dressings. Notify the team leader of unusual drainage.
6. Assist the patient if he vomits. Turn his head to the side to empty his mouth and to prevent aspiration. Use the emesis basin to catch the emesis and assist the patient to rinse his mouth. If excessive retching takes place, check to make sure the dressings and incision are intact and that suction equipment is operating properly.
7. If the patient is receiving intravenous fluids or blood, check the rate of flow and the time due for the next bottle. Check

to make sure the needle is in the vein.
8. Make sure to record accurate intake and output.
9. Turn the patient and encourage him to cough and breathe deeply as ordered.
10. Assist the patient to move or to ambulate as soon as ordered.
11. Observe, note, and report at once any unusual or alarming symptoms. Be certain that the time is also recorded. A nurse is responsible for keeping intelligent and accurate records.

## IMMEDIATE POSTOPERATIVE COMPLICATIONS

The nurse should be on the lookout for 3 serious immediate complications: hemorrhage, shock, and lowered oxygen supply (hypoxia).

### Hemmorhage

Hemorrhage or excessive blood loss at the time of surgery causes shock and indicates the need for blood transfusions or other fluid replacement. Most patients are routinely typed and cross matched before surgery so that blood will be available if needed. Prompt action is necessary in the case of hemorrhage, because excessive bleeding can cause death.

Secondary hemorrhage sometimes occurs after the patient returns from surgery; consequently, the wound dressing should be inspected frequently. If bleeding is noted, report it. However, remember that concealed bleeding is revealed mainly through the symptoms of shock.

### Shock

While shock may result from pain, fear, or other factors, it is most frequently associated with severe hemorrhage. Because the blood supply to the peripheral blood vessels is reduced and the circulation of blood becomes insufficient, the blood is unable to carry out its normal functions.

**Symptoms.** The nurse should be on constant alert for the following signs of shock:
1. Drop in blood pressure
2. Restlessness and anxiety
3. Thirst

4. Cold, moist and pale skin
5. Drop in body temperature
6. Increased pulse rate (rapid and weak or thready)
7. Deep, rapid, gasping respirations (air hunger)
8. Complaints of ringing in the ears and spots before the eyes
9. Pallor or blueness of the lips and conjunctiva in light skinned persons.

**Supportive Measures.**   The supportive measures for shock are:

1. Put the patient in Trendelenburg position unless contraindicated. Elevate the lower part of the body so that the patient's feet are higher than his head (unless he has had brain surgery or spinal anesthesia, in which case he should be kept flat).
2. Supply heat sufficient to keep the body at a normal temperature.
3. Give oxygen and drugs as ordered by the doctor to elevate the blood pressure.
4. Control hemorrhage.
5. Restore fluid balance by administering blood, plasma or other parenteral fluids. The term *parenteral* refers to injection by any method other than the gastrointestinal tract.

### Hypoxia

Anesthetics and preoperative medications sometimes depress respirations and interfere with the oxygenation of the blood, causing a condition known as *hypoxia*. Mucus blocking the tracheal or the bronchial passages lowers the amount of oxygen entering the lungs, and the patient suffers from difficult breathing and cyanosis. Oxygen and suction equipment should always be on hand for emergency use to meet these problems.

## POSTOPERATIVE DISCOMFORTS

By the time the patient has returned from the recovery room to his ward or room, he is usually awake and fully aware of a number of discomforts.

**Pain.**   Pain is the first postoperative discomfort that the patient will encounter. The competent nurse is wise enough to know the value of sufficient medication to ease pain. If the patient receives medication early and it

is spaced properly, he will be kept relatively comfortable.

**Thirst.**   Thirst is present and is usually due to a decrease of fluids preoperatively, to the loss of fluids during surgery, to anesthetic recovery, and to the dryness following the use of atropine which inhibits mucous secretion. Most patients receive fluids intravenously during surgery and immediately postoperatively. This helps to prevent thirst as does rinsing the mouth. Most physicians allow sips of water or ice chips in small amounts.

**Distention.**   Temporary paralysis of the intestinal movement of peristalsis allows gas to accumulate in the intestines and causes distention. Normal peristalsis is affected by the handling of the intestines during a surgical operation, by the lack of solid food, and by restricted body movements. Accumulated gas (flatus) causes sharp pains which often are more distressing than the pain related to the incision. Early ambulation, which permits the patient to get out of bed soon after an operation, helps the patient to expel the flatus. Small amounts of solid food also help. However, do not give ice to a patient suffering from distention. If discomfort increases and nursing measures do not bring relief, the doctor usually orders one or more of the following:

1. Application of heat to the abdomen
2. Insertion of a rectal tube
3. Intramuscular injections of neostigmine (Prostigmin), a drug which stimulates peristalsis.

If intestinal paralysis persists, a serious complication, known a *paralytic ileus,* may develop. In this case a nasogastric tube is inserted.

**Nausea.**   If the patient complains of nausea, medication should be given to prevent emesis if possible.

**Urinary Retention.**   It is important to check voiding in the new postoperative patient, because some patients have difficulty in voiding. If all else fails after 8 to 12 hours, catheterization, as ordered, will bring relief. Accurate intake and output should be continued on all new surgical patients.

**Constipation.**   Disruption of the normal diet and the daily elimination schedule may cause constipation. Usually, the routine postoperative orders will include a medication to prevent this complication.

**Restlessness and Sleeplessness.** The patient may be restless and have difficulty in sleeping. Every attempt should be made to relieve these symptoms by ordinary nursing measures. Medications to promote sleep and relieve pain also play an important part.

## PREVENTION OF LATER POSTOPERATIVE COMPLICATIONS

Much can be done to prevent the development of later postoperative complications. Attention to preventive measures, advances in medical science, and early ambulation have all gone a long way toward eliminating the hazards that once accompanied an operation. Teaching the patient before surgery is also an important factor in preventing postoperative complications.

### Respiratory Complications

The principal respiratory complications following surgery are pneumonia and atelectasis. *Pneumonia* results from an infection of the lungs and may be aggravated by inactivity (hypostatic pneumonia). *Atelectasis,* the collapse of a portion of the lung due to a plug of mucus closing one of the bronchi, will cause acute and severe symptoms. The patient becomes somewhat cyanotic and develops very rapid respirations in an attempt to get oxygen. Removal of the mucous plug (by coughing, forceful pounding of the chest, or aspiration) will relieve this difficulty.

**Turning, Coughing, and Deep Breathing.** The dangers of pneumonia and atelectasis will be greatly lessened by the technic of turning, coughing, and hyperventilating or deep breathing:

1. Support the operative area, often with a pillow.
2. Instruct the patient to take a deep breath, hold it, and then cough as hard as he can.
3. Encourage the patient to breathe with the chest muscles.
4. Have the patient repeat steps 2 and 3 5 times every hour or 10 times every 2 hours.

**Blow Bottles.** The blow bottle is simply a bottle of water with a straw in it. The patient is instructed to blow bubbles in order to expand his lungs.

**IPPB Treatments.** The IPPB (intermittent positive pressure breathing apparatus) may be done by the nurse or by the inhalation therapist. This technic will be discussed more fully in Chapter 48.

### Circulatory Complications

Thrombophlebitis and embolisms represent 2 of the more serious circulatory complications which can develop after surgery.

*Thrombophlebitis* is the formation of a blood clot in a vein and is caused by venous stasis, which is the slowing or stopping of the return flow of venous blood as a result of increased clotting, lack of activity, increased pressure of vessels, and other factors. It most often occurs in the calf of the leg.

An *embolus* occurs when a piece of a clot or thrombus breaks off and enters the circulatory system, usually ending up in the lungs and causing serious complications.

If thrombophlebitis does occur, the following supportive measures may be ordered: (1) elevate the affected body part, (2) see that the patient gets bed rest, (3) administer anticoagulants as directed, and (4) avoid rubbing the body part.

Medical opinion varies on the value and safety of elevating the extremity. The patient's physician must make the decision. Those who favor elevation point to the reduction of venous congestion and edema. Those opposed to elevating the affected body part fear that when a leg is elevated the risk of releasing emboli is increased.

One means of avoiding circulatory disorders after surgery is to apply elastic stockings when the patient goes to the operating room or when he leaves surgery.

### Complications from Bedrest

Dangers of prolonged bedrest include complications in the respiratory and circulatory systems as previously mentioned, development of pressure areas, generalized edema, contractures, and osteoporosis, difficulty in weight bearing and in balance, formation of renal calculi and scrotal edema, constipation, loss of appetite, and general mental depression and disorientation.

Thus, the sooner the patient can move about, the better. Initially the patient will merely dangle his legs over the edge of the bed, then he will sit in a chair, and finally, he will walk. Early ambulation, sometimes on the day of surgery, assists circulation, improves respiration, prevents lung congestion, and aids in voiding and bowel activity. It encourages people to eat and to sleep better, it encourages the patient to help himself, and it gives tangible evidence to the patient that he is making a quick recovery and that things are going well.

## Other Postsurgical Complications

**Wound Infection.** An otherwise unexplainable temperature elevation 2 or 3 days after an operation and a redness and swelling occurring around the incision are usually signs of a wound infection. In spite of the use of antibiotics, staphylococcal organisms persist widely, which demands an increased vigilance on the part of nurses to prevent the infection from spreading. The treatment consists of the injection of antibiotics, rest, and an adequate diet to build up resistance. If necessary, the wound is drained.

**Evisceration.** This is not a common occurrence, but it does happen occasionally when the edges of the wound separate and allow the abdominal organs to protrude. Usually the patient will describe his sensations as though "something *gave*." The most a nurse can do is to cover the protruding organs with sterile sponges which have been wet with normal saline and lose no time in reporting the incident.

## ADDITIONAL MEANS OF SUPPORTING THE PATIENT AFTER SURGERY

**Nutrition.** The patient needs to have adequate food and fluids as soon as possible. He often will be started on a progressive diet, since this is, in effect, as much as he can tolerate. He begins on clear liquid, then is given a full-liquid diet, and finally progresses to a soft or general diet. Generally speaking, the sooner the patient can tolerate food, the sooner he will begin to recover in other ways.

**Handling of Drainage.** Often the patient has a drain or a wick in place to allow for drainage which may be profuse during the first few days following surgery. In her report of the patient's condition, the nurse should note the amount, color, and other features of the drainage. The same is true if the patient has suction tubes in place. Later, we will discuss specific measures for handling drainage.

In some instances a pack is put in place during surgery. The patient's chart should inform the nurse that the pack is there and should indicate if and when she is to remove it. In any event, the nurse should observe the pack to see that it is in place and that the drainage is not excessive.

**Dressing Change.** The nurse is often asked to assist the doctor with a dressing change. There is a difference between dressing reinforcement, which the nurse can do without an order, and dressing change, which is done under the direction of the doctor or upon his order.

## PARENTERAL REPLACEMENT THERAPY

**Indications.** The importance of maintaining fluid and electrolyte balance in the body was mentioned in Chapter 11. Any disease or injury to the tissues, such as pneumonia or severe burns, which interferes with the normal metabolism of cells, may disturb this balance. As far as the surgical patient is concerned, during, after, and many times prior to a surgical procedure there is inevitably a loss of fluids and electrolytes through bleeding, vomiting, excess perspiration, and drainage. When the loss is severe, and the patient is unable to replace it by taking fluids orally, the fluids and the electrolytes are restored by injection. This process is known as *parenteral replacement therapy,* and the various methods of injecting large quantities of fluid into the body are referred to as *infusion.*

**Methods.** There are 4 available routes for the injection of parenteral fluids, namely, intravenous (into the vein); intramuscular (into the muscles); subcutaneous (into the tissues directly beneath the skin); and intramedullary (into the bone marrow cavity). However, the most commonly used is the intravenous route, referred to as the intravenous infusion (I.V.).

The solution drips slowly into the blood stream through a vein, usually at the rate of 60 to 80 drops a minute or as ordered by the physician. Some of the commonly used solutions are isotonic saline (0.9% sodium chloride solution); electrolyte solutions containing many of the electrolytes found in the intracellular and tissue fluids; glucose in water solutions (5% to 10% solutions); blood plasma; and whole blood.

### Observing the Patient

Every patient receiving parenteral replacement therapy should be observed closely for an abnormal reaction whether he is the postoperative patient, the patient who has retained fluid in the tissues as a result of malfunctioning kidneys, or the one who has experienced severe blood loss from an accident. The reaction may occur during the procedure or may be delayed as long as 24 to 48 hours after the infusion has been discontinued. Reactions due to faulty technic and equipment are becoming less frequent as a result of better methods of preparing solutions, improved sterilization, and the use of disposable equipment. However, such reactions may also occur from patient sensitivity.

During the infusion, the most common symptoms of an abnormal reaction are nausea, vomiting, chills, and an increase in the pulse rate. Should they occur, the infusion should be stopped, and a report made to the physician. Nausea and vomiting also are seen frequently in a delayed reaction and should be reported.

In addition to any adverse reactions, signs that the desired effects are being obtained are noted as well. For example, if the infusion is being administered to counteract the effects of hemorrhage, the nurse should observe the blood pressure, the rate and the volume of the pulse, and the respirations to see if they begin to return to normal. She should also note whether other signs of hemorrhage are disappearing.

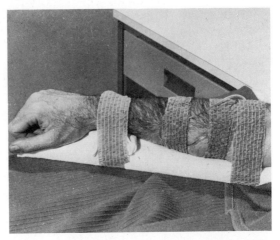

Figure 32-4. The patient who is receiving I.V. therapy is made as comfortable as possible. The needle is supported by taping the arm to an armboard. Note that paper tape is used for more comfort. The nurse should be sure to watch for possible infiltration. (Medical Products Division, 3M Company)

### Infiltration of the I.V.

As with many procedures, the nurse should observe the patient and make sure he is as comfortable as possible. She should also be able to recognize the signs and symptoms of infiltration so that she can report this complication as soon as possible and discontinue the infusion, if ordered to do so. Signs of infiltration (the needle is not in the vein and the fluid is running into the surrounding body tissues) are:

1. The area is hard and cold.
2. The patient complains of pain and burning sensation at the site.
3. Blood does not return in the tubing when the bottle is lowered below the level of the patient.
4. Later, the arm becomes white and shows a raised area.
5. Edema is sometimes noted.

In these instances, the I.V. should be discontinued as soon as possible and moist, warm packs applied to the affected area.

# 33

# Administering Selected Medications to the Patient

## BEHAVIORAL OBJECTIVES

*The student successfully attaining the goals of this chapter will be able to:*

- *discuss the importance of and method for establishing drug standards.*

- *explain the difference between the generic and trade name of a drug.*

- *reassure patients who are apprehensive about taking medications ordered by their doctor.*

- *list at least 4 factors which are known to affect drug dosage.*

- *list at least 6 methods by which drugs can be given.*

- *demonstrate an understanding of abbreviations commonly used in medication orders.*

- *state the "5 Rights of Giving Drugs" and discuss the importance of each.*

- *demonstrate a clear understanding of the proper method of giving all types of injections, including knowledge of sterile technic, and carry out such procedures as required by student's school and hospital.*

- *correctly transcribe doctors' orders if asked to do so.*

- *list 4 types of drugs which affect the skin and mucous membranes.*

- *define an antibiotic and identify desirable characteristics of antibiotics.*

- *discuss several uses of penicillin, methods of administration, potential side-effects, and the importance of a sensitivity test before administering the drug.*

- *identify and discuss, including potential side-effects, at least 2 drugs which affect the following body systems: central nervous, autonomic, musculo-skeletal, circulatory (including drugs affecting the blood), urinary, gastro-intestinal, respiratory, and reproductive; as well as drugs affecting the eye and those used to treat allergic reactions and destroy parasites.*

- *briefly describe the use of serums and vaccines as drugs.*

- *indicate the ability to check appropriate references for necessary information on specific drugs being administered to patients in the clinical setting.*

# INTRODUCTION TO PHARMACOLOGY AND DRUGS

*Pharmacology* is the study of drugs and their actions. A drug is a substance, other than food, used in preventing disease, in aiding the doctor to diagnose a disease, in treating disease, and in restoring or maintaining normal functions in the body tissues.

## Drug Standards Are Necessary

Standards for the strength and purity of drugs are essential to protect the public from the dangers of misuse or adulteration. The *Pharmacopeia of the United States of America* (usually called the U.S.P.) is a book which defines standards for the approval of drugs used in medical practice. The U.S.P. was first published in 1820, and revised editions are issued every 5 years by a committee of outstanding physicians, pharmacologists, and pharmacists.

Another publication that defines standards is the *National Formulary* (N.F.) which provides a supplementary list of drugs and is prepared and kept up-to-date by the American Pharmaceutical Association. The Food, Drug and Cosmetic Act designates the U.S.P. and the N.F. as the approved standards for listing the official drugs.

Another general reference book is called the *United States Dispensatory* (U.S.D.) and discusses both official and nonofficial drugs.

The Council on Drugs of the American Medical Association has been publishing a yearly up-to-date list for physicians on the actions, uses, and dangers of commercial drug products. This information helps to protect the public and physicians against false claims and misleading advertising about drugs and their effectiveness. This is not an official publication, but it is widely used and provides much valuable information about the newer drugs. It is called *New and Nonofficial Remedies.*

The Food, Drug and Cosmetic Act designates the Food and Drug Administration as the agency empowered to enforce drug standards (see p. 34).

## Names of Drugs

The rapid increase in the number of drugs and the variety of names for the same drug is confusing. The *official,* chemical, or *generic,* name of a drug is the one under which it is listed in the U.S.P. or the N.F. It also may be known by one or more trade names. For example, meprobamate is the official name of a drug which is also marketed under the trade names of Miltown and Equanil.

## Resources for Studying Drugs

In addition to the *National Formulary,* the *U.S. Pharmacopeia,* and *New and Nonofficial Remedies,* the *Physician's Desk Reference* (PDR) is an invaluable source of information on drugs. This book should be available in every hospital, clinic, or other medical facility and should be used whenever there is doubt about the action, side effects, or dosage of a particular drug. This book lists drugs by chemical names, by trade names, and by manufacturer and gives pertinent information about each drug.

Another book which could be very helpful to the nurse is called *Facts and Comparisons.* It is published at intervals and lists drugs under the following classifications: nutritional products, blood modifiers, hormones, diuretics and cardiovascular drugs, autonomic drugs, central nervous system drugs, gastrointestinal drugs, anti-infectives, and biologicals.

The nurse should be aware of references such as these. She must never give a drug unless she knows its action, proper dosage, and side effects. If you are in doubt about any drug, *look it up!*

## Forms of Drugs

The form of a drug, its properties, and the effect desired determine the method for giving it. Combinations of drugs are sometimes given because together they produce desirable effects which would not be possible if one of them were given alone.

Drugs are prepared in forms suitable for the various methods of administration. These forms are liquids, solids, and semisolids.

**Ampules and Vials.** *Ampules* are sealed

glass containers that usually contain one dose of a powdered or a liquid drug; powders must be dissolved in sterile water or normal saline solution before they can be given. *Vials* are rubber-stoppered glass containers which contain several doses of a drug. *Disposable syringes* containing single doses of a drug for hypodermic injection are now widely used. Another type of "disposable" (Tubex) contains one dose of a drug in a cartridge unit with an attached sterile needle which fits into a metal frame. Cartridge and needle are discarded after they are used.

## Drugs and the Individual Patient

It is not unnatural to be apprehensive about medicines. A patient may fear that a hypodermic will hurt, a medicine will have an offensive taste, or a capsule will stick in his throat. He may think he is being made a subject for experimentation, that nothing will help him, or he may simply be tired of swallowing things every 2 or 3 hours. Encourage him to talk about his feelings, and let him know you sympathize with him. Patients often conceal their real feelings because they are afraid of offending a nurse. Also, most patients want to know why a medicine is being given. If a patient is worried, it is reassuring to be told that something is being done. You can help to give him this reassurance when you give a medicine—"I've brought you something for your cough" or "to relieve your pain" or "to help you sleep."

It is important to know about the possible actions of drugs to be able to observe and report their effects intelligently. This knowledge is applied every time a medication is given in order to observe its effects on an individual patient. This is not as difficult as it seems because the science of pharmacology has given us detailed information about the actions of a vast number of drugs. This helps you to recognize both favorable and unfavorable effects. It also reminds you that drugs affect people as individuals. In other words, you are concerned about the effect of digitalis on John Gray instead of simply giving digitalis to a "heart" patient.

## Drug Dosage

The dose is the amount of a drug given as treatment. Drug dosage is regulated and described in this way:

*Minimal Dose:* The smallest amount necessary for a therapeutic effect.

*Maximal Dose:* The largest amount that can be given safely.

*Toxic Dose:* An amount that causes unfavorable symptoms or poisoning.

*Lethal Dose:* An amount that will cause death.

In prescribing the dosage of any drug, the doctor always considers certain individual differences that are known to affect drug dosage, such as:

*Age:* Children are more sensitive to drugs than adults; the effects of drugs on elderly people may be different from the effects on younger adults due to body deterioration or loss of body function.

*Sex:* Some drugs given to the mother may be harmful to the unborn fetus or to the nursing infant. However, authorities are not in agreement that sex is important in prescribing the dosage of drugs.

*Weight:* Drug dosage is often prescribed in relation to a patient's weight, especially when concentration of the drug in the blood is desirable. This usually requires larger doses for the heavier person.

*The Patient's Condition:* The nature of a disease and its severity may make a difference in the dosage. It takes more of a drug to quiet a highly disturbed patient or to control severe pain.

*Disposition:* A highly nervous person requires less of a stimulant and more of a depressant drug. The opposite is true of a less excitable or more stoic patient.

*The Method Used:* The speed with which a drug enters the circulation may affect the dosage. This, in turn, depends on how the drug is given. The intravenous method is quicker than the subcutaneous—both are more rapid than the oral method. Less of a drug may be required if absorption is rapid; with some drugs, the method makes no difference.

*Distribution:* Some drugs are distributed evenly throughout the body and reach every cell; others appear only in certain body fluids or tissues. For example, one antibiotic may enter the spinal fluid, but another may never reach it.

*Elimination:* Normally, a drug remains in the body long enough to do its work and is eliminated by the excretory organs (in the urine, feces, breath, perspiration). Some drugs leave the body in their original form; others have been made inactive by chemical changes that have taken place in their structure. If these processes are slow, it may prolong the effect of the drug for too long a time; if they proceed too rapidly, the drug may be excreted before it has a chance to do its work effectively. Chemical changes also may form substances that are harmful if the body is unable to dispose of them rapidly enough.

## Methods of Giving Drugs

The method chosen depends on the nature of the drug and the effect that is wanted. This may be *local* (at the point where the drug is applied) or *systemic* (absorbed into the circulation and carried to body cells). For local effects:

*Application to the Skin:* Antiseptics and soothing drugs are applied directly to the skin (iodine on a cut or scratch, lotion on an itchy rash).

*Application to Mucous Membranes:* Drug preparations are applied to mucous membranes of the eye, mouth, nose, throat, or genitourinary tract by swabbing, spraying, instillation, or irrigation; they are applied to the vagina and rectum in the form of suppositories. Drug-saturated packs can be inserted in body cavities.

For systemic effects there are a number of methods for introducing drugs into the circulation. Again, the choice depends on the nature and the amount of the drug to be given, the speed of its action, and the patient's condition:

*Oral:* The patient swallows the drug. This is convenient and economical, but the method has its drawbacks. Some drugs have an unpleasant taste or odor; others injure the teeth. Patients who are nauseated or vomiting cannot take drugs by mouth; some irritate the lining of the stomach, causing nausea and vomiting. Digestive enzymes destroy the effectiveness of certain drugs.

*Sublingual:* The drug is placed under the patient's tongue, where it dissolves and is absorbed. The patient must be able to understand instructions: keep the drug under the tongue; do not swallow it; do not take a drink until it is absorbed. Few drugs are given this way—nitroglycerine in tablet form is one of them.

Any method of administering a drug which is not in the mouth, or digestive tract, is called *parenteral.*

*Rectal:* This method consists of the injection of a liquid or suppository drug preparation into the rectum. It is used if a patient is vomiting, if the taste of a drug is offensive, or if the action of the digestive enzymes interferes with a drug's effectiveness. It also can be used for an unconscious patient. The drawbacks in using this method are that the patient may not be able to retain the drug, or if part of it is expelled, there is no way of knowing the amount retained. Drug preparations administered by rectum are usually given in small amounts and are preceded by a cleansing enema to empty the rectum and make absorption easier. As was stated in Chapter 29, medicated rectal suppositories are occasionally used also for their systemic effect.

*Inhalation:* Drugs that can be vaporized may be given through the respiratory tract. So much absorbing surface is available in the lungs and the bronchi that the drug is quickly absorbed and is immediately effective. This is highly important in an emergency, such as in the administration of oxygen.

Drugs may be injected into body fluids or tissues through a needle. They must be soluble, absorbable, and sterile and must not irritate or injure the tissues. Injection has the advantage of rapid action, but this can be dangerous if there should be an error made in dosage or technic. Repeated insertions of a needle may also make the tissues tender and sore; there is always the possibility of infection when the skin is pierced. Injections are given in a number of ways:

*Intradermal Injection:* A small amount of a drug is injected just beneath the outer layer of the skin, making a bump, or *wheal,* where it is absorbed slowly. The doctor uses this method in making allergy tests.

*Subcutaneous Injection:* A small amount of a drug is injected into the subcutaneous tissues (hypodermically). This method is used to give drugs that are soluble and nonirritating, often with disposable syringes and needles (a simpler and more accurate procedure for this method).

Occasionally, substantial amounts of a therapeutic solution are injected into subcutaneous tissues *(hypodermoclysis).* The fluid is injected slowly, through long needles, into loose connective tissue—usually under the breasts. Intravenous infusion has largely replaced this method.

*Intramuscular Injection:* A drug is injected into the muscle which lies beneath the subcutaneous tissue. This method is used in giving irritating drugs or larger amounts of a drug, because deep muscle tissue has fewer nerve fibers; also, absorption of the drug is faster because muscle tissue has a great many blood vessels. The injection is most commonly given in the gluteal or deltoid muscles, because they are large enough to absorb a substantial amount of a drug.

*Intravenous Injection:* A drug is injected directly into a vein. This method is used to get a rapid effect or when it is impossible to inject a drug into other tissues. If a large quantity of solution is given it is called an *infusion.* The procedure requires technical skill and is usually done by a doctor. However, in some hospitals, professional nurses now perform this procedure under a doctor's direction. Intravenous injections and infusions are commonly given for dehydration and excessive loss of blood and to dilute poisons in the blood and other body fluids and to provide electrolytes, drugs, and foods. (See Chap. 32.) If blood is given, this is called a *transfusion.*

## How Drugs Are Prescribed

A prescription is a written formula for preparing and giving a drug preparation. Physicians, dentists, and veterinarians are the only persons licensed to write prescriptions. *The nurse may give a drug preparation only on an order from a doctor.* In the hospital the doctor writes his orders in an order book or on an order form attached to the patient's chart. Sometimes orders are given verbally, in an emergency, or over the telephone. The nurse sees that such an order is written in the proper place and signed by the doctor later. *This is important*—a written order is protection for the doctor, the patient, and the nurse. It is a permanent record which cannot be disputed and always is available for reference. The nurse is responsible for carrying out an order as it is written—she is not permitted to make the slightest change. If she has any reason to question an order or does not understand it, she must consult the head nurse or the doctor about it before she proceeds. The student nurse should *never* take verbal orders.

**Prescription Drugs.** Some drug preparations can be purchased without a prescription, but Federal law now requires one for any drug that is not considered safe to use without a doctor's supervision, such as a narcotic. Such a prescription cannot be refilled without written or telephoned authorization by the doctor.

## Preparing Prescribed Medicines

The pharmacist is the only person qualified and licensed to make up drug preparations. In a hospital, the prescription is sent to the hospital pharmacy; otherwise, it is prepared by a local pharmacist. Every hospital has its own procedure for handling orders for prescribed drugs.

**The Doctor's Orders.** The doctor uses standard abbreviations in writing orders, prescriptions, and labels to be used for drugs. Some of the most common are listed as follows:

| ABBREVIATIONS | MEANING |
| --- | --- |
| @ | at |
| aa. | of each |
| a.c. | before meals |
| ad lib. | as desired |
| alt. hor. | every other hour |
| A.M. | morning |
| b.i.d. | twice a day |
| c̄ | with |
| cc. | cubic centimeter |
| ʒ (dr.) | dram |
| & (et) | and |
| dc. (disc.) | discontinue |
| Gm. | gram |
| gr. | grain |
| gt., or gtts. | drop, or drops |
| H (h) | hypodermic |
| h (hr.) | hour |
| h.s. | at bedtime (hour of sleep) |
| i.m. (IM) | intramuscularly |
| i.v. (IV) | intravenously |
| L. | liter |
| m., or min. | minim, or minims |
| mg. | milligram |
| ml. | milliliter |
| NPO | nothing by mouth |
| od | right eye |
| os | left eye |
| ou | both eyes |
| ʒ (oz.) | ounce |
| p.c. | after meals |
| per | by |
| P.M. | afternoon |

| ABBREVIATIONS | MEANING (Cont.) |
|---|---|
| p.o., (o) | by mouth (per os, oral) |
| p.r.n.* | when required |
| pt., or O. | pint |
| pulv. | powder |
| q. | every |
| q.d. | every day |
| q.h. | every hour |
| q. (2,3, etc.) h. | every (two, three, etc.) hours |
| q.i.d. | 4 times a day |
| q.o.d. | every other day |
| ℞ | take |
| s̄ | without |
| Sig or S | write on label, instructions |
| s.c. | subcutaneously |
| s.o.s.* | if necessary |
| s̄s̄ | one half |
| stat. | at once, immediately |
| t.i.d. | 3 times a day |
| tsp. | teaspoon |
| T (tbsp.) | tablespoon |
| ungt. | ointment |

**Abbreviations for Specific Drugs or Substances.**

| ABBREVIATIONS | MEANING |
|---|---|
| Fe | iron |
| $FeO_2$ | iron oxide |
| Na | sodium |
| K | potassium |
| $O_2$ | oxygen |
| Ca | calcium |
| $CO_2$ | carbon dioxide |
| P | phosphorus |
| $H_2O$ | water |
| CHO | carbohydrate |
| $KMnO_4$ | potassium permanganate |
| $AgNo_3$ | silver nitrate |
| $H_2O_2$ | hydrogen peroxide |
| KI | potassium iodide |
| SSKI | saturated solution of potassium iodide |
| KCl | potassium chloride |
| Ba | barium |

---

* Note the difference between these abbreviations: *s.o.s.* (if necessary) means for *one* dose only; *p.r.n.* (when needed, as often as necessary) means the nurse is expected to use her judgment about repeating the dose. For instance, the doctor may leave a p.r.n. order for a cathartic: if the patient has an adequate bowel movement a cathartic is not necessary on that day; 2 days later it may be needed. p.r.n. orders usually specify the frequency with which the drug may be given and usually must be rewritten at intervals in order to be considered valid.

**The Parts of a Prescription.** The doctor's prescription has several parts:

*The Patient's Full Name:* This avoids the danger of confusion with another patient having the same surname. Often the patient's room number is also included.

*The Date and the Time of Day:* This tells when the order begins. If it is for a specified number of days it also tells when the order is to be discontinued. An order for a narcotic is usually legally valid for 24 to 48 hours only. This means that the order must be rewritten if the drug is to be continued beyond that time.

*The Name (or Names) and the Amount of the Drug in the Preparation:* The use of the generic name is preferred to the trade name.

*The Dosage:* This may be stated in either the metric system (gram, cc.) or in the apothecaries system (grain, dram, ounce), depending on the system used in the individual hospital. Equivalents for fluid and weight measures are given on p. 328.

*The Time and the Frequency of Dose:* The hospital nursing service usually determines the time schedule for drug routines. For instance, for drugs to be given every 4 hours, one hospital may choose the even-numbered hours, another may choose the odd. The doctor may give other less definite directions, such as once or twice a day, before or after meals, at bedtime. Hospital policy usually sets the definite hour.

*The Method To Be Used:* Usually it is understood that the oral method is to be used if no other method is specified. Otherwise, the doctor specifies the method, especially if the drug can be given in more than one way.

*The Physician's Signature:* This is essential for legal reasons or if there is some question about the order. An unsigned order may mean that the doctor had not finished writing it.

## THE ADMINISTRATION OF MEDICINES

In most hospitals, a special unit in each patient area is provided for storing and measuring medicines. It is equipped with cupboards, a sink, running water, and work space and is usually located in the nurses' station. Wherever it is, it should not be accessible to the public, and it must provide a double-locked compartment to store narcotic drugs. Medicines should be placed on the shelves in an orderly fashion. Every drug should be plainly labeled. If a label is illegible, send the container to the pharmacy for relabeling—never label or relabel a drug yourself and never change bottles. Some drug preparations must be stored in the refrigerator or in brown bottles to preserve their effectiveness.

## The Medicine Card

Most hospitals use a card system for giving medications. A card is made out for each medication, with the patient's name, the drug, the dosage, and the time for giving the medicine. These cards are kept in a file and taken out for use when the medications are measured and given. Sometimes different-colored cards are used—each color represents a different time of day, a different route, or a different type of medication, depending on the policy of the hospital.

As each medication is measured, it is placed with its card on a tray to be carried to the patient; this identifies the medicine from the time it is measured until the patient takes it.

## Measuring Systems

Drugs are measured by both dry and liquid measures; 2 systems are used for measuring drugs—the *metric system* and the *apothecaries' system*. In addition, there is the system of *household measures* that you use in cooking; however, household measures are not accurate for measuring medicines, but can be used if other measuring equipment is not available in preparing solutions to be used externally. The measures given in the following tables are those that you will use in measuring medicines, solutions used in nursing treatments, and the fluids taken in and excreted by the patient. All hospitals may not use the same system; you may be asked to measure urine in *cc.'s* or in *ounces*. Therefore, you need to understand both systems and to know the household measure equivalents if you have to use household equipment. The units of measure are listed, with their corresponding abbreviations:

| METRIC SYSTEM | | APOTHE-CARIES' SYSTEM | | HOUSEHOLD MEASURES | |
|---|---|---|---|---|---|
| gram | Gm. | grain | gr. | drop | gtt. |
| cubic cen- | | minim | m. | teaspoon | tsp. |
| timeter | cc. | dram | dr., ʒ | tablespoon | tbsp., T. |
| liter | L. | ounce | oz., ʒ | measuring | |
| | | pound | lb. | cup | c. |
| | | pint | pt. | | |
| | | quart | qt. | | |

The following tables show these systems in their equivalent relationships:

### DRY MEASURES

| METRIC SYSTEM | APOTHE-CARIES' SYSTEM | HOUSEHOLD MEASURES |
|---|---|---|
| 1 Gm. | 15 gr. | ¼ tsp. |
| 4 Gm. | 1 dr. (60 gr.) | 1 tsp. |
| 30 Gm. | 1 oz. | 8 tsp. or 2 tbsp. |

### LIQUID MEASURES

| | | |
|---|---|---|
| 1 cc. | 15 m. | 15 drops |
| 4 cc. | 1 fl.dr. | 1 tsp. |
| 30 cc. | 1 fl oz. | 8 tsp. or 2 tbsp. |
| 500 cc. | 1 pt. (approx.) | 2 measuring cups |
| 1,000 cc. | 1 qt. (approx.) | 4 measuring cups |

(1 cc.=approx. 1 milliliter, ml.)

### MEASURING EQUIPMENT

| | |
|---|---|
| Minim glasses | Medicine droppers |
| Graduates measuring from 5 to 30 cc. or more | Glass rod |
| | Small paper containers or |
| Medicine glasses | Teaspoons |
| Drinking glasses | |

## Measuring Medicines

Routines may vary slightly from hospital to hospital, but the safety rules are the same everywhere. If you are tempted to deviate from these rules, remember that they have been set up to protect the patient and to protect you from mistakes which could have serious results.

Give your undivided attention to the job at hand when you measure and give medicines.

Read the order and check it with the medicine card and the label on the medicine; they should check exactly.

Read the medicine label 3 times: (1) when you take it from the shelf; (2) before you remove the medicine from the container; and (3) before you put back the container.

Check the medicine to make sure it is not spoiled, cloudy, or otherwise unsafe.

Measure the dose with appropriate equipment. Hold the measure at eye level when measuring liquids, with your thumbnail on the line of the desired amount. Pour liquid medicines from the unlabeled side of the bottle, to avoid soiling the label.

Never give a medicine from an unlabeled container. Labels must be clearly readable.

Shake the required number of tablets or capsules into the container you are using. Small paper cups are usually provided for this purpose. Never handle medicines with your fingers.

Assemble each medicine, with its card, on the medicine tray as you prepare it.

Be completely familiar with abbreviations and trade names, and use extreme caution with drugs which have similar names.

## Administering Medicines

---

The 5 RIGHTS of Giving Drugs:
1. Be sure you select the RIGHT PATIENT.
2. Be sure you select the RIGHT MEDICINE.
3. Give the RIGHT DOSE.
4. Give the medication at the RIGHT TIME.
5. Give the medication by the RIGHT METHOD.

---

Be sure that you are giving the correct medicine to the right patient. Check the name on the medicine card with the patient's identification band. (Do not give a medication to a patient who does not have an ID band; the bed tag *is not* sufficient identification.) If you are not sure of the patient's identity, ask him his name. He must tell you his name, not just answer "yes" or "no" to your question, "Are you Mr. Winter?" Saying a name helps to associate it with the name on the medicine card.

Stay with the patient until he has swallowed the medicine. If left alone with a medicine, patients have been known to dispose of it in various ways.

Never leave a medicine tray within the reach of patients. If you must leave the room or the ward, take the tray with you.

Chart medicines as soon as you have given them. Never chart a medicine before you give it. Record the time, the name of the drug, the dosage, and the method of giving it. Add your initials or name, so the doctor will know who gave the drug. Record and *report immediately* any unusual reaction, such as vomiting the medicine, an unfavorable change in the patient's condition, his refusal to take the medicine or inability to take it all. If you find that you have forgotten to give a medicine you must report it promptly.

Discard an unused dose of medicine—never return it to the stock container. Medicines which are discarded should be poured down the sink or flushed down the hopper.

Never give a medicine that someone else has prepared. If a mistake occurs, you will be held responsible.

Listen when a patient questions a medicine; if he has been getting a red pill and is offered a white one instead, it is not surprising if he suspects a mistake. Recheck the order, the label, and the medicine card. If a patient states that he is allergic to any medication, check before giving any medicine.

Wash equipment which is not disposable in hot, soapy water.

Be sure you are giving the right medication at the *right time*. Check the time on the doctor's order with the Kardex and with the medication card. Follow the routine of the hospital for intervals or routine times at which medications are given. You must know which types of medications are usually given 4 times a day, during waking hours, and which types of drugs are given every 6 hours, around the clock. For example, antibiotics must be given at regular intervals, in order to maintain a constant blood level.

You must give a drug within 15 minutes either way of the time for which it is ordered. Any deviation from these limits constitutes a *medication error*. Be sure you know the abbreviations for times, such as t.i.d. and b.i.d., and ask if you are not sure.

Be sure you are giving the right medication by the *right method*. Check the doctor's orders to verify the method by which the medication should be given. Some drugs can be fatal if given by the wrong method. You should be aware of the usual route for certain medications. Know the color codes of the medication cards as followed by your hospital. Whatever the codes be sure the color of the card is correct. Keep the drug and the card together by clipping them together or use a medication tray with special slots for the drug cup or syringe and the card.

Do not place different types of drugs together in a cup. For example, do not place a PRN medication with a regularly given medication and do not place digitalis with other medications. The reason for this is that the patient might not get one medication and you would not be able to identify, for certain, which was which in the cup, if they were together.

**STAT Medications.** If a medication is ordered to be given STAT, it means just that, *immediately*. Check the order, make a card, and pour and administer the medication as soon as possible. When you make the medication card from a STAT order, check it on the order sheet, so someone else will not administer the medication again. Be sure to chart STAT medications as soon as they are given, so there will be no duplication. Sometimes, it is also a good idea to tell the team leader that you are giving a STAT medication, so that she will not assign someone else to do it.

**PRN Medications.** If the patient asks for a PRN medication, be sure to give it as soon as possible. You must check the chart to make sure that the correct time period has elapsed since the last dose of the PRN medication. If there is any chance of duplication, check before giving. Be sure to chart and report immediately after giving a PRN medication.

**HS Medications.** Bedtime medications, such as sleeping pills and laxatives are often ordered PRN, (as needed). If so, ask the patient if he needs a sleeping pill or a laxative and then set up the medications. Chart these immediately *after* administering them. Be sure to use correct procedure in disposing of a medication which the patient requests and later refuses.

## Medication Errors

Occasionally, a medication error may occur. This must be reported at once, to prevent danger to the patient. In some cases, immediate emergency action must be taken to prevent death or other undesirable side-effects. Medication errors include the giving of the wrong medication, the giving of a medication at the wrong time or in the wrong dosage, or the administration of a medication to the wrong patient. This is why the 5 RIGHTS are so very important. If you have any doubt about a medication, ask before giving the medication, to prevent an error. On the other hand, if you think you might have made an error, do not hesitate to report it at once. Do not think of yourself at this time, but think about the patient and the potential dangers to his health and his life.

## ADMINISTERING DRUGS BY MOUTH

More medicines are given by mouth than in any other way. Liquid medications may be given full strength or may be diluted with water, milk, or fruit juice. You must check to see what the appropriate solvent would be. Some substances *do not* mix well. Small amounts, measured in minims, must be diluted or most of the medicine will be left in the glass. Preparations given to soothe the throat are given undiluted. Adequate water is provided to aid in swallowing tablets and capsules and to act as a "chaser" after other medicines (except when a patient is on restricted fluids). For your convenience, directions are given below:

*Liquids:* As measured, or diluted with water after measuring.

*Powders:* Dissolved in water, unless ordered otherwise—sometimes given in capsules if the amount is not too large.

*Pills:* Given as they are, unless the order directs that they should be crushed and dissolved in water, jello, or other substance. They are crushed with a mortar and pestle.

*Capsules:* Given as they are. You may sometimes open the capsule, if so directed.

Some types of medications are given in a specific way:

*Cough Medicines:* Given undiluted, to get the maximum soothing effect on the throat membranes.

*Unpleasant-Tasting Medicines:* Holding a piece of ice in the mouth before taking the medicine numbs the taste buds. Orange or lemon juice, or a piece of fruit, helps to remove the taste of oil. It helps to drink through a straw, so the medication does not touch the taste buds.

*Castor Oil:* Add orange or lemon juice to the oil—add ½ teaspoon of sodium bicarbonate—mix and give, or beat orange or lemon juice into the oil and give; usually it is a good idea to give a piece of orange after the oil also.

*Acid and Iron Preparations:* Give through a straw or a drinking tube—these medicines discolor and injure the teeth.

*Metallic Preparations:* Give through a straw because of the unpleasant taste.

## ADMINISTERING DRUGS BY INJECTION

*Injection* is a method of introducing drugs into the tissues through a needle. The word parenteral is used to describe this method of administration. Injections are given in

Figure 33-1. One type of disposable injection unit is the Tubex closed injection system. The prefilled disposable sterile cartridge-needle unit containing the medication is being placed in the reusable syringe. (Wyeth Laboratories)

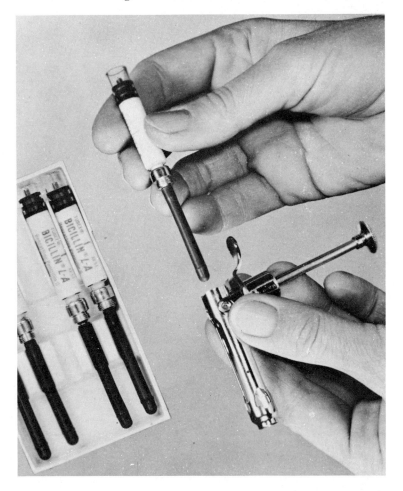

slightly different ways, but the principles discussed here apply to every form of injection. Drugs given by injection must be in liquid form. This means that if a drug comes as a tablet, it must be dissolved in sterile water or normal saline solution.

A drug may be administered parenterally for the following reasons: if it is necessary to guarantee the accuracy of the dosage of the drug injected or retained, if the patient is nauseous or vomiting, if the mental or physical status of the patient renders him unable to swallow oral medication; and if the drug cannot be absorbed via the digestive system.

The general types of parenteral injection are *intradermal* (into one layer of the skin), *subcutaneous* (just under the skin), *intramuscular* (into a muscle), and *intravenous* (into the vein, thus, directly into the blood stream). All of these types of injection are absorbed faster than are drugs administered by the oral route, and they are absorbed increasingly faster as they progress from the skin to the blood stream. The fastest method of absorption of those mentioned is the intravenous injection. There is an even faster type of injection which is used in extreme emergencies only—an injection directly into the left ventricle of the heart, so that the drug is pumped to the body with the next beat of the heart.

An injection is momentarily painful when the needle pierces the skin; therefore, the needle should be sharp and free from burrs that make its insertion difficult. An injection is less painful if the needle is inserted and withdrawn quickly. The needle should be of the smallest gauge that is appropriate to use for each type of injection. Injecting the solution fairly slowly distributes it more evenly

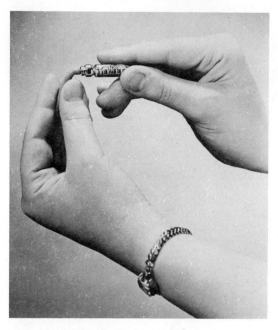

Figure 33-2. After using any disposable syringe or Tubex injection system, be sure to break the needle off the syringe. This prevents later usage in an illegal or abusive way by others. Be sure to dispose of needles and syringes in designated places to prevent any injury to the persons responsible for disposal of wastes. (Wyeth Laboratories)

in the tissues and prevents painful pressure. Gently massaging the area after the needle is withdrawn speeds up absorption of the drug.

**Sterile Equipment.** Sterile equipment is a "must" in giving injections to avoid introducing harmful organisms into the tissues or the blood stream. Sterilization under steam pressure is the most reliable method; in many hospitals all equipment for giving injections is prepared in this way in the surgical supply room, or more often, sterile disposable equipment may be provided.

**Cleansing the Skin.** It is impossible to sterilize the skin but it should be as *clean* as possible. A cleansing agent or antiseptic applied to the area of injection helps to reduce the possibility of infection. A sterile cotton ball is moistened with alcohol or Zephiran, or a premoistened sterile sponge is applied at the point of the injection and moved firmly over the rest of the skin area in a widening circle. Haphazard wiping drags contaminated material back over the point of injection.

## The Subcutaneous Injection

A hypodermic injection is the introduction of a drug into subcutaneous tissues with a needle and a syringe. This method is used (1) to obtain rapid action of a drug, (2) when the patient cannot take medications by mouth and (3) when the digestive juices would change the action of a drug. Drugs to relieve pain (morphine, codeine), stimulants (caffeine), and insulin are examples of medicines that are given by hypodermic injection. The drug may be in a vial, an ampule, or in the form of a tablet. A tablet must be dissolved in a liquid before it can be given; normal saline or distilled water are considered the most desirable solutions to use, but tap water is also considered safe (in an emergency) if it has been boiled.

**Syringes.** A subcutaneous injection is given with a 2-cc. syringe; there are special syringes for giving tuberculin and other intradermal skin tests and insulin. Some syringes, Luer or Luer-Lok, have a metal tip to ensure proper fastening of the needle. The newer types of syringes are disposable: in one type the entire unit is thrown away after one use; in another, the medication is contained in a disposable cartridge-needle unit which is clamped in a nondisposable syringe. The disposable syringe, of course, necessitates less time for sterilization, decreases the chances of cross infection, and reduces the "breakage" problem (see Figs. 33-1 and 33-2).

A syringe has 2 parts: the *barrel* and the *plunger* (see Fig. 33-3). Some syringes have metal guards to keep the plunger from falling out when the syringe is held upside down. The barrel and the plunger are ground with great precision to fit together smoothly and without leakage; the same number is stamped on the barrel and the plunger, so that the parts of an individual syringe can be matched to each other. Syringes should have good care and handling; they are expensive and are useless when out of order. A syringe that is stuck or *frozen* or one with mismatched parts may cause serious delay in giving a medication. Syringes should be cleaned thoroughly when taken apart and matched properly after they are used.

Two kinds of markings for measuring medications are stamped on the barrel of the

Figure 33-3. This illustration shows the parts of the syringe which should not be touched while they are being assembled for use. (Becton, Dickinson & Co.)

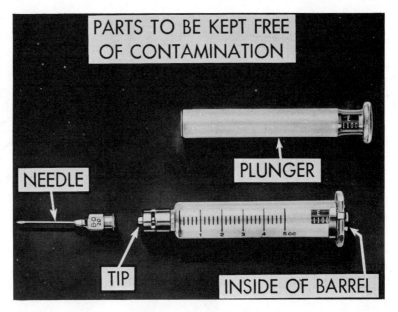

PARTS TO BE KEPT FREE OF CONTAMINATION

NEEDLE

PLUNGER

TIP

INSIDE OF BARREL

syringe. One set of markings measures 2 cc.; the other measures 30 minims. The cc.'s are also marked in *tenths*; the minims are marked from 1 to 30. You will never give more than 2 cc. in a hypodermic injection with this type of syringe. Insulin syringes are marked in units on the sides of the barrel. Generally, a separate syringe is used for U-40 and for U-80 insulin. They are marked accordingly and should not be used for the opposite type of insulin.

**Needle.** The hypodermic needle is hollow: the part that is attached to the syringe is called the *hub*; the slender pointed shaft is the *cannula*; and a wire which is occasionally threaded through the needle is the *stylet*. The stylet keeps the needle open and ready for use. The needle has a sharp point and a beveled edge, so that it can be inserted easily and with a minimum amount of discomfort to the patient. Always inspect a hypodermic needle to be sure that the point is perfect—a burr or a hook on the point will injure the tissues and cause pain. Be sure the needle, whether disposable or not, is firmly attached to the syringe.

**Handling the Sterile Syringe.** Never touch the shaft of the plunger, the inside of the barrel, or the tip or the shaft of the needle with your fingers when you are handling a sterile syringe; never handle the hypodermic tablet with your fingers—shake it into the cover of

the bottle, then into the syringe when you dissolve it. Secure the needle to the syringe by a *twist* to anchor it, or the pressure may force the needle off and the medication will be lost and the needle contaminated.

**Area for Injection.** A hypodermic is given in an area where the bones and the blood vessels are not near the surface; the areas commonly used are the upper part of the arms and the thighs. For the occasional hypodermic, the arm is the most convenient site. If a patient is having hypodermic injections regularly, you choose a different location each time; for example, use the right arm, then the left arm; the right thigh, then the left thigh. Try to find a spot in each area that has not been used for a previous injection, for at least 1 inch in all directions. The skin is cleansed with alcohol (70 per cent), or some other antiseptic such as pHisoHex or Zephiran Chloride (1 to 1,000), to prepare the area for the injection. This is a precaution against introducing harmful organisms into the body through pierced skin.

An undernourished or emaciated person has less subcutaneous tissue than a stouter person. The solution is usually injected at a 45-degree angle, but it may be necessary to vary this angle slightly—in a very fat person the short needle may not even reach the subcutaneous tissue.

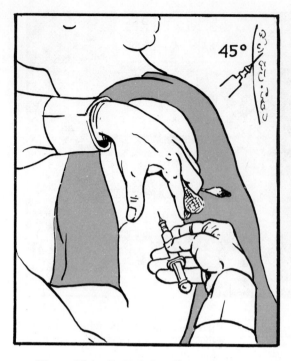 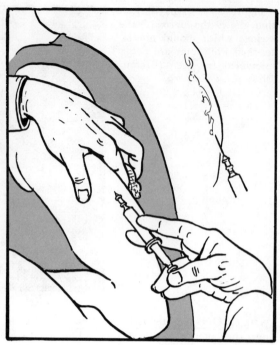

Figure 33-4. (*Left*) Subcutaneous injection. Needle introduced at an angle of 45 degrees to the skin. Little finger should be held at the end of the plunger to prevent forcing the plunger off. (*Right*) Injection of the fluid. Pressure, which is exerted on the arm with the left hand, is released when the solution is injected.

The following procedure describes the method for giving a subcutaneous injection. (See Fig. 33-4.)

### EQUIPMENT

2 cc. syringe
Hypodermic needle—¾ inch, 24 or 25 gauge
Prescribed medication
Antiseptic solution
Sterile sponges or cotton balls
Waste container

### PROCEDURE

Check the medicine card with the drug order and the drug label.

*Reason: Repeated checking prevents mistakes.*

Shake the tablet into the syringe, then dissolve, or draw up the solution to be given.

*Reason: Handling a drug with the fingers increases the possibility of infection. Solid drugs must be dissolved before they can be injected and absorbed.*

Draw the solution into the syringe; pick up the needle by the hub and attach it to the syringe with a slight twist.

*Reason: Fixing the needle firmly helps to prevent separation from the syringe.*

Expel the air from the syringe and the needle by pushing gently on the plunger until a drop appears on the needle tip.

*Reason: Injection of air into the tissues can be harmful. Loss of a minute amount does not affect the dosage appreciably, but the effectiveness of a drug depends on accurate dosage.*

Protect the needle with the plastic cap which comes on a disposable syringe. If using a glass syringe you must use a sterile, *dry* cotton ball or sponge. Bring the syringe and needle to the patient on a tray.

*Reason: Exposure to air or contact with unsterile surfaces will contaminate the needle. Wet sponges will conduct bacteria.*

Cleanse the area for the injection with a sterile cotton ball and antiseptic solution; wipe firmly from the center in circles outward.

Figure 33-5. The entire hip area or buttock has been divided into quadrants by drawing lines from the iliac crest (A) to the level of the lower edge of the buttock (C), and from the division of the buttocks (D) to the outer surface of the body (B). The needle is inserted at the shaded area (E) outside and above the point where the lines cross. This location must be determined by feeling and not just by visual calculations. This avoids striking the large blood vessels and the sciatic nerve. Intramuscular injections may also be given further to the side. This is called the ventrogluteal site. (Fuerst, E. V. and Wolff, L.: Fundamentals of Nursing, ed. 4. Philadelphia, Lippincott, 1969)

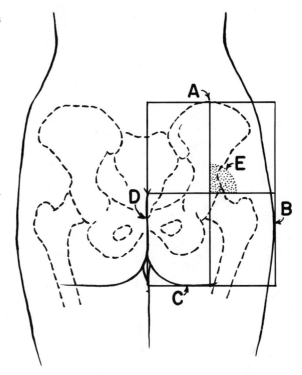

*Reason: Rubbing helps to remove contaminated material from the skin.*

With the left hand, pinch up the area around the site of the injection to form a cushion.

*Reason: Insertion into a tissue pad prevents the needle from penetrating to bone or muscle tissue.*

Insert the needle quickly at a 40-degree to 50-degree angle, depending on the plumpness of the tissue cushion (see p. 334).

*Reason: Well-nourished individuals have more subcutaneous tissue than thin or emaciated people.*

After the needle is inserted, release the hold on the tissue; pull back on the plunger slightly to see if the needle is in a blood vessel.

*Reason: Drugs injected into a blood vessel are absorbed rapidly—with some drugs this may be dangerous.*

If the blood is not evident, inject the solution slowly. If blood is evident, withdraw the needle slightly and try again.

*Reason: Rapid injection of fluid causes pressure on the nerves and pain.*

Withdraw the needle quickly.

*Reason: Slow withdrawal pulls the tissues, which is uncomfortable.*

Massage the area gently with the sponge.

*Reason: Massaging helps to distribute the drug in the tissues and aids absorption.*

## Giving an Intramuscular Injection

An intramuscular injection is given in much the same way as a subcutaneous injection, except that a longer needle is used and the drug is injected into the muscles instead of into the tissues directly beneath the skin. This method is used when a drug is irritating to the tissues and when rapid absorption is desired. Also larger doses can be given.

**Dangers in the Method.** Intramuscular injections are more difficult and dangerous to give than subcutaneous injections, for these reasons:

1. The needle must penetrate thick muscles —if the drug is injected into subcutaneous tissues, it is not absorbed quickly and may cause pain and serious irritation.

2. The possibility of striking bones, large nerves and blood vessels is greater when a longer, larger needle is used. Paralysis or

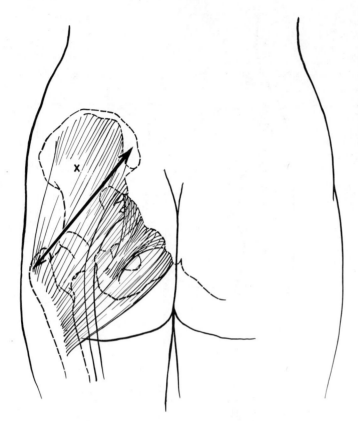

Figure 33-6. "X" indicates a second safe area for an intramuscular injection in the buttock. Note that the needle is inserted lateral and slightly superior to the midpoint of the imaginary line running from the posterosuperior iliac spine to the greater trochanter of the femur. (Fuerst, E. V. and Wolff, L.: Fundamentals of Nursing, ed. 4, Philadelphia, Lippincott, 1969)

nerve damage can result from use of an incorrect site.

Intramuscular injections are usually given in the thick gluteal muscles of the buttocks, although small injections may be given in the front of the thigh in the vastus lateralis muscle (part of the quadriceps femoris) or in the outer part of the upper arm in the deltoid muscle. The spot in the buttock can be located by drawing 2 imaginary intersecting lines to divide the buttock into 4 equal parts —the needle is inserted in the upper, outer quadrant, toward the *outside* and *above* the point where the lines cross each other (see Fig. 33-5).

Another safe area on the buttock for an intramuscular injection is found by locating an imaginary line from the posterosuperior iliac spine to the greater trochanter of the femur. The injection is made lateral and slightly superior to the midpoint of the line (see Fig. 33-6).

A third site for injection in the hip area is that of the ventral area of the gluteal muscles below the iliac crest (the ventrogluteal site).

The site is located by placing the index finger on the anterior superior iliac spine and the palm of the hand over the greater trochanter of the femur. The index and other fingers are spread out as far as possible, forming a V and pointing toward the patient's head. The injection is given between the index and second fingers and is aimed immediately below the iliac crest. If it is not possible to locate the anterior superior iliac spine, the injection can be given an inch below the iliac crest in a vertical line with the lateral thigh.

This method, also known as Hockstetter's method, is recommended by many people as safer and less painful than the traditional method. The fat is thinner in this area, while the gluteal muscle is thicker, even in very thin patients. One disadvantage is that the patient can see the administration of the injection.

Another site frequently used in giving intramuscular injections, especially in persons who are receiving frequent injections and need rotation of the site, is the lateral or anterior thigh.

Figure 33-7. (*Top, left*) The left hand is exerting pressure on the buttock, thus flattening and fixing the tissue. (*Top, right*) The needle has been thrust into the buttock. Note that a portion of the needle extends above the skin surface. (*Bottom, left*) The operator is withdrawing the plunger in order to be sure the needle tip has not entered a blood vessel. (*Bottom, right*) The solution is being slowly injected. (*Inset*) Close-up of injection.

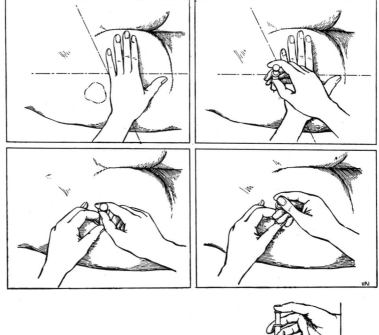

**Important Points in Giving an Intramuscular Injection.**

1. A 5-cc. syringe may be needed to give the larger amounts of some intramuscular injections, although usually no more than 2 cc. are given in any one site. The needle should always be at least 1½ inches long and 20 to 22 gauge.

2. The patient should be lying down. If he is standing, he will not be relaxed enough.

3. The injection is prepared in the same way as the subcutaneous injection; the skin preparation is the same.

4. The flesh at the site of the injection is stretched and flattened and held in this position until the needle has been inserted. It may also be pinched.

5. The syringe is held perpendicular to the skin, and the needle inserted straight into the muscle; the needle is then withdrawn slightly, and a pull is made on the plunger of the syringe to see whether or not the needle is in a blood vessel. If blood is sucked back into the syringe, the needle must be withdrawn and inserted in another spot. A drug that can be injected into the muscles without doing harm may cause a serious reaction if it is injected directly into the circulation.

6. Following the injection, the site is massaged thoroughly to promote the absorption of the drug.

The following procedure describes the method of giving an intramuscular injection in the gluteal muscles of the buttocks.

PROCEDURE (Fig. 33-7)

Place the patient in the prone position with the arms at the sides and the feet over the edge of the mattress, with the toes pointed inward. If this position is not possible for a patient, place him on his side.

*Reason: The prone position relaxes muscles—injection into tense muscles is painful and often impossible, because of resistance.*

Locate the spot for the injection in the inner angle of the upper outer quadrant.

*Reason: This point is beyond the sciatic nerve and the large blood vessels.*

Cleanse the area.

*Reason: The needle can introduce bacteria from the skin into the tissues.*

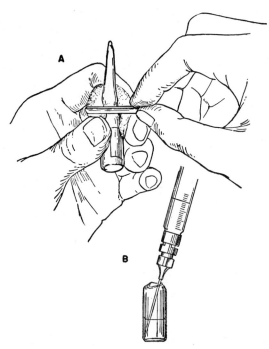

Figure 33-8. (A) The fingers are protected by cotton when the stem of the closed glass ampul is scored with a file and then broken off. (B) When the stem of the glass ampul is removed, the drug is drawn up into the syringe easily because air displaces the fluid. The sterile needle should not touch the rim of the ampul. The ampul may be tipped without losing the solution.

With the thumb and the first 2 fingers, spread the tissues beyond the site of the injection.

*Reason: Pressure flattens the subcutaneous tissues so the needle can penetrate to the muscle. In a very thin patient, it is better to pinch the tissues to avoid hitting a bone.*

Swiftly thrust the needle straight into the tissues.

*Reason: Slow motion is more painful. Force drives the needle for its entire length to enter the muscle.*

Pull back slowly on the plunger to see if the needle is in a blood vessel. If blood appears, withdraw the needle slightly and test again.

*Reason: Muscle tissue contains many blood vessels. Drugs entering a blood vessel are absorbed rapidly, which might be dangerous.*

If blood is not evident, inject the solution slowly.

*Reason: Slow injection reduces painful pressure on the tissues.*

Withdraw the needle quickly.

*Reason: Rapid withdrawal of the needle is less painful.*

Massage the area of injection.

*Reason: Massaging helps to distribute the solution in the tissues and hastens the absorption of the drug.*

If a patient must have intramuscular injections frequently, the sites should be rotated, and a notation of the site used each time should be made on the patient's chart.

## Complications of Injections

The nurse should not be afraid to give an injection, but she must realize that possible dangers do exist. The injection may enter a blood vessel, in which case the drug could be absorbed too rapidly and cause other damage. Paralysis or nerve damage may also result, as might scar formation, necrosis and/or sloughing of the tissues, embolism, and abscess or cyst formation.

## Other Considerations for Injections

**Withdrawing a Drug From an Ampule.** A drug put up in a glass ampule usually is for a single dose and must be withdrawn with a sterile hypodermic syringe and needle. The stem of the ampule may be constructed to break off easily or it may be necessary first to scratch the glass with a metal file. By grasping the stem with a sterile cotton ball as it is broken off, the fingers are protected and the open ampule is not contaminated. The drug is then drawn up into the syringe (see Fig. 33-8).

**Withdrawing a Drug From a Vial.** A vial is a small rubber-capped bottle which may hold either a single dose of a drug or a number of doses. The rubber cap on the vial usually is covered with a metal cap which is easily removed when the drug is to be given. Although the rubber cap was sterilized when the drug was prepared, it is common practice to cleanse the cap with an antiseptic before inserting the needle into the vial. In withdrawing the solution, it helps to first inject an equal amount of air into the vial; the increased pressure moves the solution up into the syringe (see Fig. 33-9).

If a vial contains several doses of a drug, the above procedure is followed, but only the amount of the prescribed dose is withdrawn.

**The Injection of Insulin.** Insulin, a drug used to control diabetes, must be given subcutaneously; it cannot be given by mouth because the digestive enzymes destroy it. The doctor prescribes the dosage according to the needs of the individual patient and adjusts it if necessary.

The administration of insulin in the treatment of diabetes mellitus will be discussed in Chapter 52.

**Observing the Patient During an Intravenous Infusion.** Intravenous infusion is a widely used method of treatment in hospitals today to restore the fluid and electrolyte balance in body fluids. You will not be responsible for giving an infusion, but you should know what to observe since you may be taking care of a patient who is having this treatment.

A needle is inserted in a vein—usually in the antecubital space in front of the elbow. To this is attached a length of tubing connected to a glass container of the prescribed solution. A clamp on the tubing regulates the flow of fluid and a dripmeter measures the number of drops per minute. A glance will tell you whether or not the solution is running properly; inspection of the needle will tell you if it is in place. Swelling around the needle indicates that the needle has come out of the vein and that the fluid is running into the tissues. If this occurs, close the clamp to shut off the flow and report it immediately. Nausea, vomiting, rapid breathing, or increase in the pulse rate are signs of an unfavorable reaction and must be reported promptly, after the flow of solution is shut off.

An infusion often necessitates keeping the arm in one position for several hours, so every effort should be made to make the patient as comfortable as possible. When the infusion is completed, the needle is withdrawn from the vein and pressure is applied over the puncture for a short time to prevent the oozing of blood.

**Intravenous Drugs.** The most commonly used intravenous solutions are dextrose in water (in 5% or 10% solution in distilled

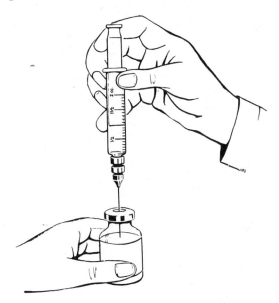

Figure 33-9. One cubic centimeter of air is being injected into the rubber-stoppered vial. Note that the forefinger is exerting pressure against the plunger, thus preventing its forceful expulsion in case there is excessive pressure within the vial.

water), called $D_5W$ or $D_{10}W$. Also used is saline solution in 5% (hypotonic saline solution) or 10% (physiologic saline solution; normal saline solution). Ringer's solution and Ringer's lactate may also be used. Many other drugs, such as antibiotics, mineral salts, and vitamins are commonly added to I.V.'s. The practical nursing student will not be asked to mix intravenous solutions. If you are asked to do this as a graduate, you will need special inservice instruction.

## OTHER METHODS OF ADMINISTRATION

Some drugs are given rectally, usually in enema or suppository form. Other drugs may be given topically, that is, applied to the skin or mucous membranes. The nurse must be careful to be sure that a drug is appropriate for mucous membrane, because if it is not, it can be very irritating. The method for administering eye medications is discussed in Chapter 53. The nurse must be sure never to place any medication into the eye which is not specifically labeled as an eye medication.

## ADMINISTERING DRUGS TO CHILDREN

Later, when you study *pediatrics,* or the care of the ill child, you will learn more about administering medications to children. However, a few brief points are in order. The nurse must remember that the child is smaller in size than the adult and therefore, can tolerate only a fraction of the adult dosage of a drug. Drug overdoses and drug errors are more apt to occur when drugs are administered to a child. Since a child is also more likely to be allergic to drugs, the nurse should be watchful for any allergic or anaphylactic reactions.

## TRANSCRIBING DOCTOR'S ORDERS

Usually a unit secretary or ward manager is assigned to transcribe doctor's orders, but sometimes the LPN is asked to do this. Several general rules will be discussed here, but the practical nursing graduate will need special inservice education in order to be proficient at transcribing doctor's orders. This is a very great responsibility and must be done with care.

The medication must be written on the Kardex in pencil and the appropriate medication cards made out. All information must be included and STAT medications must be given immediately. In many hospitals, the medication must be ordered from the pharmacy when the order is transcribed. You must write clearly and legibly, so that everyone can read your writing and no mistakes will be made. Be sure to note the date when a drug is to be discontinued. When a medication is discontinued, be sure to erase or cross out the order on the Kardex, destroy the medication card, and notify the nurse who is giving medications to that patient for the day.

Of course, if you are transcribing medication orders, you will also be transcribing other orders for treatments, blood work, x-ray examinations, etc. Hospital policy will determine the manner in which you do this.

After transcribing orders, be sure to draw a line directly under the order and sign it, usually in red, so that it can be determined who transcribed the orders. The line is drawn under the others after they are transcribed so that no more orders can be added above that line. It goes without saying that all orders must be signed by the physician.

## ANTISEPTICS AND DISINFECTANTS

An *antiseptic* is a chemical agent that slows the growth and the development of microorganisms but does not necessarily kill them. We are likely to think of antiseptics as agents that are applied directly to body tissues, especially to the skin. Many of these antiseptics have been mentioned under drugs that affect the skin. They include soaps and detergents, such as green soap preparations and pHisoHex, and Zephiran.

A *disinfectant* is a chemical agent that kills harmful microorganisms. A germicide and a bactericide are two other substances that destroy bacteria, and it has become common practice to use these terms synonymously with the term, disinfectant. It is only on rare occasions that any of the 3 are effective against bacterial spores.

## DRUGS WHICH AFFECT THE SKIN AND MUCOUS MEMBRANES

Drugs are applied to the skin to treat pain or discomfort caused by itching, to treat infections, and to soften the skin. The skin does not absorb drugs readily because a substance (keratin) in the outer layer sheds moisture just as a "weatherproof" raincoat does. Absorption is better if the skin is softened by soaking in water or by perspiration, or if the drug is applied to an area where the skin is thinner. Substances combined with alcohol or natural fats are absorbed more readily.

### Emollients

Emollients are preparations which are used to soothe irritated skin or mucous membranes or are used as carriers for medicinal substances. Some of the common emollients are:

*Oils:* Used to lubricate the skin, such as olive, flaxseed, or cottonseed oil.

*Glycerin:* Used in combination with water or rose water to soothe irritated lips and skin.

*Petrolatum (Petrolatum Jelly Vaseline):* Used as an ointment base.

*Liquid Petrolatum:* Used for medicines applied locally.

*Cold Cream:* A combination of water and oil with other ingredients. There is a nonallergic type available for those allergic to the perfumed cold cream.

*Cocoa Butter:* A solid oil, used mainly for suppositories.

*White Ointment and Yellow Ointment:* Mostly petrolatum with white or yellow wax added to make it stiffer.

*Zinc Oxide Ointment:* Vitamin A and vitamin D in a petrolatum-lanolin base.

*Lanolin:* A combination of the purified fat in sheeps' wool and water, with petrolatum added. Lanolin never becomes rancid.

*Water-Soluble Lubricant (K-4 Jelly):* Is used in certain situations where oil would be dangerous.

## Lotions and Solutions

*Aluminum Acetate Solution (Burow's Solution):* Used diluted with 10 to 40 parts of water. Aluminum subacetate solution, diluted in the same way, is used as a wet dressing. It soothes itching.

*Calamine Lotion:* A combination of drugs used for poison ivy rash, prickly heat rash, and insect bites.

## Powders

Powders are dusted on the skin to absorb small amounts of moisture; in very moist areas they cake and are not beneficial. Those containing antiseptic drugs also have a mild antiseptic action. Some commonly used powders are:

*Purified Talc:* A native magnesium silicate used to absorb moisture and soothe the skin.

*Zinc Stearate:* A fluffy white powder with a slightly slippery feel used for its antiseptic effect.

*Thymol Iodide (Aristol):* A powder containing a mixture of iodine derivatives of thymol used for its drying and antiseptic action.

## Antiseptics

It is impossible to sterilize the skin—antiseptics strong enough to destroy bacteria will injure it. Strong antiseptics cause irritation which makes it easier for bacteria to enter. Soap-and-water washing, using mild friction, followed by the application of a mild antiseptic does help to remove loose skin flakes and bacteria, thereby lessening the danger of infection.

Infectious skin lesions sometimes do occur, caused mostly by staphylococci and strepto-cocci which enter through broken skin. Certain drugs are helpful in combating such infections:

*Antibiotics:* Bacitracin is used in an ointment or powder. Tyrothricin is effective in wet dressings. Neomycin is applied to the lesion—sometimes it irritates the skin. Vioform and Xeroform are also helpful. Antibiotics are also given orally or by injection in treating such infections as boils or carbuncles.

*Ammoniated Mercury Ointment and Furacin (Ointment and Solution):* Effective preparations when applied to an infected area. Furacin sometimes causes allergic reaction.

## Antifungal Drugs

*Iso-Par:* An ointment used for fungal infections of the hands and feet and for eczemas of the ear. It is applied at bedtime and again in the morning.

*Asterol:* Especially effective for athlete's foot, for ringworm of the scalp, and for fungus infections around the nails. It is not suitable for treating young children who may carry the drug to their mouths with their fingers and so develop harmful side effects.

*Propion Gel:* A jelly used to treat vulvovaginal infections (moniliasis).

*Gentian Violet:* A dye with antiseptic properties, but it does stain clothing.

*Whitfield's Ointment:* A preparation containing a salicylic acid which is used in treating athlete's foot.

*Grifulvin and Fulvicin:* Comparatively new preparations for the treatment of fungus infections which can be taken orally at the same time ointments are being used.

## Pediculicides

Pediculicides are preparations used to kill lice (pediculi):

*Gexane and Kwell (Lotion or Ointment):* Applied to the scalp, will kill lice but will not kill nits (eggs). A 10 per cent solution of acetic acid or vinegar is effective in removing nits, with a shampoo and bath 24 hours after this application.

*Bornate:* Also effective, but since it is irritating to the skin, it must be removed after 10 minutes with a shampoo.

## Scabicides

Scabicides are drugs used in treating scabies, or itch, caused by the itch mite. The itch mite burrows under the skin and also attaches itself to clothing, especially in the seams. Therefore, to prevent reinfection after the application of scabicides, particular attention is given to sterilizing clothing and bed linen. The newer drugs are more effectve—1 application may be sufficient. More than 2 applications are almost sure to cause skin irritation.

*Gexane and Kwell:* Effective scabicides.

*Benylate and Albacide:* Preparations to be applied to the skin after it has been scrubbed with soap and water. After the first application has dried, a second one is applied to the worst areas. In 24 hours, the patient is given a warm bath, clean clothing, and clean bed linen.

Precautions which are necessary in using pediculicides and scabicides are: (1) to avoid causing skin irritation by too frequent applications and (2) to keep the preparations away from the eyes or the mouth.

## Stimulants and Irritants

Some drugs stimulate healing in skin lesions and wounds by their mildly irritating action. Tars obtained from wool or coal, such as juniper tar, cade oil, coal tar have this effect. Some of them are used in treating psoriasis. Compound Benzoin Tincture is often used for bedsores, ulcers, cracked lips, or anal fissures.

Other drugs, the *kerolytics,* are used to soften scales and loosen the outer layers of the skin. Salicylic acid and Resorcinol are used for corns, warts, fungus infections, and chronic dermatitis. These preparations are available as plasters, ointments, or combined with collodion.

## Antipruritics

Drugs used to relieve itching are called antipruritics. Progress in understanding skin disorders has given us new remedies for itching. Hydrocortisone (lotion or ointment) is an effective remedy. Other remedies that can be taken internally are small doses of barbiturates, preparations or ergotamine (Gynergen), and the antihistamine drugs (Caladryl or Benadryl).

Lotions, pastes, or ointments are effective also. Dressings wet with potassium permanganate (1 to 4000), boric acid, or normal saline solution are soothing, as are calamine lotion, starch baths, and other types of soaks.

## Protectives

Protective drugs are soothing because they form a thin film over the skin. They should be nonabsorbable and nondrying and should not soften the skin. Two effective protectives are preparations of collodion and adhesive plaster. Nonabsorbable powders are sometimes used as protectives, but they are not very satisfactory because they must be scraped off moist surfaces and will not adhere to dry surfaces.

Some water-soluble protectives (solution or ointment) are used for their soothing and deodorizing effect and for stimulation of healing in ulcers, burns, or wounds. Chloresium is such a drug.

# THE ANTIBIOTICS

An antibiotic is a substance, produced by microorganisms, which destroys other microorganisms or prevents their growth. Sir Alexander Fleming, an English scientist, made this discovery in 1928 when he noticed that a Penicillium mold on some staphylococcus organisms was inhibiting their growth. He extracted the effective substance from the mold and named it *penicillin.* Further study and experiments in using penicillin to fight disease yielded spectacular results, but they were mostly temporary because the supply of the drug was insufficient for prolonged treatment or large doses. In 1941, wartime needs for an antibiotic became so pressing that the United States began to manufacture penicillin on a large scale. Since then, many other antibiotics have been made available for the treatment of infections and are widely used. Some antibiotics can be made synthetically.

## The Action of Antibiotics

Antibiotics interfere with the nourishment of microorganisms, inhibiting their growth and weakening them so that the normal body defenses are able to destroy them. Antibiotics may also destroy bacteria outright. Antibiotics are classified as broad-spectrum, if they are effective against many organisms, and specific or narrow-spectrum, if they are effective against a few microorganisms. A microorganism may not be susceptible to the action of an antibiotic or it may develop resistance. Resistance is the power of a microorganism to "hold out" against an antibiotic—to remain unaffected by it.

Antibiotics may sensitize a patient if they are used indiscriminately for every minor ailment. Medical authorities discourage this use of antibiotics which may create a hypersensitivity and, therefore, makes it dangerous to use a drug when it is really needed for a severe infection.

## Desired Characteristics of Antibiotics

*Selectivity:* The drug should kill the microorganism and yet should not harm the patient. It is better if the drug is a broad-spectrum antibiotic meaning that it is effective against many microorganisms.

*Bacteriocidal:* The drug should kill bacteria and not just slow down the growth (bacteriostatic).

*Antiresistant:* It is very undesirable if the drug induces organisms to produce resistance. Thus, the best antibiotic is the one against which organisms will not form mutations, rendering the antibiotic ineffective. Sometimes, antibiotics are given in combination to reduce the danger of organisms building up resistance.

*Nontoxic:* The drug should be able to be given in large doses without a great number of side-effects which would harm the patient.

*Versatile:* The drug should be able to be given in all ways; oral or parenteral.

*Stable:* The drug should be able to be stored at room temperature. Many antibiotics must be refrigerated or cannot be exposed to sunlight, making it difficult to preserve and use them. It is also desirable if the drug can be mixed easily and completely. This avoids mistakes in dosage.

## Selecting the Appropriate Antibiotic

It is important not to use antibiotics indiscriminately, to reduce the possibility of organisms building up resistance to the drug. Thus, the physician usually will take a sample (*culture*) of the wound or infected area and will have *sensitivity tests* done on this culture to determine which antibiotic would be the most effective in killing that particular organism.

In this way, the organism will be killed quickly and will not have the opportunity to create resistance. Cultures may be done of blood, sputum, pus or wound drainage, urine, or mucous membrane discharge.

## Antibiotics Today

At the present time, the *penicillins, streptomycin, erythromycin,* and the *tetracyclines* are the most effective and most widely used antibiotics. In some infections, any one of several antibiotics will be effective—in others, only one will be of any value. Sometimes it takes a combination of antibiotics to control an infection. If there is a choice between several which are equally effective, usually the one given most often is the one which is the least expensive and the least toxic.

**Penicillin.** Penicillin is made from the common bluish grey mold (Penicillium) which we often find on fruit or bread. It interferes with the growth of those bacteria which are susceptible to it and kills many of them, provided that there is a sufficiently high concentration of the drug in the body. Penicillin is excreted rapidly in the urine and is remarkably free from toxic effects.

Its Action. Penicillin is most effective against the gram-positive organisms, such as streptococci, staphylococci, and pneumococci. It is also active against some gram-negative organisms, such as gonococci and meningococci and against the *treponema* which causes syphilis. However, some of the gonococci and staphylococci have become resistant to it. It is not effective against the tubercle bacillus or in viral infections or typhoid fever. It is a narrow-spectrum antibiotic.

Methods of Giving Penicillin. This drug can be given in a variety of ways. The commonly used methods are:

*Intramuscular (I.M.):* This is the method most often used to give the slower acting penicillins most widely used at the present time.

*Intravenous (I.V.):* Penicillin is given intravenously in severe infections when quick action is needed.

*Oral (O):* This is the easiest method of giving penicillin and is usually effective for all but the most severe infections. Gastric secretions destroy some of the drug, so the oral dose is larger.

## TABLE 33–1.  PENICILLIN PREPARATIONS

| Preparation | Commonly Known Names | Method of Administration | Antibiotic |
|---|---|---|---|
| Ampicillin | Penbriten, Omnipen, Polycillin | O, I.M., I.V. | (Should not be used for resistant staph. organisms.) |
| Cloxacillin | Tegopen | O | |
| Potassium Penicillin G | benzyl penicillin potassium, Crystalline penicillin | I.M., I.V. | |
| Procaine Penicillin G | Crysticillin, Duracillin, Wycillin, Lentopen, Pronapen | I.M. | (Highest incidence of allergic reactions.) |
| Penicillin G Tablets | potassium or sodium | O | |
| Benzathine Penicillin G | Bicillin, Permapen, dibenzyl penicillin | O, I.M. | |
| Penicillin O | Cer-O-Cillin, Depo-Cer-O-Cillin | O, I.M. | |
| Penicillin V | V-Cillin-K, Pen-Vee K, V-Cillin, Pen-Vee, Compocillin | O | |
| Phenethicillin Potassium | penicillin 152, Alpen, Chemipen, Darcil, Maxipen, Ro-Cillin | O | (Semisynthetic) |
| Methicillin Sodium | Staphcillin, Dimocillin, Syncillin | I.M., I.V. | (Used especially against resistant staphylococcus organisms.) |
| Nafcillin Sodium | Unipen | O, I.M., I.V. | |
| Oxacillin Sodium | penicillin P-12, Prostaphlin, Resistopen | O, I.V. I.M. | |
| Penicillin Ointment† | | | |

\* I.M.: Intramuscular.　　I.V.: Intravenous.　　O: Oral.

† Rarely used—often causes allergic reactions.

SIDE-EFFECTS. Penicillin has almost no toxic effects even in large doses, except for the person who is sensitive to it. Then it causes an allergic reaction, which may be comparatively mild, causing hives or a rash. In severe cases, it may cause anaphylactic shock. (See Chapter 54 for a complete discussion of anaphylactic shock.) Patients with a history of allergy or of previous reaction to a drug should have a sensitivity test before receiving penicillin. Sometimes a patient is sensitive to one type of penicillin but not to another.

The usual treatment for a mild allergic reaction is an *antihistamine*. In severe reactions, epinephrine, aminophylline or oxygen may be given. Penicillinase (neutrapen), an enzyme which makes penicillin inactive, is sometimes recommended in allergic reactions.

TYPES OF PENICILLIN. Pencillin preparations are available in powder, liquid, or tablet form. The dosage is measured in units, grams, or milligrams. It varies with individual needs and with the type of penicillin—rapid acting or slow acting. For instance: 200,000 units of rapid-acting penicillin, given 3 to 8 times a day, may be increased to a million units every 3 hours in a severe infection; 300,000 to 400,000 units of slowly-absorbed penicillin may be given once a day or twice in 24 hours; and 600,000 to 1,200,000 units of long-acting penicillin may be given as a single dose and not repeated from several days to a month.

PENICILLIN PREPARATIONS. Many penicillin preparations are available, some of them in several forms suitable for every type of administration and others in fewer forms. Table 33-1 does not include every penicillin preparation, but it does include examples of those most commonly used and the variety of forms in which they are available. The commonly known names capitalized are the trade names. In some cases a penicillin preparation is best known by its generic name which is not capitalized. You must remember that there are only a few of the preparations, and that scientific researchers are constantly searching for and finding new ones.

**The Streptomycins.** Streptomycin is an antibiotic obtained from a fungus. *Dihydrostreptomycin* is obtained from streptomycin. The main use of streptomycin is in the treatment of tuberculosis to inhibit the growth of the tubercle bacillus; it is also effective for infections of the urinary tract and for infections resistant to penicillin. Tuberculosis requires prolonged treatment, and during this time the tuberculosis organisms may become resistant to streptomycin. PAS (para-aminosalicylic acid) is given at the same time to delay this effect. (See p. 620). Penicillin is also given with streptomycin for certain other infections, such as subacute bacterial endocarditis (SBE).

SIDE-EFFECTS. Streptomycin may cause toxic effects in the kidney and liver. Some individuals are allergic to this drug and develop rashes, hives, nausea, and vomiting. Deafness, dizziness, and vertigo are not uncommon as a result of damage to the 8th cranial nerve. This is most likely to happen with *dihydrostreptomycin*. The patient should drink a large quantity of fluids to help eliminate the drug.

PREPARATIONS. The commercial preparations of *streptomycin sulfate* are available in the form of powders and solutions. They are most effective when given intramuscularly because the intestinal tract does not absorb them readily. The dosage is determined by the intensity of the infection and by the susceptibility of the organism to the drug. One trade name is Lincocin.

**Erythromycin (Ilotycin, Erythrocin).** Erythromycin has much the same action as penicillin, but is not as effective. It is used against organisms that are resistant to penicillin or when a patient is allergic to penicillin. It is available in tablets, sterile solutions for injection, and in oral solutions. The usual dosage ranges from 1 to 2 Gm. a day.

SIDE-EFFECTS. Erythromycin has few toxic side-effects, although in large doses it may cause nausea, vomiting, and diarrhea. Patients rarely become hypersensitive to it.

**Chloramphenicol (Chloromycetin).** Chloramphenicol is a synthetic preparation which is effective against many gram-positive and gram-negative bacteria and against certain large viruses; it is *the* antibiotic effective against typhoid fever. It is also effective against organisms resistant to penicillin, thus, it is a wide-spectrum antibiotic.

SIDE-EFFECTS. Chloromycetin may cause nausea, vomiting, and diarrhea. However, its most serious toxic effects is on the bone marrow, causing aplastic anemia. For this reason frequent blood examinations are made to detect signs of harmful effects. It may be given by injection, but is most often used orally to reduce the possibility of side-effects.

PREPARATIONS

*Chloramphenicol (Chloromycetin):* capsules, solutions, ointments, 1 to 4 Gm. daily
*Chloramphenicol Palmitate:* oral

**The Tetracyclines.** The tetracyclines are broad-spectrum antibiotics. They are effective against a wide variety of organisms, such as cocci and bacilli and certain viruses. These drugs are easily absorbed in the gastrointestinal tract and are usually given by mouth, but are also available in solutions for intramuscular or intravenous injection. They are not effective against true viruses, such as those causing the common cold or polio.

SIDE-EFFECTS. Compared with other antibiotics, the tetracyclines have a few toxic side-effects. Those which do occur are chiefly in the gastrointestinal tract, such as nausea, vomiting, and diarrhea. Giving the drug with milk or with sodium bicarbonate often reduces these effects. Symptoms of gastric irritation or vaginitis should be reported because they are signs of developing infections due to the suppression of helpful bacteria. Large doses of tetracycline may cause liver damage. Declomycin may cause hypersensitivity to sunburn or brown discoloration of the teeth in children.

PREPARATIONS

*Aureomycin Hydrochloride, Achromycin Oxytetracycline Hydrochloride (terramycin), Chlortetracycline (declomycin), Steclin, Nystatin, Panmycin, Sumycin, Tetrex* and *Declomycin Hydrochloride:* Oral, 25 to 500 mg. every 6 hours, occasionally given I.M. or I.V.

## Antibiotics With Special Usefulness

The antibiotics discussed in detail on previous pages are those which are most effective and most widely used. Other antibiotics are more limited in their usefulness but are very valuable in special conditions, such as in treating infections resistant to the commonly used antibiotics (such as penicillin). Among these less frequently used antibiotics are:

*Seromycin:* Used with other drugs in treating tuberculosis.

*Kanamycin (Kantrex):* Active against many forms of staphylococci, especially in the urinary tract, the respiratory tract, and in soft tissue infections.

*Cephalothin Sodium (Keflin):* Only used parenterally. Especially useful in patient with poor kidney function.

*Neomycin Sulfate (Mycifradin, Myacyne):* Used in serious infections which do not respond to the safer antibiotics, but only as a last resort because it has dangerous effects on the kidneys and the 8th cranial nerve.

*Novobiocin (Albamycin, Cathomycin):* Used for certain staphylococcal infections or when a patient is allergic to other antibiotics. Patients easily become sensitized to it and develop skin rashes and urticaria (hives).

*Matromycin:* Used when commonly used antibiotics are not effective.

*Cyclamycin, Spontin, Vancocin:* Especially effective against staphylococcal infections.

*Viomycin Sulfate (Vinactane, Viocin):* Used in tuberculosis infections resistant to other drugs.

*Fumagillin (Fumidil):* Used for intestinal amebic infections.

*Colistin (Colymyan):* Is a narrow-spectrum drug which is effective against gram-negative organisms. It is given I.M., and its side-effects include visual and speech disturbances.

## A Last Word

As with other drugs, you may not find that every antibiotic used to treat infections is listed here. New ones are appearing all the time. The U.S.P. and manuals on drugs will help to keep you up to date. What you should know about antibiotics in general is that:

1. Certain antibiotics are widely used because they are effective against many organisms.

2. Other antibiotics may be used because they are effective against organisms that are resistant to the commonly used antibiotics.

3. Certain antibiotics are used because an individual is sensitive to the commonly used ones.

4. The dosage prescribed depends on the severity of the illness and the resistance of the organism to the drug.

5. The side-effects of antibiotics vary; some have very few or mild side-effects; others may have side-effects that are serious and can cause permanent damage in the body. It is important to know the possible side-effects of an antibiotic and to be alert in observing and reporting them.

## THE SULFONAMIDES

Since the advent of penicillin and other antibiotics, the sulfonamides are not used as much as they were in the past. They are, however, effective against certain types of infections, and are used in the patient who is allergic to penicillin and other antibiotics. They are recommended for use in such conditions as trachoma, urinary tract infections, toxoplasmosis, malaria, and chancroid, and as an alternative to penicillin in the prevention of rheumatic fever (sulfadiazine). The sulfas can damage the kidneys, so that the patient must "force fluids" to eliminate the drug.

The commonly used sulfonamides are:

*Sulfisoxazole (Gantrisin):* A specific drug for urinary tract infections.

*Azo-Gantrisin:* a combination of Gantrisin and an antiseptic dye.

*Succinylsulfathiazole (Sulfasuxidine):* Used for antiseptic bowel preparation prior to gastrointestinal surgery.

*Sulfadiazine:* Used in meningococcal meningitis, because it can penetrate into the spinal fluid.

*Sulfamethoxypyridazine (Kynex):* Used in several types of infections. More long-acting than the previously mentioned sulfonamides.

## DRUGS WHICH AFFECT THE CENTRAL NERVOUS SYSTEM

The nervous system affects many body processes. When its functions are disturbed, certain drugs will increase or decrease the activity of the nerve centers in the brain or in the nerve pathways. *Stimulants* help to speed up certain mental and physical processes; *depressants* slow them down.

## STIMULANTS

Many drugs have a stimulating effect on the central nervous system, but only a few of them are especially valuable for that purpose. The most valuable are: (1) drugs that stimulate the respiratory centers in the brain, and (2) drugs that alleviate depression and make people more mentally alert and counteract the toxic effects of depressant drugs, such as overdoses of barbiturates.

**Caffeine.** Caffeine is obtained commercially from tea leaves, but it is also found in the coffee bean and so is present in the beverages we call tea and coffee. Actually, tea leaves contain more caffeine than coffee beans, but in this country we are likely to make our coffee stronger than we do our tea—naturally, this increases the amount of caffeine we consume, since we are a nation of coffee drinkers.

The main value of caffeine is as a stimulant to the respiratory center of the brain, but it also acts as a mild stimulant to the thinking centers, to make a person more alert and less aware of fatigue.

SIDE-EFFECTS. The side-effects of caffeine are restlessness, irritability, insomnia, heart palpitation, and some increase in the output of urine. Signs of mild caffeine poisoning often appear in people who work at night. Night nurses who habitually depend on large amounts of coffee to keep them alert when they are sleepy or physically exhausted may develop these symptoms. People who are used to drinking moderate amounts of tea or coffee ever day develop a tolerance for caffeine. Coke is also high in caffeine content.

PREPARATIONS. The most widely used preparations of caffeine are:

*Citrated Caffeine:* Powder, tablet, oral, 0.3 Gm. (5 gr.)

*Ergotamine With Caffeine (Cafegot):* Tablets, oral, 1 to 2 tablets
*Caffeine Sodium Benzoate:* Liquid in ampul, oral, I.M., 0.5 Gm. (7½ gr.)

**Amphetamine.** Amphetamine is a synthetic drug which increases energy and alertness, overcomes sleepiness, and increases muscle strength. It also stimulates the respiratory center and depresses appetite.

SIDE-EFFECTS. It is dangerous to take amphetamine regularly as "pep pills" because it can obscure signs of fatigue which may be symptoms of an underlying condition which should be corrected. It is dangerous for people with cardiovascular disease or hypertension or for those who are overly anxious or excited. It is also a habit-forming drug. It may cause mouth dryness, insomnia, and irritability.

PREPARATIONS
*Amphetamine Sulfate (Benzedrine):* Tablets, capsules, solution, oral, inj.
*Amphetamine Phosphate (Raphetamine):* Tablets, liquid, capsules, oral
*Phenmetrazine Hydrochloride (Preludin):* Tablets, oral, 25 mg.
*Dextro Amphetamine Sulfate (Dexedrine):* Tablets, liquid, capsules, oral

Two other preparations having fewer toxic side-effects are Pipradol Hydrochloride (Meratran Hydrochloride) and Methylphenidate Hydrochloride (Ritalin Hydrochloride). They are used to relieve depression and to restore a sense of worthwhileness to people who feel life does not matter any more. They are also effective in counteracting the effects of oversedation. Other mood elevators known by the trade names of Marsalid, Marplan, Niamid, Tofranil, and Nardil are used also to relieve depression. Picrotoxin, Coramine, and Metrazol are especially useful to counteract the depressant effects of overdoses of barbiturates. Strychnine, once widely used as a stimulant, is rarely used today for medical purposes. Occasionally, instances of strychnine poisoning do occur.

Some other mood elevators or antianxiety drugs commonly used are Elavil, which is often used in psychiatry to relieve depression and anxiety, and often to eliminate the need for electroshock therapy, and Parnate, Deaner,

Alertonic, Aventyl, Vivactil, Desoxyn, and Vio-Dex. The nurse must constantly be aware of the dependency-producing potential of these drugs (see Chapter 57).

## DEPRESSANTS

Drugs that depress the activities of the central nervous system are (1) *analgesics* to relieve pain, (2) *hypnotics* and *sedatives* to bring rest and sleep, and (3) *general anesthetics* to cause loss of consciousness. In addition to discussing these depressants, we will consider also some of the drugs known as "selective depressants" which are used for the symptomatic treatment of various conditions.

### Analgesics

The analgesic drugs relieve pain but do not cause unconsciousness. The patient may go to sleep because he is more comfortable, but the drug does not induce sleep.

**Narcotic Analgesics.** Opium is the hardened dried juice of a poppy which is grown mostly in China, India, Iran, and Asia Minor. It was first used in its crude form by physicians in Greece and Arabia; later, it was found that the effective component of opium was the alkaloid, morphine. This led to the discovery of other useful opium alkaloids; those most widely used are morphine, codeine, and papaverine. Morphine and codeine mainly affect the central nervous system; papaverine affects smooth muscles.

All drugs produced from opium or opium derivatives or having habit-forming effects are subject to the narcotic regulations of the Harrison Narcotic Act.

If a drug is covered by the Federal Narcotic Act, it must be accounted for properly, and kept under double lock at all times. When a dose is taken out of the medication cupboard, it must be signed out according to the patient who is to receive it, the doctor who ordered it, the time taken, and the nurse who is to administer it. It must be charted immediately after being given.

The drugs which must be counted are counted by 2 nurses at the beginning of each shift. (One of these is the nurse going off duty and the other is the one coming on duty.) The count must agree or a search is undertaken to find the missing drug.

The nurse who is carrying the narcotic keys has a responsibility to keep track of the keys and to make sure that they are turned over to the next nurse in charge. If you ask for the keys, you should wear them on the outside of your uniform, perhaps on your name tag or pinned to your collar, so that you will not forget and take them home with you. It is a good idea for the student practical nurse not to keep the keys but to return them immediately after use. In some instances and some hospitals, practical nursing students are not allowed to give narcotics.

MORPHINE (MORPHINE SULFATE). The most important function of morphine is its ability to relieve severe pain and so bring rest and sleep. It also relieves fear and anxiety and promotes a feeling of well-being. It is helpful in checking peristalsis in such conditions as diarrhea, peritonitis, or stomach and bowel surgery. It relieves apprehension before an anesthetic, and it keeps a patient quiet after pulmonary hemorrhage.

*Side-Effects.* Morphine depresses respiration—severe morphine poisoning may cause respiratory failure and death. It contracts the pupil of the eye and may cause nausea and vomiting. In toxic amounts, it lowers blood pressure and slows the heart rate. Because it slows peristalsis, it may cause constipation. Allergic reactions to morphine occur fairly frequently.

Morphine is not recommended to relieve pain when a milder drug will do as well. This is especially true of pain in a prolonged illness since habit-formation is almost sure to occur. Exceptions are such painful conditions as inoperable or terminal cancer when recovery is impossible and morphine is the patient's only source of comfort and relief. Morphine is more effective if it is given before pain becomes extreme. Nurses sometimes withhold a dose of morphine as long as possible for fear of encouraging addiction. There is little or no danger of habit formation when morphine is given for a short time to relieve severe pain, which in itself can be damaging.

*Poisoning.* Opium or morphine poisoning is usually the result of an attempted suicide. The usual dosage is ⅛ to ¼ gr.; 1 grain is a toxic dose, and 4 gr. is a fatal dose. The significant early symptoms of poisoning are *slow respirations* (less than 12 per minute), *deep sleep,* and *constricted pupils.* Emergency treatment begins with respiratory stimulants such as nikethamide, caffeine and sodium benzoate, amphetamine, or ephedrine. If breathing decreases dangerously, artificial respiration followed by intratracheal oxygen are used. The stomach is emptied if the drug has been taken by mouth and strong black coffee as hot as it is safe to give may be given by tube, mouth, or rectum.

SYNTHETIC SUBSTITUTES FOR MORPHINE. Some synthetic drugs are now available which are effective pain relievers and have fewer unfavorable side-effects than morphine. Some of these drugs are meperidine hydrochloride (Demerol), Methadone Hydrochloride (Dolophine, Adenon), Alphaprodine (Nisentil), and Oxycadone (Percodan, Eucodol). These drugs are also covered by the Narcotic Law.

DEMEROL. Demerol is used instead of morphine to relieve pain which is not severe. Demerol acts quickly, but its effect is not prolonged. It is often used before anesthesia. It is less likely than morphine to cause nausea and vomiting, and normal doses have few ill effects on respiration or heart action. Demerol is often given to obstetric patients in combination with other drugs.

*Side-Effects.* Demerol may cause dizziness, nausea and vomiting, headache, and fainting, and in toxic amounts may cause dilated pupils, mental confusion, convulsions, respiratory depression, and death. It is definitely habit-forming, perhaps even more so than morphine.

METHADONE HYDROCHLORIDE. Methadone is much like morphine in that it is an effective pain reliever and has similar lasting effects. It is slightly more effective than morphine in relieving chronic pain and is effective for cough.

*Side-Effects.* Like morphine, it may cause nausea and vomiting, itching, constipation, and respiratory depression. It is also habit-forming.

OTHER SUBSTITUTES FOR MORPHINE. Other preparations used as morphine substitutes are Nisentil, Levo-Dromoran Tartrate, and Prinadol. Some of the drugs which are used effectively in combating narcotic poisoning are Nalline Hydrochloride and Lorfan Tartrate (narcotic antagonists).

CODEINE. Codeine is a derivative of morphine, but its action is milder. It is especially effective in relieving a dry cough, but it also relieves minor irritations and mild pain. It is less depressing than morphine and less habit-forming; it is also less constipating. Codeine is a common ingredient of cough mixtures, such as terpin hydrate and codeine elixir.

PAPAVERINE. Papaverine is not a pain reliever, but is useful in relaxing muscle spasm and is less depressing than morphine.

DILAUDID. Dilaudid (dihydromorphinone hydrochloride) is prepared from morphine and has about 5 times the analgesic effect of morphine, but the effect does not last as long. The effect is prolonged if the drug is given by suppository. It causes very little drowsiness, nausea, or vomiting but does depress respiration. Dilaudid is an addictive drug.

OMNOPON (Pantopon) is similar to morphine, but is sometimes tolerated by patients who are overly sensitive to morphine.

OPIUM TINCTURE. Opium Tincture (Laudanum) and camphorated opium tincture (Paregoric) are liquids used to check peristalsis. These preparations are always given by mouth. Brown's Mixture is a compound of opium and glycerin which is used as a cough mixture.

*Preparations.* Opium preparations and average doses are:

*Morphine:* Tablet, hypodermic, 0.01 Gm. (⅙ gr.)

*Codeine:* Tablet, hypodermic, oral, 0.03 Gm. (½ gr.)

*Dilaudid:* Tablet, hypodermic, oral, rectal (suppository), 0.002 Gm. (1/30 gr.)

*Metopon:* Tablet, oral, 0.003 Gm. (1/20 gr.)

*Paregoric:* Liquid, oral, 4 cc. (1 fluid dram)

*Brown's Mixture:* Liquid, oral, 4 cc. (1 fluid dram)

**Non-Narcotic Analgesics.** There are certain drugs such as Darvon, which relieve pain but are not prepared from opium and are not habit-forming. They may be used alone or combined with other drugs as aspirin; Zactirin is such a drug.

Colchicine is a drug that is used to relieve acute attacks of pain in gout. It is also helpful in preventing such attacks.

Signs of toxic side-effects from colchicine are nausea and vomiting, abdominal pain, and diarrhea. Scanty urine and blood in the urine are signs of kidney damage. In severe poisoning, death may result from impaired heart action and respiratory failure. Some new drugs are being tested for their effects in gout (see Chapter 45).

**Narcotic Antagonists.** Certain drugs offset the undesirable effects of narcotics and are given in cases of overdose and other instances. These include Nalorphine hydrochloride (Nalline), which is also covered by the Federal Narcotics Law, and Lavallorphan tartrate (Lorfan). Both are given parenterally and are not addictive.

**Antipyretics.** Some non-narcotic drugs have the ability to both reduce fever and relieve pain. These drug preparations, products of salicylic acid or of coal tar, are not habit-forming and are comparatively inexpensive.

THE SALICYLATES. The salicylates are derived from salicylic acid and are most effective in relieving pain in the joints and muscles and in reducing fever by increasing the elimination of heat from the body. Normal doses of salicylates do not affect respiration or harm the heart. Salicylates do not cause sleep and are not habit-forming. They are readily absorbed from the stomach and duodenum and are excreted rapidly by the kidneys. Therefore, the patient should "force fluids." These drugs sometimes give the urine a brownish-green color. They will reduce the misery of a cold or influenza, but they will not "cure" it. They are specifically effective for headache, neuralgia, rheumatoid arthritis, rheumatic fever, and dysmenorrhea. The most widely used preparations of salicylic acid are aspirin and sodium salicylate.

*Acetylsalicylic Acid (Aspirin ASA).* Aspirin is a bitter drug available in tablets (plain or enteric-coated) or capsules. The usual dose for adults is 0.6 Gm. (10 gr.) every 3 or 4 hours as necessary. Candy-coated tablets or flavored chewable tablets of 65 mg. (1 gr.) are available for children. They should be kept out of a child's reach since they may be mistaken for candy.

*Sodium Salicylate.* Sodium salicylate is a powder that tastes salty-sweet and is available in 300 mg. and 600 mg. (5 and 10 gr.) plain or enteric-coated tablets. Like aspirin, it should be given with large amounts of water. It is absorbed more rapidly than aspirin, but it has similar effects. The usual dose is 0.6

Gm. (10 gr.) as often as is necessary. It is also available in ampules for intravenous injection when it is desirable to give large amounts of the drug.

*Methyl Salicylate (Wintergreen Oil).* This preparation is very irritating and cannot be used internally (except as flavoring). It is no longer considered valuable as a remedy for pain in joints or muscles when applied externally—in fact, it has poisoned children when applied over a large area of the skin.

*Phenyl Salicylate.* This is mainly used to coat tablets (enteric coating) to keep irritating drugs from dissolving in the stomach.

*Salicylic Acid.* This is too irritating to be taken orally, but it is often used in ointments and other preparations. So-called "corn removers" contain salicylic acid.

*Side-Effects.* The salicylates have remarkably few toxic side-effects, but if they are used extensively for every minor discomfort they can cause mild poisoning, with such symptoms as dizziness, ringing in the ears, hearing and vision disturbances, nausea and vomiting, and diarrhea. They may also cause skin eruptions and other allergic symptoms. Extreme reactions result in respiratory depression with labored breathing, coma, and an unsteady pulse and blood pressure. Children are especially susceptible to overdosage, and since aspirin is likely to be considered a harmless drug, it is often left where children have easy access to it. Salicylates should never be given to children indiscriminately.

**The Coal Tar Analgesics.** This group of drugs is derived from coal tar products; they are used to relieve pain and reduce fever, mainly headache and muscle aches. Headache remedies often contain one or more of these drugs.

SIDE-EFFECTS. The prolonged use of these drugs, as in taking a proprietary headache remedy, may cause poisoning. The symptoms are nausea and vomiting, sweating, skin eruption, cyanosis, slow respirations, and slow, weak pulse. Some people seem to be susceptible to these drugs while others show no ill effects from them. Some of them may damage the blood and bone marrow. Symptoms of fever, malaise, sore throat, and ulcerated mucous membranes should be reported at once.

PREPARATIONS. The most widely used preparations in this group with their average dosage are:

*Acetophenetidin (Phenacetin):* Oral, 0.3 Gm. (5 gr.)

*Antipyrine (Phenazone, Felsol):* Oral, 0.3 Gm. (5 gr.)

*Acetaminophen (Apamide):* Oral, 0.3 Gm. (5 gr.)

*Acetanilid:* Oral, 0.3 Gm. (5 gr.)

*Acetylsalicylic Acid, Acetophenetidin and Caffeine Capsules (APC Capsules):* Oral

PHENYLBUTAZONE (BUTAZOLIDIN). This is a synthetic preparation which is chemically related to the antipyrines. It is a highly potent drug in relieving pain in rheumatoid arthritis, bursitis, etc. Because of the high incidence of its toxic effects, it is usually not recommended, unless other drugs are ineffective. It may be used in acute attacks of gout and to reduce the accumulation of uric acid in the blood.

*Side-Effects.* The serious side-effects include edema, hepatis, hypertension, and a deficiency in white blood cells. Patients taking this drug are closely observed and have frequent blood examinations for signs of toxic effect. Other side-effects include nausea, skin rash, and dizziness.

SYNTHETIC NON-NARCOTIC ANALGESICS. The most commonly used drug in this classification is propoxyphene hydrochloride (Darvon), which relieves mild to moderate pain. It is sometimes used in combination with aspirin and is generally nonaddicting. Other drugs in this classification include Zactirin and Talwin.

Other non-narcotic analgesics which are also an antipyretic include Tylenol, aspirin, which has already been mentioned, and Indocin, which is a potent anti-inflammatory drug. Indocin may be used in such conditions as arthritis, although its undesirable side-effects often outweigh its beneficial effects. The side-effects include stomach ulcerations, severe indigestion and nausea, dizziness, and bone marrow depression.

## Hypnotics and Sedatives

Sleeplessness is not always caused by pain; a hospital patient may be disturbed by unfamiliar noises, lack of privacy, personal worries, or minor discomforts, such as cold feet, backache, and too much or too little fresh air; he may even be hungry or thirsty. A nurse can correct many of these irritations without drugs, but sometimes drugs are necessary to assure adequate rest and sleep. A *hypnotic* is given at bedtime and produces sleep rather quickly. A *sedative* is given in divided doses throughout the day and has a soothing, quieting effect so the patient naturally sleeps better at night. The tranquilizing drugs have effects similar to sedatives (see p. 354). Because of the possible dangers from overdose, many barbiturates and sedatives are counted by the nurses in the same way as are the narcotics.

**The Barbiturates.** The ideal hypnotic acts quickly, brings a natural sleep without "hangovers," is not habit-forming, and does not have harmful effects on the body. The search for this kind of drug has given us hundreds of barbiturates, but for one reason or another, only a few of them approximate these requirements. These drugs are widely used and can be obtained only through a doctor's prescription. Formerly, anyone could purchase barbiturates over the counter anywhere, and they were—and still are—often used indiscriminately—sometimes for suicide attempts.

Barbiturates produce sleep; they quiet restless and nervous patients; they relieve tension in patients with such emotionally-upsetting conditions as colitis or gastric ulcer; they prevent and control convulsive seizures. Barbiturates are used before anesthesia and for obstetric sedation. In psychiatry, they lessen a patient's resistance to treatment and enable him to be more cooperative.

Barbiturates are easily absorbed and can be given orally or by injection. Preparations are available for many types of action—ultrashort, short, intermediate, and long-acting.

SIDE-EFFECTS. The patient may have "hangover" reactions—he may be depressed and listless or emotionally disturbed. Sometimes a barbiturate causes a skin rash or urticaria hives or can even precipitate an asthmatic attack. It may cause restlessness and unpleasant dreams or delirium. Elderly patients, especially, are likely to become confused and need careful watching if they must get up to go to the bathroom at night or look after themselves in other ways. Severe poisoning causes a deep sleep or stupor—the patient becomes comatose, with slow or rapid and shal-

## TABLE 33–2. COMMONLY USED BARBITURATES

| Preparation | Usual Adult Dose | Usual Method of Administration | Length of Action |
|---|---|---|---|
| Barbital, N.F. (Veronal); Barbitone Sodium B.P.* | 300 mg. (5 gr.) | Orally | Long acting |
| Phenobarbital, U.S.P. (Luminal); Phenobarbitone, B.P.* | 30-100 mg. (½ to 1½ gr.) | Orally | Long acting |
| Mephobarbital, U.S.P. (Mebaral) | 400-600 mg. (6 to 10 gr.) | Orally | Long acting |
| Metharbital (Gemonil) | 100 mg. (1½ gr.) | Orally | Long acting |
| Amobarbital, U.S.P. (Amytal)* | 100 mg. (1½ gr.) | Orally | Intermediate |
| Aprobarbital, N.F. (Alurate) | 60-120 mg. (1 to 2 gr.) | Orally | Intermediate |
| Probarbital Sodium (Ipral Sodium) | 120-250 mg. (2 to 4 gr.) | Orally | Intermediate |
| Butethal (Neonal) | 100 mg. (1½ gr.) | Orally | Intermediate |
| Butabarbital Sodium, N.F. (Butisol Sodium) | 8-60 mg. (⅛ to 1 gr.) | Orally | Intermediate |
| Pentobarbital Sodium, U.S.P. (Nembutal Sodium); Pentobarbitone Sodium, B.P. | 100 mg. (1½ gr.) | Orally; rectally | Short acting |
| Secobarbital Sodium, U.S.P. (Seconal Sodium); Quinalbarbitone Sodium, B.P. | 100-200 mg. (1½ to 3 gr.) | Orally; rectally | Short acting |
| Cyclobarbital Calcium, N. F. (Phanodorn); Cyclobarbitone, B.P. | 200 mg. (3 gr.) | Orally | Short acting |
| Butallylonal (Pernoston) | 200 mg. (3 gr.) | Orally | Short acting |
| Hexobarbital Sodium, N.F. (Evipal Sodium) | 2-4 ml. 10% | Intravenously | Ultrashort acting |
| Thiopental Sodium, U.S.P. (Pentothal Sodium); Thiopentone Sodium, B.P. | 2-3 ml. 2.5% in 10 to 15 sec. repeated in 30 sec. as required | Intravenously | Ultrashort acting |

From Krug, E. E.: Pharmacology in Nursing, St. Louis, Mosby, 1963.
* Sodium salts are available.

low breathing and a weak, rapid pulse. This may lead to death from respiratory failure.

Slow poisoning from barbiturates may also occur with such symptoms as mental confusion and depression, loss of memory and incoherent speech, weight loss, gastrointestinal upsets, and anemia. The person's judgment is impaired to the extent that it is unsafe for him to drive a car or to work with machines. Poor motor coordination makes him liable to injury from falls; he may fall asleep while smoking or may turn on the gas burner and forget to light it. Also, a person may become addicted to barbiturates if he takes them every day in fairly large doses for a long period of time. Many opium addicts are also barbiturate addicts who take these drugs when they cannot get opiates—a habit which some authorities consider even more undesirable than opium addiction.

Overdosage is fairly common, due either to suicidal intentions or because a dose does not seem to be effective and the person takes more tablets when he is partially drowsy and does not know what he is doing.

PREPARATIONS. Phenobarbital (Luminal) does not take effect quickly, but its action lasts for 6 hours or more. It is useful in such nervous conditions as chorea (St. Vitus Dance), stomach and intestinal upsets and menopausal disturbances. It is also used to relieve tension before or after an operation. It is one of the least toxic drugs that can be given for epilepsy, but in doses large enough to control convulsions it is more depressing than the anticonvulsant drug, Dilantin (see p. 354). Phenobarbital is often given for a prolonged period after brain operations.

Phenobarbital sodium injection has the same uses as Luminal but is in injection form. A nurse must be careful to note this difference in these 2 preparations.

Table 33-2 lists some of the commonly used barbiturates.

**Other Hypnotics.** Some hypnotics that once were widely used have been replaced by the barbiturates. Others that are used less extensively than they formerly were are still recommended because they have the advantages of quick action and a wide margin of safety.

PARALDEHYDE. Paraldehyde is a hypnotic that depresses the central nervous system to bring almost natural sleep in 10 to 15 minutes after it is given, in spite of pain. It is especially effective in preventing possible convulsive seizures or for extreme nervous excitability in such conditions as tetanus, strychnine poisoning, delirium tremens, or maniacal behavior. It is sometimes given rectally to children before an anesthetic. The usual adult oral dose is 8 ml. (2 fluid drams), which should be given in fruit juice or in a flavored syrup or very cold wine to hide its disagreeable odor and taste and to mitigate its irritating effect on the throat and stomach. Paraldehyde can also be given by rectum and intramuscularly in a sterile solution.

*Side-Effects.* The disadvantages of paraldehyde are its unpleasant taste and odor and its irritating effect on the stomach unless it is well diluted. Paraldehyde is partially excreted by the lungs, and consequently the breath reeks of the drug; it is seldom given to patients who are up and about. It is an excep-

tionally safe drug and if mild poisoning does occur, the effects can usually be "slept off" in the same way as alcohol poisoning. The symptoms of poisoning are like those of chloral hydrate poisoning. It is possible to become addicted to paraldehyde.

CHLORAL HYDRATE. Chloral hydrate is a sedative which has a hypnotic effect in cases of insomnia not caused by pain. (Chloral hydrate is not a pain-reliever.) It is one of the best hypnotics; it acts quickly (in 10 to 15 minutes) and brings nearly natural sleep for 5 or more hours. It has a wide safety range and is inexpensive. Its disadvantages are its unpleasant taste and its irritating effect on the stomach. However, it can be given in capsule form and as a suppository. The usual dose is 500 mg., given 3 times a day.

*Side-Effects.* Taken orally, chloral hydrate may cause nausea and vomiting. Symptoms of poisoning are those of depression, profound sleep, stupor, coma, fall in blood pressure, slow respiration, weak, slow pulse, and cyanosis. Long range effects are kidney and liver damage. It is never given to patients with heart disease or to those with disturbed kidney or liver functions. Habitual users of the drug may show signs of nervous and gastrointestinal disturbances, skin irritations, and weakness.

THE BROMIDES. The bromides (especially sodium bromide) once widely used for their sedative effects have largely been replaced by more effective drugs. They are still found in some headache remedies. They have a slowly depressing effect on the nervous system.

OTHER NONBARBITURATE SEDATIVES AND HYPNOTICS. These include Placydil, Doriden, and Noludar.

## Selective Depressants

**The Anticonvulsant Drugs.** Convulsive seizures are signs of brain disorders associated with changes in the electrical activity of the brain. Anticonvulsant drugs are nervous system depressants which help to prevent or to control the different types of seizures which vary from mild to severe forms. The safest and the most effective drugs in use today are phenobarbital, Dilantin, and Tridione.

Other anticonvulsant drugs are Phenurone, Mesantoin, and Paradione, used for their specific effect on certain types of seizures. Still others now under investigation are Celontin, Mebaral, Mysoline, and Milontin.

PHENOBARBITAL. Phenobarbital (Luminal) is effective for almost all types of seizures and is one of the safest anticonvulsant drugs. However, it has one disadvantage: it must often be given in such large doses that it causes sleepiness and sluggishness.

DILANTIN. Dilantin controls grand mal seizures, but does not cause drowsiness or mental deterioration (see p. 351). It can be taken orally; the usual dose is 100 mg., 3 times a day which may be increased if necessary. Side-effects may be nervousness, dizziness, loss of muscle coordination, and blurred vision. Sometimes the patient has hallucinations and tremor, with nausea and vomiting. Dilantin is sometimes combined with other drugs, such as phenobarbital (Hydantal) or Mebaral.

TRIDIONE. Tridione is especially effective in treating petit mal seizures in children. It must be given under careful supervision because it may have serious side-effects. Nausea and vomiting, skin eruptions, blurred vision, and sensitivity to light are signs of trouble. Periodic blood examinations are made because some patients taking this drug have developed aplastic anemia.

MAGNESIUM SULFATE. This is an anticonvulsant which is most often used in emergency situations.

**Alcohol.** Although alcohol is not considered to be a selective depressant, it is mentioned here as a drug which affects the nervous system. Alcoholism as a national health problem is discussed in Chapter 57.

**Ethyl Alcohol.** Once considered a stimulant to the nervous system, ethyl alcohol (ethanol) is now known to be a depressant. It has a variety of medicinal uses which are described under the various conditions for which it is used. Its chief uses are (1) as an *antiseptic* to disinfect and toughen the skin, (2) as a *solvent* for other drugs, and (3) as a *dilator* for surface blood vessels in impaired circulation.

SIDE-EFFECTS. Alcohol dilates skin blood vessels and causes heat loss—an intoxicated person is more likely to freeze to death than a sober one. Excessive consumption of alcohol eventually causes stomach and liver disturbances and poor nutrition. Alcohol adds nothing to food but calories. In excess, it can cause kidney and liver damage, arteriosclerosis, tremors, and muscular weakness. Its prolonged use or sudden withdrawal may result in the delusions of delirium tremens, with visions of snakes or other horrors, or in insanity.

**Methyl Alcohol (Wood Alcohol).** Taken internally, methyl alcohol is a destructive poison, which causes nausea and vomiting, abdominal pain, headache, and blurred vision which may lead to blindness. Fatal doses lead to convulsions, coma, and death.

**The Tranquilizers.** The tranquilizing drugs (*ataractics*) have been an aid to troubled patients in every type of illness. They calm the anxious and apprehensive; they relax the tense; they bring rest and sleep. Troubled people, sick or well, are unable to function at their best—indeed, extreme anxiety is in itself an illness.

The tranquilizers are especially effective in behavior disorders and in mental disease. They have spectacular effects on violent behavior in mental illness, although they cannot cure it. Unlike sedatives, they do not cause stupor and coma—the patient may go to sleep because he feels calmer and more relaxed but he can be awakened easily.

RESERPINE. Reserpine (Serpasil) is derived from the roots of a group of plants called *Rauwolfia*, which grow in India and various tropical regions. In these countries the powdered roots of the plant have long been used to treat mental illness. Reserpine calms and quiets without causing drowsiness, mental confusion, or insensibility. It gives people a feeling of well-being and makes them less sensitive to small irritations. It is most effective when it is used to treat mentally ill patients who are overactive, excited, and destructive. It does not relieve pain, nor does it help the depressed and withdrawn patient. In fact, it may actually harm him.

Because reserpine acts slowly, improvement may not be noticeable for several weeks after the patient has begun to take the drug, but it has lasting effects, even after it has been discontinued. Some patients continue to take small doses of the drug indefinitely. Reserpine is very valuable in making the disturbed patient receptive to psychotherapy, which he might otherwise resist. It is useful in treating some types of hypertension (see Chapter 47). It can be given orally, intramuscularly, or intravenously.

*Side-Effects.* Reserpine seems to have few toxic side-effects, but increased dosage may cause nasal stuffiness, diarrhea, and a gain in weight. Other undesirable effects that sometimes appear are nosebleeds, insomnia, anxiety, and fatigue, with skin eruptions and stomach irritation.

Other Rauwolfia preparations, similar to Serpasil in action, are Harmonyl and Moderil.

CHLORPROMAZINE. This drug is widely used to relieve tension, anxiety, and overactive behavior in psychotic and psychoneurotic patients. With the aid of chlorpromazine (Thorazine), many patients whose behavior made it necessary to confine them to mental institutions are now able to live at home. The drug does not cure mental disease, but it changes the patient's behavior to make it more acceptable. The dosage varies according to the needs of the individual patient.

*Side-Effects.* Chlorpromazine causes drowsiness and sleep which may be a desired effect in some instances. Other side-effects may be mouth dryness, nausea and vomiting, sensitivity to light, and dermatitis. Toxic effects, such as trembling, drooling, muscular rigidity, jaundice, sore throat, and anemia are warnings to discontinue the drug immediately.

Other newer drugs resembling chlorpromazine in their action are being used; time will tell how comparatively effective and safe they are.

MEPROBAMATE. Meprobamate (Miltown, Equanil) is a calming drug which relieves anxiety and tension (thus relieving insomnia), decreases irritability, and promotes a feeling of well-being and relaxation. It is not as potent as reserpine or chlorpromazine.

*Side-Effects.* The most common unfavorable reactions are skin rash and urticaria, with itching. Sometimes chills and fever develop, with edema, double vision, and diarrhea; large doses may cause coma and a marked fall in blood pressure. A patient can become mentally and physically dependent on the drug; it is habit-forming.

Tranquilizers are not a substitute for an understanding nurse but rather help a nurse find the reasons for disturbed behavior.

## DRUGS WHICH AFFECT THE AUTONOMIC NERVOUS SYSTEM

As you have learned, we do not consciously control the activities of the autonomic nervous system—its responses take place automatically. However, certain drugs do affect these responses. Some of these drugs are prepared from natural hormones (see Chapter 20). Two important hormones are epinephrine and norepinephrine—hormones produced by the adrenal glands.

### Epinephrine

Epinephrine (Adrenalin) constricts blood vessels when applied to the mucous membrane or wounds or when injected into the tissues. It has no effect on the unbroken skin. Since digestive enzymes destroy it, it is never given by mouth. It speeds up the heart rate, raises blood pressure, constricts surface blood vessels and relaxes smooth muscles in the respiratory tract—it is the most valuable drug that can be used to relieve acute attacks of bronchial asthma. It is especially valuable in treating allergic reactions, such as anaphylactic shock, serum reactions, hay fever, and urticaria. It is a powerful heart stimulant but must be used with great care so that it does not interfere seriously with the heartbeat. As a last resort, when the heart has stopped beating, injection of adrenalin directly into the heart muscle or into nearby veins has been known to restore heart action and bring the patient "back to life."

One thing important to remember about giving adrenalin is that it is a powerful drug and is usually given in small doses. The usual injection dose is 3 to 8 minims.

**Side-Effects.** Nervous patients and those with hypertension or exophthalmic goiter who take this drug may become more nervous and develop tremor, anxiety, headache, difficulty in breathing, and stomach pain. More dangerous symptoms, resulting from large doses or intravenous administration, are dilatation of the heart, edema of the lungs, and cerebral accident. Adrenalin is unsafe for patients with heart disease or hyperthyroidism or for those who are emotionally unstable.

### Norepinephrine

Norepinephrine (levarterenol) constricts blood vessels in most of the vascular beds of the body. Levarterenol bitartrate is used to maintain blood pressure in hypotensive states resulting from such conditions as hemorrhage, trauma, and myocardial infarction.

**Side-Effects.** Excessive amounts of levarterenol may raise blood pressure in elderly people to dangerous levels and cause cerebral accidents. Like epinephrine, it can interfere with the heartbeat and must be used with caution.

## DRUGS WHICH AFFECT THE MUSCULOSKELETAL SYSTEM

Certain drugs are useful in relieving muscle spasm, as in back strain or in cerebral palsy; to relax muscles during anesthesia in surgical operations or in the manipulation of bones and joints in reducing fractures. Some of these drugs are potent, can be dangerous and must be used with great care; they may cause respiratory paralysis and heart failure.

**Curare and Related Drugs.** Preparations of curare, a drug used by the South American Indians as an arrow poison, are seldom used today because they have been replaced by safer and more effective drugs. Some preparations which are now available are Tubadil, Metubine, and Mecostrin Chloride. Other drugs now considered more effective than curare are Soma, Succinylcholine Chloride (Anectine), Syncurine, Paraflex, and Robaxin.

SIDE-EFFECTS. The side-effects of these drugs are similar. In different degrees, they tend to depress respiration and to speed up heart action. In toxic amounts, they may be fatal.

**Quinine.** Quinine is a muscle relaxant which is effective in relieving cramps in the leg muscles which sometimes trouble people at night.

## DRUGS USED IN TREATING DISTURBANCES OF THE HEART AND BLOOD VESSELS

Drugs are used for their effect on the action of the heart itself or for their effect in dilating or constricting the blood vessels. Failure of any part of heart action or circulation inter-

feres with the body's supply of oxygen and nutrients and with the removal of waste products. The heart muscle is responsible for pumping the blood through the circulatory system—it literally pumps 9 to 10 *tons* of blood through 60,000 to 100,000 *miles* of blood vessels every day. It also must maintain its own circulatory system—the coronary circulation. One common form of heart disease is circulation failure; when the heart loses its efficiency as a pump, the circulation fails. Disease or degenerating changes in the heart itself or in the blood vessels impair its efficiency. Chapter 47 discusses these conditions in detail.

### Heart Stimulants

Certain drugs will make the heartbeat faster; others slow it down but strengthen its force. Sometimes this type of drug would be needed in the case when the heart is forced to beat faster than it should to make up for the weakness of its beat and is in danger of exhaustion from overwork. Cardiac stimulants which strengthen heart action are:

*Atropine:* To strengthen the heartbeat
*Caffeine:* A quick stimulant to make the heartbeat strongly and rapidly
*Epinephrine:* A powerful emergency stimulant to the circulation

**Digitalis.** Digitalis is a drug which is obtained from the leaves of the purple foxglove. It makes the heart beat slower and more strongly, giving it time to rest between beats. This improves circulation to reduce edema in the lungs and abdomen, thus making breathing easier. Digitalis does not cure heart disease, but it helps to prevent heart failure.

The amount of digitalis prescribed for an individual patient is regulated by the dose that gives him the optimum benefits. This is usually determined by giving the total amount necessary to produce the desired effect—the *digitalizing dose*—in divided doses, over a period of 2 to 4 days. This dose, slightly reduced, is the amount he will receive every day thereafter—his *maintenance dose*. This will vary according to the needs of the individual patient. Many patients who need digitalis must take it for the rest of their lives.

SIGNS OF OVERDOSE. A patient who is receiving digitalis needs close medical and nursing observation. Accuracy is especially important in giving this drug because it is very powerful, and even a minute difference in amount can be dangerous. It is important to observe the pulse closely—it should be counted before giving each dose. If it is lower than 60 beats a minute or if there is a change in the rhythm, withhold the dose and report these conditions to the head nurse or team leader immediately. Be sure to pour digitalis preparations into separate cups from other medications, so you will know which to withhold, if the pulse is below 60. Be sure to check the pulse both apically and radially before you report any decrease in heart rate.

Other symptoms of disturbance include nausea and vomiting, headache, diarrhea, and sometimes drowsiness and blurred vision. A record of the patient's intake and output of fluids is kept and he is watched for signs of edema and breathing difficulty.

PREPARATIONS. Some preparations of digitalis that are used are:

*Digitalis Tincture:* Oral, 1 ml.
*Digitoxin (Crystodigin, Purodigin):* Oral, 0.1 mg.
*Gitalin (Gitaligin):* Oral, 0.5 mg.
*Digoxin (Lanoxin):* Oral, 0.5 mg.
*Cedilanid*

## Heart Depressants

Heart depressants make the heart less active and decrease the heart rate. Heart disease affects the rhythm of the heartbeat causing the heart to quiver without rest between beats. This affects the circulation and may lead to congestive heart failure. Some drugs steady the heart rate by increasing the rest period, which changes a rapid irregular pulse to one which is slow and regular. Quinidine is such a drug. The difference between Digitalis and quinidine is that Digitalis stimulates more power in the heart muscle, while quinidine restrains erratic heart muscle activity to slower and more regular action.

Quinidine and procainamide (Pronestyl Hydrochloride) have essentially the same effects, except that procainamide is much less toxic and its effects last longer.

PREPARATIONS
*Quinidine Sulfate:* Oral, 0.2 to 0.4 Gm.
*Procainamide Hydrochloride (Pronestyl Hydrochloride):* Oral, 0.25 Gm.

## The Effect of Drugs on the Blood Vessels

Some drugs affect the circulatory system by constricting (*vasoconstrictors*) or dilating (*vasodilators*) the blood vessels. The vasodilators lower blood pressure; the vasoconstrictors raise it. They produce their effects indirectly, by their action on the nervous system, or directly, by action on the muscle cells in the blood vessels.

**Vasoconstrictors.** The vasoconstrictors (*hypertensive agents*) are used to control superficial hemorrhage, to raise blood pressure, and to relieve nasal congestion. The most important ones are epinephrine (Adrenalin), levarterenol bitartrate (Levophed Bitartrate), ergotamine tartrate, and phenylephrine hydrochloride.

Blood vessel constricting drugs are most widely used to shrink mucous membranes and relieve nasal congestion in mild infections of the upper respiratory tract. A number of preparations are available—Neosynephrine, Privine, Vonedrine, and Benzedrex—to mention a few of them. They are comparatively safe, but taking large doses, too often, is unwise.

EPINEPHRINE. The most important use of epinephrine is as a local application to constrict small blood vessels to stop bleeding from the eye, nose, or ear or to reduce swelling in the mucous membrane of the nose. It will not stop hemorrhage from a large blood vessel, and it must be applied directly to the area to stop superficial bleeding. It is used also with local anesthetics to prolong their action, to check bleeding, and to make them safer. It relieves hives, itching, and edema in allergic reactions.

LEVARTERENOL (LEVOPHED). Levarterenol is used to raise blood pressure after surgery, hemorrhage, or shock. It is given intravenously in a solution of dextrose and saline.

ARAMINE (METARAMINAL BITARTRATE). This is another drug used to raise or maintain blood pressure in an emergency.

EPHEDRINE. In small doses, ephedrine stimulates the heart and raises blood pressure. Large doses depress heart action. Local applications reduce swelling in the turbinates of the nose.

PHENYLEPHRINE HYDROCHLORIDE (NEO-SYNEPHRINE). This drug relieves congestion in mucous membranes and is used to treat some types of shock. It raises blood pressure and stabilizes it and is used sometimes to treat allergic reaction.

ERGOTAMINE TARTRATE (GYNERGEN). Ergotamine tartrate is especially valuable in treating migraine headache; it is more effective if it is taken when the first signs of an attack appear. This drug accumulates in the body, so it must be taken cautiously. Symptoms of trouble are numbness and tingling in the fingers and toes, muscle pains and weakness, gangrene, and blindness.

**Vasodilators.** Drugs that dilate the blood vessels are used to treat peripheral (toward the surface) blood vessel disease, coronary artery disease, and hypertension. Some of them (the *nitrites*) have been used for many years, especially in an acute attack of angina pectoris or to prevent an attack, by relieving angina pain caused by spasm of the coronary blood vessels.

NITROGLYCERIN. Nitroglycerin acts quickly—in 2 or 3 minutes; when a tablet is placed under the tongue it is rapidly absorbed by the mucous membranes. Its effects last for about 30 minutes. The usual dose is 0.4 mg. (1/150 gr.) which can be repeated several times a day.

AMYL NITRITE. Amyl nitrite comes in glass ampules (pearls) covered with a thin material so that it can be crushed easily and inhaled. It has a strong and rather disagreeable odor, and 2 or 3 inhalations are a safe limit—more may cause overdosage.

Other nitrite preparations are available; some of them, such as Peritrate Tetranitrate, have longer lasting effects—up to 6 hours or more.

*Side-Effects of the Nitrites.* The patient may feel dizzy and faint from a sudden lowering of blood pressure and may have headache. Large doses of these drugs exaggerate these symptoms and also make the face and neck flushed and the pulse weak and rapid. In nitrite poisoning, the patient's head should be lowered, and he is treated for shock; administer oxygen if he is cyanotic. People who are subject to attacks of angina usually carry these drugs with them to use in an emergency, so the nurse should know what to do for a person who takes an overdose.

PAPAVERINE. Papaverine is particularly effective in relaxing spasm in the coronary, peripheral, and pulmonary arteries. The aver-

age dosage ranges from 30 to 60 mg. when given intramuscularly.

AMINOPHYLLINE. Aminophylline has some effect in dilating blood vessels and is thought to be effective in preventing attacks of angina pectoris. It is sometimes used in coronary occlusion.

ALCOHOL (ETHYL). Alcohol dilates the blood vessels in the skin and is used for this effect in some diseases of the peripheral vessels, such as Raynaud's disease. For cardiac patients, alcohol is usually given in the form of whisky, with soda, for its mildly sedative effects in producing rest and relaxation.

**Drugs That Reduce Blood Pressure (Hypotensive Agents)**

RAUWOLFIA DRUGS. The tranquilizing action of these drugs has been discussed on page 354. They also are effective in treating the less extreme forms of hypertension. They relieve dizziness and headache, lower blood pressure, and slow the pulse rate. They are sometimes given with other drugs. The most common side-effect is a stuffy nose, but they may also cause drowsiness, nightmares, and depression. Some preparations commonly used are:

*Rauwolfia (Raudixin):* Oral, 200 to 400 mg. daily
*Reserpine (Serpasil and others):* Oral, 0.25 to 1 mg. daily

APRESOLINE. Apresoline reduces blood pressure and helps to control hypertension. Treatment begins with small doses, 10 mg. taken after meals and at bedtime; the dosage is adjusted to obtain the desired effect. It often causes unpleasant side-effects which are not necessarily serious, such as headache, heart palpitation, depression, nausea, and vomiting. More serious symptoms include chills, fever, pain in the heart region, and edema of the legs and feet.

CHLOROTHIAZIDE (DIURIL). Although chlorothiazide is used primarily as a diuretic, it is also effective in lowering blood pressure in hypertension when used alone or with other drugs. It has few unpleasant side-effects. Other preparations are Hydrodiuril, Ademol Renese, and Naturetin.

GUANETHIDINE (ISMELIN). This is a powerful drug used to reduce blood pressure; its effect is more noticeable when the patient is sitting or standing up. Patients may feel weak and dizzy when they move about. It is especially important to safeguard elderly patients who may get up to go to the bathroom during the night. Other side-effects are diarrhea, fainting, and a slow pulse.

## DRUGS WHICH AFFECT THE BLOOD

We have discussed the effects of drugs on the circulation of blood. Drugs also are used to treat disturbances of the blood itself, such as anemia or leukemia, and to influence blood clotting. Blood is composed of plasma, red cells, white cells, and platelets. Red cells are made up mainly of a substance called hemoglobin, which contains iron. Hemoglobin has the all-important job of carrying oxygen to every cell in the body. (See Chapter 15.)

Normally, an adequate diet provides the essentials to form blood (iron, vitamin C, and parts of the vitamin B complex, vitamin $B_{12}$, animal protein). Some disease conditions need treatment which will get results more rapidly, and certain drugs help to do this.

### Iron

Iron is not only an essential part of hemoglobin but is also distributed throughout the body cells and is stored in the blood-forming organs. Actually, the body needs only small amounts of iron from the diet because it salvages iron from the worn-out blood cells and uses it again. Adolescents (especially girls) and women during pregnancy and the menopause need more iron than at other times; in fact, women up to and through the menopause need 4 times as much iron as men. Iron deficiency causes anemia and is usually due to a massive hemorrhage or to prolonged slow bleeding from a tumor or hemorrhoids or to profuse menstrual bleeding.

**Iron Preparations.** The market is flooded with iron preparations, but only a few justify the claims made for them. Among the most effective are:

*Ferrous Sulfate (Feosol):* Prepared in enteric-coated tablets of 3 and 5 gr. and given after meals.

*Ferrous Sulfate Syrup:* The usual dose is 8 ml. 3 times a day.

*Ferrous Gluconate (Fergon):* Tablets of 5 gr. each, usual dose is 1 tablet, 3 times a day. It is less likely to cause stomach distress than ferrous sulfate.

*Ferrocholinate (Chel-Iron, Ferrolip):* One of the newer iron preparations which is considered less toxic than some of the older products. The normal dose is 330 to 660 mg., 3 times a day.

*Ferric Ammonium Citrate:* One of the most soluble iron preparations. The usual dose is 500 mg., 3 times a day.

Iron is usually given by mouth, but preparations such as Imferon and Astrafer that can be given by injection are also available if the oral method is not feasible.

SIDE-EFFECTS. Iron taken over a prolonged period may cause loss of appetite, nausea and vomiting, headaches, stomach pain, diarrhea, or constipation. Large doses can cause poisoning, especially if taken by children.

Many iron preparations are irritating to the stomach, which is the reason why they are given after meals or with food. Solutions should be taken through a straw because they stain the teeth and because the metallic taste is unpleasant.

**Vitamin $B_{12}$ (Cyanocobalamin, Rubramin, Redisol, Normocytin).** It has been many years since 2 medical scientists, Minot and Murphy, discovered a substance in liver, vitamin $B_{12}$, that would cure pernicious anemia, which once was a fatal disease. Vitamin $B_{12}$ is necessary for the manufacture of red blood cells, but for some reason, certain people cannot absorb this vitamin from their diet and develop pernicious anemia if it is not supplied in some other way. It is thought that these people lack a substance in the stomach (the intrinsic factor) which makes it possible to absorb vitamin $B_{12}$. Therefore, the treatment is to give injections of vitamin $B_{12}$ which will arrest the disease. Since the discovery of vitamin $B_{12}$, the patient is no longer forced to consume large quantities of liver.

The patient with a marked vitamin $B_{12}$ deficiency feels tired, weak, and breathless; his tongue and mouth are sore; he has difficulty in coordinating his movements; his skin takes on a pale yellowish tinge; and he develops tingling and numbness in his extremities. The dosage is measured in micrograms; the amount depends on the seriousness of the patient's need for it. Usually it is given intramuscularly to hasten the effects. Hydrochloric acid frequently is given with the vitamin $B_{12}$ since most patients with pernicious anemia have a deficiency of this acid in the stomach. Vitamin $B_{12}$ has no undesirable side-effects.

## WHOLE BLOOD, BLOOD PLASMA, BLOOD PROTEINS

A transfusion of *whole blood* increases the number of red blood cells quickly, restores the volume of blood, and so raises blood pressure. It may save a patient's life when his survival depends on quick action. The blood must be of a type compatible with the patient's blood type.

*Blood plasma* is that fluid part of the blood which has been separated from the blood cells. It restores blood volume in shock, in severe hemorrhage, and in severe burns. It can be used as a liquid, or it can be dehydrated, concentrated, and stored for a long time without losing its effect; by adding sterile distilled water it is ready to use, without the need of considering blood groups. Plasma is obtained by processing the blood of qualified blood donors to remove blood cells.

Blood proteins are other constituents of blood plasma which can be separated from blood plasma for use. For example, albumin has the same effects as plasma in treating shock and can be administered in smaller amounts. Thrombin and fibrinogen together in a solution form *fibrin,* which can be applied locally to stimulate blood clotting, or it can be given intravenously. Other preparations are normal human serum albumin (used in treating shock) and antihemolytic human plasma (a temporary aid to the hemophiliac). Immune serum globulin (gamma globulin) is also a blood protein given to help the patient ward off a specific infection.

## Blood Coagulants

Drugs which promote blood clotting are called *hemostatics* or *coagulants.* When blood plasma lacks the elements which cause blood to clot, certain drug preparations can be used to supply this deficiency. Some of them are:

*Absorbable Gelatin Sponge (Gelfoam):* This is a form of gelatin that is used to stop capillary bleeding and can be left in a surgical wound, where it will be absorbed completely.

*Fibrin Foam:* A dry preparation of human fibrin that can be applied to a bleeding surface to stop hemorrhage. It is used in kidney, liver, or brain surgery.

*Tolonium Chloride (Blutene Chloride):* A dye which lessens a tendency for excessive bleeding from the uterus. Used for profuse menstruation for which no cause can be found.

*Oxidized Cellulose (Oxycel, Hemo-Pak):* A treated cotton or gauze pack which is absorbable and can be applied to check hemorrhage.

*Thrombin:* A preparation from plasma which is used to check surface bleeding.

*Vitamin K:* A vitamin necessary to make prothrombin, which is the substance that starts the formation of a blood clot. Vitamin K is found in many foods, but sometimes the intestine is unable to absorb it. It may be given to patients who have a prothrombin deficiency, as in jaundice, or to the newborn. Many preparations are available; among them are Vitamin $K_1$, Synkayvite, menadione, Hykinone, Mephyton, and Konakion. They are in forms which can be given by mouth, by injection, or intravenously. The dosage is measured in milligrams and varies from 0.5 to 20 mg. or more, according to the needs of the individual patient. If vitamin K is given by injection, it is given deep I.M., because it tends to be quite irritating to the tissues.

## Anticoagulants

Drugs to prevent abnormal clotting of blood are highly important, since clots in major blood vessels are one of the chief causes of death in this country (coronary occlusion and cerebral vascular accidents). Some drugs that prevent blood clotting or make it less likely to occur are:

*Sodium Citrate:* Used to prevent the coagulation of blood to be used in transfusions.

*Heparin:* This drug is especially useful in preventing postoperative thrombosis and embolism. If a patient is receiving heparin, the nurse should watch for bleeding from the wound or for blood in the urine and should report them at once. Heparin is given by injection or intravenously.

*Dicumarol:* Dicumarol is given to prevent venous thrombosis and pulmonary embolism and thrombophlebitis (inflammation of a vein). It is available in tablets and capsules and the usual beginning dose is 200 to 300 mg. daily, given by mouth. Later doses vary according to the patient's needs. This drug has few side reactions, but overdosage can cause hemorrhage. Nosebleed, bleeding into the skin, or blood in the urine should be reported. Other anticoagulants with similar action are Coumadin, Indon and Dipaxin. The patient who is receiving an anticoagulant should have regular prothrombin time or clotting time evaluations to make sure he is not becoming "over-heparinized" or subject to hemorrhage. If his clotting time becomes too long, his anticoagulant dose will be decreased.

## DRUGS WHICH AFFECT THE URINARY SYSTEM

The urinary system consists of the kidneys, the ureters, the bladder, and the urethra. The kidneys are the chief organs for excreting waste substances from the body. Excess water and other substances the body does not need are excreted in the urine. When kidney function is impaired, there are drugs which help to alleviate the problem.

### Diuretics

Diuretics are drugs used to increase the elimination of water and salts from the body by increasing the flow of urine. One way of doing this is to give the patient increased amounts of fluid. Taking in more fluid seems to stimulate an increase in fluid loss. Therefore, water is also a diuretic, although it is not a drug. When the flow of urine is inadequate, water and salts accumulate in the tissues and cause edema (retention of fluid in the tissues and swelling). An increased flow of urine reduces edema.

Caffeine, theobromine, and theophylline have a limited diuretic effect. The mercurial diuretics, such as Thiomerin, Cumertilin, Mercuhydrin, Neohydrin, and Mersalyl are among the most effective in reducing edema, especially edema caused by cirrhosis of the liver, kidney nephrosis, or cardiac edema. These drugs are given orally or intramuscularly every 3 or 4 days, preferably in the morning, so that most of the urine elimination will take place during the day. A patient may void as much as 8 or 9 quarts of urine during the day the initial dose is given.

**Side-Effects.** Signs of unfavorable reactions are inflammation of the gums, increase in saliva, diarrhea, and albumin and blood in the urine, flushing, and skin reactions. Since prolonged used of these drugs may cause kidney damage, urine specimens are examined periodically for blood cells, albumin, and casts.

Cardrase and Diamox may be used to prevent edema in cardiac patients and to increase the output of urine.

Chlorothiazide preparations are effective in relieving edema associated with congestive heart failure and hypertension and cirrhosis of the liver. Diuril and Lyovac Diuril are the commonly used preparations. The usual dose is from 500 mg. to 1 Gm. every day. The side-effects include allergic reactions, nausea, stomach discomfort, dizziness, and muscle cramps. Some of the newer drugs related to this group are longer-lasting and less toxic, can be taken orally, and are relatively inexpensive (Renese, Ademol, and Naturetin).

### Antidiuretics

In some conditions, such as diabetes insipidus, the patient excretes an excessive amount of urine. This condition is caused by the lack of a pituitary hormone. (This should not be confused with diabetes mellitus, which is caused by lack of insulin.) Pituitary extract, injected hypodermically or applied to the nasal membranes, is given to supply this deficiency.

### Drugs Which Affect the Bladder

Bladder difficulties are often caused by a frequent desire to empty the bladder or by an inability to empty it. Either way, the trouble is caused by muscle tone. Drugs which improve muscle tone in the bladder are neostigmine and bethanechol chloride (Urecholine Chloride). Hyoscyamus tincture is given to relax bladder muscle.

### Urinary Antiseptics

Urinary antiseptics are used to combat infection in the urine and urinary tract. This type of infection is often caused by colon bacilli, but it may also be caused by forms of staphylococci or streptococci. These organisms are carried easily to the urethral opening from the rectum if the proper precautions are not observed in carrying out nursing procedures involving these parts.

A number of the sulfonamides and antibiotics destroy or inhibit the growth of infectious organisms in the urine and urinary passages. The one selected is chosen for its specific effect on the organism causing the infection. This is determined by microscopic examination or laboratory culture of a urine specimen.

Some of the sulfonamides commonly used are Gantrisin, Sulamyd, Kynex, and Gantanol. The usual dosage is 0.5 Gm., daily. The use of sulfonamides is contraindicated in the patient with impaired kidney or liver function or in the patient who has severe allergies. The patient who is taking a sulfonamide should be encouraged to drink extra fluids. An accurate intake and output should be kept.

Of the antibiotics, penicillin is the least effective in urinary infections because so many of the organisms causing the infection are resistant to it. Streptomycin, erythromycin, novobiocin and kanamycin are more effective. Chloramphenicol, bacitracin, and neomycin are effective but must be used cautiously because they have certain damaging effects on the bone marrow and the kidneys. Methenamine (Mandelamine) is effective in cystitis, pyelitis, and pyelonephritis. Furacin is one of the more expensive drugs, but the dosage required is small. Pyridium is given to soothe the mucous membrane of the bladder and urethra and to relieve frequency of urination. It also helps to relieve discomfort caused by a retention catheter. The nurse must be aware that some of these drugs (Pyridium) makes the urine a bright orange color.

Other urinary antiseptics are Furadantin, Neg Gram, and Urised.

## DRUGS USED IN TREATING GASTROINTESTINAL DISEASES AND DISORDERS

Drugs affect the gastrointestinal tract through their action on muscles and glandular tissues, by stimulating peristalsis, or correcting enzyme deficiencies and excess acidity or by relieving vomiting.

### Drugs Which Affect the Mouth

Good oral hygiene to keep the mouth and teeth clean is more effective than drugs, although some drugs are mildly helpful.

**Mouthwashes and Gargles.** Drugs used for this purpose do not have a very powerful germ-killing effect because they cannot be used in strong enough concentrations without harming the tissues. They are useful as disinfectants and in removing mucus from the mouth and throat. A 1 per cent *sodium bicarbonate solution* (½ teaspoon in a glass of water) is a useful mouth wash for removing mucus. A 0.9 per cent solution of *sodium chloride* (common salt) is as satisfactory a gargle as any other mixture.

*Sodium perborate* in a 2 per cent solution is a useful mouthwash and is effective in treating Vincent's infection and pyorrhea. It is an ingredient of many tooth powders. Most hospitals use a mouthwash prepared in their own pharmacy, with directions about whether it is to be used full strength or diluted.

*Hydrogen Peroxide* may be used for mouth care in the unconscious patient, or for the patient who must breathe through his mouth. Rinse with clear water after using peroxide to remove the taste.

**Dentifrices, Tooth Powders, or Abrasives.** The usual ingredients in a dentifrice are an abrasive, a foaming agent, and flavoring materials. A safe dentifrice is one which will not harm the teeth or gums. Some dentifrices claim they contain a special ingredient which prevents tooth decay. (The Council of Dental Therapeutics investigates and reports on such claims.) Stannous fluoride is recognized as having some beneficial effects of this kind. The American Dental Association and the American Medical Association have recommended the fluoridation of drinking water as a method of reducing dental decay; but the decision to fluoridate its water supply is made by a city or community, and some cities have voted against fluoridation. A 2 per cent solution of sodium fluoride applied to children's teeth has been found effective in preventing dental caries (decay). Other ways of giving fluorides in milk, table salt, and fluoride tablets are being investigated.

### Drugs Which Affect Stomach Conditions

Certain drugs are used to control the excessive production of stomach acids, to aid digestion, to relieve gas distention, and to cause, prevent, or control vomiting.

**Antacids.** Antacids are used in treating peptic ulcer to reduce and control stomach acidity and give the ulcer a chance to heal. Two widely used and readily absorbed antacids are sodium bicarbonate (ordinary baking soda) and sodium citrate, an ingredient of proprietary drugs for relieving stomach distress. The dosage depends on the needs of the individual patient. Many people have completely mistaken notions about stomach acid, not realizing that a certain amount is necessary for the digestion of food. The habit of taking sodium bicarbonate to avoid "acid stomach" can interfere seriously with the electrolyte balance in the blood and cause alkalosis (an excess of alkali in the blood). In the eyes of the public, advertisers have made "acid" an unfavorable term—a public enemy to be fought.

Other antacids are often preferred because they are not readily absorbed and are not apt to cause alkalosis, although, in very large doses, they may severely upset the acid-base balance of the body. Some of the most commonly used ones are:

*Aluminum Hydroxide Gel (Amphojel, Creamalin, Alkajel):* In tablet or liquid form, it is given orally in doses of 4 to 8 ml. every 2 to 4 hours. It is usually diluted in a small amount of water or followed by a drink of liquid to make sure the medicine is washed down from the throat into the stomach.

*Magnesium Oxide (Light Magnesia and Heavy Magnesia):* A powder insoluble in water. The usual dose is 250 mg. It is slow-acting but has a lasting effect. It has also a laxative effect which sometimes causes diarrhea.

*Gelusil:* Contains magnesium trisilicate and aluminum hydroxide.

*Maalox:* Contains magnesium-aluminum hydroxide.

*Sippy Powders* (No. 1 and No. 2): A mixture of antacids which are given alternately with a milk and cream diet, usually on an hourly basis.

*Milk of Magnesia:* A liquid mixture, sometimes combined with other magnesium salts as Maalox; the usual dosage is 8 ml. which is given with a small amount of water or followed by a small amount of water or milk.

Other antacids are Kolantyl, Aludrox, and Phosphaljel.

**Digestants.** Digestants aid digestion in the gastrointestinal tract and supply digestant deficiencies.

Hydrochloric acid aids in the digestion of protein; it kills bacteria and helps to maintain electrolyte balance. Some people, elderly ones especially, are deficient in hydrochloric acid because too little is secreted by the stomach. This deficiency is associated with gastric carcinoma, pernicious anemia, gastritis, and other conditions. Dilute hydrochloric acid is given to remedy the deficiency. The usual dose is 4 ml., given in half a glass of water (through a tube because it injures tooth enamel). Eating food or using an alkaline mouth wash after taking it will help to kill its sharp, sour taste.

*Acidulin:* Another preparation containing hydrochloric acid which comes in capsules and is usually given before meals.

*Pepsin:* A stomach enzyme which aids protein digestion but is seldom used today because hydrochloric acid is considered more effective.

*Bile Salts:* A constituent of bile which is essential in the digestion of fats. They are used in the treatment of liver disorders to aid digestion and to increase bile drainage. Some commonly used preparations are Ox Bile Extract, Zanchol, and Decholin.

**Carminatives.** Carminatives are mildly irritating drugs which help to expel gas from the stomach and intestines. They are chiefly home remedies, such as peppermint water, and are either taken alone or are combined with brandy or whisky in hot water.

**Emetics.** Emetics are given to make a patient vomit to rid the stomach of its contents, usually as first aid in emergencies when quick action is necessary (see Chapter 35). The drug apomorphine, given by injection, causes vomiting quickly but is a depressing drug when given in large doses. Gastric lavage (washing out the stomach) is the most effective way of emptying the stomach.

**Antiemetics.** Antiemetics are given to relieve nausea and vomiting. These symptoms may be the result of a number of things—emotional distress, motion sickness, the effects of drugs, gastrointestinal disease, or reaction to x-ray or other treatments. They are sometimes relieved by simple remedies, such as a cup of tea, carbonated drinks (ginger ale, cola), sodium bicarbonate in warm water (to wash out the stomach), or gastric lavage. Quieting drugs (barbiturates) and the antihistamines are also effective. Common antiemetics are Compazine, Dramamine, Bonine, and Emetrol.

A common drug for the "morning sickness"

of pregnancy is Bendectin. This drug contains Bentyl (an antispasmodic, which quiets the gastrointestinal spasms of nausea), Decapryn (an antihistamine, which controls nausea and motion sickness), and Pyridoxine HCl (which corrects vitamin $B_6$ deficiency, which often occurs in pregnancy). This drug is specially coated so that it can be taken in the evening and its effects will be maximal in the morning. The patient may become drowsy while taking this drug.

## Drugs Used in X-Ray Procedures

Barium sulfate is used in x-ray examinations of the gastrointestinal tract, to detect peptic ulcer, cancer, and other conditions (see Chapter 49). Iodine compounds (Iodekon, Priodax, Telepaque) are useful in examinations of the gall bladder and the bile passages. These substances are used because they will show on x-ray (radiopaque).

## Drugs Which Affect Intestinal Action

**Cathartics.** Far too many people have very hazy notions about intestinal activities. To miss even one daily bowel movement is considered a catastrophe; they believe that poisons are piling up so rapidly they must get rid of them at all costs and they rush for a pill. First cousin to this notion is the firm belief that a regular daily movement is not enough —that a "good cleaning out" every so often is necessary for something they call "the system." The advertising claims for cathartics bolster these ideas. Healthy people should not need cathartics.

On the other hand, many people do suffer from true constipation, much of which could be prevented by proper diet and eating habits, attention to the impulse to defecate, and sufficient exercise. People who must lie in bed in one position, who are having drugs such as morphine or codeine, or who have impaired muscle tone which affects the colon are likely to be constipated. Constipation is also often associated with mental disorders, anemia, or sick headaches. The doctor determines when a cathartic is necessary and prescribes a suitable one.

Elderly people who have been taking cathartics for constipation for most of their adult lives may be exceptions. For one thing, it is not always possible to prescribe roughage in the diet of a person who is unable to chew it. Elderly people, like everyone else, are not likely to take kindly to the idea of changing lifetime habits. A mild cathartic taken regularly as prescribed by the doctor is not likely to be harmful.

**The Action of Cathartics.** Cathartics act in several ways:

To stimulate peristalsis by increasing the bulk or water contents of the feces
To moisten the stool
To irritate the lining of the intestine

AGAR, METAMUCIL. Dry agar, obtained from seaweed, and Metamucil, a preparation of psyllium seed, swell when moistened and give bulk to the feces. Both are given with a sufficient amount of water. Agar can also be sprinkled in such foods as mashed potatoes, cereal, or soup; it may also be combined with liquid petrolatum (Petrogalar). In spite of advertising claims, Petrogalar is an ineffective bulk producer because it contains very little agar. Other preparations used to produce bulk are Methocel, Methyl Cellulose, Carmethose, Cellothyl, and Konsyl.

SALINE CATHARTICS. Saline cathartics are the most effective ones to reduce edema, to obtain a stool specimen, or to empty the intestines in cases of food or drug poisoning or worms. They are used also to remove feces. Saline cathartics produce watery stools. Those preparations most frequently used are:

*Milk of Magnesia:* A mild cathartic and is often used for children. The usual adult dose is 15 ml. (½ fluid ounce). Milk of magnesia is also an antacid.

*Magnesium Sulfate (Epsom Salt):* A crystalline or powdery substance with a salty, bitter taste which must be dissolved in water. The usual dose is 15 Gm. (½ ounce). It should be given with fruit juice which helps to disguise the taste.

*Seidlitz Powders:* Seidlitz powders are put up separately, one in a blue and one in a white paper. The contents of each paper is dissolved separately in ⅓ of a glass of water and the 2 are combined *at the bedside* immediately before swallowing. Since the mixture is effervescent and flavored, it is easy to take.

*Magnesium Citrate:* A mild cathartic which is

easy to take because it is carbonated. The usual dose is ½ to 1 bottle (6 to 12 ounces).

MINERAL OIL. Liquid petrolatum, or mineral oil, is a petroleum product which is simply a lubricant to soften feces. It is given to prevent straining with a bowel movement after rectal operations or for chronic constipation in inactive persons, such as elderly people. Mineral oil is said to interfere with the use of vitamin A in the body, and some doctors will not prescribe it. It should be given between meals or at bedtime to avoid delaying the passage of food from the stomach. The dosage ranges from 15 to 30 ml.; only standard official preparations should be used.

Other preparations such as Colace or Doxinate moisten the feces so that soft stools are formed.

IRRITATING CATHARTICS. *Castor Oil (Oleum Ricini):* Castor oil irritates the small intestine to expel its contents rapidly to completely empty the bowel. It often produces a number of semiliquid stools in 2 to 6 hours after it is taken. This means that there are likely to be no more bowel movements for a day or two—an after-effect that sometimes worries patients. Castor oil is excreted into the milk of a nursing mother and may affect the baby's bowel elimination. Castor oil is unpleasant to take, but the taste can be disguised in various ways —for example, by giving it with fruit juices. Most hospitals determine the method to use. It is not prescribed as frequently today as formerly.

*Cascara Sagrada:* Cascara is obtained from the bark of a shrub and acts mainly on the large intestine. Like similar drugs obtained from plants, it is likely to cause cramps and acts in 6 to 12 hours. The fluid extract is flavored and easy to take; the adult dose is 2 to 12 ml. given orally.

*Compound Licorice Powder:* This is a combination of senna and other ingredients which resembles cascara in its action but is more powerful; the usual oral dosage is 4 Gm. mixed with water. Other senna preparations are senna syrup, and senna fluid extract.

*Phenolphthalein:* This is a synthetic substance which produces mild bowel irritation and does not cause cramping. It is incorporated in tablets, is not unpleasant to take, and is sold in proprietary preparations which resemble candy. They should be kept out of children's reach since they might take a fatal overdose of the drug.

*Dulcolax:* Dulcolax stimulates peristalsis in the colon and is effective for constipation and for cleansing the bowel before an operation and x-ray or rectal examinations. The average oral dose is 10 to 15 mg. in the evening or before breakfast.

*S.S.B. and C. Pills and Hinkle's Pills:* These pills are a combination of aloin and other cathartics. The usual dosage is 1 pill given orally.

**Antidiarrheics.** Certain drugs act on the intestine to soothe the mucous membrane, to form a protective coating over it, to shrink swollen and inflamed tissues, and to fight infection. The particular remedy used in treating diarrhea depends on what is causing the diarrhea.

*Kaolin and Kaopectate:* Preparations of charcoal take up poisonous substances or gas from the intestines. Kaolin dosage varies from 15 to 60 Gm. every 3 or 4 hours until the symptoms are relieved. Kaopectate is effective when given in fairly large doses of 15 to 30 ml., several times a day. The use of these preparations is questioned by some authorities on the ground that nutrients cling to them and are also removed.

*Bismuth:* These preparations have a soothing effect on irritated intestinal mucous membrane. In powder or tablets, the usual dose is 1 to 4 Gm., 4 times a day.

*Azulfidine:* Used in treating ulcerative colitis, in 1 Gm. doses every 4 hours around the clock, later reduced to 1 Gm., 4 times a day when the patient is up and around.

*Sulfadiazine:* Used in treating dysentery in doses beginning with 2 to 4 Gm., followed by divided doses of 1 Gm. every 4 to 6 hours.

*Tannic Acid:* Protects the mucous membrane and checks secretions. The usual dose is 1 Gm. given in a capsule.

*Antibiotics:* Streptomycin, chloramphenicol, and combinations with penicillin are sometimes used.

*Camphorated Opium Tincture (Paregoric) and Opium Tincture (Laudanum):* Sedative preparations for relieving diarrhea. The dose for paregoric is 4 to 8 ml. (1 to 2 fluid drams) and for laudanum is 0.3 to 1 ml. (5 to 15 minims). Codeine and morphine are also effective but are not used for chronic conditions because they are habit-forming. Belladonna tincture helps to relieve intestinal spasms, given in 10-drop doses.

In addition to drugs to check diarrhea, patients also need replacement of the fluids, electrolytes, vitamins, and food lost by the overactivity of the intestines.

## DRUGS WHICH AFFECT THE RESPIRATORY SYSTEM

Respiration, or breathing, is an essential life process for supplying the body with oxygen and for eliminating the waste product, carbon dioxide. The respiratory system involves the nose, pharynx, larynx, trachea, bronchi, lungs, the chest muscles, the diaphragm, the respiratory center in the brain, and the blood. Some drugs stimulate the respiratory system; others depress it.

### Respiratory Stimulants

The chief respiratory stimulants are carbon dioxide, caffeine, atropine, Coramine, and Metrazol. They act on the respiratory center in the brain and have been mentioned already on pages 347 - 348, under "Drugs Affecting the Nervous System." They are useful in a variety of respiratory diseases and disorders.

*Carbon Dioxide:* Carbon dioxide is a gas which increases the capacity of the lungs to take in oxygen and to expel carbon dioxide waste—it deepens breathing. It is used to relieve asphyxia (suffocation) in carbon monoxide poisoning, to prevent postoperative pneumonia and to deepen breathing when anesthesia is used. It relieves postoperative hiccough; ordinary occasional hiccoughs, as well as hysterical hyperventilation, can be relieved by breathing and rebreathing into a paper bag held tightly over the mouth and nose. Otherwise, carbon dioxide is given by using a face mask attached to a tank of the gas. Overdosage causes difficult breathing (dyspnea), greatly increased movements of the chest and abdomen, and increased systolic blood pressure.

*Caffeine:* Caffeine stimulates the respiratory center. Some authorities believe that other stimulants now available are more effective.

*Atropine:* Atropine is often given with morphine to counteract the depressing effect of morphine on the respiratory center and to check mucous secretions and prevent spasm of the larynx.

*Coramine:* Coramine stimulates the respiratory center, increases the rate and depth of respirations and constricts surface blood vessels.

*Metrazol:* Metrazol stimulates the respiratory center and is especially effective in counteracting barbiturate poisoning.

### Respiratory Depressants

Respiratory depression may occur as an undesirable side-effect from the opiates and barbiturates, or from an overconcentration of carbon dioxide in the blood. Strangely enough, carbon dioxide stimulates respiration, but too much of it has the opposite effect.

### Drugs To Relieve Cough (Antitussives)

A cough which helps to rid the respiratory passages of irritating substances is helpful and is referred to as *productive*; a *nonproductive* cough is annoying and exhausting.

*Narcotic Drugs:* Morphine, Levo-Dromoran, and dihydromorphinone are potent cough depressants, but they also depress respiration and are habit-forming drugs. Codeine and Hycodan are less effective but have fewer side-effects. Methadone is also effective but is habit-forming.

*Non-narcotic Cough Relievers:* Other drugs that relieve cough are Nectadon, Toclase, and Romilar Hydrobromide. These drugs seem to be as effective as codeine and have few undesirable side-effects.

*Cough Syrups:* These preparations relieve coughs by forming a protective coating on the mucous membrane of the throat. The most common ones are tolu, acacia, citric acid, and glycyrrhiza syrups. A plain syrup, honey, or hard candy are home remedies often used for a cough. (Liquids or food should not be given immediately after a cough syrup.) Aromatic substances such as menthol or oil of pine are sometimes added to the water in a steam inhalation for their soothing effect.

*Sprays:* Nasal sprays containing ephedrine, epinephrine, or amphetamine, relieve congestion in nasal mucous membranes. They should be used sparingly, as the doctor directs, because overspraying may force the infection into the sinuses or middle ear and do more harm than good.

### Antiseptics

Antiseptics powerful enough to kill bacteria in nasal or throat infections would injure the mucous membrane. Therefore antibiotics in the form of sprays, and sulfonamides, such as sulfadiazine, taken internally, are used instead.

### Expectorants

Certain drugs *increase* the secretion of mucus in the bronchi and help to expel sputum. Among these drugs are ammonium chloride and saturated solution of potassium iodide (SSKI), 0.3 Gm. (5 gr.), given in a syrup 4 times a day with a full glass of water. The water is important because it helps to increase the flow of mucus to protect the mucous membrane from irritation. These drugs may cause skin eruption, frontal sinus pain, or coryza if they are used for a long period of time. Ipecac syrup is a preparation that is also used, especially for children, for bronchitis accompanying croup. The adult dose varies from 1 to 8 ml. The dosage is 5 minims for infants 1 year old, increased slightly for each year of age.

Expectorants used to *decrease* secretions have a healing effect on the irritated lining of the bronchi. Terpin hydrate, an elixir, alone or combined with codeine, is such a preparation. The usual dose is 4 ml. (1 fluid dram).

Other expectorants are Robitussin, Romilar, and Benadryl.

## Cold Remedies

Many cold remedies contain atropine, which checks secretion in some types of bronchitis. Authorities are cautious about recommending the wholesale use of these antihistamine drugs, such as Benadryl and Pyribenzamine. These drugs seem to be useful in relieving the sneezing and continuous nasal discharge which accompany cold infections, that is, if they are taken when the first signs of a cold appear. The Council on Drugs of the American Medical Association cautions people about using these drugs indiscriminately because they may cause drowsiness to the extent that the user may fall asleep when driving or manipulating machinery. Prolonged use also may harm the nervous system and the blood-forming tissues.

Some authorities believe that Vitamin C is effective in preventing the common cold.

## DRUGS WHICH AFFECT THE REPRODUCTIVE SYSTEM

The female reproductive system consists of the ovaries, the fallopian tubes, the uterus, and the vagina. The male reproductive organs are the testes, the seminal vesicles, the prostate gland, the bulbourethral glands, and the penis. In both male and female the endocrine glands control the reproductive organs to a great extent, through the hormones they secrete. The pituitary gland is especially influential; the ovaries and the testes (the sex glands; or *gonads*) are also endocrine glands

which secrete hormones that influence secondary sex characteristics. This function and the reproductive function of the sex glands diminishes in middle life and finally ceases. As was stated in Chapter 19, this is the period of the climacteric which in women is accompanied by the cessation of menstruation (menopause).

As hormone production diminishes it often causes a number of unpleasant symptoms which can be relieved by *hormone extracts.* Hormone extracts are used also to supply deficiencies in hormone production which cause retarded sexual development, or to stimulate or to depress the activities of the reproductive organs.

## Drugs Which Affect the Uterus

The uterus is a muscular organ with great power to expand or contract. The drugs which affect the uterus are those that increase or decrease this power.

**Oxytocics.** The drugs used to *increase* uterine contractions are called *oxytocics.* The commonly used ones are preparations of ergot and extracts from pituitary gland hormones. Ergot is a dried portion of a fungus that grows on grain—especially on rye. Preparations of ergot are used to promote the contraction of the uterus to its normal size after childbirth and to constrict the smaller blood vessels to prevent postpartum hemorrhage. Some preparations are:

*Ergotrate:* Given subcutaneously or intramuscularly immediately after delivery; the usual dose is 0.2 mg., which may be repeated every 4 hours for 6 doses after delivery. Tablets for oral administration are also available.

*Methergine:* Resembles ergotrate in its action, but it is more powerful, has more prolonged effects, and is less likely to raise blood pressure. The usual dose is 0.2 mg. given by injection or by mouth.

SIDE-EFFECTS. Possible side-effects of these drugs are nausea and vomiting, dizziness, headache and diarrhea, and abdominal cramps. These are most likely to occur after large doses of the drug are taken, such as in attempted abortion. Severe poisoning may cause gangrene, brain degeneration, and blindness.

**Posterior Pituitary Hormone Extracts.** These preparations are given during childbirth to increase uterine contractions at the time of delivery; they may be given during a long labor when normal contractions fail to expel the fetus. They are also used to contract the uterus and reduce hemorrhage after the placenta is expressed. *Obstetrical* Pituitrin and Pitocin are commonly used preparations available in ampules. The first is given subcutaneously, the second intramuscularly. The usual dosage varies from 0.3 to 1 ml. They are rarely used in the first stage of labor. Patients receiving these drugs *during labor* must be watched closely, with frequent checks of blood pressure and fetal heart tones. Prolonged contractions of the uterus diminish the blood and the oxygen supply of the fetus.

**Drugs To Decrease Uterine Contractions.** Sometimes it is desirable to relax the muscles to quiet down uterine contractions, as when premature labor threatens or when contractions are rapid and irregular. Large doses of the barbiturates or opiates (morphine, Demerol) are effective. Phenergan relieves fear and enhances the action of morphine when both drugs are given together.

Lutrexin as well as Edrisol is sometimes used to relax spasmodic tightening of the muscles in dysmenorrhea (painful menstruation). Premenstrual tension is relieved by a drug called Pre-mens. Magnesium sulfate given by mouth acts as a cathartic, but given intramuscularly or intravenously it depresses muscle activity. It is given to ward off convulsive seizures in eclampsia.

## Hormone Extracts Which Affect the Sex Glands (Ovaries and Testes)

Certain hormone extracts affect the development and the functions of the female and the male sex glands. Three hormones made by the anterior lobe of the *pituitary gland* (FSH, LH, LTH) are thought to have a definite effect on the functions of the ovary. Two of these hormones also affect the male sex glands. Completely satisfactory preparations of these hormones have not yet been developed; consequently, there are no *officially* approved preparations listed, although some have been used with some success in treating amenorrhea and sterility.

**Placental Hormones.** During pregnancy the placenta secretes hormones which affect the development of the corpus luteum in the female and the male sex hormones, to promote the development of the accessory sex organs. The preparations Follutein and Entromone are used in treating undescended testicles.

**Ovarian Hormones.** The ovaries themselves secrete 2 important hormones which affect the activity of the sex glands. One of them, the *follicular hormone,* is made up of substances called *estrogens,* which are especially effective in relieving the discomfort of the menopausal disturbances which occur when the ovaries stop functioning. They are also used to relieve engorged breasts when it is desirable to suppress lactation. They have a limited effect in easing discomfort in inoperable breast cancer. The young woman who undergoes an artificial menopause because of surgery or radiation, will often take estrogen preparations for many years.

Estrogen Preparations. These preparations are usually given intramuscularly, in doses which vary from a fraction of a milligram to 5 mg. or more, and are given once or twice a week for as long as necessary. Available natural estrogen preparations are: Theelin, Diogyn B, Ovocyclin, Progynon, Estinyl, Depo-Estradiol, and Premarin.

The synthetic estrogen preparations are equally effective and are less expensive. Also, they can be given orally. Among those used are diethylstilbestrol, Synestrol, hexestrol, and Benzestrol.

Side-Effects. The side-effects of estrogens usually include nausea and vomiting, diarrhea, and a skin rash. When these symptoms appear, they are likely to be mild and disappear with an adjustment in the dosage, with the use of another estrogen, or with a change in the method of administration. Many doctors believe that estrogens should never be given to women who have had cancer of any part of the reproductive system or have such a family history. The reason is that estrogens are known to cause cancer in animals who have an inherited sensitivity to certain types of cancer.

**Progesterone.** Progesterone, the *luteal hormone,* is secreted by the corpus luteum which influences the conditions of pregnancy. It prepares the lining of the uterus for the implantation of the ovum and nourishment of the embryo, suppresses ovulation during pregnancy, and reduces the irritability of the uterine muscle. Sometimes it is used for uterine bleeding for which no cause can be found or for menstrual irregularity. It is used also in treating repeated miscarriages (abortion) or to promote fertility.

PREPARATIONS. Various preparations of this hormone are available, such as Progestin, Proluton, Lutocyclol, Provera, Norlutin, and Delalutin. They seem to have few serious side-effects; some patients complain of headache, dizziness, and allergic reactions. Most of these preparations are available in tablet form and can be taken orally. The dosage varies from 5 to 25 mg. or more, taken daily.

**The Androgens (Male Sex Hormones).** The androgens are essential for the development of male sex characteristics, and for maintaining normal conditions in the sex organs. Androgen preparations are given to supply a hormone that is missing. Both men and women produce male and female hormones but their effect on men is opposite to the effect on women and vice versa. They are used in treating male reproductive organ deficiencies, disturbances during the male climacteric, and, in women, for dysmenorrhea and to suppress lactation. Androgens are also used for temporary relief in advanced inoperable breast cancer.

PREPARATIONS. Testosterone can be given by injection or by mouth. The dosage varies from 10 to 60 mg. several times a week as needed.

Other preparations of testosterone or similar to it are Oreton, Delatestryl, Neodrol, and Halotestin.

SIDE-EFFECTS. Undesirable effects on a woman are the development of such masculine characteristics as a deep voice, excessive body hair, and shrunken breasts. General and more serious effects may be edema, caused by an accumulation of salts and water in the body, which may lead to heart failure in either sex. Androgens are never given to patients with prostatic cancer.

### Birth Control Drugs

**Oral Contraceptives.** These drugs are given to create temporary sterility. If the patient stops taking the drug, she is again able to become pregnant, and in fact, may be more fertile than before. The function of the ovarian hormones is to prevent ovulation by simulating a pregnancy within the body. The hormone given is that which is released when a woman is pregnant; therefore, if she takes this hormone, she will not ovulate. The drug is contraindicated in women for whom pregnancy would be physically dangerous, such as the diabetics.

A complete discussion of all contraceptive agents is contained in Chapter 51.

**Fertility Drugs.** In some cases, the woman is unable to become pregnant and drugs are given to promote ovulation. The most common of these is Clomiphene citrate (Clomid). This is a synthetic, nonsteroid compound which is administered orally and is believed to stimulate the pituitary to release hormones which, in turn, cause ovulation. It is contraindicated in women with liver disease or with abnormal uterine bleeding. The occurrence of multiple births after taking this drug is very common.

## DRUGS USED TO TREAT EYE CONDITIONS

Drugs which affect the eye are used to treat eye infections and irritations, to dilate or to contract the pupil, to prevent or to relieve pain, or to reduce pressure in the eye. Some of these drugs produce their effects through their action on the autonomic nervous system by relaxing and contracting smooth muscle; others act directly on the tissues. The drugs which dilate the pupil are called *mydriatics*; those which contract the pupil are called *myotics*.

Local anesthetics (injected or applied locally) are used to prevent pain during eye examinations or eye operations. They should not be used repeatedly for painful or irritated eyes because they will injure the cornea. Cocaine and Opthaine are some commonly used preparations.

Eye infections can be treated with whatever antibiotics are effective against the microorganism causing the infection. Some of the antibiotics used in solutions and ointments are tetracycline, streptomycin, bacitracin, neomycin, gantrisin, and others. Antiseptics are generally conceded to be of little use in eye treatments except as cleansers.

Antiseptic solutions are used for eye irrigations. Among those used are silver nitrate, metaphen, and merthiolate solutions.

Glaucoma is caused by an abnormally high production of the fluid in the eye (aqueous humor), resulting in increased pressure within the eyeball. Some drugs used to reduce the production of this fluid are dichlorphenamide, echothiopate iodide, D.F.P., Neptazane, Diamox, Cardrase, and Daranide. Some of them are given orally; others are used as eye drops.

A solution of benzalkonium chloride (Zephiran) is used in cleaning and inserting contact lenses.

## DRUGS USED IN TREATING ALLERGIC REACTIONS AND MOTION SICKNESS

### The Antihistamines

The antihistamines are most effective in relieving the discomfort of the sneezing, dripping victim of hay fever or other pollen-caused irritations. These drugs will not cure an allergy, but they do bring temporary relief and comfort.

The most common unpleasant side-effect of antihistamines, is drowsiness, which may progress to deep sleep. Other side-effects may be mouth and throat dryness, uncertain muscular coordination, and muscular weakness.

**Preparations.** Some of the most commonly used antihistamine preparations are:

*Antazoline:* Nose drops, spray, oral, 50 to 100 mg., 3 times a day (or more)

*Pyribenzamine:* Oral, spray or nose drops, 50 mg., 3 times a day

*Benadryl:* Oral, spray, 25 to 50 mg., 3 or 4 times a day (causes drowsiness)

*Coricidin:* Oral, 2 to 8 mg. (enteric-coated tablet with prolonged effect)

**Antihistamines in Motion Sickness.** Many of the antihistamines are effective in preventing and relieving motion sickness. They are also used to control nausea and vomiting and dizziness in ear conditions, such as fenestration surgery (a delicate operation for deafness) and Meniere's disease. Some of these drugs are effective against the nausea of morning sickness in pregnancy. Among those used are:

*Marezine Hydrochloride:* Oral, rectal, 50 mg. ½ hour before a trip (repeated 3 times a day if necessary)

30 minutes before departure, up to 100 mg., every

*Dramamine:* Oral, rectal, intramuscular, 50 mg., 4 hours for nausea and vomiting

*Perphenazine* is a specific drug used to combat morning sickness.

*Bendectin* is also a specific drug to combat morning sickness and has been discussed elsewhere in this chapter

## Drugs Used in Treating Asthma

Certain drugs relieve bronchial spasms (*antispasmodics*) and edema in asthmatic attacks. Ephedrine, epinephrine, aminophylline, the nitrites, and belladonna have been discussed previously under their specific therapeutic uses.

Drugs used to treat lung infections (PAS, INH, streptomycin, etc.) are discussed in Chapter 48.

## DRUGS TO DESTROY PARASITES

*Anthelmintics* (meaning, against worms) are drugs used to expel worms (*helminths*) from the body. Worms may infect the intestinal tract, muscle tissue, the blood, and other parts of the body. The successful treatment of worms depends on recognizing the type of worm that is present, and then selecting the most effective drug and observing the results.

### Aspidium (Male Fern)

Aspidium, a green liquid with an unpleasant taste, paralyzes worms so that they then can be expelled with the aid of a cathartic. It is effective for pork and fish tapeworms. The patient's dinner and supper are omitted and he is given a saline cathartic in the evening. The next day he is given the drug on an empty stomach, in divided doses an hour apart. It is usually given in enteric-coated capsules. Two hours after the last dose he has another saline cathartic, and this is followed in 2 hours by a soapsuds enema. As soon as the cathartic is effective, he can resume eating.

Every bit of stool must be saved—this is very important to see if the head of the worm has come through. If not, the worm will grow again, and the treatment will have to be repeated.

Aspidium is toxic if much of it is absorbed by the intestine, which is an additional reason for giving cathartics and enemas to remove it. This drug is not used for children.

## Quinacrine (Atabrine)

One dose of quinacrine usually eliminates a beef tapeworm; this drug is effective also for pork and fish tapeworm. It is preceded by a saline cathartic and no food. It may cause gastric irritation—usually sodium bicarbonate is given with it to prevent nausea and vomiting. Quinacrine is effective also in treating malaria, another parasitic infection.

## Piperazine Preparations

These drugs are effective in destroying roundworms and pinworms. They are more effective on the mature worms than on the newly-hatched ones; therefore, a course of treatment of a week or more may need to be repeated a week after the first one. Some of the preparations used are Piperat, Antepar, Perin, and Hetrazan. The advantages of these drugs are that it is not necessary to go without food or take cathartics while they are being given.

## Hexylresorcinol

This drug paralyzes roundworm, pinworm, hookworm, and dwarf tapeworm. Often, a single dose is effective; if necessary, the procedure can be repeated in 3 or 4 days. A saline cathartic is given before and after and no food is allowed during the treatment.

The following is a brief summary of the preparations used in treating the various types of worms:

*Tapeworms:* Aspidium, quinacrine, hexylresorcinol

*Roundworms and Whipworms:* Dithiazanine, piperazine salts, diethylcarbamazine

*Pinworms:* Hexylresorcinol, dithiazanine, gentian violet—pinworms deposit their eggs around the anus, so this region should be kept clean

*Hookworms:* Tetrachloroethylene, hexylresorcinol

## Amebiasis

Amebiasis is caused by intestinal parasites called *amebae.* They destroy tissues within the intestine and outside of the intestine, in the parts of the body where they choose to locate, such as in the liver or spleen. Drugs used to treat amebiasis in the intestine are Carbarson, Milibis, Balarsen, Diodoquin, and Vioform. The antibiotic Fumidil is also effective.

For amebiasis outside of the intestine, Emetine is the most effective in controlling amebic dysentery. It is used extensively in treating amebic hepatitis and liver abscess. Undesirable side-effects are degenerative changes in the liver, kidney, heart, and muscles. Aralen is another effective drug in treating amebic hepatitis and amebic abscess.

## SERUMS AND VACCINES AS DRUGS

The part played by serums and vaccines in preventing or treating disease has been emphasized in the discussion of immunity. The specific process of antigen and antibody reaction is also discussed elsewhere in this book. Specific serums and vaccines are mentioned also in connection with specific disease conditions in which they are used.

## Serums

There are two kinds of serums—immune and antitoxic. Immune serums are obtained from normal blood or from the blood of people who have recovered from a disease. They are used to prevent the disease in others. Examples are the human serums used to prevent measles, infectious hepatitis, whooping cough, and poliomyelitis. Examples of these serums are immune serum globulin, human gamma globulin, and pertussis human serum.

## Antitoxins (Antitoxin Serums)

Antitoxic serums are produced in the bodies of animals. They are given to neutralize the poisons produced in the bodies of people by certain diseases. These serums are the diphtheria, tetanus and gas gangrene antitoxins. They are given when the patient has been exposed to a disease and does not have time to build up antibodies.

## Vaccines

Vaccines are preparations of disease organisms (which may be live vaccines or may have been killed) that produce immunity to infectious disease. It may take several weeks for immunity to develop; sometimes, if an effective human serum is available, a dose of the serum is given first to insure immediate protection from a disease. This might be done when there is danger of immediate infection, as when many cases of an infectious disease appear in a community and individuals run the risk of being exposed to it.

Vaccines are available to prevent or to treat mumps, whooping cough, typhoid, yellow fever, smallpox, rabies, tuberculosis, influenza, and poliomyelitis. Polio vaccine (the Salk vaccine) has practically eliminated poliomyelitis in this country (see Chapter 46); however, there is some doubt about the effectiveness of the influenza vaccines now being used.

## Toxoids

Certain infectious conditions produce poisons (toxins) in the body. *Toxoids* are toxins with the poisonous effects modified to make them nontoxic but still capable of building up immunity to a disease. Toxoids are effective in building up immunity to diphtheria and tetanus. They are used separately or in various combinations with whopping cough vaccine—a combination of the three (*triple toxoid*) is the choice for immunizing children. They are given as a routine procedure, after which the patient builds up his own antibodies.

## Immunity Tests

Tests can be done to determine whether or not a person is susceptible to certain disease organisms. A small amount of the toxin produced by a disease is injected intracutaneously on the forearm. If his body has not produced enough antitoxin to protect him from the disease, a reddened and swollen area appears around the point of the injection—a *positive* reaction. *Schick test toxin* is available to test diphtheria susceptibility.

A positive reaction to a test with *old tuberculin* will show whether or not a person has had tuberculosis at some time, but it does not necessarily mean that the person has active tuberculosis at the time of the test.

## ENZYMES AS DRUGS

Enzymes are substances that speed up chemical reactions in the body, without being changed themselves during the process. Used as drugs, they help to promote the absorption of fluids or drugs, to reduce thick, purulent discharges, to thin fluids, and to dissolve blood clots. They also destroy certain toxins or allergens. Some enzyme preparations in current use are Alidase, Wydase, Trypsin (Tryptar), Varidase, and Chymar. Penicillinase (neutrapen) is effective in treating a penicillin reaction by "pulling the teeth" of the allergen which is causing the trouble.

## DRUGS USED IN TREATING CANCER

So far, no drug has been found that will cure cancer—only early surgery and x-ray will do that and, then, only if all of a cancerous growth is removed before the cancer cells have been carried to another part of the body (metastasis). However, antimalignant (antineoplastic) drugs help to retard the progress of malignant disease that has spread to another part of the body and help to make the patient more comfortable, sometimes for months and even years. These drugs are used specifically to treat malignant tumors and cancerous conditions of the blood and lymph (leukemia), the bone marrow, and the spleen. They are used only when there is no hope of recovery because they affect healthy cells as well as malignant ones; they also are harmful to bone marrow and lower the patient's resistance to infection.

Experimental work is constantly going on in search of a drug that will cure cancer. Thousands of drugs are being tested every year under the direction of the National Cancer Institute of the U. S. Public Health Service, in cooperation with hospitals, research centers, industry and government. Every year a number of drugs are approved for testing with patients, but so far, none of the drugs tested has given indisputable scientific proof that it cures cancer.

## Radioactive Isotopes

These are radioactive substances which give off rays that penetrate tissues and arrest the growth of cancer cells. They affect the cells of the ovaries and the testes particularly, as well as the lymphocytes and the bone marrow, and they act on cells in the intestinal tract to reduce accumulations of fluid. Patients undergoing this treatment may be troubled with nausea and vomiting and diarrhea.

Precautions are necessary in handling isotopes, as their rays damage normal tissues, such as the skin, and cause radiation burns. (See Chapter 43.)

## KEEPING UP WITH DRUGS

Since new drugs are constantly being tested for approval by the Federal Drug Administration and appearing on the market, you will not find every drug used in treating patients listed in this book. Some drugs already listed may be replaced by newer drugs that are more effective; others may be removed from the approved list because their continued use has been shown to have dangerous effects on health.

The nurse has a grave responsibility to her patients to be very sure of any drug which she is giving. She *must* look up any drug about which she has a question. There is *no excuse* for giving a drug without knowing the appropriate dosage, the proper form, and the possible side-effects. Therefore the nurse must be familiar with the reference books which are available and must keep up with new drugs, in an effort to give the best possible nursing care to her patients.

# 34

# Rehabilitation

---

## BEHAVIORAL OBJECTIVES

*The student successfully attaining the goals of this chapter will be able to:*

- *define rehabilitation.*
- *discuss the concept of restorative nursing care.*
- *demonstrate an understanding of the principles of rehabilitation in the clinical setting with patients with varying degrees of disability.*
- *plan possible activities for patients with cardiac disorders, diabetes, nervous system disorders, paralytic disorders, special needs following surgery, poor eyesight and deafness.*
- *involve the patient's family in the task of rehabilitation.*

---

The National Society for Crippled Children and Adults reported recently that there are nearly 22 million disabled people in the United States—an increase of over 2 million in a single year. This means that 1 in every 9 Americans must contend with some sort of handicap which requires special attention. While accidents have always been a great cause for disability, this rapid increase in the number of disabled people is partly due to modern medicine which saves afflicted babies and prolongs life to the ages when people are more likely to develop disabling conditions, such as strokes, heart ailments, and arthritis.

## DEFINITION OF REHABILITATION

The modern definition of rehabilitation is the restoration of a disabled person's former abilities or, if complete restoration is not possible, helping him to make the most of the capabilities he has. Until recently, we were accustomed to thinking of rehabilitation as attention to overcoming some very marked physical disability such as the loss of an arm or a leg. Highly trained, skillful people have worked with the big disability problems—the polio victims, the amputees, the spastics. In past years, a vast number of people with disabilities such as those caused by heart conditions, strokes, or arthritis were condemned to a life of semi-invalidism or complete invalidism because they were considered incapable of anything else.

## RESTORATIVE NURSING CARE

Rehabilitation from an illness begins with the treatment to halt destructive processes and to repair body damage. It also includes preventing further injury and restoring normal functions. This is restorative nursing—every nurse's responsibility in rehabilitation. It includes the whole person, but unfortunately we do not always do as well as we might, even with the patient's body, not to mention his emotional needs.

## The Successful Rehabilitation Nurse

The most important asset of the nurse who is working with patients undergoing rehabilitation, is that of *empathy*—not pity or sympathy. In other words, she should make an attempt to understand how the patient feels and assist him in working through his feelings.

The nurse should be a good clinical practitioner of nursing. She must be especially observant, not only of physical difficulties, but also of feelings and emotions.

The nurse must remember that the patient is concerned with himself at the time of admission to the rehabilitation unit. He has just undergone a severe blow to his self-image and is interested in helping himself. First impressions are very important, and the nurse who belittles or humiliates the patient will most likely never get another chance with that patient. The patient's defenses are very low at this time, and if hurt once, he is unlikely to open up easily.

The patient must be assisted to work through his feelings about his disability, especially if he was suddenly disabled, and must be encouraged to work toward making the most of the facilities he has available to him. Since a patient often goes through a period of depression and then hostility before he is able to adjust to his difficulties, the nurse must understand this, so that she does not react unreasonably to his demands or outbursts.

## Your Attitude

The National Easter Seal Society for Crippled Children and Adults suggests several ways in which you can make the handicapped person feel more comfortable, whether you meet him in or out of the hospital. The most important factor is that you must remember that the handicapped person is, first of all and most importantly, a *person*. He has feelings, goals, desires, and problems just like anyone else. Generally, he does not want to be treated in a special way, but wants you to treat him just like you would anyone else. He is not different, except for a physical limitation. Do not assist the handicapped person unnecessarily unless he requests help or unless the doctor has specifically ordered this. The person wants to be as independent as possible and can only become so if he is allowed to do things for himself.

## The Patient's Attitude

A patient is likely to meet the problem of a disability in much the same spirit as he has faced other problems. He may be resentful, despairing, or disbelieving or he may face a disability with the determination to do everything possible to overcome it. The nurse needs to be sensitive to the kind of person he is; she must be prepared to offer encouragement and assistance, with respect for the patient as an adult capable of making decisions. It is a mistake to treat people with body disabilities as if they were also mentally disabled, which is quite different from being mentally depressed. It may take a great deal of patience and perseverance to interest the patient in making an effort to improve his condition and to convince him that it is not hopeless. He and his family must also understand the extent of his disability and how it is possible to regain some—perhaps all—normal functions. Even in such illnesses as arteriosclerosis (hardening of the arteries), which grow progressively worse, the patient should be encouraged to help himself as long as possible.

## The Assistance of Other Disciplines

In rehabilitative nursing, the practical nurse will be working with health workers from other fields of study. These people include the Physical Therapist, the Occupational Therapist, the Recreation Therapist, the Music Therapist, and the Speech Therapist, as well as the medical doctors who are specialists in each area. You should discuss the patient with these people in an effort to determine how best to assist him in meeting his daily living needs.

## The Patient's Interests

The key to selecting activities to keep a patient interested or amused lies in his interests. With a woman who likes to sew, do not take it for granted that she is interested in reading too, if she has never read much. People like to use their minds in different ways—to direct their hands or their thoughts or both. The more things a person knows how to do and the more things he is interested in, the easier it will be to find something to divert and occupy him.

The wife and mother who loves to cook may resent illness most because it keeps her out of her kitchen. It may not be easy to sell her the idea of playing solitaire—perhaps she *would* like to take this time to copy those recipes lying loose in a kitchen drawer.

## The Patient's Limitations

Of course, it all comes back to the patient's physical condition and the things he is able to do and can do safely. Often you can persuade a patient that this is the time to relax and do something silly and amusing; perhaps this is his opportunity to learn something he never has had time for. Many of us have secret longings to do things which seem to serve no practical purpose and feel guilty about taking time for them—such as crossword puzzles or mystery stories. Some people get the most satisfaction out of making something useful.

## Planning Ahead

Determine the patient's needs and plan accordingly. A patient may need only some diversion to pass the time until he is able to get back to normal life. If he is left with some handicap, a long-range plan is needed to build up physical strength, to retrain muscles, to learn how to carry on his work with the handicap, or to learn new ways of looking after himself and making a living.

**The Cardiac Patient.** Let us look at a few suggested activities for patients. For example, the cardiac patient's activities depend on the kind of heart condition that he has. Physical activities may be permitted; they may be limited; or they may be forbidden. Perhaps he can use his hands to play solitaire or to work on a hobby, such as stamp collecting, wood carving, working with plastics, or fly-tying. Sometimes a hobby will bring in money—an additional satisfaction. If activities are forbidden, you will concentrate on making him as contented as possible. He may be able to read with the assistance of a page turner, or he may be allowed to watch television.

**The Diabetic Patient.** You always have to think of possible dangers to the patient's body. A diabetic is susceptible to infection. Never give him things that might injure his skin, such as sharp tools or rough materials, without proper instruction. His eyesight may be poor, so he must have good light in which to work. His muscles may be weak, so pay attention to his posture and do not let him get tired.

**When the Nervous System Is Affected.** Anything that affects the nervous system is likely to interfere with muscle coordination and fine movements. If the patient's mental ability is impaired, he will be unable to do complicated things. If the brain deteriorates, the activities must become more simple. Avoid the activities which require small, fine movements—they are impossible for such a patient and only discourage him when he finds that he cannot carry them out. Some conditions grow progressively worse; others improve. Begin with large movements. A patient might be able to grasp a washcloth to wash his face yet be unable to feed himself. You can work up the finer movements gradually, as the condition improves.

**After Polio or Other Paralytic Disorders.** Aside from the special training required to re-educate paralyzed muscles and to learn to use braces, these patients need encouragement. They can use their hands and minds in spite of paralyzed legs. They may need new interests, to take the place of those which are physically impossible, or help to see how they still can participate in their former interests to some extent. A youngster who cannot play football still can watch a football game; perhaps he can keep an eye on sweaters and hold wristwatches and valuables for the players. He should be encouraged to be as nearly like people of his own age as possible.

**After Surgical Operations.** Choose activities which prevent handicaps and improve physical limitations. If Mrs. Gray has had her breast removed, the breast muscles will contract, if they are allowed to and prevent her from raising her arm. The doctor will tell you how much she can do safely and when. Help her to stretch the muscles by encouraging her to powder her nose and comb her hair. When Mark comes out of his cast, think what it will mean to him to get his leg back to normal—Mark is a truck driver. Listen carefully to the directions that the doctor or the head nurse gives you and use every opportunity that you have to help Mark. Often he does not understand why he needs to be careful or to persist with certain exercises himself. As his nurse, you know that the bone that bridges the break needs protection until time hardens it; the cast protected it, but now the cast is off.

**When Eyes Fail.** The patient who is going blind is bewildered and lost. He needs to develop his sense of touch as a substitute for his eyes. Help him to experiment with finding his way around his room and around the house. He still can hear; point out that he can learn to recognize footsteps and also that he can talk with people as well as ever. He also can learn to read Braille. Help him with his food; tell him where things are on the plate, at 12 o'clock, at 3 o'clock, etc. Always try to put the same kinds of things in the same places. You can learn to help him to help himself to the extent that people will forget that he is blind. Try blindfolding yourself for a while and practice walking and eating. This will assist you in thinking of some of the things you should teach the blind person.

**The Deaf Person.** The deaf person is lonely. Companionship depends so much on hearing that the deaf person feels out of things. He sees lips move and does not know what they say. He dreads bothering people to repeat their words. A hearing aid is the answer for certain types of deafness. If a hearing aid will not help, many people can learn lip reading. Of course, the deaf person can read and do things with his hands that the blind person has difficulty in doing.

**Color and Materials.** Color is important. Some colors are soothing; others have an irritating effect. Find out what colors the patient likes and those which bother him. Some people hate the feeling of woolly things; some materials have an odor which people dislike.

**Reading Aloud.** When you read aloud, choose the parts of the newspapers, the magazine article, or the book that the patient likes. If he likes the sports page, read that. Before you read anything, learn *how* to read. Pro-

nounce the words distinctly—do not gallop but do not crawl, either. Put some expression into your reading; be interested yourself. Practice now, while you are a student, and get your classmates to criticize your performance.

**The Family Can Help.** Take the patient's family into your confidence. Explain why one activity is good for mother, or grandfather, or Johnny, and why another might be discouraging or harmful. "Isn't she doing too much?" they will say. Or "Poor Grandpa—I can't bear to see him fumbling with his washcloth. Wouldn't it be better to wash his face yourself?" Without meaning to, the family may make the patient more dependent instead of less so. Explain that pity emphasizes a handicap and makes people feel "different!"

**Watch the Results.** Watch the effect of an activity. Begin it when the patient is rested; stop before he gets tired. Notice whether he seems bored. Use an activity to fill up the empty places in the day. Encourage the patient to show his work and to talk about it.

It all amounts to this: your job really is to feel with your patient what it means to him to be a human being, to be able to enjoy himself, to work again, to accept a handicap and to learn to be independent in spite of it. You watch out for things that may cause deformities —sheets tight over the toes, lack of support under the knees, pillows that are too high, harmful body positions. You help patients to adjust appliances, to use crutches correctly, to protect themselves from accidents. And, most important of all, you build up their self-confidence by encouraging them to help themselves.

**Look and Listen.** Many patients are not in the hospital long enough to start activities which help to provide interest and keep them occupied during convalescence or a long-term illness. However, if you are alert you can learn a great deal about a patient while you are giving him nursing care. He will talk to you, perhaps will ask questions, or discuss his worries with you. This gives you an opportunity to make helpful suggestions for activities which will occupy his time and may even be useful as well as interesting. At the same time you can emphasize the importance of following orders which are a part of his treatment, such as diet regulations, medicines, and exercises. The opportunities for restorative nursing in a nursing home are almost unlimited, for we now know that many more of these patients can be encouraged to do things for themselves which once were considered impossible for them to accomplish. People who are helping themselves are likely to be happy people.

## REHABILITATIVE AIDS

The Bell Telephone System has developed many valuable aids for the handicapped. Special equipment makes it possible for a blind person to operate a telephone switchboard. A device that can be incorporated in a telephone receiver helps the hard of hearing. Shut-in students can keep up with their school work from home or hospital with speakerphones that do not have to be held or lifted. For the voiceless, an electronic artificial larynx substitutes for the vibrations of normal vocal cords.

Information about these aids is available from local offices of the Bell Telephone System.

Other health agencies will provide special services, many of which are free. For example, the local Cancer Society may lend a wheelchair when the family is unable to provide it. In some cases, the National Foundation will arrange for physical therapy treatments for the paralyzed person who is retraining muscles. The nurse must explore available community resources when help is needed and instruct the patient or his family accordingly. Many people are unaware of these special services.

Many other rehabilitative aids exist such as braces and splints, adaptive devices for the homemaker, special controls on automobiles, respiratory aids, artificial limbs and other body parts. It is even possible for the patient to learn to write or paint with his feet or to type using a special device in his mouth. Almost any patient can regain some function, using special devices and aids.

# 35

# First Aid and Care in Emergencies

---

### BEHAVIORAL OBJECTIVES

*The student successfully attaining the goals of this chapter will be able to:*

- *list 7 principles of first-aid care.*
- *state the information to be found on a Medic Alert tag.*
- *define asphyxiation and indicate the treatment required.*
- *discuss measures for controlling hemorrhage.*
- *recognize poisoning and take appropriate steps to help victim.*
- *describe first aid for burns.*
- *effectively deal with common emergencies arising in and out of the hospital.*
- *discuss legal aspects of first aid.*

---

## THE PROBLEM OF ACCIDENTS

Every year, thousands of people lose their lives in accidents—on the highway, at work, during recreation, or in the home. In the 1 to 34 age group, accidents are the first cause of death; in the 35-44 age group, accidents are second only to heart and circulatory diseases. The fatalities are approximately 100,000 per year. The injury total every year is numbered in the millions. Over 4,000,000 injuries happen in the home. The chances are greater than ever that any person may be at the scene of an accident at some time and should be able to act promptly and intelligently.

Unquestionably, many accidents could be prevented. First-aid instruction should go hand in hand with information about accident prevention. State and local governments provide public protection by means of highway regulations, fire laws, and industrial safety requirements. The National Safety Council and the state safety councils carry on a determined campaign for safety; through lectures and films they demonstate to civic groups how accidents can be prevented. Accident costs amount to staggering sums every year. These costs include medical expense, wage losses, property damage, etc., and are in the billions.

### Emergencies and Nursing Care

When an emergency occurs, you must be able to meet it. This chapter is not a substitute for a complete course in first aid, but it does tell you how you can deal with common emergencies and offers you some important information on the *legal responsibility* of a nurse during an emergency situation.

To begin with, first-aid principles tell you what to do and what *not* to do when accidents happen. In your eagerness to do something, you may do the wrong thing; sometimes the less you do the more helpful you are so far as the victim is concerned. The victim is not the only person you may have to deal with—someone among the bystanders or a member of the family may initiate hasty action, may faint or become hysterical. In a serious emergency, if you are confident, matter-of-fact, and calm, you reassure the patient and everyone else. You must make up your mind *quickly* about what you are going to do, and your attitude and your knowledge of first-aid principles will give you command of the situation.

## FIRST AID

### Principles of First-Aid Care

1. *Breathing:* Since oxygenation of the blood is essential for life, one of the first things to check is the status of the victim's breathing. You can do this by listening to the chest, by placing a mirror in front of the patient's nose (and watching for it to steam up), or by feeling the chest to see if it is expanding. If the patient is not breathing, it is imperative to establish *pulmonary resuscitation immediately*. It is also imperative to check for heartbeat immediately.

2. *Heartbeat:* Since respiration and circulation are interlocked, the patient must be breathing in order to oxygenate the blood and the heart must be beating in order to circulate that blood. You can check for heartbeat by feeling the pulse in the radial (wrist), femoral (groin), or temporal areas. Sometimes a carotid artery pulsation can be felt in the neck, even in the case of weak heartbeat. If the heart is stopped, you must begin *cardiopulmonary resuscitation immediately*.

3. *Bleeding:* Excessive bleeding must be controlled immediately in order to save the patient's life. Direct pressure over the wound with a sterile compress is the measure to try first. This will usually succeed in stopping hemorrhage. If all else fails, apply a tourniquet. Once the tourniquet is applied, do not remove it or loosen it. Be sure to mark the patient's forehead with a T, so that the doctor will be aware that there is a tourniquet in place.

4. *Shock:* Lower the patient's head (except in the case of a head injury) and cover him to maintain his body temperature, but do not overheat him. Attempt to reassure him, so that he will not become overexcited.

5. *Notify a Doctor:* If you are alone on the scene of an accident, you will need to restore breathing and heartbeat, stop hemorrhage, and treat for shock before notifying a doctor or ambulance. If someone else is on the scene, however, the ambulance should be called immediately. If you are in an unfamiliar area, call the operator and she will assist you. The local police department or highway patrol are also of invaluable aid in an emergency.

6. *Splint Fractures:* Prevent further injury by applying splints to fractures. Remember that a compound fracture must be treated as an open wound, to prevent infection.

7. *Dress Wounds:* Cleanse and apply bandages to other wounds, if you have the equipment and the time.

8. Perform other general first aid measures as needed.

### General Procedures and Follow-Up

1. *Size up the situation.* Is it serious enough to send for a doctor? A pailful of hot water upset over a child, gushing blood, a dangling arm, or an unconscious victim are signs that a doctor is needed. You can deal with excited or hysterical bystanders by giving them something to do—ask one of them to call the doctor at once. This leaves you free to give your whole attention to the patient.

2. *Examine the patient.* In minor accidents this is comparatively easy—Tommy holds up the scratched knee, and a glance tells you what has happened; even so, you must be sure that he has no other injuries. Get the victim to tell you how the accident happened and look for bumps or scratches on other parts of his body, if this seems necessary.

3. *Make the victim comfortable.* Be careful not to add to his injury by moving him too much; in most emergencies, it is best not to move the patient at all. Keep the victim lying down and comfortable. Moving a limb may displace a fractured bone still farther. Keep the patient warm; keep the crowd away.

4. *Give the necessary first-aid treatment.* This may be the only treatment that the victim needs, but in serious conditions you give emergency treatment only until the doctor arrives.

5. *Provide for safe follow-up care.* If an accident happens in public, instruct the victim

to see his doctor if a doctor has not been called at the time of the accident. Be prepared to report to the doctor or the ambulance crew exactly what was done for the patient.

6. *Report the treatment.* Medical aid is always available for emergencies in the hospital; you will always report any accident to the head nurse, no matter how trivial it seems. Hospitals have a legal responsibility for patients' safety; a prompt report and a detailed account of the accident must appear on the patient's record. In any case, every injury requiring emergency treatment *must be reported and noted on the chart.*

## The Medic Alert Tag

Every nurse must be aware of the Medic Alert tag and what it means and must always look for it in any emergency situation. This tag is worn as a bracelet on the wrist or on a chain around the neck. It signifies that the person has a health problem of some sort, which the doctor and nurse must take into consideration when administering first aid or other care. The tag is shown in Figure 35-1.

Each person who wears a tag of this type is given a number, which can be used for identification. There is also a telephone number on the tag, which can be called day or night to obtain further information about the patient, his name, the name of his doctor, and any other pertinent information which is not printed on the tag.

The types of information which are printed on the back of the tag indicate whether the patient is a diabetic, has seizures, has glaucoma, is wearing contact lenses, has a laryngectomy and is breathing through a tube in his neck, or is allergic to any of many drugs or other substances. If these factors are not taken into account and if the patient is not treated correctly, he may die.

Since other sources of information may be found on a victim's person, the nurse should also look in the billfold of an unconscious accident victim to see if any medical information is there. If the nurse finds a card indicating that the person wishes to donate one or several organs of his body for transplant after death, she should inform the doctor of this at the scene of an accident.

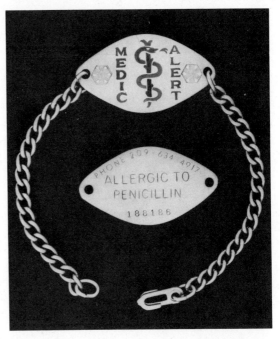

Figure 35-1. This is the standard Medic Alert tag. Take a good look at it so that you will be able to recognize it in an emergency. The phone number to call in the event of an emergency is (area code 209) 634-4917 (in the United States). (Medic Alert Foundation International)

## Asphyxiation

**Definition.** In first aid, asphyxiation refers to the inability of the victim to breathe. This may be due to several causes, but the result is the same: anoxia (lack of sufficient oxygen to sustain life) and an excessive amount of carbon dioxide in the tissues.

**Physical Causes**

  Choking or strangling on a foreign object
  Electric shock
  Drowning
  Inhalation of poisonous gases
  Compression of the chest by outside force
  Overdosage of respiratory depressant drugs

**Treatment.** The initial treatment is to ascertain the cause of the asphyxia. If a foreign body has obstructed the air passages, it must be removed to allow atmospheric oxygen to reach the lungs. If an electric current has interrupted the central nervous system response so that breathing has stopped, remove the victim from the cause of the shock by turning off the current or by moving him with a non-

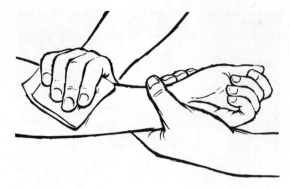

Figure 35-2. Direct pressure over wound. You can do this best by placing the cleanest material available (sterile gauze is best) against the bleeding point and applying firm pressure with your hand until a bandage can be applied. (American Red Cross: First Aid Textbook, ed. 4, New York, Doubleday, 1957)

conducting instrument (a wooden pole). Inhalation of poisonous gases (illuminating gas is one of the most common) requires that the gas be turned off and that the patient be removed immediately to a gas-free atmosphere so that proper exchange of oxygen in the lung tissues may be restored. If the victim's chest is compressed by an outside force (for example, when trapped by a landslide), you must make every effort to remove the compression in order to permit proper expansion of the chest. If the compression is by fracture of the bony cage of the ribs, never use artificial respiration by applying pressure—*puncture of the lung may result*. Instead, employ the mouth-to-mouth breathing technic. A sedative or hypnotic, such as opium, and coal-tar derivative drugs, given in an overdose, depress the respiratory center of the brain; each has its own method of treatment.

Whatever the cause of asphyxiation, the main principle of first aid is: (1) to establish an open (patent) airway and (2) to restore the normal mechanism of breathing.

The technics of cardiopulmonary resuscitation have been discussed at length in other portions of this book. (Cardiac resuscitation is discussed in Chapter 47; respiratory resuscitation is discussed in Chapter 31.) Every nurse must know the methods of restoring the patient's airway, breathing, and heartbeat. The nurse must remember that, once resuscitation

has been initiated, it cannot be discontinued until the doctor arrives and makes the decision.

## Hemorrhage

The blood is distributed throughout the body by the arteries, which branch again and again until they form the capillaries. From the capillaries, the blood returns to the heart through the veins. When any blood vessel is cut or torn, blood escapes. The amount of bleeding depends on the number and the size of the injured blood vessels. A severe injury to one large blood vessel may cause a serious hemorrhage, but an injury to many small vessels may cause damage which is equally serious. When a severe hemorrhage occurs, the body loses the red blood cells which are necessary to carry oxygen to the cells, and it loses fluid, upsetting the body's fluid balance. Therefore, the most important first-aid treatment in this case is to stop the hemorrhage. The second step is to treat shock, which always accompanies severe bleeding, by keeping the patient quiet and warm.

**Control by Pressure.** Bleeding can be controlled by applying pressure to the bleeding area or by shutting off the main arteries that supply blood to it.

The first thing to do in a case where bleeding is serious or superficial is to apply pressure: pressure at the right spot will control bleeding in most external injuries. Fold a clean dressing to make a pad and apply it to the bleeding area (see Fig. 35-2); you can use a clean handkerchief or cloth if you do not have a sterile dressing. Newspaper is also a clean substitute. Press the dressing firmly on the bleeding area; then apply a firm bandage to hold the dressing in place. Be sure that the circulation is not shut off entirely.

**Pressure Points.** You can frequently tell by the flow whether the bleeding comes from an artery or a vein: blood from an *artery* comes in *spurts,* but blood comes from a *vein* in a *steady flow.* Pressure on a large artery supplying blood to the injured part will control bleeding; the artery must lie close to a bone so that there is a firm surface to press against. The 6 main *pressure points,* (see Fig. 35-3) used to stop bleeding from the various parts of the body, and the arteries they control are:

Figure 35-3. Diagram of pressure points showing their relation to arteries and bones.

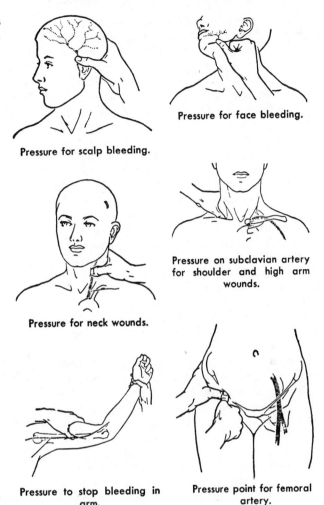

Pressure for scalp bleeding.

Pressure for face bleeding.

Pressure for neck wounds.

Pressure on subclavian artery for shoulder and high arm wounds.

Pressure to stop bleeding in arm.

Pressure point for femoral artery.

*The head and the neck*

1. The *carotid artery* in the neck, located beside the windpipe (trachea). Press *back* against the spine—pressure on the trachea will shut off breathing.

2. The *temporal artery,* in front of the ear

3. The *facial artery,* on the jawbone about an inch forward from the angle of the jaw

*The shoulder and the arm*

4. The *subclavian artery,* just behind the inner end of the collar bone, or clavicle, exerting pressure down against the first rib

5. The *brachial artery,* on the upper arm next to the body, halfway between the elbow and the shoulder

*The lower limbs*

6. The *femoral artery,* midway in the groin where the artery passes over the pelvic bone

Bleeding is usually not very extensive in a minor wound, but it is important to cover any wound with a clean dressing to prevent infection. You can apply an antiseptic before applying the dressing, if the ambulance is not coming. Apply the medication with a sterile cotton applicator. Never apply ointments or oils to a wound.

Apply a sterile dressing and secure it firmly with a bandage or strips of adhesive; if the dressing slips or slides over the surrounding skin, the dressing becomes unsterile.

A Band-Aid makes an adequate dressing for small cuts or scratches; Band-Aids come in different sizes and should be in every home medicine cabinet. Be sure never to touch with your fingers the part of a sterile dressing that covers the wound; put the dressing exactly where you want it because you cannot move it afterward without unsterilizing it. Be sure that the bandage or the adhesive is firm but not tight enough to cut off the circulation. Telfa pads are much less irritating than conventional bandages.

**Applying a Tourniquet.** *A tourniquet should be used only in case of an extensive hemorrhage which is endangering a life, and in a case which does not respond to the direct pressure method of control. This is only when a large artery has been injured or when a complete or partial amputation of a limb has occurred.*

A tourniquet must be made of materials present at the site of the accident. This can be anything that will make a flat band about 2 inches wide, or rubber tubing if it is available; a strip of inner tube makes an excellent tourniquet. You can use a stocking, a belt, or a large handkerchief folded into a cravat—never use cord or wire because it would injure the flesh. Place a compact, rolled piece of material over the pressure point of the artery controlling the blood flow to the injury. Wrap the tourniquet around this pad, tie a half knot, place a stick or similar object over it, tie a square knot over the stick, then twist the stick to tighten the tourniquet. Fasten in position. *Do not loosen the tourniquet without the permission of a doctor! Tag the patient with a note stating its location and the time of application. Transport the victim to medical aid immediately!*

A tourniquet must be tight enough to cut off the flow of blood in the artery; if it is too loose, it will only prevent the blood from flowing back through the veins and increase the bleeding. Obviously, a tourniquet is never used to apply pressure to the carotid artery, since it would strangle the patient.

Never cover a tourniquet with anything. If forgotten, it will cause gangrene by damaging the circulation permanently. Apply a sterile dressing to the wound and bandage it. Gauze helps in preserving the blood clot, and the bandage exerts pressure. Never wipe blood clots from a wound—the clot acts as a plug for ruptured blood vessels. If it breaks loose, it can cause death. Keep the bleeding part quiet and elevate it if possible.

**Nosebleed.** Nosebleed will be discussed in Chapter 48.

## Shock

Shock was discussed in Chapter 32 as a postoperative complication. Here we are considering it as a complication following an injury, but the cause and the symptoms are the same as shock occurring after surgery. The skin is cold, pale, and moist; the pulse, rapid and thready; the respirations, difficult and gasping, and there is a drop in blood pressure. Shock is usually caused by severe blood loss, externally or internally. Anything that causes or increases hemorrhage should be avoided, especially handling or moving the patient roughly.

Every victim should have preventive and precautionary treatment for shock, since these signs do not always appear immediately after injury and can occur as a result of fright. Keep the patient lying down to facilitate the flow of blood to the head and the chest (the head and the chest may be elevated if breathing is difficult). Elevate the lower part of the body unless there is a head injury, a breathing difficulty, fractures of the lower extremity, or abdominal pain.

Apply sufficient covering to retain body heat; a blanket placed beneath the body if the patient is lying on the ground or the floor is helpful. If it is necessary to use hot-water bags or heating pads in extremely cold weather, be sure that these objects are not in contact with the skin since the victim may not be conscious of a burn.

Blood, plasma, or other parenteral fluids are usually given when the patient is under medical care. If this is delayed, sips of water may be given except when the patient is unconscious or nauseated or has an abdominal wound. *Do not give alcoholic drinks.* Control hemorrhage when possible; keep the patient quiet and maintain his morale with words of reassurance.

## Poisoning

Any substance which affects health or threatens life when it is absorbed into the body or when in contact with body surfaces is a poison. All drugs are potential poisons, but many do not have poisonous effects because they are given in small doses. Poisoning is all too often the result of misreading the label on a drug, taking a drug from an unlabeled bottle, or taking a drug from a medicine cupboard in the dark.

Poisonous substances are all around us in household cleaning agents, insecticides, antifreeze, furniture polish, kerosene, and nail polish, to name a few. Accidental poisoning happens frequently, especially with children who consume colored tablets of barbiturates, aspirin, or other drugs, thinking that they are candy. Sometimes poisons are taken deliberately, with the intention of committing suicide. In this case the barbiturates are often used, or the person inhales carbon monoxide gas from an automobile exhaust.

In the case of any poisoning, if possible, call the nearest *Poison Control Center*. The responsible nurse must take it upon herself to find out where it is located.

*Food poisoning* (ptomaine) is almost always caused by eating food which has been contaminated by bacteria. The normal action of the bacteria on the food causes decomposition which, in turn, causes the formation of toxins (poisonous substances). Other causes include the accidental eating of certain fruits, berries, or vegetable materials (for example, toadstools) which contain substances poisonous to humans.

The symptoms of food poisoning include abdominal pain, nausea and/or vomiting, and diarrhea. The onset is acute (within a few hours after taking the contaminated food). The symptoms usually disappear in 1 or 2 days after the toxins have been excreted.

A more severe form of food poisoning is called *botulism*. This is caused by a specific organism, *Clostridium botulinum*. Over 45 per cent of the cases result in death. Home-preserved foods are a common cause and are most dangerous to use unless they have been sterilized at 248° F. to kill possible contamination.

The symptoms of botulinus poisoning are weakness, headache, muscular weakness, paralysis of the eye and the throat muscles and, finally, respiratory paralysis. Specific antitoxins are effective if given early; artificial respiration is essential until the antitoxin takes effect.

**The Emergency Treatment of Poisoning**
(Table 35-1)

1. Always remember that the first thing to do in case of poisoning is to call the doctor.

2. Identify the poison. Question the victim, if possible, as to the possible source. Save *all* vomitus, urine, and stools and the remains of the food or the drugs which may have been responsible.

3. Remove the poison from the stomach by inducing vomiting (except in the case of a strong acid or alkali, or if the patient is unconscious). This can be done by giving an emetic made of 1 tablespoonful of mustard in a glass of warm water, or of 2 tablespoonfuls of salt in a glass of warm water. Give this to the victim orally, followed with copious amounts of warm water until vomiting has apparently cleared the stomach of the poisonous substance.

4. Give an antidote. An antidote is a substance which inactivates the poison or keeps it from being absorbed. Common household substances that are available are milk, egg white, strong tea, coffee, or starch.

5. Give supportive treatment. Keep the patient warm by applying external heat to the body. Use artificial respiration or oxygen if the respirations are affected. Maintain the heartbeat.

## Fainting

Fainting is caused by an insufficient supply of blood in the brain. People faint when they are hungry, tired, or in close, crowded rooms. Emotional shock or the sight of blood may cause fainting. Fainting may occur after a great deal of blood has been lost or if severe pain is present. Standing for a long time may cause fainting.

It is not uncommon to have someone faint at the scene of an accident or while watching an operation. A fainting person may fall and injure himself if he does not recognize the symptoms and behave accordingly.

The signs of fainting are dizziness, blackness before the eyes, pallor, and perspiration. The victim loses consciousness, his pulse is weak, and his breathing is shallow. When someone complains of these feelings, have him sit down, or lie down, bend his head forward between his knees to put his head lower than his heart to bring more blood to the head. Keep him lying down with his head lowered or his limbs elevated; loosen tight clothing. Do not allow him to get up until you are sure he has recov-

## TABLE 35–1. POISONS: SYMPTOMS AND TREATMENT

| Poison | Symptoms | Emergency Treatment | Supporting Treatment (under doctor's orders) |
|---|---|---|---|
| Acids | Severe burning in mouth, throat, stomach. Profuse vomiting and diarrhea. Dyspnea, cyanosis, collapse | Milk of magnesia or lime water followed by milk, demulcents, etc. External acid burns—Baking or washing soda with large amounts water. Do not induce vomiting | Stimulants and external heat for collapse. Sodium bicarbonate intravenously or by rectum for acidosis |
| Alcohol (grain) | Excitement, followed by general depression | Evacuate stomach | Cold applications to head, heat to extremities. Coffee, caffeine or strychnine if necessary |
| Alcohol (wood) | Excitement, nausea and vomiting, blindness, dizziness, headache, dilated pupils, delirium | Evacuate stomach | Treat as above. Also $CO_2$ inhalations and artificial respiration |
| Alkalis | Mucous membranes of mouth soapy, swollen and white. Severe abdominal pain. Vomiting of blood and mucus. Collapse | Dilute acids: Vinegar, tartaric acid, lemon juice. Tea, milk, oil | Stimulants. Artificial heat. Opium preparations if necessary |
| Alkaloids { Atropine, Cocaine, Morphine, Strychnine } | Symptoms vary | Tannic acid, strong tea, or potassium permanganate by lavage | Support circulation and respiration, and promote elimination |
| Arsenic (Rat poisons, etc.) | Burning pain in esophagus and stomach. Abdominal pain. Nausea and vomiting. Garlic breath. Diarrhea, rice-water stools. Thirst. Scanty urine. Collapse | Evacuate stomach. Give iron hydroxide with magnesia. Sodium thiosulfate. Milk, water, olive oil. Dimercaprol (BAL) | Stimulants – caffeine, atropine, strychnine. External heat |
| Food Poisoning | Abdominal pain. Nausea and vomiting. Diarrhea. Collapse | Lavage stomach with tea or tannic acid or water | Stimulants. Rest. Warmth. Opium for pain |

## POISONS: SYMPTOMS AND TREATMENT (*Continued*)

| Poison | Symptoms | Emergency Treatment | Supporting Treatment (under doctor's orders) |
|---|---|---|---|
| Gas (Carbon Monoxide) | Drowsiness, giddiness, ringing in ears, dyspnea, loss of consciousness. Flushed cheeks, cherry-colored mucous membranes. Violent heart action. Coma | Fresh air. Oxygen with 5% carbon dioxide | Artificial respiration alternating with $O_2$ inhalations Heat. Stimulants Hyperbaric oxygenation |
| Lead | Chronic or cumulative: Anorexia Lead colic Nausea Constipation Metallic taste Anemia "Lead line" on gums Palsies | Magnesium or sodium sulfate Evacuate stomach if recent dose has been taken | Stimulants, opium, external heat for acute condition Viosterol and calcium salts for chronic condition |
| Opium { Laudanum Paregoric Morphine Codeine, etc. } | Sleep. Stupor Slow respirations (3 to 4 a minute) Pinpoint pupils Cyanosis. Slow pulse Coma | Lavage with potassium permanganate 1-2,000, or tannic acid | Keep patient awake and active Atropine 1/100 gr. q. 1 h. (by order) Oxygen and 5% $CO_2$ inhalations Catheterize. Give coffee and stimulants |
| Poison Ivy { Poison Oak Poison Sumac } | Itching swollen areas on skin, which rapidly form vesicles | Scrub skin with strong yellow soap and water Apply alcoholic solution of lead acetate, calamine solution | Sedatives if necessary Soothing lotions, e.g., sodium bicarbonate, calamine lotion, etc. Benadryl |
| Strychnine | Stiffness of muscles of face, neck, jaw. Twitching. Convulsions. Asphyxia | Tannic acid, tea, potassium permanganate solution, charcoal Lavage stomach before convulsions occur | Rest and quiet. Dark room Artificial respiration. Oxygen and 5% $CO_2$ Catheterize Paraldehyde, chloral, bromides |

ered, then get him to rise gradually, first to a sitting position, before he attempts to walk.

Most people seem to feel that everything will be all right if a person who is recovering consciousness can be made to sit up and move around. Nothing could be worse, and such treatment may be dangerous. Unconsciousness may be due to conditions more serious than fainting, such as skull fracture, concussion, shock, or cerebral hemorrhage.

## Fractures

When a person has been the victim of a fall or an automotive accident, you must consider the possibility of fractures. Because the bones which are well-padded with flesh may have an obscured fracture site, the cardinal rule of first aid is *do not move the victim.* Call a doctor, or have someone else do so for you. Question the victim (if conscious). Observe him for obviously deformed limbs. Cover him with a blanket until adequate help can be obtained. Caution the victim against moving if you are suspicious of a fracture. Splint an arm or a leg with the material available.

Never attempt to replace the ends of bones in a fracture where the skin is broken. Cover the area with a clean cloth and control excessive bleeding by direct pressure on the applicable pressure point.

**Splinting a Fracture.** The most easily applied type of splint is the inflatable plastic bag. Such splints are specially made for leg, arm, wrist, and other parts of the body.

Any hard, straight item can be used for splinting. An ideal emergency splint for an arm is a magazine which is wrapped around the arm and tied.

The first aider must be careful not to tie splints so tightly as to cut off the circulation to the limb. It is also important to remember not to change the position of a fracture. For example, if a limb is bent badly out of shape, do not attempt to reduce the fracture (do not attempt to pull it back into its normal shape). Splint it the way it is, or do not splint it at all.

## Transporting the Patient

It is absolutely vital to transport the patient with the utmost of care. Any back injury or other injury can be made more severe by care-less transportation. When moving the patient to the stretcher, be sure to keep his body straight. Sometimes, it is advisable to put the patient on the stretcher in the position in which he is lying, rather than to attempt to straighten his body out. Use as many people as you need to move the patient as effectively and as safely as possible.

**Danger of Explosions.** In the event of an automobile accident in which there is great danger of fire or explosion, the patient must be removed from the car, even though this might aggravate his injuries. Be as careful as possible, but get him out of danger.

## Frostbite

Frostbite is the freezing of tissues by exposure to extreme cold without sufficient protection of the exposed area. The body is more susceptible in a high wind because warmth is removed from the body more rapidly. Usually the frozen area is small—occurring on the nose, the cheeks, the ears, the fingers, and the toes, but it may be larger. The affected area becomes a grayish white color because ice forms in the tissues. Frozen hands or feet are painful, but frostbite in other areas is not usually painful; the victim may not know that his cheeks or ears are frozen until someone notices the color of the frostbitten spot.

*Never rub the frozen part*—rubbing bruises the frozen tissues and may cause gangrene. The victim of mild frostbite can be placed in a warm room, but he should not be near a stove, a radiator, or an open fire. Thaw the frozen part gradually in warm water or simply by exposure to air if the victim is in a *cool* room. Heat may cause blisters and is painful. Give the victim a warm drink; coffee is excellent.

After *prolonged* exposure to cold, the victim should be placed in a cool room until the circulation is restored. After chilling and long exposure in water, the temperature of the affected part should be raised gradually, but the victim of long exposure should have immediate medical attention.

## The Effects of Excessive Heat

Excessive heat may cause sunstroke, heat exhaustion, or heat cramps. The persons most likely to be affected are the very old and the very young, obese individuals, alcoholics, or people with some general disease.

Sweating keeps the body temperature normal during exposure to excessive heat, but a person loses much salt from the body in perspiration. This salt loss is the main cause of heat exhaustion, and it plays an important part in sunstroke. People working in excessive heat need to take from 12 to 15 glasses of water a day and need additional salt—at least a 5-grain salt tablet with every glass of water. The tablets should be dissolved or they may cause nausea and pain.

**Sunstroke.** Sunstroke and heat stroke are essentially the same, although one is caused by the sun's rays, and the other by indoor heat. The symptoms of sunstroke include dizziness, pain in the head, nausea, a feeling of oppression, and a dry mouth and skin; these symptoms are often followed by unconsciousness. Sunstroke kills about 25 per cent of the severe cases. The skin is dry and hot; the face, flushed; the pulse is full and rapid. The temperature often ranges from 107° to 110°, and occasionally, convulsions occur.

Get the victim into the shade and in a cool place; remove the clothing. Put the patient on his back and elevate the head and the shoulders slightly. Apply cold to the head; cool the body by wrapping it in a sheet and pouring on cold water—do this gradually. After several minutes of this treatment, observe the patient and note the effects of the treatment on the skin; go on with the treatment if the skin becomes hot again. Rub the limbs toward the heart, over the wet sheet, to stimulate the circulation. Call the doctor. Give cool drinks when the patient becomes conscious but do not give a stimulant.

**Heat Exhaustion.** Exposure to the sun or to intense indoor heat causes *heat exhaustion,* or *heat prostration.* Alcoholics and people in poor physical health are especially susceptible. The symptoms are dizziness, muscular weakness, nausea, and a blundering, staggering gait. Often the victim vomits, and he may have involuntary bowel movements. He is pale, perspires profusely, and his body is clammy and may become cold; his pulse is weak, and his breathing shallow. He may faint before he lies down. Severe cases may die without recovering consciousness.

Get the victim into circulating air. Have him lie down and cover him. Give him one half-teaspoonful of salt in one third of a glass of water until he has had a tablespoonful of salt—strangely enough, this seldom makes the victim nauseated. Give warm tea or coffee; call the doctor if the symptoms persist.

*Heat cramps* affect the muscles in the abdomen or the limbs. They are most painful and may be accompanied by heat exhaustion symptoms. Treat as for heat exhaustion with drinks of salt solution at frequent intervals.

## Giving First Aid for a Superficial Burn

Burns are usually caused by steam or hot liquids, by contact with hot surfaces, or by electricity: electric burns occur when the current or electrical flashes pass through the body. Strong chemicals also burn the tissues.

There are 3 degrees of burns:

1. *First degree*—the skin is reddened only, and the burn is superficial.

2. *Second degree*—the skin is blistered.

3. *Third degree*—the tissues are charred or cooked.

Fourth degree has also been identified by some authorities—this involves the charring of bone and other structures. Any first or second degree burn is painful because exposed nerve endings come in contact with the air. The chief dangers from severe burns are shock and infection.

**Preventing Burns.** Handles of saucepans on the stove should be turned inward so that children cannot reach them. Children should be taught not to touch hot radiators or stoves. Matches should be kept in a safe place. Electric or gas heaters should be placed where there is no danger of elderly people falling over or brushing against them. Be sure that the cords attached to electrical appliances are placed where no one will trip over them.

**Treatment.** Severe burns must have medical attention. At home, you can cut away the clothing but do not attempt to remove cloth that sticks to the tissues; outside of the home, do not remove the clothing—cover the patient, keep him lying down, and get him to the hospital as soon as possible.

Do not use boric acid solution for burns and never apply ointments of any kind to burns, because the doctor will want to see the burn. Never use absorbent cotton on burns; it will stick to the tissues, and removing it causes more injury. Blisters should be opened only by the doctor.

Chemical burns should be flooded with large quantities of water to wash the chemical away and prevent deeper tissue damage. If a chemical gets into the eye, have the patient lie down, and pour cupfuls of water into the inner eye, with the head turned to allow the water to run off.

Sunburn is usually a first- or a second-degree burn; severe sunburn may make the victim really ill and cause blistering and fever. Oils and calamine lotion are soothing for sunburn. Vinegar is soothing for sunburn and, if applied early, can prevent a great deal of blistering and pain later.

The best first aid treatment for any burn is *cold water.*

## Head Injuries

One thing the nurse must know is that any laceration of the scalp bleeds profusely, so that even the smallest wound looks very serious. However, it is important to determine the extent of the injury. If a bump on the head causes a lump to form, the patient is less likely to have a hemorrhage within the brain (which is more serious).

First aid includes lying the patient down flat, but not elevating his feet, keeping him warm, and checking for signs of increasing intracranial pressure (see Chapter 46). Serious complications are signified by such symptoms as dizziness, nausea, unconsciousness, confusion, and other symptoms of brain injury.

## Removing a Foreign Body From the Eye

The important function of the eye is *sight*; the structures of the eye are delicate and easily damaged by either injury or infection. The purpose of first aid is to preserve the sight, by preventing further damage and securing the necessary medical attention for the victim.

Foreign bodies may be particles of dust or soot or an eyelash lodged on the lining of the eyelid, or they may be particles that become embedded in the eyeball. Never attempt to remove an embedded foreign body. Anything

that lodges in the eye irritates it, especially when the eyelid is closed; a foreign body has a scratchy effect and makes tears flow. Follow these instructions to prevent serious damage:

Instruct the victim not to rub the eye—rubbing may drive a foreign body in deeper. Keep the eye shut and avoid blinking.

Never use an instrument, a toothpick, or a match to remove a foreign body.

Never attempt to remove a foreign body if there is the slightest possibility that it is embedded in the eyeball.

This is what you may do to remove a foreign body that is not embedded:

1. Pull down the lower eyelid to see whether the body is on the eyelid membrane; if so, you may be able to lift it off by touching it gently with the corner of a clean handkerchief or with a cotton-tipped applicator moistened in water—always moisten cotton before touching it to the eye.

2. Grasp the lashes of the upper eyelid with your forefinger and thumb; ask the patient to look upward, pull the lid forward and downward over the lower eyelid. Usually this dislodges the foreign body, and the tears wash it away.

3. Flush the eye with a weak solution of salt water. You can do this with a sterile medicine dropper or a small bulb syringe.

If none of these measures is successful, the patient must see a doctor as soon as possible; the longer a foreign body remains in the eye, the greater the danger of injuring the tissues.

## Removing a Foreign Body From the Nose, the Throat, or the Ear

Children sometimes put small objects in their noses; unless the object is clearly visible and at the edge of the nostril, do not attempt to remove it with a finger; a pea or a bean or a kernel of corn in the nose is likely to swell. Have the victim blow the nose gently with *both* nostrils open.

Objects often become lodged in the throat; children put coins or buttons in their mouth, and bits of food or bones can lodge in the throat or the esophagus. Do not attempt to remove the foreign body with your fingers unless it is an object that you can dislodge easily. If you are unable to see the foreign

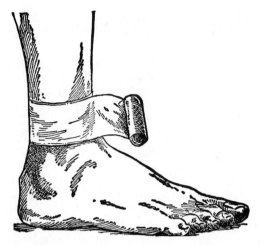

Figure 35-4. Circular turns of a bandage.

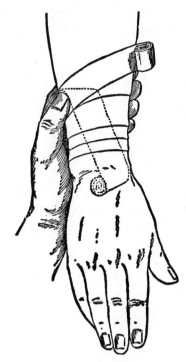

Figure 35-5. Spiral bandage.

body, but the patient is able to breathe all right, send for the doctor. You can tell by the patient's color whether or not his air supply is sufficient. If the patient is blue and distressed, hold him upside down and slap his back sharply; this may dislodge the object. By having an adult bend over, his trunk and head are upside down. Sometimes artificial respiration is necessary even though the obstruction has been removed.

If a foreign body lodges in the ear, do not attempt to remove it but call the doctor.

Always consult the doctor if a foreign body has been swallowed.

## BANDAGES

A bandage is a piece of material used to hold dressings or splints in place, to give support, or to apply pressure. The different materials used for bandages are described in the discussion of dressings, but the methods for applying bandages will be discussed here. Here is a list of rules to use when applying bandages.

1. Apply firmly but not so tightly that the circulation is cut off: after an injury the bandaged part may swell, so watch for evidence of tightness and loosen the bandage if necessary.

2. Always tie a square knot because a square knot will not slip.

3. If possible, leave the tips of the toes and

the fingers exposed so that you can tell by their color if the bandage is cutting off the circulation.

*Roller bandages* of gauze, muslin, elastic, Kerlix, and other materials come in different widths suitable for bandaging the various parts of the body. Appropriate widths are:

| | |
|---|---|
| Fingers and toes | 1-inch |
| Hand and foot | 2- or 3-inch |
| Head | 2-inch |
| Limbs | 2- to 6-inch |
| Trunk | 4- to 6-inch |

A roller bandage can be applied neatly and snugly on the extremities because it can be made to fit. Each turn of a roller bandage should be exactly as tight as the one before it; if you make the turns tighter and tighter as you progress, the bandage will constrict the part. If you let the turns grow looser, the bandage will slip and may come off. If you purposely apply the entire bandage loosely to allow for swelling, it can be anchored with strips of adhesive tape.

The *circular bandage* makes 2 or more turns around the part, each layer covering the

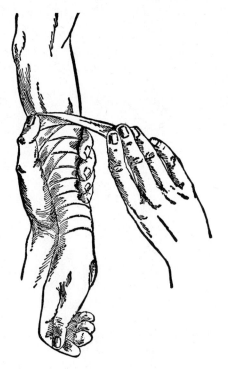

Figure 35-6. Spiral reverse bandage.

one below it. When applying any roller bandage begin with 2 circular turns to anchor the loose end firmly (Fig. 35-4).

The *spiral bandage* winds like a coil either upward or downward. Anchor the bandage with 2 circular turns, then cover the part with spiral turns slanted evenly, each turn overlapping the one beneath for half its width. Finish with 2 circular turns and fasten (Fig. 35-5).

The *spiral reverse bandage* is sometimes used to fit a tapering part. Start with a spiral until you reach a point where the layer will not lie flat on the one below it; then reverse the turn, slanting the bandage back on itself. Make as many of these reverse turns as necessary to keep the bandage flat, reversing at the same point each time (Fig. 35-6).

The *figure-8 bandage* makes slanting turns, alternately ascending and descending around the part and crossing in the middle. This bandage is used for joints, such as the ankle, the shoulder, the knee or the elbow (Fig. 35-7).

To apply a *finger spiral bandage*, make 2 circular turns around the base of the injured finger, then make spiral turns until the area is covered. If the injury is at the base of the finger, make 2 turns around the finger, carry the bandage across the back of the hand to the wrist, make 2 turns around the wrist, then carry the bandage back around the finger; repeat as many times as necessary to cover the area and anchor the bandage. To cover the end of the finger, make recurrent loops of bandage over the end in this way: hold a spiral turn at the base of the finger, on the back; bring the bandage up over the end of the finger and down over the front until the

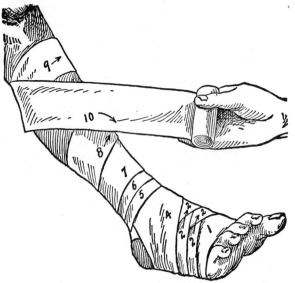

Figure 35-7. Figure-8 bandage.

finger is covered sufficiently—overlap each loop slightly and hold the loops at the base— then continue the spiral, binding down the recurrent loops and finishing with anchorage around the wrist (Fig. 35-8).

A *triangular or handkerchief bandage* is made from a square of cloth and can be fastened without adhesive tape or pins, if necessary. The 36- or 40-inch square is an adequate size. Cut diagonally through the center to make 2 triangular bandages. The triangle can be folded several times to make a strip, or a *cravat bandage.*

The triangular bandage is very often used to make a sling to support an arm. To apply a sling, use this procedure: put one end of the triangle over the shoulder on the *uninjured* side, with the point of the triangle pointing toward the injured arm and placed under it. Bring the other end of the triangle over the shoulder on the *injured* side and tie the 2 ends of the triangle together at the side of the neck. Then bring the point of the triangle forward and pin it to the sling. You can adjust the sling by adjusting the knot or by pinning a tuck in the front of the sling above the hand; the hand should be elevated 4 or 5 inches above the elbow level (Fig. 35-9).

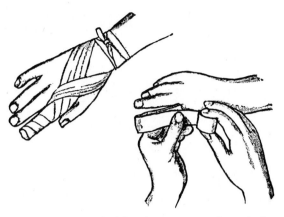

Figure 35-8. Spiral bandage to cover the end of a finger. (American National Red Cross: First Aid Textbook, ed. 4, New York, Doubleday, 1957)

## LEGAL ASPECTS OF FIRST AID

Most states have a "Good Samaritan" law which protects the first aider from legal liability, providing that the first aider acts within the bounds of good sense and reason. As long as you perform *only* first aid and do not diagnose or treat the person in any other way, you should not have any difficulty. The most important thing for the nurse to remember, if he or she practices first aid in an emergency, is to use *good common sense.*

Figure 35-9. Triangular bandage used as an arm sling. (A) Step one. (B) Step two. (C) Step three. (American National Red Cross: First Aid Textbook, ed. 4, New York, Doubleday, 1957)

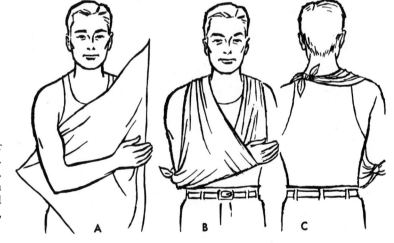

# Unit 8:

# Care of the Mother and Newborn Infant

36. *The Beginning Family — Pregnancy as a Normal Process*
37. *Assisting the Mother During Labor, Delivery, and Puerperium*
38. *Care of the Neonate*

# 36

# The Beginning Family— Pregnancy as a Normal Process

## BEHAVIORAL OBJECTIVES

*The student successfully attaining the goals of this chapter will be able to:*

- *demonstrate an understanding of the anatomy and physiology of the reproductive systems (studied earlier) by giving an oral summary of key concepts.*
- *define the terms fertilization zygote, placenta, and embryo.*
- *describe fetal circulation.*
- *explain the significance of the Rh factor to the mother and child.*
- *discuss the growth and development which occurs in normal pregnancy from the end of the 1st lunar month to the end of the 10th lunar month.*
- *state the presumptive, probable and positive signs of pregnancy.*
- *discuss prenatal care including its importance, goals and implications for maternal teaching.*
- *indicate how the normal weight gain of pregnancy is distributed.*
- *review orally general health practices during pregnancy.*
- *give 8 minor discomforts of pregnancy and indicate how each may be treated.*
- *state 5 complications of pregnancy and define each condition.*
- *discuss the special problems of the mother who is diabetic, has a heart disorder, is dependent on drugs, or must have a cesarean section.*
- *demonstrate sensitivity in working with mothers and/or fathers who are experiencing special problems, including the death of a child.*

*Obstetrics* (from the Latin *obsto,* meaning to stand by or to protect) is the branch of medicine concerned with the management of childbirth. The doctor who practices this specialty is called an *obstetrician.* In the past, women relatives or a midwife attended a woman in labor; recent figures tell us that today a physician is in attendance for 97 per cent of the births in this country. The early midwives were untrained and relied solely on experience for their knowledge. Here and in other countries, the need has been recognized for trained midwives to supplement the work of the obstetrician in isolated areas where doctors are few and far between.

A new trend in larger communities is for midwives to attend patients in the course of normal labor and delivery, thus freeing the doctor to care for patients who present obstetric problems. There is an increasing number of schools for midwives in the United States. The ultimate hope and aim of all workers in the field of obstetrics is to assist a healthy mother to produce a healthy baby with a minimum of danger and discomfort to both.

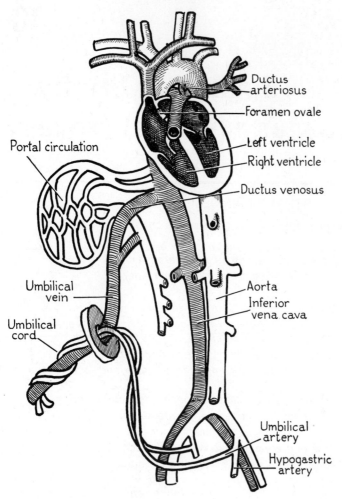

Figure 36-1. Diagram of fetal circulation. (Baillif and Kimmel: Structure and Function of the Human Body, p. 141. Philadelphia, Lippincott)

Ductus arteriosus
Foramen ovale
Left ventricle
Right ventricle
Ductus venosus
Portal circulation
Umbilical vein
Aorta
Inferior vena cava
Umbilical cord
Umbilical artery
Hypogastric artery

## PREGNANCY

*Pregnancy* is defined as the condition of being "with child." To understand pregnancy we must know how it begins, how the baby grows in the uterus, and how pregnancy affects the mother. The anatomy and the physiology of the reproductive systems may be reviewed in Chapter 19.

**Growth Underway.** The mature ovum and sperm both contain 23 chromosomes; their union (*fertilization*) produces the total of 46 chromosomes, which is characteristic of all human cells. Fertilization usually occurs when the ovum is in the outer third of the fallopian tube. After fertilization, the ovum travels down from the fallopian tube into the uterus, where it will have room to grow and be nourished. The lining of the uterus has been pre-paring for this while the ovum was ripening in the ovary.

Before the fertilized ovum (called a *zygote*) reaches the uterus, it already has begun to divide rapidly. The zygote forms 2 cells; 2 cells form 4 cells; and so on. After about 3 days the mass of cells, now called the *morula*, reaches the uterus where it starts to implant itself in the uterine lining (endometrium). Some of the cells secrete an enzyme which permits the zygote to burrow into the endometrium.

The cells continue to divide to form a hollow ball which has an inner and an outer layer of cells. Some of the outer cells send out projections (*chorionic villi*) which are the "roots" through which the developing baby receives its oxygen and nourishment from the mother. These villi eventually join with an area of uterine tissue to form the *placenta,* a vascular and glandular organ which supplies the developing baby with food and oxygen and also produces hormones. Certain cells in the inner layer of the morula continue to divide, and they begin to differentiate themselves into 3 distinct types, which ultimately will form the body structure of the fetus. Other cells making up this cavity eventually form a fluid-filled sac (the *amnion*) in which the embryo floats. (The developing baby is called an *embryo* during the first 2 months.)

**How Sex Is Determined.** There is no way that a mother can influence the sex of her child; it is determined by the sperm from the father at the time of fertilization. A female ovum carries only one type of chromosome to determine one type of sex; it is called X. A male sperm cell may carry either one of the two sex chromosomes, X or Y. If the ovum is fertilized by a sperm cell carrying a Y chromosome, the baby will be a boy (XY); if the sperm cell carries an X chromosome, the baby will be a girl (XX).

At the present time there is no way to "order" a boy or a girl; however, odds seem to be a little in favor of the boys, since there are about 106 boys born for every 100 girls.

**Old Wives' Tales.** There are many queer notions which surround pregnancy. The one that comes to mind most often is the belief that the mother can *mark* her baby or influence its mind if she sees something unpleasant or ugly. This is impossible, since there is no direct connection between the nervous systems of the mother and the baby. Nor can the mother tie knots in the umbilical cord by stretching her arms to hang curtains; the child may turn in the uterus and cause a knot, but the mother has nothing to do with it. Also, a hopeful mother's special interest in art and music cannot have any effect on her unborn infant; although he may display interest in these areas, probably it will be the result of environmental direction rather than of prenatal influence.

## Fetal Circulation

The fetus in the uterus is attached to the placenta by the umbilical cord which contains 2 arteries and 1 large vein twisted about each other (see Fig. 36-1). Circulation in the body before birth differs from the circulation in the body after birth. The unborn infant, the fetus, secures oxygen and food from the mother's blood instead of using its own lungs and digestive system. Since the fetal and the maternal blood are in separate capillaries and do not mix, there must be some place where the interchange of gases, food and wastes can take place. This occurs in the *placenta,* sometimes called the *afterbirth,* since it is cast out of the uterus following the birth of the baby. Fetal capillaries in the placenta are surrounded by maternal blood, and the exchanges take place across the capillary membranes. In this way, the mother supplies food and carries off wastes for the baby.

The fetal heart drives the deoxygenated blood to the placenta through 2 vessels, the *umbilical arteries.* The oxygenated blood is returned to the fetus from the placenta by a single vessel, the *umbilical vein.* This is another exception to the classification that all arteries carry oxygenated (bright red) blood, and all veins carry deoxygenated (bluish) blood (see p. 119). These 3 vessels are intertwined and covered by a soft jellylike substance called Wharton's jelly, the whole system making up the *umbilical cord.* The cord enters the body of the fetus at approximately the middle of the abdomen at the *umbilicus* (naval). Some of the oxygenated blood from the umbilical vein passes through the liver and some enters the inferior vena cava by way of the ductus venosus, passing on into the right atrium. The great bulk of blood is shunted to the arterial (left) side of the heart by 2 short cuts. These short cuts are an opening between the 2 atria called the *foramen ovale* and a vessel known as the *ductus arteriosus,* which connects the pulmonary artery and the aorta. Normally, with the first few respirations of the newborn child, the lungs are expanded. The foramen ovale then closes, and the ductus arteriosus becomes obliterated. Sometimes these circulatory adjustments do not take place, causing abnormalities.

## The Rh Factor

People worry needlessly about the effect of the Rh factor in marriage and pregnancy (see page 117). The only possibility of trouble is in

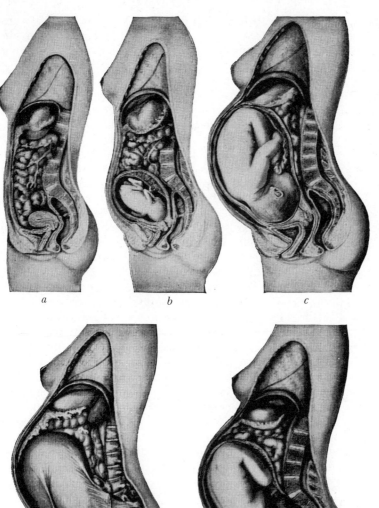

Figure 36-2. The mother's body at various stages of the fetus's growth within the uterus: (*a*) the nonpregnant uterus; (*b*) about 4 to 5 months gestation; (*c*) about 6 to 7 months gestation; (*d*) the fetus within the amniotic sac; (*e*) full-term pregnancy with the fetus "dropped" in preparation for delivery.

the case of pregnancy between an Rh+ husband and an Rh− wife. Only a small percentage of marriages have this problem. Even in this group, trouble may occur (but does not always) only if a baby inherits the father's Rh-positive blood factor. If the mother's body reacts to the baby's Rh factor as a foreign agent within her, since it is not normally present in her blood, she may produce antibodies to destroy this intruder, the Rh factor. The antibodies enter the baby's bloodstream and destroy its red blood cells. Usually, there

are not sufficient antibodies to bother the first baby, but they may produce increasing effects in later pregnancies. As a rule, such a baby is born successfully, but its life is threatened by the destruction of its red blood cells (a condition called *erythroblastosis fetalis*). If necessary, the baby can be given one or more transfusions to replace the blood which is being destroyed. Recent developments indicate this can be done even before the baby is born if its condition is severe enough to warrant such intervention.

## Development of the Baby

The fertilized ovum is called the embryo in the early stages of its growth when the cells are arranging themselves into the layers from which the tissues and the organs of the baby's body will develop. After the 5th week of development the embryo is called the fetus.

The expected date of delivery of the child is estimated by counting back 3 months from the first day of the last menstrual period of the mother and adding 7 days.

A full-term pregnancy, including the development of the fetus from embryo to birth, usually takes 280 days, which are divided into 10 months of 28 days each, or 10 lunar months. Fetal growth and development normally follow a definite pattern during each month of pregnancy. This is how that growth progresses (Fig. 36-2):

*End of 1st Lunar Month.* The eyes, the ears and the nose begin to develop, although the embryo is only about ¼ to ½ inch long.

*End of 2nd Lunar Month.* The head takes shape—it is abnormally large, because the brain is developing. Arms and legs resemble small buds. The fetus is now about 1 inch long.

*End of 3rd Lunar Month.* The fetus is about 3 inches long, excluding the legs which are very small, weighs about 1 ounce, and fills the uterus. Fingers and toes, having soft nails, appear. Sex can be determined.

*End of 4th Lunar Month.* The fetus has grown to about 6 inches and weighs from 2 to 4 ounces. Downy hair (*lanugo*) appears on the back and the shoulders, and the sex can be distinguished.

*End of the 5th Lunar Month.* The fetus is now about 10 to 12 inches long and weighs about 8 to 10 ounces. Downy hair appears over the body, and some hair has developed on the head. Fetal heart sounds can usually be heard with the stethoscope, and the mother feels the baby move.

*End of 6th Lunar Month.* The fetus is about 12 inches long and weighs about a pound or a pound and a half. Eyebrows and eyelashes appear; the skin is wrinkled and the *vernix caseosa* has begun to develop. It is extremely rare that a fetus born at this stage of pregnancy survives.

*End of 7th Lunar Month.* The fetus is now about 14 to 15 inches long and weighs about 2 to 2½ pounds. The skin is covered with a cheesy material (*vernix caseosa*); a greenish, sticky substance (*meconium*) forms in the intestines. The fetus moves freely in the uterus; if it is born now, it can breathe and cry and has about 1 chance in 10 of living.

*End of 8th Lunar Month.* The fetus is about 16 inches in length and weighs 3 to 4 pounds. A baby born at 8 months has a good chance to live.

*End of 9th Lunar Month.* The baby is about 18 inches long and weighs 5 to 6 pounds. Fat deposits underneath the skin have smoothed out the wrinkles. If born now the baby has an excellent chance of surviving.

*End of 10th Lunar Month.* The baby now is about 20 inches long, weighs about 7 pounds and is fully developed. The skin is smooth and covered with vernix caseosa; head hair is developed and dark in color. The baby is equipped to enter the world and live. His heredity and his mother's nutrition will have some influence on his weight at birth; a baby weighing 10 pounds or over is usually difficult to deliver. A baby weighing less than 5 to 5½ pounds (2500 gm.) at birth is considered as being premature; generally speaking, the smaller the baby is, the more difficult it is for him to survive.

The baby who weighs less than 2¼ pounds (1000 gm.) is called *immature* and his chances for survival are not good.

Although the bones of the baby's skull are hardened, they are not yet tightly knit together, leaving soft spots called *fontanels* on the top, the sides, and the back of the head. This makes the head less rigid and permits minor changes in shape, which is an advantage during labor and birth.

## Signs and Symptoms of Pregnancy

The signs and symptoms of pregnancy are customarily divided into 3 groups: *presumptive,* so called because while pregnancy may be presumed, these symptoms may indicate other common conditions; *probable,* because although more definite than the presumptive symptoms, they are not absolute; and *posi-*

*tive,* because these symptoms, as evidence of pregnancy, are indisputable.

**Presumptive Signs.** The presumptive signs include absence of menstruation, morning sickness, frequent urination, and tenderness and fullness of the breasts.

Other indications by which a pregnancy may be presumed are drowsiness and a tendency to fatigue easily; increased pigmentation, both of the nipples and of the *linea negra* (the dark line extending from the umbilicus to the pubis). There is also sometimes said to be a "mask of pregnancy," caused by the presence of dark brown discolorations on the face. The appearance of "quickening," known to the lay person as *feeling life,* along with *Chadwick's sign,* which is the darkening in color of the vaginal mucous membrane, are also other presumptive signs of pregnancy.

**Probable Signs.** Probable signs are designated as enlargement of the abdomen, changes in the uterus, alterations in the cervix, and positive pregnancy tests.

There are specific changes in the shape, the size and the consistency of the uterus which are important indications. The enlargement and the changes in shape should correspond to the gradual increase in the size of the fetus and the amount of amniotic fluid. Softness of the uterus at certain stages is also important to the experienced examiner. After the 6th month the fetal outline should be able to be felt or palpated; however, rare uterine tumors may so duplicate the fetal outline that this sign is not considered as being positive.

The cervix usually softens about the time the 2nd menstrual period is missed.

TESTS FOR PREGNANCY. It has been possible to develop tests for pregnancy because a hormone is present in the urine of pregnant women which, if injected into certain animals, will produce definite reactions. It is important to have a specimen of urine which has been collected in a clean, dry bottle, and to use it as soon as possible or else refrigerate it until it is used, since heat and delay make the tests less accurate.

**Positive Signs.** The positive signs of pregnancy are the fetal heart sounds, fetal movements felt by an examiner, and a roentgenogram showing the fetal skeleton.

# PRENATAL CARE

*Prenatal* refers to the period between conception and the birth of the baby, while *antepartal* refers to the period between conception and the onset of labor. Theoretically, "antepartal" would be the correct term for the discussion in this chapter. The two are often used interchangeably in obstetric literature, but since prenatal still seems to have wider usage, it will be retained here.

Good prenatal care has as its goal the maximum physical and mental fitness of the mother with the reward of an uneventful delivery and a healthy mother and baby.

Because the public has been made so aware of the value of prenatal care, today a woman goes to a doctor, privately or through a clinic, as soon as she assumes that she is pregnant. Indeed, in recent years, emphasis has been placed on *premarital* and *prepregnancy* examinations to encourage positive maternal and child health.

## Consulting a Doctor

Any one of the signs of pregnancy is reason for consulting a doctor. When one realizes what an important part the mother plays in the baby's development and future life, it is easy to understand why she needs the best advice and care from the time the baby begins its life within her body until it enters the outside world.

The doctor begins his care of the mother by taking a complete history of both the mother and the father, to learn about their past illnesses and family tendencies to diseases (such as diabetes, which may affect pregnancy). He is interested in learning whether a multiple pregnancy has occurred in either family and is particularly interested in any difficulties experienced by the mother during previous pregnancies or deliveries.

He makes a complete physical examination of the mother, which includes: examination of the gums, the teeth, the thyroid gland, and the breasts; blood tests to discover anemia or syphilis; a urine examination to determine the condition of the kidneys, which affects the ability to eliminate wastes from the body; and blood pressure and weight. He does a pelvic examination, which should include a pap smear and a test for gonorrhea. All of these are important gauges of the possible complications of pregnancy. The doctor examines the pelvic organs and takes measurements to determine whether or not the bony passageway is wide enough to permit the baby to be born, which is especially important in a first pregnancy.

A blood typing should be done and Rh factor information secured. If the mother is Rh negative, the husband's blood should be examined to discover whether he is negative or positive. If he is negative also, there should be nothing to worry about. However, if the husband is Rh positive, the mother's blood should then be tested for antibodies; this test is repeated around the 30th week of pregnancy. If antibodies are present, further tests are done regularly so that the doctor can anticipate what treatment, if any, the baby might need immediately after it is born, or before, in the case of severe antibody reactions.

The doctor advises the expectant mother about her diet and other health habits. He tells her what to observe about herself between visits and what she must report immediately. Excessive vaginal discharge or loss of fluid is not normal; bleeding should be reported at once. Swelling of the hands or of the feet and the legs, blurring of vision or spots before the eyes, headaches, and a decrease in the amount of urine voided are all danger signs.

Usually, the doctor sees the expectant mother every 3rd or 4th week for the first 7 months, every 2nd week about the 8th month and once a week during the last month. If it seems to be necessary, he will see her more often. He will ask for a specimen of urine each time, check her blood pressure and weight, and examine the abdomen. After about the 5th month, he will listen for *fetal heart tones* (the baby's heartbeat). Any other procedure will be determined by the individual patient's condition. A special treatment given to one pregnant woman may not be necessary for another.

The father should be encouraged to go with the mother on her first visit to the doctor. It might help both parents if he went occasionally, because then both of them will hear what the doctor has to say. Parenthood is a partnership in which both partners have an equal interest. Also, the mother will be helped to carry out her program if the father understands it too.

Most women adjust to the strain of pregnancy very well. Pregnancy is a normal process for which a woman's body is built. If the mother follows common-sense health rules, she ought to feel well, happy, and relaxed. To keep herself this way, she must have the right food, enough rest, some exercise and some recreation. Generally, the mother can partake in most of the activities which she did regularly before she became pregnant. However, very strenuous exercises should be avoided.

## Food for the Baby

The baby needs the same nutritional elements that the mother does, and if her diet is well balanced, he will get these food essentials. She will need to increase some foods to take care of the baby's needs in addition to those of her own. If she fails to provide these nutrients, some of them (such as calcium) will be taken from her body tissues.

**The Baby's Weight.** At one time, people believed that women would have large babies if they overate. Studies show that heavy eating does not influence the size of the baby; this is controlled by heredity or by the length of pregnancy. (Overdue babies are likely to be large; premature babies are usually underweight.) However, overeating does put an extra strain on the mother's body.

**The Mother's Diet.** In recent years, much attention has been given to the diet of the pregnant mother. Quality rather than quantity is stressed, because it is known that she supplies the building materials for her baby as well as those needed for maintaining her own physiological fitness. These are the foods required daily: 1 quart of milk; proteins supplied from meat, eggs, and fish; whole grain or enriched bread or cereals; green, yellow, and leafy vegetables; fruit (which should include citrus fruit); and butter or margarine to which vitamins A and D have been added. She should also have 6 to 8 glasses of fluid daily and extra vitamins as needed to correct any known vitamin deficiencies. If she is anemic, she may also need an extra amount of iron daily (see Chapter 22).

Changes in the mother's body during the early part of pregnancy may interfere with her appetite; therefore, special attention must be given to supplying her with proteins and vitamins. Rich foods, highly spiced foods, fried foods, and hot breads are not desirable. In the latter months, several small meals taken daily rather than 3 large ones will probably help the mother to feel better.

Obstetricians advise that a gain of approximately 20 pounds above normal weight is to be expected. The weight should increase gradually from the sixth week after conception to the end of the full term of the pregnancy. Generally, 2/3 of the weight gain occurs during the last trimester of pregnancy. Therefore, if too much weight is gained before that time, the mother will probably retain that after delivery. Twenty pounds is the usual weight loss after the baby is born; therefore, it is not regarded as being permanent.

Excessive weight gain may also add strain to the muscles of the back and the legs. Serious complications tend to occur in patients who have had an excessive weight gain.

A certain amount of weight gain is normal. This table shows approximately how this gain is distributed:

| | |
|---|---|
| The baby | 7 lb. |
| The placenta | 1½ lb. |
| Fluid around the baby | 2 lb. |
| Increase in weight of the uterus | 2½ lb. |
| Increase in weight of blood | 3 lb. |
| Increase in weight of the breasts | 2 lb. |

Additional weight gained is usually retained as fat by the mother.

## General Health Practices

**Elimination.** The mother who usually has a bowel movement every day should continue to do so. However, a movement every day is not essential if this is not her normal habit and if she is not constipated. Her diet and regular habits should be such as to encourage good elimination. If she has trouble with constipation, she should not take laxatives or an enema without consulting her doctor. If a laxative is prescribed, it is usually a mild one, such as milk of magnesia.

**Care of the Skin.** The glands of the skin are more active than usual, so a daily warm bath is important. The mother must be careful about slipping or falling in the tub or the shower. There is no proof that a tub bath is harmful at any time during pregnancy.

**Teeth.** The modern mother who eats a balanced diet and sees her dentist regularly does not need to worry about tooth damage during pregnancy. It is important to have necessary dental work done and to remove sources of infection in the mouth.

**Breasts.** Good breast care during pregnancy prepares the mother for nursing the baby. The breasts and the nipples should be washed every day with soap and water. Early in pregnancy the breasts begin to secrete a colorless liquid called *colostrum,* which may form crusts on the nipples. These crusts can be removed with cold cream. The mother should wear a brassière with wide straps which supports the breasts without causing pressure on the nipples. An underwired bra is often more comfortable for the woman with heavy breasts.

**Rest.** Rest has been defined as "the ability to relax." The pregnant woman tires more easily, and she should have enough rest to prevent fatigue. (Authorities feel that it is better to *prevent* fatigue than to have to recover from overfatigue.) The mother knows how much rest she ordinarily requires, and she should plan to have more if she needs it. Going to bed earlier, getting up later, or taking an afternoon nap may help. Many women who are employed are able to work all through their pregnancy by planning extra rest. Short daytime periods of rest will be beneficial if the mother really relaxes, even if this involves only sitting in a comfortable chair. Women are able to carry on normal household activities without harm if they avoid heavy work and get additional rest.

Later in pregnancy, postural discomforts may make it difficult for the mother to sleep. Simple measures, such as additional pillows at the back or a pillow supporting the weight of the abdomen while the mother lies on her side, will usually relieve these minor problems.

**Exercise.** Exercise improves the circulation, the appetite, and the digestion; it also aids elimination and makes the mother sleep better. Doctors feel that the customary exercises of the mother may be continued, but strenuous exercise of any kind should be avoided.

**Posture.** Because the weight of the pregnant uterus is "all in front," the mother tends to lean or tilt backward in order to maintain her balance, just as we all would do if, for instance, we carried a heavy bag of groceries. This customary posture of pregnancy is beneficial to those who ordinarily have poor posture. However, the change in body alignment causes a strain on back and leg muscles. This factor, plus the natural softening of the pelvic joints, causes many of the pains of the back, the legs, and the feet which are common in late pregnancy. Rib strains and swelling of the ankles and the feet also occur frequently. A special maternity girdle which helps to lift the abdomen up and in, while holding the back flat, will help some women by providing the necessary body support.

**Clothing.** Maternity clothing today can be most attractive and fashionable, as well as comfortable and nonconstricting. Dresses which hang loosely from the shoulder are made in becoming styles and beautiful materials. Other 2-piece fashions have expandable waistbands and a stretch section in the front of the skirt. Even amateur sewers can make maternity dresses in their own favorite colors and fashion which is an aid to the budget; these clothes do not require the usual fitting expertness and can be very successful. A becoming hair style and pretty clothes are good morale boosters at this time.

The support given by an appropriate girdle and a well-fitting brassière cannot be overemphasized. Garters should be attached to the girdle, or a special maternity garter belt should be used; round garters constrict the blood supply and add to the development of varicose veins. Panty hose are probably the most comfortable, providing they are large enough. High heels contribute to the imbalance of the body—a fashionable style from the many available walking shoes will prevent the mother from falling. Current styles in clothing and shoes are very comfortable and concealing for the pregnant woman.

**Travel.** Most women who drive continue to do so during pregnancy, at least until the last months when driving becomes too uncomfortable. (Baby, mother, and steering wheel cannot occupy the same space at the same time.) The mother must be sure to buckle her seat belt *under* her abdomen. It is probably best not to use the shoulder strap during pregnancy, but it is vital to use the lap belt.

Long trips are exhausting for anyone, but since American families are so much on the move, it frequently becomes necessary for the pregnant mother to travel also. Travel by air or train is recommended for long, tiring trips. If the mother is to travel by car, she should plan to stop every 50 miles to stretch, relax, and walk around: this prevents circulatory problems such as phlebitis. The Armed Forces have specific regulations concerning travel for the pregnant wives of men in the service. The pregnant woman must be sure *not* to fly in a small plane which is not pressurized, since the lower atmospheric pressure can cause difficulties to the baby.

It is a good idea for the expectant mother to consult her obstetrician about her travel plans, since there are special conditions and special times in pregnancy which make traveling unwise.

**Employment.** Many employed women continue to work during pregnancy; this is permissible within limits, if the expectant mother likes her work, and if her health or the baby's health is not endangered. The Women's Bureau of the United States Department of Labor, and the Children's Bureau of the United States Department of Health, Education, and Welfare have recommended standards for maternity care and the employment of mothers. In part, these recommendations specify an 8-hour day, with rest periods morning and afternoon; a 40-hour week; at least 6 weeks' leave before delivery and 2 months' leave after delivery. They rule out work involving heavy lifting, operating dangerous machines, continuous standing, or working with toxic substances.

**Marital Relations.** Sexual intercourse is not harmful up to the last few weeks of pregnancy; it should not be risked after that period, because of the danger of infection. Pregnancy diminishes sexual desire in some women, and a mutual understanding of this physiological fact by both husband and wife may eliminate the possibility of misunderstandings. Some physicians feel that sexual relations are undesirable at the times dur-

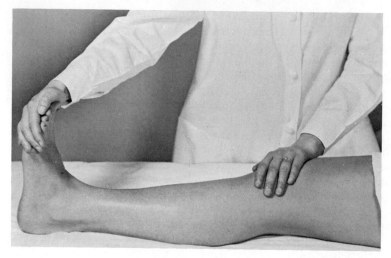

Figure 36-3. The nurse is helping the patient during a leg cramp, forcing the toes upward while putting pressure on the knee to straighten the leg. (Fitzpatrick, E., Reeder, S. R., and Mastroianni, L., Jr.: Maternity Nursing, ed. 12. Philadelphia, Lippincott, 1971)

ing the month when menstruation would normally occur. There is an increased danger of a spontaneous abortion (loss of the embryo or fetus) taking place at these times.

## Minor Discomforts of Pregnancy

Although many women who are pregnant have "never felt better," there are others who do not enjoy such optimum health. Even in normal pregnancies, many common complaints appear: these are the so-called minor discomforts of pregnancy. These disorders are not minor in the sense that they do not cause true discomfort but rather because they are not serious and usually terminate during or after the pregnancy.

Some of these discomforts are so common that they are classed as the symptoms of pregnancy, which have been discussed—frequent urination, caused by the pressure of the uterus on the bladder, during the early and the late months of pregnancy; and the occasional painful tenderness and tingling breast sensations which are temporary.

**Morning Sickness.** Morning sickness is the most common symptom and discomfort of early pregnancy. For many years it was thought that this mild nausea and vomiting was usually an emotional reaction, an unconscious response to the many changes which pregnancy and a new baby bring. However, it is now thought that there is a general reduction in stimuli to the smooth muscles accompanied by diminished gastric motility.

The symptoms may be caused by physiological changes normal to pregnancy. Many women experience this symptom before they have any idea that they might be pregnant.

Although it is called "morning" sickness, the nausea and the vomiting may occur at any time of the day, but only in a small percentage of women does it persist throughout the day. Frequent small meals, as well as dry carbohydrate foods taken before rising, often prove to be helpful, but what helps one person may not help another. There are also medications safe to use during pregnancy which control nausea and vomiting. This discomfort is usually limited to the first 3 months of pregnancy.

**Constipation.** Constipation and flatulence are not unusual in pregnancy. They are thought to be due to impaired intestinal peristalsis. These disagreeable problems are usually controlled by the diet and the mild laxatives which are prescribed by the doctor.

**Shortness of Breath.** Dyspnea (difficult breathing) or shortness of breath is caused by the pressure of the baby on the diaphragm. It is usually troublesome only in the latter weeks of pregnancy, and it is relieved spontaneously as the baby settles into the pelvis (*lightening*) or by delivery. It is naturally aggravated when the mother tries to lie down; she will rest and sleep much more comfortably if she is supported and elevated by pillows at her back.

**Leg Cramps.** Cramping pains in the calf of the leg are astonishingly painful. The general belief is that these cramps are caused by an accumulated excess of phosphorus in the body. Calcium lactate or calcium gluconate, taken before meals, or vitamin B will provide relief and prevent their recurrence. Immediate relief from cramps may be obtained by forcing the toes upward and by creating pressure on the knee to straighten the leg (Fig. 36-3).

**Edema.** Fluids may collect in the body toward the end of pregnancy, especially in the feet and the legs; elevating the legs will usually give some relief. Less salt in the diet is recommended, since salt tends to hold fluids in the body. If edema is apparent all over the body, it may be a symptom of toxemia, and the doctor should be notified at once. (See p. 410.)

**Vaginal Discharge.** In addition to the natural increase in secretions from the vaginal and the cervical glands during pregnancy, certain infectious organisms (Trichomonas vaginalis is one) or an eroded cervix may be the cause of vaginal discharge. The doctor may prescribe medicated vaginal douches except during the last month of pregnancy, when douches are never given.

**Gingivitis.** Spongy, swollen, and sometimes bleeding gums may appear, as a result of a deficiency in ascorbic acid in the diet. The condition improves when large amounts of ascorbic acid are given. An astringent mouthwash makes the mouth feel better.

**Other Discomforts.** Faintness or dizziness, nosebleed and heartburn are other comparatively minor difficulties that cause discomfort during pregnancy. Backache, due to postural changes and softening of the pelvic joints, is another symptom. Treatment of these disturbances is the same during pregnancy as at any other time.

**Varicose Veins.** Varicose veins may develop in the later months of pregnancy; they usually appear in the legs but may also develop in the groin or in the vulva. The tendency to develop varicosities is familial, and the increased intraabdominal pressure from the enlarged uterus, as well as any prolonged standing, hastens their development. The patient should not wear round garters or tight clothing which will interfere with circulation, and she should avoid being on her feet for any considerable length of time. Elevating her legs against the wall when she goes to bed will help to drain the blood back from her legs; sometimes an

Ace bandage is applied before she gets up in the morning, or she can wear nylon elastic stockings to make her more comfortable. New support-type stockings are attractively sheer.

**Hemorrhoids.** The hemorrhoidal veins in the rectum sometimes become congested (varicosed) and may be very painful. This condition is usually a result of constipation and straining to evacuate the bowels, as well as the uterine pressure interfering with the flow of venous blood. Regular bowel habits will help to prevent hemorrhoids; if this condition develops, cold saline compresses or Sitz baths will bring relief from pain. Sometimes the doctor prescribes suppositories or an analgesic ointment.

**Stretch Marks.** Some women experience such a great change in body size during pregnancy that marks occur on the breasts, thighs, and abdomen. These are called *striae gravidarum* and usually disappear after delivery. They appear as reddish or white lines and are caused by the stretching and rupture of internal tissues. Exercise seems to lessen the occurrence of stretch marks, and the less weight gained during pregnancy, the less chance that the marks will become permanent. This is, however, a highly individual thing and it is not possible to predict who will retain stretch marks and who will not. (These marks can also occur in nonpregnant people who experience a fast increase in size.)

## Some Normal Worries

**Concerns about Having a Normal Child.** It is quite natural for any pregnant woman to be concerned about having a deformed or physically impaired child. It is important to remember that most pregnancies are normal and that most babies born are normal. If the mother is unduly concerned, the nurse should inform the doctor, so that he can discuss this with the mother. It is, of course, not possible to assure every mother that she will have a perfectly normal child, since there are many conditions which cannot be predicted, and this is a particularly challenging situation if the mother has already had a child with some sort of difficulty.

**Fear about Delivery.** A great deal of the fear about delivery can be allayed by patient education. If the patient knows what will happen and what to expect, she is less likely to be apprehensive. An understanding nurse will allow the patient to verbalize and work out her concerns.

## PREPARING FOR PARENTHOOD

The idea of family-centered care can achieve its fulfillment in the preparation for parenthood. Contemporary social influences have permitted the recognition that an understanding and affectionate husband contributes tremendously to the success of making pregnancy a shared foundation in the building of family life.

Pregnancy should provide a happy experience for the prospective parents; their happiness and affection for each other should enable them to share with joy the responsibilities they will assume. But pregnancy may arouse a new set of emotions, especially in the wife. If she wants a baby, she is overjoyed at first. Then she begins to think of the months ahead, the ordeal of having the baby, and the responsibility that she faces later. She may think that perhaps the baby will interfere with her life with her husband. Baby sitters are expensive; and besides, could she trust her baby to strangers? She feels guilty because she does not seem to be filled with mother love; she longs only to eat a good breakfast without losing it immediately. There is nothing abnormal about these emotions—undoubtedly, she felt low at times before she was pregnant. When prospective parents share the experience of pregnancy, the husband understands what is happening: he can reassure his wife. On the other hand, on days when the coming responsibilities may look overwhelming to the husband, the understanding wife will provide the reassurance that he may need in their joint adventure.

**When Pregnancy Brings Problems.** Some parents may look upon pregnancy as a disaster, as a discussion of these thumbnail sketches will illustrate:

Mrs. Crane is dismayed to find that she is pregnant. Her husband has just told her that he wants a divorce, and she already has a child.

Mrs. Heath is 37 years old—she was married at 35 and is overjoyed to find that she is pregnant. But Mr. Heath is worried. He has been told that it is dangerous for a woman to have her first baby at that age.

The Martins are worried about money. They already have 4 children, and Mr. Martin has just gone into a new business.

Mrs. Norris had to stay in bed for 3 months before David was born; he was born prematurely, and she had to leave him in the hospital for 6 weeks. Both Mr. and Mrs. Norris are afraid that this will happen again; they still cannot believe that 3-year old David is really a healthy little boy.

The young Careys planned to wait until they had their own home before they had a baby. They now live in a small apartment which is crowded for two.

Problems such as these can have tragic results, and they involve some of the major social problems of our day. However, education on family living, marriage, and sex hygiene will hopefully have strong positive effects on the attitudes and the actions of the families of the future. Emphasis on education is not new in preparation for parenthood. The Maternity Center Association in New York City has been conducting mothers' classes since the early 1920's, and in 1938 it added classes for fathers, too. Classes for expectant families are now available in many communities.

**Mothers' Classes.** In these classes, mothers learn about the process of pregnancy. They learn how to take care of themselves and what to prepare for the baby; how to bathe a baby and make a formula. The importance of keeping a happy home both before and after the baby comes is explained. Mothers ask questions and get advice. (When agencies have many applicants for these classes, they try to group people with similar backgrounds.) This kind of teaching reinforces the doctor's instructions; mothers are urged to keep in close touch with their doctor.

**Fathers' Classes.** Fathers learn how to help their wives; how to choose a doctor and a hospital; how to enjoy planning for the baby. They learn how the baby grows month by month; they learn the signs of labor and how the baby is born. They practice changing, bathing and feeding a baby. These classes are intended to make a father feel that he is much more than a helpless outsider, who can only stand by and worry about his wife.

**Prenatal Classes.** Prenatal classes are often held for father and mother together. These often include discussion on anatomy and physiology of normal pregnancy and delivery and care of the newborn baby, as well as a tour of the hospital's maternity unit. The practical nurse may become involved in doing some of the teaching for these classes.

## Natural Childbirth

During the past several decades, Dr. Grantley Dick Read, an English obstetrician, became widely known for his teachings on "natural childbirth."

Dr. Read found many followers in this country. Natural childbirth classes are taught in clinics, physicians' offices, and hospitals across the nation.

Information is presented in a general attitude to eliminate fear. The anatomy and the physiology of childbearing is presented; the parents learn the process and the progress of labor and delivery, and how to cooperate with the natural process. The expectant mother is taught exercises which help to develop general muscle tone but particularly strengthen and control the muscles used in labor and delivery. Special emphasis is placed on breathing technics, which will help the mother to relax as well as to cooperate with the muscular activities involved in labor and delivery.

Many doctors feel that this type of education accomplishes many good aims. It is recognized that fear aggravates pain in any situation; therefore, to prevent or eliminate fear through education is ideal. The patients are more relaxed and cooperative; labor time is often shortened. Many doctors think that the emphasis has been distorted: the patient feels that she "does not do well" and is left discouraged, if after all her diligent and enthusiastic preparations she "fails" and requires medications to relieve the sometimes dismaying discomforts of labor. However, many patients realize that what is natural is not necessarily painless; that the measure of the success should be the patient's willingness and ability to cooperate with the normal physiological processes of childbirth, and not merely her ability to endure the process without medication or anesthesia.

The "natural childbirth" philosophy has at present reached a happy middle-of-the-road approach. The value of the classes to educate the expectant parents is clearly accepted, and improving the tone of muscles used in labor is of benefit before, during, and after delivery. Relaxing technics help the expectant mother to rest between the intervals of the hard work of labor. Nonetheless, the valued use of medications and methods of anesthesia which benefit both mother and infant are also clearly accepted. The members of the medical and nursing team recognize the contribution that they must make—the individualized care, and the attention and the support of the patient by each doctor and nurse adds greatly to the relaxation, peace of mind, and sense of accomplishment of the mother.

## PREGNANCY COMPLICATIONS

Although pregnancy is considered to be a normal physiological process, there are certain major complications which may very seriously affect the baby or the mother.

### Hyperemesis Gravidarum

This disturbance is usually connected with morning sickness, in the early months of pregnancy when the processes of digestion and elimination are slowed. If vomiting persists to the point where there is an excessive loss of weight, dehydration, and acetone in the urine, it is called *pernicious vomiting* or *hyperemesis gravidarum*. The cause of this is unknown: the disseminations of toxins into the mother's bloodstream, the endocrine and the metabolic changes of normal gestation, and diminished gastrointestinal motility are all considered as being basic factors. Some doctors feel that it is due in a large measure to a neurosis.

If the condition becomes severe, hospitalization is required. The patient is given intravenous fluids, glucose, and vitamins. Sedatives are prescribed for the general rest of the patient, which is usually badly needed. Visitors are restricted. After 24 hours, dry foods in small quantities are tried. If no vomiting occurs, the diet is gradually increased.

Fortunately, fewer patients are being hospitalized for this serious complication. Drugs that control vomiting have been found to be both safe and effective (Dramamine, Compazine, Tigan, Bendectin), and they relieve the possibility of the development of hyperemesis in a high percentage of patients.

## Toxemia

In April, 1952, the American Committee on Maternal Welfare established the following definition of toxemia:

The toxemias of pregnancy are disorders encountered during gestation or early in the puerperium, which are characterized by one or more of the following signs: hypertension, edema, albuminuria and, in severe cases, convulsions and coma.

*Toxemia* is one of the 3 major causes of maternal deaths (totaling approximately 1,000 each year in the United States) and causes at least 30,000 stillbirths and deaths in newborns yearly, primarily through prematurity. Toxemia is common, occurring in at least 1 out of every 20 pregnancies. It develops most frequently in the last 2 or 3 months of pregnancy, and it is likely to occur in young women who are in their first pregnancy. It is also more likely to occur in mothers with physical conditions, such as diabetes.

Two classifications of toxemia are *preeclampsia* and *eclampsia*. In preeclampsia, the patient who previously has shown normal progress in pregnancy develops one or more of the symptoms. In eclampsia, the patient also has convulsions.

Although the symptoms of preeclampsia most often allow the doctor to intercept it early and to prevent further symptoms, it sometimes develops explosively between visits —perhaps the day after an examination. Because of this, each expectant mother should know that she should report any of the following symptoms to her doctor immediately:

Sudden gain in weight
Edema of the fingers, the face, the legs or the feet
Spots before the eyes or blurring of vision
Severe unremitting headache
Persistent vomiting
Decrease in the urinary output

Most patients with preeclampsia respond to treatment. Very few develop eclampsia. Because eclampsia is largely a preventable condition, the preventive aspect of obstetric nursing —the importance of keen, accurate observation and reporting—must be recognized by the responsible obstetric nurse.

When the patient develops eclampsia, her preeclamptic symptoms become more exaggerated and severe, and she develops convulsions. The convulsions may occur before labor begins, during labor, or after the baby is born. After a convulsion the patient may become conscious in a few minutes, or she may remain in a coma for several hours or days. Convulsions may recur in either instance. Even if the patients are awake after convulsions, they are sometimes confused, and they may present serious nursing problems.

Eclampsia is one of the most severe complications of pregnancy. The fetal mortality from eclampsia is almost 25 per cent, and the maternal mortality ranges from 5 to 15 per cent. As the condition progresses, the urinary output lessens and albumin in the urine may increase. The pulse rate becomes very rapid, and the systolic blood pressure may hover around 200. Convulsions continue, and the coma deepens. The slushy respirations of edema of the lungs can be heard, and the prognosis is poor.

As can be seen from statistics, most patients with eclampsia survive. However, 30 to 50 per cent show symptoms of toxemia in further pregnancies. Some patients are maimed by chronic hypertension. Since the cause of eclampsia is unknown, the best treatment is prevention. The aim in the treatment is to control preeclampsia and to prevent the development of eclampsia with its convulsions which bring severe problems to both the mother and the baby. Sedatives may be prescribed to encourage rest and to limit activity. A diet which is low in salt is of prime importance. The sodium ion from salt is retained in the tissues and causes the retention of fluid which shows in the weight gain and the edema of the mother. Table salt is not used at all, and foods which are high in salt content, such as canned soups, are eliminated from the diet to reduce the edema. A diuretic (to increase urinary output) and antihypertensive medications (to reduce blood pressure) are usually ordered to control the symptoms.

If the symptoms continue and if the edema, the hypertension, and the albuminuria remain pronounced, the patient is hospitalized. The same treatment is continued, and complete bed rest is prescribed. Closer observations to help safeguard the mother and the baby are facilitated: the patient is weighed daily; the intake and the output of fluids are recorded; urine is tested daily for albumin; the blood pressure is taken at close intervals; and the fetal heart sounds are watched closely.

In severe preeclampsia, heavier sedation is

given to prevent convulsions. The patient is kept drowsy and sleepy. The room should be darkened, quiet and comfortable. Needless visits to the room and other stimuli—loud noises and bright lights—are controlled. Magnesium sulfate (I.M.) is regarded as a drug specifically used for toxemia, since it is a vasodilator, a diuretic and also a central nervous system depressant which prevents convulsions. The tranquilizing and hypotensive drugs are also effective. Preeclampsia and eclampsia develop only in pregnancy; therefore, it would seem to be logical that terminating the pregnancy would be the cure. However, cesarean sections are seldom performed for this complication of pregnancy, since experience has shown that this results in such a high mortality rate for the mother. The best therapy seems to be the conservative: to control the symptoms as much as possible and either allow labor to start normally or to initiate it when the safety of the mother and the baby permits.

Later pregnancies are usually contraindicated for the patient who has severe eclampsia.

## Abortion

If a fetus is discharged from the uterus before it is capable of carrying on its own life, the lay person usually refers to it as a miscarriage. Medically, the term *abortion* is used to describe this termination of pregnancy before the fetus is viable, that is, before it is able to survive outside the uterus. Generally speaking, this is considered to be before the twentieth week of pregnancy.

Nurses will do well to realize that the public generally associates criminal activities with the word "abortion." It has a sordid connotation for the average person. If the patient does not understand that "abortion" is the common medical term and that "miscarriage" is seldom if ever used, she may feel that the nurses and other staff think she has induced the loss of her pregnancy. She may feel very guilty when she has no reason to do so. This is another example where a few seconds of the nurses' time spent in explanation may alleviate a great deal of misunderstanding.

There are a number of common terms used to describe various causes or phases of abortion:

A *threatened abortion* is one in which the mother, early in pregnancy, has bleeding or spotting. She may also have mild cramps. The pregnancy may be saved. Many physicians will often not take extreme measures to save a pregnancy, since the spontaneous abortion is often nature's way of disposing of a malformed fetus.

An *inevitable abortion* is one in which the loss of the pregnancy cannot be prevented. Bleeding is heavier, and the cervix is dilated.

An *incomplete abortion* is one in which part of the products of pregnancy are retained and not discarded from the uterus. This usually causes intensive bleeding and usually is treated by dilatation and curettage (scraping the uterus).

*Missed abortions* are those in which the fetus has died but has not been expelled from the uterus. The dead fetus is usually expelled spontaneously within a few weeks. It may cause an infection if allowed to remain. A D&C (dilatation and curettage) is often done if the fetal remains are not expelled soon after death.

*Habitual abortion* is a problem condition in which a mother spontaneously loses several successive pregnancies. This mother, quite naturally, is usually very upset and depressed. In this case, the doctor will often make every possible effort to save the pregnancy. The doctor attempts to determine the cause of the repeated abortions and to alleviate it, if possible. Sometimes, surgery is done as, for example, in the case of an incompetent cervix.

A *therapeutic abortion* is the legal termination of a pregnancy by a physician. The Supreme Court decision of 1973 nullified the various state laws concerning abortion and generally established a more liberal basis upon which decisions for abortion may be made. Certain religions declare therapeutic abortions to be contrary to the natural law; Catholic hospitals often do not permit them to be performed.

A *criminal abortion* is the intervention in pregnancy without medical or legal justification.

Authorities estimate that approximately 1 out of every 10 pregnancies ends in a *spontaneous abortion* (one in which the process starts of its own accord through natural causes). The cause of this problem, so tragic and distressing to the parents, is presently being investigated. There is evidence supporting the theory that this is nature's method of eliminating pregnancies which would have produced abnormal babies. Some of the babies are unable to survive with their deformities. Diseases and infections sometimes lead to abortions. Hormonal problems and disorders of the reproductive tract may also be contributing factors.

The treatment in threatened abortions depends on the severity of the symptoms. If the bleeding is slight, the patient is put to bed for 48 to 72 hours; if the bleeding disappears, she may undertake limited activities. Sexual relations should not be resumed for 2 weeks. If uterine contractions occur, the prognosis is more guarded. Incomplete abortions with heavy bleeding are treated by curettage or surgical removal of the retained tissues from the uterus. If evidence of infection is present (fever, odorous discharge), strict precautions to prevent the spread to others must be carried out. If the abortion is complete, the same care is given that would routinely be given a patient following delivery. The patient is observed closely for signs of hemorrhage; her blood pressure is checked to see that it remains stable; pallor is observed; her pulse is watched for weak rapidity, which is a sign of shock. The nurse can clearly understand the alarm, the stress, and the fright of the patient in these circumstances, and she should make all possible efforts to reassure and comfort her. However, if the abortion has occurred, and the patient has been treated to the degree necessary for her safety, the presence of her husband is usually of more comfort than the presence of the nurse. Losing a baby, as well as having one, is a family affair.

## Placenta Previa

When the placenta lies low enough in the uterus to cover the internal opening of the cervix either partially or totally, the condition is called *placenta previa. Marginal placenta* is the attachment of the placenta next to the cervix but not covering it. Painless vaginal bleeding during the later months of pregnancy is the primary symptom of this complication. The treatment is usually delivery by cesarean section for complete or partial placenta previa. When possible, bleeding from marginal placenta is treated by the rupture of the membranes, which allows the presenting part to exert pressure on the placenta against the lower uterine segment, thereby slowing or stopping the hemorrhage by compression.

The dangers of placenta previa are bleeding, shock, and infection. Since the open blood vessels are low and close to the cervix, infection may develop from microorganisms in the vaginal canal. Rectal and vaginal examinations are done only in the operating or delivery rooms with personnel ready to proceed with emergency surgery if necessary. Since bleeding may be profuse, the use of blood transfusions often proves to be a lifesaving measure. Again, the constant observation by the knowledgeable obstetric nurse may prevent the development of shock.

With modern surgical methods as well as with the use of blood transfusions, the maternal mortality from placenta previa has dropped tremendously; however, it is still regarded as a serious complication. Because the separation of the placenta from the uterine wall reduces or eliminates the infant's oxygen supply, the prognosis for the baby is considered fair to poor.

## Abruptio Placenta

*Abruptio placenta* is a grave complication of later pregnancy in which the placenta separates abruptly from its attachment to the uterine wall. The bleeding may be visible, or it may be concealed because it is higher and contained within the uterus. In most cases, the patient has severe pain. The uterus becomes extremely firm and tender. Shock is often present and may seem to be out of proportion, since the bleeding is not obvious.

Of prime importance in cases of abruptio placenta is the treatment of shock; blood loss must be replaced before proceeding with cesarean section, which is almost invariably necessary. Occasionally, it is necessary to perform a hysterectomy to control the bleeding.

The treatment of abruptio placenta has been developed to the point where it is no longer fatal to most mothers. However, the outlook for the baby's survival depends on the severity of the separation and the degree to which his oxygen supply has been affected.

## Ectopic Pregnancy

The word *ectopic* means "outside" or "out of place"; therefore, an *ectopic pregnancy* is one which is attached outside the uterus. Ectopic pregnancies occur most frequently in the fallopian tubes. The symptoms begin with spotting or bleeding 2 or 3 weeks after a missed menstrual period. Often there is accompanying pain which may be quite severe. A tubal pregnancy always requires surgical removal. Rupture of the fallopian tube is a dangerous complication. Very rarely, an abdominal or ovarian pregnancy is encountered.

## Hydatidiform Mole

*Hydatidiform mole* is a condition in which certain products of conception degenerate and form grapelike clusters of vesicles. This is at first a normal pregnancy, but usually with the formation of the mole there is no fetus present. The uterus enlarges more rapidly than usual; the mother has episodes of spotting and bleeding, and frequently she is very nauseated and feels miserable. When the diagnosis becomes certain, the uterus is usually emptied by careful dilatation of the cervix and removal of the hydatidiform mole. The patient receives extensive follow-up examinations, because although the mole itself is benign, it may be the forerunner of a malignant development.

## THE MOTHER WITH A SPECIAL PROBLEM

### The Diabetic Mother

The mother who has diabetes mellitus needs special prenatal care. She is more likely to have complications of pregnancy, such as toxemia, than is the normal woman. The baby is more likely to be large and may be delivered early because of his large size. Babies of diabetic mothers may have respiratory difficulties and must be watched carefully after birth and carefully monitored before birth. It is vital to observe fetal heart tones in this mother and to report even the slightest symptom of difficulty. The nurse should also be aware that pregnancy aggravates diabetes, and she should observe the mother carefully for any signs of insulin shock or diabetic coma (see Chapter 52). The obstetrician who is following this mother will warn her of the possible complications which might occur and will instruct her to contact him in the event of any sign of complications.

### The Mother With a Heart Disorder

Women with various disorders of the heart have successfully delivered babies. In the past, it was felt that these women should be aborted, but it is now believed that it is safer to undergo a normal delivery than an abortion. If the mother has a cardiac disorder of some sort, she must be watched carefully during her pregnancy and may be delivered early to prevent a difficult labor. Documented cases reveal that perfectly normal babies have been delivered from mothers who had rheumatic heart defects, cardiac pacemakers, or other heart disorders.

### The Mother Who Has a Seizure Disorder

This woman must be watched carefully for any signs of seizures. The nurse must remember that a seizure is also a sign of eclampsia and must not confuse the two types of seizures. The most important thing in the case of the mother is to caution her to consistently take her anticonvulsive medication and to report any symptoms to the doctor. The medication may be increased while she is pregnant, since pregnancy can upset the seizure disorder. Additional measures must be taken to protect the unborn child, as well as the mother, during a seizure.

### The Mother Dependent on Drugs

The nurse should be aware of the fact that the baby born to the addicted mother will also most likely be addicted. The mother has been supplying the baby with drugs through the placental exchange before birth. The infant will usually go through withdrawal symptoms, once his supply of drugs is removed after he is born. Generally, the doctor will not attempt to withdraw the mother from drugs until after the birth of the child.

### The Mother Who Needs a Cesarean Section

In the case of *cephalopelvic disproportion* (the baby's head is larger than the vaginal opening) and in other situations, the mother may need to have a cesarean section, which involves incision into the uterus to remove the baby. This may be done as an elective procedure; that is, it is planned in advance because the doctor knows it is necessary. It may also be an emergency procedure, if some difficulty arises during labor. The actual procedure is discussed in the next chapter, but the nurse should be prepared to mentally and physically prepare the patient before the operation. The nurse must remember that the mother will not only need to recover from having had a baby, but must also recover from an abdominal operation. She needs routine pre- and postoperative care, as well as routine postpartum care.

## OTHER CONSIDERATIONS

### When the Baby Dies

Occasionally, in spite of excellent prenatal care and the best nursing care, the baby dies. This is a very unfortunate event and an excellent test of the interpersonal relationship abilities of the nurse. It is a very difficult time for the mother and father, as well as the medical and nursing staff. The nurse must be as supportive as possible and give the mother and father a chance to vent their feelings. A visit by the hospital chaplain or social worker may be appreciated, and the nurse can ask if the family wishes her to call anyone. Some hospitals believe that the mother of the baby who dies should be removed from the maternity ward, while other hospitals feel that she should stay with the other mothers. The nurse must be aware of the policy of her hospital.

### The Unwed Mother

The nurse will often come in contact with the mother who is not married. In the hospital this is often referred to as "out of wedlock" or an OW pregnancy. The nurse must remember that this mother is a person who needs physical and emotional support. She, in fact, probably needs more emotional support from the nurse than does the mother who has a husband to assist her through the childbirth process. It goes without saying that the nurse will treat this person as an individual, without making judgments and without treating her in any different way.

One consideration is whether or not the mother plans to keep her baby. Some differences exist for the unmarried mother who does not plan to keep her baby. She often does not see the baby after birth and may be in a different part of the hospital for postnatal care.

**Prenatal Care.** If the girl is very young, pregnancy is a particular strain on her body. She is undergoing the changes of adolescence as well as those involved in sustaining a pregnancy. Thus the young girl may need special dietary instructions or vitamin supplements. The danger of spontaneous abortion is fairly high in the girl under the age of 15.

Prenatal care also must include referral to a community agency, if desired. The person needs to know about continuing her education if she is still in school. She needs to know about counseling services available so that she can decide if she wishes to keep her baby or not, and she may need vocational or other educational training so that she can get a job to support herself and her baby. Or she may just need someone to talk to and to help her work through her feelings. Often, the person's parents are not helpful because they are too emotionally involved or are too upset about the pregnancy. In many instances the girl is afraid to go to her parents.

There are many community agencies which are available to assist the unmarried mother. If in doubt, the girl can contact the Salvation Army, her local church group or clergyman, the local welfare agency, or her family doctor. Financial assistance is often available through these agencies, as well as counseling and rehabilitation services.

### The Unmarried Father

The father of the child is often the forgotten man. He may feel very badly about what has happened and may wish to assist the girl, even though the couple does not wish to get married. Counseling services are also available for him, and the nurse may be asked to refer him to an agency. The same agencies which assist the unmarried mother will also assist in the counseling and guidance of the unmarried father.

### The Divorced or Widowed Mother

The mother who has recently been separated by death or divorce from her husband has special emotional needs. The nurse can offer emotional support and stay with her as much as possible during labor and delivery.

# 37

# Assisting the Mother During Labor, Delivery, and Puerperium

---

## BEHAVIORAL OBJECTIVES

*The student successfully attaining the goals of this chapter will be able to:*

- *list and recognize, in the clinical area, the signs of approaching labor.*
- *describe the 3 stages of labor.*
- *define episiotomy, indicate the purpose for performing one, and discuss care during postpartum.*
- *state at least 5 procedures which are performed when the mother is admitted to the labor room and discuss the nurse's role.*
- *list and recognize, in the clinical area, untoward symptoms which may occur during labor.*
- *describe 3 complications which may occur during labor and delivery.*
- *discuss the nurse's role in postpartum care, including both immediate care and general needs of the mother.*
- *perform or supervise a new mother during perineal care.*
- *define the term cesarean section, give 3 possible reasons for performing one, and describe the nursing care.*
- *describe 3 postpartum complications.*

---

A woman who is having her first pregnancy is called a *primigravada* or a *primipara.* (Primipara actually is the terminology after the baby is born.) These terms are not used consistently and are often used interchangeably. A woman who has had 2 or more pregnancies is called a *multipara.* A woman who has several children is called a *grand multipara.*

## LABOR

### Signs of Approaching Labor

During pregnancy the muscles of the uterus have been getting ready for their work. They have been tightening and relaxing at intervals, a process known as *contraction.* The contractions during pregnancy are usually painless, and frequently the mother is unaware of their occurring. (These are called Braxton-Hicks contractions.) As labor approaches, they may become uncomfortable; these contractions are called *false labor*.

Another indication of approaching labor is the settling of the baby lower into the pelvis. This dropping of the baby is called *lightening,* and it is usually more apparent in a first pregnancy. The mother may suddenly discover that it is much easier to breathe.

**Uterine Contractions.** True labor is characterized by rhythmic contractions of the uterine muscles. This helps to open the soft cervix and to push the baby through to the outside. The contractions occur at fairly regular intervals between 5 to 15 minutes apart, and they usually last 30 seconds or longer. The intervals between them gradually decrease, and the *show* appears. This is a pinkish or bloody mucous discharge which indicates normal changes in the cervix.

The baby lies in a membranous sac surrounded by amniotic fluid. This is called the *bag of waters.* These membranes may rupture any time during the labor. Contrary to old wives' tales, the rupturing of the membranes prior to the onset of labor, or early during the labor, does not necessarily indicate a long or difficult labor. In fact, the doctor sometimes ruptures these membranes artificially in order to begin the labor process.

**Induction of Labor.** In many instances, it is desirable to induce labor (to start the labor before the woman begins labor naturally). This may be done by administering drugs, either orally or parenterally. Some commonly used drugs are oxytocin or Pitocin.

Labor may also be induced by the artificial rupture of the amniotic membranes. This is called *amniotomy* and is carried out by the physician under sterile conditions, at times with the assistance of the nurse. After the bag of waters is ruptured by the use of a type of hook, labor usually follows very soon. If labor does not spontaneously begin, drug administration will usually follow. It is important that the delivery occur quite soon after rupture of the membranes, since this opens the uterus to a possible infection.

The function of the nurse during induction of labor consists of giving physical and emotional support to the patient and the husband, as well as assisting the doctor. It is very important to very carefully monitor fetal heart tones, since this labor may be fast and hard and may place the child in distress. Any sign of fetal distress must be reported immediately.

## Stages of Labor

**The First Stage of Labor.** Labor is nature's provision for enabling the baby to be born. He must be pushed out of his protected life in the uterus, down the bony passage of the pelvis, through the cervix and the birth canal, and out into the world. The bag of waters must break, and the cervix must open before the baby can be born. The mucous plug is expelled, along with a small amount of blood-tinged mucus. This often signals the beginning of labor. The muscles of the uterus contract to supply the pressure which stretches or dilates the cervix in the first stage of labor. For a primigravada this phase usually takes from 8 to 16 hours. The uterine contractions are involuntary, and the mother can do nothing to hurry or to control them.

Some mothers grow discouraged during this first stage of labor, as it may seem long and tedious. The process is slow in order to keep the tissues from tearing as the muscles alternately contract and relax. Labors are shorter for most multiparas, because the tissues are less resistant and stretch more easily. The first stage of labor ends when the cervix is fully effaced (or taken up), when it is fully dilated (about 10 cm.), and when expulsion of the baby begins.

**The Second Stage of Labor.** When the cervix is fully stretched, the second stage of labor begins. The abdominal muscles and the diaphragm join the uterine muscles to push the baby out. The mother may say she feels "pushing pains." (These are irresistible and the mother may describe them as being like the uncontrollable urge to defecate when a person has diarrhea.) Often a primigravada asks how she will know when to push, but when the time comes, there is no doubt. The second stage of labor is where the mother is able to help—she takes a deep breath and holds it, and then pushes with each contraction. She begins to feel the baby moving down a little farther each time, then slipping back a little as the muscles relax between contractions. If she relaxes too, she can work better when the next contraction comes. It is hard work, but it is deeply satisfying because she is accomplishing it herself, going through with a job that no one else can do. In most cases this stage takes from 1½ to 2 hours for a first baby; second and later babies take anywhere from 5 minutes to 1½ hours. The second stage of labor ends when the baby is born.

If a mother tells you that the baby is coming, *believe her* and get assistance immediately. If a delivery occurs suddenly and without advance warning and preparation, it is called precipitous delivery. A patient may "precipitate" in the labor room bed very easily if an insensitive nurse ignores her claims that the birth is imminent. The nurse can check for "crowning" (the appearance of the baby's head).

Very often during the second stage of labor, the doctor makes an incision in the perineum, which is called an *episiotomy*. This allows the infant to be delivered more easily by enlarging the vaginal opening. It helps to preserve the structure and the strength of the perineal muscles and prevents the occurrence of a jagged laceration, or extension of a tear into the anus, which would be difficult to repair.

**The Third Stage of Labor.** The third stage begins immediately following the birth of the baby and ends when the placenta and the membranes are expelled. This may take anywhere from 1 minute to 1 hour. The placenta is attached to the uterine wall; but after the baby is born, the uterine muscles contract and expel it. The doctor or the nurse keeps a hand firmly over the empty uterus until it feels firm and hard; this means that the muscles and the blood vessels are contracted and that there is less danger of hemorrhage. If the placenta is expelled with the shiny side out, this is called Schultze's presentation (about 80 per cent of the time); if the dull side is out, it is called Duncan presentation.

## In the Labor Room

Hospital procedures for the admission of patients in labor do not vary greatly, since the information needed and the care of the mother are essentially the same everywhere. The nurse asks the expected date of delivery, because if the baby is premature, special precautions are taken, and special equipment is readied. She also asks how close the contractions are and how long they last, and if the patient has noticed any bleeding. Then she can determine the approximate progress of the patient in labor. If the patient is to have a general anesthetic, the anesthetist will want to know when she last ate.

The mother is given an enema to empty the rectum of fecal material. (The doctor makes rectal examinations throughout labor.) If the bowel is not empty, fecal material will be expelled at the time of delivery and will contaminate the area and endanger the baby. The enema also stimulates uterine contractions. The pubic hair is shaved off or partially so, and the area around the vaginal opening is washed with sterile soap and water. A urine specimen is sent to the laboratory. The doctor examines the mother's heart, lungs, and abdomen and listens to the baby's heart to see if all is normal. He takes the mother's blood pressure because of the ever-present hazard of toxemia. He makes a rectal examination to see how far labor has progressed. A vaginal examination is not done unless it is absolutely necessary, because of the danger of infecting the birth canal.

**The Nurse in the Labor Room.** You may be asked to stay with the patient during labor. Your job will be to keep her comfortable and to observe her closely for any symptoms of complications which will affect either her or the baby. The waiting period for the mother should be made as pleasant as possible. Many hospitals feel that having a baby is a family affair, and they encourage the father to be with the mother as much as possible during the early part of labor. However, the nurse in the labor room has specific duties to perform for specific purposes. She listens to fetal heart tones at regular and frequent intervals. (The normal range of the fetal heartbeat is 120 to 160 per minute.) Fetal heart tones are measured with a special stethoscope called the fetuscope. The nurse should take the mother's pulse to make sure the heartbeat she is hearing is that of the baby. Irregularities, rates beyond the normal, or sudden changes may be important indications of fetal distress

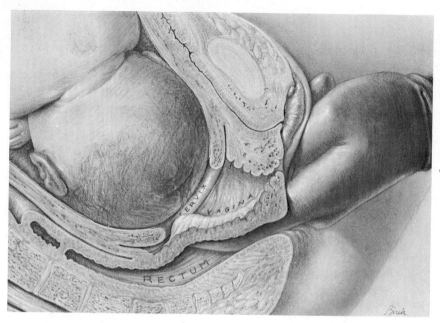

Figure 37-1. Rectal examination, showing how the examining finger palpates the cervix and the infant's head through the rectovaginal septum. (Fitzpatrick, E., Reeder, S. R., and Mastroianni, L., Jr.: Maternity Nursing, ed. 12. Philadelphia, Lippincott, 1971)

and must be reported immediately. The vital signs of the mother are also taken at intervals.

Uterine contractions are observed because they are often an indication of the progress of the patient in labor. They can be felt by placing your hand on the patient's abdomen. As the uterus contracts, the abdomen becomes hard and rigid; the uterus then relaxes, which can be felt by the softening of the muscle fibers. When contractions begin, they are usually mild, short, and far apart. As the labor progresses, they become longer, more intense, and closer together. The frequency of contractions is calculated from the beginning of one until the beginning of the next. As the patient approaches the end of the first stage of labor, she usually complains of the discomfort; the contractions often occur about every 2 or 3 minutes, last 45 to 60 seconds, and are forceful and intense. The nurse can assist the patient with her breathing exercises.

Another method to check the progress of labor is the rectal examination, usually done by the professional nurse or the doctor. The purpose of a rectal examination is to determine the size of the opening in the cervix— its dilatation. By pushing the thin anterior rectal wall (rectovaginal septum) against the cervix, the amount of dilatation can be felt (Fig. 37-1). The practical nurse can assist by seeing that the patient is draped properly.

The cervix also becomes thinner (effacement), an important part of the process.

Dilatation is measured in centimeters; the cervix is considered to be completely dilated at 10 centimeters. The patient is usually in active labor at 4 centimeters and is uncomfortable. Medications are most often given at this time, depending on the doctor's orders.

The practical nurse may be especially trained, after graduation, to perform the rectal examination to determine dilatation of the cervix. Sometimes, the doctor does a sterile vaginal examination to determine the condition of the cervix. The nurse would be asked to assist with this procedure.

The mother has to depend mostly on the nurse for comfort; do everything that you are instructed to do and a little more. Stay with her and encourage her. Sponge her face and hands occasionally; rub her back; give her a drink of water from time to time, if it is permitted. These are the comforting things that make a hot, tired person feel better. Change her gown if it becomes damp; see that the air in the room is fresh. Labor is exactly what the word says—hard work. Do all that you can to help her relax and rest between contractions. You may have an opportunity to give the father a comforting word, too.

One of the important duties of the nurse is to be sure that the patient has an empty bladder. A full bladder prevents the baby's head from descending into the pelvis and thereby slows the progress of labor. It may be necessary to catheterize the patient.

Some of the untoward symptoms during labor are: sharp unremitting pain; prolonged contractions or the failure of the uterus to relax; marked changes in the mother's pulse rate or blood pressure; change in the fetal heart tone; and bleeding. These symptoms should be reported promptly and recorded.

Water or clear fluids, such as tea with sugar, are usually allowed during the very early stages of labor. Solid or liquid foods may cause vomiting and other problems, particularly if the patient is going to have a general anesthetic. In a prolonged labor, intravenous glucose solutions may be given to maintain an adequate caloric and fluid intake. This lessens exhaustion and dehydration.

**Relief of Pain.** Almost all patients in labor are given some medication to make them comfortable and relaxed during the hard work of labor. The type of drug may vary with the locale and the physician, as well as with the condition of the patient. However, there are drugs which are given more commonly than others, for specific reasons. Drugs that relieve pain are called analgesics; and those most frequently administered for labor are Demerol and Nisentil. At times these are given in combination with scopolamine, a drug used for its amnesic effects. (It causes the patient to forget her period of labor.) Scopolamine also dries body secretions which facilitates safer anesthesia. However scopolamine is not as frequently used as it once was. Atropine is sometimes given instead of scopolamine because it also reduces secretions, but it does not cause amnesia.

A third type of drug that may be given is one that enhances the effects of the analgesic, thereby making it possible to reduce the amount of analgesic given. One such drug is Phenergan. This type of drug is valuable because almost all analgesics have some sedative effect on the baby as well as on the mother. A lesser amount of analgesic reduces the possibility of respiratory depression in the baby. These drugs are also frequently antiemetics; that is, they prevent the nausea which is considered to be a reflex at a certain stage of labor.

Most patients receive some form of anesthesia during delivery. This is usually given during the second stage of labor and may be of different types. A general anesthetic is sometimes used. A patient receiving this type of anesthesia is asleep when her baby is born.

Other anesthetics are given by injection, either into the spinal canal or into the tissues and are referred to as pudendal blocks, caudal blocks, or spinal blocks. These anesthetics affect the nerve supply to an area or a region of the body. Although the patient is awake during delivery, she has no sensation or feeling in the part anesthetized. Pontocaine, procaine, and nupercaine are agents commonly used for this type of anesthesia.

Each type of anesthesia has distinct advantages. The doctor chooses the type according to the patient's needs and wants, as well as according to facilities available.

## IN THE DELIVERY ROOM

At times the practical nurse is given training to assist in the delivery room. Her function as designated by the doctor, is to assist the mother or the doctor or to take care of the newborn baby. If you are assigned to assist the mother, you most likely will stand by her head, instructing her how to breathe and when to push and informing her of what is going on. If you are assisting the doctor, you may be asked for equipment, drugs, oxygen, or other items. If you are caring for the newborn baby you will need to make sure that he is breathing and is kept warm. You will also perform other routine procedures as described in Chapter 38.

### Fetal Presentation

While numerous types of fetal presentation are possible, the nurse should be able to differentiate between the cephalic and breech presentations. The most common presentation is the cephalic or head presentation in which the baby's chin is touching his chest. The nurse should be aware that the baby's head turns while he is in the birth canal. In a breech presentation either the buttocks or the feet (a footling) are born first. The difficulty with a breech birth stems from the fact that the head, which is the largest part of the baby's body, exits last. Whichever presentation occurs, the doctor will identify the position for the records.

## Instrument Delivery

At times, when delivery is difficult, instruments or a vacuum extractor is used to assist in the birth of the baby. If forceps are to be used, the cervix must be fully effaced and dilated, the membranes ruptured, and the bladder emptied. When a vacuum extractor is used, a gentle suction-cup device is applied to the head of the infant so that the doctor can gently ease the baby out of the uterus.

These procedures are done with extreme caution and by the physician only. The nurse's responsibility is to chart the procedure and observe the baby after birth. If there are any marks or damage from the forceps, the nurse must note them on the baby's chart.

## Complications of Labor and Delivery

One of the first duties of the nurse is to observe the patient in labor for any possible complications. Since the lives of 2 persons are at stake, this is a grave responsibility. Some possible complications of labor and delivery will be discussed here.

**Precipitate Labor and Delivery.** A precipitate labor is one which is very short and in which the contractions are usually severe. A precipitate delivery is so rapid that the mother is usually unable to be taken to the delivery room or in other ways prepared for delivery. Many times the doctor is not present. Of course, the nurse's concern is for the welfare of the patient and the baby; she must care for their needs as best she can, while preserving and applying as many of the principles of asepsis as is possible in the situation. Other problems in precipitate delivery arise from the possible trauma to both the mother and the baby from the unusual force of the labor.

**Uterine Inertia.** Uterine inertia is sometimes described as a *tired uterus*. The strong contractions which are necessary to force the baby out of the uterus are not present. Perhaps the contractions are strong to begin with and grow weaker, sometimes ceasing altogether, or they may be weak from the onset. Sometimes after the mother has been provided an interval of a few hours sleep, more vigorous labor begins.

**Abnormal Fetal Presentations.** Normally, the baby is born head first, but the fetus may assume almost any position within the uterus. Occasionally, the face is uppermost, or a hand or foot or the buttocks present first. This complication is known as an abnormal presentation. Often, the location of fetal heart tones will indicate the position of the baby. If an abnormal position is determined before labor begins, the doctor may attempt to turn the baby by manual pressure from the outside. Since some positions are impossible to deliver from below, the doctor may need to insert his hand or instruments into the uterus during labor to change the position of the baby. He may also decide that a cesarean section is necessary.

**Multiple Pregnancy.** A multiple pregnancy is one in which more than one fetus is developing in the uterus at the same time. Twin pregnancy is the most common type, although triplets, quadruplets, quintuplets, and even sextuplets or more do occur. If twins are suspected, an x-ray picture will show whether or not there is more than one fetus.

**Cephalopelvic Disproportion.** A condition in which the bones of the mother's pelvis are too small to allow the baby to pass through is known as cephalopelvic disproportion. One of the advantages of prenatal care is to discover the mother's small pelvis before labor begins. If the size of the baby and the size of the mother's pelvis are borderline, frequently the doctor will give the patient a *trial labor* before resorting to surgical delivery.

**Prolapsed Cord.** A prolapsed cord may occur if the membranes rupture and the baby's head is not low in the pelvis, allowing the umbilical cord to drop through the cervical outlet. This is a serious complication, because as the baby's head descends it may press the cord against the hard structures in the mother's pelvis, cutting off the circulation to the fetus. A prolapsed cord also may lead to infection.

**Ruptured Uterus.** A ruptured uterus is one of the most serious complications of labor. Fortunately, it is rare. In this condition the uterus splits from the strain placed upon its muscular wall. The most common cause today is a previous cesarean section, but severe labor contractions, disproportion, and the injudicious use of drugs to stimulate uterine contraction can contribute to its occurrence.

**Other Complications.** Other complications are hemorrhagic conditions, toxemia, severe chronic disease in the mother, and fetal distress. The treatments of these complications depend on the condition of the mother and/or the baby, how serious the complication is, and to what stage of labor the mother has progressed. One of the common treatments for severe complications is cesarean section.

## CARE DURING THE PUERPERIUM

The period after delivery until the genital organs and tract have returned to normal is called the *puerperium* or *postpartum*; it usually lasts about 6 weeks. During this period, the uterus returns to normal size and function, and the menstrual cycle is re-established. The length of the hospital stay for the patient with a normal delivery varies according to the policy of the physician and the hospital. The average stay is 4 or 5 days.

### Immediate Postpartum Care

Immediately following delivery, the mother experiences a feeling of extreme fatigue which is close to exhaustion, just as she would after any extremely vigorous physical activity or hard work. At the same time she is relieved and excited. She is interested in seeing and holding her baby and having a brief visit with her husband, after which she often sleeps.

While the mother is still in the delivery room, she may appear to be chilled. This is a very common and brief reaction. There is no accepted explanation, but the chill appears to be reflex in nature. An extra cotton blanket which has been closely tucked around the mother relieves this mild reaction.

The mother is observed closely for several hours after delivery for any symptoms of hemorrhage. The uterus must be checked at frequent intervals—every 15 minutes during the first hour—to see that it remains firm and contracted. If the uterus becomes soft and relaxed, the nurse cups her hand around the fundus and massages it gently until it regains its firmness. The perineal pad is checked for the amount of bleeding. The pulse and the blood pressure are noted as well. It is important to keep the mother in the delivery room long enough to be sure that her condition is satisfactory. All information about the delivery and other procedures should be recorded on her chart before she is taken to her room. This includes items such as the sex and the condition of the baby at birth, the time of birth, the time at which the placenta was expelled, the care of the breasts, and the condition of the fundus. Any medication given to the mother must be noted.

The father should not be forgotten in this interim. He goes through a severe emotional strain that is very frustrating because there is nothing he can do. Probably this is why some fathers feel the need to "celebrate" after the baby is born.

### General Postpartum Care

The general care of the postpartum patient is similar to that of other patients. The nurse observes the general comfort of the mother—her appetite, her activity, and how well she sleeps and rests. She also notes her temperature, pulse, and respiration, which in most instances are within the normal limits. In addition, there are the special needs of the patient which must be met and observations which must be made.

**Lochia.** The *lochia* is the normal discharge from the vagina after the baby is born. It consists of blood and the broken-down lining of the uterus; it lasts about 3 to 4 weeks. At first it is bright red, consisting mostly of blood, and is called *lochia rubra*. As the bleeding slows, the discharge gradually changes to a pinkish serous color and is called the *lochia serosa*. By the tenth day, the lochia is yellow or white in color, has decreased greatly in amount, and is called the *lochia alba*. If the lochia still contains blood after 10 days, the mother should notify her physician.

**Fundus.** The height and the firmness of the uterine fundus are checked several times daily. The fundus should be firm and directly below the umbilicus. Excessive bleeding or clots should be reported at once. The chart should indicate if the fundus is firm or not and how many finger breadths below the umbilicus it is located. If the fundus is not hard and firm, it should be massaged in an attempt to expel clots and restore the firmness. These procedures are also charted. The nurse must remember that a firm fundus is vital to clamp down on blood vessels and prevent postpartum hemorrhage.

**After-Pains.** For the first few days after delivery, the mother often has painful cramps as the uterine muscles contract; these are called *after-pains.* These pains are not so troublesome after a first baby, because at that time the uterine muscles have a better tone than they do after several pregnancies. Breast-feeding stimulates uterine contractions, and therefore, often brings on after-pains. An analgesic is often ordered as a PRN medication for after-pains.

**Breast Care.** The breasts contain a thin watery fluid, called colostrum, until about the third day after delivery when the milk begins to flow. The breasts often become full and hard (engorged), and sometimes painful. The baby relieves this condition when he nurses. A good supporting brassiére or binder helps to support engorged breasts. The mother who does not wish to nurse her baby is given medications to prevent milk production.

Breast care differs in various hospitals, but the trend is toward procedures as simple as possible, to prevent infection. The nursing mother cleans her nipples before each feeding. The non-nursing mother washes her breasts and nipples at the time of her daily bath. They should be bathed with a clean washcloth and towel before any other part of the body is washed.

Authorities seem to agree that most mothers can nurse their babies, barring such complications as retracted nipples, infections, or breast malformations. Exercises may be done to relieve retracted nipples. The first requirement for breast-feeding is a good supply of milk. If the mother is happy, wants to nurse the baby, and is not worried or overtired, her chances for having a good milk supply are excellent. The mother's mental attitude seems to affect both the quality and the supply of milk; her emotional upsets may affect the baby's digestion. One advantage of breast feeding is the fact that breast milk provides antibodies for the baby. However, formulas have been developed which are similar in every other way to breast milk.

Some women are unwilling to nurse their babies because it interferes with their social activities, or they believe that nursing makes the breasts sag. If a mother must work outside her home, nursing may be inconvenient or even impossible. However, there is much emotional satisfaction to be derived by her, too, from nursing her baby.

EXPRESSION OF MILK. *Expression of milk* (artificial emptying of the breasts) is sometimes necessary. The baby may be too weak to nurse, or it may have a deformity such as a cleft palate or a harelip. Sometimes the mother may produce more milk than her baby needs and can supply another baby. The electric breast pump is the best method to use for expressing milk, because the suction is controlled. Milk may also be expressed by the hands or by a hand pump. The milk is collected in a sterile bottle and kept in the refrigerator.

**Bathing.** The mother receives a daily bath or shower. It is important that the nurse give the first bed bath after delivery. This gives the nurse the opportunity to teach the mother several details of the self-care for which she will later be responsible. Some doctors do not permit tub baths for several weeks after delivery, but many permit and encourage the mother to shower after her first postpartum day. For this reason, she must be taught the procedures for breast and perineal self-care.

**Perineal Care.** Care of the perineum, the area between the vaginal orifice and the rectum, is important to maintain comfort and cleanliness to prevent odor and infection. If the mother has had an episiotomy, the healing of the stitches is promoted by keeping this area clean and dry.

Perineal care is no longer the elaborate procedure it used to be. Technics will vary from hospital to hospital, but in one respect they are always the same: cleansing is done from the pubic area back to the rectal area to avoid contamination by fecal material. This care must always be given after the patient voids or has a bowel movement. The nurse does the procedure if the patient is in bed. However, if the patient is allowed to go to the bathroom, she is taught how to give herself perineal care. She first washes her hands and then places a paper bag, a box of small cleansing tissues and a fresh perineal pad (with the clean side up, or preferably, wrapped) on a stool or a table which is adjacent to or near the toilet. The pad she is wearing is removed from front to back and placed in the paper bag for later disposal. After voiding, she cleanses herself from front to back with tissues, using fresh tissues for each stroke and discarding them in the toilet. It is important that undue pressure be avoided if the stitches of the episiotomy have not yet been removed. If she has had a bowel movement, the anal region is wiped in the same way (from front to back). The mother is taught how to handle the clean perineal pad so that the inner surface is not contaminated by her fingers, and to fasten it to the tab of the sanitary belt in the pubic area first so that it will not slip forward. The toilet should be flushed *after* she stands, to prevent any of the flushing spray from touching the perineum.

PAINFUL STITCHES. These are usually relieved by application of a soothing ointment on specially prepared pads, such as Tucks, and by warm sitz baths.

DIFFICULTY IN VOIDING AND DEFECATING. The new mother may have difficulty voiding after delivery because of the loss of muscle tone in the bladder, or because of perineal soreness or edema. The usual nursing measures should be tried, and many physicians permit the mother to go to the bathroom if she is unable to use the bedpan. A distended bladder causes the uterus to rise in the abdominal cavity and prevents it from contracting, thereby contributing to postpartum hemorrhage. Therefore, it is an important nursing responsibility to see that the mother is able to void. Occasionally, it becomes necessary to catheterize the patient if her bladder is distended and she cannot empty it. The decision to catheterize the patient should depend on the fullness of the bladder, not on the number of hours since delivery. The postpartum patient often voids more frequently than the average patient, because the extra body fluids from pregnancy are being eliminated.

The mother may be constipated for the first week or two following delivery. Diet and activity help to regulate this condition. Many physicians routinely order mild laxatives following delivery until good bowel function is re-established. If necessary, the mother will be given an enema. If hemorrhoids have bothered her during pregnancy, they may still cause discomfort; rectal suppositories or ice packs are prescribed for this condition.

**Early Ambulation.** The mother may lie in any position in which she feels comfortable. She is encouraged to lie on her abdomen for at least 2 hours every day, to bring the uterus forward. In most modern hospitals she is up the day of delivery. The following are some of the advantages of early ambulation for new mothers: muscle tone is restored more quickly to the relaxed pelvic and abdominal muscles; the flow of lochia increases, thereby facilitating the return of the uterus to normal; improved circulation aids healing; and the danger of thrombosis and embolism is decreased.

**Diet and Weight Loss.** The mother should have a normal, nutritious, well-balanced diet. If she is nursing, extra quantities of milk and other liquids may be added.

The mother loses from 8 to 12 pounds during and after delivery. This can be accounted for by the loss of the fetus, the placenta, and the amniotic fluid. She loses about 5 to 8 more pounds in the ensuing 5 or 6 weeks, due to the loss of body fluids accumulated during pregnancy. If her weight gain was not excessive, she usually returns to her normal weight in about 6 weeks.

**Postpartum Examination and Instruction.** The doctor checks the patient closely before discharging her from the hospital, which may be 4 or 5 days after delivery. She is told to return to him for a follow-up examination at the end of 6 weeks, and she is usually advised not to have sexual intercourse or take vaginal douches before that time.

The new mother is instructed while in the hospital as to the care of her baby and herself and as to feeding methods. The primipara is an excellent candidate for referral to the Public Health Nurse.

As was mentioned before, the uterus should have returned to its normal size and position at the end of 6 weeks; this process is called *involution.* Sad as it may seem to new mothers, a slim silhouette takes a while to achieve. Not only must the uterus shrink itself from approximately 2 pounds to 2 ounces, but the skin and the muscles of the abdomen are greatly stretched. If the muscles were in good condition before pregnancy, they soon begin to regain tone. The stretch marks, called *striae,* fade to faint silver lines. Exercises provide a good method to get back into shape; the doctor will usually prescribe these and tell the mother when she may begin.

Menstruation begins again in 6 to 8 weeks if the mother does not nurse her baby. If she does nurse, menstruation is delayed for 4 or 5 months or until she stops nursing. Although ovulation does not occur in most mothers during the nursing period, prolonging this period is no guarantee that pregnancy will not take place; many nursing mothers do become pregnant.

## CESAREAN SECTION

A cesarean section is a surgical procedure to deliver the baby through an incision in the abdomen and the uterus.

There are numerous reasons for doing a cesarean or C-section as it is also called: the baby's head may be too large to pass through the vaginal canal; a tumor or other obstruction may block the birth canal; the mother may have severe toxemia (although the operation is rarely done if the mother is eclampsic); the mother or the baby may be in danger from placenta previa or premature separation of the placenta or from some other cause; labor cannot be induced in a mother who is in danger.

**Preoperative Nursing Care.** While a cesarean section is frequently performed as an emergency procedure, it is often possible to foresee its need and to schedule surgery shortly before the due date. The nurse should review Chapter 32 for a discussion of the routine preoperative care of any patient about to undergo abdominal surgery. However, she must also remember that a baby is involved. Therefore she must check fetal heart tones frequently, as well as evaluate any other symptoms of fetal distress or discomfort which the mother might be experiencing.

Certain other precautions are taken such as *not* giving an enema nor administering narcotics or strong sedative drugs since the baby will also be anesthetized and his respiration possibly depressed.

Generally, the mother is given a local or a spinal anesthetic for the incision; she is not given a general anesthetic until the baby is delivered and the umbilical cord severed. In this way, the infant will not be anesthetized. Immediately after delivering the baby, the mother is given a general anesthetic and the remainder of the procedure performed. The mother should be forewarned that she will be awake for part of the procedure, so that this does not come as a surprise to her.

If a hysterectomy is to be performed, the uterus is removed at the same time that the C-section is done. Removal of the uterus (C-section followed by hysterectomy), is called Porro's operation and becomes necessary in cases of severe bleeding, sometimes in cases of placenta previa, or in cases of malignancy in the uterus.

The operating room must include preparations for the baby. This involves an isolette or incubator and resuscitation and suction equipment. A special nurse is usually assigned just to care for the baby after delivery.

**Postoperative Care.** The mother is given routine postoperative care following abdominal surgery (see Chapter 32), including early ambulation; turning, coughing, and deep breathing; probable IPPB treatments; elastic stockings; and care of the incision. The patient will also need care for the lochia and nipple discharge which follows the delivery of a baby. She may be unable to nurse her baby for a day or so, but if she desires to breast feed, her milk should be manually expressed during this time.

It may be difficult to check the fundus because of the abdominal dressing, but this procedure is very important. The nurse must remember that this mother can hemorrhage as easily as any other postpartum patient. Oxytocic drugs are usually ordered to cause contraction of the uterus to prevent hemorrhage.

## POSTPARTUM COMPLICATIONS

Some of the complications which may occur during the postpartum period should be mentioned, so that you may know about the nursing care that they require.

**Infection.** *Puerperal infection* is a condition as old as the race, and it was the main cause of maternal deaths before asepsis was known. It used to be called *childbed fever.*

Bacteria which lurk in the lower genital tract and the rectum are capable of causing infection if conditions are favorable, such as the presence of injured tissues or retained pieces of placenta, and lowered resistance. Other common organisms causing puerperal infection are the staphylococcus and the streptococcus. Since these microorganisms can be carried by hospital personnel, those who work in the labor area wear special clothing. Members of the staff who work in the delivery rooms wear caps, masks, and gowns.

Because of the many venous sinuses left open by the removal of the placenta from the uterine wall, the infection may spread through the bloodstream, causing septicemia. Fever is the outstanding symptom of infection; it may or may not be accompanied by a chill. Headache, malaise, and a foul-smelling lochia are other symptoms of infection.

The infected mother is isolated; many times she is removed from the postpartum floor. The baby is not brought to her for feeding. Antibiotics are administered and all technics to prevent the organisms from spreading to other patients are adhered to strictly.

**Hemorrhage.** Postpartum hemorrhage is a serious complication which can occur any time up to 4 weeks following delivery. Most cases occur within 24 hours after the birth of the baby; late hemorrhage is rare. Hemorrhage is usually caused by the retention of a fragment of placental tissue, which prevents the blood vessels from contracting; by tears in the reproductive tract as a result of delivery; or by the poor tone of the uterine muscle, causing the consequent lack of contraction and the delayed constriction of uterine blood vessels.

If the fundus is boggy and relaxed, massage and the administration of an oxytoxic (pituitary extract or ergotrate), which causes the muscles to contract, aids in establishing tone. If the cause of the bleeding appears to be a tear or retained placental tissue, the patient will have to be prepared for a sterile vaginal examination and treatment. If the blood loss is extensive, she may require a transfusion.

**Thrombophlebitis.** Thrombophlebitis is a condition in which there is a clot in a blood vessel with resultant inflammation. In the new mother, thrombophlebitis usually occurs in the femoral vessels in the leg. It used to be called "milk leg." Early ambulation has greatly lessened the occurrence of thrombophlebitis in mothers, but the symptoms of this complication and the necessary nursing care are fully explained in Chapter 32. In the case of a woman who has just been delivered, the anticoagulants (heparin and Dicumarol) usually administered to dissolve a clot, may or may not be given because of the danger of increasing the possibility of uterine hemorrhage. After the acute stage has passed, it is often necessary for the mother to wear a support stocking for a period of time.

**Mastitis.** Mastitis is an infection of the breast which occurs when microorganisms enter through cracked or macerated nipples. One sign of mastitis is a rise in temperature on about the tenth day; the breast becomes red and hot, and the infected area feels hard. When this occurs, the baby is not allowed to nurse. An icecap is applied to the breast, and antibiotics are given. An abscess may form if the treatment is delayed, and an incision and drainage may be necessary.

Recently, a type of mastitis has been reported as a result of infection from an epidemic strain of staphylococcus which is resistant to antibiotics. In this type, the organisms enter through the normal milk ducts in the breast rather than through nipple lesions.

**Mental Disturbances.** Mental problems occur in some postpartum patients. Pregnancy, labor, and delivery are too much to bear for these women, and they feel unable to cope with their problems any longer. The mother who is affected in this way becomes irritable and unable to sleep, she has no appetite and exhibits great anxiety. She may be depressed and dislike both her baby and her husband. This is the time to let the doctor know about these symptoms, so that early treatment may prevent a more serious mental illness from developing. If her condition is entirely the result of the imbalance in her body functions caused by pregnancy, she will recover as soon as her physical condition is normal again. Many patients have *postpartum blues,* which appears to be a normal hormonal reaction on the fourth or the fifth day.

# 38

# Care of the Neonate

---

*The student successfully attaining the goals of this chapter will be able to:*

- *describe the normal characteristics of the newborn.*
- *define the Apgar scale.*
- *properly carry out identification procedures for the newborn and chart information.*
- *evaluate respiratory status of the newborn.*
- *bathe the infant and give bath demonstration to the mother.*
- *take the infant's rectal temperature.*
- *observe the newborn and chart condition.*
- *discuss circumcision and nursing care required.*
- *explain the important principles of breast and bottle feeding, including the nursing mother's diet and the care of her breasts.*
- *perform the procedure for PKU testing.*
- *list at least 4 respiratory disorders of the newborn and discuss.*
- *describe at least 4 possible birth injuries.*
- *list at least 5 coincidental diseases of pregnancy and indicate how they may affect the baby.*
- *discuss the special needs of the premature baby.*
- *define the term postmature baby.*
- *state at least 3 important measures which can be taken during emergency childbirth.*

---

## THE BABY

### Initial Care

As soon as the baby is born, the physician removes secretions from the baby's respiratory tract, either manually or with a small soft bulb syringe or catheter; often, he holds the baby head down so that gravity can assist in removing secretions. The baby then takes his first breath and makes his first sounds. His skin has a bluish tinge at first, but as soon as the oxygen from his crying enters the circulating blood in quantity, he turns pink and rosy. Sometimes, if the mother has been medicated recently or had a long anesthetic, the baby does not breathe at once and has to be stimulated. The doctor clamps and cuts the umbilical cord. He then hands the baby over to the nurse, who has a warm blanket and isolette ready.

## Apgar Scoring Chart

| Sign | Score    0 | 1 | 2 |
|---|---|---|---|
| Heart Rate | absent | slow (below 100) | over 100 |
| Respiratory Effort | absent | weak cry, hypoventilation | strong cry |
| Muscle Tone | limp | some flexion of extremities | well-flexed |
| Reflexes<br>1. Response to catheter in nose (after airway is cleared) | no response | grimace | sneeze or cough |
| 2. Foot slap | no response | grimace | cry and withdraw foot |
| Color | blue, pale | body pink, extremities blue | entire body pink |

Figure 38-1. Apgar scoring chart.

## Normal Characteristics

Many new parents are accustomed to the pictures of infants commonly seen in magazines and are dismayed by the appearance of their newborn, by his odd-shaped head, his wrinkled skin, and perhaps his jaundiced color. Many times the nurse can reassure the parents about the normal physical characteristics of the newborn, putting their fears to rest.

The average newborn (also called a *neonate* for the next 4 weeks) weighs about 7 lbs. and is about 20 inches long. (This does not mean that a baby weighing 5½ lbs., who is 19 inches long, is abnormal—he is just not "average.") (See Chapter 8 for a complete discussion of the characteristics of the newborn baby.)

## Baptism

If the baby's condition is poor, he should be baptized at once if such action is required by the parents' religion—this is of the utmost importance to Roman Catholic parents. The procedure of baptism is important to ensure its validity. Water is poured on the baby's face or forehead, at the same time that the person performing the ceremony repeats the words: "I baptize thee in the name of the Father and of the Son and of the Holy Ghost." If there is any doubt about the baby's being alive, the baptism is given conditionally: "If thou art alive, I baptize thee in the name of the Father and of the Son and of the Holy Ghost." Whenever it has been necessary for the nurse to baptize an infant, a record of the procedure is inserted on the mother's chart on the nursing records. There should be 2 witnesses whenever possible, and their names should be recorded. Anyone can baptize; they do not have to be a Roman Catholic.

## The Apgar Scale

Dr. Virginia Apgar, a noted pediatrician, has developed a scale for evaluation of the newborn which is used in most hospitals. This chart gives the nurse or doctor a quick and fast way of assessing the condition of the newborn baby and of determining if the infant needs assistance or resuscitation.

The scale, shown in Figure 38-1, is used to measure the amount of depression (or lack of it) which the newborn exhibits. One minute after birth, the infant is evaluated. If the total score is 10, the infant is in the best possible condition; if the score is 5 or more, the infant usually does not need resuscitation; if the score is under 4, the infant usually needs immediate emergency resuscitation. About 70 per cent of all newborns score 7 or better.

### Resuscitation of the Newborn

At birth the baby must suddenly undergo a great change in his method of obtaining oxygen. He had been supplied via the placental circulation prior to birth, but must now take over for himself. If he does not breathe for a few seconds, or even for a minute, he will still receive oxygen through the placenta, which is still attached to the mother. However, if he does not begin to breathe on his own within 1 to 2 minutes, the indication is that his respiratory center is depressed, and emergency action must be taken. Most neonates breathe through their nose and not through their mouth. When not crying they breathe at a respiratory rate of 35 to 40 breaths per minute.

If the infant needs resuscitation, it must be done immediately, before he takes his first breath, if possible. The nose and mouth must be cleared of secretions, sometimes even before the rest of the body is born, because the first breath can draw secretions into the lungs and cause suffocation. Further evaluation of respiratory status will be done later because the newborn can have difficulty after he goes to the newborn nursery. When respiratory difficulties develop in the delivery room the doctor assists the infant, but the practical nurse may be the person to initiate resuscitation in the newborn nursery.

Resuscitation procedures include exaggerated Trendelenburg position (holding the baby upside-down), with the neck extended, *gentle* suction with a soft rubber catheter after the airway is opened, administration of oxygen, and sometimes administration of specific drugs. Many infants are given antibiotics as a preventive measure if extensive resuscitation has been done.

## IMMEDIATE BASIC NEEDS FOLLOWING BIRTH

### Identification

**Identification and the Chart.** Before he leaves the delivery room, the baby is given an identification mark of some kind—a name band on his ankle or wrist or a necklace of beads which spells his parents' surname; hospitals use different methods. At the time of delivery, the baby's footprints are taken, and a record of them is attached to his chart. This chart contains information which includes the sex of the baby, the hour of birth, the type of delivery, his condition, the care of the eyes, and the Rh status of the mother. The chart is made out before the baby leaves the delivery room.

Identification of the newborn is so vital, it cannot be emphasized enough. The baby should be marked in 2 places, in case one band falls off. Each foot should be footprinted; often the mother's thumb print is also added to the record before the baby leaves the delivery room.

Each time the baby is brought out to the mother for feeding, the nurse should have the mother verify that this is the correct baby, and upon discharge one of the baby's identification bands should be cut off and placed on the chart, along with the mother's signature, to make sure there is no question later.

The nurse must be especially careful in cases in which the baby has a common name. The mother's full name and the date and time of the baby's birth become especially important in such instances.

**How to Make a Good Infant Footprint.** Remove the vernix before it has a chance to dry on the bottoms of the baby's feet. Cleanse the baby's foot gently with solution specified by the hospital. Wash your hands thoroughly and hold the baby's ankle between your thumb and middle finger, placing your index finger behind his toes. Keeping the baby's knees flexed and legs close to his body, gently touch the inked Footprinter to the foot. Place the heel on the chart and "walk" the foot over the chart with a heel-to-toe motion. Remove the excess ink from the baby's foot and dispose of the Footprinter. The same procedure is used for the other foot and for the mother's thumb print.

**The Birth Certificate.** A certificate of the baby's birth must be made out and signed by the doctor who made the delivery. This must be filed with the health department for the area where the baby was born. The health department sends the mother a photostatic copy as proof that the birth has been recorded. A birth certificate is an important document which is required many times throughout one's lifetime—when entering school, obtaining a marriage license or a passport, and supplying proof of Social Security rights. The parents should be encouraged to choose a name for the baby before the birth certificate is filed, rather than resorting to an entry such as "Baby Boy Jones." This may be very confusing later in life. However, the practical nursing *student* should never witness a birth certificate.

## The Cord

A sterile dressing may be applied to the cord stump and kept in place with a binder, although many hospitals no longer use either the cord dressing or the binder. The cord stump usually dries up and separates by the end of the first week.

The nurse must remember that since the cord has been the circulatory route for some time, it is possible for the baby to hemorrhage through the cord. The nurse must watch for bleeding and make sure the clamp or ties are secure at all times. In the event that the child may need to receive a transfusion, the cord is left quite long and is kept moist with sterile saline packs.

## Warmth

Since the baby's temperature-control center is not completely developed, he may need assistance in maintaining his body temperature after birth. Usually, the neonate is placed in an infant warmer for the first few hours after birth. He is wrapped in a warm blanket immediately after delivery and is protected from drafts or chills.

## Protection Against Disease

**Silver Nitrate Prophylaxis.** To prevent infection in case the mother has gonorrhea, a 1 per cent solution of silver nitrate or a penicillin solution is instilled in the baby's eyes immediately after delivery. This is done in all states, since the gonorrheal infection can cause blindness (ophthalmia neonatorum).

The most commonly used medication is silver nitrate solution, which comes in wax, disposable ampules, and tubes. Care must be taken not to get any of the silver nitrate solution on the baby's face, since it will turn the skin black and may cause a burn. The nurse must be sure that at least 2 drops are placed in each eye. After 2 minutes, the eyes may be rinsed with a sterile saline solution to remove any excess silver nitrate.

**Other Precautions.** If the mother has some other disease, the infant may be immunized or given specific treatment. If the mother is a habitual user of drugs, the baby may need an antidote. Often, if the infant is delivered outside the delivery room, he is given antibiotics as a precautionary measure.

## Evaluation of Respiratory Status

For several hours after birth, the nurse will need to monitor the infant's respiratory status, paying extra special attention if the baby is premature.

Respiratory status is considered normal if there are synchronized movements of the upper chest. If there are retractions of the lower chest and of the xiphoid process, dilation of the nostrils, and expiratory grunts the infant is suffering from various degrees of respiratory distress. It is important for the practical nurse to observe for signs of respiratory distress and to report these to the doctor.

In addition to the aforementioned signs of respiratory distress, the nurse can also evaluate the respiratory status of the infant by his color, by his rate of respiration, and by his general activity. If the infant's respiratory rate shows a great increase during the first hour after birth, the infant is in danger and must receive treatment. The mortality rate in these infants is high.

As part of the evaluation the nurse should note on the baby's chart: the rate of respirations, (be sure to note if the child is crying or sleeping while the rate is taken), the type of respiration (amount of retraction, nares dilation, and expiratory grunt), the skin color, pulse and blood pressure, and whether or not the child is receiving oxygen.

If the nurse notices marked respiratory distress, she should hold the child upside-down, take off his shirt, administer oxygen or mouth-to-mouth resuscitation, and notify the physician immediately.

The child who is experiencing respiratory distress is often placed in a newborn intensive care unit, where he will be observed

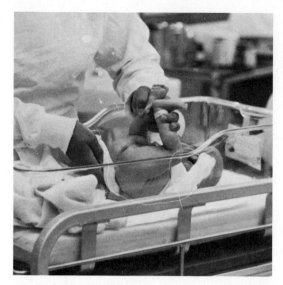

Figure 38-2. While taking the rectal temperature, it is necessary to hold both feet of the infant with one hand, while the thermometer is held with the other hand to avoid accident. Notice that the sleeves of the baby's shirt are pulled down over his hands and fastened to keep him from scratching himself. After urination or a bowel movement, the baby's buttocks must be thoroughly cleansed because the baby's skin is very sensitive and becomes easily excoriated. (Photo courtesy of Alma Johnson)

closely at all times, and where equipment is available for suctioning, administration of oxygen, thoracentesis, or other necessary procedures. This child is kept NPO until adequate respiration is established.

### The Initial Bath

Generally, the baby is cleansed with oil before he is taken from the delivery room. Sometimes, water or soap and water is used. The initial cleansing depends upon the doctor's orders. Some doctors do not want the child cleaned until he is 12 hours old. If there is a very large amount of vernix present and if a bath is contraindicated it would be well to remove some of the vernix before the child is taken to the nursery.

### Other Procedures

**Initial Observation.** Generally, the doctor will place a catheter into the baby's stomach while he is still in the delivery room. This is to make sure there is a patent esophagus and that there is no intestinal obstruction. If more than 25 cc. of fluid are present in the baby's stomach, this is strongly suggestive of intestinal obstruction.

**Weight.** The baby is weighed immediately after birth. This weight is usually recorded on the chart in grams and converted to pounds for the mother's benefit. The transfer paper is placed on the scale to avoid contamination of the scale or the baby.

**Physician's Examination.** Within 24 hours after birth, the baby must be examined thoroughly by the doctor to make sure there are no abnormalities. The practical nurse may be asked to assist with this examination.

## DAILY CARE OF THE NEONATE

### Protection for the Baby

In the nursery, every baby is placed in his own crib, which has a firm mattress and lined sides. The technics used by the nursery personnel are devised to isolate the baby from any direct contact with other babies. In some nurseries, the doctors and the nurses wear gowns and masks.

A hospital nursery can be a hazardous place for a baby if an infection is present. Epidemics of skin infection (impetigo) and staphylococcal infections, as well as a fatal type of diarrhea, have broken out in nurseries.

### Observing the Newborn

The routine daily care of the newborn involves meeting the needs of any infant for food, cleanliness, and comfort, but it also involves close scrutiny and observation for any symptoms of difficulties or abnormalities. While in the uterus, the mother's physiology supplied the baby's wants, but now he must function as an individual being. The nurse must check on his abilities to do so.

### Body Care

**Body Temperature.** The baby's rectal temperature is normally between 98° to 99° F. It tends to be slightly subnormal. However, the part of the neonate's nervous system which acts as a temperature control is still immature, so his temperature may be elevated if he is too warm or if he does not get enough liquids. The baby's body temperature must often be supported by external means for the first few days of life.

**Eyes, Nose, and Ears.** No special care is required for the baby's eyes, nose, or ears; there is no need to insert probes or applicators into these areas. However, any redness, swelling, or discharge should be reported and recorded on the chart, and the physician will prescribe the necessary treatment. There may be some reaction in the eyes from the medication used for prophylaxis against gonorrheal infection.

**Skin.** The skin of the newborn baby, no matter what its racial stock, is usually reddish and is often wrinkled, although it should become smooth and of a normal color within 2 weeks. It is very sensitive and may break out in a rash if irritated. To avoid irritation, the baby's buttocks should be thoroughly cleaned following a bowel movement (Fig. 38-2). A rash or irritated area should be reported. Many neonates have some jaundice for a few days, but this also usually disappears by the second week.

**Stools.** The very first stool, which may not be seen, is a grey or yellow, puttylike mass of matter, called the *meconium plug*. During the first days of the baby's life, his stools are dark green and tarry-looking. This is *meconium,* a waste product which is formed in the baby's intestines in the latter months of pregnancy. Then, the stool changes to a normal lighter color. The stools of breast-fed babies are bright yellow, smooth, and pasty looking; a baby fed a formula of cow's milk has a darker and more formed stool. The stools smell like sour milk. Mucus, blood, or curds in the stool as well as hard stools and any evidence of constipation or diarrhea are signs of disturbance and should be reported at once. It is very important to note the baby's first stool. If a stool does not occur within the first few hours of life, this may be a sign of an imperforate anus, a condition which must be surgically corrected at once.

**Urination.** Analysis of the amniotic fluid shows that the fetus has kidney function and voids within the uterus. He often voids immediately after birth, but care should be taken to be certain that he voids within 24 hours after delivery. At first the urine is clear; then it becomes concentrated. After the first 2 or 3 days, the infant voids from 12 to 18 times daily.

**Sleep.** Except for the time he is being fed, the newborn baby sleeps almost all the time, but not heavily. He will wake and cry when he is hungry or uncomfortable. Most authorities recommend that the baby sleep on his side, with the sides being changed frequently. However, some advise not to place him on his stomach until he can raise his head. Sleeping on the back is discouraged for two reasons: there is the possibility of his choking from regurgitation, and the soft skull bones may become flattened from the constant pressure exerted at one point.

**Taking Food.** The normal newborn baby knows instinctively how to suck and swallow. (These are reflexes present at birth.) If he takes too much food or takes it too fast, he may regurgitate it (this is simply an overflow and should not be thought of as vomiting). Food may stick in his esophagus and cause hiccups, which sips of water will usually stop. A healthy baby is eager for his food; if he refuses to nurse or to take his bottle, spits up or vomits, or has an unusual amount of discomfort from gas, the doctor should be notified. Perhaps a change in formula will relieve these digestive woes.

**Vitamin Supplements.** Many doctors will put every newborn on a vitamin supplement, especially the breast-fed baby, who might not be receiving the benefits of the vitamins and iron present in most prepared formulas. If these substances are not available in the food, they must be supplemented.

**Responses.** The newborn baby cries and tightens his muscles in response to sudden loud sounds, changes in position, the feel of something cold touching his skin, or interference with his movements. He relaxes if he is held and rocked while his skin is patted lightly.

**Crying.** A newborn baby cries a lot, especially if he is hungry or if his diapers are wet. Crying is the only way a baby can ask for help. It has been noticed that the baby who gets more care cries less.

Hunger cries are healthy, demanding cries. The baby may also put his fingers into his mouth, as an additional sign that he is hungry.

After he is fed, he is quiet unless he has swallowed air from his bottle and needs to "bubble," or he may have colic.

**Bathing the Baby.** The hospital routine for giving baths to babies varies. Some institutions order oil rubs, some use medicated lotions, and others use soap and water.

If the baby is to receive an oil or lather bath instead of a tub bath certain procedures should be followed:

The oil, lotion, or soap suds should be used to cleanse the baby, so be careful not to get the solution in the baby's eyes or on the unhealed navel area.

Wash your hands thoroughly before beginning the procedure.

Cleanse the area around the baby's eyes with clear water first, using cotton balls. If you are using soap, wet your hands and the baby's skin and then make a lather and apply it to the baby's body.

Be sure to use the corner of a washcloth or a cotton tipped swab and cleanse the outer ears. You may also use a swab to clean the outer nostrils. Use a new swab for each new part of the body.

Don't forget to cleanse the baby's head, even though he has no hair.

Cleanse the baby's genital area last, checking carefully for signs of rash or irritation. Cleanse all folds of the circumcision area.

Be sure to support the baby during the procedure so he does not become frightened. Remember that you can never leave the baby alone, so be sure to have all your equipment ready before you begin.

Today mothers leave the hospital so soon after the baby is born that you may not have an opportunity to give him a tub bath in the hospital. However, many hospitals provide demonstration baths for the new mothers. The important guide lines which apply to any bath procedure apply also to the baby bath:

Have all the equipment ready and conveniently placed before you start.

Be sure that the room is warm enough and that the baby is protected from drafts.

Check the temperature of the water carefully. It should be just warm.

Support the baby's head and body with a firm grip when you put him in the tub.

Use a soft wash cloth and towel; rinse all the soap off; dry the creases well.

Observe his body carefully for signs of skin irritation or abnormalities.

If his clothes do not open down the front or the back, put them on over his feet. A baby resists even a temporary interference with his breathing or movements.

Clean and care for the equipment and replace used supplies.

**Circumcision.** In male babies, the foreskin (prepuce) covers the glans penis or extends beyond it (see Chapter 19). The opening may be very small, a condition known as *phimosis*. A secretion called *smegma* collects beneath the foreskin, and drops of urine also may remain to cause irritation. Because of the problem it presents to cleanliness, most male infants today are circumcised—that is, part or all of the foreskin is removed. If circumcision is not performed, the foreskin must be stretched and retracted over the glans penis for cleaning, at least once every day. This may be difficult and must be done with great care and gentleness. The foreskin must be replaced immediately, because if it is tight it causes edema and pain.

If the baby is circumcised, he must be kept clean and watched closely for bleeding. A sterile petrolatum dressing is applied after each voiding for 24 to 48 hours to keep the diapers from sticking. Circumcision is usually done shortly before the infant leaves the hospital; therefore, the mother should be instructed in the care required.

## INFANT FEEDING

### Breast-Feeding

The most inexpensive, easiest, and simplest way to feed a baby is by nursing at the breast. There are no formulas to make or bottles to sterilize; the mother's milk is usually safe from harmful organisms and is always ready. Some authorities say that there are substances in the mother's milk which protect the baby from disease. Breast-feeding is also a satisfying emotional experience for both the mother and the baby.

If the mother does not want to nurse her baby, her feelings should be respected. Many mothers have definite reasons for not wanting to breast-feed their baby, and research has provided satisfactory formulas for replacing breast milk. Breast-feeding is not desirable when the mother has a chronic disease or mastitis, if the nipples are inverted, or if the baby has certain abnormalities. Exercises may be done to relieve inverted nipples so that nursing is often possible.

**Putting the Baby to Breast.** If the mother is interested in nursing the baby, she should be encouraged and assisted. It is important to put the baby to breast regularly to stimulate milk secretion, even before the milk appears on the third or the fourth day. A thin watery secretion called colostrum is present in the breasts before the milk is produced. Stay with the mother the first time the baby goes to breast to show her what to do. She puts the whole nipple in the baby's mouth, and while he is sucking, she holds the breast tissue away from his nose so that he is able to breathe. When she wants to withdraw the nipple, she presses on the baby's cheeks, or pushes back on his chin to break the suction.

Anything that makes the mother nervous or puts a strain on her body will interfere with her pleasure in nursing the baby; if the baby is uncomfortable, he may refuse to nurse as long as he should. The mother is often most comfortable when sitting up, with her back and arm supported. If she is out of bed, an armchair is best, with a pillow under her arm. Give her a footstool if she needs it; be sure that she is warm enough and protected from drafts. Wash both her hands and yours before you put the baby to breast. Some authorities say it is not necessary to cleanse the nipples before or after feedings, but others recommend it.

**The Diet for the Nursing Mother.** The nursing mother needs food not only for herself but also for the milk which she is producing. She needs extra protein, vitamins, calcium, iron, and fluids. Since milk is an excellent source of many nutrients the nursing mother should drink plenty of it. If some foods upset the baby, the mother can avoid these while she is nursing.

**Care of the Breasts.** The baby should not be allowed to suck so long that the breasts become sore and cracked. Usually, about 5 to 10 minutes of nursing at a time, at first, will help to toughen the breasts and avoid irritation. The mother should wear a nonwaterproof cotton bra. Waterproof pads keep moisture in and can cause irritation. (All new mothers should wear a bra for a short time after delivery, whether they are nursing or not. The bra or breast binder will assist the

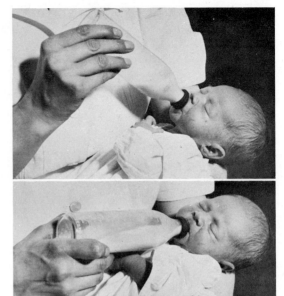

Figure 38-3. (*Top*) The right way to hold a bottle. The baby's head should be turned slightly to one side, and the bottle held so that the baby will grasp the nipple squarely. To prevent the baby from swallowing air, the neck of the bottle should be filled with milk at all times. (*Bottom*) The wrong way to hold a bottle. If the bottle is held flat, air enters the nipple, and the baby may suffer as a result of swallowing air. (Fitzpatrick, E., and Eastman, N. J.: Zabriskie's Obstetrics for Nurses, ed. 10. Philadelphia, Lippincott, 1960)

breasts to return more comfortably to their nonpregnant state.)

After the nipples have become toughened, it is permissible to wear a waterproof pad in the bra to avoid soiling the mother's clothing.

## Bottle Feeding

The basis of a formula is milk. Generally, one third of evaporated milk, two thirds of water, and 1 ounce of carbohydrate for every 20 ounces of the mixture is satisfactory. The baby takes this formula until he is 3 or 4 months old, when he can take whole milk. Most babies increase the amount they take from 12 to 15 ounces the first week to 20 ounces by the end of the second week. The amount is increased rapidly thereafter.

The same type of special care that is observed when a baby is breast-fed is also observed when a baby is bottle-fed. The

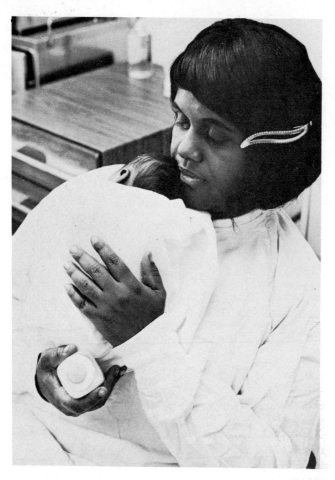

Figure 38-4. "Bubbling" the baby. While in the hospital, the mother should be taught to "bubble" her baby. Holding the baby upright against the shoulder during and immediately after nursing, gently pat his back to bring up air. Cuddly babies are sometimes difficult to put in this position. (From Blake, F. G., Wright, F. H., and Waechler, E. H.: Nursing Care of Children, ed. 8. Philadelphia, Lippincott, 1970)

mother's hands are cleansed before she is handed the baby. The rate of flow from the bottle's nipple should be checked, to make certain that it flows at a constant drip. Nipples are made with either a "cross" cut in them or with holes. If the openings are not the correct size, the holes can be enlarged by putting a red-hot needle through them.

While the baby is eating, the bottle should be tilted so that milk is in the neck of the bottle at all times to keep the baby from swallowing air. The baby should be bubbled (burped) at intervals during the feeding (Figs. 38-3 and 38-4).

The physician may prefer that the baby have a formula other than the one prepared from evaporated milk. There are many baby milk products available, each one having certain advantages for particular situations. There are even nonmilk formulas available for infants who are allergic to milk. The doctor orders these according to the infant's need. Most babies are on schedules of approximately 4 hour intervals. Smaller babies may eat every 3 hours. After the third week, the baby skips one of his evening or night feedings, usually the one at 2:00 A.M.

**Preparing the Formula.** Because bacteria thrive in milk, great care is exercised in the preparation of the infant's formula. There are 2 generally accepted methods of preparing formulas. In the first method, the bottles, the nipples, and the utensils used in the preparation of the formula are sterilized. The contents of the formula are mixed in sterile containers and poured into the bottles. In the second method, called *terminal sterilization,* the contents are mixed in clean utensils, poured into clean bottles, and placed in a large pan or sterilizer to boil for 25 minutes.

Thus the milk, the bottles, and the nipples are all sterilized at the same time.

**Premixed Formulas.** Many infant formulas come ready to use. They may be heated, the disposable nipple attached, and the baby fed. Most hospitals use these formulas for the baby who must be supplemented or who is to be entirely bottle-fed. The mother can take some of this formula home with her or can purchase it later, avoiding the bother of mixing and sterilizing the formula. Since the entire unit is disposable, this type of formula is more expensive than conventional formula, but, of course, it is much more convenient.

**Disposable Bottles.** Many nursers come equipped with plastic bags inside them which are thrown away after the feeding, thereby eliminating the need to sterilize bottles before each feeding. However, the mother must be sure that the plastic bag is securely fastened into the holder and that the baby cannot pull the end of the bag through the side of the holder.

**The Bottle-Fed Baby.** It is very important to remember that feeding does not just provide food for the baby; it also gives him a sense of security and of being loved. Therefore, always hold the baby and cuddle him while he is being fed. Hold him exactly the same as the breast-fed baby, and encourage the mother to do the same.

## Demand Feeding

Demand feeding refers to the widespread practice of permitting the infant to set his own schedule to meet his needs, rather than feeding him by the clock. Because babies cry for reasons other than food, the reason for his crying must first be ascertained. The majority of babies soon set a fairly regular schedule for themselves, with which they are seemingly happy and content. As one pediatrician stated, "Adults can go to the refrigerator or the cookie jar when they want a snack; babies can't." Babies can be on a demand schedule whether they are breast-fed or bottle-fed. Although in most hospitals it is not possible to feed all babies on a demand schedule, in hospitals where rooming-in is allowed, demand feeding is the rule.

## Supplementary Foods

When the baby is 2 or 3 weeks old he is given vitamin concentrates. Babies begin to take solid food, starting with cereal, much earlier than they used to, sometimes soon after they go home from the hospital. Some authorities believe that the time to begin such feeding is when the baby shows that he is ready for it; that is, if he will open his mouth when the spoon touches it, will depress his tongue, and will swallow. Many doctors say that he may have any of the mushy foods when he can manage them.

## PKU Testing

Before the baby leaves the hospital, he is tested for the presence of ketones in his urine (see Chapter 40). The practical nurse should know how to perform this procedure and should realize that this procedure should be repeated when the baby is brought to the doctor for his first check-up, because the test is not always valid during the first few days of life.

If the test is positive, the child must be placed on a special diet to prevent severe mental retardation.

# DISORDERS OF THE NEWBORN BABY

The first months of a baby's life are the most precarious. Before he is born he exists without making any efforts himself; he is warm and protected. As soon as he is born he has to take on the work of breathing, eating, digesting, eliminating, and stabilizing his body temperature. If trouble develops with any of these functions the baby will have a difficult time surviving. More than half of the babies who die during their first year, die in the first month. Some of these disturbances appear as soon as he is born, when his body begins to function. It is easy to see why a newborn baby needs the best of care.

## Respiratory Disorders

**Cyanosis.** The first thing that a normal baby does when he is born is to cry, which establishes breathing. If he does not breathe properly, he turns blue (cyanotic). Such respiratory difficulty may be due to a prolapsed cord (a condition in which the cord becomes compressed between the baby's head and the mother's pelvis), a congenital heart defect, faulty respiratory apparatus, a birth injury to the brain, medications, or even the anesthetic which the mother has been given.

Since the newborn infant *must* have oxygen, treatment is initiated promptly for babies who do not breathe as soon as they are born. First, it must be determined whether the air passages are clear of obstruction, such as amniotic fluid and mucus. Soft catheters and mechanical suction machines are used to remove this material. The baby's head is lowered to facilitate postural drainage. His back is rubbed gently or his buttocks patted softly to stimulate him. The baby is *not* slapped or pinched, since this causes too great a shock to the system.

If the infant fails to respond, some form of artificial respiration is instituted. In almost every delivery room today, there are modern mechanical infant resuscitators which are both convenient and effective and supply a controlled administration of oxygen at an optimum pressure. If these are not available, other resuscitation methods are used. A gentle squeezing of the chest, followed by a release, may be tried. Another method is to alternate compressing and extending the infant's body by stretching his legs and then bending them back and curving his body. Probably the oldest method used is mouth-to-mouth breathing.

**Atelectasis.** One of the causes for cyanosis in the newborn is atelectasis. Before birth the lungs are not used because the mother supplies the fetus with oxygen. When the baby takes his first breath, expansion of the lungs begins. When atelectasis is present, large areas of the lung tissue remain unexpanded, reducing the infant's oxygen supply. The prognosis depends on the extent of the atelectasis.

**Hyaline Membrane Disease.** Hyaline membrane disease is a condition in which the alveoli of the lungs become filled with a sticky protein substance which prevents aeration. The cause is not known. It is seen most often in premature infants and those born by cesarean section. The primary symptom is respiratory distress. The treatment is the administration of oxygen in an atmosphere of high humidity. If the condition does not tend to reverse itself within a short time, it is usually fatal. Other treatments involve the administration of epsom salts enemas or the steady administration of oxygen through a tube into the lungs which causes the lungs to expand and prevents the formation of the tough protein substance which keeps the lungs from expanding.

**Amniotic Aspiration.** If the first breath is taken while the baby is still within the bag of waters or while he has his mouth and nose full of fluid, he may aspirate fluid into his lungs. This is why it is so vital to clear the air passages immediately after birth.

**Bronchopneumonia.** Since the newborn is so susceptible, he may get various infections, one of the most common of which is bronchopneumonia. This is especially dangerous in the very young infant, who may choke since he is not old enough or strong enough to cough up the secretions. He is assisted to breathe by postural drainage, oxygen, and humidity. He also receives antibiotics and may be suctioned. In any type of lung infection, the older the child is, the better his prognosis.

**Choanal Atresia.** Sometimes, the nostrils are closed at the entrance to the throat so that air cannot pass through. This is one of the reasons why a catheter is passed through the nose to the stomach in the delivery room. The neonate does not breathe well through his mouth, so choanal atresia must be surgically corrected in order that he may breathe.

## Birth Injuries

Various injuries can occur to the infant during the birth process. While some of these are serious, most can be corrected.

**Fractures.** Various fractures can occur, but are rarely complicated and usually heal without difficulty.

**Brachial Plexus Palsy.** Also known as Erb-Duchenne paralysis, this condition occurs as a result of pressure on the fifth and sixth cranial nerves. It occurs when the shoulder is pulled away from the head during delivery. It may cause numbness and paralysis of the arm on the affected side. If the damage is caused by swelling and edema, it will correct itself; if it is caused by torn nerve tissues, permanent paralysis may result. Treatment consists of positioning and physical therapy treatments.

**Facial Paralysis.** This occurs when the facial nerve is damaged, usually as a result of a forceps delivery. If the nerve tissue is damaged, the paralysis may be permanent. Usually the difficulty is only on one side of the face and makes the eyelid and the mouth droop on that side. The infant's sucking mechanism may be impaired and he may need special feeding. He may also need saline irrigation or patching of the eye on the affected side, since he cannot close that eye. Plastic surgery is sometimes effective in improving cosmetic appearance. Fortunately, most cases of facial and brachial paralysis are temporary and will improve as the edema resolves.

**Other Forceps Damage.** The child who is delivered with forceps may have marks or bruises on his head, which almost always disappear and leave no scars or aftereffects.

**Molding.** This has already been mentioned as the abnormal shaping of the head during the birth process. It almost always resolves itself, with the head returning to normal within a few days. Sometimes, the infant is positioned to assist the head to return to its normal shape.

**Caput Succedaneum.** This is an accumulation of fluid within the scalp of the infant, which causes it to be puffy and edematous. It is caused by pressure to the head during delivery and disappears within a few days.

**Cephalohematoma.** This is an accumulation of blood between the bones of the skull and the periosteum (the membrane which covers the skull). It is not drained, because of the danger of infection. This condition looks very unappealing and may greatly upset the parents. They should be reassured that the fluids will eventually be absorbed.

**Intracranial Hemorrhage.** This disorder is the most common birth injury and is also the most dangerous. It may be caused by a very difficult delivery, by precipitate labor and delivery, or by prolonged delivery. The symptoms are convulsions, respirator distress, cyanosis, a shrill cry, and muscle weakness. The prognosis varies with the extent of the injury and with the treatment, which depends upon the area of the brain that is affected. The treatments are much the same as for hemorrhage in the brain of the adult patient (see Chapter 46), with the exception that the infant's brain is much smaller and more delicate than is that of the adult. In addition, the infant cannot assist with the diagnosis or with the treatment and is, thus, more difficult to treat.

The infant with a brain hemorrhage is placed in an incubator with the head slightly elevated. He is given oxygen for the cyanosis, and Vitamin K to assist in blood clotting. He may be kept in a dehydrated state to reduce intracranial pressure. He is given anticonvulsive medications, antibiotics, and sedatives. He is also fed by gavage tube because he cannot suck and because sucking would cause too much strain. Some of the complications which may occur as a result of cerebral hemorrhage are cerebral palsy, hydrocephaly, and mental retardation.

**Other Brain Damage.** Later in life, the child may exhibit behavior or learning disorders which seem to have been caused by an injury in utero or during delivery. Since these disorders are usually not detected when the child is an infant, no treatment can be carried out to prevent the later difficulties.

## Congenital Deformities

Congenital deformities are abnormalities already existing at birth and are due to the defective development of some part of the fetus. Some of the common congenital deformities are defects of the heart, cleft palate and harelip, spina bifida and neurosensory and musculoskeletal defects. These are discussed in Chapters 40 and 42.

## Gastrointestinal Disorders

**Esophageal Atresia.** In this condition, the upper end of the esophagus ends in a blind pouch so that the child cannot obtain food. Immediate surgery must be performed to correct this condition. This is another reason for passing a catheter into the baby's stomach in the delivery room. If the catheter does not pass through or if it passes into the lungs instead of into the stomach, there is difficulty.

**Tracheo-esophageal Fistula.** The atresia of the esophagus may be combined with a fistula in the trachea, which is a much more dangerous condition. Since food or mucus is then channelled directly into the lungs, this condition must be corrected immediately or the child will aspirate and suffocate. Surgery is performed immediately, with no feedings given prior to surgery. After surgery, routine postoperative care includes the administration of oxygen, intravenous fluids, or food by gastrostomy tube. A tracheostomy is often done. The child who survives the surgical procedure for a few days usually recovers without difficulty and can eat normally later in life.

**Imperforate Anus.** In an imperforate anus the rectum ends in a blind pouch causing an obstruction to the normal passage of feces. Such a condition must be corrected immediately to avoid serious complications. This is one reason for being very observant to make sure that the newborn is passing meconium after birth.

**Vomiting, Diarrhea, and Dehydration.** Vomiting can be a symptom of a congenital defect, such as esophageal atresia, or of a birth injury, such as intracranial hemorrhage. It may also be caused by an infectious process. Diarrhea most often is caused by bacteria, although it may also be caused by an incompatible formula or an allergy. Any evidence of severe diarrhea requires immediate isolation of the baby to prevent spread to other babies. The greatest concern in vomiting or diarrhea of the newborn is that of dehydration.

Dehydration occurs very fast in the small infant. He has so little excess fluid that he becomes dehydrated very fast. This can quickly become a fatal situation unless active treatment is begun immediately. He will be given intravenous fluids and probably extra oxygen and humidity. He will most likely be in the newborn intensive care unit, if there is one available.

## Coincidental Diseases of Pregnancy Which May Affect the Baby

Unfortunately, pregnancy does not provide immunity to disease. Sometimes the diseases which are present in the mother during pregnancy have an adverse effect on the fetus.

**Syphilis.** One of the common diseases which can affect the baby's physical development is syphilis. In most states, the law requires that each pregnant woman have a test for syphilis during her pregnancy. If the blood test proves to be positive, prompt treatment with penicillin early in pregnancy will prevent harmful effects on the baby. A mother with untreated syphilis can transmit the disease to her baby, since syphilis organisms are carried in the blood stream. The infant may be stillborn or may be deformed.

**Gonorrhea.** Gonorrhea is an infection which does not usually affect the pregnancy itself. However, if the organism causing gonorrhea gets into the eyes of the infant during delivery, it may cause blindness (ophthalmia neonatorum). It is for this reason that most states require the installation of silver nitrate or penicillin in the eyes of the newborn as a prophylactic measure.

**Rubella (German Measles).** Studies have shown that the virus of German measles (rubella, 3-day measles) may be very dangerous in pregnancy. Although the virus has no permanent ill-effects on the mother, it causes such defects in the infant as cataract, deafness, congenital heart defects and disease, and mental retardation. Statistics on the percentage of such defects are so variable that it is unwise to quote them, but the definite relationship between the defects and the disease is established. The best way to prevent this problem is by immunization of children, so that their mothers will not be exposed to the disease. If the mother is exposed, gamma globulin may be given to her.

**Diabetes Mellitus.** Because of the extreme alterations in metabolism during pregnancy, diabetes mellitus is a disease difficult to control. The infant death rate is higher for babies of diabetic mothers. However, modern prenatal care has increased the chance of infant survival to 90 per cent. The babies are often unusually large and may have respiratory difficulties as well as other problems. The mother requires close prenatal supervision. (See Chapters 36 and 52.)

**Thrush.** Thrush is a yeast infection which forms milklike spots in the mouth. The infected infant is isolated and treated with antibiotics, or gentian violet solution is applied to the affected area.

**Impetigo Contagiosa.** Impetigo contagiosa is an infection of the skin which is usually caused by the staphylococcus or the streptococcus. This condition is discussed in Chapter 44.

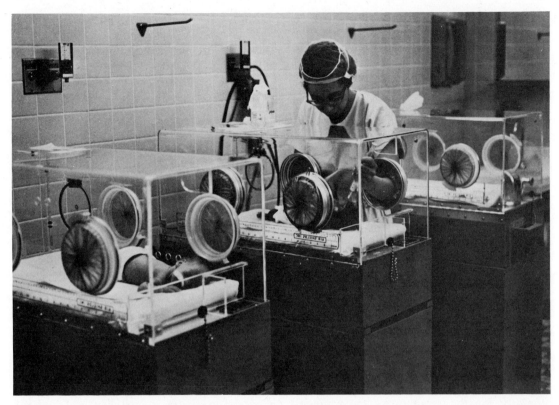

Figure 38-5. A premature intensive care unit allows several premature babies to receive expert care. The nurse is feeding the baby by means of the gavage tube. The incubator can be placed in Trendelenburg position; it has an opening through which equipment may be passed or through which humidity may be introduced. The measurements on the side of the plastic top allow the nurse to measure the baby's length without removing him from the incubator. (Ross Laboratories, Inc.)

**Staphylococcal Infections.** With the development of antibiotic-resistant strains of staph organisms, the infection rate has risen. It is dangerous to have an outbreak of staph in the newborn nursery, because it is so difficult to control. Therefore, strict nursery technic must be followed.

**Umbilical Cord Infections.** Since the umbilical cord leads directly to the blood stream of the infant, it is important to use sterile technic in cutting and tying off the cord. It should be cleansed carefully, until it falls off, to prevent infection.

## THE PREMATURE BABY

The premature baby today has more than a fighting chance to live. This happy state of affairs is due partly to the production of advanced mechanical devices, but more than anything else it has come to pass through improved medical and nursing care. How-ever, prematurity is still responsible for the deaths of about 50 per cent of the babies who die in their first month. Any baby weighing less than 5½ pounds (2500 grams) is considered to be premature, regardless of its time of gestation. Head and chest size are also used to define prematurity. Of course, the more premature the baby is, the fewer chances he has to live. There is much difference in a baby weighing 5½ lbs. and one weighing 2 lbs. The baby who weighs less than 1000 grams (2¼ pounds) is classified as *immature.*

The smaller he is, the frailer the premature infant looks. He is thin and has sharp features and weak muscles; his breathing is irregular and weak; and his temperature is frequently subnormal. Because he has accumulated so little fat, his blood vessels shine through his almost transparent skin.

Any baby who does not do well at birth is often treated as a premature baby, regardless of his weight.

Reasons for premature delivery include: multiple births, trauma to the mother, toxemia, diabetes, incompetent cervix, and infectious diseases such as venereal disease or tuberculosis.

## Care of the Baby

The premature baby must be handled as little as possible. Usually, he is not bathed immediately. Because he cannot regulate his own body temperature, he must be kept warm, his bed is warmed, and his temperature is taken often. Oxygen is supplied if necessary.

Because prematures are susceptible to infections, their contacts are limited as much as possible. Usually, only certain personnel are assigned to work in the premature nursery.

**Incubator Care.** If the baby weighs 3 pounds or less and has breathing difficulties or a very unstable temperature, he is placed in an incubator which is designed to duplicate the environment within the uterus as much as possible. The incubator is transparent so that the baby can be seen at all times. It maintains an even temperature and humidity for the premature's environment. Oxygen is given to relieve respiratory difficulties, but it is given in a concentration which is as low as possible. It was discovered that the use of concentrated oxygen was causing blindness in prematures (*retrolental fibroplasia*). Babies in incubators are covered by the incubator hoods; the nurses care for them through openings in the sides (Fig. 38-5).

**Feeding.** The feeding of prematures varies. In some instances, where small babies are concerned, no feeding is given for 36 hours, since it is believed that digestion adds to the burden of a premature's body functions. In other situations, a small amount of glucose solution is given, just as it is to the larger infant. After approximately 3 days, the baby is given milk. In parts of the country where breast-milk banks are available, breast milk seems to be the feeding of choice. In other areas, formulas are prescribed, but always in small amounts so as not to distend the small stomach or to add to respiratory distress. If the baby is not strong enough to suck, he is fed by gavage, whereby a tube is inserted into the stomach through the nose or the mouth.

**Elimination.** Because the premature baby's kidneys are not fully developed, he may have difficulty in eliminating wastes. Therefore, at times, the baby is catheterized.

**Protection Against Disease and Injury.** Since the premature is not fully developed, his resistance to disease or injuries is less than that of the full-term infant. He is kept isolated and is attended by nursery personnel who are trained to follow special aseptic technic. He may also be given antibodies or antibiotics as a preventive measure. He often has a bleeding tendency or a tendency to fracture bones and must be protected from any rough handling or injury. Generally, the premature is not dressed, so that the nurse can observe his breathing. The infant should be turned frequently.

**Observation.** It is very important to observe the premature baby very carefully and note any pertinent facts which may indicate difficulty, such as his color (cyanosis, jaundice), his respirations (retractions, rate, expiratory grunt, nares dilation), his pulse (rate, strength, regularity), the amount, frequency, and description of his stools and voidings, his general appearance and activity level, and any abnormal symptoms which he exhibits.

## Complications of Prematurity

The most common complications of the premature infant are retrolental fibroplasia and hyaline membrane disease, which have already been discussed.

Prevention is vital in retrolental fibroplasia. The oxygen content of the incubator must be checked frequently, because continuous exposure to high concentration of oxygen causes this eye defect. It is safe to give high concentrations of oxygen to the cyanotic infant, but the amount must be reduced when the cyanosis is relieved. A concentration of no more than 21 per cent above atmospheric oxygen is considered relatively safe. The nurse must continuously analyze the oxygen content of the incubator and the condition of the child and adjust the oxygen flow accordingly. Accurate charting of these factors is essential. The practical nurse would probably receive special inservice education before being asked to work in the premature intensive care unit.

## THE POSTMATURE INFANT

The baby who remains in the uterus beyond 42 weeks gestation is known as the postmature infant. Such an infant is not, as you might think, in better condition than the full-term infant. He often has respiratory problems or nutritional problems, because the placenta does not seem to be able to provide for the baby after the normal time of gestation.

The characteristics of this child are long fingernails and hair, lack of vernix caseosa, and loss of weight. He may have swallowed meconium or may have aspirated into his lungs. The postmature infant is generally treated the same as a premature baby.

If the mother is positive about her expected date of confinement (EDC), that is, the day she should deliver, the doctor may wish to induce labor about 2 weeks after that time. He will, of course, determine if the baby is large enough and will assess the general status of the baby before inducing labor. A cesarean section may be necessary to save the life of the baby, if the induction attempt is not successful.

## EMERGENCY CHILDBIRTH

Sometimes, the baby does not wait until the mother enters the hospital to be delivered. In this case, the nurse may be asked to assist at emergency childbirth, as may policemen and other rescue personnel, who are trained in this procedure. If the mother has had previous precipitous deliveries, she should carry an emergency kit with her in case of sudden delivery.

The mother's emergency kit should contain any information about the mother concerning medical problems such as diabetes or Rh negative blood incompatibilities. The regular emergency kit also contains receiving blankets, diapers, sanitary napkins, adhesive tape for identification, pencil, surgical soap, and plastic sheeting. It also may contain a sterile kit containing cotton balls, sterile gauze, sterile scissors, and cotton ties. These items are used only if absolutely necessary to tie off the umbilical cord.

An important fact to remember is that usually there are few complications in a precipitous delivery. If complications exist, you will usually have time to get a doctor or to get the mother to the hospital. However, you must follow the best aseptic technic possible. The most important thing to remember is to initiate respiration in the newborn (be sure the bag of waters is ruptured *before* the baby takes his first breath) and to be sure that the baby is kept warm. It is not necessary to tie off the cord unless you are not going to receive the services of the doctor. If you are on the way to the hospital or a doctor is on his way, the baby and placenta should be kept together. You may wish to tie off the cord, without cutting it. Cutting the cord predisposes the baby to great chances of infection and is *not necessary*. It is important to obtain medical assistance as quickly as possible, especially in the event of complications.

*Do not ever* attempt to prevent delivery. This can cause great damage to the mother and to the baby. Keep calm and deliver the baby as safely as possible. Putting the baby to breast immediately helps the uterus to contract and prevents maternal hemorrhage.

# Unit 9:

# Assisting the Child Who is Ill

39. *Fundamental Aspects of Pediatric Nursing*
40. *The Infant, the Toddler, and the Preschool Child*
41. *The School-Age Child and the Adolescent*
42. *The Handicapped Child*

**39**

# Fundamental Aspects of
# Pediatric Nursing

---

## BEHAVIORAL OBJECTIVES

*The student successfully attaining the goals of this chapter will be able to:*

- *discuss the importance of family-centered care and the role of the parents when a child is hospitalized.*
- *state the 3 phases of adjustment to hospitalization which most children go through.*
- *list at least 7 safety measures for pediatric patients and observe these measures in the clinical setting.*
- *assist with the admission of a child to the hospital, including the proper charting of all observations.*
- *carefully and gently restrain a child for necessary examination or treatment.*
- *correctly don gown before caring for child.*
- *bathe a child.*
- *give or assist with a sponge bath to reduce body temperature.*
- *give or assist with a pediatric enema.*
- *discuss pre- and postoperative care of the child.*
- *list 3 methods of administering parenteral fluids to a child.*
- *state 2 rules for determining the approximate pediatric dosage of a drug and indicate what other factors the physician may take into account in prescribing the correct dosage.*
- *demonstrate understanding of the importance of play to the child by engaging him in diversional activities.*
- *discuss the special needs of the long-term pediatric patient and the dying child, including the needs of the parents.*

---

In this chapter, we will consider the basic concepts related to the care of the child in the hospital. This aspect of nursing care is referred to as *pediatric nursing*, while the medical specialist in this field is called a *pediatrician*.

## WHEN THE CHILD GOES TO THE HOSPITAL

For many children, hospitalization presents a traumatic and disturbing experience. If it is difficult for some small children to be left with a sitter in their home, how much more terrifying it is to be left alone in a completely different environment with total strangers, and in many instances limited to one room or even confined to a bed. Often the child does not understand what is happening or why he is being taken away from his parents. If he realizes that something is wrong with his body, it may only compound his fears by threatening his body image which is so important to his sense of well being.

Even before the child is 1 year old, he becomes frightened of strangers and aware when his mother is absent. From this age through 4 and 5 years of age, he exhibits severe anxiety if he is separated from his home and family. Six- and 7-year-olds continue to show this same fear when they are ill. As a general rule, older children are able to understand the need for hospitalization and the separation from the family circle, but even teen-agers are visibly upset if no family arrives for visiting hours.

## Family-Centered Care

In the past few decades, *patient-centered* pediatric care has evolved from *disease-centered* care, and a further need has been recognized for *family-centered* patient care. Many hospitals are making great efforts to meet the emotional need of the child to remain secure as a part of his family unit.

Many articles have been written, as well as various workshops and conferences held, to help promote family-centered pediatric nursing. In the larger pediatric centers, the value of parent-child rooms and unrestricted visiting is widely accepted. However, in other areas, there is a resistance to these changes as well as to other innovations; there are those who feel that the child's family "interferes with his nursing care."

The American Academy of Pediatrics has published a booklet: *The Care of Children in Hospitals,* which encourages mothers to stay and care for their children. It states that: "In hospitals where visiting hours have been replaced by freedom to visit at any hour, parents and children are relieved of much anxiety." It also states that, "In the case of the very ill child or one for whom the separation is especially difficult, arrangements should

be made for the mother to stay in the hospital."*

## Phases of Adjustment

Robertson†, in *Young Children in Hospitals,* has pointed out that most children, particularly those up to ages of 3 or 4 years, go through 3 phases of adjustment when hospitalized: "(1) protest, (2) despair, and (3) denial," with each phase extending into the next.

The first phase is the *protest* phase in which the child's needs for his mother is conscious and sorrowful. He cries constantly and rejects all hospital staff because he is so distressed and so afraid—he wants only his mother.

In the second stage, *despair,* the child becomes very inactive and sad. His usual comfort measures, such as thumb-sucking and clutching his blanket, come into prominence. He still watches constantly for his mother, but he is quiet and withdrawn.

The third phase, *denial,* says Robertson, is often accepted by the hospital personnel as a sign that the child has adjusted to them, whereas the child is really protecting himself from anxiety by rejecting his mother. In truth, his needs for her are more intense than ever.

The impact of this anxiety carries over into the period following hospitalization. Children who have experienced separation from their parents show regression in their behavior when they return home. They do not want their mother out of their sight for a second. How long it takes the child to rid himself of this anxiety and re-establish trust depends on such factors as the length of the hospital stay and the understanding of the parents.

## Preparing the Child for Hospitalization

One way to overcome a child's fear of the hospital is to prepare him for the experience at his own level of comprehension. He should be told the truth and what to expect so that he does not feel he is being punished or

---

* The Care of Children in Hospitals: The American Academy of Pediatrics, Evanston, Ill., 1960.

† Robertson, J., Young Children in Hospitals, New York, Basic Books, Inc., 1958.

abandoned by being placed in the hospital. If possible, he should be given a tour of the hospital prior to admission to lessen his fears. It may also help, if he is allowed to help pack for the trip to the hospital when the time comes. Once the child is admitted to the hospital, the parents should tell him when they plan to visit and be there at the stated time.

## Parents Are People, Too

As the emphasis in nursing care has changed from the "disease" to the "patient," and from there to the "patient within the family," the role of the nurse has become more difficult. When parents were kept out of the hospital, the nurse gave complete care to the child. However, as Florence Erickson has stated in *Therapeutic Relationship of the Nurse to the Parents of a Sick Child,* "the modern nurse must accept the role of mother supplement, not mother substitute, and gain at least some of her job satisfaction from *supporting the mother* in her care of the child."* In other words, the nurse shares the child's care with the mother. This requires an understanding of the effect of the child's illness on the parents. The nurse must realize that when a child goes to the hospital, the family constellation changes because one member is missing. Therefore, the entire family must be considered in the care of the child, because they are so vitally interested in his well-being and in bringing him home as soon as possible.

Today's pediatric nurse must accept the reactions of parents to their child's illness and have an understanding of the reasons for parents' behavior. Blake, et al., in *Nursing Care of Children,* identify how parents react when a child is hospitalized. According to their analysis, each parent reacts in a different way, depending upon certain general psychological factors, such as (1) the seriousness of the child's illness and the immediate threat to his life, (2) the life-situation of the parent, (3) the ego resources of the parent, (4) the parent's former experiences with illness and hospital-ization, (5) the parent's individual style of coping with any threat or stress, and (6) the parent's individual beliefs and values.

Thus, the nurse must understand the threat and stress to the parent when a child is in the hospital. She must also understand that such stress affects the parent's behavior. Because the parent is no longer in control of the situation and must rely upon the nurses and other members of the health team to care for the child, the parent may feel guilty, afraid, or angry, and may vent some of these feelings upon the nurse. Or parents may be so fearful and feel so responsible that they hate to leave their child's side. Unhappily, some nurses may then expect the mother to give total care; this is a great misunderstanding of the roles of the nurse and the mother. *The parents cannot do it all.* On the other hand, the parents may feel so inadequate and helpless in meeting the needs of their child that they do not want to be in the room with him; unfortunately, many nurses have only contempt for this latter parent who is in such great need of support.

**Build a Bridge.** Your firm conviction that you *share* the care of the child with his parents is an important one. Anything you can do to help his parents to understand him is a bridge to his future health and happiness. Parents must have hope. It is difficult to reassure the ignorant, frightened mother, whose fears are intensified because there are so many things that she does not understand. The intelligent mother is comforted when the treatments and the procedures are explained to her, because she realizes all the important care that you are giving to her child, along with the reasons behind this care.

A general acceptance of the role of the mother and the role of the nurse in their relationships with the sick child will improve the quality of nursing care.

## SPECIAL ASPECTS OF PEDIATRIC NURSING

### Safety Measures for Pediatric Patients

As with all patients, the child must be protected from further injury or illness while he is in the hospital. Several general rules, designed to minimize possible danger, prevail

---

* Erickson, Florence, Therapeutic Relationship of the Nurse to the Parents of a Sick Child, Ross Laboratories, 1965.

for the care of children and are listed below. (In general, these rules are modified to fit the older child, but the nurse must use good judgement in enforcing or relaxing them.)

1. Side rails or crib sides should be up at all times to prevent the child from falling out of bed. For the older child, the bed may be put into low position when the nurse is not in the room.
2. The nurse must be aware of the fire procedure for the unit. Sometimes, this procedure is different for pediatrics wards than it is for the adult units.
3. The child must be protected from burns or shocks. Keep cribs away from heat vents, radiators, electric outlets, or electric cords of any kind. Be careful of fans or other machines, and never allow a young child to adjust the television.
4. The nurse must stay with the child when his temperature is being taken or when he is on a litter or examining table.
5. Restraints must be used on the young child when he is in a high chair or when he is left for a few minutes anywhere. The strings on the restraints must not be pinned; they should be tied to the bed frame, not to the crib sides. Remember to loosen the restraints several times a day so the child may exercise. The strings should be long enough so the child can move, but not so long that he can fall out of bed. A net should be applied to the crib of any child who jumps in bed or crawls over the crib sides.
6. All safety pins should be closed when removed from a child's clothing or diapers, even if just for a minute. Any extra pins should be taken away from the bedside. Broken pins should be thrown away. Never put pins into your mouth or into the mattress or bedding. Be careful about puncturing equipment; pins are *never* used with the Aqua-K pad or with an air mattress.
7. Discard all broken toys and check toys for removable buttons, eyes, or wheels, which could be swallowed. The child should not have toys that are easily broken. Be careful about crayons (a small child could eat them), pencils (the child can easily poke himself with them), or scissors. A child under 6 should never have these items without close supervision. No balloons or plastic bags should be allowed in the pediatric department. The child should not chew gum unless he is closely watched. It is generally best for the child to use hospital toys (unless he has a favorite which he wants to keep). In this way, the toys can be disin-

fected and taken care of. Toys should not be exchanged between children and should be disinfected if they fall on the floor.

8. Certain general precautions should be taken: only plastic glasses and dishes should be used; all broken furniture must be repaired; glass and any other objects on the floor should be cleaned up immediately; since a child burns easily care must be taken when running bath water, filling warm-water bags, and using Aqua-K pads; and the children should have their identification name tags on at all times.
9. The child is never left while he is in the tub bath, unless he is at least 10-years-old and fully alert. Even then, the nurse should check often to make sure he is all right.

## COMMON PEDIATRIC NURSING PROCEDURES

### Making Up the Crib

Usually, a waterproof pad is placed under the crib sheet. It is desirable to use a fitted or contour sheet for the bottom of the crib, so that it will stay in place better. Usually, the crib is made up with a bath blanket instead of a top sheet. A pillow is not used for the small child. (If it is necessary to prop a small child up so that he can breathe better, the infant seat, rather than pillows, is used.)

### Admitting the Child to the Hospital

The admission of the child to the hospital is much the same as the admission of the adult, except that the nurse must be especially aware of the needs of the parents and child and must realize that this is a very traumatic event for both.

The nurse must attempt to make the patient as comfortable and secure as possible. She should help him to be confident of the nursing care and to cooperate in order to receive maximum benefit from that treatment.

The parents are consulted to find out any special needs of the child, his likes and dislikes, his allergies, any special language which he uses, and any other information which would aid in the care of the child. A friendly and trusting relationship between the parents and the nursing staff is essential if the child is to be assisted.

## TABLE 39–1. AVERAGE VITAL SIGNS FOR CHILDREN

| Age | Pulse | Respiration | Systolic BP | Diastolic BP | Oral Temperature | Rectal Temperature |
|---|---|---|---|---|---|---|
| 0–1 month | 120–150 | 30–80 | | | 98.6 | 99–99.6 |
| 1 month–1 yr. | 100–140 | 20–40 | | | 98.6 | 99–99.6 |
| 1–2 yr. | 90–120 | 20–35 | | | 98.6 | 99–99.6 |
| 2–6 yr. | 90–110 | 20–30 | 60–110 | 40–75 | 98.6 | 99–99.6 |
| 6–10 yr. | 85–100 | 18–25 | 75–120 | 40–75 | 98.6 | 99–99.6 |
| 11–16 yr. | 75–90 | 16–23 | 85–130 | 45–85 | 98.6 | 99–99.6 |

### Taking the Vital Signs

*Temperature:* As with all patients, the temperature of the child is taken on admission. If he is under the age of 6 or does not seem responsible or oriented enough to hold an oral thermometer, a rectal temperature must be taken. Regardless of the method used, the nurse must stay with the patient while his temperature is being taken. The temperature is taken for a full 3 minutes; if a rectal thermometer is used, it must be held for the entire time.

*Pulse:* If the child is over 2, the pulse may be taken radially. If the child is under 2, the pulse often is not taken or may be taken apically.

*Respiration:* It is important to remember that the respiration rate will be inaccurate if the child is crying.

*Observation:* The nurse must observe the child carefully for any sign of a rash, bruise, abrasion, discharge, or any alteration in his level of consciousness. She should note any complaints of pain or other symptoms, in the same manner as she would for an adult patient.

*Blood Pressure:* Since it is difficult to take the blood pressure of an infant, the blood pressure is taken if the child is over the age of 2. Since a smaller blood pressure cuff is used for a child than for an adult, a general rule is to measure the width of the blood pressure cuff by the width of the arm. There are about 5 different widths of blood pressure cuff, each of which will affect the pressure reading. If a child's blood pressure needs to be watched closely, the cuff should be left at the bedside and the pressure taken with the same cuff each time.

*Weight:* All children are weighed on admission. If the child is small, he is weighed on an infant or child scale. To avoid contamination, a paper must be placed on the scale before the child is put on the scale. Then the scale is balanced, with the nurse using a tissue over her hand to avoid further contamination of the scale. The scale may be disinfected after the procedure if the child has a communicable disease. While the child is weighed, the nurse stays with the child during the entire procedure, keeping one hand just above the child to make sure he does not fall. After the child is weighed the paper is discarded and the weight is charted. If a cast or brace is in place, this must be charted.

*Height:* This will be recorded for the older child. The infant is measured with a tape measure.

**Dressing the Child.** The child is generally dressed in hospital clothing to facilitate treatment and to avoid losing or soiling his own clothes, which are usually sent home with the parents. Any valuables which the child may have are also sent home. If he is allowed to keep a favorite toy or blanket, it must be labeled so it does not get lost.

**Introduction.** The child and his parents should be introduced to the hospital room and to his roommates and should be made to feel as comfortable as possible. They also need

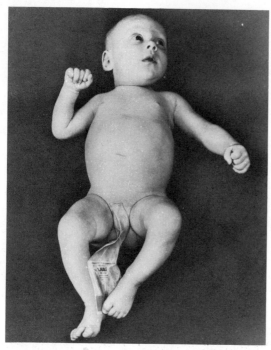

Figure 39-1. The pediatric urine collector facilitates the obtaining of a urine specimen from the child who cannot yet control his bladder. This also avoids catheterization, which could introduce bacteria into the bladder. This method of collection is convenient and safe and does not interfere with the child's activities or movements. Usually, a urine specimen is obtained upon admission to the hospital. (Hollister, Inc.)

to know the visiting hours, nap times, and other routines of the hospital. If the hospital has a provision for the parents to stay with the child, at least part of the time, this should be explained to the family.

**Charting.** The admission routines should be charted as soon as possible (Table 39-1), so the doctor and charge nurse can decide what the treatment is to be. Report any unusual findings to the charge nurse immediately.

## Pediatric Urine Collection

Since the small child cannot void on command, the pediatric urine bag is used to collect the urine specimen. The bag is disposable and has adhesive on it which is applied to the infant's skin. The adhesive is applied below the penis on the male, after the penis is inserted into the bag, and all the way around on the female. The genitals are carefully cleansed and dried before the bag is applied.

## Pediatric Venipuncture and Lumbar Puncture

If the blood sample from a very young child is taken from the jugular vein in the neck, the nurse will need to assist the doctor by holding the child in position for the venipuncture. The child is first placed in a mummy restraint and then held with head extended over the edge of a table. The child must be held very still. After the procedure any signs of swelling or bleeding should be noted around the puncture site.

Another site for venipuncture in the child is the femoral area. The nurse holds the child on his back with legs spread apart. He must be held securely while the doctor does the procedure. The nurse can easily talk to the child when he is in this position.

When a lumbar puncture is done, the infant or child is held with the back curved, while his legs are restrained with a sheet. The procedure is the same as for the adult (see Chapter 46).

## Pediatric Catheterization

The procedure is the same as for the adult patient, except that the catheter is smaller, depending upon the size of the child. Catheter sizes for children range from #8 to #10. A smaller feeding tube may also be used.

The child usually must be restrained during this procedure. The most common means of restraint is the papoose board. Usually, it is helpful to have another nurse assist in the procedure.

The catheter must be securely taped after insertion to prevent the child from pulling it out. He may also need to be restrained to prevent him from pulling on the catheter.

## Restraints and Other Safety Precautions for Children

In order to prevent accident or injury from falls, the child should be restrained. Even if he sleeps in a regular bed at home, the child is often put into a crib in the hospital. This is done not only to control the child but also to take into account the fact that a child naturally regresses to an earlier stage of development when ill. Sometimes it is necessary to enforce bedrest by applying restraints. The child should also be restrained whenever he is in a high chair or wheelchair or whenever he is up unattended. (The restraint, however, should not be substituted for good nursing observation.) Sometimes a restraint is needed to assist the doctor in doing a procedure.

The nurse must be aware of the dangers of using restraints. In some instances, a doctor's order is needed to apply them to a child. The restraint should not irritate the skin of the child or prevent him from exercising frequently. And the restraints must be checked often to make sure they are not too tight or too loose and that the strings are not too long or too short.

## Types of Restraints

*The Mummy Restraint:* The mummy restraint is used when a procedure, such as a venipuncture is to be performed. A bath blanket is folded into a triangle and the child is placed on his back, his neck even with the folded edge of the blanket. The blanket is folded over the body, encasing one arm. Then the other side is folded enclosing the other arm. The sides are pinned securely so that the child cannot move his arms. Then, the bottom is folded and pinned. In this way the nurse can assist the doctor and can hold the child with a minimum amount of effort.

*The Crib Net:* The net is placed over the entire crib in instances when the child jumps or climbs in bed and is in danger of jumping over the sides of the crib. Since the parents may object to the use of the net, the doctor should explain the reasons for its use and ask the parents to sign a release. The net is tied tightly over the top of the crib, and is secured to the mattress, not the crib sides. The ties should be placed in bows so they can be released quickly in case of emergency.

*The Jacket Restraint:* This is the same type of jacket restraint used for the adult patient, except that it is in a smaller size to fit a child. It is used when the child is up in the high chair or wheel chair and at times when he is in the crib. The jacket is applied over the pajamas to prevent skin irritation. It is tied to the back of the wheel chair or to the mattress bars on the bed, so that the equipment is not hampered by the ties. Be sure that the

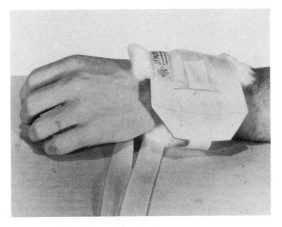

Figure 39-2. The hand or arm restraint is used in the child or adult to prevent injury to himself. The band is slipped around the wrist and then is tied to prevent it from becoming too tight. Notice the lamb's wool lining to prevent irritation of the skin. The nurse must loosen this restraint often so the patient can exercise his arm, must give meticulous skin care to prevent irritation, and must check the circulation often to make sure the restraint is not tied too tightly. (Posey Company)

ties are not too long or too short, and that the child does not become tangled in the strings. Check circulation often.

*Clove-Hitch Restraint:* Kerlix or a stockinette is used and the figure 8 is applied to one or more limbs to prevent injury or movement during treatment, such as when an I.V. is given. The commercial restraints may also be used for this purpose (Fig. 39-2). Be sure the

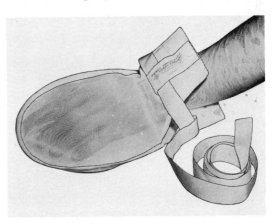

Figure 39-3. This is the glove restraint which is often used in pediatrics. Note that the hand is free to move within the glove. The wrist straps are usually tied to the bed frame to prevent scratching or pulling on tubes. (Posey Company)

restraint is not too tight and that it does not irritate the skin. Be sure that the child is allowed to exercise frequently.

*The Papoose Board or Restraint Board:* This board enables the child to be tied into any position needed and should be used only when short procedures are being done since it is uncomfortable.

*The Glove Restraint:* This restraint (Fig. 39-3) is used to prevent the child from scratching or pulling on tubes. It may be left loose or tied to the bed.

## Charting in Pediatrics

Because the child often cannot tell the nurse how he feels or how much he ate, the nurse must be responsible for recording this information as the day progresses. She must be very observant and be sure to note all information about the child, including normal behavior and reactions as well as abnormal symptoms and unfavorable signs.

*Diet:* It is important to know how much the child eats and drinks throughout the day. Intake and output for a child does not just mean fluid intake and output, it also means food intake and all kinds of output. An accurate recording is very important, because it is so easy for the child to become dehydrated. The nurse should also note if the infant spits up a great deal of the formula or if the young child does not want to eat.

*Output:* It is important to note the number, color, and consistency of stools, as well as any emesis or other drainage.

*Appearance and Behavior of the Child:* The nurse should note if the child is friendly, playful, lethargic, complaining, or listless. She should also note his color and any rash, or other noticeable signs.

*Symptoms:* The nurse should be on the lookout for any other symptoms, such as seizures, changes in vital signs, or any other irregularity.

*Comments by Parents:* It is important to note if the parents make any statements about the child's condition. They can often notice if he looks better or worse and can observe minute signs which the nurse may have missed, because she did not know the child before his illness.

## Mealtime

Generally, at mealtime the children are out of bed in high chairs or seated at a small table, if possible. The parents, if present, are encouraged to assist in the feeding of the child, since most children will eat better if their parents are there. Remember that all children must be restrained when up, and all food and fluid must be recorded after the meal.

**Forcing Fluids in Children.** It is often difficult to get the child to take fluids because he does not understand the reasons for drinking when he is not thirsty. The nurse who is kind, friendly, and understanding will have the most success in these instances. Sometimes, the child's mother will be able to assist the nursing staff. This not only helps the child obtain the fluids he needs, but also makes the mother feel helpful. Aside from actual fluids other acceptable fluid substitutes are popsicles, ice cream, jello, pop, and kool aid drinks. The use of almost any liquid will be acceptable if it succeeds in getting fluids into the child.

**Gavage Feeding by Tube.** Sometimes, the child will be fed by gastrostomy tube or by a gavage tube, which is passed down his throat. The nurse must be sure that the tube is in the stomach. Generally, the practical nurse will not pass the tube, but will assist in the feedings.

## Infant Gowning Technic

The ill infant needs to be protected from contagious illness which may spread from other infants. The nurse and family of the child under the age of 2 are usually asked to put on a gown when handling a child with a contagious disease to prevent the spread of infection from the ill child to any other child in the hospital.

A nurse's gown is hung at the bedside of each child and is used whenever he is handled. This gown should be changed at least once each shift and more often, if needed. Since the inside of the gown is considered clean and the outside is considered contaminated (it is the part exposed to the child), the gown is hung right-side-out. As in most instances when a gown is worn, the nurse scrubs before putting the gown on and scrubs thoroughly after removing it.

## Pediatric Infant Bath

The small infant is usually given a tub bath in a small bedside tub. The nurse must be sure to bring all equipment needed with her, since she cannot leave the child alone after she starts the bath. The child is weighed before his bath and covered with a bath blanket. Don't forget the infant gowning technic.

The eyes are cleansed first with clear water, from inner canthus to outer canthus; then the rest of the face is washed. The ears are cleaned with cotton-tipped swabs, but the ear canals are not probed. The hair is shampooed when needed.

The body may be bathed by placing the infant into the tub or by using the washcloth. Perineal care must be given to the female infant and genital care to the male. If the male has not been circumcised, the foreskin should be pulled back and the penis cleansed. If the baby has been circumcised, the penis should be checked for any signs of irritation.

After the bath, the hair is combed, the fingernails and toenails are trimmed, if needed, and the infant is dressed. Any signs or symptoms of disease should be reported.

## Sponge Bath to Reduce Body Temperature

Children, especially young children, often run very high fevers when they are ill. This is dangerous because it can damage body or brain tissue, and can cause seizures. Children who do not respond to regular treatment to reduce body temperature often respond very favorably to the tepid sponge.

Warm water or alcohol may be used, with ice added to the solution. Generally, the temperature of the solution is between 80 and 85° F.

The procedure is explained to the child and to the parents. The room must be free of drafts and privacy must be provided. Pajamas are removed and the child is covered with a bath blanket. Temperature, pulse, and respiration is taken before the sponge bath is begun and at intervals throughout the procedure. The patient is encouraged to force fluids during the procedure, if this is allowed.

The child is wrapped in damp towels which have been soaked in the solution. The towels are then removed and the child is fanned to allow the solution to evaporate. The axilla, groin, and popliteal areas can be sponged freely since they seem to lower the body temperature more rapidly (the blood vessels are closer to the surface in these areas).

The temperature must be taken at least every 10 minutes, and the child should be carefully observed for any signs of chilling or shivering, for any increase or decrease in pulse or for any change in skin color. If the patient has any untoward reaction, the sponge bath should be discontinued immediately and the reaction reported. The sponge bath generally is continued until the child's temperature falls to within reasonable limits (*not* necessarily to normal). If the temperature does not begin to fall within ½ hour, the doctor should be notified. The temperature should be taken again ½ hour after sponging has been completed.

The entire procedure should be charted, including time, reaction of the child, length of soaks, and the time it took for the temperature to fall.

## Routine Weighings

Since the condition of a small child can be determined, in part, by fluctuation in weight, routine weighings are a part of the nursing care of children. Generally, the child is weighed on admission and routinely thereafter. A typical routine includes daily weighings for infants under 6 months of age, weighings every other day for children from 6 months to 2 years of age, and weekly weighings for children over 2 years of age. Variations may depend upon the doctor and the hospital. The procedure for routine weighing is the same as that used for the admission weight, with care being taken not to contaminate the scale. Any drastic change in weight must be reported immediately.

## Oral Hygiene for Children

Since the child cannot always clean his own mouth, the nurse may need to assist him. The child under 3 often cannot brush his teeth, but he should be encouraged to rinse his mouth out often with water. If he can rinse his mouth and spit the solution out, mouth-wash may be used.

For the child who can brush his teeth, good oral care is urged. The tooth brush should be rinsed in cold water, left in open air to dry, and discarded when the bristles begin to soften. The brush should be kept in the child's bedside stand to prevent brushes from being mixed among children.

## Diarrhea Technic

When young children suffer from diarrhea, the main dangers are dehydration and spread of disease. Since the small child becomes dehydrated very quickly as a result of diarrhea, quick preventive measures must be taken. The nursing care includes intravenous feedings, with no food being given by mouth for a time (about 24 to 48 hours) to rest the digestive tract. When feedings are resumed, clear water is usually given first. Sometimes, saline is used, or a carbonated beverage, such as 7-up, or a popsicle is given. If this is tolerated, milk can be given, first skim milk, then whole milk. The diet progresses from strained foods, with no roughage, back to the normal diet for age.

The nursing care also includes meticulous handwashing technic to prevent the spreading of the infection. Usually, the child is placed in strict *isolation* (see Chapter 40). Stools and diapers (usually disposable) must be carefully disposed of. If possible, the skin is exposed to the air, to protect it from irritation. Placing the infant on his stomach helps to expose the buttocks to the air. Sitz baths and ointments may also be used. It is very important to chart the number and type of stools during each period of the day.

## Diaper Technic

When a child has diarrhea or has not received proper skin care, his buttocks may become very sore and irritated. The nurse must be watchful for this condition and prevent its occurrence or alleviate it once it has developed. The buttocks must be thoroughly cleansed each time the diaper is changed. Mineral oil or ointments may be used in this procedure. The proper technic is to always wipe from front to back.

## Pediatric Enemas

Enemas are given to children in the same way that they are given to adults, although the nurse must remember that the smaller size of the child necessitates using a smaller amount of solution. The amounts usually used are no more than 300 cc. for an infant and no more than 500 cc. for a child, below age 10. This, of course, depends upon the size of the child. Tap water enemas are never given to the child with megacolon. The infant may be restrained by passing a diaper under the pan and pinning it around the legs on each side.

Sometimes, the child will not be able to retain the solution. In this case, several folds of toilet tissue may be held around the tube to help the child hold the solution.

All other parts of the procedure are the same as for the adult patient.

## Suppositories

Suppositories are often given to the child, more often to administer medication than to cause a bowel movement. Drugs commonly given this way are aspirin and anticonvulsive or antiemetic drugs. The nurse must be sure to explain the procedure to the child and urge him not to expel the suppository. She should insert it and hold it in place until the child no longer feels the urge to expel it.

## Croupette and Humidity

Since many children suffer from upper respiratory infections, the croupette is a frequent sight on the pediatric ward. This device brings cool humidity and, sometimes, oxygen to the child. (The unit may be used with or without oxygen.)

The unit makes it easier for the child to breathe by liquifying the secretions so that they can be coughed up. It also lowers body temperature because ice is used to cool the air.

A rubber or plastic sheet is put under the crib sheet to protect the bed against the moisture and to prevent oxygen from escaping. A cotton blanket is placed on top of the sheet to absorb moisture so the patient will be more comfortable.

The metal frame of the croupette is fastened to the bed frame to keep it steady. The container at the back of the unit is filled with ice at intervals. Some units are now equipped with refrigeration units so that they can be operated without ice. The plastic tent is tucked securely around the crib mattress and is sealed with a folded bath blanket in the same way as the oxygen tent. The humidity jar is then filled with distilled water. The tent should be flushed with oxygen before the child is placed into the tent. The nurse is responsible for charting the procedure and noting its effects upon the child, as well as any signs of dyspnea, cyanosis, or other difficulties.

## Preoperative and Postoperative Care

The same principles prevail for the care of children who undergo surgery as for adult patients.

In addition to the child understanding what is going to be done and why, the parents should be involved, as much as possible, in the preparation for surgery. The parents often come into the hospital with the child and stay during the history and physical examination. Since they are responsible for the child, they must sign the operative release. They may stay overnight the night before surgery and may go to the operating room door with the child, depending upon the doctor and the hospital.

On the evening before the surgery, the nurse must be careful to chart any signs of an upper respiratory infection, such as fever, cough, or runny nose. These would make respiratory complications more possible and may cause the surgery to be delayed until the infection is cleared up. The nurse should also be sure to chart any open wound, rash, or other symptoms which the child might have. At this time the surgical preparation is done and often a bath is given.

On the morning of the operation, the child is asked to void and his TPR (temperature, pulse, and respiration) and blood pressure are recorded. Preoperative medications are given and any hairpins or jewelry are removed. The child should be wearing hospital pajamas as well as an identification band. The surgical preparation should be done and the nurse should check to see that all laboratory reports are on the chart, and that blood work is done. Everything, including toys, is taken out of the bed. If the patient is going to be taken to the operating room in his crib, the sheets are changed. The child is kept NPO (nothing by mouth). When everything is done the nurse should sign the chart.

Postoperatively, the nurse should prepare the room to receive the patient. She should have available an I.V. stand, an emesis basin, tissues, the blood pressure apparatus, blood pressure graph, and equipment for any other drainage or supplies needed for that particular patient. She should arrange the room so the cart from the recovery room can get in easily. She is responsible for watching the patient closely and for charting and reporting accurately, as well as notifying the child's parents when he has returned to the pediatric unit.

## Resuscitation of the Child

The nurse must remember that the child's lung capacity is smaller than that of an adult. When resuscitation is necessary, mouth-to-mouth or mouth-to-nose breathing may be used, but the breath should only be enough to expand the child's lungs. It is possible to overinflate or rupture the lung of a child if you blow too hard. To provide the best emergency care for resuscitation, pediatric Ambu-bags and child-size airways for intubation, should be present on the emergency cart in every pediatric unit.

## Administering Parenteral Fluids

Since the child's body is made up of about 80 per cent water (the adult's is about 60 per cent), the child becomes dehydrated much more easily than does the adult. If the child has diarrhea, a high fever, or difficulty in excreting urine or wastes, the fluid and electrolyte balance of the body may become upset, requiring that fluids be administered parenterally.

**Intravenous Infusion.** In this instance the child cannot take too much fluid, so a pediatric microdrip or soluset device is used to control the exact amount of fluid which the child is receiving each hour. The devices used have an extra container which will hold about 100 cc. of fluid and which is more finely calibrated than the regular I.V. bottle. Thus, the child can receive an exact amount of fluid each hour. The drops are smaller and can be regulated more closely than can the regular I.V. setup for adults.

The child may need to be restrained to prevent him from pulling on the tubes. The I.V. may be administered into the arm veins in the older child or in the scalp veins or neck veins in the younger child.

**Subcutaneous Infusion (Clysis).** Sometimes, although infrequently, the needle is not inserted into a vein, but is injected under the skin. In this instance, the rate of flow must be slow because the rate of absorption is slower than in intravenous therapy.

**Rectal Administration (Proctoclysis).** Occasionally, the fluids will be administered rectally, although the procedure must also be done slowly to prevent the patient from expelling the fluid.

## Administering Medications to Children

Most likely the practical nurse will not be asked to administer medications to children, but she must be aware that the child, because of his smaller size, will react much faster and more drastically than an adult to any medication. An anaphylactic response will be more dramatic and more likely to be fatal in a child. Thus the nurse must be constantly on the alert for drug reactions. She must realize that the child often cannot tell when he is feeling ill or having adverse effects from a drug, so she must be especially alert to any symptoms of side-effects.

Although medications are prescribed for the individual child on the basis of his condition, his disease, and other factors, there are 2 helpful general rules for determining the *approximate* dosage of a drug. The nurse should use these only as a general guide and not as an absolute measuring device for questioning the dosage of a drug.

Weight: Clark's Rule

$$\frac{\text{Child's wt. in lbs.} \times \text{average adult dose}}{150} = \text{child's dose}$$

Age: Young's Rule

$$\frac{\text{Age of child} \times \text{average adult dose}}{\text{age of child} + 12} = \text{child's dose}$$

## Diversional Activities for Children

It is important for the nurse to remember that play is an important part of a child's natural sequence of growth and development. It is especially important to give the child something to do while he is in the hospital so that he does not become too bored or upset.

Children of all ages love to be read to or to read for themselves. They all need to be talked with and to be included in the conversation. The child has a great need to have someone listen to him. The nurse should remember to spend time talking to her child patients and listening to what they have to tell her about what is happening in the new and exciting world of the hospital.

## Discharging a Child From the Pediatric Unit

The child is discharged from the hospital in much the same way as the adult, except that the child may be dressed by his mother and is taken home by his parents, who are responsible for his follow-up care. Be sure the child has been properly discharged by the doctor and has his appointment slips, medication prescriptions, and any orders from the doctor. He should be carried or taken to the car via wheel chair. The nurse or attendant must accompany the child and his parents to the entrance of the hospital. (The child is never left alone.)

## SPECIAL PEDIATRIC SITUATIONS

### The Long-Term Pediatric Patient

Some children will be in the hospital for a long time or will be readmitted often because of a chronic or degenerative disorder. These children need special nursing care and attention.

In these instances, it is especially important that a basic sense of trust be established between the child and the nurse. Thus the child should have the same nurse several times so that he will get to know one person quite well, who will answer his questions honestly and visit him often to show that someone cares and will take care of him. However, he also needs to learn to care for himself as much as possible. He can also be given duties on the ward to make him feel useful and helpful.

## The Child With a Poor Prognosis

It is very difficult for the nurse to work with the child who has a terminal illness, such as leukemia or cancer of the bone. It is especially difficult for her, because she must conquer her own feelings and emotions before she can deal with those of the patient and family.

The nurse should offer emotional support, not only to the child, but also to the parents. She can be most helpful to the patient and his family by giving a listening ear and by offering understanding support and kindness. They may not want to talk; they may just want to know that the nurse is there if they need her.

How the child, or anyone else for that matter, perceives death depends upon his age and experiences. While the very young child, under about 3, is unable to comprehend the exact meaning of what it is to die, the older child is more likely to realize what is happening and to be afraid, or worried. On the other hand he may accept it as a fact.

A great deal of controversy exists about whether or not to tell the child that his prognosis is poor. Some people feel that the child need not know; all that needs to be done is to limit his activities as his disease progresses. Others feel that if the child is older, he probably knows anyway because he can sense the change in the attitudes of those around him. Advocates of this view feel that since the child may have a distorted idea of the situation it would be better if he know the actual facts. In this way, he can verbalize his feelings and his fears and deal with them better. If he is not told that he is dying, he will have to deal with his feelings alone, which makes it more difficult for him than if he could share them with someone else.

In terms of activities, the terminally ill child should be allowed to participate in whatever ward activities he can physically stand and should be allowed to do as much for himself as possible.

## The Death of a Child

The child who is dying has several fears and concerns which must be dealt with. He is afraid of separation and of going away. He may feel guilty for something which he has done and may feel that his death is a punishment. He may also fear the medical procedures which are being done to help him and may fear that his body will be mutilated.

The greatest fear of the child or of anyone who is dying is that of being *alone*. Thus the dying child should not be isolated; he needs to feel that someone will be there.

It is helpful to answer the child's questions as honestly as possible and to treat his symptoms and make him as comfortable as possible.

**The parents.** The nurse must not forget the parent of the dying child. She must realize that because they are naturally upset and shattered, they may actually deny the fact that the child is dying, or may strike out at members of the nursing team without meaning what they say.

The most common reactions of parents are denial, then guilt, anxiety, and, hopefully, acceptance. The parents must be allowed privacy and the opportunity to mourn in their own way. It is not unprofessional for the nurse to let them know that she feels the loss, too.

**A final word.** It is a privilege and a nursing challenge to care for the dying child. It is also an excellent time for the nurse to evaluate her own feelings and motivations. The nurse should be able to handle the death of a child with empathy, reverence, gentleness, and genuine nursing skill.

# 40

# The Infant, the Toddler, and the Preschool Child

## BEHAVIORAL OBJECTIVES

*The student successfully attaining the goals of this chapter will be able to:*

- *recognize and describe normal child growth and development and deviations therefrom which cause the child to have special needs or to be unable to meet his own basic needs; demonstrate the consideration of growth and developmental patterns in planning and carrying out nursing care.*

- *effectively care for children of varying ages and with various conditions, demonstrating a knowledge of pediatric safety, of illnesses common to children, and of the feelings of the child and his family.*

- *list at least 5 special considerations in caring for or observing a child which are related to his age or size.*

- *define the term communicable disease; list 4 modes by which diseases are spread and give at least 2 examples of each mode; and review the recommended childhood immunization schedule.*

- *list at least 8 of the most common communicable diseases of childhood, including rheumatic fever; identify the deviation from normal body structure and/or function in each condition, utilizing proper medical terminology; identify the causative organism, if known; and describe the most important aspects of patient care.*

- *discuss the aspects of trauma which are peculiar to childhood; identify at least 6 common types of trauma, including that of the maltreated or battered child; and discuss the most important aspects of care.*

- *list the most common congenital and chronic disorders of the various body systems, as well as disorders of metabolism and nutrition, and neoplasms; describe each condition in relationship to normal body structure and/or function and in relationship to normal child growth and development; identify medical terms related to each condition; identify differences, if any, between this condition in a child and in an adult.*

- *identify and describe the most common parasites which invade the bodies of children; and demonstrate competency in caring for such a child.*

- *discuss the general concept of deviation from normal behavior in children; identify and describe several specific conditions; demonstrate effectiveness in dealing with children who have behavior disorders.*

- *effectively care for a child of a culture or a race different from that of the nurse.*

You have already studied the normal growth and development of the child from birth until he begins school (Chapter 8). However, it would be a good idea to review Chapter 8 before beginning the study of the disorders common to this age group.

In this chapter, we will consider the most common deviations from normal found in the child from birth to age 6. Many of these diseases or disorders are also common among adults. There are many other conditions which are found in children, but the nurse will come in contact with these so infrequently that it is not necessary to study them in a text of this type.

The nurse should also remember that many of the diagnostic, x-ray, and laboratory procedures are done for the child in exactly the same manner as they are done for the adult. If you would like to review a procedure, consult the index for its location within this book.

The deviations from normal in the child along with appropriate tests and treatments, will be discussed in terms of: (a) communicable diseases, (b) trauma, (c) congenital and chronic disorders, which affect the various body systems, (d) parasitic invasions of the body, and (e) specific behavior disorders.

Before proceeding, a word is in order concerning the nursing care of a child undergoing surgery. Several of the disorders discussed in this chapter require some form of surgical intervention. While many of the preoperative and postoperative procedures are the same for both adult and child, there are certain differences which the nurse must consider.

The nurse must remember that the child often cannot verbalize about any discomfort or symptoms which he may be experiencing. Therefore, it is the nurse's responsibility to watch the child for any untoward signs. She must also remember that the child cannot be evaluated in the same manner as the adult, because his lungs are smaller, his heart is smaller and beats faster, and his urine volume, as well as the amount of blood in his body, is smaller. Therefore, a small deviation from normal is often more important in the child than it is in the adult. For example, a small amount of bleeding in a child can be a very significant symptom, even though the same amount of bleeding in an adult would be insignificant.

The nurse must also remember to consider the child's parents. They are concerned and have emotional needs, as well as the patient himself. If the parents are included in the pre- and postoperative care of the child, both the child and the parent will be more comfortable and cooperative.

The nurse in the operating room must remember that the child will be more cooperative if he hears familiar voices and sees familiar faces. Thus a visit from the nurse or anesthesiologist the day before the operation helps relieve anxiety. It is also important that the child have as short a waiting period as possible after he arrives in the operating room suite.

## COMMUNICABLE CHILDHOOD DISEASES

The diseases that are most common to children are the communicable diseases—those which are transferred from one person to another. Although in some communities, hospitals and hospital departments or wards are set apart to care for patients with communicable diseases, many children with common communicable diseases are cared for at home.

It is impossible to keep people from being exposed to contagious diseases. Since children are often most infectious to others before the symptoms appear, it is especially difficult to control the spread of infectious childhood diseases. Methods of the spread of disease and the development of immunity to infectious diseases were discussed previously. You already know that science has discovered methods of preventing people from developing some diseases; other discoveries, such as immunization, make it possible to provide temporary or permanent protection against certain diseases. Early immunization is important to protect children when they are small.

The period between the time the child is exposed and the time required for the disease to develop is called the *incubation period*. If the disease is especially contagious the child may be placed in isolation or quarantine. *Isolation* is the practice of separating a person who has a communicable disease from contact with others. *Quarantine* prohibits anyone from entering or leaving the place where the person with the disease is kept. Except where smallpox is concerned, quarantine is not often used. If a child has a communicable disease, he should be isolated until the communicable period is passed.

Communicable diseases may be classified according to the following categories as determined by mode of spread:

1. *Respiratory:* pneumonia, diphtheria, tuberculosis, measles, polio, mumps, common cold, and "strep" and "staph" infections.
2. *Gastrointestinal:* dysenteries, diarrhea, salmonella, polio, and infectious hepatitis.
3. *Parenteral:* serum hepatitis, malaria, and syphilis.
4. *Skin and mucous membranes:* venereal diseases, impetigo, scabies, "staph" infections, the gas gangrenes, and tetanus.

Therefore, the nursing and medical management involves controlling these avenues of spread.

## Concepts in Care of Infectious Patients

There are several basic principles which should govern the communicable disease technic used in the hospital. The chief goal of communicable disease management is that of control. Since admission to the hospital is done only if the child requires hospital treatment, precautions must be taken to *prevent the spread* of the disease to other children.

For specific technics of gowning, gloving, and disposing of materials from the isolation room see Chapter 30.

**The Emotional Aspects of Being in Isolation.** The general emotional aspects of being in isolation were discussed previously, but the child suffers more from being alone than does the adult. The nurse should plan her day so that she can spend time just visiting with the patient, and should see that the patient has things to do while alone. Friends should be encouraged to write and call, and parents should be assisted in the proper technics so they can visit often.

**Upper Respiratory Infections.** Often called "URI" or LTB (larynx, trachea, bronchi), this disorder is common in children as well as in adults. It may be caused by a virus or a bacteria and usually results in a high temperature, in dyspnea with thick, tenacious sputum and mucus, and in edema of the throat. A cough may not be present, in which case, the patient is unable to cough up the secretions.

The general treatment includes antibiotics, humidity, oxygen, rest, and occasionally, a tracheostomy. The nurse must also be especially observant of the patient's respiratory status.

**Pneumonia.** Pneumonia, which is an inflammation of the lung, is another common disorder in children and adults. (See Chapter 48.) It may be caused as an initial disease resulting from an infection, or it may be secondary to another disease or the result of aspiration.

**Croup.** The basic symptoms of croup are laryngeal spasm, dyspnea, and an increased production of mucus. The child also has a harsh, seal-like cough, his chest rattles when he breathes, and he may be cyanotic. He usually has a high fever, rapid pulse, cold, clammy skin, and a flushed face.

The treatment involves placing the patient into a croupette or other humidifying device. Oxygen may be given to assist in respirations. Expectorants are often given to loosen secretions and to assist the child in coughing up the mucus. The infant is placed in an infant seat in a semisitting position to assist in breathing. The older child may be propped up on pillows.

It is very important for the nurse to observe the child carefully to see if his breathing is becoming more labored, if he is retracting (the sternum retracts or is drawn in with each breath, and the ribs can often be visualized), if he is becoming cyanotic, or if he needs to be suctioned. In severe cases a tracheostomy may need to be performed to assist the patient to breathe.

General nursing care involves giving aspirin for the temperature and sedatives to relieve anxiety (although the patient's respiratory status must be carefully determined before a sedative is prescribed) and forcing fluids. If the patient is unable to take oral fluids, intravenous fluids are given. Clear liquids, popsicles, jello, and other fluids should be offered frequently. Milk, however, is usually avoided, because it tends to form a film and obstruct breathing.

**Whooping Cough.** Whooping cough (*pertussis*) is caused by a bacillus. Infants do not receive immunity to whooping cough from their mothers; therefore, very young infants are susceptible to it. Whooping cough rarely occurs after the age of 10 years. The incubation period is from 7 to 14 days. The symptoms begin with bronchitis and a slight elevation in temperature. The cough steadily grows worse, eventually leading to paroxysms of coughing, characterized by the "whooping" sound. The child may cough so hard that it causes emesis. He may also become dyspneic. The first stage lasts about a week; the severe coughing stage, from 2 to 3 weeks. It takes about 2 or 3 more weeks for the cough to disappear, but whooping cough can last for several months if complications appear, the most serious of which is bronchopneumonia.

Isolation is practiced through the whooping period. Prevention of whooping cough is available through a vaccine which is given as early as 1 month of age. This does not provide permanent immunity, and boosters of the vaccine should be given at intervals.

The child who has whooping cough is given antibiotics and medications to relieve the coughing. The infant must be supervised closely because of his respiratory difficulties and nutritional problems.

**Streptococcal Sore Throat.** "Strep throat" is another common occurrence in young people. The most serious complication is the development of rheumatic fever and rheumatic heart disease. The strep throat is treated with large doses of antibiotics, usually penicillin, to prevent complications. (See Chapter 33 for further discussion of antibiotics.)

**Tonsillitis.** Basically, tonsillitis is an inflammation of the tonsils, caused by the streptococcus or staphylococcus organisms. The symptoms include a sore, reddened throat, with swelling and sometimes pustules on the tonsils. Swallowing is difficult, and the white blood count and temperature are elevated.

A throat culture is done to determine the offending organism, and drug sensitivity tests are run to determine the treatment of choice. Medical treatment involves isolating the patient, administering large doses of antibiotics and providing general treatment of the symptoms. For example, if the child has difficulty in swallowing, the diet may need to be altered so he can get enough food and fluids. Fluids are forced, and aspirin is given to lower the temperature and to relieve the pain. If medical treatment is unsuccessful and if the child has recurrent, severe bouts of tonsillitis, the tonsils may need to be removed.

The preoperative care of tonsillectomy involves seeing that the child has a sedative and an anticholinergic drug, takes nothing by mouth after midnight, receives an explanation of the procedure, and is given other routine operative preparation. Postoperative nursing care is directed at preventing hemorrhage, which is the most common complication. The nurse must watch to see if the child spits up a great deal of bloody sputum or vomits coffee-ground or dark substance. The vital signs must also be watched carefully, and the airway must be maintained because swelling of the throat may occlude the air passageway. The child should be kept from vomiting, if possible.

An elevated temperature postoperatively may indicate dehydration and the need for fluids to be forced. An infection is also possible, although this is not a common complication of tonsillectomy.

The patient is usually discharged the day of or the day after surgery.

**Measles.** Measles (*rubeola*) ("common measles," red measles, or 7-day measles) is caused by a virus which locates itself in the nose, the mouth, the throat, and the eyes, and in their discharges. This type of measles may be shorter in duration (7-day or "red" measles) or may be longer (hard measles). It is highly communicable and may not be recognized early because the symptoms often resemble cold symptoms. The incubation period lasts from 10 to 14 days. Measles begins with a slight temperature rise and a runny nose (*coryza*), and eyes. About the second or third day, bluish-white pinpoint spots with a red rim appear in the mouth; these are called *Koplik's spots*. Small dark red pimples appear on the head and spread gradually over the body. These pimples grow larger and group together, giving a *blotchy* appearance, which is an important difference between measles and scarlet fever. In scarlet fever, the skin appears red all over.

The respiratory symptoms grow worse. The patient sneezes frequently, his eyes are sore, and the discharge becomes purulent. Light hurts his eyes (*photophobia*). His throat is sore, and he has a hacking cough. The rash which may last for 10 days, is greatest about the fourth day. During the second week, the skin begins to flake off and continues to do so for 5 to 10 days. As a result, the patient itches all over and must be prevented from scratching.

Complications are frequent with measles. The infection may spread to the middle ear (otitis media), and pneumonia is a common development. Encephalitis occurs occasionally and may cause death. The prognosis in a measles case depends on the age and the condition of the child; it affects the very young child most dangerously.

Isolation should be practiced until the discharges from the nose and the eyes disappear and the temperature is normal, which usually occurs 5 days from the time the rash appears.

The measles itself is rarely, if ever, fatal, but the complications may be extremely dangerous. One attack, however, seems to confer immunity to the child. A specific vaccine is now available and is usually required before the child can start school. In addition to the measles vaccine, gamma globulin will afford a temporary immunity if it is given a few days after exposure; the attack will be mild if it is given later, but before the symptoms appear. However, gamma globulin has no effect if it is administered after the disease develops.

**German Measles.** German measles (*rubella*) also is another communicable disease caused by a virus, but it is mild and lasts only a short time. The symptoms are like measles but are not nearly as severe, and spots never appear on the mucous membrane of the mouth. Sometimes the rash which appears on the face is the first noticeable sign of a rubella infection. The rash spreads quickly and disappears just as rapidly; sometimes it is gone from the face and the neck before it reaches the arms and the legs. The rash is usually completely gone in 2 to 4 days. Complications rarely develop; however, two possible ones are serious. One is an infection such as encephalitis or otitis media, and the other is fetal malformations which occur when a mother contracts German measles in the early months of her pregnancy.

The most common birth defect caused by rubella during pregnancy is that of partial or complete hearing loss in the baby. It is believed that from $1/4$ to $1/3$ of all mothers who contract rubella during the first trimester (first 3 months) of pregnancy give birth to a child with some defect.

Isolation usually is very brief or not carried out at all, since the infectious stage is so short; probably there is little danger of passing on the infection after the rash disappears. One attack of rubella apparently confers lifelong immunity. A vaccine is available and should be administered to young girls before they reach childbearing age. If pregnant mothers are exposed to this disease, they are given gamma globulin.

**Measles Encephalitis.** This is a very dangerous complication which may occur after a bout of rubeola and occasionally, rubella. One out of every 6 children who have rubeola develop a complication, the most dangerous being measles encephalitis (inflammation of the brain), sometimes called "sleeping sickness." About 1 out of every 1000 cases of measles results in encephalitis, and more than $1/2$ of these suffer permanent brain damage from the encephalitis.

The disease can result in death, a more likely outcome with the younger child. For this reason, every child should have the measles vaccine. Therefore mass immunization programs are under way in this country.

It is now believed that measles encephalitis can linger in the body for some time, causing a degenerative condition. Recent research has linked the measles virus with the later development of multiple sclerosis. If this theory is definitely proven, immunization against measles will not only prevent measles and measles encephalitis, but will also possibly prevent mutiple sclerosis and other demyelinating diseases.

**Roseola Infantum (Exanthem Subitum).** This is a benign disease, which usually occurs in infants. It consists of a high fever, which lasts for a few days, followed by a rash once the temperature falls. It is believed to be caused by a virus, but is not as communicable as many other diseases. The child may have convulsions, secondary to the high fever, but other complications are very rare. One attack seems to confer life-long immunity. The treatment is entirely symptomatic.

**Chickenpox.** Chickenpox (*varicella*) is caused by a virus, which is believed to be identical to the virus of herpes zoster. The disease usually begins with a slight fever which the patient may not even notice. Then a rash appears on the face or the trunk and spreads to the extremities; spots appear and then develop into blisters surrounded by a red ring. The blisters are filled with a clear fluid which gradually dries up, leaving a flat crust, which falls off in 1 to 3 weeks. The child is usually isolated for 10 to 12 days or until all the crusts have fallen off.

The chickenpox virus is located in the nose and throat, in the blisters, and probably in the crusts. Chickenpox takes from 14 to 16 days to develop from the time of exposure. It seldom has serious complications; the most likely one to occur is infection which may develop when the blisters are scratched, leaving scars or "pock-marks." This disease sometimes is confused with a mild case of smallpox because the eruptions are somewhat alike. However, smallpox usually begins with more violent symptoms; also, the eruptions appear mostly on the face, the legs, and the arms and are deeper in the skin and have a pearly appearance.

Nursing care for chickenpox includes isolation, a normal diet, and the routine comfort care. The only child for whom smallpox is very dangerous is the newborn infant or the child who is on steroid therapy. You will need some ingenuity to keep the child from scratching and to keep him amused until the isolation period is over.

**Smallpox (Variola).** Since a vaccine is available, this disease does not occur often. It is a very serious, highly contagious disease which is also caused by a virus. It begins suddenly with severe general malaise similar to that of influenza, followed by specific skin eruptions which often result in permanent scars. Complications include hemorrhagic lesions, gangrene of the skin, eye and ear damage, and severe toxemia.

There is no natural immunity to smallpox and the vaccination is effective for only 5 to 7 years. Therefore, it is imperative to keep vaccinations up to date, for life. The vaccine may cause a mild form of the disease, which is usually not dangerous. However, the vaccination is contraindicated in the child who has eczema or a history of allergic reactions, because *eczema vaccinatum* may possibly develop and results in a high mortality rate. If the child is very allergic, he may contract this allergic reaction just by being around others who have been vaccinated. The pregnant woman also should not be vaccinated, because fetal damage may occur.

**Mumps.** Mumps (*epidemic parotitis*) is another virus disease. It affects the salivary glands, especially the parotid. Children under 2 years of age and adults seldom have mumps. A closer contact is required to transmit mumps than other contagious diseases. The incubation period lasts from 2 to 3 weeks, averaging about 18 days.

In most cases, the first sign of mumps is a swelling in the parotid gland, although occasionally, mumps may begin with a slight fever, headache, and malaise before the swelling appears. Sometimes only one of the parotid glands is affected, but both may be affected at the same time, or one after the other. The gland becomes swollen and tender and is very painful. It hurts the victim to open his mouth, but otherwise he may not feel sick. After 2 or 3 days, the swelling begins to go down and usually disappears by the tenth day. As a rule, isolation for 2 weeks is long enough.

Children seldom suffer complications with mumps, but grown men and women may. In men, mumps can cause an inflammation of the testes; in women, the ovaries, the breasts, or the external genitals are affected. The most common complication of adult mumps is permanent sterility. Gamma globulin will prevent or lessen the severity of mumps, if the serum is given a few days after the person has been exposed.

Nursing care includes isolation technics, heat applications to the swollen glands to relieve pain, and a diet which does not require chewing. Acid foods taken during the painful stage seem to increase the pain. It is difficult to keep a child in bed until the isolation period is over; modern treatment tends to let him get up if there are no complications.

A vaccine is now available against mumps and is usually given to the young person when he is about 12 years of age, if he has not yet had the disease. This gives immunity for life in most cases, and prevents the complications of mumps in adulthood.

**Scarlet Fever.** Scarlet fever is another contagious disease affecting children. It is caused by a hemolytic streptococcus, with symptoms developing after an incubation period of 1 to 7 days. Although many persons have sore throats caused by the streptococcus, not all exhibit the rash reaction. The patient has a sore throat and fever and feels very ill. Scarlet fever (also called *scarlatina*) gives the appearance of a generalized flush or redness but is really a rash of small red pinpoints very close together. Flaking of the skin (desquamation) follows the rash. The tongue also becomes coated with a white substance, which later peels off.

The complications most commonly seen are ear infections and nephritis. Arthritis, cardiac problems, and pneumonia may also occur. The treatment involves keeping the patient in bed until the symptoms disappear and administering antibiotics to which the streptococcus is susceptible. Generally, scarlet fever tends to be a milder disease than it formerly was, so that today the prognosis is for the complete recovery of the patient.

**Diphtheria.** Diphtheria is another communicable disease caused by a bacillus. It begins with a sore throat, fever, and often generalized aching and malaise. Inflammation of the throat (the disease may also appear in the nose, the larynx, or the trachea) is followed by the formation of a dirty-gray membrane which is closely adherent and cannot be removed without causing bleeding. The diphtheria bacilli produce a toxin or poison which may weaken the cardiac muscle. The patient is very ill and must be observed closely. The mortality rate from diphtheria lies between 5 and 10 per cent.

Diphtheria can be prevented by the injection of a toxin which produces a long-lasting immunity. It is usually given with the immunization injections for whooping cough and tetanus. Boosters are administered at intervals.

People who have no symptoms of diphtheria themselves may be carriers of the bacillus. Carriers are treated with antibiotics.

**Otitis Media.** Otitis media is a collection of fluid in the middle ear which may occur in the form of pus from an infection or in the form of a sterile serous fluid. The two types of otitis media are acute suppurative otitis media and serous otitis media.

In *acute purulent otitis media,* the eardrum bulges and is in danger of rupturing. There is also a marked infection in the middle ear. Usually only one side is affected. The patient is usually in a great deal of extreme pain, with a sore neck or a red, draining ear. He may also complain of nausea and vomiting and other general malaise. The very young child who cannot explain his discomfort may show the condition by rolling his head or rubbing his ear.

Ear and throat cultures are done and appropriate antibiotics or sulfonamides are prescribed. The doctor uses the *otoscope* to examine the ear and may use a *curette* to remove wax. It is very important for the doctor to examine the *tympanic membrane* (eardrum) to determine its mobility. If it does not move, then some abnormality exists. If the eardrum is bulging or ruptured and draining, this is a definite sign of otitis media. Any signs of draining pus indicates purulent otitis media.

If the eardrum seems to be about ready to rupture, a *myringotomy* usually is done to relieve the pressure. This involves puncturing a tiny hole in the eardrum, under local anesthesia. Other surgical treatments include *simple mastoidectomy* or *adenoidectomy.* Medical treatment includes inserting some warm oil into the ear, packing it with vaseline-soaked cotton to keep out the air or water, and then applying ear drops, nose drops, and warm, moist packs to the affected ear. Aspirin is taken to combat the temperature, and if the patient is over 6 years old, codeine is prescribed for the pain. Usually, the patient receives antihistamines and decongestants.

*Serous otitis media* is a collection of serous-like fluid in the middle ear, accompanied by a fluctuating hearing loss with very little or no pain. The treatment involves restoring normal function of the eustachian tube. This may be done by the Valsalva maneuver or by the use of the Politzer bag, either of which forces air into the nasopharynx and middle ear. The patient often receives decongestants, and a corticosteroid nasal spray. (Radiation therapy is no longer used.)

It is also important to restore the hearing. Sometimes, if the eustachian tubes cannot be opened, a ventilation tube is inserted to act as a temporary or permanent accessory eustachian tube. The patient with a ventilation tube must be very careful not to get water into the ears, either by swimming or by taking a shower.

There are 5 distinct clinical stages of serous otitis media: the fluid stage, the viscid stage ("glue-ear"), the adhesive stage, the recovery stage, and the stage of complications. Although the patient often spontaneously outgrows serous otitis media by age 6 or 8, there may be permanent hearing loss.

Otitis media may be caused when the ear canal is obstructed by wax or a foreign body or by blockage of the eustachian tubes. It may also be caused by congenital malformations, such as cleft palate or by a cancer. The most common organisms responsible for suppurative otitis media are viruses or bacteria, such as streptococcus. The most common cause of serous otitis media is a chronic nasal condition caused by an allergy.

The greatest complication of otitis media is loss of hearing which may be permanent. Many children suffer such a hearing loss but go undetected until they enter school. Other complications include mastoiditis, chronic otitis media, and occasionally encephalitis or meningitis.

The most dangerous of all middle-ear diseases is that of *cholesteatoma,* which may occur in any child with recurrent, chronic otitis media. While the growth is not a true neoplasm, it grows very fast, destroying tissue and bone in the process. Thus it must be treated by immediate surgery.

Surgical procedures done for otitis media and its complications are *tympanoplasty* (reconstruction of the middle ear—either with the placement of a homograft transplant of the structure or with a prosthesis) and *myringoplasty* (reconstruction of the eardrum—usually with the graft of temporalis fascia).

**Rheumatic Fever.** Rheumatic fever is both a killer and a crippler. It is the fifth leading cause of death among children and is a leading cause of heart disease in people under the age of 50. Probably more than a million people in the United States have had some form of rheumatic fever. Usually, it occurs in children between the ages of 5 and 15 years. One attack does not guarantee immunity; on the contrary, it increases susceptibility to further attacks.

Rheumatic fever belongs to a group of diseases called *collagen diseases*; that is, diseases which affect the connective tissues throughout the body. Its specific cause is still being debated, but several facts are known. Rheumatic fever usually follows streptococcal infections, such as scarlet fever or a sore throat caused by streptococci. Authorities believe that rheumatic fever results from continued infections, in which the patient becomes sensitive to the organism or develops a type of allergic response. The disease occurs in those climates where respiratory infections are most common; it also occurs more in certain families than in others.

SYMPTOMS. The symptoms of rheumatic fever vary in degree from mild to explosively severe. Children may complain of symptoms which are not always recognized as indicating this disease. A loss of weight and appetite and fatigue and irritability may be signs. Aches, pains, and tenderness in the extremities are suspicious signs which parents might ignore as "growing pains." However, there are more definite symptoms. Rheumatic fever may begin suddenly, especially after a cold or a sore throat. The patient complains of aches and pains in the arms and the legs. The fever varies, but is highest in the evening. Then the joints of the shoulders, the elbows, the wrists, or the knees swell and become excruciatingly painful. The pain travels from one joint to another and may affect several joints at the same time. This pain usually lasts from a few days to a week in each joint and then subsides gradually. Fortunately, the arthritis of rheumatic fever does not leave joint deformities; the joints usually are completely normal after the attack.

Jerky, uncontrolled movements of the face, the neck, the arm, and the leg muscles (*chorea* or *St. Vitus Dance*), are symptoms of rheumatic fever. Small, traveling nodules formed under the skin over the elbows, the ankles, the legs, the knuckles, and at the back of the head are almost certain signs. Frequent nosebleeds may also be an indication of the disease.

Another common and serious symptom of rheumatic fever is the involvement of the heart tissues; this is called *rheumatic carditis* or *rheumatic heart disease.* The nodules develop in the heart, and lesions appear on the valves, sometimes interfering with their efficiency and increasing the workload of the also affected myocardium. The symptoms of rheumatic carditis vary from mild disease to cardiac failure.

There is no specific laboratory test which is diagnostic of rheumatic fever. An increase in the sedimentation rate of the blood cells indicates an inflammatory process within the body. Electrocardiograms are valuable in diagnosing rheumatic carditis.

TREATMENT AND NURSING CARE. The course of the disease depends primarily on whether or not the heart is involved. It usually lasts from 1 to 4 months, but once the child has had rheumatic fever, he is likely to have recurrences. The keynote in the treatment of rheumatic fever is the prevention of permanent heart damage. *Complete bedrest* is ordered. Aspirin or other salicylates are given for 3 purposes: they relieve pain, they reduce fever, and, since they are also effective anti-inflammatory medications, they assist in preventing heart damage. Cortisone therapy may also be used to limit the inflammatory processes. Antibiotics, usually penicillin, are administered to combat the hemolytic streptococci. Bedrest or limited activity is continued until the disease process is inactive.

It is fairly easy to keep a child inactive when the disease is acute. Because he is very sick, he feels like being quiet and staying in bed. However, your contact with the rheumatic fever patient may come when he is convalescing, at which point regulated activity becomes more difficult to maintain. Considerable effort is required to keep a child quiet but amused over an extended period of time.

The outcome of rheumatic fever, like its progress and the treatment, depends on the involvement of the heart. The most frequent heart damage is in the valves. Neither chorea nor arthritis is likely to leave after-effects. The carditis may be fatal, or it may result in a complete recovery—even heart murmurs may disappear. Most children recover and lead perfectly normal lives.

Because the patient who once has rheumatic fever is susceptible to recurrent attacks, many medical authorities recommend that these patients be kept on a small daily dose of a sulfa drug or penicillin for life. They can also be given monthly injections of long-acting penicillin. This is continued for 5 years after the first attack, and it prevents reinfection by the hemolytic streptococci.

HEART DISEASE AND RESTRICTION OF ACTIVITY. How does heart disease affect a child's life? The following classifications of people with heart disease, prepared by the American Heart Association, show what they can do safely:

Class I—Patients who can take part in any activity—children can go to school and do anything that the other children do.

Class II—Patients who are allowed ordinary activities, but not strenuous ones—children can go to school but must not take part in competitive sports, such as races, football, basketball, or tennis.

Class III—Patients who must be moderate about ordinary activities and must avoid strenuous ones —children can go to school but should be given extra time for such things as climbing stairs.

Class IV—Patients who definitely must limit even ordinary activities—children must learn not to run and never should be allowed to become overtired; they should also have definite rest periods.

Class V—Patients who should have complete rest—children may be allowed to sit up in a chair; they may have to stay in bed.

REHABILITATION. Providing opportunities for education, better living conditions and good medical supervision is important to help children disabled by rheumatic fever to become useful citizens. Some localities have programs underway to do these things. The federal government has given money to help states set up programs for the care of children with rheumatic fever. Individual communities are making efforts to provide medical and hospital services. As with many other health programs, a great effort is being made in the research and the care of heart disease.

THE OUTLOOK. Since penicillin is usually effective in combating rheumatic fever, much rheumatic heart disease is prevented. With the advent of prophylactic penicillin given to those who are susceptible to the streptococcus, much reinfection is avoided. For the patient whose heart valves are damaged, heart surgery is often successful and offers a good future. (See Chapter 47.)

**Tetanus.** This is a highly fatal disease, caused by a specific anerobic organism, which is characterized by convulsive contractions of all the voluntary muscles. It is preventable by a tetanus toxoid, which should be given to all children and followed up by the administration of reguar booster shots. In the case of an injury, *tetanus antitoxin* is given to prevent the disease.

**Meningitis.** Meningitis is an inflammation of the meninges of the brain, which is most common in infants and may be caused by many different microbes. The infection reaches the brain via the blood stream or by way of an ear infection or trauma to the head.

Symptoms include severe headache, high fever, vomiting, twitching, and arching of the neck and back due to spasms in the muscles, (*opisthotonos*). The patient may have seizures or delerium from the high fever. A rash may occur and the fontanels in the head may bulge. Spinal fluid is obtained for culture and sensitivity, and antibiotics are started immediately.

Nursing care includes forcing fluids, accurate recording of intake and output, and very close observation. Many complications may occur, including permanent brain damage.

**Encephalitis.** Encephalitis is an inflammation of the brain. If both the brain and the meninges are involved, it is called *encephalomyelitis*. The symptoms are similar to those of meningitis, but little specific treatment is available. The care involves the treatment of symptoms and avoidance of complications until the disease subsides. It is often fatal.

## TRAUMA

The young child, especially the one who is mobile, is extremely susceptible to injury from falling, choking, or drowning or from being poisoned, burned, or caught in a moving object. Thus the mother of the young child must be constantly on the alert to prevent accidents. However, because he is mobile

every minute, it is very difficult to watch him constantly. Thus accidents occur, killing more children than all diseases put together.

### Burns

The chief nursing problems in treating burns are combating shock, alleviating pain, and restoring fluid and electrolyte balance. (See Chapter 44 for the pathology of burns.)

The nursing care involves strict intake and output (often done every hour) and forcing of fluids (which may be difficult in a child). The child should be offered popsicles, carbonated beverages, ice cream, jello, or anything else which he will take to increase his intake of fluids. Remember that the child becomes dehydrated easier than does the adult.

The nurse must also watch the child for signs of respiratory distress, and she should be familiar with resuscitation measures for a child because the airway must be kept open. The nurse must also take careful notice of the vital signs and watch closely for shock.

The child will either be on sterile technic or on open technic depending on the individual case. In either case, he will most likely receive packs of some sort. The nurse must be sure to explain the procedures to the child and his parents so that they will cooperate in the treatment.

Itching is often a problem with children who have been burned. Since young children cannot understand that they should not scratch, measures, such as restraints, must be taken to keep the child from scratching and aggravating the burn.

A later complication which the nurse should be alert for is infection. An elevation in temperature may indicate infection or dehydration. In any case, the temperature elevation must be reported immediately. An upper respiratory infection is an especially dangerous complication in the child who has been burned.

**Determining the Extent of Burns in a Child.** Since the child's body surface differs in proportion to that of the adult, a different method of determining the extent of the burn must be used. If you remember that the infant's head is larger in proportion to his body, you will gain a better perspective of the percentages of burn.

*The newborn:* The head is 18 per cent of the entire body surface, each arm 8 per cent, each leg 13 per cent, the front or back 20 per cent, genitals 1 per cent.

*The 3-year-old:* The head is 15 per cent, each arm 8 per cent, each leg 14 per cent, the front or back 20 per cent, genitals 1 per cent.

*The 6-year-old:* The head 12 per cent, each arm 8 per cent, each leg 16 per cent, front or back 20 per cent, genitals 1 per cent.

*Over age 12* (the "Rule of Nines" applies): The head 9 per cent, each arm 9 per cent, each leg 18 per cent, front or back 18 per cent, genitals 1 per cent.

## Poisoning

The average household is literally filled with poisons, which the inquisitive toddler, obsessed with putting everything into his mouth, can easily ingest. Thus it is very easy for the young child, especially the 2-year-old boy, to be poisoned from household solutions and substances.

Since many areas have a *Poison Control Center,* the nurse should find out where it is and what number to call for first-aid information in an emergency.

She should also be aware of the fact that some paints contain excessive amounts of lead and will cause lead poisoning if chewed. Since lead poisoning is often difficult to diagnose, a simple sodium sulfide test which determines the lead content of paint should be run if there is any question.

When the child is admitted to the hospital after a poisoning, generally his stomach is washed out (gastric lavage) in an effort to remove as much of the poison as possible, except if a caustic substance, such as lye or kerosene, has been swallowed, in which case vomiting is not induced, since the poison will burn as much on the way up as it did when swallowed.

However, in most cases gastric lavage is the normal method of treatment. This is an emergency procedure, which must be done quickly to keep as much of the harmful substance from being absorbed into the blood stream as possible. However, if it has been several hours since the ingestion of a drug, the stomach may not be lavaged, since the

chances are that most of the drug will have been digested already. In this case, the symptoms would be treated.

Since you, as a practical nurse, may be asked to assist with gastric lavage, you will need to assemble the necessary equipment, such as an appropriate restraint for the child, a stomach pump or Levin tube (a very large tube), fluid for lavage (usually saline), a large basin to collect the solution after lavage, and other emergency equipment and drugs.

The nursing responsibilities include assisting the doctor with the procedure, recording all pertinent information and procedures performed by the doctor and nurses, and giving support to the patient and his family. The nurse must also be ready to assist in the following procedures: suctioning the mouth and nose to prevent aspiration, administering oxygen or resuscitative measures, starting an intravenous infusion (usually done by cutdown), assisting with a tracheostomy, passing a nasogastric tube and attaching it to suction apparatus, drawing blood samples, catheterizing for urine samples, and assisting with x-rays and electrocardiograms. The practical nurse will not usually assist the doctor alone in these procedures, but will instead help the professional nurse.

After lavage, the child is generally discharged, unless much of the poison was taken into the blood stream. In this case, he is admitted to the hospital for observation. The nursing care in this case involves observing the child for any change in level of consciousness and for any signs of dizziness, nausea and/or vomiting, bizarre behavior, extreme drowsiness, or excitement. Sometimes irreversible physical or mental changes will have occurred. Surgery occasionally must be done to correct the damage from caustic materials. Sometimes, the patient will suffer from renal failure and will need to be dialyzed. The nurse must be alert to changes in vital signs and report any symptoms of toxicity immediately.

## Foreign Objects Trapped in a Body Orifice

**Aspiration or Swallowing of Foreign Objects.** The child will often swallow or aspirate a button, peanut, pin, or other object. If it is not sharp and has already entered the intestinal tract, and seems to be moving through the intestines, it will generally be allowed to pass through. The nursing care would involve close observation of the stools to ascertain when the foreign object is excreted.

If an object is aspirated into the lungs, it may be coughed out. If not, bronchoscopy or lung surgery may be necessary to remove the object, since it may cause an infection if allowed to remain in the lungs.

**A Foreign Object in the Eye.** Many times a child will get a cinder or other object in his eye and will irritate it further by scratching or rubbing. Sometimes surgery is necessary to remove the object, if ordinary first-aid measures are not effective.

**Objects in the Nose or Ears.** Many times children will put small objects, such as buttons or peanuts into their ears or noses, and then will be unable to remove them. Since a serious infection can result, the object must be removed by the doctor.

**Objects in the Rectum or Vagina.** These objects must be removed very carefully to prevent damage to the tissues.

**Prevention.** Small objects should be kept out of reach of young children as much as possible. Children should be taught never to put anything into a body orifice. The mother must be constantly on the alert for dangerous objects, many of which she would never suspect of causing harm.

## Fractures

Although children's bones are not as brittle as those of adults, children receive more blows and injuries and thus sustain a great many fractures, many of which occur when a child falls from a high chair or crib or tumbles out of a car or down the stairs. Falls are also frequent among children with nervous system disorders which impair balance and coordination. On the other hand, numerous fractures occur when a child is abused by parents or guardians. (The nursing care of the patient with a fracture is discussed in Chapter 45.)

## Lacerations, Puncture Wounds, Abrasions, and Crushing Injuries

Many children come into the emergency room with various cuts and punctures sustained by knives, forks, pencils, and other sharp objects found in the home. The obvious prevention is to keep these items out of reach of the child.

The child may also sustain a crushing injury after being caught in a wringer or a car door or under a heavy piece of furniture or a moving bicycle. The child may also suffer multiple bruises and abrasions following a fall from a tricycle, a wagon, or an automobile.

Many of these injuries are not serious enough for the child to be admitted to the hospital. They are treated by sewing (suturing) up the laceration, applying antiseptics and dressings to the abrasions, and taking x-rays of the crushing injury to determine the possible presence of a fracture. The child also usually receives a tetanus booster. Puncture wounds, especially, are watched for signs of later infection and are kept open as much as possible so they can drain. The mother may be instructed to soak the wound periodically to facilitate drainage.

## Dog Bites and Cat Scratches

**Dog Bites.** A dog bite can be very serious. Sometimes, the dog is one which the child has played with for some time, when suddenly, the dog bites the child. Frequently, the face is the area bitten. Many dog bites are very severe, requiring plastic surgery or reconstructive surgery.

The dog should be watched for signs of rabies and illness. If the dog does become ill, the child must be treated to prevent the disease. It is extremely rare for a person to survive a case of rabies, once the disease develops. Recovery has been documented on only 1 occasion, to date. When a child is bitten, he should be given a tetanus booster to make sure he is protected against that disease.

**Cat Scratches.** The most dangerous complication of a cat scratch is infection. However, more serious complications can occur if the cat scratches the child in the area of the eyes. As in the case of dog bites, the cat must be watched for signs of rabies.

## Suffocation

Suffocation may occur when a foreign object is aspirated or when a child is smothered with a plastic bag or pillow. To prevent this latter occurrence the very small child should not have a pillow because he is unable to turn his head and may very easily suffocate. Suffocation may also occur in a small infant who has an upper respiratory infection and cannot cough out the mucus which is plugging his bronchi. He may also be too small to turn over or to breathe through his mouth. Humidity usually helps to loosen secretions enough so the child can cough them up.

## Crib Death

"Crib death" is a sudden and unexplained death in a seemingly healthy infant. It occurs in about 1 out of 350 infants and seems to be more common among males than females. It also seems to be more common when the mother is very young or a heavy cigarette smoker or when the child is born at a low-birth weight. Most researchers feel that it is caused by a virus, although none have as yet been isolated. It does not seem to be due to neglect on the part of the parents.

## The "Battered Child" Syndrome

Until recently, the term "battered child" was not used in medical practice, because it was very difficult for a doctor to accuse parents of mistreating their child. More recently, legislation has been passed in most states, allowing the doctor to report suspected cases of child abuse without fear of prosecution.

In the past, it was felt that the head of the household was the ruler whom the children must obey, no matter what. It is now felt that the child also has rights which protect him against beatings and neglect. As more evidence is gathered, it is obvious that the incidence of battered children is much greater than was previously realized. It is estimated that, if all cases were reported, child abuse would be one of the leading causes of death among children in this country. About 15,000 cases of child abuse are reported each year, and the number is increasing. About 5 per cent of these children die and about 25 per cent of them are permanently injured as a result of abuse.

The definition of child abuse applies not only to the child who has been beaten and physically abused, but also to the malnourished, unsupervised, nonschool attending child, as well as the child who is denied love and medical care. For our purposes, however the definition of battered child, will be limited to physical abuse.

Usually, the children who are abused are under 3 years of age and sustain common injuries such as fractures or bruises, although some are also cut, sexually molested, burned, or choked. The most frequent offenders are the mother or father.

When the history of the battered child is examined, certain characteristic findings emerge: the general health of the child indicates neglect, the child has fractures which seem to have occurred at different times, the child often has a history of previous admissions for similar causes, and no new injuries occur while the child is in the hospital.

If the doctor reports the case as a suspected case of child abuse, the parents must understand that the purpose of the doctor's actions is to prevent further injury to the child or possible death. The child who has a history of being beaten may be placed under the care of a social agency and assigned to a foster home for care.

The recommendations for prevention of child abuse are set forth by Vincent Fontana, M.D. in *The Maltreated Child*. He states that persons in the community must be aware of their responsibilities to protect children, that governmental agencies must assist in seeing to it that the essential needs of children are met, that agencies should be set up to protect children from abuse, that troubled parents should receive assistance, and that cases of child neglect or abuse should be reported by all responsible citizens. Thus, the nurse, as a citizen, should feel responsible for reporting a suspected case of child neglect or abuse to the proper authorities.

However, the nurse must realize that the person who feels it necessary to abuse a child has emotional problems and needs treatment. These parents are often very young and immature and may be unable to accept the responsibilities and challeges of life. Or they may abuse their child because they came from a home in which abuse was the way of life and the accepted pattern of discipline.

# GASTROINTESTINAL DISORDERS

## Congenital Abnormalities

**Pyloric Stenosis (Congenital Hypertrophic Pyloric Stenosis).** In this condition, the pyloric sphincter of the stomach is unable to function because it becomes thick and narrow. Thus, as the peristalsis moves the food within the stomach, the pyloris remains closed, preventing the food from passing into the intestines. The food is then regurgitated back into the esophagus, causing severe vomiting, the most common symptom of the disorder.

The newborn usually does not show signs of this condition until he is a few weeks old. If not, it will usually be apparent by the time the child is 2 months old. Statistics show that pyloric stenosis is more common in males, in whites, and in first-born infants.

The symptoms include vomiting, which becomes projectile in nature, loss of weight, hunger, irritability, and dehydration. Often, constipation and oliguria accompany this condition. Definite diagnosis is made on the basis of a barium swallow.

The treatment may be purely medical, including gastric lavage feeding and the administration of antispasmodic and sedative drugs. The condition will usually resolve itself within the first 3 or 4 months of life. If, however, the infant is severely dehydrated or suffering from malnutrition, surgical intervention may be required. This is the most commonly followed procedure in the United States, because it gives fast relief and is usually successful. The surgical procedure is called a pyloromyotomy and involves splitting the hypertrophied pyloris sphincter down to the mucous membrane (Fredet-Remstedt procedure).

Preoperatively, the infant is given intravenous fluid therapy for hydration purposes and thickened oral feedings, usually following the administration of a muscle relaxant, such as atropine. An accurate record of intake and output is vital as well as a clear notation of the amount and type of regurgitation which occurs.

Postoperative care involves special precautions to prevent aspiration or other respiratory distress. The baby is positioned on his side, with head slightly elevated. Glucose water or plain water feedings are usually started soon after the surgery. The child usually recovers without complication.

**Chalasia.** Frequent vomiting in a newborn infant may occur because of an inadequately functioning cardiac sphincter in the stomach (chalasia), which allows feedings to be regurgitated back into the esophagus. If the baby does not become dehydrated or malnourished, he will probably not need treatment since this condition usually resolves itself. A barium swallow will indicate the precise reason for the chalasia. If the condition is caused by a hiatus hernia or an abnormally short esophagus, surgery may be necessary.

**Meckel's Diverticulum.** This congenital disorder involves a small portion of the ileum which ends in a blind pouch just before its junction with the colon. The symptoms include the passage of bloody or tarry stools without pain. Surgery is done to remove the pouch, and complications are rare.

**Hernias.** A hernia is caused when any structure does not sufficiently close at birth, allowing a portion of intestine or another structure to pass through it abnormally.

There are several types of hernias. A *diaphragmatic hernia,* which is relatively rare, occurs when a portion of the intestine passes through the diaphragm. An *umbilical hernia* involves the protrusion of a portion of the intestine through a weak umbilical ring. Since this condition usually disappears by the time the child is 3 or 4, surgery is not needed. Occasionally, an umbilical binder is applied to reduce the hernia. Strangulation very rarely occurs in these instances, although surgery may be necessary if the omphalocele (the protruding portion of intestine) is very large or if other congenital defects are also present.

In an *inguinal hernia,* which occurs more frequently in males, the intestine protrudes through the round ligament into the inguinal area and descends into the scrotal sac. If strangulation occurs, surgery must be done. If surgery is not required, the application of a support (*truss*) will often be enough to allow the muscles to strengthen and cause the hernia to disappear. When an inguinal hernia occurs in the female, the ovary or the uterus may be involved, thereby requiring immediate surgery to prevent these structures from being damaged by lack of circulation.

An *omphalocele* is a large inguinal hernia which usually does not have any skin covering. Since the peritoneum which covers the protruding abdominal contents is transparent, the contents can be visualized. The omphalocele may contain all or part of the abdominal contents. The danger of this condition is possible rupture, in which case the child would hemorrhage or contract peritonitis or a generalized septicemia. Thus, surgery is usually done early in life to correct a large hernia of this type.

**Phenylketonuria.** Phenylketonuria (PKU) is a hereditary defect in metabolism, caused by a defect or absence of a liver enzyme which is important in the synthesis of proteins in the body. If untreated, this condition leads to a severe and profound retardation, which begins during the first year of life.

PKU can be determined by a simple urine test, 5 to 10 days after birth. The test, which is most often done with a paper strip, such as the Phenistix, indicates the presence of phenylpyruvic acid in the urine, a substance not present in the urine of the normal child. Although the test will not be effective in the first few days after birth, some states require that the test be done in the newborn nursery soon after birth. Since the condition may not show up at this time and since the test may give a false positive, it should be repeated when the infant receives his 6-week check-up. However, if there is any question, the test should be repeated sooner, since treatment is more effective the sooner it begins. Once the child begins to show symptoms of PKU, the damage is irreversible, but treatment will prevent further damage. Siblings and other children in the family should also be tested to determine if they have the disorder.

The treatment is mainly dietary. Since the child cannot metabolize protein, and since the protein builds up the dangerous substances in the blood and urine, raw protein must be avoided. However, since protein is a necessary substance for normal growth, a substitute must be given. Foods which must be omitted from the diet include meats, fish, poultry, eggs, cheese, milk, nuts, and legumes. The substitute formula, such as Lofenalac, offers protein to the child in a form which can be used by his body. This diet should be started as soon as the child is diagnosed, since even a week or two can make a difference in later IQ levels.

It is not known how long the child must be maintained on this special diet to prevent retardation, although most of the damage seems to occur during the first 3 years of life. After the age of 3 or 4, the child can often return to a normal diet without sustaining damage.

## Other Gastrointestinal Disorders

**Intestinal Obstruction.** An intestinal obstruction may occur as a result of poor peristalsis, a neoplasm, an ingested foreign object, or a stricture. In any event, intestinal obstruction usually requires immediate surgery to prevent rupture and peritonitis or gangrene. Other measures which may be tried are nasogastric suction and antispasmodic and pain-relief drugs.

The patient will have nausea and vomiting, although the nausea will not be relieved by the vomiting or by food or a laxative. There may also be severe pain. The symptoms vary somewhat depending upon the cause, the location of the obstruction, and whether the obstruction is partial or complete. The newborn may suffer from intestinal obstruction simply as a result of underdeveloped or spasmodic muscles. Often this can be relieved medically, although at times surgery is needed.

**Intussusception.** Intussusception refers to the telescoping of one part of bowel into another. This is usually caused by hyperactive peristalsis in one part of the bowel compared with hypoactivity in the other part. One danger is that the blood supply may be cut off, causing gangrene. This condition is most common in infants, usually occurring in those who have been doing well. A definite diagnosis is based on a barium enema, and immediate surgery is needed to prevent complications. Pre- and postoperative care are routine, and the healthy child will seldom have complications.

## METABOLIC DISORDERS AND NUTRITIONAL DEFICIENCIES

### Malnutrition (Marasmus)

This condition is often diagnosed as "failure to thrive," and unless it is caused by a physical disorder, it serves as another example of the abused child. However, specific conditions may be caused by a lack of a certain nutrient in the diet (see Chapter 22). Examples of this are *kwashiorkor* (deficiency of protein), *rickets* (defect in calcification of the bones, caused by a deficiency of Vitamin D), and *scurvy* (deficiency of Vitamin C).

General malnutrition or starvation may occur as a result of a general systemic disease or a malabsorption problem or as a result of neglect or abuse on the part of the parents.

The symptoms of starvation (*marasmus*) are edema, lowered blood volume and blood pressure, lowered body temperature, and a general appearance of unhealthiness. The child often has a protruding abdomen and sunken eyes and is generally weak and listless. The physical growth of the child lags behind that of normal children of the same age, and mental development may also be retarded, simply because of lack of nourishment.

Nursing care involves restoration of hydration and nutrition, maintenance of body temperature, and general "tender loving care." The child usually will respond well to the treatment.

Other nutritional problems include undernutrition and overnutrition. *Undernutrition* is a condition in which the child continually receives less food than he needs to develop optimally. *Overnutrition* is evidenced by obesity in children and more often occurs in adolescence. Childhood obesity can generally be controlled by diet, unless there is a physical or glandular cause, which is rare.

### Biliary Atresia

One cause of malnutrition may be biliary atresia, a defect in the bile ducts which does not allow bile to escape. This causes a lack of bile in the body and thus, a defect in digestion as well as in elimination. In some cases, surgery must be done to relieve the obstruction.

### Megacolon (Hirschspring's Disease)

This condition involves the presence of an abnormally large colon, which may be either congenital or acquired. The congenital form is more common and is referred to as Hirschsprung's disease, which involves the nervous network that controls the movements of the colon. In the case of acquired megacolon, surgical treatment may be effective if it can remove the damaged or malfunctioning portion of the colon. In congenital megacolon, the entire colon is usually affected and palliative treatment may be necessary. For our purposes we will limit our discussion to Hirschsprung's disease, the congenital form of megacolon.

The symptoms of this disease are those caused by an accumulation of feces in the bowel, which cannot be excreted. The abdomen becomes very abnormally distended, and the child does not have normal bowel movements. He may have diarrhea, constipation, or watery stools. He may also have nausea and vomiting, with resultant malnutrition.

The diagnosis is made on the basis of medical history, x-ray studies and barium enema, and palpitation of the distended abdomen. A proctoscopy usually reveals an empty rectum and lower colon, and biopsy of the rectal wall usually shows an absence of nerve fibers.

Treatment is aimed at preventing complications. The portion of bowel which is affected may be removed, or the entire bowel may be removed and a colostomy done. If this is not possible, medical management must be used as a palliative measure. This includes prevention of constipation by means of small enemas, stool softeners, and digital removal of fecal impactions. Sometimes, colonic irrigations are done, which is much like an enema except that a larger tube is used and is passed up into the descending colon. Drugs, such as Prostigmin and atropine, which affect the parasympathetic and sympathetic nervous systems, may be given to alter the peristalsis.

With advances in medical treatment, many of these children live and are able to lead a normal life.

## Glutin-Induced Celiac Disease

The most common malabsorption syndrome in children, which results from mucosal absorptive defects, is called celiac disease. Celiac disease is thought to be congenital, although its effects may not show up for several months or years. Usually the condition shows up within 6 months after birth. (A malabsorption disorder in adults may be called *sprue*.)

Celiac disease is a chronic intestinal disorder of infants and young children and is characterized by enormous, floating, fatty stools, lack of appetite, malnutrition, distended abdomen, excess flatus, and arrested growth. A familial tendency is shown in that more than 1 child in a family may have the disorder. The disorder may vary in degree from mild to very severe. The more severe form of the disorder will be discussed here.

The basic defect in celiac disease is the inability to absorb fat and, to a lesser degree, carbohydrate. These substances are excreted in the stools, causing the stools to be fatty and floating. Malnutrition results from the lack of carbohydrate in the body. The body is specifically unable to absorb wheat and rye protein and remission in symptoms is often observed after these substances are omitted from the diet. Breast feeding seems to postpone the appearance of symptoms. Thus, because of increased use of artificial feeding, we are seeing younger children with this disorder.

**Celiac Crisis.** Usually, during the first 2 years of life, the child will display symptoms, such as large and watery stools, vomiting, and a very distended abdomen. This same child previously will have shown irregular weight gain and periods of occasional vomiting, but the crisis is suddenly more severe.

In the case of celiac crisis, the child becomes dehydrated and the fluid and electrolyte balance is severely upset. The child is treated symptomatically, as an emergency. Intravenous fluids are administered and occasionally steroid therapy is used. This condition must be differentiated from cystic fibrosis of the pancreas.

After the crisis, diet therapy is begun, which excludes all forms of starch or just wheat and rye glutin. Once diet therapy is begun, rapid improvement and weight gain often follow. The increased weight may cause the child to be slightly obese, since it is not always accompanied by a gain in height.

Many of these children do very well on the special diet and are able to live normal lives. It is believed that sprue in adults is the same condition and should be managed by the same dietary means which will most likely be necessary for life.

## Cystic Fibrosis (Collagen Disease)

Cystic fibrosis of the pancreas or *mucoviscidosis,* presents a much different picture than glutin-induced celiac disease. This condition is chronic and incurable and is managed by palliative or symptomatic means only. The child often dies as a result of complications, which occur most often in the respiratory system, as a result of the very thick, tenacious mucus. With active treatment, some children live past adolescence, and even longer.

This disease is hereditary and tends to show a familial tendency. It is rare in Negro people and absent in Mongolian races. The disease shows up first as a malabsorption syndrome with celiac symptoms and later shows respiratory or cardiac manifestations.

The child will first show very thick, sticky stools, which have a strong odor. Although he has a good appetite, he will not gain weight. He looks emaciated, although his abdomen is large. He suffers from malnutrition because he is not absorbing *fat-soluble* vitamins properly.

Diagnosis is made on the basis of stool specimens, which contain fats, and pulmonary function testing, which evaluates the respiratory involvement. Specific diagnosis is made on the basis of excessive salt in the perspiration. A sweat test is done to determine the content of the perspiration. An abnormally large amount of sodium chloride (salt) is generally considered indicative of a positive diagnosis, in combination with the other symptoms.

**Problems of Cystic Fibrosis.** The problems in the child with this disorder are caused by abnormal secretions of mucus-producing glands, whereby an abnormal amount of viscid secretions collects in the lungs, the pancreas, and the liver.

The patient is treated with massive doses of antibiotics to prevent infections, especially those of the lungs. Dietary control is aimed at improving the quality of the stools, increasing the amount of vitamins, and improving respiratory symptoms. A high calorie, high protein diet is given, with supplementary vitamins, since nutritional problems are present in 80 per cent of cases. Pancreatic extract is given, as well as salt in hot weather.

The lungs are treated actively, since respiratory involvement is present in virtually all of the cases. The patient received frequent IPPB treatments designed to liquefy mucus and prevent obstruction and pulmonary infections. The patient should sleep in a humidity tent, where a drug such as propylene glycol can be inhaled in mist form. The patient is taught exercises which will increase his lung capacity and is instructed in postural drainage. The small child may need suctioning. (Many of these procedures are discussed in Chapter 31.) Bronchodilators are given, as well as iodides to thin the secretions. The patient is usually on a prophylactic antibiotic. Physical therapy measures are used to assist the patient to cough up secretions.

The child must maintain his immunity to such diseases as measles, influenza, and pertussis. Gamma globulin given on a regular basis is not recommended but may be used if the child becomes ill or is exposed to a respiratory infection.

Surgery may be necessary to treat such problems as intussusception, intestinal obstruction, or pulmonary disorders.

The emotional aspects in relationship to cystic fibrosis are many. The child and his parents may have difficulty in accepting the necessary medical regimen, the physical and dietary restrictions, and the uncertainty of the future. The family may encounter problems with other children in the family and may have severe financial difficulties as a result of the equipment and medications needed for the care of the ill child. The adult who has the disease faces the decisions regarding marriage and children. Genetic counseling plays a part in the life of the adult cystic fibrosis victim.

With early detection, good medical care, and strict adherence to the medical treatment, the prognosis for this disease has greatly improved in the past few years.

## Diabetes

A general discussion of diabetes mellitus can be found in Chapter 52. As for diabetes in a child, the nurse must remember that, generally, the younger a child is when he shows symptoms of diabetes, the more difficult he will be to treat. He is more likely to be a brittle (hard to control) diabetic and to develop other complications. However, the child should be taught to administer his own insulin, as soon as he is old enough.

## Colic

*Colic* is a troublesome problem for the infant's mother, but fortunately is not a dangerous condition for the infant. It occurs more frequently in infants who are very small at birth, and is marked by frequent spurts of sudden crying, with the infant doubling up at times as though in great pain. These symptoms seem to be worse in the evening. Many doctors believe that the nervous mother is more likely to have a colicky baby.

Treatment involves feeding the baby slowly and using bottles with disposable, collapsible bags to reduce the amount of air which the infant swallows. Other methods, such as changing the type of formula or administering specific drugs such as antispasmodics or tranquilizers, are also used. In any event, the baby almost always outgrows the condition by the time he is 3 or 4 months old.

## NEUROLOGICAL OR SENSORY DISORDERS

### Congenital Abnormalities

**Encephalocele.** If the bones of the skull do not close correctly, a portion of the brain may protrude through the opening. The chief danger in this condition is possible rupture of the meningeal sac, leading almost inevitably to meningitis or encephalitis. The defect is surgically corrected, but sometimes not until the child is a year old. Until surgery is done, meticulous nursing care is necessary to prevent damage.

The amount of damage or defect in the function of the child depends upon the size and location of the encephalocele, as well as the presence or absence of strangulation or rupture.

**Spina Bifida.** Spina bifida ("cleft spine") is a malformation of the spine (usually the lower spine) in which a part of the vertebral or spinal column is missing or open. The condition may be asymptomatic or may cause severe paralysis, depending upon how large the opening is and upon whether or not the meninges or spinal cord herniates through the opening. There are various forms of this disorder as indicated below.

*Spina bifida occulta* is the condition in which there is an opening in the vertebral column, but no symptoms are apparent. The only way in which this defect is discovered is if an x-ray is taken or if an investigation is done because a dimple is present over the backbone or a small tuft of hair or a port-wine stain occurs in the vertebral area. Although this condition may cause problems when the child undergoes a growth spurt during puberty, it generally does not cause difficulty. It is easily corrected surgically, although even this is rarely needed.

A *meningocele* occurs when some of the meninges (covering of the spinal cord) protrude or herniate through the opening in the vertebral column.

The most serious form of spina bifida is a *meningomyelocele* (or myelomeningocele) in which the meninges and a part of the spinal cord itself protrude through the opening. In this case, the patient may be paralyzed or weakened, and may have bladder and bowel control problems. Serious complications can occur, including meningitis or encephalitis and hydrocephalus. Although surgery is usually done early in life, the nurse must handle the defect with great care because any damage which occurs cannot be reversed.

Surgical procedures may be done to prevent rupture of the sac, to prevent further damage, and to improve the cosmetic appearance of the child. In some instances the patient with a meningocele will have no after-effects. On the other hand, he may have muscle weakness and some difficulty with bowel and bladder control, although he rarely suffers from any paralysis. Generally, this child will lead a normal life after surgery.

NURSING CARE. The prevention of further damage in the child with spina bifida is a nursing challenge and should be handled with skill and knowledge. The most common effect is loss of sensation in the legs, in which case, the nurse must be sure to protect the child against possible leg injury. Careful examination is also necessary to check for pressure areas and tight clothing which can be very irritating. Good skin care must be given, and the baby must be changed immediately after voiding or defecating.

The nurse also assists in the medical and pre- and postoperative surgical management of the child. Although this child is managed much like any other patient with a neurological disorder, certain precautions must be taken, such as preventing infection, not only in the area of the defect, but also in the rest of the body. A common site for infection is the urinary bladder. Many of these children must be catheterized, which can predispose them to infection if the procedure is not properly managed. The lack of muscle control also predisposes the child to infection, even if he does not have a catheter. If kidney damage or other urinary system damage has occurred, a urinary tract diversion may need to be done. (See Chapter 50.)

Since it is important to prevent musculoskeletal deformities, the nurse must pay special attention to how the child is positioned and see that he has a chance to do range-of-motion exercises. The child usually is seen by the physical therapist who prescribes any special exercises which may be necessary. Sometimes, orthopedic surgery must be done to correct deformities, which are either congenital or acquired. The nurse also plays a great part in providing psychological assistance to the parents of a child with spina bifida. Since parents find it very hard to accept this condition, the nurse must understand how they feel and help them to verbalize their feelings.

**Hydrocephalus.** As you know, the brain and spinal cord are enclosed in spinal fluid, which circulates constantly. If something stops or slows down this constant circulation, fluid collects in the head and brain area and causes swelling of the head and damage to the brain. The condition known as *hydrocephalus* ("water head") most often develops because the brain or spinal cord is not properly developed or because a spinal cord defect such as spina bifida exists. It can also occur, however, as a complication of meningitis, head injury, or hemorrhage from a cranial blood vessel.

The symptoms of hydrocephalus include the progressive enlargement of the head as the sutures in the cranial bones open, the progressive atrophy of the brain as the pressure increases and at times the occurrence of seizures. The child becomes unable to control voluntary muscle movements and may die from respiratory complications, malnutrition, or infection.

Diagnosis is made on the basis of lumbar puncture, pneumoencephalogram, and ventriculograms. The only treatment is to surgically insert a shunt, or bypass, which will allow the fluid to circulate around the defect or the blockage. This procedure should be done as soon as is possible, because any brain damage which may occur is irreversible.

Preoperatively, the child is given good nursing care to prevent skin breakdown and gavage feedings to prevent malnutrition. Every possible precaution is taken to prevent any type of infection.

Postoperatively, the child is observed carefully for any signs of shock or hemorrhage, and the incisional area must be carefully observed for leakage of spinal fluid. Vital signs are taken and deep breathing is encouraged to prevent pneumonia.

The child is positioned on the side away from the operative side to prevent damage to the shunt valve. Accurate recording of intake and output must be done to determine if the child is retaining fluids. Usually, an intravenous feeding is given.

Since not all shunts are effective, the nurse must observe carefully for any signs of *increasing intracranial pressure,* such as bulging fontanels or changes in eye signs or level of consciousness. Another frequent complication is that of *infection,* which must be reported immediately. The parents should also be taught to watch for these complications, since they may occur at any time after shunt surgery. If the shunt is done before brain damage occurs and if it is successful, the child will be able to lead a normal life.

**Microcephalus.** The microcephalic child is one whose brain does not grow. Thus the head tends to be small because of the small size of the brain. The child will be mentally retarded to a degree determined by the size of the brain. This condition is congenital and may be caused by the mother taking drugs during pregnancy or contracting an infection, such as German measles, while pregnant.

Since no cure is known, the child is treated symptomatically and should be encouraged to do as much as possible.

**Craniostenosis.** This is a condition which occurs when the fontanels in the skull close before they should, resulting in a head which is too small to allow for normal development of the brain. If one suture closes and others remain open, various malformations of the head can occur.

Craniostenosis must be treated surgically as soon as possible to prevent brain damage, blindness, seizures, and other disorders. The surgery, which consists of opening the suture lines by means of craniotomy, is usually successful, although it may need to be repeated.

## Other Brain Disorders

**Seizure Disorders.** Seizure disorders are fairly common in children. A high fever, especially in children, may cause a seizure, although a single seizure of this type does not necessarily constitute a seizure disorder.

Childhood seizure disorders which generally show up between 4 and 8 years of age, may be *ideopathic* (without known cause) or hereditary. Seizure disorders may also be caused by *organic* difficulties, such as brain tumors or hemorrhage, head trauma, poisoning, or, as mentioned before, high fever. If at all possible the cause of the seizures should be determined so that it may be removed.

Any child admitted to a hospital with a history of seizures, as well as any child with a high fever, should be placed on "seizure precautions."

Details concerning the nursing care and diagnosis of seizure disorders can be found in Chapter 46. However, we should note here that the early diagnosis and treatment of seizure disorders in a child can prevent many problems. If the child can be maintained on anticonvulsant drugs, he may be able to live a normal life. However, the most important aspect of childhood seizure disorders is their psychological impact. The child must be assisted to develop normally and not to feel ridiculed, retarded, or exceptionally different, because of his seizures. Most states have epilepsy associations which help parents in the emotional development of their child.

**Brain Tumors.** As you know, any brain tumor is serious, whether it is cancerous or not, because the increase in size of the tumor puts undue pressure upon the brain and causes possible brain damage. Very young children are less likely to have malignant tumors than are older people. The most common tumors in children are gliomas of the cerebellum, the brain stem, or the optic nerve, pinealomas (tumors of the pituitary), and congenital tumors. The tumors seen in children are more likely to be fast-growing and are often inoperable. However, whenever possible, immediate surgery is required to prevent further complications. (For symptoms of brain tumors see Chapter 46.)

## URINARY AND REPRODUCTIVE (GENITOURINARY) DISORDERS

### Congenital Abnormalities

**Exstrophy of the Bladder.** Exstrophy of the bladder, which is more common in boys, occurs when the 2 sides of the lower abdomen fail to grow together, thereby exposing the bladder.

The nursing care of the infant with this condition consists of positioning the child on his side or back and keeping the bladder area as clean and dry as possible. Sometimes, the exposed bladder is kept moist with ointments or saline packs. Surgery is usually not done until the child is about 3 or 4 years old, at which time, the bladder is removed and the urine is diverted into the colon. The child thereafter must be assisted to learn to hold urine within his rectum.

**Hermaphroditism.** If any doubt arises about the true sex of the child, immediate studies must be done to determine if the child

is a boy or girl. The buccal mucosa or skin structure may be examined to indicate whether a female or male chromosomal pattern is present. Hormonal studies may also be done as well as anatomical studies. It is vital to the psychological development of a child to determine whether it is a male or a female, as soon after birth as possible.

Depending on the physical problem, treatment may be surgical, to revise or remove structures, or medical, to provide the appropriate hormones.

**Other Congenital Genitourinary Defects.** Hypospadias and epispadias are conditions involving the abnormal location of the urinary meatus. In *hypospadias* the urinary meatus is located on the bottom of the penis; in *epispadias* the meatus is located on the top part of the penis. These conditions can usually be surgically corrected and are not life-threatening. Minor hypospadias is quite common and is not corrected unless it becomes pronounced.

Other congenital defects can occur, such as the absence of one kidney or the presence of an extra kidney, misplacement of structures, or a closed urinary meatus.

*Polycystic kidney* (discussed in Chapter 50) is a condition in which the child has many cysts or tumors on the kidney. If the condition is bilateral, treatment is not effective.

*Cryptorchidism* or undescended testicle (discussed in Chapter 51) often occurs at birth, but usually corrects itself spontaneously. If not, surgical treatment is done in early childhood to prevent sterility.

### Other Genitourinary Conditions

**Hydrocele.** A hydrocele is an accumulation of serous fluid within the scrotal sac, which can become very large and painful. Often, the fluid will reabsorb spontaneously, but if it does not, the hydrocele may need to be excised and drained.

**Nephritis (Pyelonephritis).** Nephritis refers to an inflammation of the kidney, which can develop into a potentially dangerous condition. (See Chapter 50 for more detailed discussion.)

This condition is the most common childhood renal disorder, usually occurring in the child under the age of 3. Symptoms include high fever, anorexia, painful voiding, and abdominal tenderness and pain. The organism must be cultured and sensitivities done in order to prescribe the appropriate antibiotics. Treatment includes daily weighing, intake and output records, good skin care, forcing fluids, and measures to reduce the fever.

Generally, this condition is curable. The danger lies in the fact that if nephritis is untreated, it can lead to chronic nephritis, which can lead in turn to uremia and death.

**Acute Glomerulonephritis (Bright's Disease).** This condition is the most common type of nephritis found in young children and is a result of an immunologic reaction to infection, especially streptococcus. Damage may occur to the glomeruli of the kidneys and the urine output may decrease or stop. The condition usually subsides, but the patient may need to be maintained on dialysis. Children are much more likely to recover from this disease than are adults. However, the disease may progress to chronic glomerulonephritis, which is not curable.

**Nephrosis.** This is a condition in which the kidney actually degenerates. It occurs most often in children between the ages of $1\frac{1}{2}$ and 5 years and is characterized by a generalized edema and the presence of protein or blood in the urine. In addition, the urine output is scant and the patient has a high blood pressure and temperature. His abdomen is very distended and he is very uncomfortable. The child with nephrosis does not eat because of the collection of fluid in the abdomen and chest cavities. He is also very prone to other infections, such as pneumonia.

Nursing care involves palliative measures designed to treat the symptoms. The edema is reduced by administration of drugs and, at times, by the limiting of fluids as well as of salt intake. The nurse should encourage the child to eat and protect him as much as possible from exposure to infections. Special skin care is needed, and the child must be assisted to move about in bed. The child may be more comfortable while sitting up, because he will often have difficulty in breathing.

This child is very ill and needs expert nursing care, as well as a great deal of emotional support and kindness. Many of these children show remissions upon administration of steroids, but the disease is often not curable. Because the administration of steroids carries its own side-effects, such as the typical "moon face," the child is often concerned about his or her appearance.

With continued treatment and prevention of infection for several years, a remission of the disease may occur. The parents must be assisted to understand that the child has a chronic disease and will need treatment and follow-up for the rest of his life.

**Wilms's Tumor (Nephroblastoma).** This is a very malignant adenosarcoma of the kidney, which is most common in the child under the age of 3 and can begin growing even before the child is born. It is one of the more common neoplasms of childhood and is usually unilateral.

The tumor usually does not cause any symptoms until it is far advanced. Microscopic hematuria may be present but usually not until late in the course of the disease. As in many other kidney tumors, the prognosis is poor, because the disease is so far advanced by the time it is discovered.

Diagnosis is made on the basis of palpation of the mass in the abdomen, x-ray studies, and biopsy during laparotomy. If the tumor does not excrete I.V. dye, this means that the blood vessels of the kidney are involved, indicating a very poor prognosis.

The only treatment is immediate surgical removal, followed by irradiation not only to the site of the tumor but on both sides of the spine. In addition chemotherapy is often used. Radiation and chemotherapy may be used in cases in which the tumor is too far advanced for surgical removal.

Preoperative nursing care involves building the child up, so that he is in the best possible physical health and taking good care of the skin and mouth. The nurse should be careful not to palpate the abdomen, because this might cause the tumor to metastasize.

Postoperative nursing care is routine, with special attention to intake and output and observation of the urine. The care of the patient who is having radiation or chemotherapy is discussed in Chapter 43.

**Urinary Obstruction.** A urinary obstruction may occur as a result of a neoplasm, a stone, or a severe infection. It is important to relieve the obstruction to prevent complications, such as hydronephrosis. Usually, catheterization or administration of antibiotics will be effective, but if not, surgery is done to remove the obstruction.

**Renal Failure.** Renal failure is a very serious illness and usually must be controlled by use of dialysis or kidney transplant. It can be caused by a number of conditions, such as poisoning, chronic nephritis, and severe anaphylactic reactions. (See Chapter 50 for a more detailed discussion.)

**Enuresis.** Enuresis is generally a psychological disorder in which the child is unable to control his bladder, especially at night. The child should first be examined to determine if there is a physical reason for the problem, such as severe infections, trauma to the bladder, diabetes, small-bladder capacity, or bladder spasm. However, if there is no physical cause, the underlying emotional problem should be sought. If the condition persists into grade school, psychiatric assistance may be necessary.

## BLOOD DEFECTS

### Blood Dyscrasias

**Sickle-Cell Anemia (Sicklemia).** This is a hereditary type of blood condition which is more common in Blacks than in white people, and is caused by extensive red blood cell destruction. Since it is carried as a recessive gene, both parents must have the gene in order to cause clinical disease in the child.

Symptoms, in addition to the anemia, are jaundice, ulcerated areas around the ankles, and nausea and vomiting. The patient may also suffer from hemiplegia or other symptoms of cerebral vascular insufficiency.

The treatment is symptomatic. No cure is known, and very few people with this disease live beyond age 40. The patient should avoid high altitudes and nonpressurized planes because the decrease in pressure increases the sickling tendency.

**Hemophilia.** Hemophilia is a hereditary, sex-linked, recessive, bleeding disorder which occurs almost always in males, although carried by females. The most common type of hemophilia is called Hemophilia A and is a deficiency of antihemophilic globulin, which is called Factor VIII. The person tends to hemorrhage, even after a very slight injury, with the hemorrhage often going deep into the tissues, causing possible severe damage to tissue, nerve, or blood vessels. Often there is severe pain in the area of the hemorrhage, especially if the bleeding is into a joint.

Nursing care involves prevention of injury, attempts to stop hemorrhage if possible, gentle handling, and administration of frequent blood transfusions. In the past, many of these children died in childhood. Today, with better management, many of them live much longer.

The family must be taught to deal effectively with this disorder. They must learn to recognize the symptoms of bleeding and seek medical assistance immediately. They must also learn to protect the child from injury but not to the point of being overprotective.

**Leukemia.** Leukemia is a usually fatal disease characterized by an increased number of *leukocytes* (white blood cells) in the blood. Acute leukemia is more common in males and in children under the age of 5. The disease is a defect in the bone marrow whereby normal bone marrow is replaced by primitive cells, which are incapable of replacing red blood cells. In some cases, the excessive white blood cells actually destroy normal red blood cells. The patient is severely anemic and has bleeding tendencies. The untreated child generally does not live longer than 4 to 6 month. Chronic leukemia, which may last over a period of years, is very rare in children. It is estimated that 15,000 people die each year from leukemia in the United States.

Diagnosis of acute leukemia in the child is made on the basis of his medical history— often he becomes suddenly ill with general malaise, high fever, joint pains, bleeding from the body orifices, and enlargement of liver, spleen, and lymph nodes. The child may also become ill gradually, showing increasing weakness and pallor. The white blood count is elevated, with characteristic abnormal cells present. The patient is anemic, with a hemoglobin as low as 4 to 8. positive diagnosis can be made by means of a bone marrow biopsy. Lymph node biopsy is also done at times.

Generally, the child is managed on chemotherapy. There are 4 chief types of drugs used, none of which is curative. When the child does not respond to one, another is tried.

1. *Cortisone:* Usually the response to this

drug is fast and dramatic. It is usually reserved for the acutely ill patients, since in earlier stages of the disease, other means may be just as effective. Occasionally, the child may have more than one remission from the use of adrenocorticoids. Side-effects include edema and "moon face."

2. *Vincristine:* This drug is given intravenously and may be given alone or with cortisone. Side-effects include motor impairment. A fairly large percentage of patients will have a remission following administration of this drug.

3. *Antimetabolites:* These include the folic acid antagonists (Aminopterin or methotrexate) and the purine analog (6 mercaptopurine). These drugs are often effective in producing remission. Side-effects include ulceration of the mucous membranes and hemorrhage.

4. *Cyclophosphamide* (a nitrogen mustard derivative): This is an alkylating agent and is activated only in the human body. It is given orally and acts by depressing the action of the bone marrow. Therefore, it is usually used in patients who are resistive to other drugs because of bleeding tendencies and lack of antibodies.

In addition to the drug therapy, the patient may receive blood transfusions, or x-ray therapy. The nursing care of patients receiving chemotherapy, radiation, and blood transfusions is discussed in Chapters 43 and 47.

Much research is being done as to the causes of leukemia. Some scientists believe that a virus is responsible. If this virus is located, an immunization may be possible. The parents of the leukemic child should be assisted to accept the course of the disease but should also be allowed to live with the hope that a cure will be found in time to assist their child.

**Other Blood Dyscrasias.** Other blood disorders are *agammaglobulinemia,* which is an absence of gamma globulin in the blood, and *hypogammaglobulinemia,* which is a lowered amount of gamma globulin.

The causes for these disorders vary. If the disease is congenital, it will usually occur in males and be manifested by recurrent infections after 3 months of age. If the disease is acquired, it will occur more frequently in adults. These disorders may also occur as a result of neoplasm, or they may be ideopathic

(without identifiable cause) or physiologic (occurring between the 4th and 20th week of life when the immunity passed on to the baby from the mother is lost). Hypogammaglobulinemia may also occur as a result of irradiation therapy, excessive exposure to x-rays, or certain antineoplastic drugs.

The greatest problem is that of infection, since the natural antibody formation does not exist. Aside from taking precautions against infections, the patient may receive injections of gamma globulin. However, he should not be vaccinated against smallpox, because of the danger of infection. With better measures of protection against disease and more refined gamma globulin, the life expectancy of the person with agammaglobulinemia is increasing.

## Other Blood Disorders

**Anemias.** Many children suffer from various forms of anemia, the most frequent type being *iron-deficiency anemia.* Many doctors recommend iron fortified formula for all babies in an effort to prevent this condition. Other anemias must be treated with the administration of certain vitamins, as well as iron.

Anemia may also be the result of hemorrhage, hemolytic disease, or heredity factors (sickle-cell anemia).

**Purpura.** Ideopathic thrombocytopenic purpura (ITP) is the most commonly acquired bleeding disorder of childhood, occurring most often between the ages of 3 and 7. It is a disorder of the platelets in the blood and possibly of the small blood vessels, as well. In children, it occurs equally in both sexes, although in adults, it is more common in females. The symptoms include easy bruising, often without an obvious cause, small petechiae on the mucous membranes, frequent nose bleeds, or bleeding in the bladder or gastrointestinal tract.

In children, the disease is seldom fatal and usually runs an acute course and then is over. Most children recover within 6 weeks. The greatest risk is that of cranial hemorrhage, which occurs in 2 to 4 per cent of the cases.

Sometimes, the cause of the disease cannot be identified. However, if the mother is infected, it can be transmitted to the child through the blood stream.

Nursing care involves close observation for hemorrhage, avoidance of injury, and bedrest. The patient does not receive intramuscular injections because of the danger of hematoma formation. Sometimes, transfusions are given or the patient is placed on steroid therapy. In extreme cases, a splenectomy is done.

**Epistaxis.** Epistaxis or nose bleed is a common occurrence in children. It may be caused by a foreign object placed into the nose, by a systemic disorder, or by trauma. It usually can be stopped, without difficulty, by using pressure across the bridge of the nose, but the nose may need to be packed to stop the hemorrhage. The nurse must remember that the child's blood volume is lower than that of an adult, so the nose bleed is potentially dangerous. It is also important to remember that the bleeding may be swallowed, rather than being evident. Thus, any symptoms, such as vomiting of coffee-ground material, should be reported.

## HEART AND BLOOD VESSEL DEFECTS

### General Characteristics

Many possible defects may develop either in the heart itself or in the blood vessels. Generally, these may be divided into those which cause cyanosis and those which do not. The heart and blood vessel defects which cause *cyanosis* are further divided according to whether or not they are accompanied by pulmonary hypertension.

1. Cyanotic conditions with pulmonary hypertension
   a. Tetralogy of Fallot
   b. Tricuspid atresia
   c. Anomalous venous return
2. Cyanotic conditions without pulmonary hypertension
   a. Transposition of the great vessels

The *acyanotic* defects are also divided into 2 further categories: those which include a shunt from left to right (a right-to-left shunt produces a cyanotic condition) and those which are related to an obstruction.

1. Left-to-right shunts
   a. Ventricular septal defects
   b. Atrial septal defects
   c. Patent ductus arteriosus
2. Acyanotic conditions related to obstruction
   a. Pulmonary stenosis
   b. Aortic stenosis
   c. Coarctation of the aorta

### Diagnosis of Congenital Heart Defects

The infant with a heart defect may show signs of cyanosis, which is usually indicative of heart disorder. However, in a great many congenital heart defects, there is little or no cyanosis. In these cases, other symptoms may be present such as dyspnea, coughing or choking, pulse rate over 200, heart murmurs, failure to gain weight, difficulty with feeding, listlessness, and the general appearance of a child who is not doing well. The older child will show poor physical and sometimes mental development, low tolerance to physical activity, clubbing of fingers and toes, cyanosis in certain cases, elevated blood pressure and pulse rate, and a possibly enlarged heart. He may also need to squat or sit up to breathe.

Definite diagnosis is made by auscultation (listening for heart murmurs), x-ray, EKG (electrocardiogram), careful physical examination, and a complete history of the child's previous medical condition. At times a definite diagnosis is reached by the use of cardiac catheterization and angiocardiograms. However since these procedures are more dangerous, they are not carried out unless they are necessary to finalize the diagnosis (see Chapter 47).

A few minutes spent reviewing the circulation of blood and the anatomy of the normal heart will help you understand why some cases of congenital defects cause cyanosis and why others do not. If the body receives oxygenated blood, there will be no cyanosis, but in the cases where the blood is shunted before it can reach the lungs, the patient will be cyanotic.

It is also important to remember that cyanosis is difficult to determine in the Black person. Other symptoms will show, such as clubbing of fingers or dyspnea, but the cyanosis may go undetected for some time.

## Types of Disorders

**Tetralogy of Fallot.** Tetralogy of Fallot is a combination of several defects and is the most commonly occurring cyanotic defect. These defects usually include pulmonary stenosis (narrowing of the blood vessel into the lungs), a ventricular septal defect (an opening between the ventricles), overriding aorta (the aorta receives venous as well as oxygenated blood), and right ventricular hypertrophy (the right ventricle is enlarged because the heart must pump harder to compensate for the unoxygenated blood and to pump blood into the lungs). The patient with a very severe defect in any of these areas usually does not survive beyond 2 years of age. If he does, surgical procedures may correct some of the defects, depending upon their severity. The corrective surgery is very complicated and is usually deferred until the child is at least 6 years old. Palliative surgery may be done earlier to provide an artificial patent ductus arteriosus, by means of a shunt. This operation (the original "blue-baby" operation) increases blood flow to the lungs and thus reduces cyanosis and dyspnea.

**Tricuspid Atresia.** This is the absence of an opening between the right atrium and the right ventricle, which decreases pulmonary circulation because the only routes through which the blood can get to the lungs is through a ventricular septal defect, a patent ductus, or bronchial vessels. If no other defect exists, the child will die very soon after birth unless corrective surgery is done. Since the oxygenated blood going into the body is mixed with unoxygenated blood, the child is cyanotic.

**Anomalous Venous Return.** In this defect, the pulmonary veins empty into the right half of the heart instead of the left half of the heart, thereby bringing oxygenated blood to the wrong side of the heart. If all the pulmonary vessels empty in this way, there must be an accompanying septal defect or the child will die. If some of the vessels empty on the wrong side of the heart, the child will be cyanotic and will need surgical correction.

**Transposition of the Great Vessels.** The aorta and the pulmonary artery are changed around so that they connect to the wrong side of the heart. If no shunts or septal defects exist between the sides of the heart, the child will die very soon. Surgical correction is not very successful, but should be attempted.

**Ventricular Septal Defects.** This represents the most frequent congenital anomaly of the circulatory system and consists of an abnormal opening between the left and right ventricle. These defects are usually acyanotic because the greater pressure in the left ventricle causes a shunt from left to right, allowing the patient to receive oxygenated blood in the body. If pulmonary hypertension exists, the shunt may go the other way, in which case, the patient will be cyanotic. These defects are of various sizes and can usually be corrected in open-heart surgery by placing a patch (usually teflon) into the opening. If the opening is small and no pulmonary hypertension exists, the patient may not need surgery, or the surgery may be postponed until the child is older.

**Atrial Septal Defects.** This is an abnormal opening between the right and left atria. The large majority of these defects occur in the area of the foramen ovale. Those which occur lower in the septum are more likely to involve the mitral and tricuspid valves as well as the septum. Usually, the shunt of blood is from left to right, so that the patient is acyanotic. These defects are closed surgically unless the patient has severe pulmonary hypertension. If the valves are involved, the operation is much more complicated and may involve valve replacement.

**Patent Ductus Arteriosus.** The ductus arteriosus is a vessel between the aorta and the pulmonary artery which usually closes before birth or very soon after. When this vessel remains open (patent), a patent ductus arteriosus defect occurs. As you can see from the description of other anomalies, sometimes this patent ductus is lifesaving. The blood flow in the ductus is reversed by the higher pressure in the aorta, making it difficult to obtain enough blood in the pulmonary circuit. The correction is done by surgically ligating and severing the ductus. This closed-heart procedure was one of the first heart procedures to be done. The surgery is usually done, even if the patient does not show symptoms, because of the danger of subacute bacterial endocarditis.

**Pulmonary Stenosis.** This is an abnormal functioning of the pulmonary valve, which does not open to allow blood to go into the lungs. On rare occasions it may also consist of a narrowing of the pulmonary artery. If the defect is causing symptoms, surgical correction is done (commissurotomy). A closed-heart method may be used, whereby the surgeon attaches a sharp blade onto his finger and inserts it, freeing the cusps of the valve. If the stenosis is severe, open-heart methods may be used so the valve can be directly visualized. Occasionally, the valve is replaced.

**Aortic Stenosis.** This defect involves the aortic valve and causes the heart to work harder in order to pump blood out to the body. The treatment is similar to that for pulmonary stenosis.

**Coarctation of the Aorta.** In this defect, the aorta narrows either before it passes the ductus arteriosus (preductal) or after (postductal). The symptoms are similar to those of aortic stenosis, except that the coarctation is usually further from the heart and thus causes difficulties in the arms and head. In children, conservative medical treatment is attempted, because the surgical procedure is difficult. Surgical correction consists of either excising the coarctation and suturing the 2 ends of the vessel together, or using a blood vessel graft.

## Treatment of Congenital Heart and Vessel Defects

**Medical Treatment.** Generally, the older a child is when he undergoes surgery, the better his chance for survival. Of course, in the case of the child who is exhibiting symptoms of heart failure, pulmonary hypertension, or severe cyanosis, surgery must be done sooner.

Sometimes, palliative surgery is done so the child will be older when corrective surgery is attempted. Other times, the child is maintained on drugs and reduced activity to lessen the strain on his heart. The most common drugs given are digitalis compounds, diuretics, and antibiotics to prevent infections. Some children regularly receive oxygen. The child

is built up to the best possible state before surgery is done.

**Surgical Treatment.** (See Chapter 47 for a detailed discussion.) In some cases of large vessel surgery or open-heart surgery when the heart must be entered it is necessary to bypass the heart circulation by means of a heart-lung pump (pump oxygenator). In these cases, it is often necessary to stop the heart and restart it later. In other cases, closed-heart methods may be employed. These procedures are much safer, although any person who is undergoing open-chest surgery is subject to a serious operation.

Sometimes, surgery is done under hypothermia (reduced body temperature) or under hyperbaric conditions (increased atmospheric pressure which enables the blood to carry more oxygen).

## CARCINOMAS AND NEOPLASMS

Children are subject to several types of neoplasms, including malignant lymphoma (Hodgkin's Disease), lymphosarcoma, and other sarcomas (such as osteogenic sarcoma of the bone). However, neoplasms are not as common in children as they are in adults. Most commonly, the tumors which affect the child are those of the brain, the kidneys, and the nervous system. They are fast-growing and often go undetected until they are far advanced; thus, the prognosis in childhood cancers is often poor.

## MUSCULOSKELETAL DISORDERS AND ORTHOPEDIC CONDITIONS

### Congenital Hip Dysplasia or Dislocation

At times, one or both hips are not properly located in the ball and socket joint, the head of the femur may be displaced, or the acetabulum may not develop properly. If the disorder is unilateral, the buttock on the affected side will have an additional crease. X-rays are diagnostic. The term *dysplasia*, refers to the improper development of the acetabulum, which in turn causes *dislocation* of the hip.

Statistics show that this condition is more frequent in females, occurs at a rate of about 1 to 3 per 1000 live births in the United States, is uncommon among Black people, and occurs most often on one side only.

If untreated, the dislocation will cause deformity in later life, including a shorter leg on the affected side and limited abduction on the affected side. Later, the patient will walk with a limp and will show lordosis (concave curvature of the lumbar spine) and protruding abdomen.

**Treatment.** If the dysplasia is discovered before dislocation occurs, the condition can be treated medically. (Most infants show dysplasia without dislocation.) The child is placed in a Frejka pillow splint, which maintains the hips in an abducted position for 3 or 4 months. This keeps the head of the femur within the acetabulum.

If the hip has been dislocated, it must be replaced and maintained in that position. If ligaments or muscles have been torn, a spica cast may need to be applied and worn for 6 to 9 months. Sometimes, traction is necessary first.

If the child has been walking for several years, surgical repair is needed. Various types of procedures may be done, depending upon the damage. If the child is over 6, the prognosis for repair is poor.

**Nursing Care.** The child should be handled carefully, but should be picked up to encourage normal social development. The pillow splint or cast must be protected from soiling or wetting.

Normal rules for cast care apply, with the nurse being watchful for any signs of irritation or pressure. The child should be turned often and any parts of the body which are available should be exercised. The child should also be taken to the play room.

The parents should be instructed in the care of the child in the splint or cast. Often, it is helpful to obtain a hospital bed with a Balkan or Bradford frame so the child can move about in bed. This would be an excellent choice for referral for public health nursing.

## Clubfoot (Talipes)

The term "clubfoot" is used to describe a foot which is twisted or bent out of shape as a result of hereditary factors or an abnormal position in utero. It occurs more commonly in males and more often in multiple births than in single births. Unilateral clubfoot is slightly more common than bilateral clubfoot.

Treatment includes various stages of casting or splinting which generally are designed to correct one deformity at a time. Surgery may be necessary for older children or for those children with severe defects.

If the child has not been treated by the time he is 2 years old, he will most likely need surgery. The type of surgery done depends upon the specific defect. In young children, usually only the soft tissues need to be altered, since the bones are not yet calcified. In older children, however, the bones may need to be altered.

The usual procedures and precautions for observing and caring for a child in a cast are observed. The parents of the child are taught how to care for the child and what signs of complications to look for. They should realize that a great deal of patience is required, since the child may be in a splint or cast for several years.

## Osteogenesis Imperfecta

This condition involves a skeletal deformity due to the abnormal or imperfect calcification and mineralization of the bones. Symptoms include easily fractured bones and poor posture or body alignment. The condition may be congenital or acquired. If the child is born with the disorder, the prognosis is poor. The older the person is when the symptoms appear, the better is his prognosis. Newer medical technics improve the life span of this child.

## Wry Neck

*Torticollis* (wry neck) may be congenital or acquired. The congenital type is caused by a failure of the sternocleidomastoid muscle to lengthen as the child grows. A lump can be felt in the muscle and must be corrected or a curvature of the upper spine and an abnormal elevation of the shoulders will result.

Treatment includes passive or active exercises, surgical correction, or casting. The child must be checked until after puberty to make sure there is no recurrence.

## Juvenile Rheumatoid Arthritis

Known as Still's disease, juvenile rheumatoid arthritis is a generalized systemic disease which involves the entire musculoskeletal system. This condition can lead to deformities, such as contractures and impaired movement of body parts. The cause is unknown and girls are more likely to be affected than boys.

Many of the characteristic symptoms of arthritis are present, such as painful joint movement and subcutaneous nodules. (The condition of arthritis is discussed more fully in Chapter 45.)

Some drugs, such as aspirin, help to relieve the symptoms, but there is no known cure. Many children experience a spontaneous remission, with no recurrence of the disease.

Nursing care during the acute phase of the disease includes exercising the limbs, helping the child with activities of daily living, and sometimes applying heat in the form of a hot bath, packs, or whirlpool treatments.

## Rickets

This is a skeletal condition caused by a Vitamin D deficiency which prevents the bones from metabolizing calcium properly. However, with the advent of irradiated milk, rickets is becoming quite rare.

The child with rickets does not walk or crawl at the normal age and may be small for his age. His bones may have lumps on them, especially in the epiphyseal areas. Weight bearing bends the bones and causes characteristic bowed-legs or knock-knees. X-rays will show the abnormal calcification processes. In the adult who is deficient in Vitamin D, demineralization (*osteomalacia*) occurs, which may cause the patient's posture to change, resulting in hump back or bent legs.

Treatment involves the administration of Vitamin D and physical therapy to prevent deformity or to correct those deformities which have already occurred.

## DISORDERS OF THE EYES, NOSE, AND MOUTH

### Cleft Lip and Cleft Palate

*Cleft lip* (or *harelip*) and *cleft palate* are deformities commonly found together at birth, and result from failure of the upper lip and the palate to close completely during the second and third months of gestation.

Statistics reveal that these deformities are more common in whites than nonwhites, that left cleft lip is more common than right, that unilateral cleft lip (on 1 side only) is more common than bilateral, and that cleft lip, in general, occurs in about 1 out of every 750 or 800 births and is more common in males. Cleft palate, on the other hand, appears to be more common in females. Evidence also indicates that there is a slight tendency for familial occurrence.

Cleft palate appears as an opening which occurs in the roof of the mouth and leads into the nose. The cleft lip may be no more than a notch in the upper lip or may extend up into the nostril on one or both sides. The cleft in the lip may be *complete* or *incomplete* and may be complicated by other factors, such as a lip muscle which is separated by the cleft, skin which is thinner than normal, missing hair follicles and sweat glands, a flattened nostril on the affected side, and a missing part of the jaw, along with some teeth. We should note that mental retardation is not related to cleft lip and/or palate.

Usually, an operation to close a large cleft in the lip is done as soon as possible after the child is born. If the closure is delayed until the child is older, his physical condition may deteriorate because the deformity interferes with feeding.

**Feeding Problems.** Since part of the soft palate is missing in cleft palate; the uvula is almost always absent as well as part of the hard palate. As a result the mouth and throat are not closed off from the nose. This causes difficulty in feeding because if the baby is fed by the usual methods, the milk regurgitates out through his nose. If the child also has a cleft lip, he may have difficulty in sucking, thus requiring special feeding methods.

Some babies can be fed by using a soft nipple with large holes. The baby is held sitting up so he will not draw milk into his nose. Occasionally, a special, flattened nipple (*duckbill nipple*) or a *cleft-palate nipple,* which has a flap to cover the hole in the palate, will be used. In the very extreme case, gavage feedings may be necessary until part of the palate is corrected. In any case the nurse must be very careful to prevent aspiration.

**Oral Hygiene.** Good oral hygiene is essential in the care of these children. In the small infant, a small amount of sterile water may be given after the feeding, while the older child may be encouraged to use mouthwash or to brush his teeth often.

**Surgical Treatment.** Various procedures are necessary to repair the deformities involved in this condition.

The cleft of the lip is sutured, generally when the child is quite young. A skin graft or revision of the scar may be necessary at a later date. The scar is quite prominent immediately after the operation, but often becomes unnoticeable as the child grows older.

The palate may be repaired surgically by placement of a graft or by the use of a dental prosthesis, which is either attached to the teeth or provides the missing teeth and part of the jaw. This aids in speech by closing the hole between the mouth and the nose. The palate repair is usually done in one procedure, but may be carried out in several stages if the cleft is severe. The palate may be closed when the baby is young, but more often, it is repaired when the child is a few years old.

*Speech aids* are used to help the child to speak by preventing air from communicating between the nose and mouth. These aids are attached to the palate prosthesis and extend back into the throat. The speech aid is not moved as the uvula would move in normal speech. Instead the child is trained to move his throat around the aid so that he can learn to talk. The child may be fitted for this type of speech aid as soon as he has enough teeth to which the prosthesis can be anchored. The prosthesis is made of soft plastic and is removed and cleaned after eating. It is changed every 2 years or so to fit the child's growing mouth. Sometimes, the doctor will use a prosthetic palate until the child is older and then will do a surgical repair of the palate.

*Dental surgery* is often necessary to rebuild the missing gums and to replace missing teeth. In this case the prosthetic palate may include the prosthetic teeth. The mouth must be kept very clean, since this child is more susceptible to tooth decay than other children. Thus he must see the dentist often.

*Rhinoplasty* (repair of the nose) at times is necessary, although it is usually not done until the patient is a teen-ager.

**Cleft Lip Repair (Cheiloplasty).** If the child is a young infant, very little preoperative preparation is needed. The goal of the surgery is to restore function to the lip and to improve the child's appearance.

Immediate postoperative care is directed toward maintaining the airway, preventing shock and/or hemorrhage, using proper feeding technics, and preventing injury to the suture line.

**Cleft Palate Repair (Palatoplasty).** This is often done when the child is from 2 to 6 years old. The goals of this surgery are to restore normal speech, to avoid damage to the suture line of the lip, and to close the palate as much as possible.

The postoperative care involves preventing aspiration by positioning the child properly and by suctioning. Elbow restraints are usually used and oral hygiene is given.

**Speech Therapy.** As previously indicated defective speech is one of the problems faced by the child with a cleft palate. A cleft lip alone generally does not present speech problems.

The parent must remember that the child will not be able to produce some speech sounds until his palate is repaired. Both parents and nurse should remember to speak clearly to the child and make every attempt to understand what the child is saying. He is probably speaking as clearly as possible. Thus he should not be forced to speak distinctly, until after the palate is repaired. The speech therapist can give guidelines as to what exercises the child should practice. While most children with cleft palates are able to develop understandable speech patterns, many are able to develop normal speech.

**Hearing Difficulties.** Because the pathway is open between the mouth and the nose, the child with a cleft palate is unable to equalize the pressure in his eustachian tubes by swallowing, as the normal person can do. Since he may develop infections easier than other children, he may also suffer some hearing loss as well. Thus he should be protected from colds and upper respiratory infections. Because of the speech problem inherent in cleft palate, the nurse must remember that good hearing is essential for good speech development.

**Emotional Aspects.** How the child adjusts to a cleft lip or palate depends in large part upon how the parents react to the deformity. It is difficult for parents to have a deformed baby; often they blame themselves or feel guilty in some way. If this is the case the best type of therapy for the parents seems to be group discussion with other parents. The nurse can be the most helpful by understanding how the parents feel and by listening to them and allowing them to express their feelings.

One thing the parents should learn is that they can help the child as he grows up, not by protecting him from teasing, but by helping him to deal with it. (See Chapter 42 for a general discussion of the emotional aspects of handicap conditions.)

## Eye Conditions

**Strabismus (Squint).** This condition, commonly known as "crossed eyes," is an inability to move the eyes together. Although strabismus is usually congenital, it may develop as a result of a disease in childhood. Since the normal newborn is cross-eyed because he cannot control his eye muscles, it may be difficult to detect this condition until the child is older, even up to about 5 or 6 years of age.

There are 2 chief classifications of strabismus: *paralytic strabismus* (a condition in which the muscles of 1 eye are underactive), and *concomitant strabismus* (in which both eyes move, but the deviation of the affected eye is always the same). Other terms associated with strabismus are *convergent* (both eyes looking toward the center), *divergent* (both eyes looking outward), and *vertical* (the affected eye moves only on a vertical plane).

In concomitant strabismus, the condition may involve the same eye (*monocular*) or it can affect alternate eyes (*alternating*). The person uses the unaffected eye for vision at any particular time. If 1 eye is used for vision all the time, the person begins to disregard the vision in the other eye, because of double vision (*diplopia*), causing the eye to weaken. *Latent strabismus* is a form of strabismus in which the muscle imbalance is overcome by great effort, causing the child to complain of eye strain, headache, and diplopia.

Treatment includes patching the unaffected eye to increase the vision in the unused eye, corrective eyeglasses (which can be prescribed as early as 1 year of age), eye exercises, *miotic*

drugs (those which cause the pupil to contract), and surgical intervention. The treatment should be done as soon as possible to prevent further damage and to improve the child's appearance.

The surgical treatment involves alteration of the affected muscles to make them the same as the unaffected muscles. Often, elbow restraints are all that is needed and the child can be up and about following surgery. If he is to be on bedrest or is to have his eyes covered following surgery, he should be prepared for this preoperatively and his parents should stay with him. The nurse must remember that when a child's eyes are covered, she should speak to him before touching him, so that she will not frighten him.

**Errors of Refraction.** Often, the eye muscles in a small child are not developed enough to allow the eyes to accommodate properly. Since other factors may also be involved, the child should be examined regularly after age 3, or earlier if any symptoms appear, to determine if he is able to see properly. Such symptoms include rubbing the eyes, red, puffy eyes, watering eyes, and complaints of headache, dizziness, or double vision. It is important to determine whether vision difficulties arise from an error of refraction, which can usually be corrected by eyeglasses, or are the result of another problem, such as a brain tumor.

**Ptosis of the Eyelids.** This is usually a congenital condition in which the eyelids droop. Surgical correction, which is usually done for cosmetic reasons, involves suturing the eyelids up. However, because the surgical procedure is difficult, correction is not often perfect.

## SKIN DISORDERS

### Nevi and Hemangiomas

*Nevi* is the term used to refer to abnormal markings of the skin which may be congenital or acquired or pigmented or vascular. Numerous terms describe the many varieties of these disorders.

*Mongolian spots* are irregular dark blue-green areas which generally appear on the lower back. They are almost always present in infants of Asian extraction and occur frequently in Mediterranean and African peoples, but rarely in Caucasians. They usually disappear by about age 5 or 6.

*Pigmented nevi* (birthmarks or moles) are either simple brown spots or dark, hairy spots composed of cells containing melanin (melanocytes). Although normally harmless, they must be watched for change because they can develop into malignant melanomas, especially if they change in size or shape, become darker, or begin to bleed, ulcerate, or crust. Pigmented nevi which are constantly irritated are also more likely to become malignant, as are those appearing on the legs or mucous membranes.

There are three main types of nevi: *intradermal* (common moles), *junctional nevi* (flat or raised, found at the junction of the dermis and epidermis), and *active junctional nevi* (most likely to develop into melanoma).

Pigmented nevi are removed if there is any chance of malignancy, in which case, wide excision is done. They may also be removed for cosmetic reasons.

*Vascular nevi* (*angioma*) are localized areas of skin which have an overgrowth of vessels. If they consist of blood vessels, they are called *hemangiomas*; if they are composed of lymph vessels, they are called *lymphangiomas*.

Capillary hemangioma (port-wine stain, nevus flammeus) is a red or purple lesion, which usually does not fade. There is no known treatment.

Immature hemangioma (strawberry mark, nevus vasculosus) usually regresses and disappears, so treatment is usually not necessary. However, if ulceration is likely to occur, the lesion is treated by surgical excision, electrocoagulation, or the application of dry ice.

Cavernous hemangioma is a raised, red lesion, which does not regress. If it is very disfiguring, surgery may be done but is not too successful.

## Infantile Eczema

Eczema is a severe dermatitis which may show remissions and exacerbations. The type seen in infants (infantile eczema) is often more severe and is accompanied by a great deal of discomfort from itching, burning, and oozing or crusting. The mildest form is "cradle-cap." Eczema, which appears to be worse in the winter and seems to run in

families, is caused by allergens, some of which may be identified, but the mother often does not know what caused the disorder.

The baby with severe eczema is miserable. He cries and wants to scratch his lesions constantly. The nurse should spend as much time as possible with the child so that he will not need to be restrained for long periods. However, the child will need to be restrained at times to prevent scratching, which can lead to severe excoriation, infection, and later scarring, or to a much more fatal complication, called *eczema herpeticum.*

One effective type of restraint is the elbow restraint, used for cleft lip repair. However, the child's hands must also be tied down to prevent him from holding his arms out straight and scratching his face with them. It is a good idea to place the child in a rocking chair, so that he can move, even though he cannot scratch.

Dermatitis packs or therapeutic baths are often effective in relieving the itching. Sometimes, antibiotic or cortisone ointments are applied. (These procedures are discussed in Chapter 54.)

The diet of the child should also be adjusted to avoid any offending substances, which may have been identified as causing the eczema.

## Rash

Many small babies exhibit a rash for no known cause. The skin of the newborn is very delicate and easily irritated. If no cause can be determined, the rash should be treated symptomatically. Exposure to the air generally relieves the rash and other symptoms, such as itching.

## PARASITIC INVASIONS OF THE BODY

Many parasites which infest the body are more likely to occur in children than adults. Some parasites, such as certain types of bacteria, are necessary to digestion and serve a useful function. However, there are many parasites, such as the following, which become destructive to the body and cause various types of problems.

*Tapeworms* live in the intestine of the child and may eventually become very large. They are detected by the discovery of eggs in the stool or if the child complains of dizziness, abdominal pain, or diarrhea. Medications are usually effective in erradicating the worms.

*Flukes* are parasitic worms which may be found in polluted drinking water or in infested swimming water. Drugs are effective against flukes.

*Hookworms* usually enter through bare feet. They are then circulated through the blood stream into the lungs where they climb into the mouth and throat and are swallowed. These worms destroy red blood cells and cause the child to become anemic. The abdomen may become distended, and blood or hookworm eggs may be found in the stool. Various drugs are effective against the worms, and iron tablets or blood transfusions are used to offset the anemia.

*Roundworms* are most common in warm climates when living conditions are not clean. The eggs are swallowed and the larvae burrow into the intestine and enter the blood stream. The worms attack the lungs, the liver, or the heart and may be coughed up or appear in the stool of the child. Symptoms include diarrhea, pneumonia, and intestinal obstruction, sometimes with intestinal rupture. Drugs are specific against these worms and are usually effective. The secondary disorders must also be treated.

*Pinworms* are one of the most common infestations in children. The eggs are ingested and mature in the cecum. The hatched worms lay eggs in the anal and perineal folds and cause local itching. It is easy to infect other children or members of the family with these parasites. The child will scratch, especially in the anal region, may grind his teeth in his sleep, and often is tired, anorexic, and irritable. The worms can be visualized in the anal region or on the stool. Several drugs are specific for pinworms.

*Stool Specimen for Ova and Parasites:* The nurse will often see an order for this test. When the stool specimen is obtained (the nurse must be careful not to contaminate herself), the specimen is then examined for ova (eggs) and parasites (the worms themselves). Most kinds of worms can be identified in this manner.

*Pediculosis* is the condition of being infested with lice. The main types of lice are head lice, body lice, and pubic lice. Several drugs are available which are effective in killing the lice, but these must be used diligently on the clothes and furniture of the child and his family.

*Tinea pedis* (athlete's foot) is a common condition of children, especially those of school age. The feet itch and burn, cracks occur between the toes, and blisters may form. The child should be taught to wash and wipe his feet carefully each day and to take special precautions in locker rooms and public swimming pools. There are drugs which are quite effective against this condition, although the child may be reinfected often.

## BEHAVIOR DISORDERS

No attempt will be made in this book to define or to discuss in detail child psychiatry. However, a few of the more common childhood disturbances will be discussed here and in the next 2 chapters.

### The Hyperkinetic Child

The hyperkinetic child is one who is overactive to a point of disability. Since the child with hyperkinesia experiences increasing difficulties from infancy, by the time he reaches school age, he is impulsive and has a limited attention span and a low frustration tolerance. Because of these characteristics, he reduces any place to a disaster area. Early therapy is necessary to avoid severe personality damage, impaired learning, and serious behavior disorders. The hyperactivity, however, is generally outgrown by the middle teens.

The diagnostic signs are hyperactivity, short attention span, inability to follow orders, no sense of danger (he is very accident-prone), good gross motor coordination, but poor fine motor coordination, low frustration tolerance, and an inability to postpone satisfaction. The child is easily distracted and aggressive, shows an inability to make friends, does poorly in schoolwork, and is anxious, uncontrollable, and generally impossible to manage. Before a definite diagnosis is made, tests should be run to rule out a seizure disorder, brain damage, or any brain or learning dysfunction.

Treatment includes psychotherapy for parents and child, reducing the external stimuli in the home environment, and sometimes prescribing drugs to counteract specific behaviors. However, the side-effect of the drug given may be just the opposite of that desired; the child may become even more stimulated. In this case, the drug is changed. One drug which is contraindicated is phenobarbital which tends to intensify organic brain syndromes.

## The Hypokinetic Child

The *hypokinetic* child is the opposite of the hyperkinetic child. He is drowsy and lethargic, does not move much, and seems to be perpetually depressed, moody, and withdrawn. As a result, he is apathetic and does poorly in school.

## Behavior Problems in Children

Many behavior disorders in children are a result of extreme behavior on the part of the parents. The parent who is overprotective, overpermissive, or overly strict and abusive with his child is likely to cause the child to become insecure, upset, neurotic, or psychotic. Many times, the psychiatrist can identify the reasons for the childhood behavior problem and can alleviate the condition in the child by helping the family adjust its own behavior.

## Childhood Psychoses

**The Autistic Child.** The autistic child prefers to be alone and may show changes in activity; one minute he is overactive, the next he is not moving. He is routinistic and often will not talk. He may often laugh inappropriately, will not allow himself to be physically touched or cuddled, and avoids eye contact with other people. He has generally poor school performance, but can excel in one area, such as mathematics, if he wants. He seems to be totally interested in *things,* not people and is insensitive to pain.

It is believed that this condition is caused by overly rigid parents who are unable to accept the child. It is most common in boys and occurs most frequently in the oldest or only child.

Operant conditioning has been helpful in

some cases, although this problem is very difficult to treat. About one third of these children will grow up to be functioning adults. However, many authorities feel that they will have difficulty in forming normal human relationships.

**Childhood Schizophrenia.** Childhood schizophrenia is seen in the child who loses contact with reality, sometimes as a result of a sudden severe emotional experience or sometimes as a result of an inability to adjust to his environment. Some of these children are helped by means of play therapy, operant conditioning (behavior modification), and drug therapy. However, the child is subject to mental deterioration if the illness is prolonged. Many researchers are attempting to identify the cause of this disorder. Some believe that there may be a chemical basis to schizophrenia. If this is proven to be true, many children and adults will be helped.

# THE CHILD FROM ANOTHER CULTURE

The child from a culture which differs from that of most of the patients or nurses in the hospital presents a special problem. For one thing the child and his parents may find it difficult to accept the care you offer because you are different from them. It is also especially frightening and difficult for a child if he does not understand the language spoken in the hospital. Thus it is helpful if the parents are allowed to be with him as much as possible so they can interpret for him and explain things to him. However, the nurse must make her own effort to communicate with the child. She may use pictures in this endeavor or may ask the child to teach some words from his language to the nurses.

The nurse should use every means possible to make this child feel comfortable and relaxed in the hospital, because if he is too apprehensive, his treatment may be impeded or unsuccessful or he may not eat or sleep. The nurse must also take into consideration any religious customs or dietary differences which the child is used to. In this last regard she may try to find foods which are acceptable to the child. Generally, the imaginative nurse will be able to relate well with a child, no matter what his background or previous experiences.

# 41

# The School-Age Child and the Adolescent

---

## BEHAVIORAL OBJECTIVES

*The student successfully attaining the goals of this chapter will be able to:*

- *identify deviations from normal body structure and/or function in the school-age child or adolescent which cause the patient to have special needs or to be unable to meet his own basic needs; relate these deviations to the normal patterns of growth and development; list and define common medical terms related to each condition; describe the most important aspects of medical treatment; and demonstrate competency in assisting these patients to meet their needs.*

- *describe some of the special emotional considerations of this age group; and demonstrate effective nursing care to assist the patient to work through these conflicts.*

- *discuss special aspects of the nursing care of adolescents.*

---

## SPECIFIC DISORDERS OF THE SCHOOL-AGE CHILD AND THE ADOLESCENT

### Musculoskeletal Disorders

While postural defects are the most common type of musculoskeletal problems which develop in the early school years and during adolescence, other more serious disorders can occur during these years of growth.

**Postural Defects.** Many of the following postural defects occur during the prepubertal or adolescent ages.

Lordosis (curvature of the spine in which the pelvis tips forward)

Scoliosis (a side-way curvature of the spine which gives the spine an S-shape appearance)

Kyphosis (commonly called "hunchback")

Swayback (a combination of lordosis and kyphosis)

These problems should be corrected, if possible, or they will generally continue to grow worse and eventually become untreatable.

**Treatment of Postural Defects.** Treatment will depend on whether the cause is emotional or physical. If the cause of the defect is emotional, the person may need professional counseling or therapy. Nagging *does not* help. If the cause of the defect is weak muscles or another physical cause, treatment is usually initiated as soon as possible.

Various types of traction or braces are effective in altering the course of scoliosis and kyphosis. Sometimes, the brace is worn all the time, while in other cases traction is applied for a specified time during the day. In some instances, a plaster cast is worn. It is also possible that the patient may be required to sleep in a special bed or in a plaster mold.

There are two distinct types of scoliosis: functional scoliosis and structural scoliosis. *Functional scoliosis* is a postural defect which is due to poor posture. *Structural scoliosis* is a result of defects in the spinal muscles or bones. In the case of structural scoliosis, spinal fusion is often necessary. Several methods are used to immobilize the spine before and after fusion. One of the more common devices is the Milwaukee brace, which exerts pressure on the chin, pelvis, and the deformed part of the spine to force correction. Another method is the turnbuckle cast, which can be adjusted as the correction changes. In other instances a spica body cast is used, which must be changed periodically to allow for the correction. A more detailed discussion of the care of a person in a brace or cast can be found in Chapter 45.

**Slipped Femoral Epiphysis and Legg-Perthes Disease (Coxa-Plana).** Various disorders can occur when the epiphyses of the bones do not calcify properly. Perthes disease is a disorder in which the blood supply to the hip joint is temporarily disrupted, causing necrosis of the joint. The cause is unknown and the disorder usually remisses spontaneously. It generally affects children between the ages of 5 and 10 and usually lasts about 2½ to 3 years, occurring in stages. First, the tissues necroses, then the blood vessels begin to function again, and finally, bone growth is renewed so that the acetabulum is replaced.

The child must not be allowed to bear weight until the calcification of the joint is complete or the bones will become misshapen, causing coxa plana (flat hip). The first symptoms include pain in the hip joint and a limp. X-rays confirm the diagnosis. The treatment consists of bedrest, traction, and splinting. Passive and active range-of-motion exercises are carried out and the child is not allowed to bear any weight on the affected side. The younger child tends to recover better, and the less weight bearing which has been done, the better the prognosis for recovery.

**Juvenile Rheumatoid Arthritis (Still's Disease).** The disease of arthritis has been discussed elsewhere, but it has different effects on children. The disease, which affects girls more frequently than boys, is characterized by an inflammation and painful swelling of the joints. Sometimes, nodules form over joints

and then disappear. The growth may be stunted or malformations may occur as a result of uneven maturation of bones and joints. There is no cure, but most cases do remiss, with only about 20 per cent continuing into adulthood. Treatment is palliative, with aspirin for pain, sometimes steroids (although there are many side-effects), and physical therapy to prevent contractures and other deformities. The child with arthritis is a good candidate for referral to various community resources, such as the public health nurse or the outpatient physical therapy department.

**Orthodontic Care.** Many young people need orthodontia (correction of irregular tooth positioning and jaw deformities). The technical name for irregular tooth placement is *malocclusion*. The condition may cause facial deformities, as well as difficulty in eating and chewing. It often makes the teeth difficult to clean and, thus, leads to excessive decay. Generally orthodontic care should begin when the permanent teeth begin to erupt, about age 8 to 12, although sometimes the treatment is begun later. The nurse can encourage the young person to follow through on the treatment, since it will be to the person's advantage later in life.

## Skin Problems

**Acne.** Many young people suffer from various degrees of a skin eruption called acne vulgaris. The emotional impact of this disorder is most distressing; the young person is often very embarrassed about his appearance and will try all sorts of creams and lotions to cover the eruptions or pimples and cure the acne. Good skin hygiene and a well-balanced diet, which includes plenty of vegetables, fruits, and milk and excludes fatty foods, are often the most effective means of treating acne. Radiation is occasionally used, but very cautiously, to avoid other damage. Once the acne has subsided, the scarred skin may be removed (dermabrasion), but this procedure is done only in the most severe cases. Fortunately, most young people outgrow acne without scarring. The nurse can be helpful to the young person by reminding him that picking and pinching pimples is more likely to cause infection and scarring, than leaving the lesions alone.

**Body Odor.** If the young adolescent begins to have difficulty with body odor, he should be encouraged to use a deodorant, trying numerous brands until he finds a deodorant which is effective without irritating the skin.

## Trauma

Because the school-age child and adolescent is so active, he is subject to injury of all kinds. Thus the nurse will see many fractures, burns, and other trauma in this age group. The nursing care of these conditions is discussed elsewhere in this book.

## Genitourinary Disorders

The young person often needs assistance in dealing with disorders of his maturing genitourinary system. Although the nurse can be helpful in many instances, she must remember that the young person is especially modest and sensitive about any disorder in the reproductive or urinary organs. A tactful nurse will respect this modesty.

**Menstrual Difficulties.** The preteen and teen-age years are the time of life when many menstrual difficulties occur. (See Chapter 51 for more detailed discussion.) One such difficulty is mittelschmerz (pain on ovulation), which is more common in the woman before she has a child. As the body becomes accustomed to its adult female role, the girl may need assistance in regulating her periods or in managing the flow. The nurse will often be asked to help, since she is expected to understand the causes and cures for menstrual problems.

**Abnormal Sexual Development.** Many young people experience either precocious or retarded sexual development. In either case, it is a very embarrassing and trying time for the young person. The nurse will often be asked questions, but she should remember that she is not a doctor and should refer any patients who need assistance to the appropriate person.

**Venereal Disease.** This is thoroughly discussed in Chapter 51, but the nurse must remember that in this country a large percentage of the venereal diseases occurs in people under the age of 25. Do not hesitate to urge the young person who thinks he or she might have a venereal disease to go to the doctor. Most doctors will now treat this disorder without reporting it to the parents, so the young person should not be afraid to seek help. There are also many public and free clinics which give venereal-disease tests and advice and birth control information to young people.

## Gastrointestinal and Endocrine Disorders

The 3 most common gastrointestinal and endocrine disorders in the school-age child and the adolescent are chronic ulcerative colitis, appendicitis, and diabetes mellitus.

**Chronic Ulcerative Colitis.** This is a disorder of the large intestine which seems to be based on emotional factors. It often begins in the teen years and can continue into adulthood. If psychological and medical assistance is obtained early in the course of the disease, it may prevent surgery and other difficulties later in life.

**Appendicitis.** Appendicitis occurs most frequently during the teen-age years. Generally, an appendectomy is done and the young person usually recovers without difficulty.

**Diabetes Mellitus.** This disease is discussed at great length in Chapter 52. However, the nurse should remember that the younger the person is when he contracts the disease, the more difficult it may be to control. Although juvenile diabetes is more likely to be brittle, the young person should be encouraged to give his own injections as soon as possible and to lead a normal life and be independent.

## Cardiovascular Disorders

The 2 most common disorders of this type in the school-age and adolescent group are anemia and epistaxis.

**Anemia.** Because the body is growing so fast, the young person is often anemic. Frequently the cause in teen-agers is an inadequate diet; thus the adolescent should be encouraged to eat properly, especially girls, who often do not realize that they need more iron than boys, because of menstrual flow.

**Epistaxis.** The teen-ager is a frequent victim of epistaxis (nosebleed), because he is so active. Usually, this condition can be treated successfully and does not reoccur. However, if the child has frequent nosebleeds, he should be checked for other systemic difficulty.

## Malignancies

Young people do not usually have malignancies, but if they do, the malignancies often grow faster than in the adult.

**Osteogenic Sarcoma.** This is one of the most common and serious of the malignant bone tumors. It occurs most often in young people and is usually found in the diaphysis of long bones, although it may involve other bones. The spread is via the venous flow, with metastasis usually involving the lungs first. The only hope of cure is amputation above the lesion. Radiation is not effective and most of the antineoplastic drugs have proved to be quite ineffective. Because of these factors, the mortality rate is over 90 per cent.

Parosteal sarcoma, which is less deadly, involves the surface and not the interior of the bone.

**Ewing's Sarcoma (Ewing's Tumor).** This malignancy also involves the bones of young people, although it may affect the shaft instead of the end of the bone. This tumor is one of the most malignant and fatal of all tumors. Amputation is not often recommended, since radiation can sometimes arrest the growth and amputation is rarely done in time to be effective. The prognosis is extremely poor and the course of the disease is very short.

Both of these types of tumors are so fatal that the parents and the patient must decide whether to undergo amputation and an uncertain future or whether to forego the amputation and face certain death. The child and his parents must be given a great deal of emotional support and allowed to ventilate their feelings and fears. The person should be encouraged to live life to the fullest for as long as possible. Chapter 39 discusses many nursing aspects of the terminally ill child.

**Other Tumors.** Other cancerous tumors can occur in children, as well as in adults.

(See Chapter 43 for a discussion of cancer.) The nurse must remember that cancer is the same in both adults and children, although the treatment may be different because of the age of the patient.

## Infectious Diseases

**Acute Infectious Mononucleosis (Glandular Fever).** This is an acute infectious disease, which is characterized by infection and enlarged lymph nodes, and a characteristic heterophilic agglutinin in the blood. The disease rarely occurs after age 35 and is believed to be transmitted by droplets or air. It is common in schools and colleges, where young people are together.

The symptoms are fever, chills, general malaise, and sometimes headache, stiff neck, or chest pains and an abnormal EEG. There are three chief types of the disease: *glandular* (marked swelling of the lymph nodes), *febrile* (high fever), and *anginose* (pharyngeal symptoms). The disease is usually benign, although complications such as liver, spleen, heart, or neurological damage may occur.

The treatment is entirely symptomatic, with the person usually becoming well again within a few weeks. Fluids are forced and the fever is controlled. In rare and severe cases, corticosteroids may be given. In the case of rupture of the spleen, the spleen must be removed (splenectomy).

**Streptococcal Infections and Rheumatic Fever.** These disorders have already been discussed, but mention should be made of them here, since they often occur during the school-age and adolescent years. The young person must be encouraged to maintain bedrest and the medication regime to prevent permanent heart damage.

**Immunization Programs.** The school-age child and the adolescent must be encouraged to maintain his immunizations, since he is now exposed to many more diseases than before he went to school. Other immunizations, such as mumps vaccine, are added after the child enters school. The young person must be encouraged to keep up to date especially on his tetanus boosters, since he is so prone to injury.

## Emotional Difficulties

Since the young person in undergoing a great change in his life, he is subject to many emotional upsets, some of which are minor and can be dealt with easily. Others, however, are much more severe and require more extensive treatment.

The adolescent has several difficult developmental tasks which he must achieve before he can be considered an adult: he must become emotionally independent of his parents and yet be able to accept them; he must adjust to the role of man or woman; he must decide what he is going to do for work or education in the future; he must be able to form intimate relationships with other people; he must make decisions about his life, such as whether or not to drink, smoke, go to church, attend college, or engage in premarital sex. Some of the more common difficulties encountered by the young person are discussed here. However, while these problems generally show up in later school years, they may occur in the young school-age child as well.

**Peer Relationships.** The young person needs friendship and co-relationships with other people of his own age. It is important to have friends of both sexes, not just as dates, but also as friends, without love interest.

The person learns how to get along with others, first from his family and later from playing with other children. The child who lives in an unhealthy home relationship is most likely to have difficulties with friendships later in life. The child who is chronically ill or who has brain damage or other handicap conditions can also suffer from difficulty in making friends of his own age. Often the young person who has no friends of his own age is seen by a counselor or psychologist.

**Anorexia Nervosa and Overeating.** The young person with psychological difficulties often uses food or lack of it as a crutch to assist him in dealing with his problems.

The person with anorexia nervosa does not eat. He or she is thin and nervous, and often irritable and suffering from malnutrition. This child may be admitted to the hospital for evaluation to make sure that a physical disease is not causing the symptoms. If there is no physical cause, the young person is usually referred for psychiatric help.

The young person, especially the adolescent, is often prone to overeating or to eating types of food which add to weight. As a result many teen-agers become overweight, a condition which is difficult to correct later in life. Very few cases of obesity are caused by glandular disorders, so the young person can be placed on a reduction diet and given counseling and guidance, as well as encouragement in an effort to lose the excess weight. Often, obesity in adolescence contributes to difficulty in peer relationships, as well.

**Enuresis.** Wetting the bed has been discussed previously. However, if it continues into the school-age years, the advice of a doctor should be sought. Usually, it is caused by a psychological rather than a physical problem, and counseling or psychiatric assistance in combination with drugs, such as Tofranil, will usually alleviate the problem. The parents should not shame or belittle the child, because this may cause psychological damage which is much more harmful than the bedwetting.

**Constipation.** This may be caused by improper diet, nervousness, lack of exercise, or other factors. Often, if the adolescent is constipated, it is because of an emotional problem which can be alleviated by counseling. The young person should be encouraged not to take laxatives without first consulting a doctor.

**Sleep Disorders.** Narcolepsy (uncontrollable urge to sleep—usually for only a few minutes) and hypersomnia (uncontrollable urge to sleep, but usually for 12 to 18 hours), are the most common disorders of sleep in young people. These disorders, which usually begin in the teen-age years, must be differentiated from petit mal seizures. Sleep research is being done to determine what dysfunction of the brain causes these disorders. At times there is a definite physiological cause, such as brain damage or other physical illness. However, in other instances, sleep disorders may be a manifestation of a psychological problem; the person just wants to sleep to escape from the world.

Nightmares and sleep walking (somnambulism) are also common childhood occurrences which are usually outgrown. When dealing with a sleep walker the major concern is with his physical protection. If blood appears on the pillow after a child has nightmares, the doctor must consider a psychomotor seizure disorder. While the adult who exhibits sleep walking and night terrors (nightmares) often has a psychological problem, this is not necessarily true in children and adolescents.

Sleep talking (somniloquism) is very common and may or may not be associated with sleep-walking.

**Drug-abuse.** This subject is thoroughly discussed in Chapter 57, but should be mentioned here, since it often begins in adolescence or young adulthood. The nurse must remember that overuse of any chemical, such as alcohol, tobacco, or any other drug, is often harmful.

**Child and Adolescent Psychiatry.** A great many psychiatric units are set up in larger hospitals to deal exclusively with young people. It is usually beneficial to allow the young person to be in a separate unit, rather than to be hospitalized with adults who are having mental problems.

While behavior problems in childhood may be caused by organic factors, such as brain damage, the cause, more often, is impaired relationships with other people. Emotional problems may be manifested by withdrawn or destructive behavior or by many other behavior or speech patterns. A child who needs professional assistance may be identified if he is unable to control his impulses or his behavior as others of his age are, if he exhibits behavior which is very different from others of his age group, if he does not have friends, if he has a great deal of difficulty in learning, even though he is tested as being of adequate intelligence, if he has constant physical symptoms which seem to have no physical basis, or if he exhibits specific deviant behaviors.

One way of manifesting emotional problems is by defying the law or by being a "juvenile delinquent." Many police forces are now employing juvenile specialists or counselors to assist the young person who is asking for help by being in constant trouble with the law. The most effective means of dealing with the problem is through counseling with the family, the school, social workers, and psychiatrists and psychologists. Most young people who show deviant behavior are asking for help and will respond favorably to assistance.

**Adolescent Suicide.** Many young people commit suicide, either accidentally or on purpose. The problems of adjusting to a seemingly hostile adult world are so great that the young person often feels he cannot cope with the situation. The nurse must be watchful for warnings from the young person, because almost every person who commits suicide gives prior warnings which are not recognized by others. If the nurse can be observant and notice these signs, many adolescent deaths can be avoided. Many community agencies and telephone services are available in large cities to assist troubled young people with their problems. Many large cities also have suicide prevention centers which offer around-the-clock services to persons in need.

The problems of accidental suicide can be tackled through education. For example, many young people are unaware of the dangers of some drugs and so do not realize that they can easily kill themselves, without intending to do so. The nurse can be a teacher to her friends in many of these areas.

## SPECIFIC NURSING CARE OF THE ADOLESCENT PATIENT

The young adult needs certain special accommodations in nursing care in order to preserve his self-respect and identity. The nurse must remember that the young person does not belong on either the pediatric ward or the adult ward. If possible, a special unit should be provided for the adolescent patient. If this is not possible, the young person's roommate should be the same age and the same sex; it is usually disturbing to any child over the age of 4 or 5 to be in the same room with a person of the opposite sex. They are also embarrassed if they must share a bathroom.

The hospitalized adolescent needs to continue his relationships with his peers. Thus his friends should be allowed to visit, but their activity should be regulated so they do not overtire the patient.

### Meeting the Emotional Needs of the Hospitalized Adolescent

Since the personality of the adolescent is different from that of the child, the nurse must alter her emotional nursing care to fit the personality of the patient. The physical care is much the same, but the psychological care differs.

The adolescent should be admitted without his parents being present. He will most likely be embarrassed if they are there and may omit pertinent facts. Girls should be draped properly and examined with a female nurse present. Boys should be examined without the nurse or in the presence of a male nurse.

It is desirable to place young people of about the same age together. The person with an acute illness may be in a private room, but the long-term adolescent patient should have a roommate to talk to. Young people in the same ward should have a chance to visit with one another.

We must remember that the adolescent is interested in himself and in how he appears to others. He is very upset by a blemish or deformity. He resists efforts to tell him what to do and often rebels, because he is struggling to find his own identity and to become a person in his own right.

The nurse should remember that the adolescent is trying to grow up. He will respond best to sincere interest and will probably react negatively to demands or sarcasm. He needs personalized care. Many young people worry a great deal, especially about damage to their bodies or about death. Since they are concerned about sex, their modesty must be respected.

Since the young person is striving for independence, the nurse should attempt to include the patient in his care as much as possible. Give him a right to his opinions and ask him how he would like his care done. Treat the young person as a person and recognize his individuality as you do with all other patients.

As a nurse you should not argue with the patient or be upset by defensiveness. Do not give orders, but suggest that it is time to do something. Listen to him and trust him. Treat him like a person and he will treat you like a person.

## The Teen-Aged Nursing Student and the Teen-Aged Patient

It is often difficult for the young nursing student to care for the patient of approximately the same age, especially when the patient is of the opposite sex. It is important that the patient and nurse realize what their roles are and not overstep the bounds. It is difficult for the nurse to avoid becoming overinvolved with the patient. Be kind, be friendly, and listen to the patient; try not to forget that you are the nurse and he is the patient. The patient will usually understand that you are trying to assist him and will cooperate. If you feel confident in your role as a nurse, the patient is most likely to accept you in that role.

# 42

# The Handicapped Child

BEHAVIORAL OBJECTIVES

*The student successfully attaining the goals of this chapter will be able to:*

- *discuss the 4 major considerations in dealing with any handicapped child; and demonstrate understanding of these concepts in the clinical area.*
- *deal kindly, yet effectively, with the child who has a handicap and with his family; assist him to meet his special or basic needs by adapting nursing care to each child; and assist in teaching the child and his family.*
- *list the various types of intellectual impairment, describe each, and adapt nursing care to each individual child and his family.*
- *discuss briefly the child with special learning needs or with a behavior disorder.*
- *describe and discuss the 2 major types of neuromotor disorders, cerebral palsy and muscular dystrophy or atrophy; identify the chief symptoms of each, the types of each, and the major aspects of medical treatment; and demonstrate proficiency and understanding in nursing care and patient and family teaching, stressing the positive capabilities of each child.*
- *maintain the role of the practical nurse as regards family planning, genetic counseling, or referral to various community resources.*

## INTELLECTUAL IMPAIRMENT

The practical nurse will come into contact with many people who suffer from various degrees of intellectual impairment. This term refers to the person who is mentally retarded or mentally subnormal or suffers from a learning disability of some sort. As with any kind of handicap, you must remember that the person with intellectual impairment is more like you than unlike you, because he has basic needs, just as any other person. Of course, he probably needs more understanding and assistance, which you, the nurse, can give. You can also encourage his family to provide the emotional support which he so desperately needs.

There are over 6 million people in the

United States with some form of mental retardation and several million more with learning disabilities or special learning needs. The nurse must remember that almost everyone can learn to some degree, and she must help the person to progress as far as he can, within his capabilities. The retarded person learns more slowly than others and is limited in how much he can learn, but is otherwise like everyone else.

### Extent of Impairment

The degree of intellectual impairment varies with the individual. The person who has the ability to take care of himself with some assistance is said to be "mildly impaired;" the person who needs considerable

*499*

support and supervision in order to be self-sustaining is said to be "moderately impaired;" the person who is unable to learn to read and write, but who can do some useful work is said to be "severely impaired;" and the person who requires care to meet all of his basic needs is said to be "profoundly impaired or profoundly retarded." The trend is away from using IQ levels as the criteria of judgment, because IQ is based upon abstract concepts and reading skills, which are not appropriate for all people.

Evaluation of intellectual ability must also take into consideration any *physical impairment* which may exist. If the person has cerebral palsy, brain damage, or some other physical condition, it may be very difficult to obtain a true measure of his native intelligence, simply because he cannot respond to the questions. This does not mean that he is retarded, but simply that he cannot respond in the conventional manner to questioning. Many people with various forms of brain damage are very intelligent, but special means must be used for teaching them and for ascertaining their intelligence.

**Lack of Stimulation as a Cause of Retardation.** A very important factor in the process of growing up, especially in the first few years of life, is the degree of intellectual stimulation. In Chapter 8, we discussed the basic needs of all children, including stimulation and opportunities to learn. If these opportunities are not provided, the child will be educationally or culturally handicapped and will have difficulty in keeping up with his peer group when he enters school. The majority of retarded people in the world are so because they have not been given the opportunity to learn, not because they were not born with innate potential to learn. The understanding nurse or teacher can attempt to find within each person the level of his ultimate potential and can try to help him to reach that potential, whatever it may be. The person is "teachable" only at certain times of his life, and it is up to us to find those teachable moments and to make the best possible use of them.

## Types of Congenital Intellectual Impairment

Some types of mental retardation or intellectual impairment are congenital defects,

present at birth, and are not caused by an unstimulating environment.

**Down's Syndrome (Mongolism).** This condition occurs in about 1 out of every 600 to 700 births and can cause any degree of retardation from mild to profound. The child with this condition can often be recognized at birth, because he tends to have a flat nose and slanting eyes. There are many other characteristic features, which are more noticeable in the more profoundly retarded person with this disorder. The person often also has physical defects such as strabismus, cataract, congenital heart defects, or other congenital disorders.

It is believed that this defect occurs about the eighth week of gestation as a result of *translocation in the child's chromosomes* (either 47 chromosomes instead of 46, or extra material attached to one chromosome). Since this chromosomal defect may sometimes be seen in the chromosomes of the parents, genetic counseling is often done on the basis of chromosomal studies. The risk of having a child with this defect rises sharply if the mother is over the age of 40, especially if this is her first pregnancy. Mongolism can occur, however, in any family, regardless of race, age, or social status. The defect is more likely to be hereditary if the forty-seventh chromosome is attached (translocated), rather than if the extra chromosomal material is unattached. Since the defect may be carried as a recessive trait and may skip a generation, chromosomal studies should serve as the basis for genetic counseling in brothers and sisters of children with Down's syndrome.

*Genetic makeup* has a great deal to do with many types of congenital retardation and it would be well to review Chapter 12 and its discussion of genes and DNA and RNA and their functions in reproducing the species. If a mutation occurs at the DNA–RNA level, it can cause physical or mental defects.

**Prenatal Infections.** Sometimes, an infection or disease in the mother, notably German measles during the first 3 months of pregnancy can cause severe mental or physical handicaps. Any mother who is exposed to German measles should seek immediate medical attention. Often she will be given gamma globulin to prevent the disease.

**Drug-Induced Retardation.** Some mothers who are habitual drug-abusers or who take other drugs may have congenitally retarded children as a result of the drug's effects on the fetus.

**Other Defects.** Other defects which may cause retardation and mental impairment are hydrocephalus craniostenosis, microcephalus kernicterus, cretinism, gargoylism, Niemann-Pick disease, phenylketonuria (PKU), and Tay-Sachs disease. (See Chapter 40 for a more detailed discussion of many of these disorders.)

## Types of Acquired Intellectual Impairment

Many types of intellectual impairment are not congenital, but are acquired at or after birth. One of these, lack of infantile stimulation, has already been mentioned. Others are discussed below.

**Birth Injuries.** Sometimes, the child can be injured by forceps or by a difficult delivery, which can cause brain damage. The child may also be retarded if he suffers from anoxia for several minutes after birth. This lack of oxygen to the brain causes irreversible damage.

**Poisoning.** Many types of poison, such as lead or carbon monoxide, can cause permanent brain damage and retardation or impairment in both children and adults. Usually, these conditions are not reversible, although the child can be taught to do many things.

**Infections:** Some infections, such as encephalitis, can cause permanent intellectual impairment.

**Trauma.** A severe blow to the head, at any age, can cause permanent brain damage and any degree of intellectual impairment or learning disability.

## Nursing Care of the Intellectually Impaired Patient

There are many general concepts which relate to the care of the person with an intellectual defect. Most agencies feel that if it is at all possible, the person should live in a normal family situation, where he can receive stimulation and love from the members of his family. However, in some situations, the child will benefit more from being in an institution.

**Behavior Modification.** This concept involves giving positive reinforcement for a job well-done (see Chapter 56). This method can be used to condition or train those who are intellectually impaired to care for themselves. Many people who were completely bedridden or unable to care for themselves in any way have responded very favorably to behavior modification.

In training the retarded person, it is important to remember that he will need to repeat the skills many times before he learns them. He must be ready to learn and be interested in learning. You must repeat many times and give praise when he does the task correctly. The attention span will be short, so the task should not be very involved. The retarded person will not often be able to generalize from one situation to another, so you must teach him each specific skill, task, or behavior. The person needs a routine and needs to do things the same way each time he does them. There are specific technics for teaching dressing skills, feeding skills, toilet training, and other activities of daily living. Teaching should be done in a quiet place, with few distractions. The place should be neat and kept in the same order at all times. Remember, that patience is the most important factor in training the person with intellectual impairment. You must realize that he will progress slowly so do not push him to learn faster than he is able.

**What You Can Do.** The most helpful thing you, or anyone else, can do is to provide friendship and companionship to the person with difficulties. He needs to feel loved and accepted, often more so than other people. A state hospital in Minnesota has a program called "Foster Grandparents" which provides a friend to the institutionalized person. The visitors talk to the patients, read to them, and answer their questions. This program has proven beneficial to the patients, as well as to the senior citizens who volunteer their services in the hospital. They are _concerned_ and this is what the person with intellectual impairment needs.

## Prevention of Intellectual Impairment

Many of the causes of mental defects can be determined and eliminated. This is especially true of many diseases which can be treated if they are discovered early enough. Thus it is important to prevent certain diseases such as German measles (all children should be immunized). Other preventive steps include seeking good medical care during pregnancy to prevent congenital defects, avoiding any exposure to radiation to the ovaries or testes or to the abdomen during pregnancy, avoiding harmful drugs, obtaining genetic counseling in the event of suspected congenital defects, and generally keeping yourself and your children in good health at all times. It is important to have a newborn baby examined early in life and periodically thereafter to make sure there are no defects.

## THE CHILD WITH SPECIAL LEARNING NEEDS

There are many children who have difficulties in learning, not because they are truly retarded, but because they have some sort of brain dysfunction or brain damage which makes them unable to learn in conventional ways. Some of these disorders have been called hyperkinesia, hypokinesia, dyslexia, language disturbance, or perception handicaps. This child may demonstrate his difficulties with medical problems, behavioral problems, or educational difficulties. The causes can be hereditary or environmental. Many times, these children are considered retarded. Newer methods of diagnosis and treatment have made possible many advances for the child with special learning needs.

The child with minimal brain dysfunction or special learning needs must first be evaluated to make sure that there is no physical cause for the educational retardation, such as poor eyesight, deafness, or a severe brain disorder. After these factors have been ruled out, the child can be evaluated and trained.

The key factors in the education of this child are the processing of sight and sound into the brain (*input*), the decoding within the brain (*integration and evaluation*), and eliciting the appropriate response (brain *output*). The specific defect must be discovered and the education aimed at this defect. The keys to this education are positive reinforcement when the child does the correct thing, clues given so that the child knows what to do, practice, and individualized instruction.

Often, the parents of the child who has difficulty learning, for whatever reason, can benefit from a group-therapy session with other parents. Many times, the parents can come up with suggestions which will be helpful to each other. This group also gives the parents a chance to ventilate their feelings about their child and his difficulties.

## Cerebral Palsy

**Cause.** Cerebral palsy (congenital diplegia, Little's Disease, congenital spastic paralysis) is a comprehensive term used to describe conditions in which a person has difficulty controlling voluntary muscle activity. This is sometimes the result of an infectious disease which causes brain damage after birth. However, many cases seem to be the result of brain injury incurred during delivery or from anoxia immediately following birth. The development of the child is either stopped or becomes disorganized and abnormal.

**Symptoms.** The most frequent symptom is spasticity or stiffness and rigidity of the muscles of the extremities. Movements are not destroyed completely, but the child cannot control them. Motions are jerky, and the muscles are tense. Any part of the body may be involved—one portion or all. A generalized involvement results in a helpless child.

If the disability is severe, it may be recognized shortly after birth; more often it is recognized at the time the child should be developing normal muscular skills, such as sitting or walking. For instance, if the legs are involved, the muscle rigidity becomes more noticeable when the child begins to walk. The muscles that draw the feet and the knees toward each other are stronger than those that draw them apart, so the child walks crosslegged—his legs move like scissors.

Mental retardation or behavioral problems may accompany cerebral palsy. However, intelligence also may be normal or above normal. Because the child may have speech difficulties or difficulties communicating in any way, an adequate assessment of his intelligence is often difficult.

**Treatment.** We presently have no methods for repairing a brain injury. The problems of each child must be appraised and understood; his therapy must be based on his abilities.

The family's acceptance of their child and their willingness to assist in his development may be the greatest factor in his development. The parents should be helped to understand that much can be done for the cerebral palsied child. He needs highly individualized care to give him the same opportunities which are open to other children. The Crippled Children's Service or local Welfare Department are community agencies which make this care possible, if the parents are unable to pay for it.

One of the primary objectives in the treatment of cerebral palsy is the prevention of muscle contractures. Splints and sometimes surgery are used; muscle relaxants assist in muscle re-education. The cerebral palsied child progresses slowly. Attempts to force or hurry the child only make him tense and less able to move.

The child must be evaluated early in life and periodically thereafter, in order to determine what he can and cannot do. After the evaluation, plans can be made for his future rehabilitation.

**Protection.** The child may need to be protected from injury. The old-fashioned head helmet to protect the head is seldom seen, since more attractive protective measures are now available. Often, the girl will enjoy wearing a wig, which will cushion her head from injury. If the child tends to fall, he may practice walking on a tumbling mat. It may be necessary to restrain the child in a chair to prevent falls. Walk with the patient as much as possible to encourage movement and to provide safety.

**Feeding.** Learning to eat is sometimes a problem for the child with cerebral palsy. He should be encouraged to chew his food thoroughly and must be conscious of the act of swallowing, so he does not aspirate. Do not place food in the center of his mouth, but on the side, so he can handle it better. Encourage the child to use his lips to remove the food from the spoon, to bite off pieces of food, to move food around in his mouth with his tongue, to swallow consciously, and to suck from a straw. These actions will help greatly in the development of speech.

**Speech Development.** This is often a difficult thing for the child to master. The therapist must be very patient and encourage the child to speak and to say each word as slowly and as clearly as possible. Do not talk baby talk to the child. Encourage him to listen, and even if he cannot answer you, be sure to talk to him. Tell him what you are doing and try to anticipate questions which he might have and answer them, even if he is not able to ask them. Read to the child and allow him to look at the pictures.

**Socializing.** It is very important for the child with cerebral palsy to play and have friends. He must feel loved and a part of the family. Although it may be difficult, there are many types of toys which can be made for the child. He needs the feeling of being around other people and can be taught ways to relate which will make him acceptable to others.

**Physical Care.** There are many hints for specific care of the child. It is important to know what type of disorders the child has and to treat him accordingly. The most important factor is safety and prevention of further deformities. It is vital to provide as much mobility as is possible for this child.

**Psychological Factors.** Cerebral palsy is a handicap which creates many psychological problems for the child. The intelligent child is bound to feel frustrated, because it is difficult or impossible for him to make his body respond. He feels insecure and may be unattractive in appearance. He is incapable of doing many of the things that other children do. He may have speech difficulties, reading difficulties due to eye defects, and writing problems due to lack of coordination.

Adolescence can be difficult enough for normal children; the child with cerebral palsy feels his handicap keenly at a time when he wants to be independent, to establish boy-girl relationships, or to join in social activities. Parents and teachers must assume attitudes which will help to make other children accept him as a person. He needs to be with people his own age, to make friends, play games, and go to parties. His ambitions may go far beyond anything he ever will be able to do. It is important to begin early in childhood to guide cerebral palsied children to do the things they can learn to do satisfactorily. The child must learn to face reality and to make the most of his life in spite of his handicap.

This child would be an excellent candidate for referral to the Public Health Nurse. There are also many other community agencies which would be helpful in caring for this child at home.

## Muscular Dystrophy and Atrophy

Muscular dystrophy actually refers to a group of symptoms sometimes referred to as "the muscular dystrophies." It involves a progressive wasting-away of muscles, whereby the child becomes weaker and eventually is unable to move at all. It affects the voluntary muscles (unlike polio, which affects muscles of breathing, via nerve damage), and is usually bilateral (the same on both sides of the body). This disorder can strike at any age; adults may be afflicted with it, and may suffer with it for 20 or 30 years. In children, the disease progresses much more rapidly, so that very few children afflicted with the disease live to adulthood. There is usually no pain involved and the disease is not contagious.

Diagnosis is made on the basis of muscle biopsy, electromyelogram, and accurate physical examination and medical history of the patient.

**Treatment.** The treatment is palliative. There is no cure. The child is encouraged to move as much as possible to prevent contractures and faster progression of the disease. Physical therapy is also given, and lung exercises are done to arrest lung involvement, the difficulty which often claims the life of the patient. As the disease progresses, a great deal of nursing care is needed. (See Chapter 46 for a discussion of neurological nursing.) Extensive research is being done in an effort to find the cause of the disease and thus, the cure.

As you can imagine, a great many psychological problems occur involving both the patient and his family. As in so many other instances, the nurse can be helpful by listening to them and by assisting in referring them to the appropriate hospital or social agency. The person must be assisted to remain active mentally and physically, as long as possible, and to make the best possible use of his abilities.

**Muscular Atrophy.** This disorder can be easily confused with muscular dystrophy, since many of the symptoms are similar.

## Speech Difficulty

Many children have difficulty in speech and are not treated because the parents feel that the disorder will disappear by itself. The nurse can be helpful in encouraging the parents to seek medical assistance as soon as possible to prevent as much damage as possible. Speech disorders may be caused by physical factors, such as cleft palate, deafness, or brain damage, or by functional factors, such as emotional problems.

The most common types of speech disorders in children are dyslexia (the inability to say what one wants to say or of reversing the order of written letters), aphasia (inability to speak), and stuttering. Dyslexia has been mentioned before in terms of a special learning need. This child reverses images within the perceptual centers of his brain and is unable to interpret images as others do.

Aphasia in young children is most often caused by deafness. With great patience and perseverance the child can be taught to speak. Of course, aphasia can also be caused by trauma to the head or by a hemorrhage, a tumor, or a blood clot within the brain.

Stuttering is most often a functional difficulty. That is, it seems to be caused by emotional factors since no physical cause can be found. It is important not to label the child as a "stutterer" or his stuttering will tend to become worse. Praise him for doing well and do not force him to speak to groups. Allow him enough time to say what he wishes to say. Read to him and encourage him to read, since this might be easier for him than speaking without planning ahead. This child generally will stop stuttering if he is not ridiculed or pushed. The understanding nurse will let him know that he is accepted.

## GENERAL ASPECTS OF DEALING WITH ANY HANDICAPPED CHILD

There are several general factors involved in the nursing care of a child with any type of difficulty. The nurse must also remember that the parents must be considered, as well as the child.

Emphasize the positive; stress what the child can do and not what he cannot do. Everyone has some positive attributes and the nurse must remember to stress these. Encourage the child for the job he does well and do not punish him for mistakes.

Allow the child to be as independent as possible; don't do everything for him. Be sure to allow him to help himself, even though it may take longer. Offer him assistance in a kind way, if he needs it.

Make sure the child is allowed to develop usual social contacts for his age; it is unfair to isolate the child with a handicap from other children. Encourage him in social contacts and teach him ways of making friends which emphasize his positive points and play down the handicap.

Consider the emotional aspects of the child's development. The child must be assisted to accept his difficulties and to make the best of his life. He may need referral to a community agency or to the special interest group which is concerned with his special problem. The nurse can often give this type of information to the parent or to the child.

## GENETIC COUNSELING

In the event of a severe hereditary handicap condition, the parents may often wish to seek the advice of an experienced geneticist before having more children. Many times, in families in which a hereditary disease exists, the young people will wish to discuss the matter before marriage or before having any children.

The couple will most often wish to know if they are able to have normal children. The doctor, in discussing this probability, may need to refer to special sources of information regarding certain diseases. Generally, the agencies which are interested in specific diseases are the most up-to-date source of research information on a specific disease.

The genetic counselor also needs to know about the possibility of a congenital disorder in the event of an existing pregnancy. In this case, the mother can be managed and the newborn child examined very carefully, to rule out any disorder or to treat any disorder which does exist.

Many new technics exist for determining the possibilities of a couple having defective children. The doctor can make good use of these tests in his counseling of prospective parents.

The doctor will tell the parents the facts and let them make the decision as to whether or not to have children. The doctor is usually willing to assist in preventing pregnancy, but generally will not tell a couple definitely not to have children.

If the nurse is asked questions relating to genetic counseling, she should refer these questions to the doctor.

## COMMUNITY RESOURCES

It is very important for the practical nurse to remember that almost every distinct disease condition, especially those which involve children, has an agency which is specifically interested in that condition. The agencies often sponsor research and usually have booklets and films or other materials which are available. The patient should be referred to agencies which might answer their questions or might help them to solve a specific problem. The nurse should be aware of the agencies which exist or know how to find out about them.

# Unit 10:

# Assisting the Adult Who Has Impaired Body Structure or Function

43. *The Patient With Cancer (Oncologic Nursing)*
44. *The Patient With a Skin Disorder*
45. *The Patient With Musculoskeletal Disease or Injury*
46. *The Patient With a Disturbance of the Nervous System*
47. *The Patient With a Cardiovascular Disease or a Blood Disorder*
48. *The Patient With a Respiratory Disorder*
49. *The Patient With a Digestive Disorder*
50. *The Patient With a Urinary Disorder*
51. *The Patient With a Reproductive Disorder*
52. *The Patient With an Endocrine Disorder*
53. *The Patient With a Disorder of the Sensory System*
54. *The Patient With an Allergy*

# 43

# The Patient With Cancer
# (Oncologic Nursing)

---

## BEHAVIORAL OBJECTIVES

*The student successfully attaining the goals of this chapter will be able to:*

- *define the term cancer; discuss the emotional aspects related to cancer, identify the chief types of the disease; list and define at least 6 medical terms specifically related to cancer; and discuss some factors which are believed to predispose to the development of the disease.*
- *list the 7 danger signals of cancer as defined by the American Cancer Society.*
- *identify the most common sites for cancer in men; in women.*
- *list and discuss the 8 chief methods by which cancer is discovered.*
- *discuss thoroughly the 3 major forms of treatment for cancer; identify the situations in which each treatment might be used, the relative effectiveness of each, and the specific nursing problems related to each; demonstrate ability in the clinical area to assist patients to meet special needs by caring for patients who are undergoing various types of treatment and tests; and demonstrate ability to do patient and family teaching as it relates to cancer and in the prevention and/or early detection of the disease.*
- *demonstrate ability to assist the patient to meet special needs which are caused by cancer such as problems with the skin, diet, and odor, as well as by assisting the patient to deal with pain.*
- *be helpful to patients and others by interpreting the dangers of cancer quackery.*
- *list at least 5 research goals of the American Cancer Society.*

---

## WHAT IS CANCER?

Cancer (also known as carcinoma or C.A.) affects plants and all forms of animal life. It is a cellular disease characterized by an alteration in the role and manner of growth. The one thing which distinguishes all cancer cells from normal cells is *uncontrolled replication*. Cancer, for which no cause has been established, may involve virtually any of the body's tissues, organs, or systems.

## A NATIONAL HEALTH PROBLEM

Cancer is next to heart disease as a cause of death in the United States. It affects all areas of the body and takes thousands of lives every year. Most of the people who have cancer are 40 years of age or over, but it attacks people of all ages. Often it can be cured if discovered in time. Thus time is of the essence in the diagnosis of cancer, because untreated cancer grows worse and is always fatal.

## CANCER AND HOW IT SPREADS

Cancer is a wild, disorderly growth of body cells that undermines and spreads through normal tissues. It can be identified without doubt by examining a specimen of suspected tissue under the microscope. Not all growths or tumors are cancers. The *benign* growths are noncancerous, but the *malignant* ones are cancers. Two common forms of malignant growths are *carcinoma* and *sarcoma*. Malignant tumors usually are not confined within a capsule and can spread to nearby tissues; they also spread by *metastasis* to other parts of the body through the blood and the lymph. There is no way to tell whether or not this has happened until symptoms of a growth appear or an x-ray film reveals it. Some types of cancer grow more rapidly than others.

**The Spread of Cancer.** The spread of cancer to other parts of the body is known as *metastasis*. The place where the cancer starts is called the *primary site,* while the metastatic sites are known as *secondary sites* or secondary lesions. Cancer may spread through the body by the following routes: (1) by extending directly into nearby tissue or a body cavity, such as the abdomen and chest which are the most frequently affected sites, (2) by spreading throughout the lymphatic system, both through vessels and within the tissue where lymph circulates or the nodes where it often localizes, (3) by traveling through blood vessels to other parts of the body, especially the lungs, the bones, and the liver.

Generally, if the cancer is detected while it is in the primary site, it can be excised and cured. However, if metastasis has begun, the prognosis is usually poor. A person is considered to be *cured* of cancer if 5 years have passed without recurrence of symptoms or lesions.

## CAUSE OF CANCER

Medical science has not been able to pinpoint any one cause for cancer; authorities now are inclined to believe that it develops from a combination of causes rather than from any one thing. However, there are some predisposing factors which seem to contribute to the tendency for the disease to develop. These factors, known as *carcinogens,* include the following:

*Exposure to specific agents,* especially in industry, such as coal soot, oil, aniline dyes, or other chemicals, luminous paint, asphalt. Work with radioactive materials may present new hazards of which we are not yet aware. Over 400 agents have been identified as being carcinogens.

*Cigarette smoking:* A definite relationship has been established between cigarette smoking and cancer.

*Chronic irritation,* while not an actual agent, is another factor involved in the predisposition to the development of cancer. Included under this heading would be such things as pipe smoking, which can lead to lip cancer, ill-fitting dentures, which can lead to mouth cancer, gall stones, exposure to strong sunlight, friction on a mole from a belt, suspenders, or a brassiére strap and cervical irritation.

*Benign tumors* sometimes have a tendency to become malignant, such as growths in the mouth and the rectum, pigmented moles, ovarian cysts, and x-ray or radium irritations of the skin.

*Virus:* Some researchers now feel that cancer is caused by a virus which is present everywhere. They feel that some people have the tendency to contract it or are weak and lack resistance to the disease.

This theory is, as yet, unproven. However, if it is true, it is also possible that an immunization could be developed to combat cancer. As research continues, more hope exists for cancer victims.

*Heredity* also plays a part. Incidence in siblings is higher than that for the general population. However, it is not known if this is a hereditary or an environmental factor. If the theory of viral cancer is found to be true, the hereditary factor will be considered to be a familial weakness or inability to resist the virus. It also seems that a person who is once diagnosed as having cancer, even though he is considered cured, is more likely to have cancer again.

These predisposing causes do not always result in cancer; some people develop cancer even though they never have been exposed to any of the aforementioned conditions. There is reliable evidence that there are other predisposing causes *within* the body—this makes it seem likely that several factors working together cause cancer.

## SYMPTOMS

No one can know whether or not he has cancer without seeing a doctor. This is one of the reasons that a regular health checkup is so important. There are 7 danger signals that people can recognize; anyone should consult a doctor at once if one or more of these symptoms appear. According to the American Cancer Society the danger signals are:

1. Any sore that does not heal
2. A lump or a thickening in the breast or elsewhere
3. Unusual bleeding or discharge
4. Any change in a wart or a mole
5. Persistent indigestion or difficulty in swallowing
6. Persistent hoarseness or cough
7. Any change in normal bowel habits

Usually, pain does not appear until the later stages of cancer; unfortunately, people do not always pay attention to slightly uncomfortable sensations that serve as warnings. Pricking, tingling, tightness, or soreness are not normal feelings; if they last for any length of time, they should be investigated. Weakness and loss of weight always are danger signals—these symptoms may indicate cancer.

## WHERE CANCER OCCURS

Cancer develops in many places in the body. Statistics show that more women than men die of cancer; the reasons for this difference are: (1) there are more women than men in the population; (2) the average life span of women in the population is longer than that of men; and (3) cancer of the breast and the female reproductive organs is very common. Thousands of women die of breast cancer every year with cancer of the other reproductive organs being the next most frequent cause of cancer deaths in women. Thus a periodic and complete physical examination is very important. Women over 20 years of age should be examined once a year. Those with cystic disease or a family history of cancer should be examined twice a year.

Cancer in men occurs most frequently in the following order: the stomach, the prostate gland, the intestines, the bronchus and the lungs, the rectum, and the anus. Most cancers of the esophagus occur in men, and cancer of the stomach affects twice as many men as women. More men than women have cancer of the rectum. Other cancers include leukemia, which is believed to be cancer of the blood or blood-forming organs (the bone marrow, the lymph nodes, and the spleen), and Hodgkin's disease, which is primarily con-

sidered to be a malignant tumor of lymphatic tissue. Cancer also occurs, although rarely, in the kidneys, the bladder, the testis, and the bones.

## HOW CANCER IS DISCOVERED

Cancer is discovered through the following methods:

1. *Observation and palpation of surface lesions.* Sometimes exploratory surgery is done to explore internal lesions.
2. *Use of visualization instruments* such as the sigmoidoscope, vaginal speculum, gastroscope, bronchoscope, and laryngoscope.
3. *Radiology.* (X-Ray examination).
4. *Laboratory tests.* In some cases, such as in cancer of the prostate, there is an increased blood level of acid phosphatase. Other laboratory tests are also used to aid in diagnosis.
5. *Biopsy.* This is the most important means of detecting cancer. The pathologist studies a portion of tissue which has been removed from a patient. This tissue is obtained in 3 principal ways: excision, needle biopsy, and scraping.
6. *Frozen section.* This is done by the pathologist when a nodule or other part of the body has been excised. The tissue is flash frozen and sliced into very thin slices, which are then studied under the microscope. This method is very fast and can be done while the patient remains anesthetized. The pathologist then returns the findings to the surgeon who will then be able to decide, on the basis of the frozen section, what type of surgery to do.
7. *Cytology.* The study of cells can contribute to diagnosis, since cancer cells do not cling together as well as normal cells. A cytology examination is done on sputum, bronchial washings, vaginal secretions, prostatic secretions, pleural secretions, and gastric washings. This method is less accurate than biopsy but has proven value, particularly in cancer of the cervix and uterus.
8. *Subjective or objective symptoms reported by the patient.* These would include loss of weight, a general feeling of discomfort or a change in elimination habits or other functions of the body.

## TREATMENT

### Surgical Treatment

Complete removal of all malignant tissues before they have metastasized to other body tissues is the best treatment for most types of cancer. This sometimes involves extensive surgery, including the removal of the tumor and a wide area of the tissue surrounding it, in an attempt to include all the malignant cells which may have spread to the surrounding area. Typical of such surgery is the removal of not only the breast, in some cases of carcinoma of the breast, but also a large area of the overlying skin, the underlying muscles, the axillary lymph channels, and the lymph nodes which drain the area. Virtually any cancer can be cured if it is *localized* and *removable*.

Surgery may also be used as a preventive measure in *precancerous lesions,* such as hairy moles. This is called *prophylactic* or preventive surgery. In addition, some of the glands in the body which are known to influence the development of cancer can be removed.

## Radiation

Treating cancer by radiation involves exposing tissues to radioactive substances which destroy malignant cells. Generally, radiation is used in medicine for diagnosis, therapy, and research.

**X-Ray Theory.** Radiation affects tissues by altering the chemical structure and the behavior of atoms in the cells, a process known as ionization. Experimental evidence shows that atoms contain positively charged, negatively charged, and neutral particles which vary in number and determine the "weight" of the atom. The atoms of most elements remain intact and stable because of the neutralizing effect of the charges upon each other, i.e., the negative charges balance the positive charges. However, some of the heavier atoms, such as those in radium, have more positive and neutral charges and, consequently, become unstable with a tendency to disintegrate (fall apart). In their attempt to remain intact, they give off *rays,* a process called *radioactivity.* We call these elements *isotopes.* In addition to the natural radioactive elements such as radium, there are isotopes such as iodine and gold which are produced artificially by mechanical bombarding—smashing the atoms in special machines and changing their weights.

**Diagnostic X-Ray.** Because of their ability to penetrate and destroy tissues, these rays are widely used as a means of diagnosing and treating cancer and other illnesses. The photograph (x-ray plate) produced by the x-ray machine with which most of us are familiar is extremely important in diagnosis. The rays which penetrate the tissues and are responsible for the picture are produced by bombarding radioactive elements in the x-ray machine.

**Therapeutic Radiation.** Radiation therapy is indicated in many cases of cancer and may be used as either a therapeutic (curative) treatment or a palliative treatment (one which gives relief but does not cure). Many patients are fearful of this treatment and should be told what to expect.

Both deep and surface x-ray is used in therapy, as well as cobalt, radium, and radioactive isotopes. The cancer cells are more susceptible to radiation than are normal cells. Usually, the greater the degree of malignancy, the more susceptible it is to radiation.

Extreme precautions are taken to protect both the patient and the personnel administering radiation therapy, since healthy cells are destroyed as well as diseased cells, and there are many hazards involved in exposing normal tissues to the rays.

### General Nursing Care in Radiation Therapy

1. Adequate rest is required since the patient may be tired from the treatment.
2. High calorie, high protein diet, as well as one high in vitamins and minerals should be given. The nurse should encourage the patient to eat because it conserves the patient's strength and helps to offset the nausea and diarrhea which may occur. Sometimes, it is helpful to give the diet in several small feedings, rather than in 3 large meals. However, the patient should not be fed immediately before the radiation treatment.
3. Special skin care is needed. Avoid direct sunlight, since the skin may burn easily or may become mottled. Keep the radiation site dry and free from irritation. Use no soap and very little water, and avoid any powders or ointments, especially those containing metal. Use cornstarch or a mild ointment, such as A and D. Do not remove marks which have been applied as a guide to the radiologist. If irritation from the radiation occurs, report this im-

mediately. (Do not refer to this as a "radiation burn," because it may imply carelessness.)

4. Adequate explanation to the patient can alleviate many of the fears of radiation therapy. The patient should understand that the treatment will not hurt, that it will only take a few minutes, and that he or she will feel no heat. Do not mention "radiation sickness," as many patients do not experience these symptoms. It is wise not to mention the number of treatments the patient is to have, since this may change.

5. "Radiation sickness" is probably the most talked about side-effect of radiation therapy and is also the most misunderstood. If the patient does suffer from gastrointestinal symptoms, he should be supported with routine nursing measures. If these symptoms are too severe, the radiation may have to be discontinued.

**The Patient With an Implanted Radioactive Isotope.** In some forms of cancer, a radioactive isotope, such as radium, is implanted into the cancerous area. These implants may be in the form of "seeds" of gold containing radon or in the form of direct radium implants, which are either permanent or temporary. This is commonly done in cancer of the cervix or tongue. These measures sometimes apply in the care of the patient who has had an injection of radioactive material into the body.

The nurse, caring for a patient who has radioactive material within the body, should be aware of its presence and can protect herself by following a few simple procedures:

1. Do not stay with the patient longer than necessary to complete good nursing care. Different nurses should care for this patient so that one nurse does not become overexposed.
2. Do not stand closer to the patient than necessary.
3. Do not care for this type of patient if you are likely to be pregnant, especially in the first trimester of pregnancy.
4. Handle drainage and dressings with care since they might be radioactive.
5. Be alert in noticing if the implant is still in place. If it does fall out, do not touch it except with a long forceps. It should be put into a lead container and the radiologist notified.
6. Do not be afraid of the patient. Remember, he or she is a person and no doubt is afraid too.

## Chemotherapy

While some drugs are used to halt the progress of cancer, no drug has been found that will cure cancer. Drugs such as Aminopterin and amethopterin are sometimes given to restrain the formation of folic acid in the body and thereby halt the growth of body cells. Because of their action, these drugs are called *folic-acid antagonists.* Nitrogen mustards, also known as cytotoxic agents, which attack cells that are growing rapidly, are used in the treatment of blood and lymph cancers. Other chemical agents used include antimetabolites, such as 6-mercaptopurine, bisulfan, and 5-fluorouracil (5 FU). Adrenal hormones (ACTH and cortisone) are sometimes given for temporary relief (*palliative* treatment). Sex-related hormones are also used, since it is believed they slow down the growth of the cancer cells by making the environment less favorable.

**The Nurse and Chemotherapy.** The nurse will usually not give the intravenous *antineoplastic* (against cancer) drugs, but will often assist in their preparation. It is important to remember that these drugs kill normal cells as well as cancer cells. Thus the nurse should wear gloves when preparing them to prevent injury to herself. She should be especially careful not to allow these drugs to come in contact with the eyes or mucous membranes. If this should happen, rinse thoroughly with clear water and obtain first aid immediately.

The nurse in caring for the patient receiving chemotherapy should consider the following points:

1. Symptoms of toxicity may appear and should be reported.
2. The patient should be supported both emotionally and physically.
3. Symptoms, such as diarrhea may need attention. Give good oral hygiene and assist with personal care. Assure an adequate fluid intake.

4. The patient should have a high calorie, high nitrogen diet, to build up strength.
5. The patient may be susceptible to hypostatic pneumonia. Provide for position changes and deep breathing.
6. Personality changes may occur.
7. Sex-related changes may occur. Men may have engorgement of the breasts; women may experience a deepening voice or hair on the face.
8. Skin eruptions may occur. Use no soap and keep the skin moist and free from irritation.
9. Alopecia (loss of hair from normally hairy parts of the body) is a common symptom. Encourage the woman patient to wear a wig.
10. The patient may develop a tendency to retain fluids. Give a low-salt diet; often diuretics are given.
11. Nausea and vomiting may occur. This does not happen in all cases, although it is the most frequently mentioned symptom. Give the patient support and PRN medications for nausea.
12. Bleeding may occur. Observe, give emergency first aid, and report. Anemia is also common.
13. The major hazard is depression of bone marrow function. The laboratory tests and vital signs should be watched for any indication of infection. Since the white blood count is lowered, the nurse should attempt to protect the patient from infection.

## NURSING CARE OF THE CANCER PATIENT

### The Patient's Attitude

Patients react to illness in very different ways; cancer patients are confronted with a knowledge that they find hard to face. A nurse is bound to be faced with the patient's questions about his illness: "Do I have cancer?" or "Will I get well?" are questions uppermost in the patient's mind even if he is afraid to ask them. So much information is available to the public today that it would be unusual, in most instances at least, if the patient did not recognize some aspects of his disease.

Most cancer patients will undoubtedly face the need for surgery. In addition to the general fears which trouble any preoperative patient, the cancer patient awaiting surgery has other worries: For one thing he has no choice in the matter—it is a matter of life and death. Secondly, he has to accept the disfigurement which may result. Thirdly he has no time to adjust to the idea of having surgery, because it must be done immediately. And, finally, he has no guarantee that he will be cured even if the operation is performed.

**The Nurse's Role.** Cancer patients who have gone to a doctor in time have a good chance of being cured; you will take care of them after surgery or radiation therapy. You will also take care of cancer patients during a terminal illness—the patients in whom cancer was discovered too late. Remember that a terminal illness is difficult for the patient's family; your sympathetic care of the patient will help them through a trying time. Your role is a difficult one; to be sympathetic but not emotional; to be cheerful but not aggressively so; to be patient and kind; to understand the patient's fears and depression and to sense ways of comforting him. Sometimes spiritual consolation can be a great source of strength; contact with the hospital chaplain or with a clergyman of the patient's own religious faith may be most welcome.

For those who will get well, the hope of a satisfactory return to a normal life is the best reassurance they can have. Your cheerful encouragement of any patient to help himself restores his shaken confidence in his ability to look after himself.

### Common Nursing Problems

Several of the nursing problems which are a trial to one cancer patient affect many cancer patients. These problems are no different than those of other patients, but cancer patients are apt to have more of them at the same time and to have them more severely. For example, pain not only may be accompanied by nausea and incontinence, but also by bleeding and infection.

**Skin Care.** Some cancer patients must be in bed for months. They lose weight and become emaciated. In these instances, the skin over bony prominences should be kept clean and dry to prevent pressure sores or decubiti. Rub the skin with lotion frequently and use pads to relieve pressure. After radiation treatments for cancer of the pelvis or the abdomen, the skin over the sacrum needs special attention. If the patient is incontinent keep him dry; absorbent pads will help.

**Diet.** Cancer depletes the body proteins and affects nutrition generally. The diet should be high in body-building foods and vitamins. For colostomy patients, the amounts of fruits and vegetables should be regulated to prevent diarrhea; vitamin concentrates may be prescribed to make up deficiencies.

A cheerful, unworried patient is more likely to have a good appetite. See that his dressings are clean and that fresh air is circulating through the room at mealtime. If his appetite is poor, tempt it with small servings of food and an attractive tray. Sound the hopeful note with convalescent patients by emphasizing the normal diet they are permitted to have. Encourage every patient to feed himself if he is able; ask him to tell you what foods he likes.

**Control of Pain.** Many cancer patients have considerable pain. Follow the doctor's orders about giving morphine or other pain-relieving drugs when the patient needs them. Nurses sometimes are reluctant to give habit-forming drugs, but prolonged pain in terminal cases can do more harm than the drug. Sedatives are sufficient to keep some patients comfortable; everything you yourself do to make a patient comfortable will help to make any medication more effective.

**Secondary Infection.** In cancerous growths, if the cells are deprived of food and oxygen, they die or become necrotic. As this dead tissue sloughs, it may leave a raw open area, or *ulcer,* which may bleed if the cancerous growth involves blood vessels. This open surface provides an excellent entrance for bacteria. The odor attributed to cancer is caused by this infection. Good nursing care in keeping the wound clean by irrigations and frequently changing dressings is very important. As infection decreases, the patient's general condition may also improve. Radiation or chemotherapy may also render the patient more susceptible to infections.

**Odor.** Some cancer patients have discharge or drainage which give off an offensive odor. The thoughtful nurse will try to relieve this problem as much as possible by providing good skin care, good perineal care and good mouth care, as well as by using deodorizing agents. Changing dressings or pads as often as possible also helps to eliminate odors.

**Terminally Ill Patient.** The nurse can be most helpful to the patient and to his family by being supportive and by listening. (The care of the dying patient is discussed more thoroughly in Chapter 30.)

## CANCER QUACKERY

Millions of dollars are spent each year by frantic patients and their families in an effort to cure a cancer. Many of these people could have been cured if they had gone to a reputable physician early enough in the course of the disease. It is unfortunate that the cancer quacks are able to prey on unsuspecting people. The only way to cure cancer is to go to a doctor as soon as possible and to receive reliable medical treatment. The practical nurse can be helpful to her friends and family by educating them in this way.

## CANCER RESEARCH

Research is the key to solving the puzzle of cancer. Only by finding the cause and eradicating it can we stop the spread of the disease. At the present time a great deal of research is being done on laboratory animals in hopes of finding the cause and cure of cancer in humans.

The major goals of cancer research today, as identified by the American Cancer Society, are (1) discovering cellular trigger mechanisms that start malignant cell growth; (2) developing a means of stopping metastasis, (3) discovering chemicals which will kill cancer cells without destroying normal cells, (4) gaining insight into the possible immunization or defense mechanisms within the body, (5) conducting more research into the viral theory of cancer spread, and (6) gaining a better understanding of the chromosomal influences of DNA and RNA upon the predisposition for cancer.

# 44

# The Patient With a Skin Disorder

---

## BEHAVIORAL OBJECTIVES

*The student successfully attaining the goals of this chapter will be able to:*

- *identify, define, and correctly utilize in reporting at least 10 general medical terms which relate specifically to disorders of the skin.*
- *discuss the emotional aspects of skin disorders.*
- *effectively assist the patient to meet his needs caused by a disorder of the skin, taking into consideration his physical and emotional discomfort; and accurately and kindly administer nursing treatments which are specific to skin disorders.*
- *list, describe, and identify the symptoms and causes of the most common skin disorders, classifying each as a disorder of the sebaceous system, an allergic reaction, an infection, a parasitic infestation, a chronic condition, a manifestation of systemic disease, or a tumor; describe the most common types of medical treatment and nursing care in each case; and demonstrate ability to competently carry out nursing care.*
- *specifically describe the mechanism of a traumatic burn; describe several types of medical treatment; and demonstrate ability to safely and kindly assist the patient who has been burned.*
- *briefly discuss the concept of plastic surgery.*

---

## TERMINOLOGY

Besides basic terms such as *dermatology* which describes the study of diseases of the skin, and *dermatologist,* which applies to a doctor who specializes in this field, the nurse should be aware of certain general terms which are used in charting and describing skin disorders.

*Pruritus* (itching) is usually a symptom of some skin disease but may appear with general disease conditions such as liver ailments, cancer, diabetes mellitus, or thyroid distur-

bances. It may also occur in elderly people. Pruritis presents real nursing problems, because the patient is almost irresistibly compelled to scratch, which leads to breaks in the skin and possible infection. It is best to be practical and realize that telling the patient not to scratch probably will be futile. Try to get his mind on something else, avoid overheating, keep irritating materials away from his skin, keep his nails short, and if necessary, give him cotton gloves to wear at night. Soothing baths or local skin applications often give relief.

516

*Dermatitis* literally means an inflammation of the skin. However, the term is used in connection with specific conditions. *X-ray* or *radiation dermatitis* may occur after heavy exposure to x-rays. *Dermatitis venenata* is caused by direct contact with certain plants, such as poison ivy, poison oak, or nettles. Some drugs cause dermatitis. The general treatment for dermatitis is to remove the irritant and to use local remedies which the doctor may prescribe such as wet compresses of boric acid solution, Burrow's solution, or calamine lotion. In order to relieve the itching, these compresses are applied to the affected area. Antiinflammatory drugs, such as Benadryl, may also be given.

Various terms are used to describe the many kinds of skin lesions which may occur. Included among the lesions which *do not cause a break in the skin* are: *macules* (unraised spots on the skin), *papules* (elevations of the skin which do not contain fluid), *pustules* (elevations which contain pus), *vesicles* (elevations which contain clear or serous fluid), and *wheals* (localized areas of edema).

Among the many lesions which involve a *break in the skin* are: *scales* (thin flakes, usually of skin), *crusts* (the dried residue of an exudate), *excoriations* (a scraped area), an *ulcer* (an open area produced by sloughing of necrotic inflammatory tissue), or a *fissure* (a crack or cleft in the skin).

## NURSING PROCEDURES

### Diagnostic Tests

Since the skin is visible, it is rare that a diagnostic test must be done. However, sometimes such procedures as cultures and sensitivity tests are done, not to determine if there is a disorder, but to determine what the disorder is and what drug will combat it.

### General Aspects of Dermatologic Nursing

It should be remembered that skin lesions may represent an actual problem or may be indicative of an internal problem. In the latter case, they are merely present as a symptom of another disorder.

The nurse must be able to describe in detail what the skin disorder looks like, how it feels, how large it is, whether or not it is draining, what the drainage looks like, and other objective symptoms. She must also be able to describe subjective symptoms which the patient may tell her, such as the presence of pruritis, tingling, or pain. The patient can also sometimes tell the nurse what the cause of the skin disorder might be. The nurse may also observe such factors as an area which the patient has been scratching, an elevated temperature, or other symptoms.

### Special Nursing Skills Used in Dermatology

**Application of Moist Dressings.** Moist packs are used in many dermatological disorders in order to reduce swelling and weeping in acute dermatitis, to soften and remove exudate and crusts, and to relieve pruritis and discomfort. The dressing may be either open or closed. The *open* dressing is not covered with plastic or other firm dressings. As a result it will evaporate very fast and will require frequent changing or resoaking. The *closed* dressing is less frequently used because of the danger of tissue necrosis from lack of oxygen.

Many different solutions are used on the dressings. The doctor will specify which he wants. Often, the pharmacy will mix the solution and send it to the floor. Common solutions are saline, Burow's solution, potassium permanganate ($KMnO4$) and silver nitrate (for burns).

Before the nurse applies or changes the dressings, she should explain the procedure to the patient. The pack is soaked in the solution and applied semidripping to the area indicated. If unaffected skin is also covered with the pack, it should first be coated with vaseline to prevent necrosis. The packs are kept wet, as ordered. Generally, they are changed or resaturated at least every 2 hours. The nurse should remember to protect the bed and herself from the solution.

A bed cradle should be present if the legs or trunk are to be packed, and blankets should be provided so that the patient will not become chilled. It is also important to chart the procedure, as well as any observations made when the packs are off. The used dressings, if they are to be changed, are to be considered contaminated, unless otherwise ordered. The packs may be tied or pinned into place, under normal safety precautions. In the case of a child, the hands must often be restrained to prevent scratching which may spread or start an infection.

**Removal of Exudates or Crusts.** In some cases, the doctor will order the nurses to remove loose skin, crusts, or denuded tissue. This is a sterile procedure which is often carried out at the same time the packs are changed. Be sure to receive full instructions as to how this is to be done for the individual patient, since each case is different.

**Therapeutic Baths.** Many dermatology patients are given a special bath, which, aside from cleansing the body, soothes the skin, relieves itching, helps remove dead skin or crusts, and offers a means for applying medication to the entire body at one time. Therapeutic baths also provide an opportunity to apply warmth to the body so that physical therapy and range of motion procedures may be done to prevent contractures and other deformities.

Common substances used during these baths include detergents, oatmeal, antipruritis preparations, and other substances, such as copper sulfate, coal tar, or emollient oils.

The bath is usually given in a bathtub, which has been disinfected before the bath (and again after the bath), or in a whirlpool tank. The nurse follows the doctor's orders regarding the substance to be used, the length of time the patient is to be in the bath, and other treatments which are to be carried out at the same time.

**Fluid and Electrolyte Balance.** Fluid and electrolyte balance and general nutrition are often problems in dermatology patients because of exudates or serum lost in the inflammatory process. The nurse should be prepared to force fluids and to encourage the patient to eat. He generally will be on a high calorie, high protein diet.

**Emotional Aspects.** Skin problems are often related to emotional factors in that the skin eruption may be the manifestation of an internal psychological problem. However, once the eruption occurs, it contributes its own impact on the emotional state of the patient. For example, the problem of itching which accompanies so many skin disorders creates emotional as well as physical discomfort. If you have ever had a severe form of pruritis, you know that itching is often more irritating than pain and is often more difficult to control by medication.

Chronic skin problems present their own emotional challenges. Very often, the disorder is one which flares up at intervals throughout the life of the patient, so that he must learn to live with it. In other instances the patient must be hospitalized for a long time and often faces the problem of disfigurement or skin grafting.

The nurse can be most supportive by listening to the patient and by doing what she can to control the symptoms of his disorder. However, she will need to control *her own feelings* concerning the patient's appearance before she can help him deal with this difficulty.

## SPECIFIC SKIN DISORDERS

### Sebaceous Gland Disorders

**Sebaceous Cysts.** The sebaceous glands secrete oils and are combined in the skin with hair follicles. When a sebaceous gland becomes plugged, small, hard nodules form. They do not need treatment unless they become large and annoy the patient, in which case they are drained or excised surgically.

**Acne Vulgaris.** *Acne vulgaris* is a chronic skin disorder marked by blackheads, pimples, cysts, nodules, and scarring. It usually appears on the face, the back, the chest, and the upper arms. Often it is associated with puberty and adolescence and seems to be affected by general health, diet, and hormonal balance. Rich foods, lack of sleep, and emotional pressures are known to aggravate acne, but no single factor alone causes it. It is believed that hormonal imbalance during adolescence is partly responsible. Acne is not only disfiguring, but it also may leave permanent scars on the victim's face and personality, for it comes at a time when a young person is agonizingly conscious of how he looks and of what people think of him.

Treatment usually consists of practicing good personal hygiene (diet, cleanliness, good elimination, sunshine, and outdoor exercise). The patient should be under medical supervision to prevent the use of "quack" remedies which are inefficient and often harmful. Ultraviolet light treatments sometimes help and, when all else fails, x-ray therapy is often beneficial. Scalp treatment should be carried out if it is necessary—dandruff might aggravate acne. Surgical planing (dermabrasion) is sometimes done to remove the scars of severe acne, as well as other scars or tatoos.

**Dandruff (Seborrheic Dermatitis).** Treatment of dandruff consists of frequent shampoos as advised by the doctor (not the hairdresser). He may recommend tincture of green soap or some other cleansing solution. Sometimes medicated ointments are prescribed to alternate with shampoos, along with scalp massage and brushing. A low fat diet, exercise, and rest are also important aspects of therapy.

**Seborrhea.** Seborrhea occurs as scaling or yellow, greasy patches which appear on various parts of the body, other than the scalp, and are caused by hyperactive sebaceous glands.

## Allergic Skin Reactions

**Urticaria.** *Urticaria* (hives) is characterized by the sudden appearance of edematous, raised pinkish areas that itch and smart. Sometimes they disappear as quickly as they come, but they may remain as long as several days. In most instances, urticaria is an allergic reaction to a foreign protein substance. It may be face powder, an insect bite, a serum, or a food protein. Occasionally, it seems to be caused by emotional pressures. Edema is only a temporary annoyance, but it can be dangerous if it involves extensive and vital areas. If it should develop into *angioneurotic edema,* in which the lips and the tissues around the eyes swell tremendously, or involve the larynx, causing it to interfere seriously with breathing, it might cause death. Mild cases can be treated with soothing lotions, such as calamine lotion or with antihistamines. In some severe cases (anaphylactic shock) adrenalin may be used. (See Chapter 54.)

## Infections of the Skin

**Impetigo Contagiosa.** *Impetigo contagiosa* is an infection which is seen at all ages but

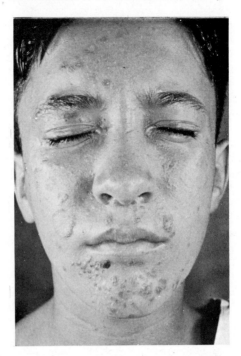

Figure 44-1. Impetigo contagiosa. Note crusts that form over lesions. (Medichrome—Clay-Adams, Inc., New York City)

most frequently in babies and children. It is caused by streptococcal and staphylococcal organisms whose natural homes are on hands, clothing, and objects. Redness appears and vesicles break open to leave a sticky yellow crust, usually on the face and the hands (Fig. 44-1). Impetigo is highly contagious, and the utmost care should be taken to isolate the patient and his equipment in order to prevent the spread of infection. It can be very serious in a nursery for newborns where, given a chance, it will spread like wildfire.

In treating impetigo, the crusts are removed with soap and water, or with mineral oil, followed by the application of any one of a number of ointments: neomycin, ammoniated mercury, or gentian violet. Severe cases may require antibiotics.

**Athlete's Foot.** *Athlete's foot* is a fungus infection that attacks the skin between the toes; watery blisters form into moist, weepy spots that burn and itch. The organism responsible for the infection lurks on the floors of public baths and showers and grows lustily in any damp place. A physician's advice should be sought concerning the treatment of athlete's foot. Many manufactured remedies are available, such as Whitfield's ointment, Desenex powder and ointment, or Lysol solution. The greatest preventive measure is to dry thoroughly between the toes after a bath or a shower and especially after swimming. Athlete's foot may recur if the skin is not kept dry and clean, since the fungus may continue to live in the shoes. Keep shoes thoroughly ventilated and expose them to sunlight and fresh air as often as possible. Alternate between 2 pairs of shoes.

**Warts.** *Warts* are small brownish or yellowish lumps which have rough surfaces and appear on the skin singly or in bunches. They are caused by a virus and may remain for years or disappear of their own accord. They are not painful, with the exception of the *plantar* type, which appears on the soles of the feet and grows inward under pressure from the weight of the body. Warts are destroyed by treatment with short, high-frequency electric sparks (electrodesiccation), by x-ray treatment, or by application of acid.

**Herpes Simplex (Cold Sore).** The cold sore is caused by a virus. There is a theory that this virus lurks in the body and pounces in the presence of a cold or a fever. Another theory claims that a cold sore may develop as the result of an emotional upset or at the beginning of the menstrual period. It generally appears on the mouth in the form of a group of small blisters, which burn and are painful. It usually does not last long and does not require treatment. If this lesion appears inside the mouth, it is called a *canker sore.*

**Herpes Zoster (Shingles).** *Herpes zoster* is caused by a virus that affects the nerves. It is caused by the same virus which causes chicken pox in children. Groups of vesicles appear along the course of a sensory nerve, usually on the face or the trunk of the body. The blisters are preceded by fever and malaise, followed by neuralgic pains that may be quite severe, especially in elderly persons. Sometimes this neuralgia persists for weeks after the eruption has disappeared, which usually occurs within 3 to 5 days. Treatment is designed to keep the patient comfortable with analgesics and to soothe the painful lesions with calamine lotion.

**Furuncle, Carbuncle, Furunculosis.** A *furuncle* (*boil*), is an acute infection of a hair follicle. A *carbuncle* is composed of several boils in a cluster. *Furunculosis* is a condition of many recurrent boils.

These conditions are caused by staphylococcal infection; when boils keep recurring it usually means that the patient has poor general health, an inadequate diet, and a lowered resistance.

A furuncle is a whitish, tender, painful spot in the middle of a reddened area, which after a few days discharges pus and finally a *core.* A carbuncle is a large swollen area, frequently occurring on the back of the neck. It is very painful and has pus draining from several openings. Furunculosis, characterized by many boils, may be accompanied by fever and weakness.

Boils usually are caused by bacteria that enter the skin through areas that have been broken through rubbing or scratching and sometimes through the pinching or squeezing of a pimple. It is dangerous to pick or squeeze a boil since this may spread the infection to the surrounding tissues and possibly to the blood stream. Hot wet dressings or soaks are used to *localize* or center the infection at one point. Antibiotics, such as penicillin or tetracycline, help to control the infection. It is sometimes necessary to incise a boil to allow the pus to drain. If the patient has frequently recurring boils, it is safe to assume that his general health needs to be investigated. An *autogenous vaccine* (a vaccine made from the organisms causing the boil) is sometimes given if boils persist.

## Infestations by Parasites

**Scabies.** *Scabies* (7-year itch) is caused by itch mites that burrow under the outer layer of the skin. A month or more after they enter the body, the skin begins to itch, especially when it is warmly covered. Red spots with a row of blackish dots from $1/8$ to $1/2$ inch long appear with tiny blisters and depressions, especially between the fingers. Since the parasites get into bed clothing and personal garments, special precautions are necessary to keep scabies from spreading. Ironing or boiling clothing kills the parasites. The usual treatment recommended is a bath to open up infected spots, followed by the application of a prescribed ointment, such as benzyl benzoate, to the entire body. The infected person puts on clean clothing and uses clean bed linens and does not remove the ointment for 24 hours.

**Pediculosis (Lice).** There are 3 forms of lice which infest humans: head lice, body lice, and pubic lice. They are very difficult to eradicate, since their eggs, or *nits,* can live for a long time on clothes or bedding or in overstuffed furniture. Symptoms include extreme pruritis and the presence of nits. The disease is most common in children, especially girls, with poor personal hygiene being a contributing factor.

**Bedbugs.** This insect lives in clothing or bedding and is quite difficult to eradicate. When it bites a person, usually on the legs and feet, it causes itching and burning.

**Parasites and the Practical Nurse.** When a patient comes into the hospital with various forms of parasites, it is important that the nurse not impose her personal values and aversions upon the patient or treat the patient with disrespect.

## Chronic Conditions

**Vitiligo.** *Vitiligo* is a condition in which areas of the skin do not produce the pigment (melanin) that gives the skin its normal color. As a result, the pigment-deficient areas appear as light-colored patches. No really effective remedy has been found for this condition, although the use of drugs called *psoralens,* followed by exposure to sunlight or ultraviolet light, has been found to offer temporary relief. The treatment is prolonged and time-consuming and must be done under the close supervision of a physician. The use of cosmetics designed to cover birthmarks is a practical solution to the problem of vitiligo.

**Eczema.** There are many kinds of *eczema,* all of which are more or less chronic and look and behave alike. Eczema appears as small blisters on a reddened and itchy skin; sometimes these vesicles burst and ooze, after which, crusts form in the affected area. Perpetual irritation and scratching make the skin leathery and thick. Eczema usually appears in the folds of the elbows and the knees and on the face and the neck; it may spread to other areas. It may disappear completely for months, sometimes for years. Unfortunately, it may recur at any time.

Eczema has a definite relation to heredity and allergy and also to emotional stress. In one type of eczema, the patient's family history usually shows allergy in some of its members—this may be in the form of hay fever, asthma, or eczema. As a person grows older, emotional factors seem to aggravate eczema. The treatment consists of applying soothing ointments, such as hydrocortisone, wet dressings or starch baths for inflamed skin, and sedatives or tranquilizers to relieve tension and itching. Remember that emotional tension unknown to you may be affecting the patient, and you must try to relieve that tension. Be on the alert to protect him from allergens to which he is sensitive. Reassure him about his condition—tell him that eczema can improve and even disappear.

**Psoriasis.** *Psoriasis* is a chronic disease that affects young adults and people in early middle age. Men suffer from it more often than women. The cause of psoriasis is unknown, although it is sometimes attributed to heredity or a metabolic disorder. It is characterized by red patches covered with silvery scales which have a tendency to shed. These patches usually appear on the extensor surfaces of the elbows and the knees, on the scalp, and on the lower back.

Treatment of psoriasis is not very satisfactory. Ointments containing ammoniated mercury or salicylic acid are used. A low fat diet may also be tried, and ultraviolet light and x-ray therapy may help.

## Systemic Diseases With Skin Manifestations

**Lupus Erythematosus.** Lupus erythematosus occurs in 2 forms: the discoid type and the systemic type. *Discoid lupus erythematosus* is a chronic, although nonfatal, condition which appears on the skin as disc-like patches with raised, reddish edges and depressed centers. *Systemic lupus erythematosus* is an acute or subacute febrile disease, which occurs primarily in women, and causes widespread collagen damage to many organs and systems. It is marked by remissions and exacerbations and is often fatal. It causes a characteristic skin rash with butterfly formation around the eyes and rash over other parts of the body.

**Other Conditions.** Several other conditions manifest skin disorders, such as the nodes of rheumatic fever, the rash of diabetes, and the ulceration of circulatory disorders.

### Tumors

**Nonmalignant Tumors.** Various nonmalignant tumors, such as warts, cysts, angiomas, and keloids appear on the skin. *Moles* are also known as pigmented nevi and are usually benign, although they may become cancerous, especially if they are very dark, hairy, and highly elevated. Thus any suspicious looking mole should be biopsied. An *angioma* (birthmark) is a vascular tumor involving the skin and underlying tissues, as well as blood vessels. Some are difficult to remove such as the port-wine angioma, but most are not very noticeable or dangerous. *Keloids* are benign scars which may be treated with plastic surgery for cosmetic reasons.

**Skin Cancer.** Skin cancer is the most common form of cancer and is also the most curable. Because the lesion is visible, the patient usually seeks early treatment. The 2 most common types are the squamous cell carcinoma and the basal cell epithelioma. Most skin cancers are slow growing and are treated by x-ray or excision.

Malignant melanoma is another form of skin cancer which is more difficult to treat. It looks like a mole, but is faster growing, changes color, and frequently bleeds. It is often metastatic, either as a primary site or as a secondary metastasis. The prognosis is guarded.

### THE PROBLEM OF DISFIGUREMENT

Skin troubles make people uncomfortable and irritable, but perhaps one of their most damaging effects is on appearance.

Plastic surgery may be done for its *cosmetic effects* or to *repair defects* that are congenital or the result of accident or injury. Improvement in plastic surgery opened up a whole new world of hope for the wounded of World War II. It is now possible to replace parts of the body with plastic prostheses so natural looking that no one can detect them.

A nurse sometimes worries about what she should say to a patient who has had plastic surgery. In the first place, most plastic surgery looks rather hopeless immediately after the operation, when swelling and black-and-blue spots predominate. The nurse can explain this and warn the patient against expecting too much too soon. The doctor has told the patient what improvement to expect, but sometimes the nurse can give further reassurance.

**Skin Grafts.** Skin grafts are a means of covering areas where skin has been lost through wounds, burns, or infections. They are transplants of skin from another part of the patient's body or of skin from another person. It is a painstaking procedure which may be prolonged for many months, depending upon the size and the number of areas to be covered and the success of each operation. Every surgeon has his own preferred method of caring for the plastic surgery area; it usually includes scrupulous attention to aseptic technic and protection of the grafts.

## THE PATIENT WHO HAS SUFFERED A BURN

The best first aid for a burn is the immediate application of sterile cold packs. (See Chapter 35 for more detailed discussion.)

### What Does a Burn Do to the Body?

A burn kills the cells making up the tissues of the body because it damages the protein in the cells.

**Degrees of Damage.** Burns are classified in terms of degree of damage: The *first degree burn* which appears as redness of the skin is superficial and not usually dangerous. The *second degree* burn involves a destruction of the outer layer of skin and the formation of blisters. Skin healing can usually take place without grafting, even in large areas of second degree burn. *Third degree* burn involves destruction of the skin, fat, and muscles and presents an emergency which requires immediate hospitalization and treatment. Healing will not take place without skin grafting. *Fourth degree* burn is not always defined as such, but is a type of burn involving the bone. This type of burn which is experienced in plane crashes and close range explosions, is usually fatal. *Combinations* may occur in degrees of a burn.

**Amount of Body Involvement.** The "Rule of Nines" is used to determine the percentage of the body involved (Fig. 44-2). One arm is 9 per cent, one leg is 18 per cent, the head is 9 per cent, the back is 18 per cent, the front is 18 per cent and the neck (or genitals) is 1 per cent. Therefore, a person with a burn of the back and one leg would be considered to have suffered a 36 per cent burn.

## Nursing Care of the Burn Patient

**Vital Signs.** Since the burn patient is very subject to shock, his vital signs should be taken often. The nurse should also be alert to any change such as tachycardia, which can be very dangerous, or a rise in temperature, indicating dehydration or the beginning of an infection.

**Respiratory Status.** It is very important that the burn patient be watched for respirations, since he often has inhaled smoke and may have sustained burns of his lungs. Frequently this is a cause of death in the patient who is not noticeably burned externally. Because of possible respiratory complications a tracheostomy tray should be kept at the patient's bedside. The nurse should begin immediately with precautions to prevent hypostatic pneumonia. Blood gasses and pH are measured frequently to determine respiratory status and general body status.

**Renal Function.** The urine output is very important because often the kidneys slow down or stop completely after the body has undergone a severe shock, such as a burn. The urinary output is measured, at least hourly, for the first few days, with attention paid to its specific gravity. A very high or a very low urine output is significant. If the output is too low, dialysis may need to be done. Acidosis is a frequent complication.

**Fluid Intake.** Since the patient is losing body fluids constantly from open wounds, these must be replaced. The patient usually will have an I.V. and will receive fluids and plasma, as well as oral fluids. The nurse must be sure that accurate intake and output are recorded.

**Electrolyte Balance.** The electrolytes are

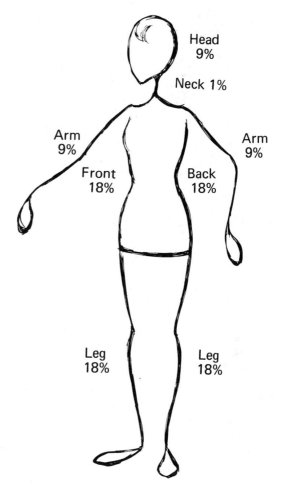

Figure 44-2. "Rule of Nine" chart for calculating per cent of body burns in the adult. (Actual values have been modified for practical purposes.) (From Brunner, L. S., *et al.*: Textbook of Medical-Surgical Nursing, ed. 2. Philadelphia, Lippincott, 1970)

lost through seepage from the wounds and because of impaired kidney function. The laboratory does daily determinations and the electrolytes are controlled by administration of appropriate medications.

**Bowel Function.** Often stool softeners are given to avoid straining.

**Dietary Management.** Good nutrition is vital to the burn patient who needs as many as 6000 calories a day to rebuild the tissues which have been destroyed. The diet should be high calorie and high protein and usually is supplemented by vitamin preparations. The

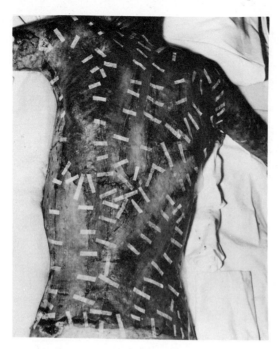

Figure 44-3. Multiple skin grafts have been applied to this patient's back following a severe burn. Notice that tape is used instead of suturing. Taping is easier to do, more likely to hold, and more comfortable for the patient. This patient recovered from his injuries and has normal movement of his extremities. (Medical Products Division, 3M Company)

patient must be forced to eat, because it is so important in his recovery. He cannot rebuild the tissue without eating.

**Prevention of Infection.** The patient may be put into "protective isolation" which means that he is isolated in an attempt to keep organisms from reaching him; he is very susceptible to infection because of his lowered resistance and because of the many open areas on his body. The patient will also receive antibiotics and probably antibacterial body packs.

**Management of Pain.** While the patient with a first or second degree burn is in a great deal of pain, the patient with a third degree burn is not in so much pain because the nerve endings have been destroyed. Since morphine is the drug usually given to relieve pain, the nurse must be alert for symptoms of respiratory depression, which is a side-effect of morphine.

**Dressings.** Several types of dressings are used including sterile dressings, gauze impregnated with an antibiotic or other drug, and moist packs, soaked most commonly in silver nitrate solution.

Sterile dressings are not commonly used except in protective isolation. If they are used, the nurse should follow routine sterile technics in applying and removing them.

External medication is often applied in the form of gauze-impregnated strips. The most common drug in use today is Sulfamylon, although Furacin and vaseline are also used. The nurse may or may not be asked to change these dressings. Sometimes they remain in place under moist packs. If the practical nurse is asked to remove gauze strips, she should be as careful as possible to avoid tearing or ripping the viable tissue. Often when the dead tissue is removed it pulls on the viable tissue, causing great pain for the patient. The thoughtful nurse will offer a pain medication a few minutes before the dressing change.

When moist packs are applied, the most common solution used is 0.5% silver nitrate solution. This is an antibacterial substance which seems to have a very striking effect on burns. It usually eliminates the need for the patient to be in protective isolation. Usually, these packs are kept moist all the time, but they may be applied intermittently. They are not sterile, but clean.

The nurse should be aware that silver nitrate will turn everything black. She should take measures to protect herself, as well as the floor and the bed to prevent permanent staining. The patient should be told that the black color is part of the effect of the drug so he will not become alarmed.

All dressings or packs removed from the patient should be considered contaminated and disposed of accordingly.

**Debridement.** The debridement of eschar (burned tissue) must be done to expose the viable tissue so that grafting may be done successfully. The packs and external medications assist in loosening and softening the eschar. If the nurse is asked to remove the eschar she should have special instructions.

**Reconstructive or Cosmetic Surgery.** Sometimes a part of the face or body is totally burned off. In this case, the plastic surgeons will rebuild that part using skin from other parts of the patient's body.

Skin grafting is done to replace tissue which cannot heal by itself because of the extensive damage (Fig. 44-3). It is also done for cosmetic reasons to limit the amount of scarring. If the patient has enough skin area which was not burned, an *autograft* is done. When healing begins to take place and the eschar is completely removed, the plastic surgeon slices paper-thin slices of skin from an unaffected part of the patient's body and places these grafts on the affected area. If the patient's own skin cannot be used, cadaver skin or skin from another person may be used. This is called a *homograft*. Sometimes, antirejection medications must be given so the patient's body will accept the skin from a foreign source. Skin grafts are very delicate and care should be taken not to disturb them so they may attach themselves to the live tissue underneath and grow.

**Prevention of Contractures.** Since the burn patient is often in bed for some time, special care should be taken to provide passive or active range of motion exercises as soon as possible to prevent contractures or other deformities. The patient is often very reluctant to move because of the pain or fear of pain, so he needs to be encouraged.

If the burn has occurred in the area of a joint, contractures are more likely to form and may need to be released surgically.

**Physical Therapy.** The patient is often taken to the physical therapy department for whirlpool treatment and exercises. The whirlpool serves several purposes: it helps clean the body and often assists in removing eschar; it can provide external medication; it gives warmth so that the patient can exercise with less pain; and it helps to stimulate the viable tissue. When the whirlpool treatment is completed the physical therapist then exercises the patient's extremities to prevent contractures.

**Occupational Therapy.** The burn patient is often in the hospital for a long time and needs diversional activity. He also may need counseling or job retraining after he is released from the hospital. The woman, if she has suffered any deformity from the injury, may need assistance in learning how to take care of her home. Occupational Therapy can be planned to exercise those muscles which need it most, thereby preventing deformities.

**Social Service.** Because of the long-term nature of a severe burn, the patient may need assistance in arranging for the care of his family while he is in the hospital.

**Emotional Aspects.** The patient often becomes discouraged, as do many other people who are hospitalized for long periods of time. He may become demanding because he has become accustomed to the extensive attention he received when he first was admitted. If he is in isolation, he faces the added problem of loneliness. He also is frequently concerned about his appearance. The nurse can be most helpful by listening to him and by encouraging him to do as much for himself as possible.

**The Outlook.** Although the course of treatment is long and difficult, as well as dangerous, the new technics available today have given many patients a chance to live. Many burn patients are saved and return to normal lives after their course of treatment. The practical nurse is a vital member of the health team which provides this treatment.

# 45

# The Patient With Musculo-skeletal Disease or Injury

---

BEHAVIORAL OBJECTIVES

*The student successfully attaining the goals of this chapter will be able to:*

- *describe some of the common deviations from normal body structure and function of the musculoskeletal system, keeping in mind the normals studied in Chapter 13.*

- *discuss the relationship of x-ray, laboratory, and physical examination to the diagnosis of musculoskeletal disorders.*

- *briefly list, define, and discuss at least 5 specific musculoskeletal disorders, including osteomyelitis; identify the causes and considerations for medical management of each; demonstrate competence in assisting the patient to meet special needs caused by a musculoskeletal disorder.*

- *thoroughly discuss the arthritic disorders; identify 4 possible causes of arthritis; describe symptoms of each type of arthritis; discuss the major considerations in medical management; and demonstrate competence in assisting the patient, keeping in mind the goal of rehabilitation to as great an extent as is possible for each person.*

- *discuss common traumatic disorders of this system; list, diagram, and define at least 8 types of fractures; discuss and demonstrate competence in immediate first aid in the case of injury.*

- *discuss and demonstrate competence in the nursing care of a patient in a cast; list at least 7 complications which might follow a fracture; list and describe at least 6 signs of pressure or infection; and demonstrate competence in the physical and emotional care of a patient in a cast and in the care of the cast itself, as well as in assisting with the application or removal of a cast.*

- *list and define 3 methods of immobilizing a body part, other than the use of a cast; and identify the situations in which each might be used.*

- *identify and discuss at least 6 special considerations in the nursing care of the patient in traction.*

- *describe and demonstrate 4 types of crutch walking; identify situations in which each might be used; demonstrate ability to assist in the adjustment of crutches and in teaching the patient.*

- *discuss amputation in terms of physical and emotional needs of the patient; and demonstrate ability to meet the physical and emotional needs of the patient and his family during recovery.*

---

Disturbances of the muscles and the bones often require a combination of medical and surgical treatment. The branch of surgery that treats diseases and injuries of the bones and joints and corrects deformities of this type is called *orthopedics*. The surgeon who specializes in this field is an *orthopedist*.

## WHAT CONSTITUTES MUSCULOSKELETAL DISEASE OR INJURY

Bones give structure to the body—anything that interferes with their firmness puts health off balance. Soft, displaced, broken, or infected bones weaken the body framework, interfere with movement, limit body activity, and may deform the body permanently.

Muscles serve to move the bones and joints. Any defect in muscle function also upsets the functioning of the musculoskeletal system.

### Diagnostic Procedures

Since the structures of movement or locomotion, which compose the musculoskeletal system, are inside the body, several means are used to determine their status and functioning.

**X-ray.** This is by far the most common method used to determine the structure and sometimes the function of bones. It is simply a means of visualizing the bones and other internal structures of the body in an effort to determine if there is any deviation from normal.

**Laboratory Tests.** There are several laboratory tests which can determine the condition of bones and muscles, such as the mineral level of calcium and phosphorus in the blood.

**Electromyelogram.** This is a test of electrical conductivity, similar to the electrocardiogram or the electroencephalogram. It measures the reaction of muscles to electric impulses. In this way, the physician can determine whether or not the muscles are responding appropriately.

**Reflexes.** The doctor, in doing an examination, tests the reflexes of the body. This not only determines the ability of the muscles to react to nervous stimuli, but also measures the function of the nervous system.

## SPECIFIC MUSCULOSKELETAL DISORDERS

### Rickets

*Rickets* is a nutritional disease that comes from a lack of vitamin D in the diet. It affects the hardening process in bones and is brought about through the faulty absorption, from the gastrointestinal tract, of calcium or phosphorus needed for bone structure. The bones stay soft and are distorted until they finally harden in this deformed state. *Bowlegs* is a good example of the effect of rickets on the bones. Children with rickets are slow in learning to walk and in cutting teeth; they are pale and irritable and inactive. We have reason to be concerned about the large numbers of undernourished children in this country who develop rickets. Rickets is prevented and treated by regular doses of cod-liver oil and exposure to sunshine, both of which provide vitamin D. Any extensive calcium deficiency can cause a rickets-like condition of the bones.

### Bursitis

Bursae are sacs filled with synovial fluid that act as pads on bony prominences in joints. *Bursitis* is inflammation of a bursa. In diseases of the bursae the amount of fluid in the sac increases and distends it. Eventually, the wall of the bursa hardens and becomes calcified. One type of bursitis is the result of long-continued irritation or friction in a joint. It is comparatively painless and does not cause disability. The usual treatment for bursitis includes heat and rest of the affected part. Chronic inflammation of a bursa may result in calcification, which causes pain and tenderness in the joint and interferes with its motion. X-ray treatments often relieve this condition; if these are not effective, the bursa must be excised.

### Tenosynovitis

*Tenosynovitis* is the inflammation of a tendon. It may be caused by a gonococcal infection, which particularly affects the wrist or the ankle. The infected tendons swell and cause pain and disability and can be treated by heat and antibiotics. Tenosynovitis may also develop from an infected wound or from infection in nearby tissues. Sometimes it comes from a bloodstream infection. The treatment indicated here is surgery and antibiotics. Noninfectious tenosynovitis is caused by strains or blows or by the prolonged use of a particular set of tendons. Examples of overuse are extensive piano playing or typing. The symptoms are pain and tenderness, especially when there is motion. (Incidentally, this is not the same thing as "writer's cramp.") The treatment includes resting the sore part, applying heat, and changing to another activity which does not involve the affected tendons.

### Ganglion

A *ganglion* is a "bump" caused by a distended synovial sac, which appears under the skin near a joint, usually at the wrist. Strains or bruises, especially if they are repeated, may cause a ganglion. Usually it is painless. Sometimes the sac ruptures, often as the result of a blow, and the bump disappears.

### Bone Tumors

There are 2 kinds of bone tumors: those that start in a bone and those that travel to a bone from somewhere else in the body. They are usually malignant and, if metastatic, are very difficult to treat. The symptoms of a bone tumor are pain and swelling. The treatment consists of surgical removal of the primary tumor. The procedure may be extensive, including the removal of a limb. X-ray therapy is also used but not always successfully. The prognosis of cancer of the bone is very poor. The nursing care is centered on making the patient as comfortable as possible.

### Osteomyelitis

*Osteomyelitis* is infection of a bone. It is a very serious condition which may develop as the result of a compound fracture, which exposes the bone to outside infection, or by organisms such as the staphylococcus or the streptococcus which are carried by the blood to the bone from infection somewhere else in the body. The first signs of trouble are fever and pain, often accompanied by nausea and

headache, with an increase in the white blood cells and tenderness and swelling in the affected area. Then pus forms in the shaft of the bone, gets under the covering (periosteum), and separates it from the bone. Fragments of dead bone loosen and have to be removed.

**Treatment.** The treatment consists of:

1. Surgical drainage to remove the pus. The surgeon may drill a number of small holes in the bone.
2. Antibiotics, placed directly in the wound, along with a catheter inserted for irrigation purposes and to provide for drainage.
3. Rest and good nutrition to build up the body's defenses.

**Nursing Care.** Osteomyelitis is so painful that the affected part is sensitive to the slightest movement. Thus it should not be moved any more than is absolutely necessary. When it must be moved, support it, splint it with a pillow, and lift and move it as you move the rest of the body. Sandbags, a cast, or a brace helps to immobilize the limb. Again, extreme care should be taken to avoid jarring the bed.

The prescribed diet is high in proteins, calcium, carbohydrates, and fats, to build up the patient's resistance, and high in fluids as well.

Swelling, redness, or pain in some other region may be signs that the infection is spreading to another bone and should be reported. Pathologic fractures may also occur and may not be recognized because the pain of the fracture is eclipsed by the greater pain in the infected area. A growth of new bone may lengthen the infected bone; bone destruction may shorten it. Careless aseptic technic in changing dressings could introduce outside organisms into the wound. Osteomyelitis tends to become chronic, and the wound may drain for years. The patient may develop muscle spasms because he is inactive; he often becomes thin and weak, and eventually it may be necessary to amputate his limb. Antibiotics have greatly increased the chances for recovery from osteomyelitis.

## ARTHRITIS

This disease is as old as time itself. It is one of a group of rheumatic diseases that cause more disability in the United States than any other ailment. *Arthritis* is inflammation of a joint. You will remember that a joint is the place where 2 or more bones meet and are held together by ligaments and tendons. A joint is enclosed in a capsule lined with a synovial membrane which secretes a lubricating fluid (synovial fluid).

**Causes of Arthritis.** Some causes of arthritis are:

Infection—caused by an organism such as the tubercle bacillus or the streptococcus
Direct injury
Tissue degeneration
Disturbances of metabolism

Nobody knows *exactly* what causes arthritis, but everything on the above list seems to play a part in its development.

**Infectious Arthritis.** Infectious arthritis is caused by an organism that enters a joint and causes pain and swelling as the result of an increase in the synovial fluid. A culture of the fluid will tell what the offending organism is. The antibiotics that are most effective against this organism are then given; sometimes they are injected directly into the joint. Antibiotics have practically eliminated infectious arthritis.

**Traumatic Arthritis.** This condition is the result of a blow on a joint, a sudden twist, or a repeated series of small blows.

**Common Forms of Arthritis.** The most common forms of arthritis include: *rheumatoid arthritis,* which is the most serious, the most painful, and the most crippling form of arthritis; *osteoarthritis,* also called degenerative joint disease, which generally comes with aging as a result of wear and tear on the joints; *ankylosing spondylitis,* which is a chronic inflammatory arthritis of the spine; *rheumatic fever,* an acute systemic disease which is caused by the streptococcus organism and is usually found in children (see Chapter 40); and *gout,* a painful disease which attacks small joints.

## Rheumatoid Arthritis

*Rheumatoid arthritis* is one of the 2 chief causes of arthritic disability. It occurs all over the world, although some people believe that it is less common in hot climates. It affects 3 times as many women as men.

## How Rheumatoid Arthritis Develops

Nobody knows exactly what causes rheumatoid arthritis. Whatever the cause, inflammation makes the joints swell, destroys cartilage, and forms a tough tissue that interferes with joint motion. If this tissue becomes calcified, the joint is obliterated and movement becomes impossible (ankylosis). The process may go on for years before ankylosis occurs. In some patients, nodules appear under the skin and over pressure points, such as the spine or the elbows; these are usually painless, unless pressure is put on them.

In general, rheumatoid arthritis begins gradually. The patient notices painful twinges and stiffness in one or more joints when he gets up in the morning. As time goes on, some joints, particularly the fingers, become swollen, red, and sore. Gradually, other joints are affected. Sometimes these symptoms disappear for a time, only to return later. The patient does not feel well; he tires easily, has fever, and loses weight. He becomes more than usually sensitive to changes in temperature and is anemic.

**Body Changes.** The muscles around the affected joints become wasted. The finger joints next to the hand swell; fingers and toes feel cold and moist and look bluish. The joint ligaments relax, and the joints become distorted and may even become dislocated. All of these symptoms develop gradually, and although they may disappear suddenly, they almost always return. This process may go on for years, but every new flare-up of the disease causes more joint damage. Without treatment, and sometimes in spite of it, the joint is destroyed in 10 to 15 per cent of the victims.

As calcification increases, the joint becomes immovable and stiff. The pain is less, but the discomfort from lost motion remains. The purpose of the treatment is to lessen the inflammation before the joint is permanently damaged.

**General Treatment.** Arthritis cannot be cured, but early treatment will do much to lessen joint damage. This includes measures to build up body resistance, such as rest and a good diet. Consistent exercise helps to prevent immobile joints and wasted muscles. Deep breathing also helps to strengthen body tone.

**Drug Therapy.** Drugs will not cure rheumatoid arthritis, but they do help to reduce pain and sometimes slow down inflammation. Narcotics are avoided because this is a long-drawn-out disease. Salicylates are used to relieve joint pain. *Aspirin* (acetylsalicylic acid) is the first choice as a pain reliever and seems to reduce inflammation. It must be taken daily, even if the symptoms have subsided. Gold salts are also used because they reduce the inflammation. However, they are toxic and must be carefully given. Other drugs used are phenylbutazone and antimalarial drugs, as well as Indomethacin (Indocin). Cortisone and related steroids are used, although they present special problems. Even though they cause immediate remission of the symptoms, they often cause very serious side-effects. And while they relieve the symptoms, they do not stop the disease process; they merely disguise it.

**Exercise.** Exercise is important to keep the joint functioning, to maintain muscle tone, and to prevent contractures and deformities. Exercise is planned to alternate with rest. Gentle stretching is beneficial, especially if the patient does it himself rather than being "stretched" by someone else. Deep breathing should be practiced several times a day, with frequent changes of position. Braces or splints help to prevent deformities in painful joints. Excessive strain on a joint, caused by poor posture, can be relieved with a corrective corset. *Heat* combined with exercise is also very effective and may be applied by means of paraffin dips, whirlpool therapy, and hot packs.

**Surgery** is sometimes used as a last resort, to manipulate a joint, transplant tendons, or even to build a new joint (arthroplasty). If a joint is very painful, and if there is no hope of making it useful again, the surgeon may ankylose, or solidify, it. Joint motion is lost, but the pain is also gone. "Frozen" joints may also be surgically released.

**Arthritis Fads and Fallacies.** Some patients can avoid being crippled by paying strict attention to diet, rest, exercise, medication, and physical therapy. However, they still have to contend with constant pain. Thus many of them become discouraged and turn to anything that promises a cure. Quacks are quick to take advantage of the fact that rheumatoid arthritis often does disappear for a time; they claim that these let-ups are the result of taking their remedies. Desperate arthritics spend millions of dollars every year on such products as vibrating pillows, copper rings, and radioactive earth.

## Osteoarthritis

*Osteoarthritis,* a degenerative joint disease, progresses slowly in a series of destructive changes. Unlike rheumatoid arthritis, it never lets up and is not accompanied by fever. It may begin in the middle 30's, but it usually afflicts middle-aged and elderly people, both men and women. Osteoarthritis in the joints of fingers and toes is common in women during the climacteric. Obese people are more likely to develop this disease because of the effect of the extra weight on their joints. As the disease progresses and the tissues harden around the joints, the cartilage that covers the ends of the bones becomes thin and uneven and loses its movement. The result of this process is pain and limited movement in the affected joint, although it does not become fixed or ankylosed. There is some evidence that heredity and possibly altered metabolism play a part in the development of osteoarthritis.

**Symptoms.** Osteoarthritis develops slowly; its victims first notice joint stiffness in the morning. This is more marked when the weather is damp or after unusual activity. Any joint may be involved—the spine, the hips, and the knees are most commonly affected. At first, the patient is merely uncomfortable, but eventually movement is painful. The joints are not swollen, and the muscles remain firm. Warmth, rest, and aspirin make the patient comfortable as long as he does not exercise the affected parts. As times goes on, motion becomes more and more limited. Osteoarthritis seldom cripples. Unlike rheumatoid arthritis, it often localizes in one area, rather than spreading to other parts of the body.

**Treatment.** Rest of the affected joints is important. Exercises in moderation are also helpful, although care must be taken to avoid strain. Heat is comforting, and aspirin relieves the pain. Weight loss is recommended for obese individuals. Belts, braces, crutches, and canes give support and relieve strain on the affected joints. Sometimes traction is used to give relief.

## Rheumatoid Arthritis of the Spine

Sometimes called *rheumatoid spondylitis* or *ankylosing spondylitis,* this disease is an inflammation of the joints of the spinal column, accompanied by increasing stiffening and pain. It mainly afflicts young men and almost always appears before the age of 50. Rheumatoid arthritis of the spine begins gradually with aches and pains which alternately disappear and reappear in the lower part of the back (sacro-iliac area). As the inflammation moves upward it interferes with chest expansion. The stiffening spine eliminates the lumbar curve and causes a humpback curvature in the chest area. Stiffening of the neck makes it impossible to turn the head, and the patient has pain and muscle spasm.

**Treatment.** Salicylates are given to relieve the pain, and moist heat helps to relax muscle spasm. Steroids are not helpful, except in acute attacks. Phenylbutazone is sometimes given. Exercises are important to keep the spine as movable as possible and to aid chest expansion. During an acute attack, the patient remains in bed, and attention is centered on relieving his pain and keeping him as comfortable as possible.

## Gout (Hyperuricemia)

In the process of protein digestion substances called *purines* are produced. If the body is unable to metabolize these substances, uric acid accumulates in the bloodstream and forms crystal deposits (tophi) in the joints. This condition is called *gout.* It usually appears in the big toe, the instep, the ankle, or the knee, but it may appear in any joint. It attacks periodically, causing swelling and excruciating pain and eventually limits motion in the affected joint. Other pathology includes renal damage, and vascular damage (especially atherosclerosis).

**Symptoms.** An attack of gout begins with agonizing pain, swelling, and redness. It lasts from 3 to 14 days, after which it disappears

as suddenly as it came. It may return anytime from a month to a year later; in the meanwhile the joint gives no trouble. The slightest touch or weight is unbearable during an attack. As time goes on, repeated attacks damage the joint permanently. The list of things that may set off an attack is a long one: alcohol, allergy, an emotional upset, surgery, injury, infection, nitrogenous or fatty foods, a reducing diet, antibiotics, liver extract, vitamin B, or a mercurial diuretic. Most gout attacks are brought on by emotional crises or by changes in the patient's surroundings, although individuals react differently to such things as food and alcohol.

**Treatment and Nursing Care.** Gout cannot be cured, but the attacks can be controlled and prevented. However, the patient must stick to the routines set up for him and must see his doctor regularly to be advised about changes that will be necessary as the course of the disease changes.

Diet comes first and foremost in the treatment, especially in preventing pain. Except for restrictions in high-purine foods, the diet is not restricted rigidly unless gout is severe. The high-purine foods to be avoided include liver, kidneys, sardines, bacon, goose, mackerel, salmon, turkey, and leguminous vegetables, such as peas and beans. The patient may have such low-purine or nonpurine foods as breads, cereals, spaghetti, fruits, eggs, milk, and nonleguminous vegetables.

A bed cradle to protect the affected joint is a necessity. Preventing the affected part or the bed from being bumped or jarred is so important that a sign warning everybody to be careful may be necessary. Gentle application of warm or cold compresses is sometimes ordered, and elevating the affected joint may make the patient more comfortable. Exercise should begin as soon as the pain and the redness are gone, to prevent the joint from stiffening.

Colchicine is a drug that works wonders in relieving gout. If it is given early enough, it relieves the pain in 12 to 24 hours, along with the other symptoms. The side-effects are nausea, vomiting, and diarrhea. ACTH, Indocin, and phenylbutazone are also effective.

Of all the arthritic diseases, the control of gout is the most successful.

## Long-Term Management of the Arthritic

A patient with arthritis should be told how arthritis progresses and how important it is to prevent deformities. He needs to know the effects of fatigue and how to avoid it by spaced rest periods. He should know that much depends on his own efforts—that if he persists faithfully in his treatment, much can be done to prevent crippling deformities. Many things can be done to make things easier for him. He should have a flat, firm bed, the same height as the seat of his chair, to make it easier for him to move from one to the other. Any chair that he sits in should be 3 or 4 inches higher than an ordinary chair, to prevent overbending at the hips. Using pillows in a lower chair only tends to force him into a hunched position, which is tiring. In their anxiety not to be a trouble to anyone, some arthritic patients overexert themselves and need to be cautioned about this.

**Medications.** Aspirin can be given safely in fairly large amounts, although large doses sometimes cause nausea and vomiting, ringing in the ears, and deafness. It may also affect kidney function; usually, the fluid intake is stepped up for patients who are having large doses of aspirin, to prevent renal calculi (kidney stones).

Phenylbutazone (Butazolidin) helps in about 50 per cent of these patients. A 10-day to 2-week trial period will show whether or not it is effective. Some patients have uncomfortable side-effects, such as nausea, visual disturbances, dizziness, abdominal pain, fever, and a skin rash. Edema may appear if the patient has any cardiac difficulty. Periodic blood counts will tell whether or not he is anemic.

Antimalarial drugs (Atabrine, chloroquine, Plaquenil) are sometimes used to control inflammation. Occasionally, nausea or a skin rash appear as side-effects.

Recent studies have shown that gold salts definitely are effective in treating rheumatoid arthritis. However, in some patients, gold salts cause a mild skin rash. More serious side-effects are jaundice, hematuria, hepatitis, change in urinary output, and severe intestinal upsets.

**Steroids.** These hormones relieve pain and stiffness quickly but when used over a long period, their side-effects cause more disability than would have occurred without them.

The *cortisones* are synthetic reproductions of the adrenal cortical hormone *hydrocortisone*. This hormone strengthens the body's ability to stand strain and regulates metabolism and fluid balance. The preparations commonly used are prednisone (Meticorten, Deltra, Deltasone), prednisolone (Delta-Cortef, Meticortelone, Hydeltra, Sterane), and cortisone (Cortogen, Cortone).

Corticotropin (ACTH, Acthar) has the same effect as cortisone. It cannot be given orally, because it is destroyed in the intestinal tract.

SIDE-EFFECTS OF THE CORTISONES. Cortisones often cause toxic effects, because they are given over such long periods of time. They reduce inflammation, and consequently infection may go untreated because the patient has none of the symptoms. Therefore, it is important to report even a slight elevation of temperature or a minor discomfort, since they may be signs of really serious trouble. The patient who is taking cortisones may gain weight and develop edema as well as the characteristic "moon-face." A daily weight check and a continuous weight record should be kept.

The steroids increase the amount of glucose in the bloodstream which might lead to overproduction of insulin with symptoms of insulin shock. They can also cause peptic ulcers—symptoms of stomach distress should be reported. Sometimes skin disturbances appear, menstruation may cease, and the patient may be mentally depressed. The symptoms disappear when the patient stops taking the drug. After a course of steroid treatment patients seem to be able to carry on without these remedies.

**Physical Therapy.** Physical therapy is excellent for improving the condition of an arthritic patient. The warmth of infrared heat and diathermy on inflamed joints relaxes muscles and relieves pain. Heat also increases the flow of blood to the affected part. Massage is helpful if the joint is not acutely inflamed.

# MUSCULOSKELETAL INJURIES

## Sprains

Sprains are injuries to the ligaments around a joint which cause the ligaments to be stretched and torn. Sprains are painful but seldom serious; they cause swelling and interfere with movement. Rupture of the nearby blood vessels makes the skin black and blue. The usual treatment is to elevate the injured part and to provide a firm support for it, such as an elastic bandage.

## Dislocations

When a ligament gives way so completely that a bone is displaced from its socket, the joint is said to be dislocated. This causes pain, an abnormal position of the bone, and inability to manipulate the joint. Following an x-ray examination, the doctor is able to put the bone back into position. This is sometimes done under anesthesia by stretching the ligaments and manipulating the joint. He then applies a splint or elastic bandage to immobilize the parts until they heal. It may take several weeks to allow the joint capsule and the surrounding ligaments to return to normal position.

## The Patient With a Fracture

Any break in a bone is called a *fracture*. Since bones can break in a number of ways, there are several classifications for fractures:

*Greenstick:* The bone bends and splits but does not break completely. This is common in children because the bones are still soft and pliable.

*Complete:* The fracture goes all the way through the bone, transversely or in a spiral direction.

*Comminuted:* The bone is fractured in several places.

*Impacted:* One portion of the bone is driven into another portion of it.

*Simple:* No open wound exists.

*Compound:* The bone breaks through the skin, causing an open wound and exposing the patient to infection. This is a more serious condition since it is necessary to consider both the fracture and the danger of wound infection.

*Complicated fracture:* This is a fracture in which there is also injury to nerves, blood vessels, and joints.

*Spontaneous (pathologic) fracture:* This type occurs without force or injury sufficient to break a normal bone. It may occur in such conditions as certain types of malnutrition, porous bones (osteoporosis), and cancer and as a side-effect of cortisone and ACTH therapy.

*Compression:* The bone is dented and pushed inward.

*Transverse:* The fracture runs across the bone.

*Oblique:* The fracture runs in a slanting direction across the bone.

*Spiral:* The break coils around the bone.

*Longitudinal:* The break runs the length of the bone.

**Causes of Fractures.** Accidents are the chief causes of broken bones. Fractures may occur when hard surfaces are struck accidentally or by falls in sports activities, automobile accidents, and accidents with machinery. Up to the age of 45, more men than women have fractures; after this time, more women are affected. Elderly people in particular are susceptible to home hazards, such as slippery floors and bathtubs, loose rugs, and dark stairways or corners.

**Symptoms.** The most pronounced symptom of a broken bone is pain which becomes more severe with movement of the part and with pressure over the fracture. Pain is accompanied by loss of function and deformity (an unnatural position of the part). Other symptoms are swelling over the part and discoloration due to bleeding in the tissues. First aid for fractures is described in Chapter 35.

**Treatment.** The next step after first aid has been given for a fractured bone is to take an x-ray of the injured area in order to find the extent of the fracture and the position of the fragments of the broken bone. The doctor then takes steps to restore the bone so that it can resume its original function. The method he chooses will depend on the place and the extent of the break and the condition and the age of the patient. His object is to bring the fragments back into place (*reduction*) and to hold them in that position (*immobilization*) until the break is healed. There are 2 kinds of reduction: closed and open. In *closed reduction* the bone ends are realigned through external manipulation. In *open reduction* the realignment is accomplished through surgery. There are also different types of immobilization: internal fixation, traction, splints, and casts (plaster or synthetic).

**Complications.** *Nonunion of the bone ends* is one of the common complications of fractures and may be due to: (1) poor physical condition, including nutrition, (2) poor circulation, or (3) age. The speed with which bones generate new growth varies with individuals.

*Nerve damage* may occur if the fractured bone presses on or cuts into a nerve, or if a cast is applied poorly, is dented, or is too tight.

*Blood vessel damage* may also occur in the same ways as nerve damage.

*Kidney stones* may form as a result of poor nutrition or the healing process of the bone or as a result of inactivity or overmedication with salicylates.

*Contractures, footdrop, and external rotation* may also occur.

*Embolism* presents an emergency situation and is most likely to occur when a long bone has been fractured.

*Constipation* can be a problem accompanying recovery from a fracture because of the patient's age, inactivity, or eating habits.

*Wound infection,* in compound fractures, interferes with healing and may cripple the patient permanently if the bone itself becomes infected. It will prolong the patient's illness and necessitate wound dressings.

*Confusion,* especially in the elderly, is not uncommon. The patient may try to get out of bed, disarrange apparatus, and tear off the bed coverings—usually at night. Side rails provide some safety.

## The Patient in a Cast

The most common method of immobilizing a fracture is by means of a cast. A cast is a solid material which is applied to a limb and must remain in place until the bone ends have joined together.

**Nursing Care.** The nurse's chief concern in observing a patient in a cast is to watch for signs of *pressure*. Undue pressure of any kind can cause the most serious kind of damage to nerves and blood vessels and death to the tis-

sues. Signs of pressure include the following symptoms:

1. *Edema:* Swelling appears at the edges of the cast and in the parts beyond, such as the fingers or the toes
2. *Blanched or cyanotic skin color:* Fingers and toes must be inspected frequently to note any signs of circulatory impairment. (This is difficult to determine in the Black patient.)
3. *Temperature of fingers or toes colder than on the unaffected side:* Compression of nerves and blood vessels can do a great amount of damage. A loss of oxygen to the tissues over an extended period of time results in tissue death and gangrene. The patient should be able to wiggle his fingers or toes and should be aware if you touch his toes.
4. *Odor:* A pressure sore may develop without the patient's knowledge. The only indication of this would be the odor emitted by decaying tissue.

*Patient's complaints:* Since a cast is not very comfortable, a patient may have many complaints to make about his general discomfort. However, it is well to listen and report repeated complaints about the same thing. *Never* ignore a complaint of pain or pressure from a patient in a cast!

A patient in a *spica* (body) cast needs special attention. For one thing he must be turned frequently. This procedure may cause apprehension at first, because he is helpless and naturally afraid of falling. Specific attention must also be given to elimination and the area near the buttocks. In hot weather, this patient is very likely to be uncomfortable and to complain of itching and burning. Smith and Gips in *Care of the Adult Patient* suggest slipping a corset stay wrapped in cotton and dipped in alcohol under the cast to soothe the itchy spot.

The doctor often puts a loose piece of stockinette inside the cast so the nurse can scratch the patient's back. The nurse should be sure that no crumbs or other foreign substance get inside any cast.

The patient should be encouraged to exercise as much of his body as possible to promote good circulation. Make it as easy as possible for him to do things for himself, even though it takes more time to arrange the necessary equipment. When a patient is made to feel adequate rather than helpless, it helps his morale. It is less boring to be able to stretch and exercise when doing things for himself than it is to exercise mechanically.

The patient with an arm cast who is up and about should support his arm in a sling. If the cast is on the leg, the patient can get about in a wheelchair which can be adjusted for leg support.

Finally, *report any abnormal symptoms* to your charge nurse, especially any signs of *embolism.* An emergency situation occurs if the patient develops a fatty embolus which may go to the brain, heart, or lung. Symptoms are consistent with blockage of blood supply to that area.

**Care of the Cast.** If a plaster cast has been applied, the practical nurse must care for it properly so that it will accomplish its intended purpose—immobilizing the injured part wihtout further damage or injury.

After application, the cast will be wet for 24 to 48 hours. Since it must be allowed to dry in the same shape as it was when it was applied, the cast should be supported with pillows in the same contour as when applied. It should be kept uncovered and the patient should be turned to dry all sides of the cast (as well as to prevent complications). The wet cast should be handled with the palms of the hands only and not with the fingertips, as the fingers may dent the cast and create a pressure point. Bind all rough edges with tape, padding them first, if needed. This is called *petalling* the cast. Protect the cast from moisture if it is in the genital area. Remember, that even after the plaster cast is dried, it cannot get wet or the plaster will dissolve.

Newer types of material are being used for casts which do not require this type of care. A light, synthetic material is available which is dried under a special lamp, within a few minutes following application. After it is dry, the patient can bathe and function normally. In addition, it is a fraction of the weight of a plaster cast, although somewhat more expensive.

**Removal of the Cast.** The cast is removed with a cast saw. Since this is a very frightening experience for the patient, explanation from the nurse beforehand is very helpful. The saw oscillates back and forth, although it gives the appearance of going around. The blade only moves a fraction of an inch and even if it touches the skin, it will not cut the patient because the skin also is able to move that far. If the patient can realize that there is no danger from the removal of the cast, he will be able to stand the noise and the plaster dust.

## Internal Fixation

Another method of immobilizing a fracture is internal fixation, whereby a device is put into or onto the bone to keep it reduced or immobilized or both. Internal fixation is almost always done as a surgical procedure, in *open reduction,* so the surgeons can see the bones and determine exactly how to put them back together. It is the treatment of choice in fractures such as those of the hip, where casting is generally impossible.

Internal fixation is accomplished with a variety of devices:

*A nail* or long spike may be driven the length of the bone. Although usually done surgically, this is the only form of internal fixation which may be done by closed reduction. This method is used most frequently in the long bones of the leg, in which case, it is called an intermedullary nail. Usually it is done if there is more than one transverse fracture or if the patient's history indicates that fractures do not align or heal easily by the cast method.

*A metal plate* may be applied with screws to the outside of a bone to remain in place permanently. This is often done if the bone is fractured in several places.

Screws are sometimes inserted to hold the bone fragments in place without the use of a plate.

Wires may be used to wire the fragments of the bone together.

**Nursing Care in Internal Fixation.** The nurse must remember that since the patient has an open wound, she must watch for signs of infection and treat the dressings as she would any other surgical dressing. The patient also has the added pain of the surgical procedure.

The nails, screws, and plates used are of a special metal alloy which should not irritate the body or set up a rejection reaction. However, since an adverse reaction occasionally occurs, the nurse must be aware of this possibility.

The patient who has had a fracture immobilized by internal fixation may not have any other visible form of immobilization, in which case the nurse must be aware that he does have a fracture and handle him carefully. However, internal fixation will often be combined with another form of immobilization, such as traction.

## Splint

A third method of immobilizing a fracture is through use of a splint. This procedure is most often done as a first-aid measure until a cast can be applied or internal fixation established. Often, a cast cannot be applied until the swelling reduces, in which case, a splint would be applied. As discussed in Chapter 35, any firm straight item can be used in emergency first aid.

In the hospital, a commonly used splint is the half-cast, whereby a full cast is applied and then half is sawed off. Sometimes, both halves remain in place with a crack in between; other times just the bottom half is used. Half-casts are applied to the leg with an elastic roller bandage, which may also be used after healing begins, to give support. It may be taken off at intervals and reapplied or it may stay in place for the full period of immobilization.

Another type of splint which should be mentioned is the inflatable splint. Although most often used in emergency first aid, it may also be used in the hospital. It consists of a plastic bag within another plastic bag, with a zipper on one side. It comes in sizes to fit different parts of the body such as leg, ankle, and arm. If it is to remain in place for some time, a light stockinette is loosely applied to the arm, after which the splint is applied, zipped up, and inflated. It is inflated just enough to immobilize the part. It is comfortable for the patient because it is light, and is very convenient for the doctor and technicians because it is transparent and does not need to be removed when x-rays are taken. Obviously, the nurse must be careful not to puncture the bag. Another splint is the Thomas splint or the ring splint which is often used in combination with traction.

## Traction

A fourth means used to immobilize a fracture is traction (which is also used for other purposes). Traction may be used alone or in combination with other means of immobilization, such as internal fixation.

Traction means *pulling*; it is used in fractures to keep the bone fragments in a good position to heal properly. The strength of the pull on the bones, by means of weights, must be enough to counteract the over-all pull of the muscles. For an adult, 8 to 10 pounds is usually sufficient.

The traction is controlled by principles of physics. The direction of the pull and the extent of the pull is controlled by the weights, by the location and number of pulleys, and by counterbalance measures. A Balkan frame, which is attached to the bed, holds the traction pulleys and equipment. A *trapeze* should also be attached so the patient can pull his head and shoulders off the bed.

There are 2 distinct types of traction: skeletal and skin traction. Skeletal traction involves attaching the traction directly to the bones. Skin traction means external traction in that the equipment pulls on the outside of a leg or other part of the body. Under each type of traction there are specific classifications:

**Skeletal traction**

1. *Skull Traction or Head Traction:* This is a form of skeletal traction which is accomplished by inserting a device such as a Vincky or Crutchfield tongs into the skull bone. It is used to reduce a fracture of cervical vertebrae. The Circ-o-lectric bed or Strycker frame may be used in combination with the tongs.

Nursing care includes caring for those spots where the tongs were inserted, since they go through the skin. Thus good skin care is important. The nurse should make sure that the patient is straight in bed at all times so that the traction will be able to accomplish its function.

2. *The Steinmann Pin or Kirshner Wire.* Either of these devices are driven through the

Figure 45-1. The Russell method of treating a fracture of the shaft of the femur. A small spring scale sometimes is inserted between the pulley and the traction block so that the amount of traction may be estimated accurately. (Brunner, L. S., *et al.*: Textbook of Medical-Surgical Nursing. Philadelphia, Lippincott, 1964)

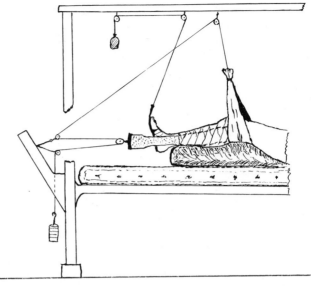

end of a bone (commonly used in leg fractures) and is then attached to traction.

**Skin Traction.** Tape or rubber is applied to the skin and then attached to traction. The traction on the skin transmits the pull to the musculoskeletal structures. There are 3 main types of skin traction:

1. *Pull in One Direction:* Examples of this kind of traction are Buck's extension, in which the leg is wrapped and the pull is directly downward over the end of the bed, and Russell's traction (Fig. 45-1), in which the pull is both down toward the end of the bed and up at the knee.

2. *Balanced Traction:* In the balanced form of traction, the pull is equalized in both directions. That is, the heaviest pull is toward the foot of the bed, but a counterbalance is also pulling toward the head of the bed. The patient in this type of traction is able to move about in bed much more easily because he will not upset the pull of the traction by changing position.

3. *Pelvic Traction:* A belt is applied under the pelvis, with most of the pull directed upward. The belt should be around the hips and not the abdomen. It is used in herniated intervertebral disc or muscle spasms in the back muscles. It is usually applied intermittently: on for 2 hours, off for 2 hours. Weights on the traction are increased gradually. The nurse should never remove or change the weights without orders.

## Nursing Care of the Patient in Traction

Some doctors order the leg supported with pillows; others believe that pillows create pressure behind the knee, which may cause thrombosis. If pillows are used, they should be covered with oiled silk to eliminate friction and should support only the entire thigh and calf, *not* the heel. In order to prevent *footdrop* (contraction of the foot into an abnormal position) keep the foot in a normal position with a footboard. This gives the patient something to push against and keeps the covers from pressing on his toes. Encourage him to exercise by pushing against this board and tell him to point his toes "in" while he is on his back. Every effort should be made to prevent the deformity of footdrop. Watch the pulleys and the ropes because ropes sometimes slip out of their grooves. If the footpiece is touching the pulleys at the bottom of the bed, report it at once. Be sure that the weights are swinging free. *Never remove the weights without an order.* When adding weights, or attaching traction, release the weights gradually. Note the color and test the feeling of the hand or the foot. Watch the patient's elbows for irritation and apply lanolin. Also observe the buttocks for redness and signs of irritation.

**Body Alignment.** Keep the patient's body in good position. See that he does not slump, with his chin resting on his chest.

**Skin Condition.** Be sure that the tape is not irritating the patient's skin. It is often helpful to shave the leg or arm before applying the traction. If internal fixation or skeletal traction has been used, be sure to care for the incision site as you would any other incision.

**Elimination.** Use the fracture bedpan, which is a small, flat bedpan which can be slipped under the patient's hips more easily than the large conventional pan.

**Ambulation.** If the break is such that a walking cast can be applied, the patient will be able to get around out of bed with the help of a cane. Otherwise, the patient must use crutches when he is allowed to get up following a leg fracture.

The doctor determines the amount of movement allowed. One nursing problem is getting enough movement in the elderly patient to counteract the danger of *hypostatic pneumonia* (congestion in the lungs). A method to prevent this is by deep breathing exercises, which can be carried out by blowing up balloons or by blowing bubbles into a glass of water through a straw. However, any movement that interferes with the traction pull must be avoided.

## Hip Fractures

The hip may sustain one of several types of fractures, including fractures of the head of the femur, or fractures of the neck or the trochanter. These fractures heal poorly because nutrition is interrupted by the healing process. They often occur in older people whose bones heal slower. The treatment includes reduction of the fracture by traction or internal fixation, known as hip pinning. The patient is up in the chair as early as the first postoperative day. Routine postoperative measures, such as turning, coughing and hyperventilating, and good nutrition, are very important.

The procedure for turning the patient is as follows: Turn the patient to the unaffected side with a pillow between the knees to provide good alignment. Position the patient comfortably and make sure to support the patient with pillows or sandbags and trochanter rolls so that his body is in correct alignment and so that he does not suffer contractures. Passive and active range of motion exercises are important also.

Good back and skin care are necessary because the patient is in bed a great deal. Since the patient with a fractured hip is often older and has nutritional difficulties his skin is more subject to breakdown.

Crutch walking is begun early without weight bearing on the affected side. Weight bearing begins in 3 to 5 months.

**The Hip Prosthesis.** Sometimes a part of the hip is replaced because the pieces cannot be realigned. This is done by the use of a metal prosthesis, which usually includes the head of the femur and part of the neck and shaft of the femur. Most patients are able to walk again after a prosthesis is inserted.

## CRUTCH WALKING

The first steps in using crutches come *before* the patient tries to use them to stand or to walk. Reconditioning exercises prepare his body for action; he dangles his legs over the edge of the bed, sits in a chair, and learns to stand by the side of the bed. As he does this he is learning good posture—head and chest up, abdomen in. If his disability allows, he may be encouraged to press his feet down on a footstool to get the feeling of standing again; or, with his arms extended, he may be shown how to press his palms down on the bed to exercise his arm muscles.

Now for the crutches: they must be right for him. If they are too long, they cause pressure in his axilla—if they are too short, he slumps. Crutches are measured for length in several ways; for one method, the patient lies straight in bed and is measured from the front axillary fold to a point 6 inches out from the side of the foot. The placement of the hand bar is just as important; it should be at a height that allows the patient to extend his arm almost entirely when he leans on his palms. Even if the crutches are the correct length, individual arm lengths are different. Shortening the crutches more than an inch usually means the position of the hand bar must be changed.

A crutch tip should be made of a good rubber that will wear well; it should fit snugly

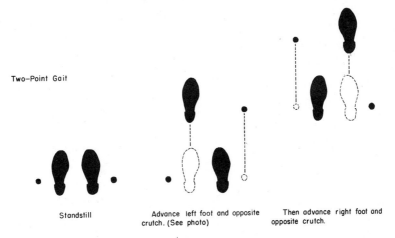

Two—Point Gait

Standstill

Advance left foot and opposite crutch. (See photo)

Then advance right foot and opposite crutch.

Figure 45-2. Two-point gait.

and not move when the weight is placed on the crutch. A large vacuum tip now available is almost a necessity for the severely disabled person who must place his crutches wide apart to provide a firm base. This tip sometimes gives a patient more confidence, even if the ordinary tip is perfectly safe for him.

It should not be necessary to pad the top of the crutch; if the crutch fits and is used properly, there is no pressure under the arm. A patient may tend to lean on his crutches if the tops are padded. Once he learns how to use his crutches, rubber pads can be used to protect his clothing; sponge rubber covered with some soft material or rubber pads made to fit the crutch are inexpensive. Properly fitted crutches are comfortable to use.

The patient should wear a shoe that fits well, with a low, broad heel and a straight inner border. An old pair of good, comfort-able shoes is excellent. Bedroom slippers give no support and may damage the foot seriously.

## Technic of Crutch Walking

The patient's strength and disability determine the best method of crutch walking for him. He should use and improve as many muscles and joints as possible. There are 4 types of crutch walking:

1. TWO-POINT: The patient puts his weight on one leg and the *opposite* crutch, brings the other crutch and leg forward together, and shifts his weight to them; then he brings the other leg and crutch forward (Fig. 45-2). This gait is faster and less boring for the patient; as his muscle power improves he can change to it.

2. THREE-POINT CRUTCH WALKING WITH BOTH CRUTCHES AND ONE FOOT ADVANCED AT

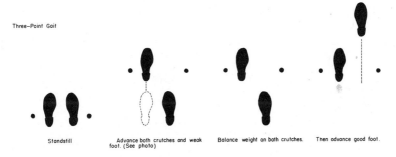

Three—Point Gait

Standstill

Advance both crutches and weak foot. (See photo)

Balance weight on both crutches.

Then advance good foot.

Figure 45-3. Three-point gait.

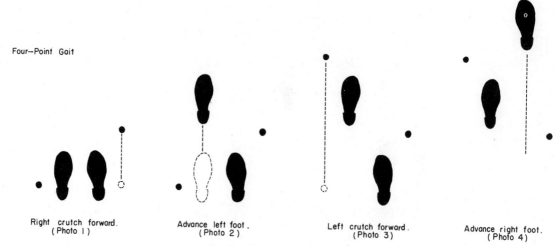

Four—Point Gait

Right crutch forward.
(Photo 1)

Advance left foot.
(Photo 2)

Left crutch forward.
(Photo 3)

Advance right foot.
(Photo 4)

Figure 45-4. Four-point gait.

THE SAME TIME: The weak leg and *both* crutches are advanced together, the weight is balanced on them, and the *good* leg is advanced (Fig. 45-3). Equal-length steps are important, as well as equal timing without a pause before the good leg is advanced. This method is used when one leg is disabled but the other is strong enough to bear all the patient's weight.

3. FOUR-POINT: One crutch is placed forward, and the *opposite* foot is advanced; the second crutch is brought forward, and the opposite foot follows (Fig. 45-4). Rhythm and short equal steps are important; counting helps to develop rhythm: ONE—right crutch forward; TWO—advance left foot; THREE —left crutch forward; FOUR—advance right foot. This is the easiest gait and the safest— the patient always has 3 points of support. He must be able to bring each leg forward and clear the floor with each foot. Polio paralytics, patients with fractures of both legs, or arthritic patients can use this gait.

4. SWINGING OR TRIPOD WALKING: The patient stands on his good leg, puts both of his crutches the same distance in advance, rests his weight on the palms of his hands and swings himself forward slightly ahead of his crutches; he rests his weight again on his good leg and gets his balance for another step (Fig.

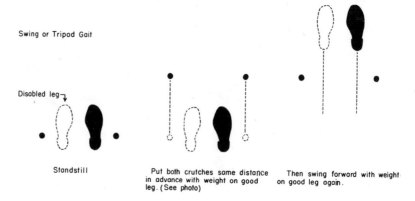

Swing or Tripod Gait

Disabled leg

Standstill

Put both crutches same distance
in advance with weight on good
leg. (See photo)

Then swing forward with weight
on good leg again.

Figure 45-5. Swing or tripod gait.

45-5). Since this is a fast gait, the patient should not attempt it until he has learned balance. The patient who is allowed to put his weight on one leg and must hold the other up should bend his *knee* (not his hip). This gives him better balance. This is the best method for an amputee, a patient with a recent fracture, or a patient with little power in his legs. Bending the knee is tiring—the patient should rest frequently, with this leg elevated. (A leg strap or sling may be used.)

When the patient is able to progress to using only one crutch, he places it on the *strong* leg side. Later he may use a cane; it should have a curved handle, not too well-polished in order to provide a secure grip, and a good, well-fitted rubber tip. It should be long enough to allow the patient to bear his weight on his palm with his arm almost completely extended.

## THE PATIENT WITH AN AMPUTATION

Once amputation was the only remedy for a compound fracture, because otherwise the patient died from wound infection. Modern treatment makes amputation unnecessary in most cases unless the blood supply to the limb is permanently cut off as the result of a severe injury or gangrene. Cancer or an extensive infection may also make amputation necessary. It may be desirable to remove a useless or deformed limb to replace it with a useful prosthesis (artificial limb).

### Nursing Care of the Amputee

Two primary dangers following an amputation are hemorrhage and infection. A tourniquet always should be within reach in case of hemorrhage. This means watching the dressing for signs of bleeding and using aseptic technic in changing dressings. Usually, the stump is elevated on a protected pillow for the first 24 hours after surgery but no longer, for fear of causing hip contractures. For the same reason his mattress should be firm. Skin traction is applied to the stump as soon as the patient returns from the operating room; it can be manipulated to allow the patient to move and turn and to be out of bed in a wheelchair.

**Exercises.** The patient begins to get ready to walk almost as soon as he recovers from the anesthetic. The physical therapist begins exercises to maintain muscle tone and directs the nurse in helping the patient to prevent contractures. Usually, the patient is helped to sit up on the edge of the bed by the second or the third postoperative day and soon progresses to a wheelchair. He should go back to bed and lie down at intervals; prolonged sitting may also cause contractures.

**Care of the Stump.** Elastic bandages are applied to the stump in order to shrink it as soon as the incision is healed. It shrinks rapidly at first, but usually some shrinkage is evident for a year or more. Two sets of bandages are needed, because the bandage is changed at least twice a day—more often if the patient perspires freely. The patient and some member of his family are taught how to apply the bandage. The nurse must also watch for skin irritation.

Massage and exercise are physical therapy procedures that are usually started immediately after the operation. If a bed cradle and electric bulbs are used, see that the temperature is no higher than 96° F. This is especially important if the patient is a diabetic or has a vascular disease, because these patients burn easily. The physical therapist may show you how to help the patient carry out some simple exercises.

**Phantom Limb.** The *phantom limb* is an annoying complication that often afflicts patients after an amputation. The patient will tell you that it feels as if the amputated limb were still there, and he feels pain in it. Sometimes a patient hesitates to mention this for fear everybody will think he is mentally ill. If he seems to be disturbed and uneasy for no apparent reason, encourage him to tell you what is bothering him. Then you can explain that this often happens after an amputation and is caused by the nerves in the stump and that it will gradually disappear. If the pain persists, it may interfere with fitting a prosthesis. The doctor can inject the nerves with alcohol, which will eliminate the painful sensations temporarily.

## The Prosthesis

As soon as possible after surgery, the patient is fitted with a prosthesis. Sometimes, a permanent prosthesis is attached while the patient is still anesthetized. The patient should be encouraged to care for his own prosthesis and should be taught how to put it on as soon as possible. This is an emotionally trying time for many people, and they need to verbalize their feelings.

Skirts and trousers hide a leg prosthesis which has a shoe that is exactly the same as its mate on the opposite foot. An arm prosthesis is more conspicuous, since the hand end of it cannot be covered and still be useful. Besides, it is difficult to make an artificial or "dress" hand look real. A practical prosthetic hand is fashioned with a mechanical hook consisting of metal prongs placed opposite each other which take the place of fingers. The amputee works the prosthesis by means of a harness which extends around the opposite shoulder; a wire connects the harness to the hand. The amputee thrusts his shoulder forward to open the prongs and relaxes it to close them. The shoulder movements are barely noticeable, but the patient learns how to make them very effective.

**Aid for the Amputee.** Assistance for the amputee is available from the American Rehabilitation Committee, from the Division of Vocational Rehabilitation in your state, and often from local voluntary agencies. Their services include medical and financial aid, counseling, and job placement.

# 46

# The Patient With a Disturbance of the Nervous System

---

## BEHAVIORAL OBJECTIVES

*The student successfully attaining the goals of this chapter will be able to:*

- *describe common deviations from normal structure and function of the nervous system, keeping in mind the normal relationships studied in Chapter 14.*

- *identify and describe the components of a neurological examination and assist the doctor with this examination; effectively evaluate the neurological status of a patient; and quickly identify and report pertinent change in this status.*

- *describe and state reasons for performing procedures such as the lumbar puncture, radiological studies, and the EEG; and assist patient and doctor before, during, and after such procedures.*

- *define and discuss common disorders of the brain which result from trauma, tumors, or disease; identify the cause of each disorder, the major symptoms, medical treatment and nursing care; and demonstrate nursing competence in the clinical area by assisting the patient to meet special needs or basic needs which he cannot meet because of his condition.*

- *discuss special considerations in the event of a brain tumor; demonstrate understanding of nursing care by safely and compassionately assisting the patient who has brain surgery.*

- *describe general seizure precautions; demonstrate ability to assist the person who is having a seizure, either in or out of the hospital.*

- *define cerebral vascular accident; identify causes; describe symptoms and the stages of hemiplegia possible; discuss medical treatment and nursing care; discuss special emotional aspects of CVA; and display effectiveness in assisting this patient to meet his needs, emphasizing rehabilitation.*

- *identify at least 3 common degenerative nerve disorders, including Parkinson's disease; describe the symptoms; discuss the medical and nursing care; and demonstrate ability to assist this patient to meet his needs.*

- *discuss the result of disease or injury to the spinal cord, with emphasis upon the symptoms of a noncontinuous cord at various levels; describe available treatment; discuss special emotional needs of the patient; and demonstrate ability to assist patients to meet their basic and special needs.*

---

## THE NERVOUS SYSTEM

The nervous system controls every mental and physical adjustment that must be made to meet any situation. It controls reasoning and thinking, body movements, and body processes. The central and the peripheral nervous systems, which consist of the brain, the spinal cord, and the cranial and spinal nerves, control voluntary actions. The autonomic nervous system consists of a specialized group of peripheral fibers which regulate involuntary processes, such as heart action. (See Chapter 14 for discussion of anatomy and physiology of nervous system.)

## THE NEUROLOGIC EXAMINATION

The neurologic examination includes a number of special tests to estimate the status and function of the nervous system. It establishes a base to which further observations may be compared. The nurse should watch for and report any changes in this base-line level in order that the doctor may know if the patient's condition is deteriorating or improving.

**General Health.** The doctor will test movements, muscle strength, vision, hearing, taste and smell, and sensations of pain, heat, and cold.

**Time and Place Orientation.** The doctor will test the patient's ability to reason and his knowledge of where he is and what is going on around him. For example, he might ask who the governor of the state is, a question that almost anyone normally could answer.

**Level of Consciousness.** During the examination, the patient's state of consciousness will be tested. The variations from normal consciousness are:

*Profound coma:* The patient gives no response in this coma which often leads to death.
*Coma or semicoma:* The patient responds only to the most painful stimulus.
*Stupor:* The patient can be partially aroused momentarily with great difficulty.
*Delirium:* The patient is disoriented, restless, and has no real idea of where he is or what he is doing.
*Confusion:* The patient seems to know vaguely where he is and has difficulty in remembering.
*Lethargy:* The patient is slow to respond.

Whatever the patient's state, always remember that although the patient may not be able to speak or respond, this does not always mean that he cannot hear, so be very careful never to discuss his condition with other people if he is helpless.

**Behavior and Emotional State.** Patients with neurologic disease often have little control over their emotions—they may be deeply depressed one minute and wildly happy the next, for no apparent reason.

**Reflexes.** The doctor will use various means to test the patient's physical responses to stimuli. Common reflexes tested are the knee-jerk (quadriceps) whereby the patient's lower leg will involuntarily kick when the nerve below the knee-cap is stimulated by a tap with a percussion hammer, the corneal reflex (eye-blink), and the plantar reflex (the foot will demonstrate plantar flexion when the sole is stroked from heel to toe). In the normal patient these reflexes occur automatically. Since the patient cannot control his reaction to these stimuli, the reflexes can serve as a measure of the function or status of the nervous system. Presence of abnormal reflexes or absence of normal reflexes indicates some neurological difficulty.

**Eye Signs.** The doctor or nurse can test the function of the nerves which serve the eyes. Pupil accommodation is checked by shining a flashlight quickly into the eye. The pupil should contract immediately and dilate when the light is removed. Each eye should be checked separately. To test coordination, the patient is instructed to follow a moving object with his eyes, both of which should be able to follow the object. In general appearance, the pupils of the eyes should be round, regular, and equal (both pupils the same size). The common phrases used for eye signs are "round, regular, equal" and "react to light" (RRE and React to light).

Often the nurse is ordered to record the eye signs and level of consciousness at regular intervals.

**Motor and Sensory Evaluation.** The doctor will ask the patient to walk so that he may observe his gait, posture, and balance. The patient will also be asked to stand with his feet together and his eyes closed. If his sense of balance or the sensation to his feet and legs are affected, he will probably fall. As a test of coordination, the patient will be asked to touch his nose with his forefinger, while his eyes are closed. Some patients cannot do this even with their eyes open.

Sensory tests involve a pin prick or other stimulation to various parts of the body to determine numbness or paralysis. Some patients who are paralyzed still have sensation in the part of the body stimulated. This is most often true in the patient who has suffered a cerebral vascular accident.

**Color and Temperature of Skin.** The patient's extremities will be tested to see if the color and temperature of the skin are the same. Cyanosis may be noted, especially in the Caucasian or Oriental person, by a greyish or bluish color in the nail beds. The blood pressure may be lower in the affected arm of a person who has had a cerebral vascular accident.

**Evaluation of Cranial Nerves.** The doctor will often ask the patient to identify odors, read an eye chart, and move his tongue. He will also test the patient's hearing ability.

## Special Tests

**Lumbar Puncture.** The brain and the spinal cord are enveloped in the *cerebrospinal fluid,* which acts as a cushion to protect them from injury and to maintain an even pressure within the parts of the brain. At times a lumbar puncture is done to: (1) obtain a specimen of the spinal fluid for laboratory examination; (2) inject a drug (spinal anesthetic); (3) measure the pressure of the spinal fluid; (4) withdraw spinal fluid to relieve excess pressure; and (5) inject a radiopaque dye before taking roentgenograms of the brain and the spinal canal.

Many neurologic disorders produce changes in the spinal fluid. These changes assist the doctor in determining the cause of the patient's difficulty. In testing the spinal fluid the doctor may find: (1) disease organisms, such as the tubercle bacillus, the spirochete of syphilis, and other organisms; (2) pus, which may indicate an inflammation of the membranes surrounding the brain and spinal cord; (3) increased pressure of the spinal fluid, which may be caused by an increase in intracranial pressure and may be a sign of a cerebral vascular accident or brain tumor; (4) low-

ered pressure, which may indicate that something is obstructing the flow of spinal fluid; or (5) the presence of blood which may indicate cerebral hemorrhage.

PROCEDURE. The Lumbar Puncture is done by inserting a special needle into the space between the third and fourth lumbar vertebrae. This particular spot is chosen because the spinal cord does not extend this far down, and there is no danger of injuring it. The pressure is measured by the manometer, which is attached to the needle; the manometer estimates the pressure of the spinal fluid by measuring the level of the fluid which flows into the manometer against the resistance of atmospheric pressure. Specimens of the fluid are collected in sterile test tubes and examined in the laboratory.

### EQUIPMENT

Labeled sterile test tubes
Manometer and sterile manometer tubing
Sterile lumbar puncture needles
Sterile rubber gloves
Sterile sponges
Sterile towels
Sterile anesthetic solution
Sterile syringe—for withdrawing fluid
Sterile hypodermic syringe for injecting the anesthetic solution into the skin
Sterile hypodermic needle
Sterile medicine glass—for the anesthetic solution
Antiseptic solution—to cleanse the skin
(These items often come in a prepackaged, disposable kit.)

Notice that sterile equipment is used in this procedure. The 2 main reasons for this are to prevent introducing any organism into the spinal fluid specimen and to protect the patient from infectious organisms that might enter his body from the punctured skin or by means of the other equipment used in the procedure. Use the technic required for handling any sterile equipment.

NURSING ASSISTANCE. If it is necessary for you to assist with this procedure, you can bring the equipment to the bedside. Explain to the patient that the doctor is collecting some spinal fluid to get information that will help him (the patient). Tell him that the doctor will use a needle after anesthetizing the spot of the puncture; explain that lying on his side makes the procedure easier and quicker.

Figure 46-1. Position of the patient for a lumbar puncture. The patient is placed on his side at the edge of the bed. His knees and head are flexed acutely in order to spread the vertebrae and to provide the widest possible space for easier insertion of the needle. Small pillows are used to maintain a horizontal position of the spine. The diagram in the upper right shows the separation of the vertebrae and the point of insertion of the needle. The dotted line follows the normal curvature of the spine without flexion of the knees and head. (Brunner, L. S., et al.: Textbook of Medical-Surgical Nursing, ed. 2. Philadelphia, Lippincott, 1970)

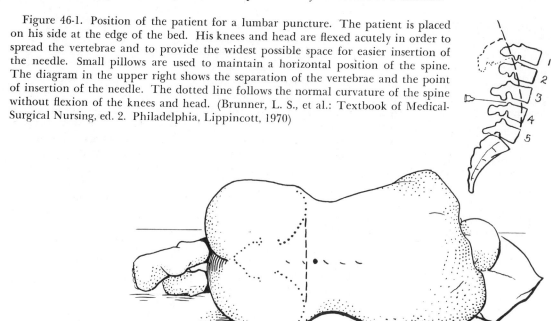

Put the patient in the proper position (on his side), with the lower part of his back at the edge of the bed, his knees well drawn up toward his chin, and his back arched outward; this position increases the space between the vertebrae and makes it easier to introduce the needle (Fig. 46-1).

During the procedure, you can reassure the patient and encourage him to cooperate. You may need to assist the patient by holding him in position. You may remove the stoppers from the test tubes, hold the tubes for the doctor, hold the stoppers to keep them sterile, and restopper each tube. You can apply strips of tape or a Band-Aid to hold the dressing in place over the puncture wound.

When the procedure is over, replace the bedclothes and make the patient comfortable. Keep him in bed, with his head low, for several hours. Explain to him that this prevents severe headache. The *postpuncture headache,* which is usually caused by leakage of spinal fluid at the puncture site, may be severe, but is usually relieved by lying flat.

Remove and care for the equipment and see that the specimens are labeled properly and taken to the laboratory.

**Cisternal Puncture.** The procedure for a cisternal puncture is the same as for a lumbar puncture with the exception that the puncture is made between the lower part of the occip-

ital bone in the skull and the first vertebrae. It is not done as frequently as the lumbar puncture.

**Pneumoencephalography.** This procedure is done to discover lesions or growths of the brain. It consists of a lumbar puncture to withdraw spinal fluid, followed by the injection of filtered air which rises through the spinal canal to the ventricles of the brain. X-rays are then taken to show any abnormal condition, such as a tumor.

PREPARATION OF THE PATIENT. The patient has regular preoperative preparation for this procedure: an enema and a sedative the night before; a sedative before the procedure the next morning, and nothing by mouth for 6 hours prior to the procedure.

NURSING CARE. Sometimes pneumoencephalography is followed by a severe headache. Nausea and vomiting may occur and sometimes shock, convulsions, or breathing difficulties. The patient lies flat in bed for about 12 hours, during which time he should be bathed and fed. He should avoid turning his head, since this increases his discomfort. An ice cap applied to his head, and codeine or aspirin may be ordered to relieve pain. Usually, his blood pressure is taken every 15 or 30 minutes for a few hours immediately after the procedure. The patient may be allowed up in a day or two but should be assisted to sit up gradually before he stands and walks.

**Ventriculography.** *Ventriculography* is similar to encephalography, except that the air is injected through holes drilled in the skull. This procedure is only used when it is impossible to do pneumoencephalography. The preoperative preparation is the same, with the addition of shaving the area on the skull where the holes are to be made. The aftercare is the same.

**Cerebral Angiography.** A radiopaque substance is injected into the carotid artery, and x-rays are taken of the blood vessels in the brain, to discover a tumor or abnormal conditions in the blood vessels. Usually, an ice cap is applied to the neck after this procedure to reduce edema and oozing from the puncture in the carotid artery. Sometimes the patient shows signs of muscular weakness in the face or in the extremities, or he may have respiratory difficulties. A tracheostomy set is kept at hand.

**Myelography.** When a *myelogram* is taken, a lumbar puncture is made, and a radiopaque substance is injected into the spinal canal, the patient is positioned so the dye will flow into the spinal cord instead of the brain; then x-rays can be taken to discover tumors or a ruptured intervertebral disk. The dye is drained off after the roentgenograms have been taken to avoid irritation of the meninges. The patient is kept in bed for a few hours after this test and observed for signs of irritation, such as a stiff neck or pain when he bends his head forward.

**Electroencephalography (EEG).** This test records the electrical impulses generated by the brain and is used frequently in the diagnosis of seizure disorders. The *electroencephalograph* is the machine that makes the graph (encephalogram) of these impulses. It is connected to electrodes which are placed on the patient's scalp by paste or by the insertion of many tiny needles. The procedure is relatively painless and has no after-effects—it takes about one half to 2 hours to do the test. The use of electrical equipment may frighten the patient unless its use is explained beforehand and he is assured that there is no danger of an electric shock.

**Arteriography.** A radiopaque dye is injected into the common carotid artery and x-rays are taken. This procedure allows visualization of the cerebral arterial system. It may be done by the *open method,* in which the artery is exposed, or by the *closed method,* in which the dye is injected via needle, through the skin, into the artery.

**Radioactive Brain Scan.** A radioactive substance is injected, after which a scintillator is used. The rationale is the same as that of the thyroid scan, that is, a site of pathology will accumulate the radioactive isotope to a greater degree than normal brain tissue.

## SYMPTOMS OF NEUROLOGIC DISORDERS

### Headache

*Headache* is associated with many diseases and difficulties. It is not a disease in itself but it often appears with such conditions as eye strain, sinusitis, brain tumor, increased intercranial pressure, hypertension, or emotional tensions. Many of us have an occasional headache that disappears after taking an aspirin tablet. This should not be confused with a persistent pain that drives the victim to take headache remedies every day. Such headaches are caused by some more serious condition which needs the attention of a doctor.

Sometimes, frequent headaches are caused by emotional upsets. These are called *tension headaches* and may be treated with a mild tranquilizer, a muscle relaxant, or an analgesic.

**Migraine.** *Migraine headache* is thought to be the result of constriction, followed by dilatation, of the cerebral arteries. No single cause of it has been determined, but emotional strain seems to bring on an attack, and it appears to run in families.

A migraine attack usually begins with fatigue and irritability. Before the actual pain begins, the patient may have visual disturbances, such as the presence of spots or a sort of "ric-rac" pattern before the eyes. Pain usually begins on one side but may spread over the entire head during the attack. The pain is intense—a throbbing, bursting feeling—which is aggravated by light. The patient may be nauseated and vomit. Sometimes the attack lasts for several days, in which case the patient can only lie quiet in a darkened room until the pain subsides. *Ergotamine tartrate* brings relief if it is taken immediately, when the signs of an attack first appear; sometimes it will prevent an attack from developing.

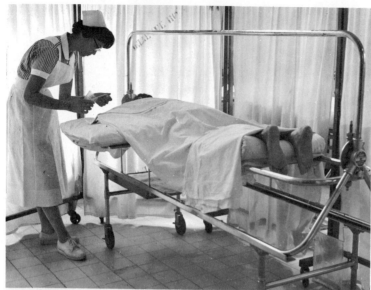

Figure 46-2. (*Top*) The Stryker frame. The patient is resting on the frame in the prone position. (*Below*) These nursing students are about to turn him to the supine position. The frame on which the patient will lie has been placed over him and tightly secured. After turning, the patient will be lying on his back on the frame, which is now over his body. (Smith, D. W., Germain, C. P., and Gips, C. D.: Care of the Adult Patient, ed. 3. Philadelphia, Lippincott, 1971)

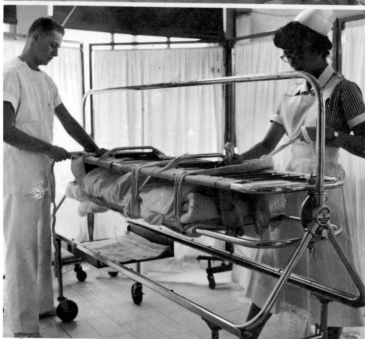

Nausea and vomiting and muscle cramps are possible side-effects of this drug. People who are subject to migraine should avoid emotional upsets, since these can trigger an attack.

## GENERAL NURSING CARE FOR NEUROLOGIC PATIENTS

In addition to assisting with and doing some of the diagnostic procedures, the nurse will face several general problems in assisting many neurologic patients.

## Loss of Motor Function and Movement

The patient will often have some difficulty in moving. He may be totally confined to bed or to a wheelchair. He may be on a special bed or frame to maintain his alignment or to assist in his care. The nurse needs to review the basic technics of good bed-to-chair trans-

Figure 46-3. The CircOlectric bed. The bed turns vertically by electricity, making it possible to put the patient in an upright position or on his stomach. (Smith, D. W., Germain, C. P., and Gips, C. D.: Care of the Adult Patient, ed. 3. Philadelphia, Lippincott, 1971)

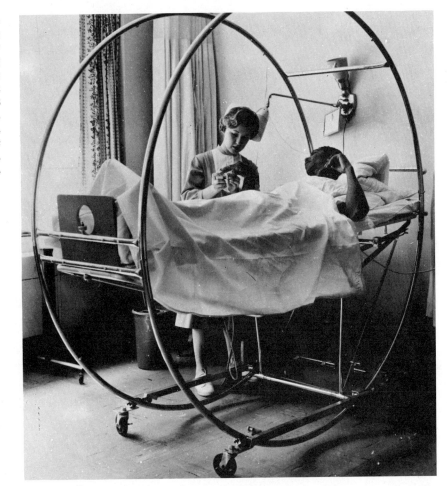

fer or good bed-to-stretcher transfer and utilize these technics in the care of the patient. The nurse must also remember the technic of good body mechanics to avoid injury to herself when moving patients.

It is important to stress that the patient should be allowed to do as much for himself as he possibly can. He should be assisted in the rehabilitation process to become as self-sufficient as possible.

**Clothing Adaptations.** It is often necessary to make adaptations in the patient's clothing so that he can dress himself. Examples are: clothes which are larger in size than usual, large buttons, zippers with a ring on the pull, velcro fasteners, stretch fabrics, elastic shoelaces, buttonhooks, or garters on a string to assist in putting on stockings. Patients are taught special technics for putting on clothing, such as hooking a bra in the front or keeping the knot in a necktie when it is taken off.

**Other Adaptations.** Other adaptive devices are used, such as the spork (combination spoon and fork), a long plastic drinking straw, an electric page-turner for reading, a bath mitt with soap in it, a spoon holder, or a plate holder.

## Special Equipment for Body Alignment

**The Stryker Frame.** Many patients are placed on this type of special bed to maintain good alignment (Fig. 46-2). It is important for the nurse to remember that this frame is very narrow and that the patient must be placed carefully in the middle so that he will not fall off. In addition, the frame must be securely anchored after each turning. *Never* turn a patient in a Stryker frame by yourself. *It takes 2 people.* The person at the head of the patient gives the instructions and the commands as to which way the patient will be turned and what the signal will be for turning. The ac-

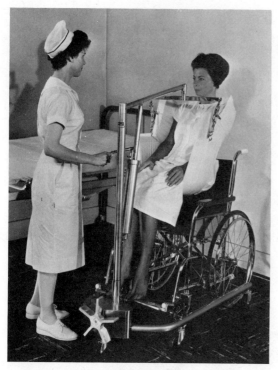

Figure 46-4. The hydraulic patient-lift is being used to move the helpless patient from bed to wheelchair. It is easy for one nurse to move a patient, although care must be taken to prevent the patient from falling. Many different attachments are available to accommodate any size patient or to meet any patient need. (Porto-Lift Company)

Braces are applied to the legs, either in the form of short-leg braces or long-leg braces. If he is able, the patient is taught by the physical therapist to put on the brace and to remove it. Then, the nursing personnel reinforces what the therapist has taught the patient. If the patient is a quadriplegia he may also have a neck brace.

**The Circle Bed** (Fig. 46-3). General nursing care of a patient in a circle bed is much the same as it is for a patient in the Stryker frame. It is possible, although not advisable, for one person to turn a patient in a circle bed. The circle bed can also be placed at any angle between the flat-lying position and the standing position. It is used to gradually accustom the patient, who has been in bed for some time, to assuming a standing position again. As the bed is turned, it can be stopped for a few minutes or seconds in the standing position.

**The Patient Lift.** A hydraulic lift is available to lift the completely helpless patient (Fig. 46-4). It can be used to lift the patient from bed to wheelchair or into the bathtub. The nurse must be careful to see that all the slings are correctly fastened and that the patient is properly restrained so that he or she will not fall.

tual turn should be done as quickly as possible.

If the patient is encumbered with tubes, I.V. equipment, or catheters or is in skeletal or skin traction, precautions must be taken before he is turned so that nothing will be disconnected or twisted. Both people involved in the procedure should check the patient after turning him to make sure the bottom of the frame is fastened so that it cannot turn accidentally. They should also make sure that the patient can breathe freely and that he has his call bell if he needs anything.

**Braces and Splints.** Many patients with neurologic problems make use of special braces or splints to give support to the affected limb or place it in correct position. Splints are available in 2 forms: there are resting splints, which keep the hand from becoming contracted, and there are dynamic hand splints which enable the patient to function better than he could without the splint.

## Loss of Bladder and Bowel Control

Many patients with a disorder of the nervous system suffer from incontinence of bladder or bowel function. The patient may have a catheter for a while, but often mechanical bladder and bowel retraining can take place. Retraining is vital to the health and emotional status of the patient. If he can be retrained, he will avoid a possible source of contamination, as well as a great deal of embarrassment. It is possible for many patients to establish regular habits if everyone concerned will take the time and the effort necessary to make these habits automatic.

**Bowel Retraining.** The vital factors are (1) timing (the elimination should be done at the same time each day), (2) fluid intake (a high fluid intake is recommended), (3) diet (a diet which will assist in maintaining a fairly solid consistency, without causing constipation is recommended), and (4) physical activity (the more exercise the patient receives, the more likely he is to be able to achieve bowel control).

The nurse can assist by:

Providing a large amount of liquids and bulk foods in the diet, such as fresh fruit and vegetables, and avoiding those foods which have been found to produce loose stools.

Establishing a regular time for giving the patient the bedpan or taking him to the toilet each day. If possible, get him to the bathroom, because moving helps to stimulate a bowel movement and also gives the patient the satisfaction of feeling less helpless.

If the patient must have enemas at first, they should be given at the same time every day. Later, a suppository at this time may be all that is necessary to stimulate a bowel movement, until finally the patient needs neither of these aids.

Manual pressure may also be applied to assist in the evacuation of the bowels.

A problem exists in giving an enema to this patient, because he will not be able to retain the enema solution. One device which has been effective in helping the paralyzed patient to retain an enema is to pass the enema tube through a hole which has been made in a hard rubber ball, and to press the ball against the anus while administering the solution.

**Bladder Retraining.** Here again, timing is essential, as well as plenty of fluids and exercise. The bladder must be emptied the first thing in the morning and the last thing at night. Sometimes pressure is applied above the bladder area (*credé procedure*) to encourage the beginning of voiding. The bladder eventually becomes trained to empty at regular intervals with the assistance of manual pressure.

*Bladder incontinence* is more difficult to control, but with patience and perseverance control can be established for many patients. At first, the patient has an in-dwelling catheter to prevent retention of urine and to provide a constant urine drainage into a disposable plastic bag. The catheter sometimes is irrigated at intervals to keep it open, for which sterile normal saline, distilled water, or perhaps Renacidin solution is used. Later, the catheter is clamped off, with the clamp being released every 1 to 2 hours to accustom the bladder to holding and emptying urine as

it does when it functions normally. The length of time between releases is gradually lengthened to 3 or 4 hours, until finally the catheter is removed, and the patient is encouraged to void every hour. At first, an hour is usually as long as he can retain urine, but this period can be lengthened gradually to 2, then to 3 or 4 hours. During the night, the male patient wears a rubber sheath over the penis which is attached to tubing and a disposable plastic drainage bag. Women must wear absorbent pads and rubber pants.

Be prepared for accidents during the training period by protecting the bed with a waterproof sheet and pads. Assure the patient that bladder control takes time, that accidents are to be expected and are by no means a sign that he has failed. Applying pressure over the pubis often helps the patient to urinate at the scheduled time. A careful record is kept of the fluid intake and output to be sure that they balance and that urine is not being retained.

Complete bowel and bladder control is not possible for every patient, but many do accomplish it. Bladder control is especially important because a permanent catheter in the bladder greatly increases the danger of bladder infection, which is a dreaded complication for paraplegic patients. Male patients with a catheter can attach the tube to a rubber urinal strapped to the leg, which can be concealed by their clothing. Women are not so fortunate. This sometimes drives women to make greater efforts toward control.

## Aphasia

Many patients who have suffered disorders or injury to some part of the nervous system are unable to speak. This can be very frustrating and frightening to the patient, because usually his mental functioning is unimpaired. The patient may also have a more complicated disorder in which he cannot say what he means. This is more difficult to deal with.

The 2 major nursing goals in aphasia are assisting the patient to communicate nonverbally while he is aphasic and retraining the patient to speak, if at all possible.

The patient may be able to write, to point to key words on a board, or to use a spelling board to spell out what he wants to say. This is a very tedious process, but it is vital that the nurse be patient and try to understand what the patient is trying to say. If the patient cannot write, it helps to write out key words and phrases on a chart so that he can point to a whole phrase, instead of spelling out each word individually.

If the patient cannot move at all, usually a system can be set up whereby the patient blinks, perhaps once for "yes" and twice for "no." He may be able to move a finger or in some other way let you know that he understands what you are saying to him. It is vital that a communication system be established. It is frightening enough for the patient if he is not able to speak, without feeling that no one is trying to communicate with him.

It is also important to talk to the patient, even if he cannot answer or can only answer yes or no. Almost all patients can still understand even though they cannot speak. Thus it is very important never to talk about him to another person in his presence. And do not talk down to the patient. Try to realize how he must feel and talk to him accordingly.

Once progress has been made with basic communication, speech therapy should begin as soon as possible. While the speech therapist decides what procedures to use, it is important that the nursing staff reinforce what the speech therapist is trying to teach.

In short, do everything that you can to make the patient want to speak. Help him in his attempts, by encouraging him and reward him when he does well. Include him in his care as much as possible and talk to him about things which interest him. Even when you have nothing to say, spend some time with him.

## Personality Changes

Many neurologic patients undergo personality changes, which may be either functional or organic. The *functional* type of changes occur as a result of frustration, such as not being able to speak or to walk, or as a result of other people's attitudes. In either case he may feel that he is useless or unwanted. The *organic* changes may result from blockage of blood supply to a part of the brain, which often occurs in stroke (CVA) patients. In this

instance, the patient may be prone to crying or excitement, which he cannot control.

The nurse must be aware of these possibilities and deal with them in a kind, understanding manner. The patient needs, most of all, support and reassurance, not rejection or scolding. He needs to feel accepted just as he is *right now*. And he needs to feel that you will help him as much as you can to regain his former powers.

## Physical Problems

**Contractures.** Contractures can be prevented if the patient receives the proper kind of exercises and is positioned properly in bed.

RANGE OF MOTION EXERCISES. These exercises may begin within 48 to 72 hours following the onset of paralysis. At first, the exercises will be passive—Passive Range of Motion (PROM)—which means the nurse moves the patient's body since he is not able to do so himself. Later the range of motion exercises will become active (Active Range of Motion), in that the patient does the exercises with the nurse's help until he is able to do them by himself.

POSITIONING IN BED. The patient must be in good body alignment at all times and should be positioned as though he were standing. Pillows, sand bags, or rolled towels should be employed to support him in this position. He should have a foot board, as well as a bed board under the mattress. Don't forget that his hands should be supported in an open position.

Positioning may also be necessary to prevent edema of the affected limb.

**Special Skin Care.** Skin care is vitally important for any person who is paralyzed or has suffered any loss of sensation. Because the patient is unable to feel pressure or pain, he can develop decubiti without knowing it. Good nursing care must be directed at the prevention of this problem. Once a decubitus develops, it is very difficult to cure, so nursing care must be directed at prevention. Sometimes surgical correction is necessary. *No patient should be permitted to rest on one body surface for more than 2 hours* at any time.

Good skin care must be given regularly. The best substance to use is powder or oil.

Alcohol is not recommended because it is an astringent and may cause the skin to lose blood supply. Soap generally should not be used on bony prominences because it tends to dry out the skin. The nurse must also remember to use hypoallergenic tape to prevent skin irritation.

Other body functions and systems also affect the condition of the skin. Good nutrition contributes to good skin health as does good fluid intake, while incontinence adds to the danger of infection or skin breakdown and increases the need for good skin care.

If a pressure area does develop, cleansing agents, antibiotic ointments, saline, or other substances may be used to assist in the healing process. Specific substances used to treat pressure areas and their actions are listed below:

A & D ointment—stimulates tissue growth
Alcohol—toughens skin around ulcer
Antibiotic ointments—combat infection
Tincture of Benzoin—promotes healing
Elase ointment—removes necrotic tissue
Collodion—protects tissue
Hydrogen peroxide—cleanses area
Sugar—promotes healing
Saturated salt solution—promotes healing

SPECIAL PADDING. Frequently special padding is applied to the bed or wheelchair of the paralyzed patient as a further effort to prevent pressure areas. Lamb's wool is often used because of the lanolin in the wool. Other commercial products are available, such as foam rubber or special floatation pads.

The floatation pad is far superior to foam rubber, because it adjusts its volume to support the patient and reduces pressure and friction. The pad is somewhat heavy and is filled with a gel-like substance. It is placed under the patient at the area of most pressure, such as under the buttocks. The floatation pads come with washable covers and a carrying sling. The nurse should also clean the pad with soap and water or occasionally with alcohol. A floatation pad large enough to cover the entire bed is available, but is quite expensive. The paralyzed person who sits in a wheelchair all day needs some sort of padding in the seat of the chair.

Often, the bed patient is further protected at points of pressure, such as the elbows or the heels with lamb's wool, cotton, or a commer-

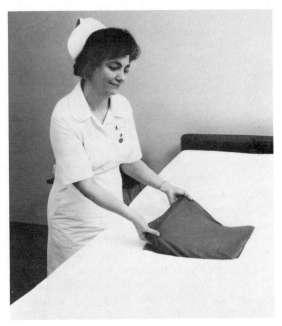

Figure 46-5. The floatation pad is inserted into a special foam rubber mattress to prevent pressure on usually high-pressure areas. This is also used to pad the seat of a wheelchair for the patient who sits up all day. This is a very effective means of protection for the patient, although he must still be turned and moved by the nurses or taught to change his position himself. A floatation pad is not a substitute for good nursing care, but is designed merely to assist in the care of the patient. (Medical Products Division, 3M Company)

cial foot elevator or elbow protector. Other body areas requiring attention are the ears, the head, and the pelvic crests.

**Special Eye Care.** Many patients who have some form of paralysis, are not able to blink their eyes. They need special eye care to keep the cornea moist and prevent ulceration. Sterile saline irrigations are often ordered for the patient who cannot blink his eyes, and the lids are kept lubricated with a tiny amount of mineral oil. The doctor will check the eyes often to detect any signs of irritation or ulceration.

In emergency situations, certain precautions must be taken to prevent eye injury or ulceration, such as removing an artificial eye or contact lenses from patients who are unconscious or semiconscious. Tiny suction cups are available for removing contact lenses in just such an emergency. As added protection, these patients should wear identification tags, so that medical personnel will know they are wearing contacts, in case they are admitted to the hospital in an emergency situation.

**Special Mouth Care.** Many unconscious patients or patients with facial paralysis breathe through their mouths, which causes the buccal mucosa to become exceptionally dry and makes the patient very uncomfortable. The easiest way to maintain mouth care for these patients is to use 2 tongue blades wrapped in gauze, although applicators may also be used. Peroxide and mouthwash are often used to clean the mouth and mineral oil is applied to the lips. Great care must be taken in maintaining oral hygiene for the unconscious patient to prevent aspiration of the liquid or damage to the mouth, teeth, or lips.

Oral care should be done several times a day. The patient may assist in this if he is conscious. Be sure to remember to clean the dentures often, if the patient is unable to do so. (The unconscious patient should have dentures removed.)

**Care of the Hair.** The patient should have regular shampoos, and women patients should be given attractive hair styles, so they will feel more pride in their appearance. The man should be shaved daily and should have regular haircuts.

**Care of the Nails.** The fingernails and toenails should be cared for by the nursing staff, since the patient cannot do so himself. Check the nails for any sharp corners and hangnails which need trimming. Soak hands and feet in warm, (not hot) soapy water and trim nails straight across with a blunt scissors.

## The Dangers from Physical Inactivity

The nurse must be aware that certain dangers can arise as a result of the patient's inactivity. One of the most common problems is respiratory difficulty such as hypostatic pneumonia. To prevent this type of complication the nurse should turn the patient often and give IPPB treatments when ordered,

To counteract circulatory problems such as thrombophlebitis or embolism, elastic stockings or elastic bandages may be worn. To guard against infection, antibiotics are often administered as a prophylactic measure. If the patient is catheterized, meticulous care must be given the catheter.

## Diet and Fluid Requirements

The patient needs a good well-balanced diet, which is high in proteins so that damaged tissue can be rebuilt and tissue breakdown prevented. The patient usually receives additional vitamin supplements.

Fluids should be encouraged for any patient who is in bed a great deal or who has difficulty in moving, in order to prevent such complications as renal calculi, bladder infections, constipation, and dehydration. Adequate fluid intake also helps establish bladder and bowel routine. A careful record of intake and output (perhaps of both food and fluids) should be kept.

The patient may be subject to edema, in which case, he would probably be on a low sodium diet and diuretics.

**Feeding the Semiconscious Patient.** Some neurologic patients have difficulty in swallowing, in which case they should be given a semiliquid diet. In some instances the food is blenderized into a semiliquid consistency and fed through a tube. If the patient has difficulty in swallowing, it is important to feed him very slowly and make sure that he is swallowing properly so that he does not choke or aspirate the fluid into his lungs.

An asepto syringe can also be used in feeding the patient. However, be sure to put a rubber tubing on the end of the syringe, so that if the patient bites down, he will not break the glass.

When giving a liquid diet, it is best to have the patient turned to his side and his head elevated, so that any fluids which are not swallowed will flow out of his mouth. He should also be encouraged to swallow with each part of the feeding. If the patient cannot swallow, he is fed by nasogastric tube feedings (see Chapter 49).

## Pain

Generally, there is very little pain associated with such disorders as cerebral vascular accident. There may, however, be pain associated with spinal cord injury, due to the damage to the nerves. If this cannot be controlled by medication and physical treatments such as heat and physical therapy, the patient may have to undergo surgical treatment. A lobotomy will relieve the pain because it interrupts those pathways which transmit pain. A rhizotomy or cordotomy may also be done. Another surgical procedure called a *spinothalmic tractotomy* often gives dramatic relief.

Pain following spinal cord injury may be aggravated by other problems such as infection, bladder calculi, fecal impaction, or emotional upsets.

The pain may be in the affected extremities, in which case, it is called *referred pain*. In a spinal cord injury, the pain may occur in ring-like fashion at the level of the injury, in which case it is called *girdle pain*. Temporary relief may be obtained by the injection of a local anesthetic.

The patient, with a spinal cord injury or one who has suffered a cerebral vascular accident may also suffer from autonomic disturbances such as perspiration or gooseflesh above the level of the injury or on the side of the injury. He may also have dilated pupils, high or low blood pressure, or headache. Disturbances of this type are sometimes treated with atropine-like drugs.

## Emotional Adjustment

Any neurologic disorder has a traumatic effect on the patient. Prior to the disorder he was able to care for himself, but now finds himself helpless. To help reduce his sense of frustration the nurse should allow the patient to do as much for himself as possible. She should also show patience, sympathy, and tact. In some instances, group-therapy sessions prove helpful.

The most difficult situations arise with degenerative disorders. Because these disorders grow progressively worse, it is difficult to deal with the patient and his family. The nurse can be most helpful by allowing the patient and his family to express their feelings and anxieties.

## Diversional Activities

As with any patient who is hospitalized for an extended period of time, it is important to find activities which will occupy his time and give him a feeling of worth. The Occupational Therapy Department will not only assist the patient to find activities which are interesting, but will also initiate exercises for those muscles which need exercise so as to prevent deformities. They will also help the patient to move about and thus, prevent such difficulties as hypostatic pneumonia, decubiti, thrombophlebitis, and constipation.

## The Unconscious Patient

Excellent nursing care is required to maintain the life of an unconscious patient. Several of the considerations have been mentioned previously in relation to the semiconscious patient. Of prime importance is the maintenance of the patient's airway. In severe cases, a tracheostomy may be required or an oral airway inserted into the patient's mouth. In less severe cases, an adequate airway can be maintained by properly positioning the patient. The patient should *never* be on his back because of the danger of aspiration and because when the head is flexed forward, the airway is closed. To further facilitate breathing the patient is often suctioned to remove secretions and mucus which collect because the patient cannot swallow or cough.

As previously mentioned, the patient's temperature, nutrition, and skin must also be maintained by good nursing and medical management, and he must be given good eye and mouth care. He should also be protected from infection, aspiration, and injury. As a protective measure side rails should be used.

The unconscious patient is the truest test of nursing skill and offers the nurse the best opportunity to practice all those skills she has learned.

## DISORDERS OF THE BRAIN

### Intracranial Pressure

An increase in intracranial pressure often causes changes in the base-line of the neurologic examination. Increased intracranial pressure may cause loss of consciousness, slowed reflexes, or inability to speak. It may also cause other autonomic changes, such as poor respiration, slow pulse rate, and increased blood pressure and temperature. The pulse pressure (difference between systolic and diastolic readings) widens, which is considered a dangerous sign.

The temperature control center may also be affected by an increase in intracranial pressure, so that body temperature may need to be regulated by outside means such as the hypo/hyperthermia blanket, aspirin, alcohol sponges, ice packs, or drug therapy to reduce the temperature to below normal (Thorazine, Demerol, and Phenergan may also be given in combination to control body temperature.)

The nurse must be aware that, generally, increasing intracranial pressure is a dangerous symptom, which should be reported immediately.

## Brain Injuries

The brain is protected from injury from minor blows by the thick bones of the skull. However, severe blows to the head can affect the brain. A blow on the head may cause hemorrhage and edema of the brain, creating intracranial pressure which may result in brain damage.

**Concussion.** A blow on the head may shake the brain violently and cause a *concussion*. It may also cause unconsciousness, which lasts for varying lengths of time, depending upon the individual case. As the patient becomes conscious, he may be nauseated and vomit. He might complain of headache or dizziness, and sometimes he may become restless and irritable. Some patients seem to recover from a blow on the head with no apparent ill effects, although symptoms of concussion may appear later. Patients with head injuries should be observed closely for at least 24 hours, especially for signs of increased intracranial pressure. If slow internal bleeding is taking place, the patient becomes drowsy and then comatose, but these symptoms may not appear for some time after the injury. Prolonged unconsciousness may be a sign of extensive internal bleeding, and a surgical operation may be necessary to tie off the bleeding vessel and to remove the blood clot.

**Depressed Skull Fracture.** A severe blow on the head may break the bone and force the broken edges to press in on the brain. The symptoms of a *depressed skull fracture*

vary according to the location of the brain injury. For example, if the fragment is pressing on the area of the brain that controls speech, the patient will be unable to talk until the pressure is relieved. Many skull fractures are minor, being no more than cracks in the bone, which heal without trouble. However, any fracture at the base of the skull may injure the nerves entering the spinal cord or interfere with the circulation of the spinal fluid, or it may damage the control center, the cerebellum, an especially dangerous situation.

TREATMENT. *Every patient* who has had a blow on his head needs watching until it is certain that the injury has not damaged his brain. As you can see, the symptoms of damage do not always appear immediately. The patient who is conscious should be watched for headache, dizziness, blindness, deafness, or signs of bloody drainage from his ears, nose, or mouth. He should also be watched for increased or decreased blood pressure, change in eye signs, and other indications of increasing intracranial pressure. The hospitalized patient is checked frequently for level of consciousness, eye signs, or personality changes, as well as nausea or dizziness. A patient released after receiving first-aid treatment following a head injury should be told to consult a doctor immediately if he has a dizzy spell, suddenly feels drowsy, or begins to see double.

## Brain Tumors

Even a benign brain tumor can be fatal, because the pressure it makes as it enlarges causes brain damage. Only a small percentage of brain tumors are malignant and usually are the result of metastasis from some other part of the body. Brain tumors occur in all age groups.

**Symptoms.** Increased intracranial pressure, causing headache, sudden projectile vomiting, and eye signs, will appear. The area of the brain affected by the pressure determines other signs; for example, if the motor area is affected, numbness or twitching in the arm may occur. A tumor on the frontal lobe of the brain causes changes in the person's personality and affects his memory or his ability to reason. If greatly increased intracranial pressure near the brain stem is not relieved, it will cause severe respiratory difficulties and possible death from respiratory failure. With all growing brain tumors, the symptoms get progressively worse.

**Treatment.** The only cure for a brain tumor is surgical removal. The success of the operation depends upon the location of the tumor and whether it can be removed without damaging the brain. (Sometimes it is impossible to remove a tumor without causing brain damage or ending the patient's life.) The operation is called a *craniotomy* (making an incision through the skull) or a *craniectomy* (removing part of the skull). Brain surgery is successful in about half of the patients.

**Preparation for Craniotomy.** Prior to a craniotomy, routine preoperative preparation is done, including bowel preparation and withholding of food and fluids before surgery.

Since the patient's head will be shaved, he should be informed of this before it is done, because it may have a traumatic effect on him. The hair is saved and put into a paper bag and labeled. Thus in the event of death the hair can be used to prepare the body for viewing.

If the patient is to remain awake during a craniotomy, he should be informed of this before the operation. It would be very upsetting for the patient to go to the operating room and then find out that he is not to receive a general anesthetic. However, he may receive heavy sedation. On the other hand, if he is expected to assist the doctor in ascertaining the functions of the brain, he will not be sedated heavily. Thus, when the surgeon stimulates various parts of the brain during the surgery, the patient can respond. In this way the surgeon can be sure that he is operating on exactly the right spot. The patient should also be told beforehand, if he will be expected to answer questions during surgery. He should also be told that there is very little pain involved in brain surgery, because the skin is locally anesthetized. He must realize that the surgeon will saw out a part of the skull bone, which will be noisy and uncomfortable. However, since the brain itself has no sensory nerves, he will not feel any pain in his brain.

**Preoperative Nursing Care.** A patient may have come into the hospital before the operation with only slight symptoms of a brain disturbance, or he may be unconscious or in a coma. If he has only slight symptoms, he is almost certain to be apprehensive and perhaps frightened by the very thought of an operation on his brain. Your interested and competent preoperative care will help him to feel that he is in good hands, ready and able to give him whatever help he needs.

His family will be anxious too; they are probably trying to conceal their feelings from the patient, but they are uncertain about what to say to him. The operation will be a long one; most brain operations take from 3 to 6 hours. Anything you can do to make the waiting period more bearable for the family will be helpful. Just taking time to say a few words to them at intervals will let them know that they are not forgotten.

**Postoperative Care.** Following the operation, the patient requires expert observation and nursing care during the immediate postoperative period. Comparison must, again, be made between his present condition and the initial neurologic examination in order to note any changes, such as signs of increasing intracranial pressure. The patient should also be positioned on his side and his dressings should be checked for bleeding—especially in the back and on the side, since the blood will run down.

During his convalescence he will need encouragement and understanding of his difficulties—for example, he may find that it takes time to regain control of his bodily movements. He may spill food and drop things and become dizzy when he walks. Assurance that these difficulties are to be expected and are a part of getting well will lessen his discouragement with what seems to him to be slow progress.

**Emotional Aspects of Brain Surgery.** Most people are very apprehensive about having brain surgery. They are afraid of being disabled, either physically or mentally, after the surgery. This, certainly, is a possibility, since the brain is such a delicate organ. It is best to listen to the patient and allow him to express his fears. While it is not possible to promise success from every brain operation, the nurse should be as encouraging as possible, yet realize that the patient has a justifiable right to be apprehensive.

Sometimes, if the patient is extremely apprehensive, the surgery may be postponed, unless it is an emergency procedure; the fear may cause untoward effects, which the surgeon cannot control. However, if the operation is carried out as scheduled, additional problems may arise, since an extremely frightened patient will not be able to cooperate in the operating room.

## Brain Abscesses

A *brain abscess* is usually caused by the spread of an infection in the middle ear. Fortunately, antibiotics have practically eliminated this possibility. It may also be the result of an infection carried to the brain in the bloodstream. The symptoms of brain abscess are the same as for a brain tumor, with the additional appearance of fever followed by drowsiness or stupor and sometimes convulsions. Surgical treatment is necessary to drain the abscess. The patient may be left with some brain damage, or he may be completely cured.

**Postoperative Care.** Strict aseptic technic is maintained to prevent meningitis. As part of this precaution, the patient may be put into protective isolation. Since it is necessary to build the patient up, a high calorie, high protein diet should be given.

## Convulsive or Seizure Disorders

**Epilepsy.** The most common type of seizure disorder is epilepsy, which is probably as old as the human race—Hippocrates described this disease as early as 400 B.C. As recently as 100 years ago it was believed that it was caused by good or evil spirits. Although modern treatment has done away with many of the superstitious beliefs about epilepsy, there are still many people who think of it as a mysterious, dreadful, and shameful disease. We know now that it is a disease that can be treated and controlled, and that many people who have epilepsy are otherwise perfectly healthy and normal. Epilepsy is a condition which causes a temporary loss of consciousness during which convulsive movements of

the body may occur. An epileptic attack is commonly referred to as a *seizure*. (Head injuries, brain infections, body disturbances, brain tumors, high fever, and emotional upsets also can cause seizures.)

Nearly 4 million people in this country have this disorder, which may be acquired or genetically related. Whatever the cause, diagnosis is made on the basis of history, physical examination, laboratory tests, and electroencephalogram.

The electroencephalogram is especially important because scientists have found that the electric waves given off by the brain of some persons follow a different pattern from those of most healthy persons; people with these "different" brain waves seem to be susceptible to epilepsy. The EEG pattern of these brain waves is called *dysrhythmia* and indicates that there is an excessive neuron discharge in the brain. This irregular brain wave pattern (known as seizure disorder) seems to run in families, although not every member of the family may have seizures. In most cases, the disease shows up in childhood and early adulthood.

The patient sometimes has a warning or *aura* before an attack especially in grand mal type seizures. He may see a flash of bright light, smell a peculiar odor, or hear a queer sound. If this happens long enough before an attack to give the patient time to lie down, he can avoid falling and hurting himself when he becomes unconscious.

### Types of Seizures.

GRAND MAL ("BIG SICKNESS"). In this type of seizure, the patient cries out and falls down unconscious, with his body muscles contracted in a rigid spasm (the *tonic stage*). Spasm of his larynx and chest muscles temporarily interferes with his breathing, and he may be cyanotic for a few seconds; then breathing resumes. This is followed by jerky movements caused by violent alternate contraction and relaxation of the muscles all over his body (the *clonic stage*). Saliva froth appears on his lips and he may bite his tongue. He perspires freely and may void involuntarily during the convulsion. After the seizure, he usually does not remember anything about the attack but may have a headache; he feels exhausted and often sleeps for some time.

PETIT MAL ("LITTLE SICKNESS" OR PYKNO-LEPSY). This involves only a momentary loss of consciousness (5 to 30 seconds), sometimes with a slight twitching of the head or the eyes that is hardly noticeable. Petit mal is most common among children.

STATUS EPILEPTICUS. This is a condition in which the patient has one seizure after another, either grand mal or petit mal, without regaining consciousness in between. If the seizures are grand mal, an emergency situation may exist requiring that the patient be treated with oxygen and large doses of sedatives and anticonvulsants, and protected from injury. If these seizures are petit mal, the patient may be very confused for a long period of time and the difficulty may be hard to diagnose.

PSYCHOMOTOR ATTACKS (TEMPORAL LOBE SEIZURES). These attacks are temporary mental disturbances during which the patient does not know what he is doing and does not remember anything. The patient behaves erratically for no apparent reason, and he usually behaves the same way during each attack. It is useless to try to stop this behavior, because the person has no idea of what he is doing and pays no attention to anyone. Such actions do no harm, unless the person becomes aggressive when he has an attack. Some patients have this type of epileptic attack instead of grand mal seizures.

JACKSONIAN SEIZURES. These convulsions are caused by a brain tumor or a lesion in the brain, and they affect the side of the body opposite the side on which the brain is afflicted. The seizure starts with jerky movements of one part of the body, which spread to include every part of that side. The manner of progression is always the same. The patient may remain conscious during this type of seizure and be able to describe the attack in detail.

**Treatment of Seizure Disorders.** Seizures that are caused by a lesion in the brain (usually acquired after birth), sometimes can be cured by removing the cause if this is possible. Otherwise, there is no positive cure for the attacks. Sometimes, they may disappear of their own accord, especially in the young, but in most cases continuous treatment is necessary to control seizures.

DRUGS. Anticonvulsants increase the pa-

tient's resistance to seizures and sometimes do eliminate them.

THE TELESTIMULATOR. This is a new electronic device which can be implanted into the patient's brain. It is used in cases of seizure disorders, tic douloureaux, and other disorders caused by erratic nerve impulses. The telestimulator, programmed to cut off stimulation to certain nerves, is activated by the patient at the beginning of a seizure. This device can also be used to initiate nerve impulses in the person who is paralyzed. Its use is still largely experimental, but it offers hope for a more normal life to many people.

**General Seizure Precautions to be Observed in the Hospital.** If a patient is admitted to the hospital with a history of seizures, he is usually put on "seizure precautions," which simply means that special steps are taken to assure that he will not be injured as a result of a seizure. Equipment used in these precautions include the following: (1) side rails, which should be up at all times and (2) restraints, which are used while the patient is up in the chair or if he is prone to grand mal seizures, (3) a padded tongue blade, which should be at the bedside at all times, and (4) a suction machine, which also may be kept at the bedside.

The nurse also should be careful to keep the electric bed in low position, take rectal temperatures rather than oral temperatures, and cover the mattress with waterproof cover.

CARE DURING A CONVULSION. One convulsion is not proof of epilepsy. Drugs can cause convulsions, and high fevers in children are also frequent causes. In any case, it is important to protect the patient from injury. If he has fallen, do not attempt to restrain him or move him, but protect him from striking against harmful objects. If possible, insert a soft pad between his teeth to keep him from biting his tongue; a padded wooden tongue depressor is ideal but a folded handkerchief will do. *Never* use your finger. Be careful not to injure his teeth. The attack is usually over quickly, lasting only a few minutes. The nurse is responsible for observing and recording the course and description of the seizure. It is very important that all the facts about the seizure be recorded, as they will aid the doctor in his diagnosis. He needs to know: how the seizure began, the body parts involved and how they were involved, the size of each pupil, the presence of unconsciousness or incontinence, the length of the seizure, and the appearance and activity of the patient afterward.

**Identification.** It is most important that the person with a seizure disorder wear an identifying tag so that hospital personnel will know what is wrong if he is admitted. It is also important for the person to tell the doctor about his disorder if he comes in for an unrelated disorder. For general safety precautions, the person must be well-controlled by medication in order to operate machinery or to drive a car.

# NERVE DISORDERS

## Trigeminal Neuralgia (Tic Douloureaux)

Sometimes, generally in older people, the 3-branched facial (*trigeminal*) nerve becomes very painful. Nobody knows why this happens, but the pain is excruciating and comes in spasms that last from 2 to 15 seconds. The pain may be triggered by the slightest touch to various parts of the face or by a breeze, strains of music, a change in temperature, or a mouthful of food, depending upon where the tigger zone is. The patient lives in constant dread of an attack of searing pain.

Some drugs—Bartine, or Dilantin, for instance—may help temporarily, but surgery is the most satisfactory treatment. Partial removal of the nerve roots eliminates the pain permanently, although it sometimes leaves burning, tickling sensations for a time. Injecting alcohol into the nerve to paralyze it brings relief for about 6 months, after which the injection must be repeated. If the patient is elderly and surgery is not desirable, this treatment can be used.

After surgery, the patient may have some eye irritation or experience difficulty in eating until he gets used to a certain amount of numbness. Usually these seem like minor problems compared with the agony of the previous attacks of pain.

## Bell's Palsy

Bell's palsy is a very emotionally upsetting condition for the patient. It produces a paralysis of part of the face, usually on one side, and gives the patient a lopsided look. The eye on the affected side will not close, so that special eye care may need to be given. Nor can the mouth on the affected side be controlled or turned up when the patient smiles. This lack of control often causes the patient to drool. A Bell's-palsy-type syndrome may occur as the result of a brain lesion. However, true Bell's palsy may be caused by a sudden chill. It is treated with heat and massage. Usually, the symptoms subside gradually but may take months to do so.

## Shingles (Herpes Zoster)

Shingles is an acute inflammation of nerve cells which produces severe and constant pain, followed by a rash. The pain may last for some time after the infection is arrested, and some scarring may occur. The infection may invade the eye and cause a possible loss of sight in the affected eye (ophthalmic zoster). Generally the disorder occurs in adults and is believed to be caused by the same organism which causes chickenpox in children. Gamma globulin has been partially successful in preventing the disease in persons who have been exposed to the virus.

## Neuralgia

The term neuralgia literally means pain in a nerve and is often applied to fleeting pains in the shoulder and upper arm which are caused by angina, spinal tumor, or herniated intervertebral disc, as well as by other conditions.

# VASCULAR DISORDERS

## Aneurysms

An aneurysm is a "ballooning-out" at one spot in the wall of a blood vessel. In most instances, an aneurysm in cranial vessels develops slowly, and the symptoms do not appear until it becomes greatly enlarged. Blood may leak slowly from a puncture in the wall of the aneurysm, or it may burst and cause severe hemorrhage and pressure on the brain. The hemorrhage may be subdural or subarachnoid or intracerebral if it occurs within the brain. If possible, the aneurysm should be removed surgically, before it breaks. About 45 out of 100 patients survive an aneurysm of the brain, and of those who live, about one third suffer some brain damage.

## Cerebral Vascular Accidents (CVA)

The brain receives its supply of food and oxygen from the blood. A sudden interruption of the blood supply to some vital center in the brain is known as a *cerebral vascular accident* (usually abbreviated to CVA). It is also known as apoplexy ("shock" is the term often used in New England). It may be caused gradually by *cerebral thrombosis* or suddenly by a *cerebral embolism*. It may cause complete or partial paralysis or death. More than 250,000 people die in the United States every year as a result of CVA, and millions more become partial or total invalids.

**Causes.** The direct causes of CVA's are:

*Cerebral hemorrhage or aneurysm:* an artery in the brain bursts, due to a rise in blood pressure or to arteriosclerosis.

*Cerebral thrombosis:* a blood clot blocks an artery that supplies some vital center in the brain, usually as a result of arteriosclerosis.

*Cerebral embolism:* a blood clot breaks off from a thrombus somewhere else in the body and is carried to the brain, where it gets stuck in a blood vessel and shuts off the blood supply to some part of the brain. A thrombus may form anywhere in the body as a result of infection, or it may be the result of an obstruction in the coronary arteries (coronary thrombosis).

**Symptoms.** With a cerebral hemorrhage, the CVA happens suddenly with very little, if any, warning; sometimes the patient feels dizzy or has a strange sensation in his head just before he collapses. He becomes unconscious, his face is red, and he breathes noisily and with difficulty. His pulse is slow, but full and bounding. His blood pressure is elevated, and he may be in a deep coma which becomes deeper and deeper until he dies, or he may gradually regain consciousness and eventually recover. Patients who are comatose for a long period of time are less likely to recover.

The patient who is not comatose may have a poor memory or inconsistent behavior; he may be easily fatigued, may lose bowel and bladder control, or have poor balance. Often he is paralyzed on one side, with loss of movement or sensation, or both.

The extent of the damage to the brain determines a patient's chances for recovery; if it was slight, he will recover more rapidly and completely. (Some elderly people have a series of "little strokes," caused by thrombi in small blood vessels in the brain, which only cause dizziness or a slight temporary paralysis. If this happens frequently, it may lead to eventual mental deterioration or senility.)

Occasionally, a young person suffers a stroke. In such cases, the chances of recovery are good because the other vessels in the brain are better able to compensate for the interrupted circulation. (The circle of Willis is involved in this compensatory mechanism.)

**Degrees of Consciousness.** A patient may be in a *semicoma,* which means that he may not move but may groan and be aware of painful sensations. As part of her nursing duties, the nurse is responsible for noting any changes in the patient's level of consciousness, as well as any changes in the other neurological findings indicated in the initial examination.

**Brain Damage.** The most common result of a CVA is *hemiplegia*—paralysis of one side of the body. You will remember that the nerves from one side of the brain cross over to the opposite side of the body; if the *left* side of the brain is injured, the *right* side of the body will be paralyzed or incapacitated in some way. For example, if vision is affected on one side, the patient may not be able to see on that side or may see double. Other functions may also be involved such as hearing, general sensation, and even circulation. It all depends on what part of the brain is affected. If the speech center of the brain is damaged, the result may be *aphasia,* which is the loss of the ability to use or understand spoken or written language. This means that the patient has trouble in reading, writing or speaking. He cannot name an object correctly, or if he is able to speak, he does not say what he thinks he is saying. Many patients recover some speech, but others never do. Sometimes, the other side of the brain is able to take over, but not always.

*Hemiplegia* generally progresses through 3 stages:

1. *The flaccid stage:* the patient is limp and weak on the affected side.

2. *The spastic stage:* the muscles are con-

tracted and tense. Movement, passive or active, is difficult.

3. *The recovery stage:* therapy and rehabilitation can begin.

**Treatment and Nursing Care.** Heparin, an anticoagulant, is sometimes given to prolong the clotting time of blood and to prevent further blood clots from forming. Dicumarol or Coumadin may be given for the same purpose. Any of these drugs must be used with great care because of the danger of hemorrhage.

Some attempts have been made recently to surgically remove blood clots collected on the brain in the hope that the brain would recover once the pressure was removed. It is too soon to recommend this procedure as being generally effective; so far it has not been widely successful.

The general care of the patient who has had a CVA includes many of the procedures described for the care of any bed patient. Note every sign of improvement, no matter how slight; also note the lack of it. Turn the patient often, at least every 2 hours, keeping his body in good alignment and supporting it with pillows. As the patient recovers, the doctor specifies the amount of activity that he wants the patient to have. If a physical therapist is available, he assumes the initial responsibility for these activities. The exercises may be passive at first, but the patient should be encouraged to do them himself as soon as possible. Exercise prevents muscle contractures and keeps the muscles strong and ready to be used when the patient needs them.

## Stages of Patient Care in CVA

**The Emergency Phase.** When the patient is admitted to the hospital, he often is unconscious and needs the type of nursing care required by any unconscious patient. (See page 555.)

**The Rehabilitation Phase.** As the patient begins to recover, he is ready to begin on the road back to as much self-care as is possible.

The quality of nursing care given during the emergency phase will often have a very great bearing upon how much rehabilitation is possible and upon how fast it can be accomplished. If contractures were prevented, the patient can learn to walk again just that much faster. If the skin was kept intact, the patient will not have to contend with ulcerations and infections. If bowel and bladder training were begun, the patient will be well on the way to independence. The goal of all rehabilitation is that of returning the patient to as much self-care in the activities of daily living (called ADL) as possible.

**Assistance with Activities of Daily Living.** There are many textbooks on the subject of rehabilitation, but a short discussion here will be helpful. The patient should be taught, as soon as possible, such skills as transferring himself from bed to chair or to toilet and dressing and feeding himself. These tasks are easier for the hemiplegic, such as the stroke patient (only paralyzed on one side), than they are for the paraplegic who has no control over his lower extremities. The hemiplegic usually has control over one leg and may also have partial control over the affected leg. However, the hemiplegic does have the disadvantage of one disabled arm.

LEARNING TO MOVE. The patient should be taught first how to roll over in bed, then how to sit on the edge of the bed and to lie down again, and then how to move into a wheelchair. In all types of movement the emphasis is on moving the affected leg with the good leg and putting the weight on the unaffected leg. The nurse can be of assistance by putting support under the patient's weak arm, by supporting him under both arms, or by supporting his good leg, holding his body, and pivoting him around.

Next, the patient learns to stand from his wheelchair. He can also learn to transfer onto the toilet or into the bathtub at this point. It is helpful if support bars are installed in the bathroom so the patient will have something to hold on to for support. The toilet seat can be elevated so that he can sit down easier, and the bathtub may have a support or grab bar, a good suction mat on the bottom, and a seat or chair so the patient can sit in the tub without having to stoop all the way down.

LEARNING TO DRESS AND WALK. The patient is taught to dress the affected side first and then pull the shirt or pants onto the unaffected side. The patient may also learn to *walk* with the assistance of crutches (discussed in Chapter 45) or canes or a walker. The physical therapist and occupational therapist are most helpful in teaching the patient to perform those skills which he will need after discharge from the hospital.

**Nursing Contact.** In all her dealings with the patient, the nurse must realize that hearing and vision, on the affected side, are often impaired. Therefore, to avoid embarrassing the patient needlessly by having to repeat, the nurse should approach the patient from the nonaffected side.

**Speech Therapy.** Speech therapy should be begun as soon as possible for the aphasic patient. The patient should first learn to hear sounds, then to imitate them, to remember them, to enjoy speaking, and finally to realize that he needs to speak and wants to speak. This progression increases the chance of successful speech therapy. The role of the nurse is to encourage the patient in his progress.

**The Patient's Family.** When it comes to the rehabilitation process, the patient's family plays a vital role. The family needs to know what the patient can do and how to reinforce this after he is discharged from the hospital. They should also understand that the patient may act differently after a stroke because of brain damage. Whatever the patient's handicap, the family should realize his emotional needs and how important it is to make him feel worthwhile and wanted.

**The Patient's Point of View.** It is difficult for a well person to realize the despair and the discouragement of a person who suddenly finds that he is unable to do even the simplest things for himself. As his mind clears, he begins to realize that neither he nor anyone else knows to what extent he will recover. However, one never can tell just how much can be accomplished by perseverance. Although some indication of his limitations should be apparent after 6 months, the patient should not give up his exercises or allow his muscles to become flabby and his joints to become stiff.

## DEGENERATIVE DISORDERS

### Parkinson's Disease

*Parkinson's disease,* also known as *paralysis agitans* and *shaking palsy,* is a disease of the basal ganglia of the brain that grows progressively worse. The patient's muscles stiffen, his movements are slowed, he becomes weak,

and his muscles develop fine rhythmic tremors that go on constantly, even when the muscles are not being used. It also affects automatic movements such as blinking, eating, talking, walking, and maintaining posture. However, Parkinson's disease does not affect thinking ability.

**The Causes.** It is estimated that probably $1\frac{1}{2}$ million people in the United States have Parkinson's disease. The exact cause is unknown, but it may be due to cerebrovascular disease and often follows encephalitis, poisoning, or severe electric shock. It affects more men than women, and usually it appears in the 50's or the 60's. People with arteriosclerosis or syphilis sometimes have the symptoms of Parkinson's disease. Following the Spanish influenza epidemics in the early 1920's, many people were left with Parkinsonian symptoms as a result of the encephalitis which accompanied the flu.

**Symptoms.** The symptoms appear gradually and become worse so slowly that it may be years before the patient becomes alarmed and consults a doctor. The tremors are regular, but they are so fine that they are scarcely noticeable. Sometimes these tremors affect only one side of the body, from which they spread to the other side; this may happen immediately or after as long a period of time as 15 years. The tremors disappear when the patient is asleep, except in the final stages of the disease. They may start in the fingers, then extend to the arm and finally spread to the entire body. Severe tremor is constant—about 2 to 5 shakes in a second, with the thumb beating against the fingers in a sort of "pill-rolling" movement. The tremors become worse if the patient gets excited, but if he makes a voluntary movement, the shaking may cease. All of the patient's body muscles become rigid; he keeps flexing his limbs slightly; and all his movements are slowed. The disease affects his spine and neck, and he sits or stands in a stooped position. His arms no longer swing when he walks, and he is unable to shift his position quickly in order to keep his balance. Therefore, he shuffles along when he walks, in order to keep from falling. If he is pushed a little, he loses his balance and goes faster in the direction of the push. Movement in the small muscles that control changes in his facial expression is affected—he cannot blink his eyes or smile, and his face has a masklike look. He has a problem with drooling, and special mouth care must be given often. He stands tense and stiff, bending his body forward.

**Treatment and Nursing Care.** Parkinson's disease progresses very slowly; it does not shorten life or affect the mind. Continued efforts are being made to find new and more effective treatment. The Parkinson's Disease Foundation and the National Parkinson Foundation, both of which are located in New York City, are devoted to research and to the service of patients with Parkinson's disease.

Many drugs now in use do decrease muscular spasms, tremor, and sluggishness. Among the drugs most commonly used are Artane, Benadryl, and Dexedrine. A patient may be taking a number of drugs at the same time, each for a different symptom. The most effective drug found to date is L-Dopa (levodopa). It is effective because these patients lack an amine (dopamine) which aids in synaptic transmissions in the brain.

Physical therapy helps to keep the patient active and helps him to feed and dress himself and get in and out of bed or a chair. The patient can be taught how to do leg and finger exercises, how to keep his balance, and how to keep his neck muscles from contracting. Exercises do not help the tremor, but they are valuable in preventing rigidity.

Because of difficulties in eating, chewing, and swallowing, the patient with Parkinson's disease often does not eat enough. To counteract this problem, the patients are given vitamins and put on a high calorie, high protein diet. They are also given a stool softener to prevent constipation.

SURGICAL TREATMENT. The most effective surgical treatment for Parkinson's disease is to purposely produce a lesion in the thalamus, by means of cryosurgery (freezing), electrocoagulation, or the injection of alcohol. The procedure is done under local anesthesia so the surgeon can find the exact spot where the lesion should be placed in order to stop the palsy.

**What the Family Can Do.** The patient's family should have some instruction on how to be helpful. They should encourage the patient to do everything he possibly can for himself and should be patient with his slow speech and movements. The family should also protect him from strain, fatigue, and anxiety, all of which tend to aggravate his symptoms.

## Myasthenia Gravis

*Myasthenia gravis* is a disease that greatly weakens the muscles. This weakness is especially noticeable after the affected muscles are exercised. It usually attacks young adults and the middle-aged, but it is not a common disease. The cause of myasthenia gravis is not known; however, it seems to be related to the conduction of nerve impulses to the muscles. This may be due to an endocrine, metabolic, or viral disorder. The muscles and nerves are normal; the difficulty occurs only at their junction—acetylcholine, which is normally present there, seems to be absent.

**Symptoms.** Myasthenia gravis usually comes on gradually; usually the patient notices that certain muscles seem to be very weak immediately after using them, but muscle power comes back after a rest. The muscles of the face may be affected, especially those used in chewing, swallowing, coughing, and speaking as well as the eye muscles. The patient looks sleepy, his face is expressionless, as his eyelids droop (*ptosis*), and he has double vision (*diplopia*). His facial muscles become flabby and weak. If the muscles of respiration are affected, he finds it difficult to breathe. If he is unable to expectorate the respiratory secretions, he may develop pneumonia.

**Treatment.** Neostigmine relieves the symptoms quickly, but it will not cure the disease. X-ray treatment or surgery may also be tried, along with drugs such as germine diacetate and ACTH. However, studies are still being conducted on these drugs.

Myasthenia gravis may persist for years, or it may become fatal rapidly. In the mild form, the patient can be active as long as he avoids activities that are very tiring. In the severe form, he will have to have everything done for him—he may need tube feeding if he cannot swallow, and suction may be necessary to remove respiratory secretions.

## Multiple Sclerosis ("Many Scars")

Multiple sclerosis, also called *disseminated sclerosis*, is a disease that destroys areas in the covering of many nerves (the myelin sheath). It leaves scars in the white matter of the brain and the spinal cord which affect the connections between the brain and certain muscles and organs of sense. Several parts of the body may be affected—for example, a person might become a paraplegic and might also be blind. This disease usually causes a slow paralysis and a slowly developing disturbance of speech and vision. It begins with a few symptoms which gradually increase and become more serious. Sometimes, the symptoms disappear in the beginning of the disease, and the patient may seem to be absolutely well for years. However, each time the symptoms reappear they are more severe and of longer duration. In other words, the disease is marked by remissions and exacerbations.

**Symptoms.** Nobody knows what causes multiple sclerosis. However, cold weather seems to aggravate it. Often it is difficult for the doctor to diagnose this disease until certain symptoms appear together, demonstrating a widespread disturbance of the nervous system. Some common symptoms are:

Weakness and clumsy movements
Tremor when using the hand
Blurred or double vision or blindness
Slurred speech
Paraplegia
Bowel and bladder incontinence or retention

Sometimes, the patient is euphoric; on the other hand he may be dizzy and have nausea and vomiting; or he may have spastic paraplegia and muscle tremors.

**Treatment and Nursing Care.** Multiple sclerosis cannot be cured, but attempts are being made continually to find a cure or to discover ways to slow the progress of the disease by various drugs and diets. The National Multiple Sclerosis Society is sponsoring research in an attempt to isolate the cause and thus, find a cure for multiple sclerosis.

Authorities agree that it is important to build up the patient's general health by providing him with plenty of rest and a good all-around diet, and by having him avoid excitement and exposure to infection. A patient may live 20 years or more after he is known to have the disease; however, he gradually becomes disabled in some way, with other disabilities developing. Paralysis may appear, and eye disturbances may progress to total blindness. The patient may have sudden emotional upsets, becoming either depressed or exuberant. His body becomes wasted, making him susceptible to decubitus ulcers. He is also susceptible to infection, especially pneumonia; if he is confined to his bed, his position must be changed frequently, and he should practice deep breathing. Paralysis and weakness can cause body deformities; therefore, attention should be given to maintaining good body alignment.

Sometimes, a high dose of a corticosteroid is helpful during an acute phase of the disease.

THE PATIENT AT HOME. Unless it is physically necessary, the patient does not need to stay in bed; instead, he should be encouraged to live as nearly normal a life as possible. The multiple sclerosis victim can live at home as long as he does not require physical care that he cannot carry out himself or which cannot be provided. Sometimes work can be found which he is able to do at home until the advancing disease makes this impossible. He should be encouraged and helped to learn to make the most of each day as it comes.

## Huntington's Disease (Chorea)

Huntington's disease, also known as chronic, progressive chorea, involves a combination of physical and mental symptoms which usually start with fidgeting, jerking, and spasms. The personality changes include irritability, loss of judgment, and carelessness. The symptoms generally do not appear until the patient is past 40 (and has probably already passed on this hereditary disease).

**Treatment.** No cure is known at present, although some drugs, such as Pronestyl, help symptomatically. Research is continuing on the finding that the cerebrospinal fluid of the patient with Huntington's disease differs from that of the normal person. As in so many chronic diseases the nurse can help by being understanding and tactful when dealing with the patient and his family.

## INFLAMMATORY CONDITIONS

### Meningitis

*Meningitis* is an inflammation of all or part of the membranes that cover the brain and the spinal cord. Infection can travel to the meninges from nearby structures, such as the sinuses or the middle ear, or it may be carried by the bloodstream. The infection may be caused by viruses, fungi, or bacteria such as the pneumococcus, the streptococcus, the staphylococcus, the meningococcus, the tubercle, or the influenza bacillus. Meningitis is a serious disease to which children are particularly susceptible.

**Symptoms.** Meningitis usually attacks suddenly, accompanied by a high fever, a painful and stiff neck, headache, nausea, and vomiting. The patient may be in a stupor or a coma and may have convulsions.

**Treatment and Nursing Care.** After a lumbar puncture has been done to determine the causative organism, the appropriate antibiotics, such as sulfadiazine or streptomycin, will be administered. The patient is very ill: cooling sponges may be ordered for his high fever, and he will be given intravenous fluids and nourishing liquids. Tube feedings may also be necessary. Side rails should be in place for the patient's protection. Since meningitis is a communicable disease, isolation precautions should be carried out.

Antibiotics are highly effective in treating meningitis in adults, but if the infection is exceedingly virulent, the drugs may prove useless and the patient may die. Sometimes the nerves of sight and of hearing are damaged as a result of a meningitis attack.

### Encephalitis

*Encephalitis,* sometimes called *sleeping sickness,* is an infection of the central nervous system which is caused by viruses, bacteria, or chemical poisoning. It destroys nerve cells and may be a consequence of vaccination or a viral infection, such as measles or smallpox. Encephalitis seems to be more prevalent after influenza epidemics. The disease may be transmitted by mosquitoes and ticks. The insect bites an infected person, then bites a healthy person, thereby passing on the infection.

**Symptoms.** *Viral encephalitis* attacks suddenly, causing violent headache, fever, nausea, and vomiting and drowsiness. The patient may show muscular weakness and he may have tremors, convulsions, or sight disturbances. Some types of viral encephalitis are more lethal than others; the death rate has varied from 5 per cent to 70 per cent, depending on the cause of the infection.

**Treatment and Nursing Care.** No drug specifically effective for treating encephalitis has yet been found. The treatment consists of reducing the fever with cooling sponges and maintaining a quiet environment with subdued lighting. Tube feedings are necessary for the comatose patient; hot moist packs may be ordered to relieve muscle spasm. Side rails should be in place.

Many patients who recover from encephalitis are left with mental changes or convulsive disorders or with Parkinsonian symptoms which become increasingly disabling.

## ADULT CEREBRAL PALSY (CP)

As the term implies cerebral palsy involves a lack of muscle control due to dysfunction of the brain. While it is considered to be a disorder which occurs primarily among children (see Chapter 41), many adults are afflicted with it. There are 5 chief types of cerebral palsy, which may occur singly or in combination. The most common form is *spastic cerebral palsy* which is characterized by tense contracted muscles. The other 4 forms are: *athetoid,* which is characterized by a constant uncontrolled motion; *rigid,* in which the muscles resist movement, *ataxic,* noted primarily by a poor sense of balance, and *tremor,* in which the victim shakes.

The cause of cerebral palsy is unknown in a great many cases, although some cases are due to birth injury or Rh incompatibility. Treatment includes physical and occupational therapy, speech therapy, and general vocational rehabilitation. Research continues to search for more answers into the cause and cure of this disorder.

## DISORDERS OF THE SPINAL CORD

### Poliomyelitis

**Poliomyelitis.** Poliomyelitis is caused by a virus that attacks the nerve cells, affecting the motor nerves that run from the brain or the spinal cord to the muscles. The virus usually enters the body through the mouth or the nose and travels along the nerve fibers to the nerve cells connected with a group of muscles. It may damage the cells only temporarily or it may destroy some of them. If enough of the nerve cells are destroyed, the muscle becomes paralyzed.

The first big step toward success in conquering polio was the discovery of the virus that causes it. This achievement was followed by the perfection of a vaccine, given by injection (*Salk vaccine*), to prevent the disease; later Dr. Albert Sabin developed the oral vaccine. A trivalent form of the vaccine provides immunization (in the form of a live virus) against 3 strains of the polio virus. When the vaccine is taken in monovalent form, the progression of shots is given in the order of Type I, Type II, and Type III.

The polio triumph does not mean that we can relax our efforts to prevent the disease. Each new generation must be immunized, and each person's present immunity must be kept active by the required "booster" doses of vaccine. Education programs informing the public about polio and immunization must be continued, so that public support may be enlisted for the immunization programs.

## Trauma to the Spinal Cord

Injury, either permanent or temporary, may be sustained by the spinal cord through an accident or a disease, such as cancer. In the case of pressure on the spinal cord, once the source of the pressure is removed, the return of funtion will depend on whether the spinal cord was severed or damaged irreversibly. In the case of injury, the spinal cord may be injured, but not severed, in which case, the patient may suffer only *temporary paralysis,* with function returning as the edema and infection subside. In the event that the spinal cord is severed completely (total cord transection), *permanent paralysis* will occur below the level of the injury. There is no way, at the present time, to reconnect a severed spinal cord. A great deal of research is being conducted in this area with the hope that some day it will be possible to reconnect the severed cord and restore mobility to all persons who have sustained a spinal cord injury.

## Pressure on the Spinal Cord

Pressure on the spinal cord can either lessen sensation or remove it altogether. It can cause muscular weakness, paralysis, or muscle spasms. Those parts of the body which are below the area of pressure will be affected. For example, pressure in the cervical region could paralyze the body from the neck down, while pressure in the lumbar region might affect the nerves that control movements in the lower extremities but would not affect nerves above that point.

**Causes of Pressure.** Pressure on the spinal cord may be due to an injury which fractures a vertebra and pushes the broken bone into or against the cord or severs it completely. When the cord is severed, it causes permanent paralysis below the level of the injury because the spinal nerves cannot repair or replace themselves. Pressure on the spinal cord may also occur when the disk of cartilage located between 2 vertebrae becomes weakened and presses against the spinal nerves (*herniated disk*). Tumors, caused by metastasis from a malignant growth somewhere else in the body, may also cause pressure on the spinal cord.

**Medical Treatment.** Skeletal traction may be applied with Crutchfield tongs or by skin traction in which a headsling or Buck's extension is used.

A herniated disk may be treated by providing rigid support beneath the spine with a bed board, or by placing the patient on a Stryker frame which allows the patient to be turned without twisting his body. Muscle spasms may be relieved with traction or with antispasmodic drugs, such as Artane. If the patient is immobilized, exercises are started as soon as possible. Ambulatory patients may wear a lumbosacral corset or brace to keep the body in good alignment. If none of these measures helps, surgery will be necessary.

**Surgical Treatment: Laminectomy and Spinal Fusion.** Spinal cord injuries are treated surgically by removing the cause of the pressure, if possible. The surgeon removes a portion of the vertebra to expose the spinal cord and takes out the bone fragment, the herniated disk, the tumor, or the clot which is pressing on the cord. This operation is called a *laminectomy*. Sometimes the weakened vertebra is strengthened by grafting a piece of bone, taken from the tibia or somewhere else, onto the vertebra and the sacrum. This is called a *spinal fusion*. When the graft heals, the spine will be stiff in that area.

**Immediate Postoperative Care.** Attention is given to routine postoperative care, plus management of pain. Since the spinal cord area is very sensitive, the operation may be

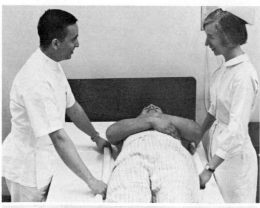

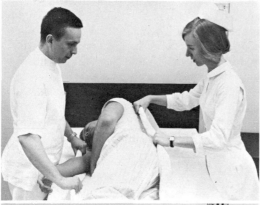

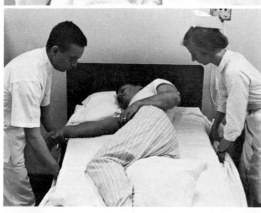

Figure 46-6. Turning the patient who has had a laminectomy. Two nurses are required. This procedure is known as logrolling, because the patient is turned as a whole. A turning sheet or a drawsheet is kept under the patient to facilitate the rolling. (*Top*) The pillow is removed from beneath the patient's head. Each nurse grasps a side of the drawsheet and the patient is moved to the side of the bed. His arms are folded across his chest. (*Center*) The patient has been rolled like a log by pulling the sheet upward on his left side. (*Bottom*) The turning sheet is straightened and anchored. The patient is made comfortable, with his body put in good alignment by the use of pillows.

very painful. To relieve pain, medications and frequent turning help.

The nurse must also watch very closely for signs of bleeding or shock caused by trauma to the spinal cord. It is very important to observe sensation and mobility in the legs, because of possible damage during surgery. Any complaints of tingling, numbness, or difficulty in moving the legs should be reported immediately. Edema is also a possible complication and may cause pressure on the spinal cord or edema in the legs.

**Postoperative Care of a Laminectomy Patient.** Rest for the back is most important. This does not mean that the patient must lie in one position without moving. He can be taught to help the nurse turn him by making his body as rigid as possible and keeping his arms straight at his sides. The nurse *rolls* him over in one motion, keeping his body in line. Two nurses may work together in a procedure known as *log rolling* in which a turning sheet is used to roll the patient over (see Fig. 46-6).

The patient should never be lifted but should be rolled onto a brace or the bedpan. A fracture pan is easiest to use, because it is smaller. He should be taught that during convalescence, he should never reach or stretch for objects on his bedside table or elsewhere.

Frequently, the patient is allowed out of bed in 3 to 5 days following a laminectomy, usually wearing a brace or a corset to give support to his back. When a brace is applied, a thin cotton shirt is put on first to protect the skin. The nurse should be sure to remove all wrinkles. Then, with the patient on his side, the middle of the brace is placed over his spine and the patient is rolled onto it. After the brace is fastened, he is helped to the edge of the bed, so that his legs will fall over the side when he sits up; then he is assisted to sit up slowly.

After a *laminectomy*, the patient will gradually be allowed to do light work, but he must always be careful to avoid heavy lifting. In fact, he should use caution when doing lifting of any kind for at least a year after the operation. A nurse has many opportunities to emphasize the importance of sticking to this rule, pointing out to the patient during his convalescence that even one instance of disregarding this safeguard may cause him harm.

If a *spinal fusion* has been done, the patient must remain in bed longer. Sometimes, the nurse is not permitted to turn this patient without special equipment, such as a brace or a halter or a Stryker frame. Never attempt to move a patient after a spinal injury or operation unless you have been given permission and have been taught how to do it in each instance. The patient who is paralyzed also needs care appropriate to the degree of paralysis.

## Paraplegia and Quadraplegia

Paraplegia is the paralysis of both lower extremities due to a spinal cord injury. It may result from a trauma, such as a gunshot wound or other injuries, or an automobile accident; or it may be caused by a disease, such as poliomyelitis or multiple sclerosis. It may occur suddenly, or it may develop gradually. It will cause disability depending on the injury to the spine and its severity.

A spinal cord injury may have some or all of the following damaging effects in varying degrees:

*Loss of sensation*—varying from tickling, burning, and numbness to partial or complete paralysis of any one or more parts of the body

*Loss of movement*—varying from muscle weakness to partial or complete paralysis

*Loss of mental functions*—varying from confusion to coma and often involving loss of speech, sight, or hearing.

The disability is greatest when the cervical vertebrae are injured—the victim then usually has paralysis of all 4 extremities (*quadriplegia*). A lumbar vertebrae injury affects only the lower part of the body. When the injury occurs in the lower cervical region, the chest muscles will be affected but diaphragmatic breathing is still possible. If the spinal cord is only partially damaged, some function may still be possible, but if the cord is severed, function below the level of the injury cannot be restored (see Table 46-1).

The most severe injury involves a broken neck and complete cord transection. This injury is often fatal, because of the many body functions which are affected. (See Chapter 35 for emergency first-aid treatment.) The patient first suffers from abdominal distention, because his stomach and intestines are not functioning. The distention, in turn,

### TABLE 46–1. LEVEL OF SPINAL CORD INJURY AND CONTROL LOST

| Spinal Nerve (from head down) | Function Lost |
|---|---|
| Cervical $C_1$ | Neck and diaphragm (Severe quadraplegic) |
| $C_5$ | Deltoid and biceps |
| $C_6$ | Wrist extensors (Some arm movement) |
| $C_7$ | Triceps and wrist extensors |
| $C_8$ | Hand |
| Thoracic $T_2$ to $T_7$ | Chest muscles (Paraplegic with arm and hand movement) |
| $T_9$ to $T_{12}$ | Abdominal muscles |
| Lumbar $L_1$ to $L_5$ | Legs |
| Sacral $S_2$ and below | Bowel and bladder (ability to walk with assistance) |

causes respiratory difficulties because the diaphragm cannot move. The diaphragm is almost totally paralyzed, but with the distention pressing against it, abdominal respiration becomes impossible. The patient has no chest expansion to assist in breathing, as well as no cough reflex to get rid of secretions. Nursing care involves preventing abdominal distention by means of a nasogastric tube, assisting the patient to cough by means of IPPB and suctioning, and providing postural drainage. Sometimes a respirator and/or a tracheostomy is necessary. Because of medical advances, many patients now survive who would previously have died during the acute phase of their injury. In addition to all the physical care these patient need, they have special psychological problems which also must be dealt with.

**Treatment of Paraplegia.** Treatment begins with taking care when moving the victim immediately after the injury has occurred, to prevent further damage. The patient with a spinal injury should be kept flat on a firm surface; he should be moved by rolling and never lifted by the head, the shoulders, or the feet, since this will bend the spine. He may also need treatment for shock and hemorrhage. After an x-ray has been taken to determine the extent of the injury, the proper treatment is prescribed. Surgery may be necessary to remove a part of a vertebra pressing on the spinal cord, or traction by a head halter or Crutchfield tongs may be applied.

**Surgical Treatment.** Sometimes surgical exploration is done to determine if the cord is severed. In some instances a laminectomy is carried out to remove a source of pressure. If the spinal column is not stable, spinal fusion is done to prevent further damage to the spinal cord and to enable the patient to have more mobility later. Prior to any thought of surgery, the doctor first must determine the exact reason for the paraplegia; is it pressure on the cord or is it a transected cord? Was the onset sudden or gradual? He determines these things by x-ray procedures and by physical examination. If surgery is indicated, it should be done as soon after the injury as possible, especially if the mobility or other neurologic symptoms are getting worse. If the motor and sensory paralysis was immediate and total, surgery is usually not done, because if the cord was totally transected, surgery would only endanger the patient's life further.

**Improvements in Treatment.** Most of the paraplegics are young people with injuries resulting from accidents or diseases such as *multiple sclerosis*. Many other paraplegics are veterans of World War II, and Viet Nam, but the number of disabled civilians is far greater than those crippled because of war. However, since World War II, tremendous strides have been made in the rehabilitation of paraplegics. In the first place, many more lives were saved during the war by improved treatment for shock and by antibiotics. Also, rehabilitative technics have improved, and the importance of physical medicine is now widely recognized.

**Available Treatment.** One patient alone may need the services of many specialists: a psychiatrist, a neurologist, a physiotherapist, or an occupational therapist. For the most part, these services are available in special institutions and in large medical centers. The Veterans Administration provides treatment for disabled veterans and civilian hospitals now have physical medicine and rehabilitation units. State health departments have also extended their efforts toward establishing centers for rehabilitation.

**Nursing Care.** The following directions apply to the patient who is powerless to help himself or to control his body functions: (However, the patient should be encouraged to do as much for himself as he can.)

1. His position must be changed frequently to prevent pressure sores and pneumonia. The Stryker or the Foster frame or the CircOlectric bed may be used to turn helpless patients (Fig. 46-3). Cleanliness, massage, and change of position help to prevent pressure sores. A footboard helps to prevent footdrop.

2. He will have to be fed; in some instances the only way a patient can be given food or fluids is intravenously or by tube. He needs a high protein diet to keep his body tissues healthy, and a high fluid intake to prevent urinary tract infections.

3. He will have urinary incontinence; usually, a retention catheter is inserted into the bladder to drain the urine. If disposable pads are used, special attention must be given to keeping the skin clean and dry, in order to prevent pressure sores. Teach the patient to apply his own appliance or to irrigate his own catheter, if this is to be permanent; force fluids, teach the patient the warning signs of genitourinary infections. Various kinds of appliances are available to avoid the use of a catheter. Bladder training should be done, if possible.

4. The patient will have fecal incontinence and may have fecal impaction. A daily enema or stool softener may be ordered to prevent these conditions.

5. Passive exercises to preserve any remaining muscle function and to restore all possible function will be needed. Paralyzed muscles that are limp at first may later develop spasms; exercises sometimes help to relieve them. Breathing exercises, if they are possible, will help to prevent pneumonia.

**Psychological Effects Upon the Patient.** The shock to the patient who is able to realize what has happened to him can be terrific. Gradually, as he becomes stronger, he visualizes his future, perhaps as a life of inactivity and helplessness. It is not always possible to give the patient the encouragement that he hopes for—a severe quadriplegic, for example, may be completely helpless for the rest of his life. It is mistaken kindness to foster false hopes of complete recovery, but the patient should be encouraged to make every effort to improve his condition. Fortunately for the paraplegic, improvement can be expected, but he has a long, hard road to travel before he can accomplish even the simplest task, which even then will be possible only through his own will power and perseverance. Without these efforts no amount of assistance will do the job. Often, he will be discouraged, and a nurse helps most by letting the patient express his frustration and discouragement, and by acknowledging these feelings, rather than constantly reminding him that he should be glad he is alive. Just to be able to let go and say how he really feels may be a great relief for him from always trying to keep up a brave front. Knowing that no one blames him for being discouraged may renew his courage to go on.

**Rehabilitation.** The rehabilitation of any patient with paralysis is centered on preventing his disabilities from increasing and on strengthening and making the most of whatever powers he may have. It begins immediately with preventing such disabilities as decubitus ulcers or foot drop, and with exercises to develop muscle strength and movement. It is true that the degree of the patient's success does depend on the nature and the extent of nerve damage, but we now know that success, through the use of modern physiotherapy and the patient's own perseverance, often is much greater than was once thought

to be possible. In spite of paralysis, many patients become able to move about and to look after themselves to some degree.

**The Paraplegic at Home.** With care and thoughtful planning, adjustment can be made in the home that make it possible for the paraplegic to be more independent. A toilet stool can be built up to the level of the wheelchair seat so that the patient can go to the bathroom without help. The bed height can be adjusted similarly; with the aid of an overhead bar the patient can transfer himself to and from the bed and the wheelchair. A ramp enables the paraplegic to wheel his chair out-of-doors. The kitchen equipment can be arranged so that it is accessible and convenient for the paraplegic or hemiplegic housewife.

**Most Likely to Succeed.** Any degree of rehabilitation is worth all the time and the effort that it takes to accomplish it. Anything that makes the patient more independent of others and more self-sufficient, perhaps even to the extent of holding a job, is worthwhile. Encouragement and perseverance are the keys to success. In a paraplegic ward, some patients will have greater disabilities than others, which tends to be discouraging. On the other hand, a paraplegic may be more willing to accept his disability when he sees other people with greater ones. Remember that, in general, paraplegics are more than usually sensitive to any action that looks like favoritism. Because a patient tries harder or seems to accomplish more, you must avoid seeming to be partial to him. Progress is so discouragingly slow at times that a patient may think that you are critical of him for not progressing faster.

# 47

# The Patient With a Cardiovascular Disease or a Blood Disorder

## BEHAVIORAL OBJECTIVES

*The student successfully attaining the goals of this chapter will be able to:*

- *identify deviations in cardiovascular structure and function, using Chapter 15 as a basis; list and define at least 5 general symptoms of disorders; discuss the 3 major diagnostic procedures and at least 5 laboratory tests which are used to determine abnormality; and demonstrate ability to perform such procedures as blood pressure and pulse and venous pressure and to assist with more complicated procedures such as blood culture and EKG.*

- *describe and discuss common ischemic heart disorders including angina, MI, and congestive heart failure; describe symptoms and medical and nursing care of each; demonstrate ability to assist the patient to meet his needs; and demonstrate ability to carry out a coronary nursing care regimen.*

- *define heart block, arrhythmia, fibrillation, and cardiac arrest; identify the signs of sudden death (cardiopulmonary arrest); demonstrate ability to recognize a need for and to initiate emergency resuscitation; and to assist the emergency rescue team.*

- *define and discuss infectious heart conditions, including rheumatic fever; identify the symptoms; discuss the medical treatment and nursing care; and demonstrate ability to carry out the appropriate nursing measures to assist the patient to meet his needs.*

- *identify and describe at least 4 peripheral vascular disorders; discuss the symptoms and medical treatment of each; and demonstrate ability to assist the patient to meet his basic or special needs.*

- *discuss at least 4 lymphatic or blood dyscrasias, including symptoms, medical treatment, and nursing care; and demonstrate competence in assisting such a patient and his family to meet their needs.*

## CARDIOVASCULAR DISEASE

Cardiovascular disease as presented in this chapter includes those conditions which interfere with the heart as a pump, those which disturb the blood flow in the blood vessels supplying it, and those peripheral vascular diseases which disturb the blood flow in the vessels in some localized area such as an extremity. These conditions are the leading cause of death in this country in people over the age of 25—the number of deaths from cardiovascular disease in the older age groups increases every year. It not only kills but it disables more people after 65 than any other disease and ranks second as a cause of disability to younger people.

## HEART DISEASE

To most people, heart disease, the most common of the cardiovascular diseases, has a sinister sound. A person's attitude toward heart disease can have a tremendous effect on his chances for recovery. Some people are so frightened that they are almost afraid to move and give up every activity, when all they need to do is to be more careful. Others, on the other hand, disregard orders about diet, rest,

or smoking. Understanding heart disease begins with a good general understanding of how a normal heart works. (See Chapter 15.)

**Signs and Symptoms.** Some forms of heart disease can be cured, while others can be controlled and made bearable by treatment. Certain symptoms can be expected to appear in almost every form of heart disease. In general, signs of heart difficulty of some kind are:

Changes in the rate, the quality, and the rhythm of the pulse
Rise or fall in blood pressure
Edema, especially in the feet and the ankles (faulty heart action causes the collection of fluids in the tissues)
A gain in weight from excess fluid in the tissues
Difficulty in breathing, and the presence of a cough or cyanosis, due to lack of oxygen in the blood and circulatory difficulties

**Diagnostic Tests.** Tests help to determine the particular form of heart disease in each case.

Electrocardiogram (EKG or ECG). An *electrocardiogram* is a record made on a graphic sheet by the action of the electric currents generated by the heart muscle; it gives the doctor information about heart action and heart damage. A technician takes this test by placing lead electrodes on the skin

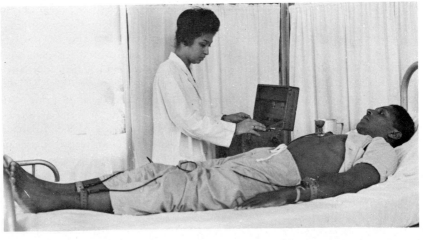

Figure 47-1. (*Top*) Technician taking an EKG. Leads have been placed on the arms, the legs and the chest. (*Bottom*) A sample of the graphic record obtained by electrocardiography. (Smith, D. W., Germain, C. P., and Gips, C. D.: Care of the Adult Patient, ed. 3. Philadelphia, Lippincott, 1971)

(on the chest, wrists, and ankles) and connecting them to a machine, the *electrocardiograph,* which measures and records these currents. The test may be done at the patient's bedside or in a room set aside for this purpose. The patient should be told that the test is painless. The graphic sheet is placed on the patient's chart; it usually is returned with both a detailed statement and a brief summary of what the test shows. The patient does not usually require any special treatment either before or after the test. (See Fig. 47-1.)

ANGIOCARDIOGRAM. An *angiocardiogram* is the record of a test to show abnormal conditions in the heart and the large blood vessels. A radiopaque dye (Diodrast or Urokon) is injected into a vein, and x-rays are taken to record the course of the dye from the heart to the lungs and back again and out through the aorta. It is used only as a last resort to get necessary information, because it is uncomfortable and sometimes dangerous.

The patient's breakfast is omitted on the morning of the test, and he is given a sedative an hour before the test is scheduled. The test is given in the x-ray department. The patient may have an allergic reaction to the dye and must be watched for signs of a delayed reaction after he returns to his room. The dye is irritating if it gets on the skin, and sometimes the point of injection becomes swollen and painful.

CARDIAC CATHETERIZATION. The purpose of this test is to get information about congenital defects in the heart. A long, flexible catheter is passed into the heart and the large blood vessels. The pressure is measured as the catheter passes through each part, and blood samples are taken in each one. These blood samples are analyzed to find out how much oxygen and carbon dioxide each contains. It is a delicate procedure which includes a cutdown (cutting down on a vein), fluoroscopy, and x-rays. It is carried out by a team of physicians, professional nurses, and technicians and takes from 1 to 3 hours. Cardiac catheterization is comparatively painless but somewhat uncomfortable.

The patient may be understandably apprehensive about the procedure; thus it will help to tell him that it is really not painful, although he may be a little uncomfortable. If he is told that the test is always done by a team that routinely does these tests he is less likely to be alarmed when he sees the number of people required to carry out the procedure.

Cardiac catheterization usually has no complications, but it is not entirely without danger. The patient's pulse is checked every 15 minutes for an hour after the test and frequently after that for several hours. A rapid or irregular pulse is reported immediately. Some doctors keep the patient in bed for the rest of the day; sometimes he is allowed to go back to his normal activities.

## BLOOD TESTS

*Circulation Time.* A drug (Decholin) is injected into an arm vein, and the time is measured until it reaches the taste buds of the patient. The patient must cooperate and tell the doctor when he tastes the substance. circulation time may be prolonged in certain heart disorders, such as cardiac failure.

*Blood Volume.* A test is usually done to determine the amount of blood in the patient's body.

*Prothrombin Time ("Pro Time").* Measurement of the prothrombin level in the blood indicates the ability of the blood to clot. Initially, the prothrombin time is 100 per cent, but after anticoagulant therapy, the level drops. It is important to measure the "pro time" level daily in a patient who is receiving anticoagulant therapy and to report the findings to the doctor. The nurse should also watch for bleeding in the patient who is receiving anticoagulants.

*Clotting Time.* It is important to measure the length of time it takes for the patient's blood to form a clot, especially if the patient is receiving an anticoagulant. A balance must be maintained between the formation of a clot and the possibility of bleeding.

*Sedimentation Rate ("Sed Rate").* Sedimentation rate is the length of time it takes cells in the blood to settle in an anticoagulant solution. The normal rate is about 5 minutes per millimeter. The rate increases in some diseases, such as rheumatic fever. This test is used to follow the course of a disease. It also helps to determine when physical activity may be increased, primarily in infectious diseases.

*Other Laboratory Procedures.* Other tests to evaluate cardiac function or blood condition measure the levels of blood pH and SGOT (transaminase) and reveal other facets of blood chemistry. The most common blood test is the CBC (*complete blood count*) which is done on all patients admitted to the hospital and includes the red and white cell counts, hemoglobin, and hematocrit determinations.

*Central Venous Pressure (CVP)*. This is a measure of right atrial function. It is influenced by blood volume, cardiac action, and vascular alterations. Blood pressure which is measured externally identifies the pressure within the arteries, while central venous pressure measures pressure within the veins. The venous pressure procedure is done by inserting a small catheter through a needle into a vein, usually the superior or inferior vena cava, and attaching this to a 3-way stopcock on an I.V. setup. The I.V. keeps the needle open, when the venous pressure is not being measured, by dripping very slowly. The 3-way stopcock is adjusted either to allow the fluid to drip into the veins or to allow the venous pressure to push the fluid into the manometer.

Venous pressure is taken by filling the manometer above the expected level and then noting the lowest level to which the fluid falls and stays. This level is recorded as the central venous pressure reading. It is important that the patient be lying down when this procedure is done and that the manometer be at the same level as the patient's body.

*Blood Culture*. This procedure is done to determine if any organisms are present in the blood of a patient or to determine what antibiotics are most effective in combating a specific organism. The practical nurse may be asked to assist with this procedure or the laboratory may do the entire procedure without assistance from the nursing staff. If the doctor asks you for assistance, the following description will help you to understand the procedure, although each hospital has its own specific methods.

The blood should be obtained while the patient is experiencing the most severe symptoms which have brought him to the hospital. That is, if he is in the hospital for a fever of unexplained origin, the culture should be taken when he has a fever. Remember, that it is the blood which is to be cultured, so that the skin and the equipment must be sterile to avoid outside contamination.

## Predisposing Factors in Heart Disorders

The nurse should understand that several factors interact and contribute to disorders of the heart and blood vessels—atherosclerosis leads to arteriosclerosis, which in turn leads to hypertension and other complications.

**Atherosclerosis and Arteriosclerosis.** When yellow, fatty deposits accumulate on the walls of arteries, the result is atherosclerosis—hardening of the wall, fibrosis, and narrowing of the lumen of the vessel. This disorder may also affect the valves of the heart.

Cholesterol seems to be a contributing factor in atherosclerosis, although the exact relationship is not known. Since the body manufactures cholesterol, some researchers feel that if the person does not eat foods high in this substance, the body will manufacture it anyway. Others feel that by controlling the amount of cholesterol in the diet, the person can control the onset of atherosclerosis. It is known that cholesterol is present in the blood of persons, whether they eat foods high in this substance or not, and that some people seem to metabolize it in different ways than others. One theory implies that the sugar and carbohydrates in the diet contribute to the cholesterol level, since cholesterol is a by-product of carbohydrate metabolism.

At any rate, cholesterol is the substance which is deposited on the walls of the vessels, causing atherosclerosis, which together with arteriosclerosis, leads to many other disorders of the blood vessels and heart. In treating the disorder, the doctor will periodically determine blood cholesterol levels and may attempt to control the amount of cholesterol by diet, and exercise.

*Arteriosclerosis* refers to the thickening of the walls of the arteries, primarily in the arterioles. These 2 conditions, atherosclerosis and arteriosclerosis, usually are interdependent; that is, they occur together, each aggravating the other. They are often predisposing factors to other diseases such as hypertension or coronary artery disease.

**Hypertension.** *Hypertension* is high blood pressure. Although not considered as a heart disease, hypertension can lead to serious conditions, such as congestive heart failure and cerebrovascular accident, often referred to as CVA. A consistently high blood pressure leads to heart damage. As people grow older, blood pressure tends to rise, although the reasons for this are not completely clear. One thing is certain: the condition of the heart and the blood vessels has the greatest effect on blood pressure. The range in normal adult blood pressure can vary from 100/60 to 130/80.

Hypertensive heart disease or high blood pressure is predominantly a disease of the small arterioles. Spasms in the arterioles increases the blood pressure and actually increases the development of arteriosclerosis. One condition makes the other worse. Since the heart must pump harder to force the blood through the arteries, the result is hypertrophy of the heart muscles. A blood pressure of 140/90, consistent with other symptoms, indicates hypertension. Hypertension may also result from a long-standing valvular disorder.

Symptoms are headache, fatigue, failing vision, pain on exertion, and signs of uremia.

Hypertension generally occurs between the ages of 25 and 50. For 75 per cent of persons with high blood pressure, there is no known cause. In others, it may be caused by kidney failure or other diseases. Predisposing factors can be obesity, excessive smoking, and extreme continued emotional tension.

TYPES OF HYPERTENSION

*Essential Hypertension.* Symptoms, other than elevated blood pressure, may not occur for years. No restrictions are imposed until other symptoms occur. The patient is encouraged to avoid excessive exercise, observe moderation in eating, and avoid tension and anxiety. He is advised not to smoke or to drink alcohol, tea, or coffee.

*Malignant Hypertension.* This form of hypertension (which is not a cancer) occurs in younger people. Onset is very sudden, progresses very rapidly, and results in death. It is often difficult to determine the cause. If the cause cannot be found or if the disorder is irreversible, it is fatal. The treatment attempts to deal with the symptoms and includes medications such as Serpasil, which lowers the blood pressure and relieves the headache and dizziness, or Aprescoline.

TREATMENT AND NURSING CARE. Hyperten-

sion cannot be cured, but treatment will help to lower the blood pressure. The treatment includes:

Reducing weight and avoiding overweight
Reducing the amount of extra salt in the diet
Building up good health habits for sleep, rest, and relaxation
Avoiding emotional upsets, such as angry outbursts or violent enthusiasms
Taking drugs with a tranquilizing effect

Reassuring the patient is an important part of his care. It may be a great shock to him to learn that he has high blood pressure. He may think that his active life is over and death is just around the corner. He can be told that many patients with blood pressure problems live for many years by following orders. The patient's family must learn how important his diet is and how rest and peace of mind help to keep his blood pressure within a safe range.

If a patient has been treated for high blood pressure for a long time, he may have been taking his blood pressure at home. Therefore, he may be justifiably resentful if not allowed to know what his blood pressure is when a nurse takes it in the hospital. Should this situation occur, the doctor should be consulted.

## CORONARY ARTERY DISEASE (Ischemic Heart Disorders)

People over 50 are the most common victims of coronary artery disease, but it may occur also in younger people. During the early middle years more men than women are affected; after the menopause the number is about the same for both sexes. There seems to be a tendency in some families to develop the disease. However, it is believed that coronary artery disease develops over many years, and precautions to prevent it should begin early in life. More attention is given now to discovering the disease early, before an attack has occurred and before atherosclerosis has severely damaged the heart.

### Angina Pectoris

*Angina pectoris,* usually referred to as angina, literally translated, means angina (pain) in the chest (pectoris). Angina occurs suddenly when extra exertion calls for an increase in the blood supply to the heart which the narrowed arteries are unable to provide. Consequently, the heart muscle suffers. In addition, if a fragment from fat and calcium deposits in the arteries lodges in one of the coronary arteries, the blood supply to the heart is shut off completely (*myocardial infarction*).

Angina is a *temporary* loss of blood supply to the heart (anoxia). If this loss of blood supply becomes permanent, the result is *ischemia* (prolonged deficiency of blood) or *myocardial infarction* (blockage of a vessel).

**Types of Angina.** There are 3 types of angina: nocturnal, decubitus, and intractable. As the term implies, the pain of *nocturnal angina* occurs at night. In *decubitus angina,* the pain occurs when the patient is lying down and is relieved when the patient sits up. *Intractable angina* does not respond to therapy and occurs so often that it prevents gainful activity.

**Symptoms of Angina.** Angina is most severe over the heart, although it may spread to the shoulder and the arm on the left side or to the jaw. (It is more likely to be felt in the left arm because this is the direction of the aortic branching. It is here that the blood loss is felt first.) The patient is pale, feels faint, and is dyspneic. The pain is over in less than 5 minutes but is intense while it lasts. This is a warning that the heart is not getting enough blood, and the victim who ignores this warning is risking serious illness or sudden death if he does not put himself under a doctor's care. He may have recurrent attacks of angina, but treatment lessens the danger of a fatal attack. If the pain of angina lasts for more than 15 minutes, it is considered to be a myocardial infarction until proven otherwise. Repeated attacks of angina can lead to myocardial infarction.

Diagnosis is made on the basis of an EKG and symptoms. If nitroglycerin relieves the attack, it is considered angina.

Angina is often precipitated by "the 4 E's": exercise (or exertion), eating, emotions, and exposure. It may also be caused by an overdose of insulin in a diabetic.

**Treatment and Prevention.** The patient who is under a doctor's care knows what to do for an angina attack. For one thing, he must quit smoking because it constricts the cor-

onary arteries. He has also been instructed to always carry nitroglycerin tablets with him and to dissolve a tablet under his tongue as soon as the attack begins. Nitroglycerin brings quick relief by dilating the coronary arteries. Patients use this drug safely for many years with no ill effects. Amyl nitrite is equally effective in relieving angina. It comes in ampules that are broken in a handkerchief and inhaled.

Aminophylline and peritrate are drugs that may be given to prevent attacks of angina. These drugs also dilate the coronary arteries; however, they do not help everyone.

When a patient knows that certain things bring on an attack he can learn to be more careful. If the attacks become more frequent and more severe, he may have to curb his activities. The patient who has angina never knows when he may have an attack; he may live for years or may die suddenly. The best he can do is to follow the rules for his treatment, learn what he can and cannot do, and live accordingly.

**Prognosis.** When the underlying disease is coronary atherosclerosis, the prognosis may be more encouraging than when other causative factors are involved. The earlier the age of onset, the poorer the prognosis.

## Myocardial Infarction (Coronary Occlusion)

Also known as MI, heart attack, or coronary thrombosis, myocardial infarction is the sudden blocking of one or more of the coronary arteries. If it involves an extensive area, death will result. If less extensive, it will result in necrosis of heart tissue and subsequent scarring. Other vessels can take over for the injured area, if the area of scarring is not too extensive. Myocardial infarction occurs most commonly in men, 90 per cent of whom are over age 40.

**Symptoms.** The attack begins suddenly with a sharp severe pain in the chest, sometimes radiating to the left arm and shoulder. It is like angina but lasts longer and is more severe; exertion may have nothing to do with bringing it on. Also, unlike angina, it does not go away with rest, and nitroglycerin or amyl nitrite do not help. Because it simulates indigestion or a gallbladder attack with abdominal pain, diagnosis is difficult. In general, the patient is restless, paces, and has a feeling of impending death; his skin is ashen, cold, and clammy; he is dyspneic, cyanotic, and has a rapid, thready pulse; and his blood pressure drops (the patient is actually in shock). Later, the patient's temperature will rise, because around 4 days after the attack, scar tissue begins to form around the injured tissue.

The patient's prognosis is guarded for 3 to 4 weeks, although the first 2 weeks are the most dangerous.

**First Aid.** Everyone should know what to do for the victim of a coronary heart attack. Much harm has been done by well-meaning but misguided ministrations in this emergency. If chest pains persist in a person suspected of having a heart attack, insist on keeping him quiet and call a doctor. This means *complete rest; do not* take off his shoes or try to undress him or get him into bed, *no matter where he is when this happens.* However, loosen any tight clothing so that the patient can breathe easier. Cover him with a blanket or coat; something under his head will help him to breathe more easily. If he shows signs of shock, keep him flat. Do not allow him to sit up or move around before the doctor has seen him, no matter how much better he says he feels. Even if this is not a coronary attack, it is better to be safe than sorry. Since cardiac arrest may also occur, be prepared to initiate resuscitation.

**Treatment and Nursing Care.** Tests will help to determine the nature of the attack. First, an electrocardiogram will be taken. Then blood tests will be done for the presence of an enzyme (SGOT or transaminase) which always appears in greater amounts after a coronary occlusion. Tests of the sedimentation rate of the red blood cells almost always show that it is higher after a myocardial infarction.

Coronary nursing care stresses the following points:

Rest comes first. The injured heart must have time to repair its injuries. The damaged spot in the heart takes from 3 to 6 weeks to heal. After about 8 weeks, tough scar tissue has formed.

The amount of activity the patient is permitted will depend on the severity of the attack. He may not be allowed any activity—not even to wash his face or feed himself, although the male patient is usually allowed to finish his bath. Some patients are permitted to do things for themselves and may be up in a chair for a short time each day. Some may be allowed to use a commode at the bedside or go to the bathroom once a day for a bowel movement. The commode is preferable to a bedpan, because the patient is more likely to strain on the bedpan. To prevent any unnecessary straining, stool softeners are also given. Many doctors want a patient to exercise his feet and legs gently to prevent thrombophlebitis.

The patient should not sit up because this cuts off the circulation to the legs and puts a strain on the heart. He may lie in bed or stand with less strain. If the patient needs to sit up in order to breathe, he should be propped so that his head is up, but with his hips flexed as little as possible. Sometimes the patient can lean on a pillow placed on the overbed table and rest in that position. If he has a great deal of difficulty in breathing, he may sleep in this position.

Prevent the patient from exerting himself, such as straining with a bowel movement or reaching for things on the bedside table or picking them up from the floor. After giving him his bath, let him rest for a little while before making his bed. The patient with breathing difficulties is sometimes more comfortable in an upright position with a backrest built up by pillows and supporting pillows for the arms and knees.

See that his family or visitors do not stay too long or talk too much, especially about things that might upset him. Also consider the family's anxiety in these situations. They are understandably upset and concerned. They need to be reassured that everything possible is being done for the patient. No doubt, the patient will need similar assurance.

A narcotic, usually morphine, is given, as well as anticoagulants. If the "pro time" is less than 10 percent, there is always the possibility of bleeding. Observe the patient for bleeding from any body orifice.

Watch his pulse, measure his intake and output, and note any sign of pain or difficulty in breathing or fatigue. Take his blood pressure regularly.

**Complications.** The major complications of myocardial infarction are arrhythmias and cardiac standstill. The nurse should be prepared and able to initiate resuscitative measures immediately in the event of a cardiac arrest.

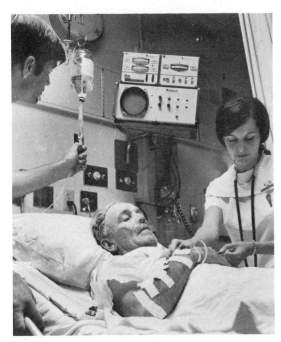

Figure 47-2. The modern coronary care unit (ccu) is specially designed and staffed to care for the acute coronary patient. This illustration shows built in oxygen, suction and blood pressure equipment, hypothermia blanket, continuous intravenous administration, cardiac monitor, as well as specially trained staff. Notice that the patient's head is slightly elevated to facilitate breathing and that he is receiving nasal oxygen. A large stop-clock on the wall can be instantly activated in the event of an emergency. (Public Information Department, Hennepin County, Minnesota)

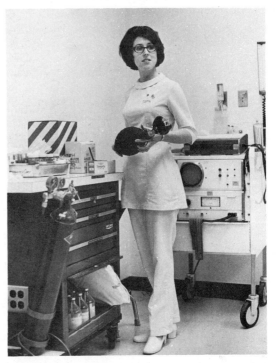

Figure 47-3. The nurse must always know where the emergency equipment is kept. Whenever you go to a new station, locate the ambu bag and other equipment, such as the "crash cart" shown. The nurse is holding the Ambu bag which is used to provide artificial ventilation in cardiac arrest. Also in the picture is oxygen equipment, the cart with emergency drugs, and the cardiac cart, which includes the cardiac monitor and the electrical defibrillator. On the back of the crash cart is usually a board to put under the patient for firmness when closed chest cardiac massage is given. (Public Information Department, Hennepin County, Minnesota)

**The Outlook.** The patient after a myocardial infarction can live a normal, useful life and can often go back to his previous employment. The recovered patient is not nearly as restricted as once was the case.

## Functional Heart Disease

Although nothing may be organically wrong with the heart, anxiety can bring on many of the symptoms of heart disease, such as pain over the heart, shortness of breath, and exhaustion. If a thorough examination shows no physical abnormality, tranquilizers or sedatives may be prescribed to lessen the patient's anxiety. Every effort should be made to find out what is causing these symptoms and to help the patient to realize that his heart is normal. Occasionally, this patient will be diagnosed as having functional heart disease and will later suffer from an infarct.

## The Modern Coronary Care Unit

Many hospitals now have a special unit designed for the care of the coronary patient. The staff is specially trained in coronary care and emergency measures. Practical nurses may be trained to work in this unit.

Training for the coronary care unit includes the following areas of study: the normal anatomy and physiology of the heart, EKG readings, both normal and abnormal, important laboratory tests and their meanings, emergency drugs and resuscitation measures, use of special equipment, and the special emotional aspects of coronary care nursing.

Some of the special equipment found in the modern coronary care unit includes oxygen equipment, heart monitors, defibrillators, resuscitation equipment, and emergency drugs. The nurse in this unit can care for more than one patient because the patients are placed close to one another and because all the necessary equipment is close at hand.

## Congestive Heart Failure

*Congestive heart failure,* also known as cardiac decompensation, cardiac insufficiency, or cardiac incompetence, means that the heart is failing and is unable to do its work. It is a term used to describe a syndrome (a group of symptoms), the key word of which is *congestive.* Heart failure affects individuals in different ways and to different degrees—one person may go about his business as usual, showing no signs of heart failure. Another person may be seriously ill. The heart will try to keep up with the demands made upon it; treatment will help it to make a satisfactory adjustment. Abnormal conditions in the heart may make continued treatment necessary or signs of heart failure will appear again.

When the heart is failing we say it is *decompensated.* After treatment, when it is able to carry its normal load, we say that the heart is *compensated.*

**Causes.** Congestive heart failure is the result of strain on the heart which may be caused by heart disease, blood vessel disease, hypertension, renal insufficiency, congenital defects, or other diseases, such as hyperthyroidism which speeds up heart action or rheumatic fever which damages the heart valves. Older people are subject to heart failure because the blood vessels lose their elasticity (arteriosclerosis).

**Symptoms.** The first sign of a failing heart which the patient may notice is excessive fatigue; he may have to rest part of the way up the stairs. He may also need 2 pillows at night and may develop a persistent cough (which indicates the start of pulmonary edema). His ankles might swell during the day, and although this swelling disappears overnight, it comes back as soon as he is on his feet again. When he gets on the scales he finds that he has gained weight, which is actually due to an accumulation of fluid in his tissues (edema). When he presses on a swollen part his finger leaves an indentation which lasts for a time (pitting).

Pulmonary edema is the most common symptom of heart failure and is caused by left-sided heart failure. The failure of the left ventricle to pump is characterized by congestion in the pulmonary system. The symptoms are cough, loose and moist rales (gurgling or bubbling sounds in the lungs), dyspnea, nocturia, palpitation (the patient can feel his heart beating in his chest), asthmatic breathing or paroxysmal dyspnea, followed by blood-streaked sputum and prostration. These symptoms are treated with morphine and oxygen.

Failure of the right ventricle to pump results in congestion in the systemic circulation. The main cause of right-heart failure is left-heart failure. Symptoms are edema of the feet and legs, numbness or tingling in the fingers, albuminuria, cyanosis, engorgement and visible pulsation of the neck veins, and engorgement of the liver with or without jaundice. The heart attempts to compensate by dilation, hypertrophy, and tachycardia.

Heart failure is not a disease in itself, but is a symptom of other pathology. If a patient has failure of one side of the heart, he will eventually have failure of the other side.

**Tests.** The usual tests for detecting heart disease are taken, such as the electrocardiogram, x-ray examination, and cardiac catheterization. Circulation time, and arterial and venous blood pressure are measured. Arterial pressure is determined by "taking the blood pressure." The venous pressure is always increased in congestive heart failure or pulmonary edema.

The urine output is diminished (oliguria), the specific gravity is elevated, and albumin (albuminuria), blood (hematuria), and casts are found in the urine. Blood chemistry shows nitrogen retention—elevated B.U.N. (blood urea nitrogen), uric acid, and creatinine.

**Treatment and Nursing Care.** In heart

failure, the heart is laboring under difficulties, and the treatment and the nursing care are designed to make its work easier. Some important aspects of therapy are:

Rest, including sedation if it is needed

Digitalis to slow the heart rate, to increase the force of the systole, and to decrease the heart size

Diuretics, such as Mercuhydrin, Diuril, or Lanoxin, which are administered to help the body to rid itself of excess fluid and salts

Paracentesis or thoracentesis (puncture of the chest with a needle) to drain off excess fluid

Oxygen, if the blood is not getting enough from the lungs

Use of a footboard alternately with the gatch knee rest, which allows the patient to move his legs and promotes circulation; also rocking beds and elastic stockings help

Rotating tourniquets, which are applied with pressure cuffs to 3 extremities at a time and rotated every 45 minutes; to reduce the amount of blood which must be circulated by an overtaxed heart

Phlebotomy to actually withdraw blood so as to reduce the amount in circulation and relieve the heart

Massage and a foam rubber pad for the patient's buttocks, since he usually sits up much of the time

Restriction of salt in his diet

Recording the patient's weight at the same time every day (the patient wears the same amount of clothing for each weighing)

Measuring intake and output.

DIGITALIS. The amount of digitalis administered is larger at first than it will be later. The dosage is gradually decreased until the amount needed to stabilize the heartbeat is found. If the amount is too large the patient will have undesirable side-effects. When the heart rate is slowed down sufficiently, we say that the patient is *digitalized*. Sometimes a patient has to continue taking digitalis for the rest of his life.

In administering digitalis the nurse should take the pulse of the patient for 1 full minute. If the radial pulse is below 60, take an apical pulse. Do not give the medication if the pulse is below 60 and report this immediately. (For this reason, digitalis should always be poured into a separate medicine cup in case it needs to be discarded.)

*Side-effects of digitalization* include gastrointestinal symptoms such as nausea and vomiting, headache, and blurred vision which gives a yellow appearance to everything. Bradycardia also occurs when the digitalis slows the heart too much.

## Arrhythmias

An arrhythmia is an irregularity in the rhythm of the heartbeat. It is a complication of myocardial infarction, as well as of other heart and circulatory disorders. It may also be caused by severe trauma or electric shock. Arrhythmias may be classified as follows:

*Sinus tachycardia:* Heartbeat is 100 or over. (Remember that this rate is normal in children.) It can be present in instances of high fever, extreme emotion, overactive thyroid, exercise, and shock.

*Sinus bradycardia:* Heartbeat is 60 or less. May occur in athletes and with overdigitalization.

*Paroxysmal tachycardia:* refers to intermittent spells of tachycardia. It is characterized by sudden onset and relapse. Symptoms are faintness, weakness, and shortness of breath. It may be precipitated by smoking, drinking, or severe gastrointestinal disorders. It is treated with quinidine and Pronestyl.

## Heart Block

*Heart block* means that the contractions of the heart are weakened and do not have enough force to send the blood from the auricles into the ventricles. It is characterized by a marked drop in pulse rate to 30 or 40. This is a disturbance of the nerve impulses from the auricles to the ventricles. With the failure of normal electrical transmissions, the heart sets up an alternate stimulus for heart beat. If the contractions are only weakened, heart block is *partial*; if they cease altogether, it is *complete*.

Heart block is not a disease in itself but it is associated with many kinds of heart disease, especially disease of the coronary arteries or rheumatic heart disease. The toxic effects of digitalis may also cause heart block. In complete heart block, the patient dies unless the contractions are started again. Epinephrine is given immediately; in a prolonged attack it is injected directly into the heart. At the beginning of an attack the patient becomes unconscious and may have convulsions.

The *electric pacemaker* is a machine which is used to stimulate heart contractions by means of wires connected to electrodes which are applied to the chest. Sometimes the electrodes are inserted into the heart. Patients who experience frequent difficulty with heart contractions may use this device all the time. A portable pacemaker about the size of a small transistor radio is now available. The patient wears it underneath his clothing. Still smaller models can be implanted surgically underneath the patient's skin. For some patients (who have *temporary heart block*), the pacemaker can be discontinued gradually, but others cannot live without it.

## Auricular and Ventricular Fibrillations

Fibrillation is a twitching of the heart, which does not result in an organized heart beat, so that the blood is not circulated. The most dangerous type of fibrillation is ventricular fibrillation, and when the doctor mentions fibrillation, this is usually the type he is referring to. *Ventricular fibrillation is an emergency situation and is fatal if not treated.* (It leads to cardiac arrest.) The treatment is external or internal cardiac massage or electrical defibrillation (cardioversion), which is done by the physician or a specially trained coronary care unit nurse. An electric shock of high voltage is passed through the patient's body in an attempt to shock the heart back into a regular beat. The nurse must be very careful not to touch the patient or the bed while this procedure is being done or she, too, will receive the shock and be fatally injured.

## Cardiac Arrest

*Cardiac arrest* means that the heart has stopped beating. Cardiac arrest may be caused by electric shock, drowning or other asphyxia, anaphylactic shock, central nervous system trauma, drug overdose, ventricular fibrillation, coronary heart disease, or general anesthetics. Treatment is useless unless it is given at once, and it should be started by the staff or people who are nearest to the victim. Two things are vital: to keep the patient breathing and to restore the heartbeat (*cardiopulmonary resuscitation*).

**Cardiopulmonary Resuscitation.** Several definitions are vital in the discussion of cardiopulmonary resuscitation.

*Sudden death* occurs when there is a sudden and unexpected lack of respiration and an absence of circulation of the blood. This is cardiopulmonary arrest. The key words are "sudden" and "unexpected."

*Clinical death* occurs at this time if no resuscitation is begun.

*Biological death* begins to occur 4 to 6 minutes after clinical death. This is the situation of irreversible damage to the tissues of the body, especially those of the brain. This is a most important consideration in such situations as transplantation of organs and in deciding whether or not to attempt resuscitation. Biological death may also be indicated by a *flat electroencephalogram,* which indicates the absence of brain activity.

Not every patient should be resuscitated!

### Steps in Dealing with Sudden Death

1. *Recognize the problem:* First, determine if respirations are present and if air is being exchanged. If respiratory arrest occurs first, the heart may beat for several minutes. Second, determine if there is a *heart beat* in the carotid or femoral areas. If circulatory arrest occurs first, respiration stops within ½ to 1 minute. Third, determine if the *pupils* are dilated. Dilation begins 45 seconds after circulation ceases and is complete in 2 minutes. If there is no respiration, no circulation, dilated pupils, the patient is in CARDIOPULMONARY ARREST.

2. *Begin resuscitation immediately:* First, provide *artificial ventilation.* Mouth-to-mouth resuscitation is the most effective method and is discussed in Chapter 35 on First Aid. An Ambu bag is available in most hospitals and is more sanitary. Second, make sure the airway is open. You may need to intubate the patient. Third, provide *artificial circulation.* Closed chest cardiac massage is most often used.

One person can do these 2 procedures until help arrives. Keep the attempt going until a doctor arrives. Once you begin resuscitation, you cannot stop without orders.

**Closed-Chest Cardiac Massage.** This is another method of resuscitation. The patient should be lying on a flat, firm surface (never on a mattress). His airway should be unobstructed. The operator kneels beside the patient and places his hands on the center of the chest, one on top of the other and at right angles to each other. He presses downward, using the heels of both hands, depressing the sternum 1 to 1½ inches, and releases the pressure briefly. He repeats this process—press, release, press, release—about 60 times a minute, until the patient responds or until a doctor pronounces the patient dead. These procedures can save a life if they are started *immediately*—if necessary, it is imperative to start them without waiting for a doctor to arrive. Mouth-to-mouth resuscitation is given at the same time.

**Assisting the Physician.** As soon as medical help arrives, the nurse's role becomes that of assisting the physician. First, obtain the necessary emergency equipment: crash cart, Ambu bag, emergency drugs, heart monitor, stethoscope, equipment for blood pressure, oxygen, I.V., and suctioning, tracheotomy tray, and oral airways. Call any other persons who are needed to assist in the emergency procedures. Make sure that you keep a record of the entire procedure, including what time the arrest was discovered, your estimation of how long the patient had been clinically dead, what emergency measures you took, what time the doctor arrived, what procedures were done from that time on, what drugs were given, in what dosage and at what time, what responses were made by the patient, and what laboratory work was done, as well as EKG's, x-rays, and other tests. Finally you must note the outcome of the resuscitation efforts and the succeeding nursing care, if any.

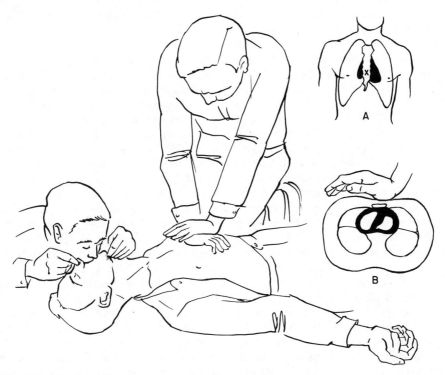

Figure 47-4. Technic for cardiopulmonary massage. One rescuer gives mouth-to-mouth resuscitation. The other massages the heart by pressing downward on the patient's chest approximately 60 times a minute. Insert (A) indicates the area where pressure should be applied. Pressure must be applied on lower half of sternum to prevent the ribs from being fractured. Insert (B) shows manual pressure on the chest, compressing the heart and forcing blood out of it. One person may do both activities simultaneously, alternating 15 compressions, 2 breaths, 15 compressions, until help arrives. The patient may be moved while the procedure is being done. (American Heart Association, Inc., New York City; adapted from Kouwenhoven, W. B., et al.: Heart activation in cardiac arrest, Modern Concepts of Cardiovascular Diseases 30[2]:642)

**Open-Chest Cardiac Massage.** In some cases of cardiac arrest, the doctor may perform open-chest cardiac massage by making a surgical incision in the anterior chest wall and exposing the heart. He grasps the heart in the palm of his hand and then carries out rapid cardiac pumping (80 to 100 times per minute), avoiding putting finger pressure on the heart. This is sometimes effective in restoring the heartbeat. However, it is rarely done, except in the operating room.

**Other Means of Resuscitation.** Two other methods of resuscitation can be used to combat cardiac arrest: injections of *Adrenalin* and *quinidine* or *procaine amide*.

**Successful Resuscitation and Subsequent Nursing Care.** If the resuscitation measures are successful, the pulse will be felt, the pupils will constrict, the patient's color will improve, and he will begin to breathe, cough, or move. Once the patient is resuscitated, he may need to be maintained on a resuscitator or given I.V. therapy or vasopressor drugs. He will need to be closely watched in case another emergency resuscitation is required.

## Aneurysms

An *aneurysm* is an outpouching of a blood vessel. Although it may occur in any vessel, the most common site is the aorta. When an aneurysm develops in the aorta or a cerebral vessel it represents an extreme emergency. If this outpouching, or aneurysm, ruptures, surgery is performed at once. If the aneurysm is discovered before it ruptures, it is treated by surgical repair or removal of the aneurysm. Usually, a synthetic graft is substituted for portion of the vessel affected by the aneurysm, although sometimes an autograft (a part of a blood vessel from another part of the person's body or from another person's body) is used.

Aneurysms may be congenital, may occur after trauma, such as an automobile accident, or may develop as a result of arteriosclerosis.

## INFECTIOUS HEART DISEASES

### Rheumatic Fever

*Rheumatic fever* is the cause of 90 per cent of organic heart disease in people under the age of 50. It often leaves the victim with heart damage which leads to chronic rheumatic heart disease. Although young adults may contract rheumatic fever, it usually is found in children between the ages of 5 and 15 years. (Acute rheumatic fever is discussed in Chapter 40.)

**Chronic Rheumatic Heart Disease.** In adults, the aftermath of childhood rheumatic fever may be malfunctioning heart valves. This chronic condition usually does not show up until about age 40. Symptoms include myocarditis, or endocarditis, or pancarditis (the entire heart is inflamed).

The most common cause of *chronic rheumatic heart disease* is a narrowing of the mitral valve between the left auricle and left ventricle of the heart. This is called *mitral stenosis*. Blood collects in the chambers of the heart and enlarges them, causing congestion in the lungs. The left side of the heart is the first to be affected. The condition progresses to the right side and leads to heart failure.

Surgical treatment involves mitral commissurotomy whereby the leaves of the mitral valve are broken apart. It is a closed heart procedure and is usually successful in relieving symptoms, although more pronounced symptoms may occur later.

**Symptoms.** The first signs of this trouble are a difficulty in breathing, a cough, and sometimes cyanosis and the expectoration of blood. If the condition grows worse, the patient's feet and ankles swell, his liver enlarges, and his abdominal cavity fills with fluid—unmistakable signs of heart failure. There may also be a lowering of the systolic blood pressure. Another complication is subacute bacterial endocarditis (SBE).

**Prevention of Recurrence.** The best protective measures are to avoid exposure, colds, and streptococcal diseases, keep up resistance, get adequate sleep, and eat a balanced diet. Complications may be activated by a tooth extraction, oral surgery, or major surgery. As a precaution against streptococcal infections, many patients with rheumatic fever take daily prophylactic penicillin which is provided at a reduced rate through the American Heart Association upon the recommendation of a physician.

**Treatment and Nursing Care.** Aside from its physical effect, rheumatic heart disease can be emotionally upsetting. Because bedrest is required for months or even years, the patient is often deprived of friends and activities and needs diversional activities to keep his mind active. The patient often has much resentment and can become overly concerned with his health. An effort must be made to assist the patient to maintain normal social development. However, the adult patient must learn to limit his activities.

Heart surgery provides relief for many of these patients. However, it is not always necessary, and an operation is performed only when the patient has such serious changes in his heart and lungs that nothing else will help him.

### Bacterial Endocarditis

The heart is covered and lined with membranes. The membrane that lines the chambers and the valves of the heart is called the endocardium. Infection of this membrane causes inflammation, a condition known as *bacterial endocarditis* or subacute bacterial endocarditis. This is a serious disease which was once nearly always fatal. Although antibiotics have changed this gloomy picture, bacterial endocarditis is still a common health problem. However, modern treatment helps to control it and to keep it from disabling the patient.

People with damaged heart valves are more susceptible to infection, especially those who have had rheumatic fever or have congenital heart defects. The extraction of an infected tooth, childbirth, or an upper respiratory infection may release disease organisms into the bloodstream which attack damaged heart valves. The streptococcus is a frequent offender.

**Symptoms.** One of the first signs of bacterial endocarditis is a low-grade fever, which gradually increases. The patient has chills and perspires, he loses his appetite and loses weight. His face has a brownish tinge, and tiny reddish-purple spots (petechiae) appear on his skin and mucous membranes. Usually, he is anemic. As the diseases progresses, the signs of congestive heart failure appear. Blood cultures will show what organism is causing the trouble.

The course of the disease is rapid and, if untreated, can result in death. However, 90 per cent of the patients treated can be cured without ill effects.

**Treatment and Nursing Care.** Large doses of antibiotics, to which the causative organism is sensitive, are given. The nursing care consists of conserving the patient's energy while he is a bed patient and making him as comfortable as possible. The rate and quality of his pulse should be noted frequently, and he should be observed closely for fluctuation in body temperature and for any symptoms of complications. For example, hematuria (blood in the urine) or pain and impaired circulation in an extremity might be the result of a blood clot (embolus) which originated in the diseased valve.

## SURGICAL ASPECTS OF HEART CONDITIONS

Some patients with heart disease may be helped or cured by heart surgery. If the surgeon actually enters the heart in any way, this is considered heart surgery. *Closed-heart surgery* refers to surgical procedures which may be done without stopping the heart. *Open-heart surgery* involves opening the heart in such a way that the heart must be stopped and the circulated blood oxygenated by an external pump, such as the *pump oxygenator*. This is known as *extra corporeal* (outside the body) *circulation*. The pump oxygenator or heart-lung pump is a complex machine which operates outside the patient's body. As the blood circulates through the machine, carbon dioxide is removed and oxygen added through a process of osmosis, filming, or bubbling. It also keeps the blood warmed to body temperature. A specially trained technician, the cardiopulmonary technician, maintains the machine and determines if the blood is being properly oxygenated. A patient can be maintained for several hours on the heart-lung oxygenator, the longest period of time occurring in a heart transplant.

**Emotional Aspects of Heart Surgery.** Many patients welcome the heart surgery as a new chance at life, because often there is no other treatment which can help them. They look to the heart surgery, even with its risks, as a chance to recover from what has usually been a long illness. New methods of treatment and new surgical technics are giving many people, who would not have survived in previous years, a chance to live a normal life.

## Types of Heart Surgery

Various types of heart and blood vessel surgery may be done with the use of the pump oxygenator. These include grafting blood vessels, implanting new blood vessels, revising or transposing the vessels that exist, correcting septal (wall) defects within the heart or valve damage, replacing valves within the heart, correcting multiple defects in the heart or vessels, and transplanting the entire heart. The pump oxygenator is also used as a support device in other types of surgery. If a *hyperbaric chamber* exists in the hospital, heart surgery is often done there to provide the patient with a greater ability to absorb oxygen.

## Preoperative Preparation

Usually, the patient comes into the hospital for several weeks before the operation. This allows time to prepare him physically and emotionally for this experience and provides an opportunity to show him that he can have confidence in the people who are caring for him.

The physical aspects of preoperative preparation include providing good nutrition, extra oxygen for the body which has been deprived of an adequate oxygen supply, vitamin therapy, anticoagulant therapy in some cases, antibiotic therapy, and routine preoperative procedures such as laboratory and x-ray examinations, heart catherization, electrocardiograms and practicing of deep breathing and coughing.

## Postoperative Care

Professional nurses are usually responsible for the immediate postoperative nursing care following heart surgery. Postoperative care is essential for the heart surgery patient, perhaps more so than for almost any other type of postoperative patient. More open-heart patients die in the first 2 days after the surgery than die on the operating table. The patient has not only had major chest surgery, he has also had surgery on a very delicate and very vital part of his body, his heart. Postoperative care includes such routine postoperative measures as checking vital signs (more than the routine measurements will be done), running blood tests, encouraging coughing and deep breathing, giving inhalation therapy, giving nutrition or fluid and blood transfusions, and maintaining drainage, suction, and other special equipment.

## Heart Transplant

Until recently, many problems prevented the transplantation of a large organ, such as the heart. First, the surgeons needed to develop successful methods of suturing blood vessels, a very delicate and difficult procedure. Then, they had to tackle the problem of oxygenating the blood while the heart was being replaced, a problem which was solved by the pump oxygenator. Other problems still exist, such as how to store the hearts or how to stimulate a heart so that it will resume beating and continue to beat. In addition moral and ethical questions are still being debated.

The greatest problem in the transplantation of any organ is the *rejection* by the body of any foreign object or protein substance. This is the mechanism which the body uses to fight off infection, but in the case of transplantation, it works against the well-being of the patient. The body's antibody response must be offset by drugs or the body will not accept the new heart. Antirejection or *immunosuppressive drugs,* that is, drugs which suppress the body's immune response, are given. With added research and improvement of surgical technics, as well as improvement of antirejection drugs, we can expect heart transplantation to become a successful means of treating many cardiac patients, for whom there was formerly no effective treatment.

# PERIPHERAL VASCULAR DISORDERS

## Thrombophlebitis

*Thrombophlebitis* is the inflammation of the wall of a vein, in which one or more clots form. It is caused by pressure or by prolonged inactivity, such as might occur after surgery or in any illness when the patient remains in one position for long periods of time. Thus the legs are most likely to be affected. Since early ambulation in illness has become an accepted routine, there is less chance for this difficulty to occur.

Figure 47-5. The nurse is explaining to a member of the family how a padded board at the foot of the bed prevents pressure on the affected limb of a patient with thrombophlebitis. This is more satisfactory than a bed cradle because there is less danger of the patient striking it with his foot or leg and dislodging a blood clot.

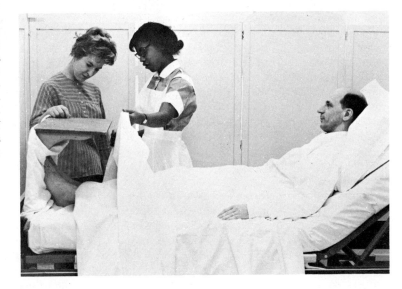

Elderly patients or people with heart disease or varicose veins are prone to develop thrombophlebitis. Prolonged sitting may also cause it. Older people especially should know that it is important to change position frequently. Other causes include trauma or pregnancy.

**Symptoms.** The symptoms of thrombophlebitis include pain in the affected leg, redness and swelling, fever, and the symptoms that usually go with fever, such as fatigue and loss of appetite. *Homan's sign* is a specific test for thrombophlebitis: the pain in the calf of the leg is greatly increased when the foot is flexed.

**Treatment and Nursing Care.** Opinions differ about the treatment for thrombophlebitis; some doctors want the leg elevated, with complete rest; others recommend exercises to promote circulation. If exercise is ordered, wriggling the toes, bending the knees, and turning the ankle back and forth are simple exercises that the patient can do himself.

Certain surgical procedures may be carried out to combat the danger of embolism (a loose clot which can travel to other blood vessels and block circulation). If the embolism is located in the femoral vein the blood vessel is ligated at that point (femoral ligation) so the embolism cannot break off. Sometimes the vena cava is made smaller or a net inserted (vena cava ligation) to prevent clots from moving to the heart.

Nursing care is directed at making the patient comfortable and preventing embolism. In caring for a patient with thrombophlebitis, the nurse should follow the set of rules listed below:

1. Prevent the patient from coughing vigorously or breathing deeply because of the danger of embolism.
2. Try to keep the patient from straining when defecating. Stool softeners are usually given for this purpose.
3. If directed by the doctor, apply continuous warm moist heat to the limbs at a low temperature to avoid overdilation of the blood vessels.
4. Check the doctor's orders before elevating the limbs.
5. If the patient is on anticoagulant therapy, follow the general nursing precautions and procedures designed for this type of therapy.
6. If the patient is to wear an elastic stocking or an elastic bandage, these should be applied with even pressure from the toes up to the knee.
7. The patient may have to stay in bed for several weeks. If so, help him progress gradually from complete bedrest to the time he is allowed to walk again.

## Embolism

*Embolism* is an often tragic complication of thrombophlebitis. You will remember that an embolus is a blood clot that may be carried in the circulation to some vital spot, such as the heart (*coronary embolism*) or the lungs (*pulmonary embolism*), and can lodge in a blood vessel. If the obstruction occurs in a large pulmonary blood vessel (the most common site for embolism from the legs), it may cause sudden death. The obstruction of a small vessel may not be so damaging; the patient is liable to complain of chest pain and breathing difficulty and may cough and become cyanotic. The immediate treatment is oxygen and complete rest. The patient may also be given anticoagulants, such as heparin or Dicumarol.

**Embolism and Thrombosis in a Limb.** An embolus may completely obstruct a blood vessel in an arm or a leg and cause thrombosis. The effects are serious, because if it happens in a large blood vessel it shuts off the main blood supply below the obstruction, and the tissues die. The affected area becomes white, cold, and unbearably painful, and the pulse disappears—soon the limb is numb, and the patient is unable to move it. Immediate treatment is imperative or the limb may have to be amputated. The first thing to do after calling for help is to keep the patient warm.

## Varicose Veins

Varicose veins result from a weakening of the walls of the blood vessels, especially in the legs. (Hemorrhoids are also a form of varicose veins, as are esophageal varices.) Actu-

ally, it is caused by a weakening of the valves of the veins so that the blood pools in the legs. Normal veins fill from below because of the valvular action. Varicose veins fill from the top and are not able to drain out the blood. Ten per cent of the population in the 30 to 40 age group have varicose veins, with women more likely to be affected than men. Predisposing factors are heredity, weakening of the vein walls by prolonged standing, poor posture, pregnancy, round garters, obesity, tumors, high blood pressure, and chronic diseases such as those of the liver or kidneys. Varicose veins may also occur as an aftermath of thrombophlebitis.

**Symptoms.** The main symptom is the appearance of dark, torturous superficial veins which become more prominent when the person is standing and show up as dark protrusions in the legs. These superficial veins can sometimes rupture, causing a *varicose ulcer.* Internal or deep varicose veins cause symptoms such as pain, fatigue, a feeling of heaviness, and muscle cramps. The symptoms are much more severe in hot weather and in high altitudes.

A *diagnostic test* involves putting the patient into Trendelenburg's position to test blood drainage. If the legs do not drain normally, this is a sign of varicosities.

**Treatment and Nursing Care.** Treatment includes elevating the legs and avoiding con-

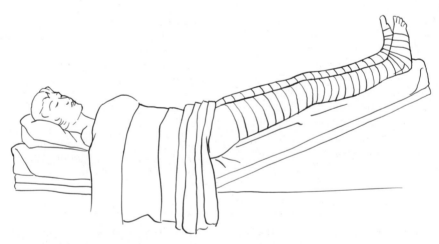

Figure 47-6. Postoperative positioning in surgery for varicose veins. The feet and the legs are elevated to aid venous return. Elastic bandages from the feet to the groin were applied in the operating room. (Smith, D. W., Germain, C. P., and Gips, C. D.: Care of the Adult Patient, ed. 3. Philadelphia, Lippincott, 1971)

striction, excessive standing, and restrictive clothing. The patient should also wear support stockings. Drugs may also be taken to sclerose (harden) the veins.

Most commonly, *surgical ligation* and *stripping* of the veins is done: the larger veins are surgically ligated, or tied off, and the smaller ones are stripped, or reamed out.

POSTOPERATIVE CARE. Elastic bandages are supplied to the leg postoperatively, and the foot of the bed is elevated to encourage the return of venous blood (Fig. 47-6). The patient may experience considerable pain and stiffness in his leg at first, and analgesics may be ordered.

Early ambulation to promote circulation is important after this operation; often the nurse is instructed to get the patient out of bed to walk as soon as he recovers from the anesthesia. The patient may be alarmed by this procedure so soon after his operation while his legs are so stiff and sore, and he will need reassurance and an explanation of the need for moving around.

Usually the patient is allowed to go home in 2 or 3 days, with instructions to elevate the leg while he is sitting, to walk but not to stand still for any length of time, to avoid sitting for long periods, and to avoid wearing anything tight around his legs. If he is obese, he may be put on a reducing diet. Before he leaves the hospital, he learns how to apply the elastic bandage (see Chapter 29).

## Buerger's Disease

*Buerger's disease (thromboangiitis obliterans)* is the result of inflammation which causes obstruction of the veins and the arteries of the extremities, especially in the legs. It is more common among men than women, and heavy smokers especially are affected. It is aggravated by chilling.

Usually the first sign that the patient notices is cramps in the muscles in the calves of his legs. Cramps are brought on by exercise but disappear when the patient rests. Other symptoms include tingling, burning and numbness of the legs, as well as edema, which may develop into *pitting edema*. The patient also develops hardened, painful areas along blood vessels. When the feet and legs hang down they become a mottled purplish red; when they are raised they become abnormally pale. Ulcers may develop which could result in gangrene. As the disease progresses, pain continues even when the patient is resting.

**Treatment.** The patient must be careful to avoid the things that make this condition worse, especially chilling of his hands and feet. Tobacco in any form is forbidden because it constricts the blood vessels. While the disease is not curable, it may be arrested, if the patient stops smoking. The patient may exercise mildly if it is not painful. Tight clothing is avoided. The Buerger-Allen exercises consist of alternately raising, lowering, and resting the legs. The smooth, seesaw motion of the electrically operated oscillating bed, or rocking bed, is beneficial. If heat is used, it must be regulated thermostatically and never be above body temperature. As you would expect, antibiotics and analgesics may be necessary for infection and pain. *Drugs,* such as Priscoline and Dibenzyline, may be given for blood vessel spasm.

Sometimes a *sympathectomy* is performed, whereby the sympathetic nerves, which innervate the smooth muscles, are cut, thus relieving the venospasms. If ulcers become infected, gangrene may develop and make an amputation necessary.

## Raynaud's Disease

*Raynaud's disease* is a condition caused by the spasmodic constriction of the arteries which supply the extremities. It especially affects the fingers and the toes. Often only the fingers are involved. Nobody knows exactly what causes Raynaud's disease, but it seems to be related to exposure to cold and to emotional tensions. It affects more women than men, especially young adults.

**Symptoms.** The symptoms of the disease are distressing. The patient's hands are blanched and cold, perspire, and feel numb and prickly. Later they become blue—especially the fingernails—and are painful. As heat brings the blood back, the hands become red and warm. In the early stages of the disease, these symptoms disappear after an attack, and the hands seem to be normal again. Later, as it grows worse, cyanosis remains between attacks, and ulcers which are slow to heal may develop on the fingertips. The skin looks tight and shiny, and the nails become deformed. The disease may lead to gangrene of the fingertips.

**Treatment.** The most important treatment for Raynaud's disease is to avoid chilling at all times. This means always wearing warm clothing out of doors in the winter, such as wool gloves, socks, and overshoes. An electric blanket at night provides steady warmth. Emotional upsets and tensions of any kind should be avoided. Smoking is definitely contraindicated. Drugs to relieve spasm of the arteries, such as Priscoline, Dibenamine, and papaverine to dilate the blood vessels, provide considerable relief. At times a sympathectomy is performed.

## Smoking and Vascular Disease

Smoking is contraindicated in *all* vascular disease, since nicotine causes spasm of the peripheral arteries. The connection between arteriospasm and smoking is so definite that some doctors feel that it is useless to try to treat the patient unless he *stops smoking!*

# BLOOD AND LYMPH DISORDERS

## Diagnosis of Blood Disorders

The most common practice is, of course, to do various determinations in the hospital laboratory. There, many tests can be done to determine the numbers and types of cells and their condition. The laboratory may also report the presence of abnormal cells or other substances in the blood. (See page 574 for a discussion of blood tests.)

**The Sternal Puncture or Bone Marrow Biopsy.** Also called a bone marrow aspiration, this procedure involves the injection of a large needle into the sternum (breastbone) or the iliac crests in order to withdraw a sample, or biopsy, of the bone marrow. (The *sample* is aspirated, while the *biopsy* is cut or reamed out.) This is done to determine whether or not the bone marrow is functioning normally. (This procedure can also be used for the injection of a drug.) This test is done most often in blood disorders such as leukemia and anemia.

The doctor will need very little assistance other than the equipment needed for the procedure. The patient will, however, need a great deal of support. He needs to have an explanation of what is being done, and he should be forewarned that he will feel a sharp, grinding pain at the moment the needle enters the sternum, as the bone actually gives way to the needle. He may also feel some discomfort as the marrow is aspirated. Since the entire procedure takes only a very few minutes, the patient will be relieved to know this in advance. Nursing care involves support of the patient during the procedure and observation following the procedure. Very few complications occur, but the patient might have some bleeding or an infection at the site of the puncture. He should rest for a few minutes following the procedure.

## Anemia

*Anemia* is a condition in which there is a reduction in the number of red blood cells and/or a deficiency in hemoglobin in the blood. It may be caused by a loss of red blood cells in hemorrhage, by the destruction of red blood cells in certain types of infection, or by interference with the production of red blood cells, such as is caused by injury to the bone marrow. Anemia is also caused by cancer, rheumatoid arthritis, and many other diseases.

**Symptoms.** There are several types of anemia, but the symptoms are essentially the same for all types: pallor, fatigue, faintness, and loss of appetite. Symptoms of congestive heart failure are also common, as are gastrointestinal complaints. Jaundice may occur. The pulse is rapid because the heart is rushing the reduced number of blood cells to the tissues and trying to circulate them faster. The anemic person is likely to feel chilly most of the time.

**The Course of the Disease.** The seriousness of the disease will depend upon such factors as the speed of onset, whether or not it is chronic, and the overall general health and nutritional status of the patient. The more rapidly an anemia develops, the more serious it is likely to be.

There are three main types of anemia: (1) anemia which results from a severe blood loss, such as may occur with an ulcer or in an automobile injury; (2) anemia which results from a failure of the bone marrow to produce red blood cells or in which the red blood cells are unable to carry oxygen; and (3) anemia resulting from the destruction of the red blood cells by the body or by a foreign substance or disorder in the body.

**Diagnosis of Anemia.** The simplest method of diagnosing anemia is determining the hemoglobin content of the blood. If the hemoglobin is below 14 grams for men or 12 grams for women, the person is usually said to be anemic. Anemia most often is a symptom of another disease, rather than a disease in itself.

**Anemia from Blood Loss.** Hemorrhage or continued slow bleeding will cause anemia. If the loss of blood is chronic, as for example from an ulcer, the treatment begins by determining and treating the cause of the bleeding. The usual treatment is to replace the lost blood by transfusions and sometimes to administer iron supplements.

The patient who is hemorrhaging as a result of trauma is more likely to show symptoms than is the person who is bleeding slowly. The patient with a massive hemorrhage will, of course, also show symptoms of *shock*.

**Iron-Deficiency Anemia.** Young people are prone to develop this most common type of anemia—it may begin with dieting or hurrying meals. When anemia actually results, a poor appetite follows. If it is caused by bleeding, the remedy is to stop the bleeding. This deficiency can be remedied easily by taking extra iron and by eating foods which are high in iron. Under certain conditions the body needs more iron, such as during adolescence or pregnancy. Women also need more iron than men because of the blood lost in menstruation.

The nurse who is administering iron should be aware that iron is irritating to the gastrointestinal tract and should be given with milk or meals. Oral iron preparations often have a very unpleasant, metallic taste and are easier to take with food. The nurse should also explain to the patient that iron will make his stools black, so that he will not become alarmed.

**Pernicious Anemia.** The patient with *pernicious anemia* lacks a substance in the gastric juice, the *intrinsic factor*, which is necessary to enable the body to absorb vitamin $B_{12}$ from food. Diet cannot help this patient; he must have vitamin $B_{12}$ supplied to him because he cannot use it as it comes in food, probably because of a defect in the synthesis of DNA. A

pernicious anemia patient has to take vitamin $B_{12}$ (cyanocobalamine) the rest of his life, but an injection every 2 or 3 weeks enables him to live normally. Vitamin $B_{12}$ is a water-soluble vitamin and may be given either orally or intramuscularly. Initially, it is given intramuscularly, followed by oral maintenance doses. The symptoms of pernicious anemia include digestive disturbances, sore mouth, diarrhea, and numbness and tingling in the extremities which are signs of nerve damage. The patient is often irritable or depressed.

**Sickle Cell Anemia.** *Sickle cell anemia* is a disease in which the red blood cells are destroyed more rapidly than usual and in which an abnormal type of hemoglobin is present. This is a hereditary condition which is found chiefly among Negroes. The symptoms are similar to those of other types of anemia and may also include leg ulcer, fever, and pain. Transfusions can be given, and although the patient seems to improve for a time, sickle cell anemia shortens life expectancy.

**Aplastic Anemia.** *Aplastic anemia* is caused by a disruption in the bone marrow's ability to produce red blood cells, white blood cells, and blood platelets. It appears at times as a toxic side-effect of such drugs as streptomycin and nitrogen mustard. Nobody knows exactly what causes aplastic anemia because sometimes it appears without an apparent cause. A patient becomes very weak and tired and short of breath on the least exertion; he has a tendency to bleed and is extremely susceptible to infection. Extra precautions, such as the administration of antibiotics, are taken to protect the patient from infection. The patient will also receive many transfusions. If the bone marrow is so damaged that it is unable to produce the needed blood cells, the patient will die. Specimens of the bone marrow are examined to determine its activity. Aplastic anemia is a very serious condition, and obviously any patient with it is extremely ill.

## Agranulocytosis

In *agranulocytosis*, malignant neutropenia, the production of white blood cells is decreased, causing leukopenia. One cause of this condition is the toxic effects of drugs, especially barbiturates, tranquilizers, and sulfonamides. The signs of this disease are chills and fever, headache, and ulcers on the mucous membranes in the mouth, the nose, the throat, the rectum or the vagina. It is frequently the result of self-medication with "sleeping pills," taken for a long time without advice from a doctor. The treatment begins by removing the drug that is causing the trouble. Since the patient's white cells are low, he is more than normally susceptible to infection, and extreme care is taken to protect him from exposure.

## Leukemia

*Leukemia* is a fatal disease in which the white blood cells (leukocytes) increase in an abnormal abundance. We usually think of an increase in white blood cells as a sign that the body is fighting disease, but this is not true in leukemia. The increase is so abnormal that it reduces the number of other cells in the blood, including blood platelets, and erythrocytes, which are essential if bleeding and anemia are to be prevented.

According to the American Cancer Society, leukemia is "cancer of the organs which manufacture blood"—the lymphatic system and bone marrow.

Statistics show that every year 1 in every 14,000 Americans dies of leukemia. It affects both children and adults. Next to accidents, leukemia is the second most frequent cause of death among school-age children. And next to lung cancer, leukemia is the most rapidly increasing lethal disease. Some authorities think that leukemia may be caused by infection, but there is a growing belief today that the cause of leukemia is linked in some way to cancer. Leukemia is sometimes called cancer of the blood or blood-forming organs (the bone marrow, lymph nodes and the spleen). It is the most common form of childhood cancer. Scientists hope that their attempts to identify a virus as the cause of cancer will help in the fight against laukemia, because many believe that this virus, or a similar one, may also cause leukemia. However, we still lack definite proof that this theory is correct even though a leukemia-type virus was grown in a laboratory in 1971. So far, no cure for leukemia has been found—only ways of delaying death.

The increase in the number of cases of leukemia is attributed to several factors: it may be that because people live longer there is a greater chance for the disease to develop. Also, it has been discovered that people whose work exposes them to considerable radiation run a greater risk of developing leukemia.

Leukemia is more common in whites, Jewish people, and men. It seems to reach its peak in winter and early spring.

**The Course of Leukemia.** Leukemia may be acute or chronic and may occur at any age. *Acute leukemia (acute lymphatic leukemia)* is more common in people under 25 years of age; after the age of 40, *chronic leukemia—chronic myelogenous (marrow) leukemia—*is more common. A form of chronic lymphatic leukemia also exists. With treatment, people with acute leukemia may live for a year or longer. Chronic leukemia victims may live for 2 or 3 years after the disease begins or, as sometimes happens, it may be 8 or 10 years before death finally occurs. It is believed that drugs and x-rays double the life span of a child who has the disease. The life span for the average child with leukemia is now about 8 to 10 months, or more. Advances in treatment not only prolong life but also make the victim happier and more comfortable. With longer time to live, the patient can always hope that ways will be found to prevent and cure this now fatal disease.

### Acute Leukemia.

SYMPTOMS. Acute leukemia symptoms appear suddenly, often with an acute respiratory infection. Unless the patient is admitted to a hospital for treatment where a blood count will be part of the admission routine, the unusual increase in the white blood cells may not be detected. The blood count will also show that not only are the white blood cells numerous, but many of them are not fully developed.

Sometimes the symptoms disappear temporarily, perhaps for several months, but usually they grow steadily worse.

MEDICAL TREATMENT. Treatment, aimed at relieving the symptoms, consists of:

*Blood transfusions* to give the patient more red blood cells, hemoglobin, and platelets.
*Drugs:* Aminopterin and A-Methopterin are given to slow down the rapid production of leukocytes. These drugs must be used cautiously because they can interfere with the production of

all blood cells and have toxic side-effects, such as nausea and vomiting and diarrhea. Frequent blood counts are made when the patient is having one of these drugs. Antibiotics are given for secondary infections. Other drugs, such as nitrogen mustard, are being used with some success. Folic acid is also effective in poisoning leukemia cells because they take up the folic acid (a B vitamin) faster than do normal cells. Many other drugs are used as palliative measures. These include cortisone, busulfan (Myleran), and new drugs such as vincristine. The drug therapy must be balanced so that it does the most damage to the disease and the least damage to the patient.

*Radiation:* The problem here is trying to destroy the leukemia cells while preserving the developing normal cells. One method, which has had limited success involves transplanting bone marrow. Bone marrow is withdrawn from the patient prior to radiation or from another person who is donating the bone marrow. This marrow is then transplanted into the leukemic person. It must be remembered, that radiation is also believed to be a cause of leukemia. There is a very delicate balance betwen using radiation to cure and using too much radiation.

THE PROGNOSIS. In spite of treatment, the time comes when nothing seems to help the patient, and he grows steadily worse—his life then is a matter of only a few weeks.

## Chronic Leukemia.

SYMPTOMS. Often the first signs of chronic leukemia are swollen lymph nodes in the neck, the axilla, or the groin or a swelling in the upper left side of the abdomen which makes the victim's abdomen feel heavy. This swelling is caused by the enlargement of the spleen. The patient has all the symptoms of anemia plus difficulty in breathing if the spleen is enlarged. Treatment will help this patient to live perhaps 5 years or longer. Eventually, he becomes very weak, bleeds easily, and has fever. He is susceptible to secondary infections, such as pneumonia, and treatment no longer helps him.

TREATMENT. As in acute leukemia, the treatment includes transfusions and antibiotics. In addition it includes:

*X-ray therapy* and *drugs,* such as 6-mercaptopurine, to slow down the production of leukocytes, and chlorambucil, a derivative of nitrogen mustard which is poisonous to all growing cells and must be used cautiously. Busulfan, a similar drug, depresses the bone marrow and it, too, is used with caution lest it cause anemia. Radioactive phosphorus is also used. The general purpose in prescribing these drugs is to slow down the processes that cause the disease and those that aid its development.

## Nursing Care in Leukemia.

*Fatigue:* Since the patient with leukemia is often exhausted, the nurse should plan nursing care so as to conserve the patient's strength and to provide rest periods. For added strength the patient should eat a high protein diet.

*Bleeding Tendency:* During a bleeding episode, the patient should be put at rest and gentle pressure applied to the bleeding site. Cold compresses should be applied where indicated. When injections are given, very small gauge needles should be used.

*Mouth Care:* To avoid discomfort and injury, avoid irritating foods or beverages, use a soft toothbrush, and keep the lips moist with oil. Give frequent oral hygiene, especially before and after meals.

*Pain:* Pain occurs most frequently in the bones and joints. For relief, the patient should have a bed cradle to prevent the bed linens from exerting pressure on the extremities.

*Fever:* To combat any fever which may occur, antipyretic drugs are given in combination with cool sponges. In addition, the patient's room is kept cool.

*Pruritis:* If pruritis occurs in combination with petechiae, keep the patient's fingernails short to prevent self-injury from scratching. Use lotion to keep the skin as moist as possible. (Use soap sparingly.) Good skin and back care are vital.

Improvement in the patient with leukemia after treatment is often spectacular. In 2 weeks he may be ready to leave the hospital. It is hard to believe that he is the same person who required almost constant attention and alert observation.

Above all, this patient needs an *understanding* nurse, a nurse who, although she knows his improvement can be only temporary, will rejoice with him in his transient recovery and encourage him. It is generally agreed that the leukemia patient should be encouraged to return to his normal life insofar as this is possible. Activity will not harm him, and complete rest will not halt the progress of the disease. A determination to live is all-important, for there is always the possibility that a cure may be found. If he is a young person, he may have important decisions to make, such as getting married or planning his career. The circumstances in every individual case will determine whether or not he should know that he has a fatal disease. He will make regular visits to his doctor and no doubt will return to the hospital many times for treatment which brings temporary improvement, although each time it is of a shorter duration.

The leukemia patient's final illness is a very difficult time for his family, who must stand helplessly by as he grows steadily worse and finally slips into unconsciousness. The death of a child or a young person is especially difficult to accept. To the family, life means hope, and they need the reassurance that everyone is doing everything that can possibly be done in the way of treatment and comfort.

## Hodgkin's Disease (A *Lymphoma*)

The cause of *Hodgkin's disease* is not known—it may be due to infection or to a malignant tumor in lymphatic tissue. Whatever the cause, it begins with a painless enlargement of the lymph nodes in the neck (cervical) and in the groin (inguinal). It affects more men than women, usually young adults, and is almost always fatal. People with Hodgkin's disease may live 10 years or more. It is diagnosed by examining tissue from an affected lymph node under the microscope.

**Symptoms.** The disease begins with the enlargement of one or more lymph nodes. This is painless at first, but as the nodes become larger they may press on the surrounding tissues and cause pain. The patient loses a great amount of weight, has a poor appetite, and feels weak and tired. Often he has chills and fever and complains of itching. He may develop anemia and a tendency to bleed. Treatment seems to help for a time—sometimes months or even years and, perhaps, permanently.

The specific diagnosis of Hodgkin's disease is based upon the identification through a bone marrow biopsy of a gigantic, malformed cell, called the "Sternberg-Reed cell."

**Treatment and Nursing Care.** The patient may be treated by x-ray therapy, and *nitrogen mustard* may be used intravenously. *Chlorambucil* may be prescribed and antibi-

otics given for infection. The nursing care is similar to the care for leukemia.

**Radiation and Hodgkin's Disease.** Recently, massive doses of x-ray have proven effective in arresting and possibly stopping the disease process. This is based upon the fact that until the final stages of the disease Hodgkin's disease usually confines itself to the lymphatic system which can tolerate larger doses of radiation than the rest of the body. Therefore, it is believed that this disease can be cured by radiation, if discovered in the early stages.

### Stages of the Disease.

*Stage I:* The disease is limited to a single node and surrounding structures. (Radiation has been most effective at this stage.)

*Stage II:* The disease involves more than a single node, but is confined to one side of the diaphragm.

*Stage III:* The disease is present both above and below the diaphragm, but does not extend beyond lymph node chains, spleen, or the mouth, nose, and throat areas.

*Stage IV:* The disease has extended to the bone marrow, lung, skin, and/or other areas of the body.

## Bleeding Disorders

There are 2 chief types of bleeding disorders: the platelet-deficiency disorders and the clotting defects. Thrombocytopenic purpura is an example of a platelet-deficiency disorder, and hemophilia is an example of a clotting defect.

**Purpura.** *Purpura* (thrombocytopenic purpura) is the term used to describe small hemorrhages in the skin, the mucous membranes, or the tissues under the skin. Sometimes they appear as tiny red spots (*petechiae*), or they may extend over larger areas. These hemorrhages are caused by lack of platelets in the blood or by damage to the blood vessels. They are signs that the patient has a tendency to bleed, and he may bleed from the nose, the mouth, or the intestinal tract. The treatment may include administration of ACTH and cortisone, transfusions of *whole* blood, or removal of the spleen. Some patients recover without treatment.

In the nursing care of a patient with purpura it is important to watch for signs of internal bleeding, such as unusual pallor, rapid pulse, and restlessness. Care includes protecting the patient from bruises that might be caused by falls or bumping into objects.

**Hemophilia.** *Hemophilia* is an inherited condition in which the blood is slow to coagulate, due to the lack of prothrombin in the blood plasma, a substance that makes blood clot. Unchecked bleeding may be severe; in hemophiliacs, even a pinprick may cause prolonged oozing of blood. The most minor surgical procedure is often risky and is usually preceded by a transfusion. Prothrombin and pressure on the bleeding can be applied, and antihemolytic human plasma can be administered as a temporary measure to curb the bleeding. Hemophilia can shorten life, and many children with this disease die young. Women are not susceptible to this condition, although a mother may inherit the trait and pass it on to a son who then develops hemophilia. The trait is not passed on by the father. (See Chapter 40 for further discussion.)

## Surgical Treatment of Blood Disorders

Certain surgical measures, such as bone marrow transplant and bone marrow aspiration, have been mentioned as part of the treatment for blood disorders.

Another procedure is *splenectomy* (removal of the spleen), which is sometimes done as a palliative or therapeutic measure. Since the spleen is involved in blood formation, as well as the destruction of old red blood cells and the storage of red blood cells, and also exerts an influence upon antibody formation in ininfection and on bone marrow, its removal may sometimes slow down the disease process. This is especially true if the spleen has been hyperactive. In some types of disease, such as Hodgkin's disease and hemolytic disease, removal of a hyperactive spleen may slow down the progression of the disease. In other conditions, when a hyperactive spleen is the actual cause of the disease, its removal will cure the disease.

# 48

# The Patient With a Respiratory Disorder

---

## BEHAVIORAL OBJECTIVES

*The student successfully attaining the goals of this chapter will be able to:*

- *identify and define at least 9 aspects of respiration which are observed in all patients, utilizing descriptive and accurate medical terminology; and demonstrate the ability to accurately observe and report these.*
- *identify and describe at least 5 laboratory tests, 2 x-ray or direct visualizations, and 1 skin test used to determine respiratory status.*
- *describe at least 6 nursing procedures used in care of patients with disorders of the respiratory system; demonstrate competence in performance of these procedures; and demonstrate ability to assist with more complex procedures, such as thoracentesis.*
- *diagram the principle of closed chest suction; describe the precautions involved; identify the situations in which suction might be used; and demonstrate ability to care for a patient with chest suction.*
- *identify 4 common disorders of the nose; describe the symptoms and medical treatment of each, keeping in mind the normal structure studied in Chapter 16; and demonstrate competence in assisting a patient with a nasal disorder, either in the hospital or in an emergency situation.*
- *review the procedures for emergency pulmonary resuscitation and demonstrate competence in the use of the Ambu bag or mouth-to-mouth breathing.*
- *identify and define 2 disorders of the throat; discuss the related medical and nursing care; and demonstrate competence in assisting patients with these disorders.*
- *name and describe at least 4 chronic respiratory conditions and the medical treatment of each; and demonstrate ability to carry out appropriate nursing measures.*
- *identify and describe at least 7 infectious respiratory conditions, including pneumonia and TB; describe the deviation from normal structure and/or function in each and the major aspects of medical treatment and nursing care; and demonstrate competence in assisting the patient to meet his needs, with rehabilitation being the major goal of all care.*
- *discuss cancer of the lung, its predisposing factors and common medical treatment; and demonstrate ability to assist a patient with lung cancer to meet his needs.*
- *demonstrate ability to assist a patient who has surgery of the lung.*
- *describe the emergency measures which must be taken in the event of a traumatic injury to the chest.*

---

## FUNCTION OF THE ORGANS OF RESPIRATION

The role of the respiratory system is the *exchange of gasses*; that is, the delivery of oxygen to the cells and the removal of carbon dioxide from the cells. If body cells are deprived of oxygen, they quickly die, so the respiratory system is vital to the functioning of the rest of the body. The respiratory system, together with the cardiovascular system, must be functioning in order for life to continue.

The respiratory tract begins in the nose, passes through the pharynx (the throat), the larynx, the trachea, and into the lungs. Breathing may take place through the mouth, as well as the nose. The lungs are the place where the actual exchange of gasses occurs, through the alveoli, via the process of osmosis.

The breathing mechanism is dependent upon a negative pressure within the chest cavity. The diaphragm moves downward, creating a vacuum (or negative pressure) within the chest cavity. This causes air to rush into the lungs from outside the body and is called *inspiration*. When the diaphragm moves up, it forces the air out of the lungs and is called *expiration*.

## COMMON RESPIRATORY SYMPTOMS

**Cough.** A cough is the contraction of the muscles in the pharynx as a result of irritation. If material is expectorated after the cough, we say that the cough is *productive*. A cough may be loose or dry, it may be occasional, or it may come in spasms that are frequent or prolonged. Note the color of the patient's face when he coughs—a bluish tinge indicates an obstruction in the air passages.

**Expectoration.** This is another term related to coughing; it refers to the material which is coughed out.

**Hemoptysis.** This term refers to blood in the sputum. It should always be considered a serious symptom and should be reported.

**Dysphagia.** Dysphagia means difficulty in swallowing.

**Sputum.** Sputum is material expectorated from the mouth. It may be coughed up from the bronchi or the lungs or may be a discharge from infection of the nasal or the throat cavities. Discharge from infected sinuses also drains into the throat at the back of the nose. The amount expectorated varies and should be noted; usually this is estimated as "small," "medium," or "large." It can be estimated more accurately by filling an identical container with water to the same level as the sputum, then measuring the water. Sputum is characteristic of such conditions as tuberculosis, pneumonia, and lung injuries.

CONSISTENCY AND COLOR. Sputum may be thin, watery, thick, or purulent. Expectorated mucus is colorless. Sputum is yellow when pus is present, or it may be gray or black. In pneumonia, sputum has a rusty color and is thick and tenacious; it may also be streaked with bright red blood. In lung abscess and cancer of the lungs, the sputum may be green. Sometimes sputum has no odor. In other instances, it may have an unpleasant odor—in lung abscess the odor is very noticeable. Precautions should be taken in the care of sputum in infectious conditions.

**Dyspnea.** *Dyspnea* refers to difficult breathing and was discussed more completely in Chapter 31. Dyspnea is defined in terms of what causes it (cardiac dyspnea), or how it occurs (paroxysmal dyspnea—occurring sometimes, but not always). *Orthopnea* refers to difficult breathing when lying down.

**Uneven Chest Movements.** If one side of the chest moves when the patient breathes, and the other side does not, this is a sign of malfunction of one lung, either of pneumothorax or a blocked bronchus on the unmoving side.

**Breathing Sounds.** The doctor, by listening to the chest with a stethoscope, can hear if the breathing sounds are normal or not. A commonly used term to describe abnormal respiratory sound is *rale*. A *clicking rale* is a sticky sound, heard in early tuberculosis of the lung; a *dry rale* is a whistling or squeaky sound, heard in asthma and bronchitis; and a *moist rale* is a sound produced by fluid in the bronchi. In examination, the doctor will often ask the patient to take a deep breath and hold it, or let it out fast, while he listens.

**Hyperventilation.** Hyperventilation refers to a condition in which the patient breathes abnormally fast or deeply. This can cause an accumulation of oxygen in the body, which may require treatment. The usual cause is anxiety or overexcitement. This condition may also be referred to as *hysterical hyperpnea*. The patient may have muscle spasms, dizziness, or faintness.

In cases of hysterical hyperventilation, the patient may be given a carbon dioxide mixture to reduce the oxygen content of the blood to normal. A first-aid treatment for this condition is to have the patient breathe in and out of a paper bag, so that he receives a higher concentration of carbon dioxide than is normally found in room air.

**Spontaneous Pneumothorax.** Occasionally, a person's lung will collapse (atelectasis) as a result of air entering the pleural cavity or accumulating between the pleura and the chest wall. The patient generally experiences a sudden, sharp pain in the chest, accompanied by dyspnea and cyanosis. He may sit up in bed and be anxious. The chest does not move on the affected side and moves more than usual on the unaffected side.

## DIAGNOSIS OF RESPIRATORY DISORDERS

### Laboratory Tests

**Sputum Specimen.** Tests are run on a sputum specimen to determine if any organisms or blood are present in the sputum. The nurse should collect the specimen early in the morning, because it most likely will contain true sputum, rather than just saliva. Explain the procedure to the patient and ask him first to rinse out his mouth with clear water to remove any food particles and then to cough deeply. Since the container used to collect the sputum will be clean (not sterile), tell him to be careful not to soil the outside of the container. (Wipe his lips with tissues.) The nurse should note the amount, consistency, and color of the sputum collected.

*Caution:* The nurse must use careful handwashing technics when collecting a sputum specimen, since the test is often done in a case suspected of infection.

**Sputum Culture.** The same procedure is used for collecting a sputum culture as is used to collect a sputum specimen, except that the container is sterile and the culture must be sent to the laboratory immediately. It will take about 2 days for the results to be returned.

**Throat Culture.** A sample of the mucus and secretions from the back of the throat are obtained on a wooden stick and applied to a slide or culture media. These are then incubated in the laboratory to determine what organism is causing the throat disorder in question. *Drug sensitivity* determinations may also be done to determine which drug will kill the organism most effectively. This method should be used in all sore throats, since many organisms cause the same symptoms, but are not all effectively killed by the same drug.

**Gastric Washing for Culture.** The purpose of this procedure is to obtain and culture sputum which the patient has swallowed. The stomach contents are removed, via nasogastric tube, and are cultured. The procedure, which is usually done 3 days in a row is most frequently carried out in cases of suspected tuberculosis. While the doctor is usually responsible for carrying out this procedure, the nurse will often assist.

**Blood Gas Determinations.** The laboratory can analyze a sample of blood and determine the relative amounts of oxygen and carbon dioxide in the blood, as well as the pH (hydrogen ion concentration) of the blood.

**Pulmonary Function Tests.** The pulmonary function test (or Tidal Volume Determination) measures the amount of air taken in (inspiration) and out (expiration) in one breath and determines the patient's general respiratory status. Many large hospitals have pulmonary function laboratories in which these tests are done. Various measurements can be taken, such as the tidal volume, the inspiratory volume, the expiratory volume, the residual volume, the total lung capacity, and the vital capacity. The ratios between specific measurements can then be determined. The machines used for these tests are called the spirometer or the vitalograph.

The pulmonary function test is used both to diagnose and to determine the result of therapy on the respiratory patient. The test helps the doctor determine pulmonary pathology at an early stage and indicates whether the patient is suffering from cardiac or respiratory disease. The test can evaluate the effectiveness of such therapy as IPPB (intermittent positive pressure breathing), bronchodilator drugs, antibiotics, and respirators and can indicate the surgical risk involved with many patients, since respiratory function is so vital to life and is often involved in postoperative complications.

## X-Ray and Fluoroscopy Examinations

**Chest X-Ray.** An x-ray is usually taken for every patient admitted to the hospital and will reveal lung cancer or tuberculosis of the lung, as well as heart abnormalities.

**Planograms.** Planograms are x-rays taken from different angles and of different planes or sections of the body.

**Bronchoscopy and Bronchogram.** This examination involves a surgical procedure which is done after the throat is anesthetized. Sometimes it is done under general anesthesia. The bronchoscope is passed through the mouth and pharynx into the trachea and bronchi. The purpose may vary from visually observing the tissue to taking a biopsy, removing mucous plugs or foreign objects, or obtaining a specimen of secretions. The bronchogram may be done at the time of the bronchoscopy. A radiopaque oil is injected into the trachea and bronchi and the patient is tilted into various positions so that x-rays can be taken.

*Postoperative care* after the procedure includes preventing the patient from taking anything by mouth until gag reflex returns, keeping the patient on his side to facilitate drainage, and watching for swelling of the throat or difficulty in breathing.

**Esophagoscopy.** This is a procedure similar to a bronchoscopy and is used for viewing the esophagus.

## Skin Tests

**Mantoux Test.** A skin test called the Mantoux test is given to determine if the patient has ever been exposed to the tubercle bacillus. About 0.1 cc. of the serum is injected intradermally forming a wheal. Two days later the injection site is examined for edema. The finding of a positive Mantoux test does not necessarily mean that the person has tuberculosis; it simply means that he has been exposed to the bacillus.

If a person has a positive reaction to the Mantoux test, he should have a chest x-ray to determine if the lungs are affected. Once the Mantoux test is positive, it almost always remains so for life.

**Tine Test.** Another method of tuberculin testing is the tine test (also called the Health Test), which is simply a different method of injecting the tubercle bacillus in a very small amount.

The substances used for injection are PPD (purified protein derivative) and OT (old tuberculin).

**Histoplasmosis Test.** A skin test, as well as blood tests, may be done to determine the presence of the histoplasmosis fungus.

# COMMON NURSING PROCEDURES IN RESPIRATORY DISORDERS

## Oxygen Therapy

Many patients with disorders of the respiratory system need to receive extra oxygen to sustain life or to make them more comfortable. Since this was discussed in Chapter 31 it might be wise to review that chapter in preparation for caring for the patient with a respiratory problem.

The methods of administering oxygen vary with the patient and with the severity of his oxygen needs. The nurse must be able to recognize the signs of oxygen want and report these so that the patient may receive assistance, if possible. In some instances, the initial, and perhaps only, procedure will be to assist the patient in clearing his airway so that he can obtain the oxygen needed for life. Several of these procedures will be described in the following pages.

## Relieving Breathing Difficulties

**Postural Drainage.** Postural drainage employs gravity to assist the patient in coughing up secretions and mucus from his lungs. The patient adopts a head-downward position (see

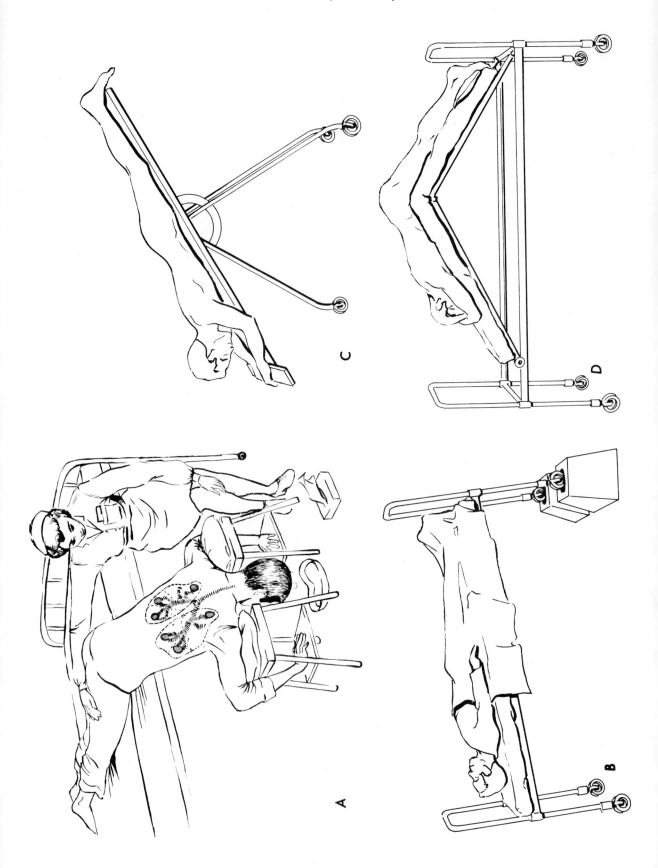

Fig. 48-1) and allows the secretions to run far enough into the trachea from the bronchi, so that he can cough them out. The exact position of the patient depends upon the portion of the lung to be drained. The nurse may assist by striking the patient between the shoulder blades with cupped hands or by "vibrating" the patient, to help loosen the secretions.

Often, this procedure is done in combination with IPPB (intermittent positive pressure breathing) treatments, in order to make the IPPB even more effective in loosening and bringing up secretions from the lungs and in preventing respiratory complications.

It is possible for the patient to gag or choke while coughing up mucous plugs, so it is advisable to do this procedure before the patient eats, to prevent vomiting or aspiration. The nurse must remember to offer the patient good oral hygiene after postural drainage.

**Positioning to Assist Breathing.** Many patients will not be able to breathe unless they are in a sitting or semisitting position (*orthopneic position*). The nurse should position this patent with pillows so that he is supported. Sometimes, it helps if the patient leans on the overbed table while in this position, since he may have to sleep sitting up.

**Turning, Coughing, and Hyperventilation.** The importance of turning, coughing, and deep-breathing was stressed in Chapter 32. This procedure is vital for any patient who is bedridden for a long time. Lung complications will occur in anyone who is immobile and will occur more quickly in the person who has an underlying respiratory problem. To prevent such complications, it is vital to see that the patient continually ventilates his lungs and expands his lungs as much as possible.

**Breathing Exercises.** Often, the doctor will order breathing exercises to help the patient build up his respiratory capacity. Blowing bubbles into water is commonly done for this purpose. As a first step, the patient is given a cup of water and a straw and is asked to blow bubbles through the straw. When he can do this without difficulty, he graduates to a regular *blow bottle,* which is a large bottle with a 2-holed stopper. Into one hole is placed a long glass tube which extends below the level of the water and is attached on top to a rubber tubing. The other hole serves as an outlet for the air. The patient is instructed to blow bubbles in the water for about 15 to 20 minutes, several times a day. The deeper the tube is inserted into the water, the more exercise the patient will receive, because of increased resistance.

The patient may also be instructed to blow out a candle at various distances or to do other exercises which will increase his respiratory capacity and function. He may be taught the technic of *abdominal breathing,* which involves moving the abdominal wall up when breathing to cause inspiration. The chest should not move at all, thus resting the chest muscles.

**Throat Irrigations and Gargles.** In order to encourage coughing and loosen secretions, the doctor may order the patient to gargle several times a day. Mouthwash or warm saline may be used.

**IPPB Therapy.** (Intermittent Positive Pressure Breathing.) This procedure is commonly used in patients with respiratory disorders, as well as in most postoperative patients (see Chapter 32). A respirator, set to trip at a certain pressure (generally about 15 to 20 cm. $H_2O$) is used to deliver a bronchodilator drug or saline to the patient to loosen secretions, increase ventilation, and reduce bronchospasms. Since the oxygen and the nebulized solution are forced into the lungs, the patient is forced to thoroughly expand his lungs. The patient is instructed to breathe as deeply as possible, using his diaphragm instead of

Figure 48-1. Positioning for postural drainage. (A) This position for postural drainage is good for the lowest lobes, fairly good for the middle lobe, but inadequate for the upper lobes. (B) This head-low position is good for drainage from the lower halves of each lung; (C) A tilt table can be used for draining the lower halves of each lung and is particularly useful in draining posterior lesions. (D) When the patient's bed can be adjusted to provide this position, it is comfortable; however, it is effective in draining the lower lung only and inadequate for the upper lobes (Brunner, L. S. et al.: Textbook of Medical-Surgical Nursing. Philadelphia, Lippincott, 1970)

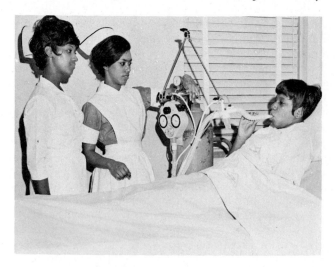

Figure 48-2. The instructor and student are assisting the patient, who has chronic obstructive lung disease, with an IPPB treatment. During the treatment the nurse encourages the patient to breathe slowly and evenly to facilitate maximum ventilation of the lungs. (Freedmen's Hospital School of Nursing) (From Brunner, L. S., et al.: Textbook of Medical-Surgical Nursing, ed. 2. Philadelphia, Lippincott, 1970)

his chest muscles. He then holds his breath as long as possible and expels it with some force. Sometimes, the patient is instructed to breathe slowly, deeply, and evenly throughout the treatment. This treatment generally takes 15 to 20 minutes and is stopped when the prescribed amount of medication is gone. The nurse must be aware that bronchodilators may speed up the heart and lead to complaints of dizziness, palpitation, or nausea.

**Thoracentesis.** This procedure involves puncturing the chest wall in order to remove excess fluid from the pleural cavity. It is done for diagnostic purposes or to relieve breathing difficulties in patients with tuberculosis, cancer of the lung, ascites, pulmonary edema, and chest injuries.

The doctor, using sterile technic, inserts a *trocar* (large needle with obdurator) into the pleural cavity and withdraws fluid. As the needle is withdrawn, the nurse should have a sterile container at hand to collect the specimen, and a graduate to measure the amount of fluid withdrawn. The specimen is then sent to the laboratory for analysis. The nurse must remember that the fluid is considered to be contaminated and should take the appropriate measures.

Throughout the procedure, the nurse will assist the patient and offer support. The patient will be most comfortable if he is in a sitting position and leans on the overbed table. The physician will need very little assistance but the patient will need a great deal of emotional support. Generally, after the procedure the patient is able to breathe better since the pressure of the fluid, which often causes respiratory distress, has been relieved. Rarely, infection or fluid leakage may occur at the puncture site. The nurse must be watchful for these complications, as well as for any complaints of pain, which can usually be relieved by an analgesic. Another possible but rare complication is pneumothorax.

**Paracentesis.** Paracentesis, although actually referring to the puncture of any body cavity for the purpose of aspirating fluid, usually refers to the puncture of the abdominal cavity. Removing fluid from the abdomen can relieve breathing difficulties because abdominal distention can immobilize the diaphragm and interfere with breathing.

**Oral-Nasal Suctioning.** Many patients with respiratory problems must be suctioned to remove excess secretions and mucus from the airway. This helps them to breathe easier and prevents aspiration and possible hypostatic pneumonia. The unconscious patient or the patient with an inactive cough reflex is the most likely candidate for this procedure.

The suctioning is accomplished by introducing a catheter into the trachea, either through the nose or through the mouth. It is usually done through the nose, although the catheter can be irritating to the mucous membranes and may cause nosebleeds. If the mouth is used, it is often necessary to hold the tongue with a 4 x 4 gauze pad. The catheter will stimulate the weak cough reflex, so that the secretions can be suctioned out.

However, the suction should not be applied while the catheter is being introduced. Once the catheter is in place, intermittent periods of suctioning can begin, about 10 seconds being the maximum time for suctioning without a rest. The catheter is slowly withdrawn in a rotating motion while the suctioning continues. Suctioning should continue until the mucus is gone, with the patient given time to rest and catch his breath between suctionings. While the patient rests for a few seconds, the catheter can be left in place with the suction off.

A solution to liquefy secretions, such as sterile saline, may be injected and then suctioned out, but great caution must be used to prevent aspiration.

## Chest Suction

**Closed Water-Seal Drainage.** After chest surgery, the lungs must be reinflated and kept inflated. As previously mentioned, the breathing mechanism operates on the principle of *negative pressure*; that is, the pressure in the chest cavity is lower than the pressure of the outside air which causes the air to rush into the lungs. Thus, a vacuum must be applied to the chest, after it has been opened, in order to re-establish negative pressure. In addition, secretions and blood which might have accumulated in the chest cavity must be removed. The most common method of re-establishing negative pressure is through the system of closed water-seal drainage. In this procedure, one or more catheters are inserted into the chest cavity. If more than one catheter is inserted, each catheter may be connected to separate suction setups, or they may all be joined together and attached to one suction setup.

The term "closed" means that no air is allowed to enter the chest cavity, or the lungs will collapse. By putting the drainage tubes under water, air is prevented from backing up into the chest.

### Precautions.

*Preventing air leakage:* Never disconnect the chest tubes! These provide the suction which keeps the lungs inflated. If they are disconnected the lungs will collapse. Clamps or hemostats should be kept with the patient, either clipped to the bedding or the patient's gown, in case the tubes are accidently disconnected. Should this happen, clamp the tubes and summon assistance immediately. If you plan to measure the drainage, the tubes must be securely double-clamped. Do not do this procedure without assistance, until you are sure you understand the principles and procedures involved.

To further safeguard against air leakage, never use pins to fasten the tubes to the bed (you may use tape) and never change a chest dressing (you may reinforce it). Never take the plugs out of the bottles without assistance and never pull on the chest tubes. Finally, tape all connections to make sure they are airtight.

*Keeping the tubes open:* The tubes must be kept patent (open). This is done by "milking or stripping" the tubes with special chest-tube rollers, called chest-tube strippers, which fit on either side of the tubing and can be rolled down the tubing, away from the patient, milking the drainage and clots down into the drainage bottle. Be sure to hold the tube in place, so you do not pull on the tube while you are milking or stripping it. (This procedure is frequently ordered on the new postoperative patient.)

If the tube becomes kinked, it will not drain properly. If this happens, report it immediately. To prevent kinking, the tube may be taped to a tongue blade at the point where it enters the drainage bottle. The tubing should be so arranged that the patient has enough room to move in bed and the tube hangs straight down from the edge of the bed to the drainage bottle. This can be done by wrapping a piece of tape around the tube and then pinning the edge of the tape to the edge of the bed, allowing the tube to hang straight down into the bottle. The rest of the tubing is in the bed with the patient so he can move. However, be sure the patient does not lie on the tubing.

*The water level:* In simple water-seal drainage, the level of the water should go up and down as the patient breathes. If the water in the water-seal bottle does not go up and down, this could indicate that all air and drainage has been evacuated from the pleural cavity or that the drainage is malfunctioning.

*Caring for the bottles:* The bottles must remain lower than the level of the patient at all times. If the bottes are higher than the patient there is danger of aspiration or backflow of fluid. If the bottles are sitting on the floor, they must be fastened to the floor so they will not tip or break. Usually, a stand is provided for the bottles to assure their safety. Sometimes they hang in a rack which is provided for this purpose and is attached to the bed. Remember that if a bottle breaks, the closed system will be disrupted. This is an emergency situation! Clamp the chest tubes immediately and summon help.

*Observing and reporting:* The nurse is responsible for accurate observation and reporting. The amount, color, and consistency of the drainage is vital information. It is most important to the doctor if a drastic change takes place. Be sure to observe for excessive bleeding or for sudden absence of drainage.

The nurse should put a piece of tape on the drainage bottle and record the level of the drainage at intervals so that she can note the amount in any period of time.

*Turning the patient:* The patient should be turned often to facilitate drainage and to prevent hypostatic pneumonia and other complications. Remember, that the wound will drain the most when the patient is lying on his affected side, so he should be turned to that side often. Be sure that he does not lie on the tube when he is in that position.

*Nursing care:* Good general nursing care is vital. The patient must be turned, coughed, and encouraged to breathe deeply. This is especially important in chest surgery. It is also vital to observe any signs of respiratory distress, which might indicate that the chest suction is malfunctioning.

It is possible for the patient to be up in the chair while the chest suction is operating. If the patient is to be up walking, generally the tubes are clamped and sometimes disconnected. Never do this without assistance and remember that the tubes must always be *double-clamped.* If the patient is up walking with his tubes and drainage bottles, the hemostats must go along too.

Abdominal distention can cause difficulty in breathing, so it is important to observe the patient to make sure he is passing flatus and that he is not having gas pains or distention difficulties.

**Complications.** The most serious complication in any patient who is undergoing chest drainage with tubes is the possibility of *pneumothorax* (the presence of air in the pleural cavity or between the pleura and the chest wall, usually causing the collapse of a lung). This is an emergency situation in which the tubing should be clamped immediately and a doctor called.

*Tension pneumothorax with resultant mediastinal shift:* This condition is caused by faulty drainage apparatus and is evidenced by dyspnea (rapid, shallow breathing), with cyanosis and puffiness of the skin. The laryngeal area becomes deviated toward the unoperated side. This is an emergency situation and the nurse should notify the doctor immediately and then check the tubing to see if she can locate the trouble. In this situation, too much drainage and/or air is present in the pleural cavity because the suction is not working properly. Clamping the tubing would only aggravate the situation.

*General items to watch for:*

1. Leakage of air into the drainage system, whether in a simple water-seal type or a mechanical suction type, is indicated by a *constant bubbling* in the water-seal bottle.
2. If the patient shows signs of cyanosis or dyspnea, or complains of chest pain, investigate the situation *immediately.*
3. In mechanical suctioning, when the suction motor is turned off, the tubing should be disconnected from the suction machine, to provide a vent for intrapleural air.
4. If the suction machine is operating properly, the *regulator bottle* or vacuum-control bottle (the one next to the suction machine), should bubble constantly.

## Exercises Following Chest Surgery

Since a great many muscles are incised during chest surgery, the patient must exercise soon after surgery to prevent "frozen shoulder" and other complications. Full range of motion exercise must be provided for the operative shoulder and arm. At first, the nurse carries out passive range of motion exercises for the patient. Within a few days after surgery the patient can do his own exercises. It is important that the exercises not overtire or overextend the muscles; the movement should be stopped at the point of pain or great resistance.

## DISORDERS OF THE NOSE

**Deviated Septum.** The nasal septum was described in Chapter 16 as a partition made of bone and cartilage, which divides the nose into right and left cavities (*nares* or *nostrils*).

The septum rarely is absolutely straight, but unless the deviation is marked it usually gives no trouble. An unusually crooked septum can interfere with drainage in one nostril. An injury that causes a deformity in the septum should have the attention of a doctor; if it is not corrected, it can cause sinusitis. The operation to correct such a deformity is called a *submucous resection.* Following the operation, which is done under local anesthesia, the patient's nostrils are packed with gauze, which is removed in 24 to 48 hours. A *mustache* dressing—a Vaseline-gauze pad held in place with strips of adhesive—is applied beneath the nostrils to catch the drainage.

POSTOPERATIVE CARE. The patient is often uncomfortable because of the surgery and because he must breathe through his mouth. He needs frequent oral hygiene and should have the head of the bed elevated to facilitate breathing. The nurse should watch for postoperative bleeding, which may occur. A fairly large amount of mucous drainage is to be expected, however.

**Hemorrhage After Nasal Surgery.** The nurse must remember that, in any surgery of the nose or in nosebleed, the blood may run down the throat and be swallowed by the patient. Nausea and coffee-ground or dark emesis or frequent spitting of blood are an indication of bleeding, as well as the presence of blood on the dressings. Since the nose is a vascular area of the body, a great deal of bleeding may occur. The nurse should be on the alert for symptoms of shock after any nasal procedure.

**Nosebleed (Epistaxis).** The irritation or injury of a small mass of capillaries on the nasal septum may cause bleeding. It can also be caused by hypertension, in which case the bleeding is more likely to be severe and not as easily controlled. It may also develop in connection with certain blood conditions, cancer, or rheumatic fever. Nosebleed is a fairly common occurrence but if it is severe it can be frightening and may be dangerous. First aid for nosebleed is simple: with the patient sitting down, apply pressure by holding the nose firmly between the thumb and the forefinger. The patient is less likely to faint in this position, and elevating his head lessens the flow of blood to the nose. Cold compresses on the bridge of the nose sometimes help. If the bleeding persists or is profuse, call a doctor. He may insert cotton pledgets saturated with epinephrine solution or a vasoconstrictor such as phenylephrine (Neo-Synephrine) in the nostril. If this is not effective, he may pack the nasal cavity with gauze to create pressure on the bleeding area or he may cauterize it. The packing is accomplished by passing a string through the nose and bringing it out the mouth. Then, the pack is tied on the string and pulled until it is in the back of the nasal cavity. Other methods are also used.

The bleeders in the nose may also be painted with silver nitrate or other solutions which tend to stop bleeding.

**Nasal Polyps.** Polyps are tumors that look like small bunches of tiny grapes. Nasal polyps obstruct breathing and sinus drainage. They are removed easily under local anesthesia, but unfortunately they have a tendency to return, and the operation has to be repeated. A biopsy of the tissue should be done to determine if the growth is malignant.

**Plastic Surgery of the Nose.** Plastic surgery of the nose (*rhinoplasty*) may be done to correct deformities resulting from injury, or for cosmetic reasons.

**Rhinitis.** Rhinitis is an inflammation of the mucous membranes of the nose. At times it is the result of allergic reactions, but more often it is caused by an infection, such as the common cold.

**Sinusitis.** *Sinusitis* is the inflammation of one or more of the sinuses located in the head. A maxillary sinus (*antrum*) is the one most frequently affected by an infection spreading from the nasal passages. If the patient's resistance is low, he is more susceptible to sinus infection. Although a sinus infection may not be fatal, it is most uncomfortable, and it is especially annoying to

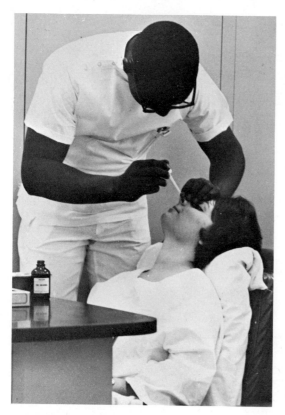

Figure 48-3. When instilling nose drops, the patient's head is tilted back to allow the solution to flow into the nostrils and is maintained in this position for a few minutes afterward to prevent the solution from draining out. The patient is instructed to expectorate any solution that may drain down into his throat.

people who live in climates where respiratory infections tend to occur. The presence of an allergy, frequent colds, or a nasal obstruction of any kind make people more susceptible to repeated attacks of sinusitis. If it is neglected, sinusitis becomes chronic and damages the mucous membranes, making treatment less effective. Of all the possible complications of sinusitis, infection of the middle ear or the brain are the most serious. Sinusitis may also lead to bronchiectasis or asthma. Early treatment is important to prevent these complications.

Acute sinusitis begins with the presence of pain and pressure, usually over the maxillary or the frontal sinuses. Pain is felt in the cheek or the upper teeth if the maxillary sinuses are affected. Frontal sinus pain occurs over the eyes. The patient has a low-grade fever, fatigue, and a poor appetite. A purulent nasal discharge appears, accompanied by a postnasal drip which irritates the throat. Sinus congestion will show up in an x-ray picture. The treatment usually prescribed includes bedrest, forced fluids, and salicylates to relieve the pain. Nose drops containing phenylephrine (Neo-Synephrine) and ephedrine are often used to shrink the swollen turbinates and to encourage drainage. Antibiotics to fight the infection may be given. Inhalation of steam or application of hot moist packs to the forehead are also effective.

If drainage is obstructed in an acute sinus infection, the sinus is irrigated with warm saline solution, which is a comparatively painless procedure. However, it may become necessary to puncture the bony wall between the nose and the sinus cavity (a Caldwell-Luc procedure), or to enter the frontal sinus through the inner aspect of the eyebrow. These procedures are quite painful for the patient; he may become frightened and feel dizzy or faint. The doctor always performs these procedures.

Chronic sinusitis is characterized by repeated flare-ups of the infection in spite of treatment. In most cases, the methods of therapy include measures to build up the patient's resistance and treatment for the cause of the infection. Occasionally, a suction apparatus is used to instill an aerosol form of a drug, such as an antihistamine, into the sinus, after which suction is applied. This is quite painful and results in only temporary relief. It is not used frequently today, since oral antihistamines are usually just as effective. A relatively simple operation to make a new sinus opening may be necessary. Many people suffer needlessly and are under the impression that nothing can be done for sinusitus, thereby allowing it to become chronic.

## Common Nasal Treatments

**Nasal Spray.** Sometimes a nasal spray is used to apply medications. Usually this is done with a hand atomizer, with the patient generally allowed to do it himself. He sits up and, holding up the end of the nostril, inserts the atomizer tip just inside, pointing it backward. At the same time, he closes the opposite nostril by pressing it with his finger. The force of the spray should be just enough to spread the solution over the nasal membrane. Too much force may force the solution into the sinuses or the eustachian tubes.

**Nose Drops.** Some people use nose drugs far too often. As a result, the medications lose their effect and eventually cause a swelling of the turbinates, the condition they are supposed to prevent. Many nose-drop preparations are sold over the counter without a prescription, and their prolonged use can be damaging. People with hypertension should never use nose drops.

A medicine dropper, paper wipes, and the prescribed solution comprise the necessary equipment for administering nose drops. The following points should be kept in mind when carrying out this procedure:

1. A sitting or lying position, with the head tilted back, allows the solution to flow into the nostrils.
2. A piece of soft rubber tubing placed over the tip of the dropper prevents injury to the nasal membrane and is necessary if the patient is an infant or is irrational.
3. Keeping the head tilted back for a few minutes afterward prevents the solution from draining out and preserves the effect of the medication.

**Nasal Irrigation.** When a purulent discharge forms crusts in the nose, a nasal irrigation may be used to remove them. The irrigating solution flows into one nostril and out through the other. The important point to observe in giving a nasal irrigation is to use the correct amount of pressure—too much pressure may force the fluid into the sinuses and the eustachian tubes, thus spreading the infection.

## DISORDERS OF THE THROAT

The throat (pharynx) is the muscular tube which communicates with the nasal cavity (nasopharynx), the oral cavity (oropharynx), and the laryngeal cavity (laryngopharynx). Two disorders, common in children, but occuring occasionally in adults are tonsillitis and streptococcal sore throat (see Chapter 40).

## Aspiration of Foreign Bodies

If the airway is totally blocked as a result of a foreign object being aspirated into the trachea or bronchi, an immediate tracheostomy must be done to save the patient's life (see Chapter 31). Usually, however, a sharp blow between the shoulder blades while the patient's head is down, will dislodge the foreign body. Mouth-to-mouth resuscitation may be necessary if the airway has been cut off for a minute or two.

If the particle is small, it may be aspirated into the lung without causing asphyxiation. In this case, however, it will cause an infection and must be removed. Generally, it can be removed by bronchoscopy procedures. However, if it is deep in a bronchus, open-lung surgery may be performed.

## Laryngitis

The larynx (voice box) lies below the pharynx and contains the vocal cords. *Laryngitis* is an inflammation and a swelling of the larynx. It often accompanies respiratory infections, or it may be the result of overuse of the voice or excessive smoking. The patient has a cough, is hoarse, and may lose his voice. Talking and smoking are prohibited, and steam inhalations are given to soothe the mucous membranes of the throat. If laryngitis is a complication of another infection, antibiotics may be given.

Chronic laryngitis may be a complication of chronic sinusitis or chronic bronchitis, or it may be the result of repeated attacks of acute laryngitis. Continued irritation of the throat by public speaking, smoking, or irritating gases are common causes. The recommended treatment is to abandon the activities that are causing the trouble and to get rid of any infection that may be contributing to it. The patient with a chronic laryngitis must be carefully checked for cancer.

## Cancer of the Larynx

Cancer of the larynx is most likely to occur in people over 45 and affects men most frequently. It seems to develop in people who have chronic laryngitis, strain their voices or are heavy drinkers or smokers. It is also believed that hereditary tendencies have something to do with its occurrence. The symptoms are chronic hoarseness and sometimes the inability to speak above a whisper. If it is detected early, radiation is effective in many cases, or surgery is often successful in effecting a complete cure. The operation consists of either removing the part of the vocal cord which is involved in the tumor (*thyrotomy*) or of removing the entire larynx (*laryngectomy*), if the cancer has spread beyond the vocal cords. (About 2000 people have this operation in the U.S. each year.)

When the larynx is removed, air must enter and leave through the trachea. Provision is made for this by inserting a tube in the trachea through an opening in the lower part of the neck (*tracheostomy*). Sometimes a *radical neck dissection* is done if the cancer has begun to spread beyond the vocal cords, possibly involving the lymph nodes. This may be very disfiguring and may present problems, such as carotid artery involvement or involvement of other structures in the neck.

**Preoperative Preparation.** Before a laryngectomy, the patient not only faces the knowledge that he must breathe through a hole in his neck, but also that the tumor may be malignant. He may fear that he will choke and perhaps die, or that if he lives, he will never speak again. The nurse can reassure this patient, by emphasizing the fact that, although he will lose his natural voice, voice training (esophageal speech) will make it possible for him to carry on ordinary conversation.

Reconstruction of the esophagus is necessary, so the patient should be told that for a time he may be fed through a tube in his nose, but that this arrangement is not permanent. However, he should know that the tracheostomy opening *will* be permanent, but that he will be taught how to take care of it himself.

**Nursing Care.** Immediately after a laryngectomy, the patient requires expert care. The respiratory passages become irritated, and the secretion of mucus increases and must be removed frequently by suction. A suction machine is constantly beside the bed of a laryngectomy patient, and he is never left alone. Remember that he may be terrified of choking or of not being able to breathe. However, the practical nurse will usually not be asked to assume this responsibility for immediate postoperative care. Another postoperative complication is hemorrhage, so the nurse must be especially watchful for hemoptysis.

The patient probably will be allowed out of bed the next day, and he soon will be taught how to suction the tube and take care of it himself. Everybody concerned with his care should know how to perform this procedure. When the airway becomes obstructed, the patient becomes cyanotic very quickly, and he may die within a few minutes if the obstruction is not removed. In this emergency, call for help and suction the tracheostomy opening. Unless the doctor has previously instructed the head nurse as to what emergency procedures to use, he should be consulted in all cases to see if the tracheostomy tube can be removed as an emergency measure. The patient's call light should always be within easy reach and should be answered with all possible speed, since he may be in trouble.

The patient usually loses his sense of smell temporarily after surgery, but this will begin to return as he learns to breathe through his laryngectomy tube. However, the sense of smell will be recovered best in the patient who learns esophageal speech.

**Esophageal Speech.** As soon as possible, training in esophageal speech should be started. The technic of esophageal speech consists of swallowing air and using the air to make speech sounds while regurgitating it. It takes patience and constant practice to learn how to do this, but patients sometimes learn the technic in 2 or 3 weeks. Some patients use an artificial larynx, an electronic device which the patient holds against his throat.

**Identification.** It is absolutely vital that the patient wear an identifying tag so that others will know that he breathes through an opening in his neck. This is especially important if he has not yet learned to speak, since he could not explain his situation to others. If the opening is plugged, he will die of asphyxiation.

**Nasogastric Tube Feedings.** The patient is often fed through a nasogastric tube for about a week after a laryngectomy. The

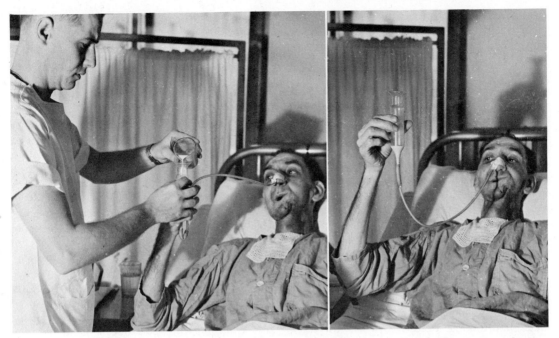

Figure 48-4. (*Left*) The nurse is pouring the tube feeding into an Asepto syringe, which is being used as a funnel. The tube is kinked while the syringe is being filled. Note the mesh square that the patient is wearing over his tube. Facial deformity has resulted from the extensive surgery that was necessary to treat his condition. (*Right*) The feeding is permitted to flow through the tube by gravity. Before the syringe is empty, more of the feeding will be added. The patient is encouraged to help with the procedure. (Smith, D. W., Germain, C. P., and Gips, C. D.: Care of the Adult Patient, ed. 3. Philadelphia, Lippincott, 1971)

amount, the type, and the frequency of the feedings are prescribed by the doctor. They are warmed to body temperature, and they flow into the body by gravity through a funnel or an Asepto syringe (Fig. 48-4). Oral medications may also be crushed, mixed with water, and administered through the tube. However, it is important to rinse the tube with water following the medication to be sure that the patient receives the entire amount. (This procedure is discussed in more detail in Chapter 49.)

**Community Resources.** Most communities have a laryngectomy club for persons who have had their vocal chords removed. (The one in Minnesota is called the "Lost Chord" Club.) The patient should be encouraged to join this club because the other members can give much encouragement and help to the new laryngectomee. Since members of the club often are willing to visit the new laryngectomee while he is still in the hospital, the nurse may suggest this. The visit often gives the patient the encouragement he needs to begin his rehabilitation process.

**Rehabilitation.** The patient should be encouraged to live his normal life after discharge from the hospital. To conceal the opening, a necktie or crew neck shirt can be worn by the man and a scarf or jewelry can be worn by the woman. Care must be used to allow free entry of air and to prevent aspiration of foreign objects. Anyone who has a tracheostomy must always be careful to prevent water from getting into the opening. He must never swim and must use caution when taking showers.

## CHRONIC RESPIRATORY CONDITIONS

### Allergic Rhinitis (Hay Fever)

*Hay fever* is the name most commonly given to *allergic rhinitis,* an inflammation of the mucous membranes of the nose, caused by an allergic reaction to some protein substance (see Chapter 54). It may be due to pollens from weeds, flowers, or grasses at certain seasons of the year or may be a reaction to dusts, feathers, or scales from the skin of animals. Contact with these foreign substances causes edema, itching, and a watery discharge from the eyes and the nose. People with an allergic background (a family history of allergy) are more susceptible to hay fever, as are people who have asthma or eczema. The number of people with a hereditary tendency is fairly high, including about 10 per cent of the population. All ages are affected, and it may appear suddenly at any age and may disappear as suddenly.

**Symptoms.** It is a most disagreeable and inconvenient disease. The victim's nose itches, he sneezes endlessly, and is tormented by a profuse, watery discharge from his nose and eyes. It is aggravated on windy days and is worse in the morning and the evening. It takes painstaking detective work to track down the cause, and detailed questioning and many skin tests are needed to find the offending substance. Sometimes several substances are the offenders.

**Treatment.** The first step in the treatment of allergic rhinitis is to avoid the substance that is causing the allergy. This may mean eliminating an offending food from the diet, avoiding cats, or curtailing drives in the country. Air-conditioning also helps. Antihistamines relieve the symptoms; desensitization may do away with them entirely (Chapter 54). Sometimes cortisone and ACTH are given for severe attacks. An untreated allergy of this kind may lead to asthma or sinusitis.

## Bronchial Asthma

*Asthma* is a bronchial spasm, accompanied by swelling of the membrane which lines the bronchi and by a thick, mucous secretion. The spasm imprisons the air that is in the alveoli and shuts out fresh air. An asthma attack is a frightening experience for the patient as he struggles to get air into his lungs. He becomes pale, and sometimes in a severe attack becomes cyanotic. He also perspires and wheezes. As the attack subsides, he coughs up thick, white mucus. It can be equally frightening to a nurse who never has seen an attack of asthma before.

**Causes.** Allergy, infection, and emotional tensions are the chief causes of asthma. A person may develop asthma from a combination of all 3 of these factors, which makes it difficult to trace the cause of any one attack. Attacks may occur only occasionally, or they may be frequent. Frequent attacks of asthma may lead to emphysema. People who have hay fever or bronchitis are especially susceptible; it can occur at any age and at any time. Asthmatic children have fewer symptoms as they grow older, but the symptoms of adults grow worse with age.

**Treatment.** The most important aspect of treatment during an asthmatic attack is to relieve the breathing difficulties. Doses of Adrenalin are given to dilate the bronchi. Adrenalin is a powerful and dangerous drug that brings immediate relief; it also has distressing side-effects if the dose is not measured exactly. Aminophylline, given intravenously, has a similar effect, as does ephedrine to a lesser degree. Long-term treatment of asthma consists of treating the allergy and other difficulties.

## Bronchiectasis

*Bronchiectasis* is an abnormal dilatation of one or several bronchi. Saclike cavities may form and fill with pus. The main cause of this disease is infection, frequently following tuberculosis, influenza, or pneumonia or chronic sinusitis. Often it begins in young adulthood and progresses slowly over a long period of time. In a child, it may be a complication of whooping cough or measles. It is rarely fatal, but may have serious complications. It is usually chronic, causing the patient to adopt a different life style.

Any type of obstruction in the bronchial tubes can cause bronchiectasis. People with this condition are subject to acute bronchitis and pneumonia and care must be taken to prevent these complications.

**Symptoms.** The characteristic symptom of bronchiectasis is a cough, which produces greenish-yellow sputum with a foul odor. The cough is most severe when the patient gets up or goes to bed. As the disease progresses, the amount of sputum increases, and sometimes blood is coughed up. The patient loses weight and has chronic fatigue and a poor appetite.

Bronchiectasis will show on an x-ray picture of the bronchial tree after a radiopaque substance (Lipiodol) has been instilled into the bronchi.

**Treatment and Nursing Care.** Drainage of the purulent material is part of the treatment. This is accomplished by *postural drainage,* a position with the head lower than the chest. The patient is encouraged to cough and to breathe deeply. Antibiotics are given to control the infection. Good nutrition and rest are also important. Special mouth care is needed, because the sputum leaves an offensive taste and breath odor. Attention to the patient's comfort helps to promote rest. Prompt attention to such conditions as bronchial asthma and bronchitis helps to prevent bronchiectasis. If only a small part of the lung is affected, surgery to remove the diseased area will cure bronchiectasis. Nothing will bring damaged bronchi back to normal.

**Prevention.** Because bronchiectasis can be prevented, we are seeing less and less of the disease. Some means of prevention are: (1) vaccinating children against whooping cough (pertussis) and measles, and adults against flu, (2) providing good nursing care in other lung disorders such as pneumonia to prevent complications, (3) maintaining good general health, and (4) giving prompt attention when a foreign object is aspirated into the lungs.

## Bronchitis

*Bronchitis* is an inflammation of the bronchial tubes—it may be acute or chronic.

**Acute Bronchitis.** Acute bronchitis often follows a respiratory infection, especially during the winter months. A dry cough is an early symptom; later, the cough produces mucus and pus. Other symptoms are fever and malaise.

TREATMENT AND NURSING CARE. Rest in bed, a nutritious diet, and plenty of fluids are the usual prescribed treatment. Humidifiers help by moistening the air—dry air aggravates bronchitis. Antibiotics help to control the infection, and precautions are taken to prevent it from spreading. Salicylates are sometimes given. As in any respiratory disease, the patient is instructed to cover his mouth when coughing, and the sputum cup is kept covered and the contents disposed of in a way that will not endanger others. Every hospital has its own method of disposing of infectious wastes. Acute bronchitis, if untreated, will develop into chronic bronchitis.

**Chronic Bronchitis.** Chronic bronchitis is a more serious condition which often develops so gradually that the victim disregards its most significant symptom, a chronic cough. Consequently, the disease is firmly established before the patient decides that he needs treatment. Repeated attacks of acute bronchitis may lead to a chronic condition, or it may develop after an acute respiratory infection, such as influenza or pneumonia. Cigarette smoking is undoubtedly one of the most common causes of bronchial irritation; air pollution may also be responsible. People who are exposed to irritating dusts or chemicals seem to be more likely to develop bronchitis. It affects all ages but is most common after 40, probably because people wait before seeking treatment, even though they should have had treatment earlier.

SYMPTOMS. Chronic bronchitis begins with a dry cough, also known as "smoker's cough," which is most severe when the patient gets up in the morning. As time goes on, he coughs up mucus and pus and sometimes streaks of blood. Shortness of breath becomes apparent with exertion; as the disease progresses it persists even when the patient is quiet. The patient's history of a cough and of his living habits helps the doctor in making a diagnosis. He is also aided by x-rays of the chest, fluoroscopic examinations, and sputum tests.

TREATMENT AND NURSING CARE. Treatment is a long, drawn-out process; there are no drugs that will work a miracle. However, treatment will reduce the symptoms and prevent complications. Untreated, the disease may progress until the bronchioles of the lungs are permanently damaged, or it may lead to asthma, emphysema, or heart failure. It is important to build up the patient's general health and to use precautions to avoid exposure to respiratory infections. He should have plenty of rest and be free from emotional pressures. He may have to change his job if his work exposes him to dust or bad weather. If he is a cigarette smoker, he has to face the fact that the habit is definitely harmful for him. Antibiotics will help to clear up additional respiratory infections, but such infections will aggravate the bronchitis.

## Emphysema

*Emphysema* is overdistention of the alveoli of the lungs which causes loss of elasticity and destroys alveolar tissue. To review the structure of the lungs briefly: the branches of the bronchi, the bronchioles, end in millions of tiny air sacs called alveoli. It is in the alveoli that the exchange of carbon dioxide and oxygen takes place. When air becomes trapped in the alveoli, the patient is unable to breathe out, the lungs become distended and the muscles suffer from lack of oxygen. This condition becomes worse as more and more air is imprisoned in the alveoli, and the heart works harder and harder to push the blood through the body, trying to get oxygen to the muscles and other body tissues. The end result of emphysema is often congestive heart failure.

**Causes.** Authorities believe that chronic bronchitis is the direct cause of emphysema. It may also follow chronic bronchial asthma and bronchiectasis. Evidence seems to be clear that the increase in the number of cases of emphysema in the last 10 years is also due to air pollution and cigarette smoking. A report by The Advisory Committee to the Surgeon General of the U.S. states that "cigarette smoking is the most important of the causes of chronic bronchitis in the United States." It also states that "the smoking of cigarettes is associated with an increased risk of dying from pulmonary emphysema." It is estimated that this disease now affects more than 7 million people in this country; nearly 10,000 people die of emphysema every year. Men over 40 are the group most frequently afflicted.

**Symptoms.** The first symptom of emphysema is difficulty in breathing after exertion. As the condition progresses difficulty in breathing occurs at all times. Other symptoms are wheezing and a chronic cough, with the expectoration of mucus and pus. The victim is pale and drawn and is afraid of choking. He does not dare to lie down and sits up, leaning forward and contracting the muscles of his neck with every breath. In the advanced stages, as carbon dioxide accumulates in his blood, he becomes listless and drowsy. The disease runs its course over a period of many years.

**Treatment.** Until recently, emphysema was considered to be a hopeless disease for which there was no help. However, modern treatment is proving that patients can be helped with intensive treatment. Preventive treatment is most important to correct the conditions that cause emphysema, because changes in the lung tissue or in the blood vessels of the lungs are irreversible. This means, for one thing, alerting the public to the danger signs, such as morning cough or smoker's cough.

The treatment includes:

Drugs such as Adrenalin, aminophylline or ephedrine, which dilate the bronchial tubes and relieve breathlessness. IPPB treatments also help.

Expectorants and postural drainage to remove secretions. Sometimes suction is needed.

Antibiotics to control infections. Respiratory infections should be prevented if possible.

Administration of oxygen with caution (it may be dangerous if there is a high concentration of carbon dioxide in the blood).

Breathing exercises to use the diaphragm more effectively and to relieve the chest muscles.

Blowing exercises to improve breathing.

Bedrest should be discouraged. The patient should be encouraged to keep active.

The emphysema patient must be faithful in carrying out his breathing exercises, because his life depends on staying active at all costs. He must limit his activities to whatever his heart and breathing power will stand. He can choose to be an invalid or to lead a fairly active life.

## Dust Diseases (Pneumoconioses)

These diseases are caused by repeated inhalation of certain heavy, harmful dusts. The most common disease is silicosis which occurs among miners and comes from breathing silica, or quartz dust. Other dust diseases are asbestosis, berylliosis (caused by inhaling beryllium dust), anthracosilicosis (caused by breathing a combination of coal dust and silica), bagassosis (caused by inhaling the dust from pressed sugar cane), and stannosis (caused by inhaling the dust of tin ore). Some of these diseases, such as asbestosis, berylliosis and silicosis are more serious than others.

As these dusts are inhaled, they eventually slow down or stop the ciliary action in the nose. Thus, the dusts are allowed to enter the lungs. Some dusts, such as household dust, are not dangerous. However, the dangerous dusts can cause irritation, allergic reaction, or chemical reaction.

**Symptoms.** Usually the first symptom is dyspnea. Later, the patient develops a chronic cough, and when the disease has advanced further, he will experience chest pains. Serious complications include other lung disorders such as tuberculosis, pneumonia, chronic bronchitis, and lung cancer, as well as emphysema.

**Treatment.** Prevention is the goal, since these diseases are very difficult to treat once they have affected extensive areas of the lungs. About the only treatment which exists at the present time is that of lessening the exposure to the dust. There is no way to reverse the damage which has been done to the lungs.

## INFECTIOUS CONDITIONS

### The Common Cold

The *common cold* is classed as a minor respiratory infection, yet it is one of the minor respiratory diseases that causes more than half of all illness every year, results in the loss of many work days, and restricts many activities. The average loss per person in a year from respiratory disease is estimated as 4 days—more than half of these losses are caused by minor respiratory infections, such as the common cold.

Colds are caused by one or more filtrable viruses and are spread by talking, coughing, or sneezing. If the body's resistance is lowered by fatigue, chilling, or gases that continually irritate the nasal membranes (smog), the body is more susceptible to the virus. The usual symptoms of a cold are sneezing, a scratchy throat, and headache. These conditions are followed by a sore throat, general malaise, nasal discharge, a cough, and sometimes a slight fever. This unpleasantness usually lasts from 5 days to 2 weeks.

**Treatment.** The most important treatment for a cold is bedrest, if the patient has a fever. This has the added advantage of keeping the afflicted person from infecting others. (A nurse with a cold *must* stay at home.) Rest is especially important where babies or elderly, weakened people are concerned, to prevent the development of more serious complications. The administration of plenty of fluids aids recovery. Strict attention to washing the hands and using disposable tissues to prevent spreading the infection are essential. Aspirin relieves discomfort. Nose drops should be used with discretion, because many of them have harmful effects on the body. (Antibiotics have no effect against the virus that causes a cold.) Vitamin C may be helpful, but this is not yet proven. Antihistamines may relieve the allergic reactions.

**Complications of a Cold.** If the symptoms common to a cold indicate more serious illness, the patient should consult a doctor, especially if he has a fever for more than 2 days, severe headache which is unrelieved by aspirin, and severe coughing, earache, and chest pains, and coughs up a dark-colored sputum. The patient with a chronic respiratory condition, such as asthma, should consult a doctor at the first sign of a cold.

### Influenza

*Influenza* (commonly called "flu") is an acute, contagious, respiratory disease caused by one of several different strains of a virus: Types A, B, and C. Influenza breaks out in epidemics, which occur periodically and are usually caused by Types A and B. (Type C is almost never seen.) In 1957, a virus similar to Type A was the cause of an epidemic that was almost world-wide. In 1918, at the close of World War I, an influenza epidemic took many lives in this country as well as abroad. Most patients recover, but others die as the the result of complications, such as heart disease, encephalitis, or the harmful effects on pregnant women. Influenza also frequently causes death among elderly people. Patients may develop parkinsonism many years after having had flu.

**Symptoms.** Influenza attacks suddenly: the patient becomes very ill, suffering from muscular pains, fever, headache, sensitivity to light or burning eyes, and chills. Also, he may sneeze, cough, have a nasal discharge, and complain of sore throat. He often has nausea and vomiting. Fever is high (100° to 103° F.) and lasts for 2 to 3 days, but the other symptoms, especially the cough, last longer. The patient may have a cough for several weeks after having had the flu. In its severest form, influenza may cause the patient to collapse.

**Treatment and Nursing Care.** The influenza victim is given quantities of fluids, including fruit juices and milk-and-egg drinks for their nutritional value. As soon as he feels better he may have a regular diet. He is kept in bed and given aspirin to relieve headache, fever, and muscular pains. Codeine may be given to relieve a cough. The patient is isolated to prevent spreading the infection while it is acute. He should be kept warm and avoid exposure to other diseases. He is watched for signs of secondary infection, such as pain in the chest, purulent or rust-colored sputum, or a rise in temperature and an increase in the pulse rate.

Polyvalent vaccine can be given as a protection against influenza. The U.S. Surgeon General stated that this vaccine is "70 per cent effective in preventing the disease." However, vaccination only protects people for about 6 months, so it is not possible to give it much in advance of an epidemic, and there is very little time to develop a special vaccine after an epidemic strikes. Moreover, some authorities doubt the effectiveness of influenza vaccines. An effort is made to give this protection to health workers and military personnel and to people who are very susceptible, such as the elderly and people with chronic disease, such as TB, emphysema, heart disease, and hypertension. Pregnant women are also often vaccinated. During an epidemic people are urged to stay away from crowds—sometimes all public gatherings are suspended.

**Complications of Flu.** The most important complication of influenza is pneumonia. The patient is particularly susceptible to any lung disorder after the flu, since the body is weakened and many viruses seem to settle in the lungs. Other complications are chronic disorders such as bronchitis, sinusitis, or ear infections.

## Acute Empyema (Pyothorax)

*Empyema* is a collection of pus in the pleural cavity. It is a secondary infection and may follow tuberculosis, lung abscess, or pneumonia. It may also spread from an infection of the chest wall or other surrounding areas or may be introduced directly by a wound of the chest or by surgery. Before antibiotics were developed, empyema was a frequent complication of pneumonia. Now antibiotics subdue the infection in the lung before it spreads to the pleura. Since it is almost always a secondary infection, empyema is difficult to diagnose because its symptoms are usually masked by the primary infection.

**Symptoms.** The symptoms of empyema are chest pain, fever, dyspnea, and a generally toxic feeling. If empyema is suspected, more decisive information can be obtained by a chest x-ray and by aspirating a specimen of the chest fluid (thoracentesis).

**Treatment and Nursing Care.** The treatment starts with antibiotics to combat the infection and with measures to remove the pus collected in the pleural cavity. This may be done by closed drainage (*thoracentesis*), in which case, an antibiotic is often injected into the pleural cavity. Sometimes, enzymes are injected to liquefy thick pus. If this is not successful open drainage is done, but is only necessary if the pus is thick and heavy. Then soft rubber drainage tubes are inserted in the wound, and large, absorbent dressings and pads are applied. Usually, the drainage is profuse at first, and it will be necessary to change the dressings frequently. As soon as drainage begins, the patient's temperature falls to normal or near-normal, and his condition improves. In open drainage, usually a rib is removed, and the patient may experience some pain. If untreated, acute empyema may become chronic empyema, which is much more difficult to treat.

**Chronic Empyema.** This may be a complication of acute empyema, or may be caused by bronchopleural fistula, osteomyelitis of the rib cage, or an aspirated foreign body. It may also be a complication of tuberculosis or fungous infection of the lungs.

## Lung Abscess

A *lung abscess* is a localized area of infection in the lung, which breaks down and forms pus. It can be caused by a foreign body in the lung or by aspirating respiratory secretions, or it may follow pneumonia.

The *symptoms* of a lung abscess are chills and fever, with a loss in weight and a cough which produces purulent sputum with a foul odor. It is treated by establishing drainage, which may require surgery to open the chest wall. If the cause of the abscess is an aspirated object, bronchoscopy usually is effective in removing the object. Antibiotics usually are effective in treating the disease, after the offending cause is removed.

## Pneumonia

*Pneumonia* is an acute infection or partial solidification, of the lung in which the air sacs fill with fluid and affect breathing. There are 3 general types of pneumonia—*bacterial* pneumonia, which is caused by bacteria such as the pneumococcus or the streptococcus, *hypostatic* pneumonia, which develops when a person lies in one position for prolonged periods and the lung tissues fill with fluid, and *aspiration pneumonia,* which develops when fluid gets into the lungs of an unconscious patient through the epiglottis, which does not close completely when the patient does not swallow. The nurse must be careful when a patient is recovering from anesthesia, to drain or suction out fluids that accumulate in the mouth and the throat, to prevent them from getting into the lungs. Breathing exercises and changing a patient's position frequently help to prevent hypostatic pneumonia.

Pneumonia may also be caused by exposure to a *chemical irritant* or by a *virus,* which for some reason does not respond to the usual treatment. Viral pneumonia is seldom fatal but leaves the patient feeling weak and ill for a long period of time after the attack.

**Who Gets Bacterial Pneumonia?** Certain groups of people, such as those who are not in good general physical health, older people, and people with chronic lung disorders, seem to be more likely to become ill and get pneumonia. The chronic alcoholic is particularly susceptible to the disease and is very difficult to cure.

**Symptoms.** Pneumonia affects the lobes of the lung (*lobar pneumonia*) or the bronchi (*bronchial pneumonia*). It is most prevalent in the winter and spreads through droplets in the air. The pneumococcus is often found in the throats of well people where it does no damage unless their resistance is lowered.

*Bacterial pneumonia* starts suddenly with:

A severe sharp pain in the chest and a chill, followed by fever which may go up to 105 or 106° F.

A painful cough, with rust-colored, tenacious, sputum and pain on breathing.

A rapid pulse and sometimes cyanosis. The patient feels very ill.

Rapid respiration with difficult expiration. Orthopneic position not only helps the patient to breathe, but also assists him in coughing up mucus.

A high white blood count.

Possible mental changes, such as delerium or anxiety.

**Treatment and Nursing Care.** Blood cultures are taken, and the sputum is analyzed to find out what organism is causing the infection. And sensitivity tests are done to determine what drug will be most effective. An x-ray of the chest will show what part of the lung is affected and to what degree. Antibiotics have revolutionized the treatment of pneumonia. In 2 days the fever usually disappears and the other symptoms improve dramatically. In some instances, the organisms causing the disease are not affected by antibiotics. The antibiotics that are commonly used in the treatment of bacterial pneumonia are:

*Penicillin,* for pneumococcal and streptococcal pneumonia. It seldom has unpleasant side-effects unless the patient has had penicillin before or is sensitive to it. A skin rash is often the first sign of an allergic reaction. The patient should be carefully evaluated before a large dose of the drug is given, to prevent anaphylactic shock.

*Streptomycin* is effective against some of the organisms that cause pneumonia. It is more toxic than penicillin and may produce such side-effects as nausea, abdominal pain, skin rash, and fever. Sometimes it causes damage to a nerve in the brain—signs of this effect are dizziness, ringing in the ears, and deafness, which should be reported immediately.

*Tetracycline* may be used when a patient is sensitive to penicillin or does not respond to penicillin. It may also be used when the organism causing the disease cannot be identified. It has few side-effects.

*Chloromycetin* is effective in atypical pneumonias or in cases when penicillin has no effect.

*Erythromycin* has effects similar to chloromycetin.

The usual treatment to build up body resistance is given, along with rest and administering large amounts of fluid, including fluids with nutritious value. Codeine may be given for the cough. If breathing is markedly difficult, oxygen is administered usually by placing the patient in an oxygen tent. Sedatives may be necessary to promote rest, and aspirin is usually given for fever. Morphine is contraindicated because it depresses the respiratory center. If the abdomen is distended, Prostigmin may be given to stimulate peristalsis. Points to observe in nursing care are:

Adjust patient's position so as to aid in breathing and to calm his fear of choking. A pillow placed lengthwise under his back helps to expand the chest. A blanket around his shoulders makes him more comfortable during chills.

Take the temperature, pulse, and respiration every 4 hours. A rapid increase in the pulse rate and increasingly labored respirations are signs that the disease is advancing.

Measure intake and output.

Change his bed linen when necessary if he perspires profusely.

Give mouth care frequently.

Encourage him to cough and bring up the excessive secretions. Splint his chest when he coughs.

Put side rails on the bed if he becomes delirious.

Observe isolation technic during the acute stage of illness.

Give small amounts of liquid foods frequently.

Keep the patient quiet. Instruct him not to talk or exert himself in any way.

Give IPPB treatments if the patient is strong enough to tolerate them.

Prevent abdominal distention, because it interferes with breathing. Use a rectal tube, suppository, or small enema (often a Fleet enema) to alleviate distention.

With antibiotics, the patient usually improves rapidly—in 48 to 72 hours he is markedly better. However, he is still weak, and remains in bed for several days after his temperature is normal. Then gradually he is allowed more activity and convalesces slowly while his resistance is built up. An x-ray is taken to make sure that the infection in the lungs has cleared up completely. Complications from pneumonia seldom occur today, since antibiotics control the disease before it has time to spread and affect other parts of the body. Complications which were seen frequently in the past were empyema, endo-

carditis, or arthritis. If the infection spreads, it also may cause inflammation of the middle ear (otitis media), sinusitis, or bronchitis.

Colds and influenza lower resistance and make people more susceptible to pneumonia, especially in alcoholics or older people who are less active. A nurse who is taking care of elderly people should remember this fact.

**"Walking Pneumonia."** Sometimes, the patient experiences pain in his chest, but does not feel ill enough to go to bed. After several weeks, a chest x-ray may be taken to determine the cause of the chest pain only to reveal that the patient has pneumonia. Usually, "walking pneumonia" clears up with antibiotic therapy, but may leave the patient weak and tired for a while.

## Pleurisy

*Pleurisy* is an inflammation of the pleura, the double membrane that covers the lungs. If only a small amount of fluid accompanies the infection it is called *dry pleurisy*. On the other hand, the amount of fluid may be so great that a large amount collects in the space between the 2 layers of membrane and creates enough pressure to collapse the lung and affect the heart. This is called *wet pleurisy* or *pleurisy with effusion*. If purulent exudate (pus) exists, the condition is called *empyema*.

Dry pleurisy usually occurs as a complication of pneumonia by infection spreading from the lungs. Wet pleurisy may be the result of tuberculosis, lung cancer, heart and kidney diseases, and general infections. The pleura becomes thickened, and the 2 membrane surfaces rub together, causing sharp pain with every breath. Later, as fluid forms, the pain diminishes, and a dry cough takes its place, accompanied by shortness of breath and exhaustion after the least effort.

Pleurisy may be primary or secondary, although it is usually secondary. Since so many patients diagnosed as having pleurisy later develop tuberculosis, symptoms of pleurisy should arouse suspicion of tuberculosis, until proven otherwise.

Pleuritic pain may occur with other diseases such as rheumatic fever, lupus erythematosus, and polyarteritis.

**Treatment and Nursing Care.** The treatment of pleurisy is very much like the treatment for pneumonia: bedrest and the restriction of activity. The patient is encouraged to cough; since this is painful, applying a tight chest binder or putting a heating pad over the area or having the patient lie on the affected side may help to make him more comfortable. Sometimes *thoracentesis* (chest tap) is necessary to remove excess fluid. Usually, pleurisy heals as the condition that caused it improves.

### Histoplasmosis

Because this disease is an imitator of the "summer flu," it is often misdiagnosed. It is also often mistaken for tuberculosis. The disease is caused by a fungus, *Histoplasma capsulatum,* which floats in the air with dust and is breathed into the lungs, where it actually grows as a fungus. Since it spreads as a spore and needs warmth, moisture, and darkness to grow, the lungs are a perfect place for it to settle. The disease is often harbored in such places as chicken houses, barns, and caves.

The persons who are most likely to get the disease are very young children and old men. They are especially susceptible to the form of histoplasmosis which spreads from the lungs to other parts of the body. The lungs become inflamed from the invasion of the foreign material, which causes damage to the lymph glands and lungs. As a result, scar tissue and calcium deposits may form.

**Symptoms.** Symptoms are much like those of the flu. Many people get the disease and never know it because the symptoms are so mild. Patients usually recover after a few weeks. In more severe cases, the symptoms include weight loss, weakness, and a very long convalescence. The chronic form of "histo" spreads throughout the body and may cause organ enlargement or anemia. It is occasionally fatal.

**Diagnosis.** Histoplasmosis is diagnosed by a skin test, similar to the Mantoux test, or by a blood test or chest x-ray.

**Treatment.** For the mild form of the disease, treatment is similar to that for the flu. Usually, the symptoms go away by themselves. In more severe cases a drug, such as ampho-

tericin B, is given. Since the drug must be given intravenously for several weeks the patient must be hospitalized. Surgery is done when the lungs are extensively involved. It is believed that a person who has been cured of histoplasmosis, will be immune for life.

## TUBERCULOSIS

In the early 1950's, people were rejoicing about the discovery of isoniazid, a drug that promised an end to tuberculosis. However, tuberculosis is still the most common infectious disease in this country. Large cities are reporting an increase in the number of cases; in some instances, the increase is quite alarming. This may be the result of a "letting up" on the war against tuberculosis. Public health officials tell us that we know how to control this disease if we will only use our knowledge. Also, we must renew our efforts to find and treat every case. An official of the National Tuberculosis and Respiratory Disease Association attributes the recent rise in the number of cases to a general relaxation of control measures by federal, state, and local governments and to reductions in funds formerly appropriated for tuberculosis control.

**Who Gets Tuberculosis?** Although the death rate from tuberculosis has gone down dramatically in the last 50 years or so (in 1900 it was the first cause of death, today it is 13th), it is still the cause of much disability in this country. In many of the underdeveloped countries it is a major health problem.

**What Causes Tuberculosis?** Tuberculosis, also known as TB, is caused by the *tubercle bacillus* which was discovered in 1882, by Robert Koch who later learned how to prepare tuberculin.

THE TUBERCLE BACILLUS. The *tubercle bacillus* is enclosed in a waxy coating, making it difficult to destroy. Many people have tubercle bacilli in their bodies but do not have active tuberculosis. The disease develops if the body's resistance is lowered by poor nutrition or lack of rest, when the organisms multiply and become active. It is possible to arrest the disease to the point where it is not infectious and remains inactive. There are several types of the tubercle bacillus; the 2 types we are most concerned with are the *human,* and the *bovine* which affects cattle and can be transmitted to people. Bovine tuberculosis is well under control now through the testing of milk-producing cattle and the pasteurization of milk. The human type is spread mainly by contact with people who have tuberculosis in an active form.

The bacillus lives in dried particles of sputum but can be destroyed by a few hours of exposure to direct sunlight. Ordinary disinfectants have little effect on it, because they are unable to penetrate its waxy coating. Some drugs do have an effect on the bacillus, although some strains are becoming resistant.

**Vaccination Against TB.** Vaccination against tuberculosis is not dependable. However, it is given where people work with or are exposed frequently to persons with the disease. It is given only to persons who have negative Mantoux tests. BCG (Bacille Calmette-Guérin) has also given some protection, but also is not very reliable.

**Preventive Drug Therapy.** Tests have shown that active TB can be prevented from developing in many people who have been exposed to the bacillus, by long-term administration of isoniazid, or a similar drug. Some physicians believe that all positive reactors, or at least those of a high-risk group, should be on isoniazid as a preventive measure.

**How Tuberculosis Spreads.** Tuberculosis spreads by inhaling infected droplets (*droplet nuclei*), which have been released into the air by a person who has an active infection. It also spreads by kissing an infected person, or by coming in contact with contaminated utensils or equipment used by them. Isolation measures are taken for a patient with an active infection—with "positive" sputum. When the tubercle bacilli are no longer present in the sputum, the urine, or the feces, isolation technic is unnecessary.

**Where Tuberculosis Attacks.** The tubercle bacillus most frequently attacks the lungs, but sometimes the blood carries the TB organism to other parts of the body, such as the kidneys or the bones. Organisms in the lungs may start a small infection which is not enough to produce any symptoms. It heals, and the person never knows that this minor infection was

there. However, it will show up in a chest roentgenogram as a small scar and is a sign that at some time there were active tuberculosis organisms in the body. This scar is the end result of the white blood cells attempting to surround and engulf the bacilli. The bacilli become enclosed into a lump, called a *tubercle.* This tubercle may remain inactive for life, but if the person's resistance is lowered, the encasement breaks down and the person becomes actively ill.

**Tuberculosis of Bones and Joints.** The bloodstream may carry tubercle bacilli to the bones and the joints. This is more common in children, where it affects the spine (Pott's disease), the hips, and the knees. In the spine, the vertebrae collapse, which causes a pronounced spinal curvature (*kyphosis*), or humpback. These patients have the same treatment as does any tuberculosis patient, with the addition of devices to prevent motion in the joints, such as casts or traction. Sometimes surgery is done to immobilize the joints.

**Tuberculosis in Other Organs.** Infection may spread to the fallopian tubes, the ovaries, and the uterus, and it may be necessary to remove the diseased organ surgically. Infection may also appear in the gastrointestinal tract, the kidneys, or the meninges.

**Skin.** Tuberculous lesions (lupus vulgaris) may appear on the skin as yellowish or red spots, most commonly on the face.

## Detecting Tuberculosis

**Tuberculin Tests.** Tuberculin tests will show whether or not TB organisms have ever been active in the body. A *positive* reaction to the test does not mean that a person *has* tuberculosis—it means that at some time he *had* a tuberculosis infection. There are about 25 million persons in this country who have TB germs in their bodies. A small percentage of these will develop active disease.

MANTOUX TEST. A minute amount of tuberculin (PPD) is injected into the skin of the forearm. If the person has ever had any tuberculosis infection, the area around the point of injection becomes reddened and hard. Everyone having a tuberculin test in a health examination needs to have this test explained, especially if the reaction is positive, or he may think that he has active tuberculosis. A positive reaction should be followed by a chest x-ray to be sure that this was an old infection and to determine its extent.

PATCH TEST (VOLLMER). A patch containing tuberculin is placed on the skin and removed in 48 hours; if the skin is reddened the test is positive. A similar test is the *scratch test* (Von Pirquet), in which the surface of the skin is scratched, and tuberculin is applied to the spot.

**The Chest Roentgenogram.** The x-ray of the chest is our most helpful aid in detecting tuberculosis. Used with or without a preliminary tuberculin test, chest x-rays of community groups have been most successful in finding cases of tuberculosis, many of whom were people who were apparently well. A chest roentgenogram has one great advantage: people can receive treatment while the disease is in its early stages. Such a program also reveals the more advanced cases. In addition to the advantages of early treatment, by finding cases of tuberculosis we prevent people from spreading the disease. Authorities say that every person who has a positive tuberculin test should also have a yearly chest roentgenogram.

## An Overview

Tuberculosis is a long-term illness; there is no way of telling how long. The patient's determination to get well and to stay well has an influence on the outcome of treatment. The tubercle bacilli usually enter the body through the nose and mouth and actually "eat up" lung or other living tissue. This is where the early name, *consumption,* originated. The disease usually develops comparatively slowly, in contrast to an acute disease such as pneumonia. There is an absence of pain due to the absence of sensory nerves in the lung tissue. The presence of pain may indicate an extension of the disease to the pleura. Cough, with expectoration of sputum, is nature's way of ridding the lung of foreign material, caseous material, and other debris. Sputum is always considered potentially infectious, until proven otherwise.

When the disease is active, the sputum may or may not be positive for tubercle bacilli. Generally, the patient cannot infect others after a few weeks of chemotherapy. Patients can be taught to control cough except when raising sputum. A sputum examination helps the doctor determine how infectious the patient is and what the status of the disease is in that patient.

Under modern drug therapy, complete bedrest is seldom prescribed by the physician. Periods of rest and relaxation are ordered considering the needs of each patient. An elevation of temperature in the afternoon may indicate a reactivation of the disease process. Hemorrhage may be of minor or major importance. If it occurs absolute rest and attendance of a physician are indicated.

Sunshine is an effective agent in killing dry bacilli in the air. Therefore, a sunny room for the patient is highly desirable, although the patient should not be exposed to the direct rays of the sun for a long period of time. Air should be free from dust and smoke, if possible, to prevent the introduction of other irritating substances. It should be fresh in order to provide the blood with the oxygen necessary to create energy and improve the general condition of the patient. Circulating fresh air also protects other patients from dry bacilli which may be present in the air.

## Symptoms

The symptoms of tuberculosis appear so gradually that sometimes the disease has a good start before they are noticed. They are often mistaken for signs of ordinary fatigue, with some loss in weight and perhaps a cough so slight that the patient ignores it. Then other significant symptoms appear, such as a slight rise in temperature in the afternoon and the evening and night sweats. The patient begins to cough up thick and sometimes blood-streaked sputum as well as blood. As the disease advances, the patient becomes weak and emaciated and may have chest pains, causing difficulty in breathing.

**If a Tuberculosis Infection Becomes Overly Active.** If the body resistance is low and a person is exposed to repeated contacts with tuberculosis, the spot of infection grows larger and breaks down into cheesy material. Later, this may slough away and leave a cavity in the lung, or it may enter a bronchus and cause tuberculous bronchopneumonia. Sometimes the bloodstream carries this material to other parts of the body to start up many small infections, a phenomenon called *miliary tuberculosis.*

## Treatment

**Chemotherapy.** Drugs have done miraculous things for tuberculosis patients. They speed recovery and help to arrest the disease in the more advanced stages. Drugs do not *cure* tuberculosis—they do slow the growth of tubercle bacilli and give the body a chance to build up resistance. They have 2 drawbacks—some of them have toxic effects, and the continued use of a combination of drugs may make the tubercle bacillus resistant to them.

*Streptomycin* was the first drug to be used effectively in the treament of tuberculosis. It has some unpleasant side-effects, such as nausea and vomiting, fever, dizziness, deafness, and sometimes a rash.

*Isoniazid (INH)* has fewer toxic effects, although it may cause voiding difficulty and constipation and sometimes neuritis and muscle twitching. Isoniazid and streptomycin are the 2 main drugs used in treating tuberculosis.

*Para-aminosalicylic acid (PAS)* is often combined with one of the above drugs to make them more effective and less likely to build up the organism's resistance to them. A number of other drugs occasionally used are Viomycin Sulfate, tetracycline, and kanamycin sulfate.

Other new drugs, such as etham butol, have been developed and are being tested.

These drugs must be taken for a long period of time without interruption in order to produce results. If a drug is stopped and resumed, it is not as effective as it would have been if continued. The goal of drug therapy for tuberculosis is to arrest the growth of the tubercle bacillus so that the natural body defenses can take over and kill the disease. These drugs do *not cure* the disease.

**Rest.** Rest is still the most important "first" in treating tuberculosis. Effective as drugs are, they cannot do the job without the patient having his rest. He may need complete bedrest, or he may be allowed bathroom privileges and may sit up for prescribed lengths of time every day. Complete bedrest which lasts for weeks is not considered necessary. Patients do well if they are allowed to increase their activity as they improve. However, a definite amount of rest is still important, because the lungs are less active when the patient is resting and so have a chance to heal.

Most young people are naturally active when they are well and rebel at having to rest when they begin to feel so much better and consider themselves cured.

**Diet and Environment.** The diet is planned to maintain the patient's normal weight (Chapter 24). It is no longer considered essential for the patient to gain weight beyond a normal level. He does not burn calories rapidly unless the disease is acute and he has fever. It is important to provide him with plenty of protein and with vitamin A and vitamin C, since the use of these vitamins is interfered with in tuberculosis. *Cold* air is not necessary but *fresh* air is. Pleasant surroundings help the patient's morale; since he is likely to be in the same environment for a period of time, everything that makes him comfortable and contented will help to speed his recovery. If he can be at home, with his own things around him, so much the better.

**Surgical Treatment.** Surgery is sometimes needed in advanced tuberculosis or if medical treatment is not effective. An operation may be performed to remove part of the affected lung (partial pneumonectomy). Or a procedure known as *artificial pneumothorax* may be carried out to collapse and rest the lung by introducing a measured amount of air between the layers of the pleura. Sometimes some of the ribs on the affected side are removed by *thoracoplasty,* an operation to collapse the diseased part of the lung permanently.

Surgical procedures are the only sure way to remove the tubercle bacillus involving the lung, and thus prevent relapse. The bacillus must be localized in order to effect a cure through surgery. Procedures used are: pneumonectomy, lobectomy, wedge resections, and artificial pneumothorax, rarely done today.

## Complications

**Spontaneous Pneumothorax.** Air in the pleural cavity between the chest wall and the lung causes the lung to collapse. The effects are severe pain, dyspnea, rapid drop in blood pressure, and rapid pulse, and a lack of chest movement on the affected side. Other symptoms are diaphoresis and anxiety. Treatment includes bedrest, quiet, thoracentesis, and drainage tubes and suction.

**Hemorrhage.** *Hemorrhage* may appear as a complication of tuberculosis, especially in the advanced stages. The signs are streaks of blood in the sputum, but a massive hemorrhage may happen suddenly. It is not likely to cause immediate death, but a severe hemorrhage may speed up the advance of the disease and cause anemia. The patient must be kept quiet; usually, a mild sedative is given, and he is disturbed as little as possible for routine personal care. Transfusions or other fluids are given to replace the blood loss.

**Recurrence.** The tuberculosis patient who has been pronounced "cured" should be examined periodically for the rest of his life, since he is prone to recurrence of the disease.

## Nursing Care

The nursing care of the tuberculosis patient is centered on building up his resistance, preventing the spread of the infection to others, and helping him to adjust to his treatment. Therefore, it will include:

Attention to his diet, to make sure that he is eating enough of the food he needs.

Making him comfortable before his rest periods, and watching to see that he does not overexert himself or stay up too long if his "up" periods are limited.

Seeing that his medications are given on time if you are responsible for their administration.

Carrying out isolation technic if the infection is active. Keep the sputum cup covered and dispose of the sputum safely according to the method used in any individual institution. (It is always safe to wrap it securely and burn it.)

Teaching the patient to keep the sputum cup covered and to wash his hands frequently.

Teaching the patient to cover his mouth with a disposable tissue when he coughs. If the patient is too ill to do this, wear a face mask yourself. Change the mask frequently—if it becomes moist it can give organisms a home instead of keeping them away. A mask should not be left dangling around a nurse's neck but should be discarded when it is not in use.

Give the patient something interesting to do.

## Rehabilitation

Rehabilitation begins as soon as the patient discovers that he has tuberculosis. The patient needs to accept the fact that he has tuberculosis and must realize that if he follows instructions, he can recover.

The National Tuberculosis and Respiratory Disease Association (The Christmas Seal Association) is a national organization which is interested in research and education regarding TB and other respiratory diseases.

The patient may also need the services of vocational rehabilitation, social service, or other agencies or community resources.

## One Last Word

Contrary to what you may have heard, tuberculosis is by no means obsolete. It is dangerous to think that we can relax our efforts to detect and treat tuberculosis and to educate the public about this disease. As a citizen, each one of us has a responsibility for supporting any program to protect the health of all citizens in the community—especially the health of groups which are known to be susceptible to tuberculosis, such as children, young people, and the elderly.

## NEOPLASM OF THE LUNG

### Cancer of the Lung

Lung cancer has increased markedly during the last 20 years. It appears in most instances after the age of 40, or at least it is not discovered until then. It affects 6 times more men than women. Several reasons are given for the increase in deaths from lung cancer. One of these is the increasing pollution of the air. Also, the report of the Surgeon General's Advisory Committee found that in the majority of lung cancer deaths the victims were cigarette smokers. There are more older people in the population today, which may account partly for the high incidence of lung cancer, since it is not a disease primarily of young people.

**Symptoms.** It is hard to detect lung cancer in the early stage because the symptoms do not appear until the disease is well advanced. Lung cancer is a malignant tumor which usually appears in the bronchi and shows no symptoms until it enlarges. The first indication of trouble generally occurs when the patient begins to cough up mucus and blood-streaked sputum. Even then he may think that he is smoking too much and simply resolves to cut down. Later, he begins to feel tired, loses weight, and experiences chest pains and difficulty in breathing. When he finally consults his doctor, bronchoscopy and a sputum examination help to confirm the diagnosis of lung cancer. If the lung is the primary site for the cancer, which is the most common case, the cancer may be curable, if it is localized. If the lung tumor is a metastatic one, the prognosis is usually poor if not always so.

**Treatment.** The only possible cure for lung cancer is surgery to remove the malignant tissue. Even this is not likely to be effective unless it is performed in the early stages of the disease. The operations that are performed are *segmental resection* (removal of a segment of a lobe), *wedge resection* (removal of a wedge of lung tissue), *lobectomy* (removal of a lobe of a lung), or *pneumonectomy* (removal of a portion of the lung tissue or one whole lung), depending upon the size of the tumor and its location in the lung.

Radiation therapy sometimes helps to arrest the spread of the disease temporarily and to make the patient more comfortable. Chemotherapy may also be helpful. The mortality rate from lung cancer is high. Metastasis to the other lung or to the esophagus may have occurred by the time the disease is discovered.

The final days for a patient with terminal lung cancer are most difficult for the patient's family, as he is in such evident physical distress. The nurse is most helpful who gives compassionate attention to the patient's comfort and shows the utmost regard for the feelings of his family. She should explain any new procedure that has been introduced and show concern for their comfort by suggesting rest or a cup of coffee.

## Benign Tumors of the Lung

A benign tumor, or cyst, may also be present in the lung and is characterized on x-ray by smooth edges and sharply defined margins. It is difficult to differentiate between x-rays showing tuberculosis, benign or malignant tumors, lung abscess, or a foreign body in the lung. Bronchoscopy and biopsy are usually done to determine which of these disorders is causing the abnormal x-ray shadow on the lung.

## Nursing Care Following Lung Surgery

Generally, when surgery of the lung is done, as small a portion of the lung as possible is removed. The postoperative care is routine, with special attention directed at preventing respiratory complications. It is easier for the patient to cough if the incision is splinted with a pillow or is held tightly with both hands. In this way he can cough as much as possible. The patient must be encouraged to breathe deeply and should be given IPPB treatments to assist in the expansion of his lungs.

The 2 most serious postoperative complications are hemorrhage and pneumothorax (atelectasis). The nurse must be watchful for any signs of shock, dyspnea, or pain in the chest and must report these symptoms immediately.

## CHEST INJURIES

Accidents, such as a blow, a fall or an automobile accident which fracture ribs, are the most common cause of chest injuries. Fractured ribs may injure adjoining parts of the body, by puncturing a lung or tearing blood vessels. If there is none of these further complications, fractured ribs can be treated by immobilizing the chest with an elastic bandage or by strapping it with tape, which is applied firmly to lessen the pain which breathing causes.

Compression of the chest as the result of an explosion may rupture a lung and cause death from hemorrhage or suffocation. Wounds that penetrate the chest are very serious and may require chest drainage or surgery.

Emergency action must be taken in any puncture wound of the chest, since this allows air to enter, thus upsetting the negative pressure required for breathing. The *hole must be plugged* in any way possible, and the lungs must be re-expanded. Since the patient usually comes in as an emergency, surgery is performed immediately in order that chest tubes may be inserted for continuous closed water-seal drainage.

In a first-aid situation, do not remove the article which is puncturing the chest, if it is still in place. Bring the patient to the hospital with the object in place. If the hole is present without anything plugging it, plug it at once. Oxygen may also be helpful and mouth-to-mouth resuscitation may be needed. In this case, the hole in the chest should be unplugged on inspiration and plugged on expiration.

## AIR POLLUTION AND RESPIRATORY DISORDERS

Today, we are hearing more and more about air pollution and its deleterious effects upon our health. Not only does it sting the eyes and irritate the nose, but it also affects our breathing. It is particularly dangerous to the person who is old and subject to hypostatic pneumonia or to the person with a chronic respiratory disorder. However, everyone, sick or healthy, must work harder to get enough oxygen, when the pollution is exceptionally bad. Much research is being done in an attempt to prevent air pollution and its complications.

# 49

# The Patient With a Digestive Disorder

## BEHAVIORAL OBJECTIVES

*The student successfully attaining the goals of this chapter will be able to:*

- *discuss some of the most common digestive symptoms, utilizing proper medical terminology; and demonstrate effectiveness in dealing with these symptoms and in reporting them in the clinical area.*
- *discuss at least 8 special diagnostic procedures related to the digestive system, including a discussion of endoscopy, describing the various types; thoroughly discuss various x-ray examinations to determine digestive disorders; and demonstrate efficiency in assisting the patient and/or the medical team during such procedures.*
- *describe and discuss special nursing procedures related to digestive disorders, including a thorough discussion of gastric suction, tube feedings, and special procedures such as enemas and digital removal of feces which assist with elimination; discuss the psychological and physical aspects of the colostomy or ileostomy and its care; and demonstrate competence in providing nursing care.*
- *briefly discuss the 3 major symptoms of cancer in the digestive tract; differentiate between the symptoms of upper GI cancer as opposed to lower GI cancer.*
- *list 5 of the common disorders of the mouth, including trauma to the mouth or jaw; discuss medical and nursing care of the patient who has a disorder of the mouth or who has had mouth surgery; and demonstrate the ability to assist this patient.*
- *describe and discuss: at least 2 disorders of the esophagus; the most common disorders of the stomach, including ulcers and cancer; at least 8 disorders of the small and large intestine, including ulcerative colitis, appendicitis, and abdominal hernia; at least 4 disorders of the sigmoid or rectum, including hemorrhoids; and at least 6 common disorders of the liver, including cirrhosis and hepatitis; identify the major symptoms of each of these disorders; discuss the medical and surgical treatment in each case; and demonstrate the ability to assist the doctor and the patient in each situation.*
- *briefly discuss cancer of the liver, including physical and emotional implications.*
- *identify and discuss the 2 major disorders of the gallbladder; describe the symptoms and medical treatment of each; demonstrate the ability to assist patients with these disorders to meet their needs, whether treated medically or surgically.*
- *briefly discuss disorders of the pancreas.*

## THE DIGESTIVE SYSTEM

The digestive system is very important in the maintenance of normal balance within the body. Disease and disorders of the digestive tract may affect the mouth, the throat, the stomach, the intestines, or the rectum. (See Chapter 17 for a review of the anatomy and physiology of the digestive system.)

### Common Digestive Complaints

As noted in Chapter 30, the most common digestive complaints include nausea, vomiting, loss of appetite, heartburn, belching, stomach pains, and diarrhea or constipation. While the causes for these difficulties vary considerably, it is the nurse's responsibility to observe and record their occurrence. For instance if the patient has vomited, the nurse, aside from providing nursing care, would note a thorough description on the chart, including the amount, color, consistency, and odor, of the vomitus and if the vomiting was projectile in nature or not. In other instances, the nurse may be required to examine and describe the feces depending on the gastrointestinal disorder involved.

### Diagnostic Tests

The *special* tests commonly used in diagnosing gastrointestinal difficulties include laboratory examinations of vomitus, stomach contents and feces, visual examination or palpation of various parts of the digestive tract, and x-ray studies. The nurse's part in these procedures is to collect specimens, assist the doctor with examinations, prepare the patient and reassure him during procedures that are often tedious and uncomfortable.

**Stool Specimens.** Laboratory examination of stool specimens is a method for discovering disease organisms, parasites, and eggs, and occult (otherwise invisible) blood. The procedure for collecting a stool specimen is discussed in Chapter 29.

**Guiac Test.** The practical nurse may be asked to perform a guiac test upon feces or other excreta to ascertain the presence of blood (*melena*). It is simple to do and is often done on the nursing station or in the laboratory. The testing solutions must be poured on the stool specimen in the correct order; if a blue color shows up, this indicates the presence of blood. The instructions are usually kept with the testing kit. Tablets, test paper, and sticks are also available.

**Gastric Analysis.** One way of obtaining information about stomach difficulties is by analyzing the stomach contents in order to find out how much free hydrochloric acid is present—too much may point to peptic ulcer; too little could be a sign of cancer or pernicious anemia. Other significant facts can also be determined by this method. This analysis can be done by examining a specimen of vomitus or a portion of the stomach contents which has been aspirated by a syringe attached to a nasogastric tube inserted into the stomach.

**The Test Meal.** Digestive system disturbances do not always cause vomiting. The doctor may want an analysis of the stomach contents because other symptoms indicate trouble in the digestive system. One method of securing a specimen of the stomach contents is by the test meal. A test meal is given to stimulate the secretion of gastric juice in the stomach; then small amounts of the stomach contents are withdrawn at intervals and analyzed. The stomach contents are withdrawn in the morning because the patient has not had anything by mouth since midnight. Thus the test meal is given when the stomach is empty.

PREPARING AND SERVING A TEST MEAL. The doctor orders the type of test meal that he considers suitable for giving him the information he wants. It may be bread or toast (without crusts) given with water or tea (without cream and sugar). After the stomach is emptied, the patient eats the test meal.

**Removing Stomach Contents.** Prepare the patient by explaining that the test meal will give the doctor information about his stomach and digestion. Explain that the procedure need not be uncomfortable if he follows directions. Explain that the tube has nothing to do with the breathing apparatus; the doctor will guide the tube. The patient will be asked to swallow, then to breathe through his mouth to keep from closing his lips and teeth on the tube and obstructing it. Tell him what the food will be, to remove fears about disagreeable tastes; explain that it is important to eat it all to get the best results from the test.

In assisting with this procedure, you can put the towel under the patient's chin, wipe his mouth, encourage him in following directions, and hold the container for the stomach contents. You can remove and care for the equipment when the procedure is finished, label the specimens, and see that they get to the laboratory.

PROCEDURE. The usual procedure followed in gastric analysis is:

1. No food or fluids are given for 12 hours before the test. This order means that nothing is allowed by mouth after midnight for an 8 A.M. test.
2. Insert the nasogastric tube. Instruct the patient to avoid swallowing saliva, if possible, during the test.
3. Withdraw the specimen. Clamp the tube after this withdrawal to prevent air from entering the stomach.
4. Withdraw the other specimens at the prescribed intervals (if ordered).
5. Label the specimens according to the order in which they were obtained and the time.
6. Withdraw the tube, give mouth care, and serve the patient his breakfast.

Sometimes histamine is given subcutaneously after the first specimen has been collected in order to stimulate gastric secretions. Since some people are sensitive to histamine, these patients should be watched closely for signs of shock. Pallor, sweating, and a weak and rapid pulse are danger signals. Some doctors leave an order to give epinephrine immediately if shock occurs.

**Examination of Stomach Contents.** Stomach contents may be examined for bacteria (such as tuberculosis), blood, free hydrochloric acid, combined hydrochloric acid, and organic acids and acid salts. Some of these tests are done after fasting and some after a test meal has been eaten or a drug administered. One method of determining the presence of free hydrochloric acid in the stomach is by the oral administration of a dye, *azuresin*. Azuresin will color the urine blue if it is acted upon by hydrochloric acid.

**X-Ray and Fluoroscopic Examinations.** The development of x-ray photography (roentgenography) and the fluoroscopic screen (fluoroscopy) have made it possible to photograph or view conditions anywhere within the gastrointestinal tract. This is done by means of a radiopaque substance, usually barium sulfate, which is given orally or rectally, depending upon which area is to be investigated. The progress of this substance through the gastrointestinal tract is noted on films at suitable intervals and on the fluoroscopic screen. The doctor observes how long it takes the barium to pass through and notes any abnormalities in the shape of the organs or the passages that might indicate ulcers or tumors. Hard bone tissues contain mineral salts that the x-rays do not penetrate easily, so the shape of bones will show on the film. The stomach and the intestines are soft tissues—in order to see their shape, it is necessary to give the patient another kind of test meal containing a substance that x-rays will not penetrate (barium).

BARIUM BY MOUTH OR RECTUM. Barium salts are heavy and are used most commonly. For examinations of the stomach and the duodenum, an upper gastrointestinal series or "upper G.I." is done, in which the patient drinks a preparation of barium (in buttermilk or chocolate milk or a similar drink). The preparation is given by rectum if the colon is to be examined (lower gastrointestinal series or lower G.I.). Sometimes both series of tests are given in a combined upper and lower G.I. series.

The area to be examined is under the fluoroscope as the patient drinks the fluid, and the outlines of the stomach and its outlet and the intestinal tract are observed. X-rays are taken at definite intervals afterward, to photograph the outlines of the stomach and the intestines and to note the progress of the material through the digestive tract.

PREPARATION FOR X-RAY EXAMINATION AND AFTER-CARE. The entire alimentary tract is prepared for the examination by emptying it as thoroughly as possible. This is done by the use of cathartics and enemas. The patient is not allowed to have food preceding the examination or for some time afterward. The doctor leaves definite orders about the time when food may be given; this is usually some time after the first follow-up x-ray picture has been taken. It is important to be alert about the orders for patients who are having a series of stomach and intestinal or other x-ray investigations.

ASSISTING WITH X-RAY EXAMINATIONS. Be sure the area around the rectum is clean before the patient goes for the examination. You may be asked to take him to the x-ray department—he will go on a stretcher or in a wheelchair, depending on his condition at the time. Stay with him until someone in the x-ray department takes over; he has had no food and may become faint or fall from the stretcher or wheelchair if left alone. If you are required to stay during the examination, you help the patient out of and into the wheelchair or assist in moving him to and from the x-ray table and the stretcher. (It is important for the nurse to remember to protect herself, during the procedure, from x-rays, by wearing a lead apron. If the nurse is in the first trimester of pregnancy, she should not assist with x-rays of any kind.)

*The Nurse's Responsibility.* This series of pictures is often called a *G.I. series.* The nurse prepares the patient, looks after him during the series and after it has been completed. Her responsibilities are:

To see that the patient has no food or fluid preceding x-rays of the upper gastrointestinal tract.

To give the laxative and the enema (or enemas) prescribed in preparation for x-ray studies of the large intestine.

To check with the x-ray department, to make sure that the series has been completed before giving the patient something to eat.

To note bowel movements and whether or not barium is passed—often a cathartic is necessary to eliminate it, and is usually prescribed as a part of the routine orders. A hard mass of retained barium might cause a bowel obstruction. The nurse must be very alert for symptoms of constipation, following a G.I. series.

To provide emotional support. The patient is likely to be afraid of the procedure and may dread the results or be afraid of the large x-ray equipment. He should be reassured and supported as much as possible. The patient may also be embarrassed about the positions he must assume during the procedure. The nurse can be helpful by teaching the patient before the procedure and by allowing him to verbalize his feelings.

**Endoscopy.** Certain hollow instruments, or *scopes,* make it possible to look at different parts of the gastrointestinal tract by means of tiny electric bulbs and mirrors within the instrument. According to the part which is being examined, the most common of these procedures are called *esophagoscopy* (esophagus), *gastroscopy* (stomach), *proctoscopy* (rectum and anus), and *sigmoidoscopy* (sigmoid colon). The nurse carries out the prescribed preparations for these procedures but the examination itself is usually performed in an operating or examining room. The patient may be apprehensive and tense beforehand and in need of reassurance. Because this type of examination is often uncomfortable and may be painful, a sedative may be ordered for the patient both before and after the examination.

A foreign object, such as a pin, may be removed during endoscopy, especially esophagoscopy. A pincher-type apparatus or an electromagnet may be used.

**Abdominal Paracentesis.** This refers to the puncture of the abdominal cavity in order to obtain a specimen or to drain off excess fluid. Depending on the purpose, the procedure may be called a *diagnostic* abdominal tap or puncture (fluid is examined microscopically or cultured), or a *therapeutic* abdominal tap or puncture (to relieve pressure in the abdomen).

A diagnostic puncture is done when bleeding or infection is suspected. It is not done if the bowel is obstructed or distended or if the patient has a blood clotting defect.

In preparation for the procedure the abdomen is shaved and scrubbed. It is very important for the patient to void immediately before the procedure to avoid rupture of the urinary bladder. Sometimes, fluid is obtained from each of the four quadrants of the abdomen and is examined and compared to determine the location of bleeding or infection.

Therapeutic abdominal tap is done when the patient is distended (*ascites*). Since he may also have difficulty in breathing, the removal of fluid will assist him. The patient is usually sitting for the procedure and the fluid is obtained from the lower portion of the abdomen. Sometimes, a catheter is inserted into the abdominal cavity for continuous drainage.

It is important for the nurse to support the patient during the procedure. She is also responsible for measuring the amount of fluid obtained and for seeing that the appropriate specimens are taken to the laboratory. A therapeutic tap may need to be repeated at intervals.

**Liver Biopsy.** The liver biopsy (needle biopsy of the liver) is most often done to verify a case of suspected cancer of the liver or to determine other disorders of the liver. However, the liver biopsy is not done in the patient who has a bleeding tendency, since the liver is a very vascular organ. A small piece of liver tissue is obtained by means of a long needle with an inner cutting cannula. The needle is inserted, with the assistance of a stylet, so that it is not hollow. The stylet is then withdrawn and the inner cannula is inserted beyond the end of the needle and rotated to obtain a specimen. This is then withdrawn. (A sample may also be obtained by suction.) The sample of tissue is examined microscopically to determine the presence of microorganisms or cancer cells.

The skin is anesthetized before the large needle is inserted, and the patient is instructed not to breathe while the needle is being inserted into the liver. The nurse should explain the procedure and assist the patient to maintain proper position while the procedure is being done. It is very important to observe the patient after the procedure for any sign of bleeding, either into the abdomen or from the puncture site itself.

## COMMON NURSING PROCEDURES

### Suction Drainage (Gastrointestinal Decompression)

The patient with a small rubber or plastic tube extending from his nostril is a fairly common sight on hospital wards. The inner end of this tube may terminate in the patient's stomach (Levin tube), or if the tube is longer (Miller-Abbott, Cantor, or Harris tubes), it may extend into the intestine. The outer end may have a clamp attached, or a glass connection may link it to longer tubing attached to one or more bottles at the bedside (Wangensteen apparatus). Suction operates when a vacuum is created by means of an electric machine, a built-in wall attachment, or through the specific arrangement of the tubes and the bottles. Suction can also be created by drawing on the end of the tube with a syringe.

Suction is used for periodic or continuous drainage in gastrointestinal conditions in order:

1. To get a specimen of stomach or intestinal contents for examination
2. To treat intestinal obstruction
3. To prevent and treat distention after surgery by removing gas and toxic fluid materials from the stomach or the intestines
4. To empty the stomach prior to emergency surgery or after swallowing poisons
5. To protect the suture line following gastrointestinal surgery.

**Nursing Care.** Special points to observe in the care of a patient with suction drainage are:

Be sure to explain the procedures to the patient.

Measure and record fluid intake and output, *including drainage,* because it is important to keep a careful check on the patient's fluid balance.

Give soothing mouth rinses and apply a lubricant to the patient's lips and nostril, and K-Y jelly to the catheter where it touches the nostril. Because he must breathe through it, the patient's mouth becomes dry and parched. If he is able, let him brush his teeth himself but tell him to rinse his mouth well and not to swallow. A humidifier is often ordered.

Check to see that the drainage is flowing into the bottle and that the nasal catheter is in place. Check the level of the fluid in the drainage bottle; it should be emptied when it reaches a designated mark.

You may not be responsible for irrigating the nasal catheter, but you should know that in order to keep the tube open, small amounts of water or saline solution are injected through it from time to time. The tube should be taped securely so that it cannot be pulled out and does not pull on the patient's nose. Generally, it is taped under the nose or to the nose and, again, to the patient's cheek or forehead. Hypoallergenic tape should be used, since it is less irritating. The skin may be prepared with tincture of benzoin before applying the tape. The tube is then attached to the bed so that it will run in a straight line from the bed to the drainage bottle. The patient must be allowed enough tubing so that he can move about in bed. When the patient gets up, the suction apparatus can go along, or if the doctor has ordered, it can be disconnected.

If the tube is irritating, the patient may need soothing medication for his throat. Sometimes an ice collar or chewing gum offers relief. Small sips of water are sometimes given, even though it will be returned with the drainage. (Be sure to measure this and subtract from the drainage amount.)

INSERTING THE NASOGASTRIC OR GASTROINTESTINAL TUBES. The practical nurse generally is not asked to insert the nasogastric tube but may often be asked to assist the doctor or professional nurse with the procedure. The practical nurse should *never* insert a nasogastric tube unless she is carefully instructed and checked in doing the procedure.

The nurse must have ready the tube, ice, if needed, water-soluble lubricant for the tube, a syringe or bulb (for inserting air to see if the tube is in place or for withdrawing solution), an emesis basin, proper draping for the patient, tape, and a stethoscope or glass of water. The tube is passed through the nose (or mouth, if absolutely necessary) after being lubricated with water-soluble lubricant. Sterile, disposable tubes are now used, to prevent cross-contamination. The person inserting the tube may wear gloves, but this is not necessary. However, good handwashing must be observed both before the procedure to prevent gross contamination of the patient and after the procedure to prevent infection of the nurse or doctor. The tube is inserted while the patient swallows. Small sips of water through a straw may help. It is vital to be careful not to insert the tube into the trachea or the patient will aspirate. This water must not be given until the tube is past the trachea. The location of the tube in the stomach may be evidenced by aspiration of stomach contents or by placing the tube in a glass of water. If it bubbles, it is in the lungs and must be removed immediately. Sometimes, the doctor will quickly inject a syringe-full of air and listen to the stomach. If the tube is in the stomach, he will be able to hear the rush of air. The danger of aspiration cannot be overemphasized; it is a fatal complication.

Other complications of using nasogastric tubes may include otitis media, infection of the stomach or small intestine, inflammation of the nose or mouth, or ulceration of the nose or larynx. The nurse must keep in mind that the nasogastric tube is potentially dangerous and must be alert for complications.

IRRIGATING THE NASOGASTRIC TUBE. If the nurse is asked to irrigate the tube, a small amount of fluid, usually saline, is injected into the tube after which suction is reapplied. The nurse usually does not draw back on the syringe, because of the danger of damage to the gastrointestinal tract. The gastric contents should return freely. The nurse must observe the nature and amount of the aspirant, as well as the fact that the tube is or is not *patent*. A plugged nasogastric tube can be a very serious complication and should be reported immediately. The nurse must remember to chart or record the amount of irrigating solution used, so that this can be subtracted from the amount of drainage.

*The Suction Machine.* The nasogastric tube will be connected to a 3-bottle-suction apparatus (Wangensteen suction) or to a mechanical suction machine, such as the Gomko suction. The nurse must be alert to any failure of the mechanical apparatus and report this. It is also important to watch the 3-bottle suction and make sure to change the bottles as soon as they are empty.

REMOVING THE TUBE. Usually, the tube is clamped for a few days before it is removed, to make sure that the patient can tolerate its absence. It is removed, simply by pulling it out, slowly at first, and rapidly when the patient begins to cough. Resistance is very seldom encountered. The nurse should be sure to remove any tape marks from the patient's face. Be sure to conceal the tube after removal and to give good mouth care to the patient. A small diet is started and the nurse must be alert to any complaints of discomfort, distention, or nausea.

Types of Tubes. There are several commonly-used types of tubes. The *Levin tube* is made of either rubber or plastic. If made of rubber, it may need to be placed in ice before being inserted, so that it will be stiffer. This is not necessary with a plastic tube. This tube may be placed into the stomach for aspiration or into the esophagus for feeding. The *Wangensteen tube* has several holes near the end and is used for aspiration of the stomach.

The *Miller-Abbott tube* is longer and may be used for decompression of the small intestine. This tube has 2 lumens, one for irrigation and for removal of gastrointestinal contents and one for inflation of a balloon at the end of the tube. It is important to check the balloon before insertion to make sure that it will inflate properly. It is also important to be sure that the balloon is entirely deflated before insertion. The tube is radiopaque and may be visualized by x-ray, so that the doctor can tell exactly where it is located. It is generally advanced a few inches every hour after entering the duodenum, until it reaches the desired location within the small intestine. It is important to tape or fasten the tube each time it is advanced, so that it will not be pulled out. If it is taped, adhesive tape should not be used, because traces of tape will be left on the tube. It is also important to mark the end of the tube which leads to the balloon, so that irrigating solution will not be injected into this lumen by mistake. Occasionally, this can cause great difficulty in the intestinal tract.

The *Cantor tube* has mercury in the balloon and has one lumen, used both for irrigation and aspiration. This tube is marked "S," "P," and "D," which indicates the various lengths which will reach the stomach, the pyloric area, and the duodenum. The normal peristalsis will assist in advancing the tube, but when it has reached the desired location, the peristalsis on the mercury will continue, which may cause a pull on the tube.

REMOVING LONG TUBES. The doctor will generally do this procedure, taking caution to prevent perforation of the bowel. The tube should not be removed if there is any resistance. Generally, if difficulty is encountered, a repeated attempt, in an hour or so, will be successful. Occasionally, though rarely, if it is impossible to remove the tube, it will be cut at the nose and allowed to pass through the gastrointestinal tract.

**Tubes to Compress Esophageal or Gastric Varices.** A tube may be inserted and balloons inflated to stop bleeding from varices or from an ulcer in the cardiac area of the stomach. The most common tube for this purpose is the Sengstaken-Blakemore tube, which has 3 lumens. One is for irrigation and aspiration of the stomach and has several openings at the end of the tube. The second leads to a small balloon which is placed just inside the stomach and puts pressure against the cardiac area of the stomach. The third leads to a long, thin balloon which, when inflated, presses against the walls of the esophagus, to compress varices and stop massive hemorrhage. These holes must be carefully labeled. An x-ray indicates proper placement of the tube. The balloon lumens are clamped off and the aspiration lumen is connected to suction. Nasotracheal suction is often necessary for this patient, since he cannot swallow. Great care must be taken to prevent aspiration into the lungs.

## Tube Feedings

**Nasogastric Feedings.** If the tube is inserted for the purpose of feeding the patient, the feedings are given in the same way as for gastrostomy feedings. (See next section and Chapter 48.) While the gastrostomy is an operation to create a permanent feeding opening into the stomach, the nasogastric feeding tube is a temporary measure.

**Gastrostomy Feedings.** *Gastrostomy* is a comparatively simple operation in itself; it is not performed as often as it once was now that the treatment of esophageal diseases and difficulties has improved. A temporary or permanent gastrostomy may still be necessary to treat conditions that cause esophageal obstructions. The operation consists of making a small incision in the upper abdomen and inserting a catheter into the stomach. The catheter is then sutured into place. The tube is clamped between feedings. Special attention is given to the care of the skin around the tubes because gastric contents are very irritating. For this purpose, ointments may be applied (petrolatum, zinc oxide). Tube feeding technic is discussed under cancer of the larynx (Chap. 48). The principles and the technics which apply to the nasogastric tube also apply to the gastrostomy tube.

After sufficient healing has taken place, the tube is removed after feedings and reinserted each time. A permanent plastic button in the opening (stoma) has a removable plug which keeps the stoma closed when the tube is removed. As soon as he is able, the patient is taught to feed himself and learns how to insert and remove the tube, using clean technic.

## Special Procedures for Elimination

**Enemas.** The patient with a disorder of the digestive system may need an enema, either to prepare for a diagnostic test or surgery or to alleviate symptoms of constipation or distention. An enema may also be given to administer specific medications and fluids or to stop bleeding. (See Chapter 29 for previous discussion.)

**Digital Removal of a Fecal Impaction.** This procedure has been discussed previously, but will be reviewed here, since it is frequently done for severely constipated patients, such as elderly persons who have not been receiving adequate medical attention and come into the hospital with fecal impaction. The digital removal of an impaction is done only after attempts have been made to remove the fecal mass by use of stool softeners or enemas (most often, oil retention enemas are used).

A fecal impaction may be confusing in its symptoms, since the most frequent symptom is that of diarrhea. The impaction stays in place, but diarrhea occurs when liquids pass around the impaction. The alert nurse will report the symptoms of diarrhea, which, in this case is very watery and is accompanied by rectal pain and cramps. An impaction may occur also after barium enema and should be considered as a possible complication of the procedure.

Digital removal of fecal impaction (also called manual fragmentation or disimpaction) is accomplished by the doctor or nurse, depending upon the severity of the impaction and the condition of the patient. Sometimes, anesthesia, either local or general, must be used to relieve pain. It is a good idea to offer the patient his pain medication before the procedure is done.

If the nurse is to manually remove an impaction, she should wear gloves, explain to the patient what she is going to do, and position the patient so he is most comfortable. Usually, the patient lies on his left side with knees drawn up as far as possible. He will be most comfortable if he takes panting breaths during the procedure. The impaction is removed as carefully as possible. In the case of a woman, a sterile gloved finger may be inserted into the vagina to assist in removing the fecal mass.

### The Patient With a Colostomy or Ileostomy

Many of the diseases or conditions that affect the intestinal tract require surgical treatment which may include a *colostomy* (an opening into the colon) or an *ileostomy* (an opening into the ileum). The purpose in this operation is to provide an artificial outlet for feces when irritation or obstruction of the intestinal tract makes it necessary to divert fecal material from the normal rectal outlet. An incision is made in the abdomen and a loop of intestine is brought through the incision and opened to allow for the drainage of feces.

A colostomy or an ileostomy may be only temporary, if treatment to eliminate or relieve the condition that made it necessary is successful. If this is the case, an operation to close the intestinal and abdominal openings is performed, and the feces are allowed to resume the normal outlet through the rectum. If treatment necessitates the removal of the colon or the rectum, the colostomy will be permanent.

**After the Operation—The Colostomy.** The colostomy opening, or *stoma,* is separate from the incision through which the operation was performed. (It is usually on the left side of the abdomen.) When the patient returns from the operating room, the stoma is covered

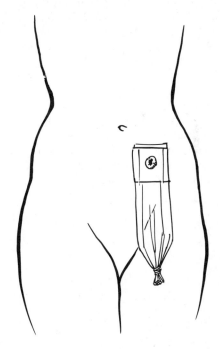

Figure 49-1. A plastic ileostomy (or colostomy) drainage bag. The bag is held snugly around the stoma by adhesive. The bag can be emptied from the bottom by removing the elastic bands. (Smith, D. W., and Gips, C. D.: Care of the Adult Patient, p. 903, Philadelphia, Lippincott, 1963)

by gauze dressings or by a plastic disposable bag or pouch which is held in place by double-faced adhesive or special skin glue. This bag fits tightly, to catch the drainage—the end is held firmly by elastic bands to make it leak-proof (Fig. 49-1). These bands are removed to empty it, and the contents are allowed to drain into an emesis basin or into the toilet or bedpan. The bag is replaced by a clean one whenever this is necessary. Later, when the stoma has shrunk, the bag may be replaced by a permanent appliance. If dressings are used, a combination of gauze fluffs and cellulose pads held in place by Montgomery straps (tapes) is applied to absorb the drainage. The adhesive ends of the straps are placed on the skin (which has been painted with compound benzoin tincture) well away from the stoma, while the other ends remain free with the sticky sides covered. Tapes passed through eyelets on the free ends are tied over the dressings to secure them. This prevents the skin from becoming irritated because adhesive will not have to be removed every time the dressing is changed.

The constant discharge of liquid feces at first after the operation makes it necessary to change the dressings or empty the bag frequently. This also helps to reduce odor and to prevent irritation of the skin around the stoma. Clean, rather than sterile, technic is adequate in changing the dressings, because the opening is contaminated by the bacteria that are always present in feces. However, it is important to avoid contaminating anything else by the soiled dressings.

The essential equipment for this procedure often is kept by the bedside. It consists of:

| | |
|---|---|
| Dressings or plastic pouches | A skin lubricant |
| Montgomery straps | Basin for soap and water |
| Newspapers or bags for soiled dressings | |

**Changing the Dressings.** Remove the soiled dressings or pouch to the newspaper; wash the skin around the opening with mild soap and warm water. Use only water if the skin is irritated. If necessary, apply whatever lubricant is ordered—petrolatum gauze, aluminum paste, or Amphojel. Remove the lubricant from the skin often enough to inspect it for irritation. Put on the dressings

or pouch; if a pouch is used, fit it snugly to prevent leakage around the edges. The skin must be dry, or the adhesive will not stick. The ambulatory patient will need an elastic belt to support the pouch.

THE IMPORTANCE OF CLEANLINESS. Cleanliness is of the utmost importance. The patient is likely to feel soiled enough without having to be conscious of a soiled gown or bedclothing and saturated dressings. Be careful to change everything that becomes soiled, trying to do this before mealtime approaches in order to avoid affecting the patient's appetite. Be gentle, but professional about everything you must do for the patient.

TEACHING THE PATIENT. Before the patient can learn how to change his dressing himself, he must be ready to accept the idea of doing it. It may be some time before he can even look at the colostomy opening or shows any interest in how you change the dressing. Eventually, he must learn to do this himself, and the nurse has to decide when he is ready to be taught. As he gradually learns to accept his condition, he responds to things more calmly and begins to take an interest in what is being done for him. A nurse can always help to stimulate his interest by casual, but encouraging, comments about his progress, such as: "Having more to eat makes the drainage more like a regular bowel movement. It looks as if you might be ready for your permanent colostomy arrangement before too long."

When the patient begins to show signs of being interested in his dressing, you can explain each step of the procedure, telling him why it is done. Let him watch you several times, then let him help by holding the equipment and handing you supplies. Encourage him to try doing the dressing himself after a while, assuring him that you will stand by to advise and help him. Do this enough times to be sure that he is ready to try doing it on his own. This does not mean that after he takes over you will abandon him. You must make it a point to watch him periodically to see if he remembers how to do the procedure correctly and to check on the drainage and on the condition of the skin around the stoma.

**The Colostomy Irrigation.** The irrigation may be given with the patient in bed but it is better to give it in the bathroom as soon as he is allowed up, since he can sit on the toilet and the drainage can go into the toilet. While he is still in the hospital he should learn to perform the irrigation himself. At first, he may be upset at the prospect of having to accept this as a procedure that he must carry out every day or so for the rest of his life. It may take a little time before he is convinced that, compared with the embarrassment and the inconvenience of fecal leakage and soiled dressings, it is well worth the effort. With a controlled low-residue diet and well-established regular evacuation, some patients do not need an irrigation every day. However, this depends on the needs of the individual patient.

The patient may be afraid to attempt the procedure on his own; he should have enough practice to give him self-confidence before he leaves the hospital, with sufficient supervision to ensure a correct performance.

The procedure for a colostomy irrigation takes about 20 to 30 minutes and consists of alternately injecting warm tap water (or other prescribed solution) into the bowel and allowing the fluid and feces to return through an outlet into the toilet bowl. This procedure is repeated until the return flow is clear of fecal material. Continuous irrigation is also possible with the use of a colostomy irrigator tip.

### EQUIPMENT

A No. 16 or a No. 18, French catheter
Irrigating set with tubing, adaptor, and clamp
Lubricant
Toilet tissue
Newspaper or bag for soiled dressings
Solution as ordered
Provision for hanging up the irrigating can
Colostomy irrigator (can be obtained from a surgical supply house—several makes are available). This is a special tip which prevents the colon from being punctured. An irrigating sleeve or trough is also available through which the solution may be channelled after it leaves the stoma.

### SUGGESTED PROCEDURE

Remove the bag or pouch gently. The solution is injected by inserting the irrigating tip or catheter into the stoma, attaching the catheter to the irrigating can tubing, and allowing the solution to run into the bowels. (The tube should be filled with fluid first, so that air will not be inserted into the bowel.)

*Guide: Lubricate the catheter.*

The amount of solution will vary—500 cc. or more may be given until the patient complains of a full feeling or cramps.

*Guide: Control the rate of flow by raising or lowering the can.*

The feces and the fluid drain into the toilet through the irrigator outlet or irrigation sleeve, which hangs down between the patient's legs.

*Guide: More solution is given when the return flow stops.*

Continue the irrigation until the return flow is clear.

*Guide: The total amount for this irrigation may be anywhere from 1 to several quarts.*

Stimulate peristalsis by using warm solution, by using sufficient fluid to distend the bowel, by massaging the abdomen, and by exercise (instruct the patient to stand up a few times).

*Guide: Peristalsis moves the feces through the intestines.*

When the return flow is clear, the inflow tubing and the outlet into the toilet bowl are closed off, and the catheter is withdrawn.

*Guide: Prevent soiling by leaving the catheter in place until the last of the fluid has been expelled.*

When the catheter is removed, the area around the stoma is washed with soap and water and dried to prevent irritation, and the stoma is covered with a clean dressing.

If an irrigation sleeve is used, it may be rolled up and left in place for $\frac{1}{2}$ to 1 hour, to prevent accidents.

IF THE PATIENT IS CONFINED TO BED. The procedure for an irrigation if the patient is not allowed out of bed is the same as for the ambulatory patient, with these exceptions:

The patient lies on his side near the edge of the bed.

The outlet tube for the drainage must be long enough to reach into a bedpan at the bedside.

**The Regulated Colostomy.** Generally, after a few weeks or months, the colostomy will become regulated enough so that the patient will only need to wear a small dressing or bandage to cover the stoma. It is a good idea to put lubricant on the stoma so the dressing will not stick. He will most likely need to irrigate only every other day. Very few accidents will occur if the patient follows the irrigation instructions and the diet prescribed for him.

**The Colostomy Diet.** Foods which cause gas or stimulate bowel movements, such as high-bulk foods, are eliminated, especially at first. The goal is a mildly-constipating diet, which will help regulate the colostomy. After about 6 weeks, the patient can begin to eat more foods, until he is eating a normal diet. However, he should avoid any foods which cause irritation or diarrhea. The foods which are most likely to cause difficulty are onions, cabbage, beans, cauliflower, chocolate, fatty foods, fresh fruits, and dried fruits such as raisins, dates, and prunes. The nurse can help the patient select a helpful diet and can remind him that all food should be chewed well in order to cut down on roughage.

**Differences between an Ileostomy and Colostomy.** An ileostomy differs in several ways from a colostomy. For one thing in an ileostomy, the colon is removed. The stoma also is smaller and is usually on the other side of the abdomen (right). The discharge will be much more watery than that of a colostomy (although it will become thicker), because the large intestine, which does most of the water absorption, is missing. Thus a collecting pouch must be worn at all times to collect the discharge and should be emptied at 3- or 4-hour intervals and changed every day or two.

Immediately after surgery, the stoma will be swollen and may bleed occasionally. As its size decreases, appropriate holes are cut in the disposable bags which are applied. After about 6 weeks, the stoma can be measured for a permanent appliance. It is important that the appliance fit properly or it will leak. The patient should be advised to purchase 2 appliances, so that one can be aired while the other is worn.

The appliance or pouch is applied by means of a karaya gum washer and sometimes an adhesive disc. It is important to center the stoma to prevent irritation. The pouch is taped (preferably with hypoallergenic tape, such as Micropore) so that it cannot leak. The bottom is closed with a clip, so that air and drainage can be released at intervals. The skin must be carefully cleansed to prevent irritation. If the skin is not completely dry, the appliance will not stick. The ileal drainage is much more irritating than the colostomy drainage, so special attention must be given to skin

care and protection. Cement solvent is usually used to remove the pouch, since it is attached to the skin. The pouch is gradually removed, with care being taken not to pull or tear the skin. (All the solvent must be washed off or it will cause irritation.)

The appliance is thoroughly cleaned and aired after removal, while the other appliance is worn. Care must be taken to allow air to circulate through the bag and appliance. The adhesive disc and karaya gum washer are discarded each time the bag is changed.

**The Ileostomy Diet.** Most patients will need to follow a special diet for a few weeks following surgery and can then gradually progress to a general diet. The prevention of diarrhea is even more important for the ileostomy patient than for the colostomy patient, because diarrhea is more likely to occur. Thus it is very important to chew food well. If, as occasionally happens, a food is eliminated in a completely undigested state, this food should be omitted from the diet. Other foods, such as nuts, whole-kernel corn, popcorn, coleslaw, and many Chinese foods, must be omitted because of the danger of obstruction. Fruits with seeds are often avoided because of their high residue content, as are gas-forming foods since the patient has no control in expelling gas.

**General Consideration in Colostomy or Ileostomy.** Good skin care has already been mentioned. The patient should be careful to prevent diarrhea, and should seek medical attention if it occurs. Since sodium and potassium will be lost should diarrhea occur, foods high in these electrolytes should be eaten.

Odor can be a problem, but is usually controlled by diet and by keeping the appliance or dressing clean. Tablets, containing charcoal, chlorophyll, or bismuth preparations, can be placed in the appliance or taken orally to help prevent odor. Aspirin tablets also may be placed into the pouch after emptying to eliminate odor.

Traveling is no problem if the patient remembers to take his supplies along. However, he should take a diarrhea medication along, since a change in food or water may cause an upset. Abdominal hair should be cut with a scissors, not a razor, to prevent cutting the skin.

**The Patient's Reactions.** The patient who learns that he is to have a colostomy or ileostomy must face a readjustment, especially if the "ostomy" is to be permanent. The doctor is not always able to assure the patient before his operation that this will be only a temporary arrangement. One never knows exactly what a patient is thinking or how many fears he is keeping to himself. Naturally, he wonders how much of his life will be disrupted, perhaps imagining it as beset by offensive odors, discharges, and soiled dressings. He may be worried about the effect on his marital relationships, about his care, and the possibility of becoming repulsive to his family and friends. He dreads the thought of being "different" and may think that bulky dressings or an awkward appliance will affect his appearance.

THE EFFECT ON HIS FAMILY. The implications of a colostomy can have a very disturbing effect on the patient's family, who will worry about many of the same things that bother him—they may be especially concerned about the care that he will need and how it will affect their home life. Also, they may be afraid that they will find a colostomy revolting and worry about concealing their feelings from the patient.

HELPING THE PATIENT. The patient should be encouraged to talk about his worries and to ask questions about the things that trouble him. This provides an opportunity to unburden his mind and to get correct information that will give him reassurance about his future. He must be shown that a colostomy does not necessarily mean that he is condemned to a useless, unhappy life. However, this point of view will not be achieved in a day. The patient will need time to come to terms with this revolutionary change in his life—to feel that it will be possible to learn to live with it. Therefore, he may not be ready mentally or physically to accept detailed instruction about the care of an "ostomy" before his operation. One thing that helps to prepare a patient for a hopeful outcome is to have him talk with someone who has a colostomy and is living a normal, active life. "Ostomy clubs" throughout the country arrange for this type of contact which also provides an opportunity to benefit from the experience of others in caring for a colostomy. Finally a referral to the public health nurse may prove helpful to the patient.

# CANCER IN THE GASTROINTESTINAL TRACT

Cancer occurs within the gastrointestinal tract in the mouth, the esophagus, the stomach, the large intestine, and the rectum; however, cancer is rarely seen in the small intestine. The general symptoms are the same as for cancer in any other part of the body: fatigue, loss of weight, weakness, and anemia. Unfortunately, pain does not appear in the early stages. Cancer of the mouth, the esophagus, the stomach, and the rectum affects more men than women; however, more women have cancer of the colon.

**Symptoms.** The specific symptoms of cancer of the gastrointestinal tract are:

1. Digestive disturbances, such as loss of appetite, indigestion, changes in bowel habits
2. Interference with the passage of food, fluids, and flatus
3. Bleeding, colored either bright red or dark brown (coffee grounds), appearing in vomitus or in tarry stools

Cancer of the gastrointestinal tract is detected by the appropriate tests and examinations, including *biopsy*—the microscopic examination of a piece of the suspected tissue.

# DISORDERS OF THE MOUTH

Mouth disorders may not seem to be dangerous, but they are uncomfortable, often painful, and at times disfiguring or cosmetically unattractive. They may also interfere with nutrition or lead to other undesirable or more serious conditions.

**Vincent's Angina.** Vincent's angina (*trench mouth*) is a mouth infection which is highly communicable and can be spread from person to person, although some people are not susceptible to it. Small ulcers appear on the mucous membrane of the mouth and are sometimes accompanied by fever and the enlargement of the lymph nodes beneath the jaw. Sometimes trench mouth is associated with dental caries or abscessed teeth. Two organisms are its immediate cause (*Bacillus fusiformis* and *Barrelia vincentii*). The gums swell and ooze blood, and the tissues become necrotic. Without treatment, the infection may destroy parts of the bone. The most effective treatment is hourly mouth washes with a sodium perborate solution. Penicillin is also effective.

**Dental Caries (Tooth Decay).** This is an erosive process which breaks down the tooth enamel and later invades the pulp of the tooth itself, causing discomfort and often necessitating removal of the tooth. The chief cause of dental decay is the growth of mouth bacteria which are nourished by food particles left on the teeth as a result of faulty brushing. The decay and how successful it is in invading the teeth depends upon the following factors: the acids in the mouth and how well they can destroy bacteria; the presence of plaques on the teeth, which predispose to bacterial growth; the susceptibility of the teeth to decay; and the length of time between brushings or removal of wastes from the mouth.

Good toothbrushing is essential to the development of a healthy mouth and the prevention of tooth decay, as is fluoridation of water which helps develop stronger tooth enamel which resists the invasion of bacteria. Professional dental care is also important. The child should see the dentist at least twice a year from the time he is about 3 years old, because the detection and repair of early cavities prevents development of serious decay. Attention to the baby teeth (deciduous) is important because they lie next to the permanent teeth and can cause infection in the permanent teeth.

**Dentures.** Many people put off having infected teeth removed because they dread replacing them with dentures which they fear will be unsightly or uncomfortable. Meanwhile, they are exposing themselves to disorders in some other part of the body, such as arthritis or heart disease. So much more is known today about the dangers of infected teeth, and so much improvement has been made in the appearance of dentures that people are losing some of their dread of wearing them. Dentures are bound to be slightly uncomfortabe when they are first fitted, but the dentist can remove sources of irritation. The only way to become accustomed to dentures is to wear them all the time. This also helps to preserve the normal shape of the face.

**Stomatitis (Foot-and-Mouth Disease).** *Stomatitis* is a contagious virus disease of animals with cloven hooves. It is transmitted to humans by contact with the infected animals and their milk. The symptoms are fever and an eruption of blisters in the mouth and the throat which break and leave ulcers. The treatment is a mouthwash of potassium permanganate and the application of silver nitrate to the ulcers. Communicable disease technic is observed.

**Herpes Simplex Infection (Cold Sore, Fever Blister).** Many people are often plagued with cold sores, which usually will remiss spontaneously, without scars and without treatment. Sometimes, they are made more comfortable by the application of a specific medication.

**Canker Sores.** *Canker sores* are small, white, painful ulcers that appear on the inside of the mouth. No one knows exactly what causes them, but there is some reason to believe that they are caused by the same virus that causes cold sores. No effective treatment has been found, and they usually disappear in a few days. Peroxide or camphor may be effective in drying up or in relieving the pain of a canker sore.

**Peridontal Conditions.** *Peridontal disease* affects the bones and the tissues around the teeth. It may be the result of poor oral hygiene, inadequate dental care, or poor nutrition. Teeth become loosened when crooked teeth do not meet evenly (malocclusion) or when an accumulation of tartar eventually loosen them. Good dental care is a preventive measure.

**Trauma.** Many accidents cause injury to the mouth such as a fracture of the jaw, laceration of the lips, or the traumatic removal of teeth.

In the case of lacerations of the lips, simple suturing is usually effective, because the lips have good blood supply and usually heal without complications. However, if the entire lip is severed, the patient may have difficulty later in smiling, in applying lipstick, or, occasionally, in speaking distinctly.

If the jaw is fractured, usually the two jaws are wired or fastened together so that the jaw will heal without the fracture becoming dislocated. The nurse must always remember that the patient cannot open his mouth and must be ready to assist him in an emergency. A wire cutter must be kept *with the patient* at all times, so that in case of severe coughing, or vomiting, the wires which connect the top jaw to the bottom jaw can be cut immediately. Otherwise, the patient will choke.

The patient with a fracture and immobilization of the jaw must also be assisted to eat. He will be able to eat only those foods which he can suck through a straw or from a spoon. If his lips are severely injured, it may be difficult for him to suck on the straw, in which case, the patient will receive intravenous or nasogastric tube feedings.

Good oral hygiene is very important, not only for asthetic reasons, but also to prevent infection to the teeth and damaged tissues. It is impossible to brush the teeth, but the mouth can be suctioned out and mouthwashes can be used. Sometimes, hydrogen peroxide is used, although its taste is rather unpleasant. Oil must be applied to the lips to prevent cracking.

The patient can usually communicate, even though his jaw is wired shut. If he has difficulty, provision should be made for him to write.

**Precancerous Lesions.** The most common of these is *leukoplakia buccalis* (smoker's patch), which frequently occurs in middle-aged men and appears as a creamy, white patch on the mucous membranes of the mouth or on the tongue. It is most common in people who smoke or have many dental caries. It often disappears if the patient stops smoking.

**Cancer of the Mouth.** The chances for a complete cure are excellent if the malignant tissue is removed in the early stages of cancer of the mouth. And early treatment is very possible because the disorder can be seen readily. If the surgery is extensive, edema may interfere with breathing and swallowing, so that tracheostomy or nasogastric feedings are necessary.

*Surgical Treatment.* The malignancy is removed, with as wide an excision as is necessary to remove all infected structures and lymph nodes, if possible. The most extreme surgical procedure is called a *radical neck dissection* (see Chapter 48).

*Postoperative Nursing Care.* Suction is used to remove secretions from the mouth, and the head of the bed is elevated to make breathing easier. The patient is instructed to cough and to breathe deeply, as the nurse supports his head by placing her hands on either side. If the patient becomes cyanotic it may be necessary to perform a tracheostomy—equipment for this procedure should be ready at the bedside.

*Medical Treatment.* Cancer of the mouth is treated also by radiation, which may be carried out by placing radium in the malignant tissue or by administering deep x-ray therapy.

*General Nursing Care.* Mouth care is important, for comfort and the prevention of odors. Liquids are given through a nasogastric tube until the patient is able to swallow. This may take a long time if the surgery was extensive. As soon as the patient is able, he is encouraged to give himself his feedings.

*Emotional Aspects.* This patient has many special problems to which he must learn to adjust. How quickly and easily he adjusts can depend, to some degree, on the nurse. For example, she can provide a pad for him to write on, so that he can express his wishes. Many hospitals provide a "Magic Slate" for these patients. The nurse can provide the patient with an adequate supply of disposable tissues to take care of drooling, and she can take special pains with his personal grooming. Above all, she must never do anything to make the patient think that he is repulsive. This operation is often followed by plastic surgery to correct facial defects; the wisdom of letting the patient see the result of a disfiguring operation before it is corrected may be debatable and is a decision which the doctor should make.

Since the patient may need to return to the hospital many times for plastic surgery, it is especially important to give him the kind of reassuring care that allows him to come back with confidence.

## DISORDERS OF THE ESOPHAGUS

**Esophageal Varices.** These are outpouchings of the blood vessels of the esophagus and most often occur as a secondary effect of cirrhosis of the liver. They are very dangerous and if untreated, may lead to a massive hemorrhage and death. This condition is discussed more completely in connection with cirrhosis.

**Esophageal Diverticulum.** This is an outpouching of the esophagus, usually at the

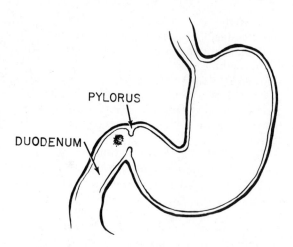

PYLORUS

DUODENUM

Figure 49-2. A peptic ulcer in the duodenum. (Smith, D. W., Germain, C. P., and Gips, C. D.: Care of the Adult Patient, ed. 3. Philadelphia, Lippincott, 1971)

point where the esophagus passes through the neck area. The patient first complains of bad breath which is caused by a collection of food in the diverticulum. The condition cannot be treated medically and thus must be corrected surgically.

**Cardiospasm.** A cardiospasm is a spasm of the cardiac sphincter and the lower end of the esophagus, which will not allow food to pass into the stomach, causing the patient to vomit and become emaciated.

Treatment may include dilation of the cardiac sphincter by means of *sounds* (dilators), also called *boughies,* or by inflation of a balloon. If this is not successful, surgery will have to be performed to loosen the stricture so that food can pass into the stomach. This has been discussed more fully in Chapter 40.

**Cancer of the Esophagus.** Cancer of the esophagus is most common in men (80%) and more common in persons who smoke. It is very distressing for the patient, because any attempts at swallowing causes food to be regurgitated, creating a disagreeable taste and odor in the patient's mouth. Often he needs parenteral fluids. Surgery is the only effective method of treating this disease if the patient is to eat normally once again. Otherwise, he faces slow starvation or being fed through a tube in his stomach for the rest of his life (gastrostomy). The malignancy is often not curable, because it may be in an inoperable

area or is discovered after metastasis has occurred as a result of the closeness of the esophagus to other vital structures.

TREATMENT. There have been rapid advances in the treatment of cancer of the esophagus in recent years, which are mostly the results of modern developments in chest surgery. In this procedure, 1 or 2 catheters are positioned in the chest for postoperative drainage and withdrawal of accumulated fluids. Surgery consists of removing all the malignant tissue, which may cure the disease if the treatment is early enough. Even if it is impossible to completely remove all the tissue because the disease has spread, surgery often can be performed so that the patient can eat normally. A palliative procedure may also be done, which involves creating a bypass for food and fluids.

NURSING CARE. After surgery, the patient is fed intravenously for several days. The nurse watches for signs of bleeding in the drainage from the nasogastric tube. A small amount of blood may be evident immediately after the operation, but after this disappears the drainage should soon be the yellow-green color of normal gastric secretions. If the patient has had chest surgery, special attention should be given to promote deep breathing and coughing. Oxygen is administered, and care is given to the chest drainage area. The patient, tubes and all, is often allowed to sit up in a chair the next day and walk a little to encourage deep breathing and to improve circulation. After several days, the patient progresses from taking small amounts of water to soft foods and a normal diet.

## DISORDERS OF THE STOMACH

### Peptic Ulcer

*Peptic ulcers* usually occur in the duodenum, but they may appear in the stomach or at the lower end of the esophagus (Fig. 49-2). The action of acid gastric juice and pepsin on the lining of these organs causes peptic ulcer. The reason why some people have ulcers and others do not seems to be related to the emotional pressures of individuals, which stimulate an excessive secretion of gastric juice which in turn creates an oversupply of hydrochloric acid in the stomach.

People with an abnormally low supply of hydrochloric acid do not have ulcers. Secretion of hydrochloric acid is also stimulated by alcohol, caffeine, and spicy foods. People tend to think that ulcers are a disease of executives when really they affect people of all classes all over the world. The increase in the number of ulcer victims is, rightly or wrongly, often attributed to the pace and the pressures of modern living. The nervous person who does not verbalize his tensions is more prone to having ulcers.

**Symptoms.** The symptoms are:

1. Burning or gnawing sensation in the stomach, usually occurring from 1 to several hours after eating. The pain may be seasonal, occurring in the spring and fall. It always begins in the same place, but may then radiate. (Milk, or other protein foods, relieve the pain.) Sometimes the victim becomes nauseated and is relieved by vomiting.

2. Tenseness and irritability: the recurrent pain causes sleeplessness and inability to work.

**Diagnosis.** Gastric analysis, gastroscopy, and x-rays help to diagnose peptic ulcer and to differentiate it from a cancerous lesion.

**Medical and Dietary Treatment.** The main purposes in ulcer treatment are to eliminate the irritation of the ulcerous lesion, to reduce the amount of acidic secretions, and to lessen the amount of mobility or activity in the stomach and intestines. The acids are neutralized by protein foods, such as milk, cream, eggs, and custard (*a bland diet*). A *low-residue diet* is also given to decrease the mobility of the digestive tract.

The *Sippy diet,* given while the illness is acute, consists of 30 to 90 cc. of milk and cream taken every hour, (alternating with an antacid on the half-hour). The cream is given because it stays in the stomach longer and thereby prolongs relief from distress, since ulcer pains appear when the stomach is empty. As the patient improves, his diet is gradually expanded to include soft foods, such as custard, gelatin, or soft-cooked eggs (see Chapter 24). The patient progresses from the hourly feedings to 3 to 6 meals a day, as his condition permits. (The food uses up the acid so it cannot attack the ulcer.) There is a tendency among some doctors today to allow a more liberal diet in treating peptic ulcer, encouraging the patient to stay away from troubling foods but to try to get back to as normal a diet as is possible.

Antacids, such as Amphojel, Gelusil, or Maalox may be given as acid neutralizers. Sippy powders, Number 1 and 2, made up of sodium bicarbonate, with magnesium oxide and bismuth subcarbonate, are also used. These preparations are given between the hourly feedings or between regular meals. Side-effects of these drugs include constipation and an upset in the acid-base balance in the body. Baking soda should not be used on a regular basis, since it upsets the acid-base balance even more.

Tincture of belladonna and atropine, drugs given to decrease acid secretion, are being replaced to some extent by the newer drugs Banthine and Pro-Banthine. All these drugs have similar side-effects, including dryness of the mouth, dilation of the pupils, and blurred vision, although the newer drugs produce them to a slightly lesser degree.

Antispasmodic drugs, such as Lomotil, are often given to reduce the hyperactivity in the bowel following gastric surgery.

Most ulcers can be controlled without surgery. Rest is an important part of ulcer treatment, although it does not necessarily imply rest in bed. Relaxation is even more important, and for this purpose doctors like to begin ulcer treatment in the hospital, where the patient is away from disturbing outside influences that aggravate his condition. Tranquilizers are also often prescribed. Once the course of treatment is firmly established, the patient may be able to maintain his routines at home. However, the ulcer patient who thinks that he is cured must remember that an ulcer has a tendency to recur and that it behooves him to follow instructions.

**Emotional Aspects.** The patient should be assisted in recognizing and avoiding as much as possible those situations which upset him. To further reduce emotional stress, the patient must be encouraged to verbalize his feelings, his fears, and his irritations. In this way, he will not internalize his upset feelings so much. It is helpful for the patient to become engaged in some physical activity which he can use to "work off" some of his excess energy and irritation. He can also counterattack stomach acidity by eating something if he does become upset.

**Complications.** *Hemorrhage* is one of the most serious and most frequent complications of peptic ulcer. It occurs when the ulcer eats through a blood vessel. If the blood vessel is small, the bleeding may be so slight that it is not noticed. Vomiting blood or passing tarry stools is evidence of more extensive hemorrhage; if the bleeding is massive, all the signs of shock appear: pallor, weak and rapid pulse, faintness, and collapse. A very significant sign is coffee-ground emesis, evidence of bleeding. The treatment is rest, enforced by sedatives, transfusion, and intravenous fluids. If bleeding continues, surgery is necessary to tie off the bleeding blood vessel. Above all, the patient must be kept absolutely quiet and should be assured that everything possible is being done to control the bleeding and replace the lost blood. Occasionally, the patient who has a bleeding ulcer and is a poor surgical risk, is treated by means of the iced saline lavage. It is done in an attempt to stop the bleeding without resorting to surgery. A large nasogastric tube is inserted, into which large amounts of ice cold saline solution are instilled. The solution is allowed to remain in the stomach for a few minutes and is then withdrawn. This procedure is repeated until the returns are free from blood. The nasogastric tube is then attached to constant suction and is watched constantly for reappearance of bleeding. A balloon filled with a circulating coolant solution may also be used to accomplish the same purpose.

If these medical procedures are not effective, surgical treatment is necessary.

*Perforation* occurs when an ulcer penetrates the wall of the stomach or the intestine, allowing the contents to escape into the abdomen and cause peritonitis. The symptoms of perforation are startling—a sudden viciously sharp pain in the abdomen that makes the patient blanch and drenches him with perspiration. His abdomen literally becomes as hard as a board and is tender and painful. He breathes rapidly, with his knees drawn up in an attempt to relieve the pain: later, his face is flushed and he becomes feverish. This condition demands immediate emergency surgery to close the perforation, since the patient will die if treatment is delayed. One important thing to remember is that a perfora-

tion can occur without warning and may not be preceded by marked signs of digestive disturbance.

*Obstruction* may occur when the scar tissue builds up to the point where it obstructs the passage of food through the duodenum. The symptoms include vomiting of undigested food and stomach pain which is relieved only by vomiting (*not* by food).

**Nursing Care.** The patient will have a Levin tube inserted to which suction is attached. He will have nothing by mouth for at least 24 hours and will be given fluids intravenously. Massive doses of antibiotics will be given to counteract abdominal infection. Continued distention, without passing flatus or feces, is a sign of serious interference with peristalsis causing intestinal paralysis (*paralytic ileus*).

**Surgical Treatment.** *Gastrectomy* is a surgical operation to remove an ulcer when other treatment fails. The lower one half to two thirds of the stomach are removed (*subtotal gastrectomy*), and the portion that is left is joined to the jejunum (*gastroenterostomy*). Sometimes, a total gastrectomy must be done. The most common procedures are the various Bilroth technics. (Gastrectomy for the treatment of cancer of the stomach is discussed on p. 641.) *Vagotomy* is the division of the vagus nerves, which reduces the stimulation to secrete hydrochloric acid and gastric motility.

PREOPERATIVE NURSING CARE. Often, antibiotics or sulfonamides are given preoperatively to free the bowel from bacteria and to lessen the danger of postoperative infection. Preoperative teaching is very important, since the patient must realize that he will need to follow a dietary regime for some time following surgery. The patient should be encouraged to talk about his feelings and should be as relaxed as possible before he has surgery. Perhaps, the hospital social worker can assist the patient in meeting financial obligations or in solving family problems, so that his worries will be lessened.

Nutrition is very important and the patient should be encouraged to eat what is offered to him. Often, he will be given vitamin and mineral supplements. He should be encouraged to practice good oral hygiene, as dental decay can contribute to infections in the digestive tract.

POSTOPERATIVE NURSING CARE. The patient returns from the operating room with a Levin tube in his stomach, where it usually remains for 2 or 3 days. Suction is attached and operated according to the doctor's orders, to keep the field of operation clean and to eliminate pressure from accumulated fluids. It is absolutely *vital* to keep this tube open at all times. The drainage is noted carefully. It may be tinged with bright red blood at first; if the amount of red increases or persists it should be reported. Normal drainage should go from dark or brownish red to greenish yellow, the normal color of gastric secretions, mixed with bile.

The patient will not be allowed anything by mouth for the first day. On the second day he may be given a small amount of water (30 cc.), which is increased to 60 cc. and then to 90 cc. in the next 2 days. He gradually progresses from liquid to soft and solid food which is given frequently in small amounts.

POSTOPERATIVE COMPLICATIONS.

*Hemorrhage.* The suture line is quite delicate and may rupture, causing hemorrhage. The signs of shock will appear as will massive hemorrhage. The nurse must watch the gastric drainage very carefully for signs of bright, red blood. It is vital that the nasogastric tube be operating properly, to avoid distention.

*"Dumping."* If the patient tries to eat too much or to eat foods which are not allowed, he will usually encounter immediate discomfort. This can be a dangerous situation, especially soon after surgery, since it can rupture the suture line. If this happens, another surgical procedure must be done to repair the damage. Symptoms of "dumping" include palpitation, sweating, faintness and excessive weakness, as well as severe diarrhea and/or vomiting. A dry meal will usually lessen this problem. Antispasmodic drugs also help, although the patient may be tempted to overdo these and upset his acid-base balance. The patient must gradually learn what foods he can eat and what foods will cause dumping.

*Evisceration.* Evisceration or the protrusion of the abdominal contents out of the body through the suture line, is a possible, although rare, complication following any abdominal surgery. If it does occur, the nurse should notify the doctor quickly. Immediate first aid consists of applying a large sterile compress which has been soaked in saline. Sterile technic must be observed! The nurse should *never* attempt to push the abdominal contents back into the abdomen.

*Diarrhea.* Some patients, especially those who have had a vagotomy, are prone to diarrhea, which may become chronic. This patient is treated symptomatically, with Kaopectate or similar drugs.

## Cancer of the Stomach (The "Silent Neoplasm")

The treatment of cancer of the stomach often requires surgery in order to completely remove the stomach and join the esophagus to the jejunum. If the tumor is small, only part of the stomach may need to be removed.

**Symptoms.** The most important symptom is that of sudden *dyspepsia* (indigestion), which is not relieved by eating. In addition there is unexplained weight loss and general weakness. "Coffee-ground" emesis and absence of free hydrochloric acid in the stomach are other significant signs. A "pap" smear of gastric contents may show cancer cells, while other routine laboratory and x-ray studies confirm the presence of a neoplasm and its exact location. The only treatment is surgical removal.

**Gastrectomy.** Removal of the entire stomach is called *total gastrectomy*; removal of part of it is called *subtotal gastrectomy*. In either case, the spleen is removed also, because metastasis to the spleen is a common occurrence in cancer of the stomach. The nursing care for subtotal gastrectomy is essentially the same as for peptic ulcer. For total gastrectomy there are these differences:

1. Since the chest cavity must be opened, procedures similar to those following any chest surgery must be carried out.

2. Drainage from the nasogastric tube is very small, because this drainage normally comes from the stomach secretions.

The prognosis is not usually good, because the neoplasm often has progressed to the point of metastasis before it is discovered.

## DISORDERS OF THE SMALL AND LARGE INTESTINES

### Irritable Colon

This condition is also known as *mucous* or *spastic colitis*. The large intestine becomes greatly overactive, causing cramps and diarrhea which, if they continue, can cause a loss of weight, an upset in acid-base balance, and dehydration. Emotional upsets can trigger an attack, and the treatment begins with an effort to get the patient to realize that his attacks are related to his emotions. His diet during attacks is regulated to avoid irritating and gas-forming foods such as raw vegetables or baked beans. It is important for the patient to realize that no particular food causes his attacks, or he may build up false notions about his diet which will interfere with his nutrition.

Opinions differ about what constitutes the most suitable diet for these patients. Some doctors prescribe milk; others limit it. Some impose no diet restrictions and encourage the patient to work up gradually to a tolerance for all foods. (See diet suggestions in Chapter 24.) Kaopectate or bismuth and paregoric may be given to check diarrhea. Belladonna, sedatives, and tranquilizers may also be prescribed to quiet bowel activity.

### Chronic or Acute Constipation

Constipation is a condition in which the patient has infrequent bowel movements, which are very hard and are accompanied by mucus. Sometimes, the patient will suffer fecal impaction or will have accompanying diarrhea. This condition may be caused by cancer, drug addiction, or mechanical obstruction. It may also be a psychosomatic disorder.

The patient should be encouraged to drink a great deal of fluids, take prune juice or eat bran, increase the amount of bulk in his diet, and follow a regular schedule for defecation. The patient should be educated to evacuate the bowel when he feels the urge, instead of postponing the act, which serves to desensitize the bowel to the presence of feces.

Since acute constipation or *obstipation* (absence of bowel movements) is often a sign of serious difficulty, such as intestinal obstruction or paralytic ileus, it should be acted upon immediately to determine the cause. The patient should also be encouraged not to strain while having a stool. Often, placing a footstool under the feet while sitting on the toilet will help to lessen the strain on the muscles.

### Diarrhea

Many patients complain of diarrhea, in which the diarrhetic stool is often light-colored, foul-smelling, and accompanied by severe stomach cramps and a large amount of flatus. The stool also contains undigested food and mucus. In addition to the stomach cramps, the patient often experiences severe anal cramps or spasms (*tenesmus*). The patient should be treated as infectious and isolated until the cause of the diarrhea is determined.

### Ulcerative Colitis

In *ulcerative colitis* the lining of the intestine becomes inflamed and ulcerated. As in colitis, it is difficult to determine the exact cause of this condition, but there is evidence that it occurs most frequently in people who have emotional problems. It is most likely to affect young adults or the middle-aged, both men and women. Typical symptoms are diarrhea, with blood and mucus in the stools, abdominal cramps, fecal incontinence, loss of appetite and weight, and nausea and vomiting. Ulcerative colitis may come on gradually or in a sudden attack. In its severest form it may cause death from hemorrhage or peritonitis. People with ulcerative colitis are more likely to develop cancer and should have periodic examinations of the digestive tract.

**Emotional Aspects.** The patient with ulcerative colitis often is a nervous person who is attached to his or her mother, even though the patient may be an adult. It is believed by many to be a psychosomatic disorder, although the symptoms are physical.

**A Nursing Challenge.** The patient with ulcerative colitis will challenge the ability of any nurse. He is weak and miserable and often frightened by his condition, since he has a serious illness which could be fatal. He has many problems to contend with—emotional tensions, dietary restrictions, diarrhea, incontinence of stool, and perhaps an ileostomy, if the colon must be removed. Procedures that are necessary in his care may also precipitate emotional crises. It takes infinite patience and understanding to handle the daily problems that arise.

*Incontinence* is a major difficulty. If possible, a bedpan should be handy to forestall soiling the bed. The patient should have the necessary help to keep the rectal area clean and to wash his hands. Since the area around the rectum may become sore, a soothing ointment, such as petrolatum, or Tucks may be applied. If the patient is incontinent, disposable pads can be used to absorb the fecal discharge. It is important to maintain an adequate fluid intake and to record it faithfully. The patient should be encouraged to take an interest in his surroundings and to see his family and friends as his condition permits. A fresh point of view often helps to build up his morale.

**Medical Treatment.** The treatment in most instances centers around resting the bowel and obtaining good nutrition through a bland, nonirritating diet. Ice is contraindicated. Vitamin supplements are often given because the restricted diet may not contain some of the essential nutrients. Vitamin K, so important in blood clotting, is often given because the intestinal tract is not absorbing it properly. The patient must rest in bed while the illness is acute. The treatment may include drugs that slow down peristalsis (atropine, tincture of belladonna) or soothe irritation (kaolin, pectin), and sedatives or tranquilizers. Penicillin or streptomycin may also be given. ACTH and cortisone often provide amazing relief, but they must be used cautiously, because they are known to have potentially damaging side-effects. If anemia develops, blood is given. Topical medications or suppositories are used to relieve rectal irritation or pain.

**Complications.** There exists the very real threat of a perforation of the intestine, causing hemorrhage and peritonitis, a condition which requires drastic surgery to remove the colon and open the ileum onto the abdomen (ileostomy). This operation may also be performed as a last desperate measure to bring relief after all other treatment has failed.

**Surgical Treatment.** The most common surgical procedure done is that of *total colectomy* (removal of the entire colon) and an *ileostomy*. The patient is prepared for the surgery as is any person who is about to have rectal or colonic surgery.

**Postoperative Nursing Care.** The psychological aspects of postoperative nursing care are vital. The patient must accept the fact that he has a permanent ileostomy. Since he may be depressed, the nurse should give him an opportunity to express his feelings. She should also see that the patient learns to care for his ileostomy in order to assure him a feeling of independence and of being worthwhile.

The patient should be referred to the local affiliate of the Ostomy Association or to the United Ostomy Association Incorporated (1111 Wilshire Boulevard, Los Angeles, California, 90017). He will receive a great deal of assistance from talking with other "ostomies." This patient is often a good candidate for a Public Health Nursing referral. But the head nurse or doctor should be consulted before any recommendations are made to the patient.

## Appendicitis

The appendix is a slender blind tube about 3 to 4 inches long which opens out of the tip of the cecum. Nobody seems to know why it is there, and people get along perfectly well without it. However, it may become obstructed by a hard mass of feces, which is followed by inflammation, infection, and gangrene, and possible perforation. A ruptured appendix is serious, because intestinal contents can escape into the abdomen and cause peritonitis or an abscess (Fig. 49-3).

**Symptoms.** An acute attack of appendicitis usually begins with progressively severe generalized pain in the abdomen, which later localizes as pain and tenderness in the lower right quarter, at a point midway between the umbilicus and the crest of the ilium (McBurney's point). Usually "rebound-tenderness" is present; that is, when the abdomen is palpated, the pain is greater when the pressure is released than it is when the doctor pushes

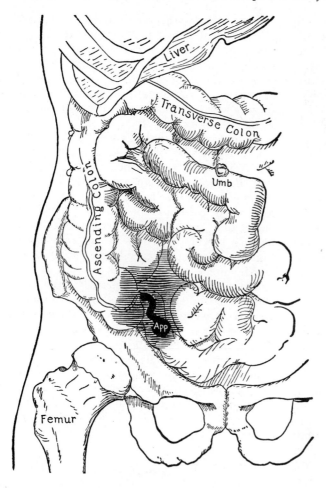

Figure 49-3. Acute appendicitis, gangrene of the appendix, perforation and spreading peritonitis. In this case, the appendix was not removed, and the inflammation spread to the surrounding loops of bowel. An abscess will form in the shaded area, or the inflammation may spread through the entire peritoneal cavity. (Brunner, L. S., et al.: Textbook of Medical-Surgical Nursing, ed. 2., Philadelphia, Lippincott, 1970)

down. Usually, the pain is accompanied by fever, nausea and vomiting, and an increase in white blood cells—a sign of the body's resistance to infection. An attack of appendicitis may subside and recur later (recurrent appendicitis).

**Treatment.** Prompt surgical treatment is necessary to remove the appendix, if possible, before it ruptures. If the patient has eaten recently, spinal anesthesia is used. In most instances, the patient recovers rapidly; he is permitted fluids and food and allowed out of bed the day after the operation and may go back to work in 2 or 3 weeks, with cautions to avoid heavy lifting and to "take it easy" for a while. If the appendix has ruptured, treatment for peritonitis is necessary, which will include an incisional drainage tube (see p. 645). This is a serious complication which can cause death. However, modern treatment, with suction devices, intravenous fluids, and antibiotics has greatly reduced this danger.

**To Prevent Complications.** Abdominal pain, nausea, and vomiting are more or less common occurrences. It is easy for the victim to mistake them for a temporary intestinal upset, probably due to "something I ate," for which he takes a cathartic or an enema as a remedy. Everyone should know what to do and more especially what *not* to do for severe abdominal pain:

*Do not* take an enema or a cathartic. They increase peristalsis, and the result may be a perforated appendix and peritonitis. If an enema is ordered as a preoperative preparation, it must be given low and very slowly.

Take nothing by mouth—even water may make matters worse. Call a doctor for any attack of severe pain or for pain that persists.

*Do not* apply heat to the abdomen.

*Do not* give morphine, because it tends to mask the symptoms.

## Peritonitis

*Peritonitis* is inflammation of the *peritoneum,* the membrane that lines the abdominal cavity and covers the abdominal organs. In the upper abdomen it is usually the result of a perforation of the intestine, which permits intestinal contents to escape into the abdomen. Since the intestinal tract is normally filled with bacteria, the result of a perforation may be inflammation and infection of the peritoneum. The most common causes of perforation are appendicitis, ulcer, or a malignant growth. *Pelvic* peritonitis may be the result of an infected fallopian tube. Peritonitis may be generalized, extending throughout the peritoneum, or it may be localized, as an abscess.

**Symptoms.** Peritonitis often develops suddenly, with severe abdominal pain, nausea and vomiting, and a gradual rise in temperature, with a weak, rapid pulse and low blood pressure. The patient's respirations are shallow, because breathing hurts the abdomen; he tries to avoid moving his abdomen and draws his knees up to prevent pressure from the bedclothes and to relieve the pain. The abdomen is tense and boardlike and becomes very distended; flatus and the intestinal contents are stationary in the intestinal tract, and paralytic ileus may develop. If the infection does not respond to treatment, the patient grows weaker; his pulse is thready, his breathing becomes more shallow, his temperature falls, and death follows.

**Treatment.** Surgery is sometimes necessary to close the perforation and promote drainage, although the perforation may close by itself. Postoperative treatment centers on replacing fluids and electrolytes and fighting infection by administering massive doses of antibiotics and analgesics, such as Demerol, to relieve pain and to provide rest. The head of the bed is elevated (Fowler's position), to promote drainage. The patient must be watched closely, with the nurse observing the pulse and temperature, vomiting, the amount of drainage through the gastrointestinal tube, the amount of intake and output of fluids, abdominal distention, and whether gas and feces are passing through the rectum. The nurse must also observe the incisional drainage, recording the amount and type.

Special attention is given to mouth care because the patient has no fluids by mouth; fever and the gastrointestinal tube make his mouth dry and parched. Side rails on the bed may be necessary to prevent him from harming himself if he becomes disoriented. Above all, everybody concerned with his care must proceed gently. The least movement or jarring of the bed intensifies his pain. Lifting and moving are agony for him, and he suffers intensely from even the slightest pressure on his acutely sensitive abdomen. The most common complications are evisceration and abscess formation.

Fortunately, fewer people develop peritonitis today than in the past, and recoveries are more frequent. This is largely due to improvements in surgery and to the use of antibiotics, which are often used in solution form to irrigate the abdominal cavity and have proved more effective when combined with the hyperoxygenation available in the hyperbaric chamber.

## Diverticulitis

*Diverticulosis* refers to the appearance of many pouches in the intestine or esophagus. *Diverticulitis* means an inflammation of these diverticuli. The cause is not known, except that a weakness in the wall of the intestine or esophagus has allowed the diverticuli to form. This condition usually affects the middle-aged or elderly person and is benign. It usually causes no symptoms unless it becomes impacted with intestinal material, in which case it becomes irritated, inflamed, and infected.

Symptoms are nagging pain in the left, lower quadrant and temperature elevation. Treatment includes a bland diet and stool softeners and occasionally, mineral oil.

Complications include a rare perforation, in which case a colostomy (usually temporary) must be done.

## Abdominal Hernia

*Abdominal hernia* is a protrusion of the intestine through the abdominal wall; the layman's name for this condition is *rupture.* The abdominal wall is weak in spots, and it is at these points that a hernia develops. Often it is possible to push the intestines back by lying down and pressing on the abdomen, thus *reducing* the hernia. Another method of control often used by the hernia victim is to wear an appliance called a *truss,* which places continual pressure on the spot. If it is impossible to reduce the hernia by these methods and the condition is allowed to go on, the intestine becomes constricted, and the blood supply is cut off. This is a *strangulated hernia,* a serious condition which requires emergency surgery to save the patient's life.

**Causes of Hernia.** Congenital defects are responsible for a large number of hernias; therefore, a hernia may appear in infants (see Chapter 40). Hernias may occur also in young adults from such strains as heavy lifting, pregnancy, or coughing or sneezing. Later in life, obesity and muscle weakness may cause hernia. The most common types of hernia are the incisional, the inguinal, the umbilical, and the femoral.

**Surgical Repair of a Hernia.** A hernia can be repaired by surgery. If it has gone unrepaired for many years, a repair may not hold, since the tissues are weakened and do not heal as easily. Hernia repair is likely to be neglected, since hernia is not a painful condition, and the victim puts up with the discomfort. A hernia may interfere with getting a job, especially in strenuous types of work.

The operation for the repair of hernia is called *herniorrhaphy.* It consists of closing the defect in the abdominal wall. Usually, the nursing care is not complicated; the patient is allowed out of bed the day after the operation and can have food and fluids. He may be allowed to stand up to void, if voiding is a difficulty, immediately following the operation. In a male, the scrotum becomes swollen and painful, and an ice cap and a suspensory support may be ordered for relief. Every precaution is taken to avoid sneezing or coughing, and the patient is instructed, if he should sneeze or cough, to press his hand firmly over the area of the incision. He is encouraged to move about, but cautioned to avoid movements that cause strain, such as lifting. The bed should be adjusted to its lowest position or a footstool provided to avoid strain when he gets in or out of bed.

Under normal conditions, the patient is out of the hospital in a week, with cautions to avoid strenuous activity. His return to work depends on such things as the nature and the extent of the hernia, his age, and his weight. It also depends on the type of work that he does—if it is very strenuous he may have to change to a lighter type of work. When a patient realizes that he must change his type of work, he may be worried or upset and may even need assistance in finding a job. This should be called to the attention of the head nurse, who can take the proper steps to direct him to assistance, which may be available through the social service department of the hospital.

## Intestinal Obstruction

*Intestinal obstruction* occurs when intestinal paralysis (*paralytic obstruction*) or a tumor or other blockage (*mechanical obstruction*) interferes with normal peristalsis and blocks the movement of gas and bowel contents through the intestinal tract. Mechanical obstruction may include adhesions (often scars from previous surgery), *volvulus* (twisting of the bowel), a foreign body in the bowel, *intussusception* (telescoping of the bowel), or a high fecal impaction. Paralytic obstruction may result from peritonitis, postanesthesia paralysis, or toxicity. A vascular obstruction, such as atherosclerosis, can also cause a gradual cessation of peristalsis, because of decreased blood supply. Sometimes a loop of intestine pushes through the abdominal wall and becomes pinched off; this is a *strangulated hernia* and is another cause of obstruction. The blockage may be partial or complete; complete obstruction necessitates emergency surgery, to prevent gangrene.

**Cancer.** Cancer is a common cause of this condition—a tumor within the intestine becomes larger and larger until it finally blocks the passage. If the obstruction is high in the gastrointestinal tract, vomiting occurs. Since the stomach contents are unable to pass the obstruction, this is Nature's way of emptying the stomach of accumulated digestive fluids. As these materials continue to accumulate, the vomitus becomes thick, dark, and foul-smelling, because the number of bacteria normally present in the digestive tract increases. Vomiting may not appear if the obstruction is farther down. The patient becomes dehydrated and is unable to take fluids by mouth. Surgery may consist of temporary relief through a colostomy. When the patient's condition is improved, the portion of the bowel containing the tumor may be removed and the ends of the bowel rejoined. Then the temporary colostomy is closed. This is not possible if the malignant process is too extensive. Suction is used to relieve distention; intravenous fluids are given, and antibiotics may also be prescribed.

### Cancer of the Colon

Cancer of the colon requires surgical treatment with the hope of removing the cancerous tissue. The ends are sutured together, thus re-establishing normal function in the gastrointestinal tract. Sometimes the tumor is too extensive or the patient's condition will not permit this procedure, in which case the obstruction is relieved by a temporary or a permanent colostomy.

## DISORDERS OF THE SIGMOID COLON AND RECTUM

### Hemorrhoids

*Hemorrhoids* are swollen (varicose) veins of the anus or the rectum. *External hemorrhoids* protrude as lumps around the anus. They are painful, especially if the patient is constipated and is in the habit of straining to produce a bowel movement. They may alternately appear and disappear. Usually, external hemorrhoids do not bleed but may become so large as to be painful and itchy. *Internal hemorrhoids* develop inside of the anal sphincter; they may bleed but are less likely to be painful if they do not protrude. Signs of bleeding may be no more than a drop on toilet paper, or bleeding may be so extensive and continuous as to cause anemia. Internal hemorrhoids almost always protrude with defecation, but at first they can be pushed back with the finger; later as the masses grow larger, this is no longer possible and they discharge blood and mucus. Bleeding is one of the signs of cancer, and this symptom should never be ignored. The proctoscope makes it possible to inspect the inside of the rectum.

**Causes.** The pressure of the uterus on the rectum during pregnancy, intra-abdominal tumors, constipation, or infection from feces are the chief causes of hemorrhoids.

**Medical Treatment.** Sometimes hemorrhoids disappear without treatment. Often they can be relieved by warm sitz baths or anesthetic ointments, such as Nupercaine. Correction of constipation may both prevent and eliminate hemorrhoids.

**Surgical Treatment.** If surgery is necessary, the veins are either tied off and excised, *hemorrhoidectomy,* or a cautery is used. Sometimes a solution is injected to shrink the tissues.

PREOPERATIVE PREPARATION. A cleansing enema is given on the night before and the morning of the operation. The rectal area is cleansed and shaved, in addition to other prescribed routines.

POSTOPERATIVE CARE. When the patient returns from the operating room he may be placed on his abdomen to prevent pressure on the operative area. He is given an analgesic for pain, preferably as soon as he awakens, or when the local anesthetic wears off. Demerol may be ordered, to be repeated at stated intervals. He will be allowed a liquid diet for his first meal after the operation, then a full diet for the following meals. He is allowed to sit up—this will be painful, and a rubber ring under his buttocks will help to relieve the pressure on the operative area. The next day the doctor may permit him to get out of bed and may order daily sitz baths to relieve pain and soreness. He must have assistance with getting in and out of the tub and should never be left alone, since the effort he must make might make him faint. He stays in the bath for 20 minutes, with the temperature of the water at 110° F. It is best if the water is circulating.

POSTOPERATIVE NURSING PROBLEMS.

*Hemorrhage.* Since the removal of hemorrhoids is actually the excision of portions of blood vessels, bleeding is possible. The nurse must be alert to any signs of bleeding, either on the dressings, or as evidenced by symptoms of faintness, weakness, or lowered blood pressure and other signs of shock.

*The First Bowel Movement.* The patient is naturally apprehensive about the first bowel movement after the operation. The nurse tells him what is being done to make it easier: that he will be given mineral oil or a stool softener, twice a day to soften the stool, so it will pass more easily, and that he will have some pain but probably much less than he imagines. When he feels that his bowels are going to move, she tells him she will be just outside the bathroom door to be sure that he is all right and reminds him not to use toilet paper. The anal area must be cleansed with moist cotton balls and dried carefully. This is a good time to give the sitz bath because some pain is inevitable after the first bowel movement.

Never underestimate the patient's pain and discomfort after rectal surgery. It may seem to be a very minor operation, but the effects on the patient can be very distressing.

## Anal Abscess and Anal Fistula

Infection of the tissues around the rectal area causes *anal abscess.* This condition is very painful and may be accompanied by fever and chills. The abscess is usually cut open and drained, or it may rupture spontaneously. Often an unfortunate result of an anal abscess is the formation of an *anal fistula,* which is a small tunnel in the tissues which discharges pus through one or more openings onto the skin. Surgery is necessary to open up the fistulous tract; then it is packed with gauze to keep the edges of the wound apart. This allows the tissues to fill in, granulate, and eliminate the fistula.

**Nursing Care.** In general, the nursing care for an anal fistula is similar to the care given to any patient after rectal surgery, with these differences:

1. The fistula wound is packed with petrolatum gauze which is changed every day.

2. The drainage from the abscess is profuse, purulent, and foul smelling. The gauze dressing on the wound and cellucotton pads need to be changed frequently.

## Anal Fissure

An anal fissure is an ulcer in the skin of the anal wall which causes severe pain with defecation and sometimes slight bleeding. The patient may dread the pain so much that he delays defecation to the extent that he becomes constipated.

Sitz baths and local anesthetic ointments are the treatments commonly used for anal fissure; mineral oil may help to soften the feces. The only cure for this condition is surgery to remove the ulcer.

## Pilonidal Cyst (Pilonidal Sinus Tract)

A pilonidal cyst is quite common in males and often exists for many years without causing any trouble. It is a closed fistula, usually containing hair follicles. If it becomes infected, opens, and drains, it is surgically excised. There are often several sinus tracts, all of which must be excised. In many cases, the area of the incision is large and must granulate from the inside out. Postoperative management is aimed at the prevention of pain by positioning, sitz baths, or medication and at early ambulation to prevent complications. Since pilonidal cysts may reoccur, some men may have to have several operations.

## Cancer of the Rectum

If the cancerous growth is in the upper part of the rectum, it can be removed without removing the rectal sphincter, so that ultimately the bowel will continue to function normally. If the tumor involves the rectal opening, a dual operation is necessary—through the abdomen from above (including a colostomy) and through the perineum from below, *abdominal perineal resection.* The danger of shock following this extensive surgery is very great.

**Nursing Care.** This patient requires an almost incredible amount of nursing care. It includes caring for a colostomy, the administration of parenteral fluids (including blood transfusion), the use of suction, caring for bladder drainage (a Foley catheter is usually inserted in the bladder), and irrigating and caring for drainage from the perineal wound. The patient must be turned frequently to prevent respiratory complications and thrombophlebitis; it is difficult for him to find a comfortable position. If his condition permits, he gets out of bed in 2 to 4 days after the operation. He will need much assistance to accomplish this. Despite a long and trying convalescence, a patient can recover if all of the malignancy has been removed and if he learns to accept the inconvenience of a colostomy.

## DISORDERS OF THE LIVER

The liver is not only the largest organ in the body but it is also the busiest. The body could not function without the liver. Some of the many activities of this vital organ are listed on page 136.

### Jaundice (Icterus)

*Jaundice* is a symptom of liver difficulty. It is the result of an abnormal concentration of bile salts in the bloodstream, which causes a yellow discoloration of the tissues. When something interferes with the work of the liver or obstructs the flow of bile into the intestines, *bilirubin* accumulates in the bloodstream. Signs of jaundice are a yellowish color in the whites of the eyes and in the skin. This is easiest to observe in the Caucasian patient, and is very difficult to determine in the Oriental person. A blood test (icterus index) will show how much bilirubin is in the bloodstream. A shortage of bile in the intestines interferes with fat digestion, causing the stools to appear pale and fatty and have a disagreeable odor. The bile salts that have escaped into the tissues make the skin itchy; the urine is dark and discolored. Lack of vitamin K causes a tendency to bleed.

**Diagnosis.** The *treatment* of jaundice begins with finding out the cause of the condition and then doing whatever is necessary to correct it. This includes a number of tests:

Examination of the feces and urine for bilirubin (which is more evident before jaundice appears). Clay-colored stools may suggest biliary obstruction.

Serum transaminase (SGOT) determinations.

Prothrombin time and serum globulin level are increased.

Liver function tests, which include injecting a dye into the bloodstream (bromsulphalein) to estimate the amount of liver damage and the cephalin flocculation determination.

Glucose tolerance tests to see how well the liver is doing its work (see Chap. 52).

Sometimes a surgeon performs a biopsy of the liver. Since this procedure involves cutting into the liver, it is important to watch for signs of bile or bleeding on the dressing and for abdominal pain. These signs indicate that bile or blood may be spilling into the abdominal cavity.

### Treatment and Nursing Care.

1. The nursing care includes measures to relieve itching. Starch baths or calamine lotion may be prescribed; tepid sponges also are comforting. If calamine lotion and cotton are placed at his bedside, the patient can apply it to itchy spots himself and prevent scratching.

2. Watch for signs of bleeding in the stool and the urine or when the patient brushes his teeth. Look for black-and-blue marks on the skin. After the needle is withdrawn at the end of an intravenous procedure, exert pressure on the puncture for a longer time than is normal. This prevents a hematoma from oozing blood which would make it impossible to use the vein again. This is important, because people with liver conditions need frequent blood tests.

3. Explain to the patient that jaundice is not unusual with his ailment.

### Liver Failure
### (Episodic Stupor, Hepatic Coma)

The patient shows a syndrome which is characterized by tremors and mental changes, including stupor or coma. It may occur after massive gastrointestinal hemorrhage, some surgical procedures, and after massive infections. It occurs most commonly after overdose of drugs including quinines, barbiturates, and opiates. It also occurs in the patient with cirrhosis. Treatment is symptomatic, including removal of precipitating factors, if possible; control of bleeding; enemas to remove blood from the large intestine; a low protein diet; and careful management of the fluid and electrolyte balance. Antibiotics may be given, and in some cases, adrenocortical drugs are given. The prognosis is guarded and the possibility of successful treatment decreases with each episode of hepatic coma.

### Cirrhosis (Laennec's or Portal Cirrhosis)

*Cirrhosis* is a condition which destroys the liver itself and thereby interferes with liver functions. In the effort to repair itself, the liver may become so enlarged that the blood vessels going into and out of it are obstructed. This can cause such disturbances as indigestion, vomiting blood, blood in the stool, constipation, fluid in the abdomen, and an enlarged spleen. It may also cause enlarged veins (esophageal varices) to form in the esophagus, an extremely dangerous condition. These disturbances show that the liver is not working properly and are signs of interference with blood clotting, with metabolism, and with the elimination of waste products.

**Causes.** Alcoholism is blamed for more than half of the cases of cirrhosis in this country. Drinking leads to poor eating habits, and good nutrition is essential to keep the liver working properly. Yet doctors are puzzled to find that the alcoholics who do have good eating habits also have cirrhosis; most of them agree that nobody knows the exact cause. One source claims that the foods eaten *with* the alcohol are responsible. Cirrhosis is more prevalent among men than women. It occurs most often between the ages of 45 to 65. Whatever the cause, liver disease is increasing. It may be that the stepped-up use of such drugs as the aureomycins and the sulfonamides is partly responsible. These drugs are excreted by the liver, and the added burden may be more than it can carry.

**Diagnosis.** Diagnosis is made on the basis of symptoms, and liver damage is evaluated in terms of circulatory disturbances, disturbances in bile drainage, and actual damage to the functioning liver cells.

**Symptoms.** Cirrhosis may develop so gradually that the patient may not realize that anything is wrong nor have any signs of the disease. He may not be aware of a low-grade fever or notice a loss of weight because the weight loss is offset by an increase in abdominal fluid. As the disease advances, the fever increases, the patient has abdominal pain, his pulse becomes rapid, and breathing becomes difficult because of his enlarged abdomen. He tends to bleed easily: blood appears in vomitus or as nosebleed, and veins become dilated because of portal hypertension. He is jaundiced, and his skin is dry; he feels weak and mentally dull and confused. Some of these symptoms are signs of 2 dangerous complications:

*Hemorrhage:* His tendency to bleed is increased. Esophageal varices often rupture, causing massive *hematemesis* (bloody emesis). The insertion of a Sengstaken-Blakemore tube will stop the bleeding temporarily, although 60 per cent of these patients die within one year of the first episode.

*Infection:* His body defenses are reduced, and he is more susceptible to outside infections. A nurse should always come to this patient with clean hands, no matter what she does for him, and should prevent visitors with colds or other infectious conditions from seeing him.

**Treatment and Nursing Care.** All treatment for cirrhosis of the liver is aimed toward helping the liver to repair itself. It does this by:

*Adequate bedrest:* Since body comfort aids rest, frequent care must be given to the patient's mouth and skin, since he is annoyed by itching. Soothing baths may be ordered.

*Transfusions* to combat anemia.

*A diet high in vitamins, and proteins, moderate in carbohydrates and fats, and low in sodium.* If these essential nutrients are not supplied, the body burns up its store of protein, thus increasing the accumulation of ammonia (a waste product) in the blood. Since the liver must transform ammonia into urea for elimination by the kidneys, this accumulation puts an extra burden on the diseased organ. Alcohol, tobacco, and very fatty foods (pork, bacon, gravies, pastries) are forbidden. Small liquid or semisolid meals given frequently will be more appealing to a poor appetite. The diet is often supplemented by Brewer's yeast, multivitamins, and extra vitamin $B_{12}$.

*Diuretics and reduced sodium intake* to reduce edema and fluid in the abdomen (ascites). Aldactone, a recent drug, may be given with other diuretics such as prednisone, Thiormerin, Diuril, or Mercuhydrin. *Paracentesis* (aspiration of fluid with a syringe and a needle) may be necessary to relieve ascites.

*Transfusion* of concentrated human serum albumin.

The patient should be told that his treatment may take a long time, so he knows what to expect and does not become discouraged if his progress seems to be slow. In the patient with liver failure, at least 2 months are needed before an improvement can be noted. With careful attention to diet and the omission of alcohol, the cirrhosis patient may live for many years. Unfortunately, many patients do not take proper care of themselves, and liver damage becomes so extensive that they are beyond help. *Uncontrolled* cirrhosis may result in *hepatic coma*. Drugs to counteract the destructive processes can be given and may help temporarily, but death will eventually follow.

**Surgical Treatment.** A palliative procedure, called the portacaval venous shunt may be performed to prevent bleeding and to relieve portal hypertension. These patients are often very poor surgical risks and the operation is not always successful.

## Viral Hepatitis
## (Infectious Hepatitis, Hepatitis A)

*Viral hepatitis* is a liver infection that has become very common since World War II. This increase is attributed to poor sanitation, crowded conditions, malnutrition, and to the difficulty in recognizing carriers of the disease. It may also be that people are becoming more susceptible to hepatitis or do not develop an immunity to it. It primarily affects children or young adults, and more white people than nonwhites. It occurs most frequently in the fall and the early winter.

**Causes and Types of Hepatitis.** Two different viruses cause hepatitis: Virus A and Virus B. *Virus B* is found in the bloodstream (*serum hepatitis*). *Virus A* is found in the bloodstream and also in the gastrointestinal tract (*infectious viral hepatitis*). These viruses are tough—they can survive the extreme temperatures that kill most organisms, although autoclaving can kill the virus.

Viral hepatitis (virus A) is transmitted by an infected food or water supply, by infected food handlers, and by the rectal thermometers, the bedpans, or the feces of a person with the disease.

**Symptoms.** The patient loses his appetite and is nauseated and feels sick all over. His head aches, and he has chills and fever. His stools are light-colored, and his urine is dark; he may become jaundiced. His *liver enlarges* and he has abdominal pain. Laboratory tests will tell which type of hepatitis he has.

**Treatment and Nursing Care.** It is important first to determine the cause of the jaundice. (Many other disorders can cause jaundice.) If the patient has infectious hepatitis, he must be put into strict isolation (see Chapter 30), at least while the disease is active. Generally, the patient is noninfectious about 1 month after he becomes ill, although it is a disease in which a person may be a carrier.

No adequate protection against this carrier is known. (A healthy carrier is a person who is harboring the virus but has no symptoms of the disease.)

A person who has been exposed may be given gamma globulin as a prophylactic measure. This does not usually prevent serum hepatitis but is quite effective against infectious hepatitis (hepatitis A).

Bedrest is important during the acute phase of the disease, that is, while the patient is jaundiced and complains of abdominal pain and while his liver function tests are abnormal. He may have bathroom privileges (BRP), and he is given a high protein, high carbohydrate diet. Some patients receive corticosteroids.

The only treatment that has any effect on hepatitis is centered around building up the patient's resistance. No drug is known to affect the virus directly. Much depends on good nursing care. A comfortable position is important for rest, and the nurse can explain to visitors the need for rest. The patient needs a nutritious diet but is likely to be revolted by the thought of food. His food should be served in small quantities and as attractively as possible. He needs plenty of fluid, especially if he has jaundice, in which case he should try to take about 3,000 cc. every day. The nurse's strict attention to hand-washing before doing anything for the patient will help to protect him from other infections. A complication is that of acute yellow atrophy.

**Homologous Serum Jaundice (Inoculation Hepatitis, Hepatitis B).** *Serum hepatitis* is also a liver infection. It is transmitted through the bloodstream from one infected person to another. The chief causes are the use of unsterile needles in injections or the administration of blood from an infected person. The use of disposable needles and syringes has eliminated one former source of infection. However, there is a rising hepatitis problem among persons who are drug abusers and who inject their drugs (see Chapter 57).

Since the incubation period is usually several months, it is often difficult to trace the exact cause or source of the disease. The symptoms are the same as those of infectious hepatitis A. Serum hepatitis is more likely to occur in people over age 30. This disease is more severe and its mortality rate is higher than that of infectious hepatitis, perhaps because the patients are older or more likely to be physically run-down.

Treatment and nursing care is the same as that for infectious hepatitis A.

**Convalescence.** The patient must avoid overexertion when he begins to feel better. Too much activity too soon is very likely to bring on a recurrence of his symptoms. This may be a boring time for him, especially if he was a very active person before he became ill. The news that his convalescence may take up to a year will not be received with enthusiasm. However, he has to be told what the situation is—that he must follow instructions or he will have a relapse. He should also be warned that he must *never* donate blood. During his stay in the hospital there are many opportunities for him to ask questions and plan with his family for his convalescence. As he gradually recovers, he will feel stronger and not as depressed, and can discuss the restrictions he must accept.

Blood banks must be very cautious about drawing blood from a person who has had serum or infectious hepatitis, since the disease will be transmitted in the blood, even if the person is no longer ill.

**Toxic Hepatitis.** Toxic hepatitis is the result of the action of certain chemicals on the liver, such as fumes from cleaning solutions and insecticides. The liver is either destroyed by the chemical or collects in the body, because the liver cannot excrete it. The treatment is much the same as for viral hepatitis. I.V. dextrose may be helpful.

## Massive Liver Necrosis (Acute Yellow Atrophy, Icterus Gravis)

This is a disease which, for some unknown reason, affects middle-aged women. It is a destructive condition which seems to be precipitated by the hepatitis virus, by poisons, or by a drug. Alcoholism, malnutrition, and pregnancy may also be predisposing factors. The symptoms are the same as in hepatitis, although the onset is more sudden. In spite of treatment the patient grows steadily worse, with the presence of coma, hemorrhages, and convulsions. A characteristic symptom is the

fishy odor on the victim's breath. The liver is *smaller* than normal in this disorder.

This disease is usually fatal within 2 weeks, although the patient may live, in which case, the disease continues, either as subacute, or chronic ("healed"), yellow atrophy.

## Liver Abscess

Liver abscesses are caused either by the spread of infection from some part of the intestinal tract, perhaps from the appendix or from the gallbladder, or by amebae in the intestines. The symptoms of a liver abscess are chills, a temperature that shoots up and down (*intermittent fever*), extreme loss of weight, nausea and vomiting, and abdominal distention. Jaundice frequently appears. Pain over the liver is a later symptom. If the abscess bursts, it scatters infection through the abdominal or chest cavity. Antibiotics are given, and the results depend upon how successful they are in combating the infection. Sometimes drainage is attempted by puncturing the liver with a trochar and establishing drainage. The nursing care includes precautions in caring for equipment and drainage, to prevent spreading the infection.

## Liver Injuries

Frequently, the liver is injured in an accident. Extensive damage is likely to be fatal, and the patient may die from hemorrhage before he reaches the hospital. Sometimes surgery is done for liver injuries to control the bleeding or to remove a portion of the damaged liver. One great danger accompanying liver surgery is the occurrence of shock. This is because the liver is such a vascular organ. Nursing care for this patient will include assistance with treatment for shock, preventing infection and observing the color of the wound drainage for indications of bile or blood. A large percentage of the patients with a rupture of the liver die.

## Cancer of the Liver

Cancer rarely begins in the liver, but it is often the result of metastasis from a cancerous growth elsewhere in the body. A cancer that does begin in the liver can be removed by a surgical operation to remove part of the liver. This procedure may prolong the patient's life for 5 years—he would not live that long without the operation. If cancer is the result of metastasis, an operation is out of the question; the patient usually is treated palliatively with radiation or chemotherapy.

## Liver Transplants

Liver transplants are attempted in some cases, especially those in which the patient is healthy except for the liver damage, as in the event of trauma to the liver. This operation is still in experimental stages, but some successes have been documented. However, the procedure should not be attempted unless no other course is available. The problems of transplantation in general have been discussed elsewhere in this book.

# GALLBLADDER DISORDERS

## The Liver-Gallbladder-Bile Combine

The gallbladder lies on the undersurface of the liver; it is the storage reservoir for the bile, which the liver manufactures continually. A small amount of bile is always retained in the gallbladder, ready for release at the next meal. Fat digestion cannot take place without bile.

As was described in Chapter 17, the flow of bile in the biliary apparatus proceeds through the hepatic duct from the liver into the cystic duct leading to the gallbladder for storage. Upon hormonal stimulation, the gallbladder contracts, releasing the bile back through the cystic duct which, with the hepatic duct, enters the duodenum as the common bile duct.

## Two Common Diseases

Two common forms of gallbladder disease are the inflammation of the gallbladder (*cholecystitis*) and gallstones (*cholelithiasis*). These conditions often occur together, and each makes the other worse. Infection causes stones; stones block the duct which leads out

of the gallbladder and imprison bacteria in its wall, which in turn causes infection. Stones may injure the wall, which also leads to infection. The most likely victims of gallbladder disease are obese women over 45; frequent pregnancies also seem to make women more susceptible. People from the Orient seldom have cholecystitis or cholelithiasis.

**Cholecystitis.** The symptoms of cholecystitis or cholelithiasis are:

*Indigestion,* due to the lack of bile. The patient complains of feeling "full" after eating. Fatty foods make this condition worse.

*Light-colored stools,* because bile pigment is missing. These stools float, because they contain fat (which must be broken down by bile).

*Fever and malaise.*

*Jaundice,* caused by stones obstructing the bile passages or by a spasm of the common bile duct. Bile backs up in the gallbladder; the liver stops manufacturing bile, and the bilirubin it would normally use in this process goes into the bloodstream.

*Gallstone colic,* a sharp pain over the gallbladder, which sometimes extends to the back or to the right shoulder. The pain usually comes on suddenly a few hours after a heavy meal, when the gallbladder is trying to contract to send bile into the intestine to help digest the food. If this effort forces a stone into the cystic duct the pain is excruciating. Usually, the patient vomits, which causes further distress instead of relief. If gallstones are very small, a person may be only slightly uncomfortable at times, or they may never give him any trouble.

*Symptoms of biliary obstruction:* Skin changes, including jaundice; yellowing of the sclera of the eyes; the urine becomes very dark because it contains bile which has been excreted rather than being used for digestion.

**Tests.** An x-ray study (*cholecystogram*) will show stones and their location in the gallbladder. The patient is given a fat-free supper the night before the roentgenogram is taken, and a dye (Priodax, Telepaque, Cholografin) is given by mouth or intravenously. The liver excretes this dye into the bile, which then goes to the gallbladder. The patient has nothing to eat for the next 12 hours, to give time for the dye to concentrate in the gallbladder. The x-ray will show the outline of the gallbladder and the stones, if they are present. Then the patient is given a fatty meal, and another picture is taken which will show how well the gallbladder is contracting. This test may not be used if the patient is jaundiced, for fear of further damage to the liver by subjecting it to the additional strain of the test.

A blood coagulation test helps to determine liver damage. If the coagulation time is dangerously slow, vitamin K can be given; this is important to lessen the danger of hemorrhage if an operation is to be done. Tests for bile pigment in the blood are the *van den Bergh* and the *icterus index*.

**Medical Treatment.** The diet is restricted to nonfatty foods (see Chapter 24). Such foods as cheese, cream, greasy fried foods, fatty meats, and gas-forming vegetables are forbidden. The patient may have lean meat (never fried), plain, mashed or baked potato, or rice. Alcoholic beverage are forbidden. Immediately after an attack he is given liquids only.

Heat to the abdomen and a plain enema help to relieve pain in a mild attack. If the attack is severe, Demerol is usually given, since morphine may increase the spasm. Pro-Banthine may be given for the spasm.

**Surgical Treatment.** Usually the most effective treatment after an acute attack of cholecystitis is to remove the gallbladder (*cholecystectomy*). Although this procedure is frequently done, complications can occur as a result of injury to the common bile duct or to the blood vessels which supply the liver.

**Postoperative Nursing Care.** The postoperative treatment and the nursing care for a cholecystectomy are essentially the same as for any major surgical operation, with an additional provision to care for bile drainage from the wound. The patient is expected to turn and cough, to prevent pneumonia from congested lungs. The nurse helps the patient by placing her hands firmly on either side of the incision, making a "splint" when the patient coughs.

If a T-tube is present, it is removed after approximately 1 week. The nurse notes the amount of bile on the dressings; if the amount does not diminish in a few days, it may be an indication that the bile is not entering the intestine properly.

THE T-TUBE. Some surgeons will place a tube into the wound for drainage following surgery. Others will allow the ducts to readjust and take over the bile drainage spontaneously. If the patient has a drainage tube, (most often called a T-tube), the drainage bottle is first placed above the patient or at bed level. This would serve only to release pressure of excess bile collection. Later, the bottle is lowered, until it is on the floor. The level of the bile bottle is noted on the Kardex as a doctor's order, and the nurse must be careful to keep the bottle at the level indicated. The amount of the bile should be measured and recorded. If the patient is losing too much bile, he may need to drink the bile again.

After the bottle has been lowered to the floor without discomfort, it may be clamped for a day or 2 before it is removed. The nurse must observe for signs of jaundice or discomfort when the bottle is lowered or the tube is removed.

Since there may be a great deal of drainage from the drainage site after the tube is removed, the skin should be protected, since bile is very irritating. (It literally digests the skin.)

The stools of the postoperative patient should be observed for the presence or absence of bile. The bile should disappear and the stools should become the normal color and consistency again, as function returns.

THE PATIENT'S DIET POSTOPERATIVELY. Most doctors will put the patient on a low-fat diet for several months. However, later, these patients in most instances have no trouble in digesting fats. The patient may want to talk over what he sees as problems after he has been told that he must keep on with a low-fat diet for some time. He may be referred to the dietician for counseling.

Generally, the patient with a disorder of the gallbladder cannot eat any fatty foods without extreme discomfort. Thus the diet should be high in protein and carbohydrate and devoid of alcohol and gas-forming foods.

**Complications of Cholecystitis.** Sometimes the infected gallbladder fills with pus and may rupture, causing peritonitis. Chronic gallbladder disease may also permanently damage the liver.

## Cancer of the Gallbladder

Often cancer of the gallbladder is not treated early enough because it is not easily detected in the early stages. In the advanced stage, treatment comes too late. Surgery may be tried in the *early* advanced stages. More women than men develop cancer of the gallbladder.

## THE PANCREAS

### Pancreatitis

The pancreas, a gland immediately behind the stomach, secretes pancreatic juice, which aids digestion. The pancreas also contains the islets of Langerhans, groups of cells which secrete insulin. Bile is not supposed to enter the pancreas, but sometimes it does, producing *pancreatitis,* a process that destroys pancreatic tissue and leads to hemorrhages, edema, and severe pain. Pancreatitis is also caused by infection. This condition can now be treated without surgery. Demerol is given to relieve pain; nitroglycerin may be administered to relieve muscle spasms. Banthine may also be used to reduce pancreatic activity in producing pancreatic juice. The prescribed diet is low in fat and high in protein and carbohydrates.

If the islets of Langerhans are affected, treatment for diabetes is necessary. Rest and freedom from emotional strain and upsets are important. Because the pain is so intense, narcotics are given frequently and may lead to drug dependency if acute pancreatitis becomes chronic.

### Cancer of the Pancreas

Jaundice is sometimes the first symptom of cancer of the pancreas, in addition to other symptoms of biliary obstruction. The only hope of cure is to remove the cancerous growth. Before the operation, attention is concentrated on building up the patient's resistance. He may need to gain weight, but his appetite is poor—an obstacle which takes patience to overcome. He needs rest, yet he must have so many things done for him that rest is hard to attain. By the time the cancer has extended to the tail or the body of the pancreas, an operation is useless. (Tumors of the pancreas are most often malignant.)

After surgery (*pancreatectomy*), the patient must be observed for symptoms of hypoinsulism. If only a portion of the pancreas is removed (subtotal pancreatectomy), the patient may show signs of hyperinsulinism, because of the stimulation of the islets of Langerhans (see Chapter 52).

# 50

# The Patient With a Urinary Disorder

---

## BEHAVIORAL OBJECTIVES

*The student successfully attaining the goals of this chapter will be able to:*

- *describe some of the common deviations from normal body structure and function of the urinary system, keeping in mind the normals; briefly discuss the relationships between circulatory, kidney, and reproductive disorders.*

- *describe some of the common nursing procedures used in urologic nursing; demonstrate ability to perform these procedures to assist in the evaluation of the patient's urinary status; demonstrate the ability to observe the urine for abnormalities and to report these.*

- *describe at least 5 common laboratory procedures, and at least 4 x-ray procedures utilized to determine urologic function or dysfunction; describe the cystoscopic examination; discuss the nursing care involved in each of these procedures; and demonstrate the ability to assist the patient with physical and emotional needs, as well as to assist the doctor to perform the procedures.*

- *describe the common symptoms of urologic disorders, utilizing proper medical terminology; and demonstrate ability to observe and report these symptoms.*

- *discuss the nursing care of the patient with a urinary catheter; describe the procedure for insertion of the catheter; demonstrate ability to care for the catheter after it is inserted, as well as skill in inserting it.*

- *briefly discuss other types of urinary diversion.*

- *discuss the nursing care of the patient with urinary incontinence.*

- *describe at least 3 common infectious urinary conditions; discuss other common disorders such as obstruction, trauma, and tumors; and discuss the special nursing care involved when the patient has surgery on the bladder or kidney.*

- *discuss the concept of kidney failure in relationship to normal urinary function; describe the nonsurgical treatment, including dialysis; describe the surgical treatment; discuss kidney transplantation; and describe the major nursing and medical considerations in each case.*

---

## THE URINARY SYSTEM

A review of the urinary system will remind you that it is composed of the *kidneys,* which secrete urine; the *ureters,* which carry urine from the kidneys to the bladder; the *bladder,* which is the urine reservoir; and the *urethra,* which is the outlet tube from the bladder through which urine is voided. This is the system of the body which removes some of the waste products from the blood left after the body burns food, and eliminates them in the urine. The kidneys process the blood, collect the wastes, and pass them on through the ureters into the bladder. The bladder outlet into the urethra is closed tightly until about 200 to 300 cc. has collected, at which time the nervous system signals that the bladder needs emptying. Interference with the operation of this system causes disease or disorder, which should be treated by a urologist who is a specialist in urologic disorders (and who may also treat disorders of the male reproductive system, since the 2 systems are closely related).

**Circulation Disorders and Kidney Disease.** Kidney disease and arterial disease are closely related. For example, the patient who has atherosclerosis is very likely to suffer renal changes, while the patient who develops renal shutdown will invariably have hypertension. Most kidney diseases are circulatory diseases which are caused by renal vascular insufficiency. Severe shock caused by hemorrhage can also cause irreversible kidney damage, if not corrected immediately.

## DIAGNOSIS OF URINARY DISORDERS

### Procedures Performed by the Nurse

There are several diagnostic procedures which the nurse may perform to evaluate urinary function. These include tests such as the clinitest (for sugar) and the acetest (for acetone) and measurement of urine volume and specific gravity (to determine how concentrated the urine is. (Some of these procedures have been discussed elsewhere.) Another test media, called Bili-Labstix (put out by the Ames Company) provides information about "urinary tract and kidney status, carbohydrate metabolism, and liver and biliary tract status." It is a paper strip which when dipped in urine yields readings within 30 seconds on urine pH, sugar, protein, ketones, blood, and bilirubin.

Negative readings in any of the aforementioned tests indicate that many of the body processes are functioning properly. Positive findings may indicate several disorders. For example, if the urine shows an abnormal pH (normal urine pH ranges between 4, 5 and 8) such conditions as gout, calculi, or infections might be suspected. If protein is present in the urine (*proteinuria* or *albuminuria*), the doctor could suspect glomerulonephritis, renal circulatory difficulties, infection, or possible toxemia of pregnancy. If sugar is present in the urine (*glycosuria*), the doctor could suspect diabetes mellitus, shock, or a possible head injury. The presence of ketones (*ketonuria*), could also indicate diabetes, as well as starvation or digestive disturbances, such as faulty fat metabolism. Bilirubin could indicate liver dysfunction or biliary obstruction or hepatitis. Blood in the urine (*hemoglobinuria* or *hematuria*), could indicate infection, calculi, cancer, trauma, overdose of an anticoagulant, or a bleeding disease. Thus, you can see that the urine is an excellent indicator of the *internal environment* of the body.

**Nursing Observations.** The nurse should observe the urine for amount, color, clarity, and odor. It is also important to note if any blood, pus, or sediment is present. Aside from these specific factors, the overall intake and output record is important in assessing urinary disorders: if the urine output is excessive, the patient is said to have *polyuria;* if the output is very small, he is said to have *oliguria;* if there is no output, the patient has *anuria.*

**Residual Urine Volume.** Sometimes the the doctor will order the nurse to check the residual urine volume of the patient. As a first step the patient voids as much as he can. Then, he is immediately catheterized with a *straight catheter* (one which will not stay in place) to collect whatever urine remains in the bladder. This is called the *residual* urine volume. If the residual volume is greater than 150 to 200 cc., the patient usually has a disorder of the bladder which is causing him to retain urine, and the doctor may order that a catheter be left in place, in which case a retention catheter should be used.

## Laboratory Procedures

**Routine Urinalysis.** *Urinalysis* gives much information about the condition of the kidneys and how well they are working. It tells whether disease is interfering with the function of the different parts of the kidneys (*renal tubules, nephrons, glomeruli*); it shows whether disease organisms are at work in the kidney; and it shows whether food materials which should go to the body cells are escaping into the urine.

The urine is collected by the nursing personnel and sent to the laboratory for urinalysis. The urine collected may consist of a single specimen or a 24-hour collection and may be collected as a clean voided specimen or a midstream specimen or by catheterization. (Methods for collecting and observing urine are discussed in Chapter 27.) Routine urinalysis (UA) includes tests for pH, specific gravity, sugar, acetone, and albumin.

**Urine Culture.** A urine culture is done by placing some urine on a special substance and allowing it to incubate to see if any organisms are present in the urine. The nurse must be very careful not to contaminate the specimen with any outside organisms so that a true culture of only the patient's urine will be obtained. Generally the urine is collected by catheterization although a midstream specimen may also be used. Once the urine is collected it must be sent to the laboratory immediately.

**Sensitivity Test.** If a urine culture reveals that an organism is present in the urine, the organism is tested with various drugs to see which one, usually an antibiotic or a sulfonamide, is most effective in combatting the organism. That drug is then given to the patient.

**Urea Clearance Test (Creatinine Clearance).** This test shows how efficiently the nephrons are filtering *urea,* a waste product, from the blood. A fasting blood specimen is taken, and the patient voids. He drinks several glasses of water, and after 1 hour he voids again. A comparison of the amount of urea in each specimen shows whether or not the kidneys are removing urea from the blood at a normal speed.

**Blood Chemistry.** This test is an analysis of a specimen of blood to find out how efficiently the nephrons in the kidney are removing the waste products BUN (blood urea nitrogen) or NPN (nonprotein nitrogen) from the blood. If the amounts found in the blood are higher than normal, they indicate kidney damage or disease. If the BUN or NPN is greatly elevated, the nurse must observe the patient for signs of disorientation, confusion, or seizures.

Blood chemistry may also indicate the amounts of other electrolytes, such as potassium, calcium, and sodium, in the blood, which reflect the overall fluid and electrolyte balance of the body and help determine renal and liver status.

**Phenosulfonphthalein Test (PSP).** When this red dye is injected into a vein it is excreted by the kidneys. For the test, the patient drinks a measured amount of water and then voids in 15 to 20 minutes. The urine is examined for redness and is then discarded. The doctor injects the dye, and 15 minutes later the patient is asked to void, and again in 30 minutes, in 1 hour, and in 2 hours. A retention catheter may be inserted to facilitate obtaining the specimens. The entire specimen is saved each time and labeled with the time it was voided: the first specimen is also labeled with the time that the dye was given. The specimens are sent to the laboratory to be analyzed. The percentage of dye in each specimen indicates how normally the kidneys are performing. The dye will come through more slowly in kidney disease.

It is obvious that when a patient is having one of these tests, the test would be ruined if a specimen is discarded or if the patient is allowed to take something by mouth. In addition the test results will not be valid if the patient is taking pyridium which colors the urine red.

**Other Laboratory Tests.** The laboratory will also test the urine for casts (cylindruria), for crystals (crystalluria), and for pus or white bloods cells (pyuria) which would indicate infection. Urine calcium may be measured to help determine bone disease; high amounts of calcium would indicate degeneration of bone tissue.

## X-Ray Procedures

**K.-U.-B. X-Ray.** A combined kidney-ureter-bladder x-ray, commonly referred to as a K.-U.-B. plate, provides an overall view of the urinary system.

**Intravenous Pyelogram.** This is a series of x-ray pictures taken after a radiopaque dye has been given intravenously; they show the outlines of the kidneys, the ureters, and the bladder. The patient has nothing by mouth for 12 hours before the test, but he is given a cathartic the night before and an enema the morning of the test.

*After-Care:* Note if the patient reacts to the dye by complaining of tingling, numbness, and palpitations. Force fluids for 24 hours to help remove the dye and to relieve any dehydration which may have resulted from the patient not having anything by mouth prior to the test.

**Cystogram.** A *cystogram* is an x-ray of the bladder and the urethra, made by injecting a dye directly into the bladder through a catheter. It will show the outline of the bladder. An x-ray can be taken to show the outline of the urethra while the patient is voiding (*voiding cystogram*).

**Renal Arteriogram.** Contrast dye is injected, via catheter, into the aorta at the level of the renal blood vessels. In this way, the blood vessels of the kidneys may be visualized to determine the presence of a pathologic condition.

**Retrograde Pyelogram Studies.** "Retrograde" refers to the upside-down position of the patient during the procedure. After the bladder is outlined, smaller catheters are inserted into the kidney pelvis and dye is injected, after which retrograde x-rays are taken, showing both kidneys and ureters. This procedure is done in combination with cystoscopy.

**Radioactive Renogram and Renoscan.** Sometimes the kidneys are tested by means of radioactive substances. If a lesion is present, it will tend to pick up more of the radioactive isotope than does normal tissue.

### Other Diagnostic Procedures

**Cystoscopy ("Cysto").** A *cystoscopic examination* allows the physician to view the inside of the bladder through a tubular instrument, the *cystoscope,* which has a mirror and an electric light on the end of it.

The cystoscope is passed into the bladder through the urethra. This examination will detect bladder inflammation or a tumor in the bladder which may be causing blood to appear in the urine. The openings of the ureters into the bladder are also visible; fine opaque wax catheters can be threaded into these openings to collect separate specimens of urine from each kidney in order to determine which kidney is diseased. The cystoscope may also be used just to view the ureters, while *sounds* (dilators) are passed through the ureters to treat ureteral strictures.

This procedure may also be done for the purpose of implanting radon seeds to treat cancer, for removing a polyp or a tumor, for doing a biopsy, or for removing kidney stones (calculi). Electrosurgery (*fulguration*) may also be performed through a cystoscope to remove small tumors or to coagulate any small bleeding blood vessels.

The patient should force fluids before the examination, and be given an enema if x-rays are to be taken. Usually he is also given a sedative, since the procedure is uncomfortable and may be painful. Sometimes a local or general anesthetic is necessary.

*Postcystoscopy Care:* The urine specimens are examined in the laboratory. Voiding may be uncomfortable for a day or two after the examination—sometimes sitz baths are ordered for comfort. The urine has a reddish tinge at first; if this lasts more than 24 hours or increases, it should be reported. Chills and fever are signs of infection that should also be reported. The patient is encouraged to drink fluids.

## COMMON PROBLEMS OF UROLOGIC PATIENTS

While there are many different types of urologic diseases and conditions, most of the patients with these disorders share many of the same problems, the most common being: edema, a dry, itchy skin, headache, nausea and vomiting, infection, an inability to wait to void (*urgency*), frequent urination (*frequency*), pain and burning (*dysuria*), urine drainage—especially after surgery (*incontinence*)—boredom with enforced bedrest and inactivity, and irritability.

The *treatment* and the *nursing care* of urologic patients can be expected to include: diuretics and antibiotics, attention to skin and mouth care, measured intake and output of fluids, observation of urine, forced fluids, a modified diet, such as low-sodium or high-fat

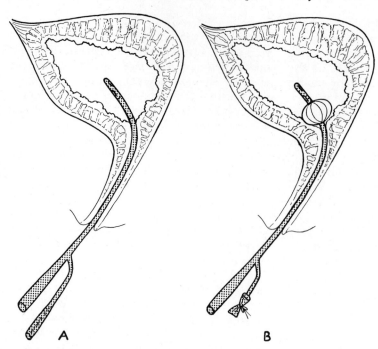

Figure 50-1. Foley catheter. (A) The catheter is inserted into the bladder. (B) The inflation of the bag prevents the catheter from leaving the bladder. The inner tube that leads to the balloon is tied (a rubber band is often used). Smith, D. W., Germain, C. P., and Gips, C. D.: Care of the Adult Patient, ed. 3. Philadelphia, Lippincott, 1971)

and high-carbohydrate, and bed exercises for the bed patient. A male patient may be embarrassed by having a woman carry out some of the procedures that are necessary. If a male nurse is available, so much the better. However, a male patient should never be exposed to the risk of incompetent treatment at the hands of an inexperienced orderly just because he (the patient) is a man. To a nurse, the patient's welfare comes first. This helps her to carry out any procedure calmy and matter-of-factly.

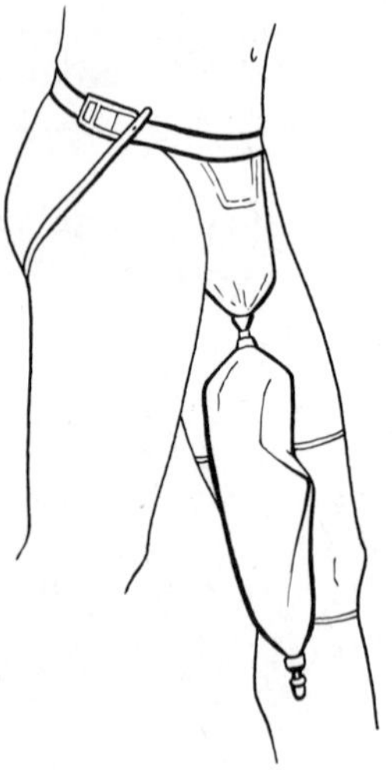

## GENERAL NURSING CARE OF UROLOGIC PATIENTS

### The Patient With a Catheter

After surgery, a retention catheter is usually inserted for urinary drainage. The Foley catheter is frequently used, although there are several other types of catheters such as the male cat 4-wing catheter or the mushroom catheter. The Foley catheter has a collapsed bag attached, which can be inflated like a small balloon after the catheter is inserted and holds the catheter in place (Fig. 50-1). A length of tubing is connected to the catheter, and the urine drains into a bottle at the patient's bedside. To prevent pulling, the catheter is taped to the leg, in a female patient, or tied and taped to the penis, in a male patient. Tape is wrapped around the catheter and is then pinned to the bed so that the tube

Figure 50-2. A rubber leg urinal placed over the penis and held in place with a belt. This device may be improvised, using a rubber condom and a catheter. (Smith, D. W., Germain, C. P., and Gips, C. D.: Care of the Adult Patient, ed. 3. Philadelphia, Lippincott, 1971)

will hang straight from the bedside to the drainage bag (straight drainage).

**Care of the Catheter.** The catheter is considered a closed, *sterile* system. Generally, if the catheter is to be changed, the entire drainage set should be changed. The nurse must be sure that there is no pulling on the catheter and that the tubing is not kinked. The tubing should go over the patient's leg when he is in bed.

**Insertion of the Catheter.** While the method of inserting a catheter has been described previously, the nurse must remember that this is a sterile procedure which must be performed with utmost care to avoid introducing bacteria into the bladder. A sterile, disposable catheterization tray, which contains everything needed is generally used. Frequently the drainage bag is already connected to the tubing, to avoid contamination. If the catheter is introduced sterilly, there will be no chance of contamination when the drainage bag is hooked up. The drainage bags today are plastic and lightweight and can be fastened to the patient's gown while he is up (Fig. 50-2).

**Catheter Irrigation.** If the doctor orders catheter irrigations, the nurse must remember that the bladder is a sterile organ and that any solution injected into the bladder must be sterile and must be inserted with sterile technics. Both ends of the drainage tubing must be kept sterile when disconnected, because organisms can travel up the tubing into the bladder after the tube is reconnected.

Catheter irrigation is usually done to remove clots, to fight infection (by using an antibiotic or bacteriostatic agent), or to make sure that the catheter is patent. The solution is usually injected and then allowed to drain out under the force of gravity. Sometimes, the doctor will order the nurse to withdraw the solution into the syringe. However, it is less traumatic to the bladder to let the solution run out naturally, but the nurse must observe to make sure that the solution is draining. The urine should be observed for sediment, blood clots, or other abnormal findings.

The patient may complain of pain when the solution is instilled into the bladder, because the bladder is accustomed to being empty. On the other hand, the solution may be too cold, thereby causing cramps.

Unless the solution was withdrawn and discarded, remember to indicate the amount of irrigating solution used on the intake and output sheet, so that the amount of solution can be subtracted from the total daily output.

**The Suprapubic Cystocath.** This is a type of bladder drainage which is often used after gynecological and other types of surgery. The catheter is inserted surgically through a small incision just above the pubic bone. It is inserted through a body seal to prevent drainage around the catheter. It is then connected to a drainage bag. The advantage of this type of catheter is the fact that the patient can void naturally while the catheter is still in place. In this way, recatheterization is avoided. The patient also does not feel any annoying irritation from the catheter in the urethra. If perineal surgery has been done, this type of catheter eliminates urinary drainage which could contaminate the surgical area. As in any other instance in which a catheter is inserted into the bladder, sterile technics and precautions are observed.

## Other Types of Urinary Diversion

In some instances of cancer of the prostate or urethra, other types of tubes are placed in the bladder for urine drainage. At times the tubes are left in place permanently. If the bladder must be removed, sometimes an *ileal conduit* or *Bricker procedure* is carried out, whereby a loop of bowel is connected to the ureters and brought out through the skin. In another procedure, called a ureterosigmoidostomy, the ureters are connected to a loop of bowel, the sigmoid colon, so that the urine can drain out through the rectum. In other procedures, a tube may be placed into the kidney and brought out through the skin (*cutaneous nephrostomy*), placed in the ureter and brought out through the skin (*cutaneous ureterostomy*) or placed in the bladder and brought out through the skin (*cutaneous cystostomy*).

These patients share the same problems: infection must be prevented, an appliance must be worn at all times to catch the continuous urine drainage, and there may be leakage and/or odor. Since the urine drains onto the skin, special skin care must be given.

## The Patient With Urinary Incontinence

Two muscles, called the *sphincter muscles,* control the voiding of urine. The *internal* sphincter controls the opening of the bladder into the urethra; the *external* sphincter controls the opening at the outer end of the urethra. When sufficient urine collects in the bladder, it stimulates nerve endings which cause a desire to void. An unconscious or paralyzed patient does not feel this stimulation, so that the sphincters relax involuntarily. Disturbances or damage to the urinary system or interference with the spinal nerves deprive the sphincters of their control over voiding. Many times the bladder can be mechanically "trained," as was discussed in Chapter 46.

**Establishing a Routine.** Often it is possible to control incontinence by establishing a voiding routine. This project will take patience and some experimenting, but it can be successful. Start by keeping a chart, noting when the patient's bladder empties—it may follow a pattern. See that he is given the bedpan or goes to the bathroom just before these times. This sets up a routine for emptying his bladder and keeps him dry.

**Appliances.** Appliances for collecting urine are available for the male patient. Such an appliance consists of a rubber bag that slips over the penis and is attached to a belt. The patient wears the appliance under his clothes. The bag has an outlet at the lower end which can be opened.

The problem of urinary incontinence is greater for a woman, since no similar appliance is available for collecting urine. She can wear a perineal pad; although perhaps a better solution is the plastic protective pants, with absorbent material and a liner inside. The liner is made of nonabsorbent nylon and is placed next to the skin; it dries very rapidly after the urine passes through it, so it protects the skin and prevents irritation. In any case, it is important to wash the buttocks and the genitals frequently with soap and water and to dry them well. An antiseptic may be applied to the skin to prevent irritation. Cleanliness and prompt attention to removing soiled pads help to eliminate urine odor. Any appliance or protective device should be washed thoroughly inside and out with soap and water at least once a day.

**When the Patient Goes Home.** Many patients go home from the hospital with the problem of incontinence. This then becomes a family problem as well, since members of the family may dread the odors, the wet pads, and the laundry. The nurse has an opportunity to give the family some practical help in dealing with this problem. She can show them how to keep the patient dry without changing the entire bed every time, by using absorbent pads covered by a liner next to the patient. The pads can be changed easily, and the liner helps to prevent irritation. Disposable pads should be used when possible. If the patient has established a routine for voiding, the nurse should be sure that the family understands how important it is to keep to that routine. She should also emphasize the importance of fluids, diet, and cleanliness.

## Other Problems Facing the Urologic Patient

**Dehydration.** Since many urologic patients will become dehydrated, special attention must be paid to forcing fluids. Since the mouth may become dry and sore, appropriate oral hygiene should be given.

**Pain.** To offset pain and discomfort, the doctor may order sitz baths or warm, moist packs. Forcing fluids will also help to dilute the urine and lessen the burning sensation which accompanies inflammatory conditions.

**Complications.** Aside from the general complications which can arise from extensive bedrest, the nurse should be aware of more serious problems related to urologic factors, such as hemorrhage and shock and variances in blood pressure.

## INFECTIOUS CONDITIONS

### Cystitis

*Cystitis* is inflammation of the urinary bladder. Normally, the inside of the bladder is sterile, but bacteria may enter it from infected kidneys and lymphatics or from the urethra. In this last instance, women are more susceptible than men, because the urethra is shorter. As indicated earlier, one reason for using sterile technic in catheterization is to prevent the introduction of bacteria into the bladder. Cystitis is usually the result of infection somewhere else in the urinary tract or in the reproductive system. Systemic disease may make a person more susceptible to bladder infection.

**Symptoms and Treatment.** The patient with cystitis has a desire to urinate frequently, although the bladder does not need emptying. Thus very small amounts are voided each time. Urination is accompanied by a painful, burning sensation; sometimes there is blood in the urine and the patient complains of a "heavy feeling" in the abdomen or perineum. Antibiotics or sulfonamides are given, with forced fluids. Sometimes a drug (potassium citrate or sodium bicarbonate) is prescribed to alkalize the urine if it is markedly acid. Cranberry juice is often given to increase the amount of potassium in the urine. Warm sitz baths help to make the patient more comfortable. Cystitis is common when the prostate is enlarged. Many women contract cystitis when they are first married.

The nurse should remember to remind female patients to wipe from front to back after going to the bathroom, to help prevent recurrence of cystitis.

## Pyelonephritis

*Acute pyelonephritis,* or inflammation of the kidney, is the most common form of kidney disease. It is usually caused by infection by organisms from elsewhere in the body. These organisms (usually *Escherichia coli* or Klebsiella) reach the kidney through the bloodstream, causing inflammation, edema, and sometimes many small abscesses. Early treatment of acute pyelonephritis is important to prevent permanent kidney damage.

**Symptoms.** The patient is very ill, with pain, pus in the urine, chills, fever, nausea, and vomiting. If the bladder also is infected, he will have a desire to urinate frequently, although burning will accompany voiding. A urine test reveals bacteria in the urine, as well as white blood cells and casts.

**Treatment and Nursing Care.** Bedrest, plenty of fluids, attention to mouth and skin care, nourishment, and change of position are important. Antibiotics or sulfonamides are given for the infection. Every effort is made to prevent this condition from becoming chronic, by eliminating the infection and building up good health. Pyelonephritis can usually be treated and controlled, although sometimes it becomes chronic, in which case, it can lead to hypertension, uremia, or septicemia and death.

*Chronic pyelonephritis* may develop if the infection recurs or an obstruction interferes with the passage of urine. The kidney becomes permanently damaged, and nothing will replace kidney tissues. The patient may develop hypertension or uremia. The treatment consists of continued efforts to prevent more damage. Sometimes, if hypertension develops, the kidney may be removed by surgery, provided that the other kidney is functioning normally. This is rarely done, however. Today, a kidney transplant is more likely and the damaged kidney is left in place.

## Nephritis (Bright's Disease)

*Nephritis* is a group of diseases in which the kidneys are damaged and partly destroyed by inflammation in the *glomeruli.* Often the signs of *acute* nephritis (acute glomerulonephritis) appear about 2 or 3 weeks after an upper respiratory infection, or after scarlet fever or chicken pox. The organism is usually the same streptococcus which causes "strep. sore throat." The patient himself may not notice the symptoms at first—it may be his family that senses something is wrong as they become aware of his pale, puffy face and swollen tissues. He is getting up many times in the night to void, his head aches, and he is noticeably irritable. Without treatment, uremia and congestive heart failure may be the next and fatal development.

**Treatment.** No single drug or special treatment will cure acute nephritis. The goal is to restore the function of the kidney, as much as possible. The patient must stay in bed, sometimes for several weeks. He is given as much fluid as he can tolerate and is placed on a diet which is low in protein and sodium but high in carbohydrates. Vitamins and iron are often used to supplement the diet. In cases of edema and congestive heart failure, salt is restricted. He receives antibiotics to counteract any infection he may have. Accurate intake and output and daily weighing are a must. Fluids are given to balance output.

With treatment, almost all patients recover from acute nephritis; they are not considered as being well until the urine has been free of albumin and red blood cells for some time.

Although most patients with acute glomerulonephritis recover, the patient may develop chronic glomerulonephritis.

## Chronic Nephritis

Chronic nephritis (*chronic glomerulonephritis*) is another story—it damages the kidney permanently by destroying nephrons and interfering with kidney functions. The symptoms are much the same as in acute nephritis, with marked edema all over the body. The disease flares up at intervals, but the patient usually feels very well between attacks. However, if uremia develops, the patient may die very quickly.

**Complications and Treatment.** Chronic nephritis can have serious complications—pulmonary edema, increased blood pressure, anemia, cerebral hemorrhage, and congestive heart failure. In the advanced stages of the disease, vision may become blurred, followed by blindness. Nosebleeds and gastrointestinal bleeding are not unusual in the terminally ill patient. However, a patient may live for years if he protects his health and builds up his resistance to infection. He cannot afford to risk catching cold, for it may lead to uremia. When signs of a flare-up of the disease appear, he must go to bed, lower his salt intake, and regulate the amount of protein in his diet. He must avoid exposure to infection of any kind. He will have transfusions if he needs them for anemia, and sedatives if he needs them for headache and insomnia. With this treatment, the symptoms usually subside in about 3 weeks, and the patient gradually returns to his normal routines.

However, the prognosis in this disease is often poor and symptomatic. Nursing care is all that is possible. The patient is put into orthopneic position to assist in breathing and is given fluids as tolerated. Digitalis is often given for cardiac failure.

## Other Infectious Diseases

Other organisms and infections which may infect the urinary system are tuberculosis, gonorrhea, or other organisms such as staph-ylococcus, streptococcus, or the trichomona and monilia organisms which commonly cause vaginal infections in women.

# NONINFECTIOUS DISORDERS OF THE URINARY SYSTEM

## Urinary Obstructions

Obstructions in the urinary system may be caused by a stone, a growth, a spasm of the ureter, or a kink in the ureter. An enlarged prostate gland in older men may interfere with the passage of urine. Urinary obstructions can eventually damage the kidneys and cause them to become enlarged with dammed-up urine (hydronephrosis). As a result waste products accumulate in the blood, causing uremia. An obstruction in the urethra causes an accumulation of urine in the bladder, where it becomes stagnant and provides a favorable place for infection to develop. Bacteria also reach the urethra through the bloodstream and from the outside. The first step in treating urinary obstructions is to establish urine drainage and later to remove the cause of the obstruction.

**Stones or Calculi.** The urine is full of salts such as uric acid, calcium, and oxalate, which, if they do not dissolve, form stones, a condition known as lithiasis. Stones form primarily in the kidneys and descend through the urinary passages. No one knows exactly why stones form, although some authorities believe that infection, dehydration, or urinary stasis, help to cause them. Sometimes people who have a tendency to form stones are allowed only a limited amount of milk, since milk is high in the mineral, calcium. Patients with a long-term illness that keeps them in bed in a more-or-less fixed position, seem to have a tendency to develop stones. Bed exercises and plenty of fluids help to prevent this condition.

SYMPTOMS. The signs of stones are *blood* or *pus* in the urine from irritation or infection; *retention* of urine, if the bladder opening into the urethra is blocked; *pain* in the region of the obstruction; and *colic,* which is an excruciating pain that comes in waves as the ureter tries to force an obstructing stone to move on. This pain is violent and unbearable—only a strong sedative will relieve it. If the stone is very small, the spasm may move it along, allowing the patient to pass it. Urine containing gravel or small stones should be saved for laboratory examination. If colicky attacks recur, surgery is usually necessary to remove the obstruction.

NURSING CARE. Nursing care involves giving medications, applying warm packs for pain, and forcing fluids. When a patient is admitted with a possible diagnosis of calculi, his urine should be strained. The nurse or the patient can do this by pouring the urine through gauze, cheesecloth, or a strainer. Usually, the urine itself is discarded, while the material which is strained out is saved for the doctor to see or for laboratory tests.

SURGICAL TREATMENT. If the stone does not pass through the urethral channels spontaneously, it must be surgically removed. A stone in the bladder may be removed by cystoscopy (the stone is crushed, *litholapaxy*, and allowed to pass out with the urine), by *cystotomy* (incision into the bladder), or by *nephrotomy* (incision into the kidney). If an incision is made into the ureter to remove a stone, the procedure is called a *ureterolithotomy*; when the bladder is incised to remove a stone the procedure is called a *cystolithotomy*. The actual removal of the stone is referred to as a *cystolithectomy*.

POSTOPERATIVE MANAGEMENT. The patient who has a tendency to form stones, is urged to force fluids, strain his urine at home, limit the foods which may have caused stones to form, and report any symptoms to the doctor.

**Urethral Strictures.** Fibrous bands may form anywhere along the urethra to narrow it and interfere with the passage of urine. Stagnant urine in the bladder leads to infection. With a urethral stricture, the patient has difficulty in voiding. He has a desire to void frequently (frequency), but voiding is accompanied by an intense burning sensation (dysuria). A urethral stricture can be stretched by inserting metal instruments (*sounds*) of graduated sizes into the urethra, beginning with the largest size that will go past the stricture and gradually increasing to larger ones. Since strictures have a tendency to tighten up again, the patient will have to return to the hospital periodically to have this *dilatation* process repeated. Sometimes surgery is necessary to cut the constricting bands.

**Acute Hydronephrosis.** Hydronephrosis is a distention of the kidney, caused by an obstruction blocking the normal flow of urine. The obstruction may be in the form of cancer, stones, or other obstructions, which causes the urine to dam up, resulting in pressure on the kidney. If the obstruction is in the ureter, only one kidney will be involved; if it is in the urethra, usually both kidneys will be affected. Hydronephrosis may be gradual, partial, or intermittent. Generally, acute hydronephrosis is reversible, but the cause of the obstruction must be removed as soon as possible. If the condition is allowed to continue, chronic nephrosis will result.

**Chronic Hydronephrosis.** This is a destructive process that goes on in the renal tubules, as a result of continued damming up of urine. It interferes with the blood flow to the kidneys and may lead to the suppression (stoppage) of urine and, eventually, to uremia. The treatment is centered on keeping the patient alive until the kidneys repair themselves and function normally again. A low-sodium diet is prescribed, diuretics are given for edema, and ACTH or adrenocortical hormones may also be given. The patient's intake and output is carefully watched and recorded and he is weighed daily. He is also frequently checked for edema (fluid collection in the tissues). If there is no improvement in kidney function, and if death from uremia is imminent, *dialysis* may be used.

In the past, this disorder was seen only in children. Now, with dialysis and transplantation of kidneys, we are seeing adults with chronic hydronephrosis. Since a great deal of research and experimentation is being done in this area, many people are able to live fairly normal lives with the assistance of new medical technics. However, because these are relatively new approaches to the problem, we do not know what complications to expect as these people grow older.

### Trauma to the Kidney or Bladder

When a person with a full bladder is involved in an automobile accident there is a danger that the bladder may be ruptured. If the bladder is ruptured, immediate emergency surgery is required to prevent septicemia. Trauma to the kidney can also be dangerous because the kidney is such a vascular organ. Since a small laceration can cause massive hemorrhage, the patient will need immediate surgery to correct the lesion and to ligate the blood vessels. Occasionally, the damaged kidney must be removed to prevent further hemorrhage.

## Tumors of the Urinary Tract

**Tumors of the Kidney.** Tumors of the kidney are almost always malignant and frequently are the result of metastasis from a cancerous growth somewhere else in the body. If the kidney is a primary site and the cancer is caught early enough, the kidney may be removed (*nephrectomy*), and the patient may be cured. Often, this patient is treated with irradiation as an added protective measure. If the malignancy of the kidney is a secondary or metastatic, lesion, or if metastasis from the kidney has occurred, generally, the kidney will be left in place and the patient will be treated with palliative measures.

The tumor is usually well developed before signs of it appear. The first sign may be blood in the urine (*painless hematuria*). Other symptoms are fever, loss of weight, and malaise; pain may appear later. After x-rays have confirmed the diagnosis, surgical removal of the kidney may be done if the other kidney is healthy.

*Cysts* of the kidney may be multiple (*polycystic disease*) or single (*monocystic*). These cysts are often not removed unless they are large or are causing difficulty.

**Tumors of the Bladder.** Tumors may be imbedded in the bladder wall or may be like small warts on the inside surface. The tumors may or may not be malignant. Superficial tumors can be removed by an electric cautery (*fulguration*) or may be cut out with an instrument called a *resectoscope,* which can be inserted into the bladder through the urethra. Patients with this type of tumor return at 6-month intervals for a check-up by cystoscopic examination to see if the tumor has recurred or if new ones have developed. Larger tumors are removed through an incision made in the bladder.

Most tumors of the bladder can be removed by cystoscopy, as discussed previously. Occasionally, the bladder must be removed and the urine flow diverted through a diversion such as the ureterostomy (see p. 661).

## KIDNEY FAILURE

### Uremia

*Uremia* is failure of the kidneys to remove wastes from the blood and the body cells and to excrete them in the urine. It may be defined as a toxic condition, associated with renal insufficiency and retention in the blood of nitrogenous substances. This may be the result of kidney disease or of urinary tract disturbances, or a result of scarlet fever. It may also be the result of acute glomerulonephritis, drug poisoning, severe transfusion reactions, and other severe shocks to the system. It may also result from an injury that decreases the blood supply to the kidneys.

**Symptoms.** Uremia may develop suddenly, but it usually comes on so gradually that the patient is not aware of it. He may pay little attention to his mild headaches, occasional intestinal upsets, and a tired feeling. He may be irritable or show other emotional or personality changes. Early signs are headache, dizziness, blurring of vision, and slowness of mental processes (from an increased blood pressure). Later symptoms include oliguria (below 500 cc. per day), with *low* specific gravity, increase in NPN or BUN determinations; pallor, and marked edema *or* dehydration, (depending on which part of the kidney is not functioning).

Gradually, these symptoms become more pronounced—the headaches are more persistent, the patient feels nauseated and vomits and is thirsty and air-hungry. These are signs of *acidosis,* which means there is an accumulation of waste products in the body. The breath of the patient assumes an unpleasant odor, and *uremic frost,* a white substance which is actually an accumulation of waste products which the kidneys are not excreting in the urine (urea and salt crystals), may occur around the patient's mouth and nose. He may also have itching or a body odor which smells like stale urine.

Although he may be restless, the patient is more likely to become comatose and may have convulsions. If he does not respond to treatment, inevitably the signs of heart failure will appear.

**Treatment and Nursing Care.** Everything is done to treat the primary cause of uremia and to treat the symptoms as they appear. Keep the patient in as normal a state as possible, and attempt to prevent further kidney damage. Sedatives are given for restlessness, transfusions for anemia, and digitalis for heart difficulty. Fluids are restricted because the kidneys are not excreting urine, (urge the patient to spread his fluid allowance throughout the day). Alkaline solutions are given for acidosis, and the patient is put on a diet high in fat and carbohydrates and low in protein, sodium, and potassium. It is very important to attempt to maintain fluid and electrolyte balance. Frequent blood chemistry studies will be done, and the nurse must be sure the doctor gets the reports as soon as possible.

Very accurate records of intake and output are vital. Good skin care and special mouth care are also very important. Chilling and exposure to infections should be prevented, and respiratory or cardiac complications should be watched for.

If the condition which is causing uremia cannot be improved, the patient will die. (By the time be actually becomes uremic, his prognosis is very poor.) However, the kidney has a remarkable ability to recover from insult.

The nurse must realize that in the severely ill patient, the nursing care may be supportive and not curative.

## The Artificial Kidney (Dialysis)

The artificial kidney is an apparatus which takes over the work of the kidney temporarily when (1) a damaged kidney is not filtering wastes from the blood and excreting them in the urine and when (2) the kidneys cease all operations as a result of acute kidney disease, shock, or lethal doses of poison. This procedure is used as a last resort, when everything else has failed to restore kidney function. Many people are maintained on intermittent dialysis.

There are two chief types of dialysis: *peritoneal dialysis* and *hemodialysis,* both of which function on the rationale of removing body wastes through a semipermeable membrane by the process of osmosis.

**Peritoneal Dialysis.** This type of dialysis uses the intestinal wall as the semipermeable membrane. A catheter is inserted into the visceral cavity through which the dialysis

solution, most often a dextrose solution, is instilled into the abdominal cavity. The solution is allowed to remain in the peritoneum for a length of time specified by the doctor and then is drained out into a bottle on the floor. This process may be continuous or repeated intermittently. Peritoneal dialysis is used most often in the *acute patient,* such as a person whose kidneys have shut down because of an overdose of a drug, (such as a barbiturate).

It is not usually used in a chronic case. Most often, if the patient will need dialysis for more than 2 or 3 days, cannulas are inserted and hemodialysis will begin.

NURSING CARE. Since the practical nurse may be asked to do this procedure, she must know the basics relating to nursing care. She will receive specific instructions at the time she is assigned to the case. The nurse is responsible for keeping records of the dialysis process, including patient intake and output through normal body orifices, as well as a complete record of the dialysate solution. She must record what solution was used, what drugs or electrolytes were added, and what time the solution was instilled and drained out. She is responsible for recording vital signs of the patient including temperature, apical pulse, respiration rate and blood pressure, as well as daily weight, level of consciousness, and eye signs. She must see that the patient is turned, breathes deeply often, and is given good skin care and oral hygiene. She should also be sure that the puncture site and dialysis fluid are kept sterile. She should watch for signs of drug reactions, as well as distention, abdominal pain, bleeding or shock, respiratory problems, infection, and leakage around the catheter which leads into the peritoneum.

**Hemodialysis.** If the patient is a person who will need chronic renal dialysis, it is more desirable to use the artificial kidney or dialysis machine. In this case the semipermeable membrane is a cellophane substance within the machine. Dialysis is carried on within the machine, by means of blood flow from the patient. An artery-to-vein shunt (A-V shunt), is performed, with the radial artery and a vein in the forearm used most often. This shunt remains in place, because this patient needs dialysis 2 or 3 times each week, to maintain life. Hypoallergenic tape should be used on the cannula, to avoid skin irritation, and heparin is usually instilled to prevent clotting.

Patients maintained on this type of dialysis are generally classified as *pending* (those awaiting transplant of kidney), *acute* (cases of poisoning or a one-time transplant), or *chronic* (those needing to continue dialysis on a regular basis for life).

COMPLICATIONS OF CONTINUED DIALYSIS. Since the practical nurse may be trained to work in a renal dialysis unit, she should know about the complications which may occur in hemodialysis.

1. The A-V shunt can come out, in which case the patient can bleed to death. He can also bleed because the cannula is heparinized.
2. The cellophane within the dialysis machine can rupture, in which case the patient can hemorrhage.
3. The machine can be set up with the wrong chemicals or the chemistry determinations of the patient can be done incorrectly in which case the fluid and electrolyte balance of the patient would be even further out of balance than before.
4. Since the blood pressure for most patients on dialysis is high (because of the renal damage), a patient may go into shock when connected to the machine.
5. The blood used in the machine must be warm or the patient can suffer cardiac arrest from the shock of cold blood.
6. Infection is always a possibility. Since this patient has especially low resistance, infection can be very dangerous.
7. The cannula can clot and cause phlebitis.
8. Men often become impotent, although this may improve as the chemistry of the body stabilizes.

NURSING CARE. The nurse must watch for the complications which have been mentioned. In addition, the patient usually is on a low-sodium, low-protein diet, with limited fluid intake. The patient cannot drink any alcohol; it will not be excreted by the kidneys and the patient will remain drunk until the next dialysis. The dialysis unit is kept as homelike as possible, and the staff is specially trained in interpersonal relationships as well as in excellent nursing skills. The aim is rehabilitation of the patient. Some patients have units in their own homes and do their own dialysis at night. In this case, a family member must be trained to assist and to recognize complications. Travel is now possible for this patient because there are satellite units around the world. The alternative for many dialysis patients is a *kidney transplant*.

As you can imagine, the patient must be very emotionally stable to undergo chronic renal dialysis.

# SURGICAL PROCEDURES IN KIDNEY DISORDERS

## Nephrectomy and Nephrotomy

As indicated earlier the removal of a kidney is referred to as a *nephrectomy*; bilateral nephrectomy is removal of both kidneys. A *nephrotomy*, on the other hand, is an incision into and/or a repair of a kidney.

**Preoperative Nursing Care.** The patient is prepared preoperatively, if possible, to attain maximum kidney function before surgery. Fluids are forced to assure maximum flushing action through the kidneys.

**Postoperative Nursing Care.** Routine care is given as for any patient with abdominal surgery. Although the patient must breathe deeply and cough, he will have difficulty with this, because the incision is close to the diaphragm. IPPB (intermittent positive pressure breathing) treatments are usually ordered. Pain medications should also be prescribed, so that the patient may cough and move after surgery.

Since the patient should have a large amount of fluids, an accurate record of intake and output is very important. If the patient has more than one catheter, output from each should be measured separately. Since urine may drain out of the wound, the nurse should know if the patient has a drain or wick in place.

The most dangerous complication, and the most possible complication following kidney surgery, especially nephrotomy, is that of hemorrhage. The kidney is a very vascular organ, and incision into it may lead to excessive bleeding. Often, clamps are left in place, because it is very difficult to tie off each bleeder during surgery. These clamps should not be disturbed by the nursing staff. The nurse must watch carefully for signs of hemorrhage and shock and report these at once, since they may become fatal in a short time.

## Kidney Transplants

*Organ transplants* are a comparatively new development that is causing something of a sensation in the medical world. In this new field of surgery, doctors take an organ, such as a *kidney,* from a well human being or a cadaver and transplant it to the body of another to replace a diseased organ. The chief difficulty with transplants is that the body does not like foreign materials, and its natural response is to reject them. This seems to be less of a problem if the transplant is from the body of an identical twin. Currently, many antirejection medications, such as Imuran, greatly increase the chances of retention of the transplanted kidney. The kidney is also "typed" before transplant; that is, it is matched as closely as possible to the blood structure of the recipient, to lessen the chance of rejection. Some patients may have repeat transplants (being maintained by dialysis in between), if they reject donor kidneys. (The rejection process was discussed in Chapter 47.)

Medical authorities pioneering in this field make it plain that a kidney transplant should be attempted only when experts think that it has a chance to succeed and when everything else has been tried to save the dying patient. Even then, they emphasize that this is not a procedure for general surgeons but should be attempted only by doctors who have had special training and study. Enough kidney transplants have been successful to encourage medical scientists to go on with research in this kind of surgery.

**Other Aspects of Kidney Transplant.** The kidney is transplanted more often than all other major organs together. One reason for this is the fact that this surgery can involve a live donor. In addition, the patient can be prepared more carefully over a long period of time and can be maintained by renal dialysis. The surgery itself is much easier than other transplants and the kidney can be matched to the recipient.

There are, however, a great many psychological and moral aspects involved in any situation of this type. The doctors must decide who will be transplanted and who will not. The psychological attitude of the patient must be excellent, in order for him to undergo the physical and emotional stress involved. The nurse must understand and support the patient during this very complicated and demanding procedure. She must be an understanding and supportive person, as well as an excellent practitioner of nursing.

# 51

# The Patient With a Reproductive Disorder

## BEHAVIORAL OBJECTIVES

*The student successfully attaining the goals of this chapter will be able to:*

- *describe some of the common deviations from normal body structure and function of the female reproductive system, keeping in mind the normal structure and function previously studied.*
- *assist with a gynecologic examination, being helpful both to the doctor and to the patient; discuss the components of the examination, including the Pap smear; discuss the reasons for various procedures and the conditions which might be disclosed; and assist in interpreting the importance of this examination to patients and others.*
- *discuss the D&C and culdoscopy; describe the medical treatment; and demonstrate ability to assist the doctor and the patient in each situation.*
- *discuss other examinations, such as x-ray and various breast examinations; and discuss the emotional and physical aspects of each.*
- *describe special procedures related to women, such as the douche or perineal care; discuss reasons for these; and demonstrate ability to assist the patient with these procedures, as well as to teach them.*
- *identify some common menstrual disorders; identify some common disorders related to the menopause; describe each condition; and discuss the major aspects of nursing and medical care in each case.*
- *list at least 10 other conditions of the female reproductive system, including P.I.D., tumors, and breast diseases; describe each condition; discuss the major considerations in medical and nursing care; and demonstrate the ability to assist the patient in each case.*
- *discuss the special considerations in cancer of the reproductive organs, including special emotional considerations; and demonstrate the ability to assist a patient with this condition.*
- *describe some of the common deviations from normal in the male reproductive system; and discuss the special emotional needs of the patient.*
- *describe some common disorders of the male reproductive system, discuss the symptoms and medical treatment of each; and demonstrate the ability to assist the patient to meet his needs.*
- *discuss the concepts of fertility and infertility, of sterilization, birth control, abortion, and venereal disease; and discuss the particular physical and emotional aspects of each.*

## THE FEMALE PATIENT

A review of the reproductive system reminds us that the female reproductive organs consist of the *ovaries,* the *fallopian tubes,* the *uterus,* the *vagina,* the *external genitals,* and the *breasts.* Diseases and disorders of this system are often allied with urinary system difficulties. The branch of medicine that is concerned with genitourinary conditions in women is *gynecology.* The specialist in this field is the *gynecologist.* These disorders usually occur during adult life, but occasionally, during early adolescence, menstrual difficulties require the attention of a gynecologist.

## The Gynecologic Examination

**The Emotional Side.** Women are likely to be emotionally upset by a gynecologic disorder for various reasons. Perhaps a woman may be afraid that it will interfere with having children, that it will disturb marital relations, or that it may mean cancer or venereal disease. Whatever the cause, a nurse should remember that a gynecologic disorder is likely to be emotionally disturbing, and she should listen to what the patient says for a clue to her feelings. Often the nurse can tell the doctor about a particular worry which only he can relieve. When the doctor discusses the situation with both husband and wife, it gives them an opportunity to ask questions about matters that they do not understand and prevents needless worries. The first consideration in the treatment of gynecologic conditions during the child-bearing years is to preserve the ability to have children, if this is possible without endangering the patient. For women past the child-bearing years, it is equally important to correct difficulties for the sake of the patient's health and comfort, as well as for her emotional well-being.

Many women dread the ordeal of the gynecologic examination (the *pelvic examination*). They may worry about exposure or embarrassing questions and shrink from knowing what they fear will be "the worst." The patient will be relieved if the nurse assures her that she will be covered during the examination and that the nurse will be with her during the entire procedure. The patient should be encouraged to tell the doctor every-thing about her difficulty—she should feel that nothing is too unimportant to mention. If she has a vaginal discharge, she may be distressed because she is not allowed to have a douche before the examination. Explain that the doctor will want to see the extent of the discharge and perhaps will want to have a smear of the discharge examined in the laboratory.

**Procedure.** Have the patient empty her bladder and strip to the waist. Position the patient on the examining table with her buttocks as far down to the foot end as possible. Ask her to put her heels into the stirrups and then cover her with a draw sheet. Tell her that she will be most comfortable during the examination if she can spread her knees and relax her legs and hips. If she has discomfort when the speculum is inserted, advise her that it helps to take a few fast, panting-type breaths.

**Equipment.** You will need a clean or sterile vaginal speculum of the appropriate size, a water-soluble lubricant such as K-Y Jelly, a flashlight, gloves for the doctor, and tissues for the patient to use to wipe herself after the examination.

Ethical rules of medicine indicate that a female nurse or attendant should be present in the room whenever a male doctor is doing a pelvic examination on a patient. The nurse can be supportive to the patient during the examination, as well as being of assistance to the physician.

**Test for Cancer (Papanicolaou Test).** A malignant growth in the uterus sometimes drops its cells into the uterine and vaginal secretions. By examining a smear from these secretions microscopically, it is possible to detect these cells before the actual symptoms of cancer appear. This examination is known as the *Papanicolaou test.* Through this early detection, no time will be lost in starting treatment to prevent a malignant growth from advancing. *Cancer of the cervix* is one of the most common forms of cancer in women. If the test is positive, or the cervix looks suspicious, a biopsy of the suspected tissue can be done.

The practical nurse will often be asked to assist the physician with the *Pap smear* (Papanicolaou test). The procedure for positioning the patient is the same as for any routine pelvic examination. The equipment needed for the Pap smear, in addition to the equipment for the pelvic examination, includes glass slides, a bottle of media (alcohol and ether), into which the glass slides are placed after the smear is obtained, and the wooden stick which is inserted through the speculum and is used to obtain a smear of cervical mucosa.

RESULTS OF THE PAP SMEAR. The pathologist examines the smear and interprets the findings, as recommended by Dr. Papanicolaou, according to the following classifications:

*Class I:* Absence of abnormal cells
*Class II:* Atypical cytology, but no evidence of malignancy
*Class III:* Cytology suggestive of, but not conclusive for malignancy
*Class IV:* Cytology strongly suggestive of malignancy
*Class V:* Cytology conclusively that of malignancy

If the patient has an abnormal Pap smear, this does not necessarily mean that she has cancer, except in the case of Class V. However, the abnormal findings do indicate that she should have further tests done to determine whether or not she does have a malignancy, and if so, what type it is and what the recommended treatment should be. The further examination might consist of a cervical biopsy, dilatation and curettage, or exploratory surgery.

The patient should understand the necessity of early diagnosis and treatment if there is a malignancy. She should also know that in many cases, an abnormal Pap smear does not reveal a malignancy.

**Other Procedures.** The doctor can also do a biopsy of the cervix during a pelvic examination, or he can cauterize a portion of the cervix. The pelvic examination offers the physician an opportunity to visualize the cervix, the vagina, and the perineum. He can also *palpate* the uterus by inserting a finger into the rectum, and he can palpate the ovaries abdominally. Every woman past her teens should have a complete pelvic examination, including a Pap smear, at least once a year, and more often if any pathology is present or if there is a strong family history of pathology.

**Culdoscopy.** Culdoscopy provides direct visualization of the uterus and *adnexa* (accessory organs, such as the ovaries and tubes),

achieved by passing an instrument (the endoscope) through the vaginal wall behind the cervix. The procedure is usually done in the operating room with the patient in a knee-chest position. The patient may have local, spinal, or general anesthesia. Usually, no sutures are involved, and routine postoperative care is given.

**Dilatation of the Cervix and Curettage of the Uterus.** In addition to serving as a therapeutic measure, dilatation of the cervix and *curettage* (scraping) of the uterus are also done to find the cause of abnormal vaginal bleeding. The uterine scrapings are examined in the laboratory for evidence of malignant or nonmalignant growths. Sometimes a "D & C" is done just before the menstrual period in an effort to find the cause of sterility. It may also be done after an abortion; and it is always done after an incomplete abortion. A D & C is frequently done for endometrial hypoplasia, menorrhagia or metrorrhagia or in order to do a biopsy as a follow-up on a positive Pap smear.

NURSING CARE. The preoperative preparation is as for any patient about to receive general anesthesia. Perhaps a cleansing douche is also given. Postoperatively, the patient usually makes an uneventful recovery. She will wear a perineal pad and require perineal care as long as a vaginal discharge persists. Any minor discomfort is usually relieved by a mild analgesic, such as Darvon or aspirin. She is often out of bed the same day and goes home in a day or 2, unless she has lost much blood. Sometimes the vagina is packed with gauze at the time of the operation, which may make voiding difficult; but usually the pack is removed the next day.

**X-Ray Examinations.** Several x-ray procedures are done to determine patency of the uterine or fallopian tubes or the presence of abnormalities in the uterus and tubes. The most common of these is the hysterosalpingogram in which the uterus and tubes can be visualized following an injection of contrast dye. The ovaries may also be visualized.

## Breast Examinations

**The Breast Self-Examination.** The American Cancer Society recommends that each woman examine her breasts monthly, immediately following the menses, to determine if there are any lumps or nodules. Each woman should also have her breasts examined by a doctor at least once a year and more often if she has a cystic disorder or a family history of pathology.

The breast self-examination is done in several steps. First, the woman stands in front of a mirror with her arms at her sides. She then looks for change in size, shape or for any puckering, dimpling, or inversion of the nipples. She should also note any discharge or change in the nipples. Then, she should raise her hands over her head and look again. The breasts should still be the same size and shape. In a lying position, she should feel for a lump or thickening of each breast first with her arm at her side and then with the arm raised above her head. Each portion of each breast should be examined carefully. The entire procedure is described and pictured in a booklet put out by the American Cancer Society and called *Self-Examination of the Breast*.

**Examination of the Breasts by the Doctor.** A woman should have a breast examination at least once a year. However, if any unusual symptoms appear the woman should have her breasts examined immediately by the doctor. He will do essentially the same palpation examination and may do other procedures as well.

**Diagnosis of Breast Lesions.** Malignant lesions are more likely to be irregularly shaped and hard and often show secondary signs such as enlarged lymph nodes in the axillary area, asymmetry, retraction of the nipple, discharge or bleeding, dimpling, or elevation of the breast. Benign lesions are more likely to be round or oval, with a smooth border and show no secondary signs. They are more likely to be movable, while malignant lesions are often attached to the surrounding skin or breast tissue.

MAMMOGRAPHY. This is an x-ray examination of the breasts, which is done in situations which require a more definite diagnosis. Sometimes a mammography is done in the person who is very frightened of cancer or in a person who has previously had cancer or has a family history of cancer. The procedure is simple and does not require the injection of dye. However, specially trained radiologists must interpret the mammary x-rays.

BIOPSY. A biopsy is the most definite means of determining if cancer is present. It may be done by withdrawing some of the tissue into a syringe or by cutting out a node and freezing a section for examination. If the doctor suspects cancer, usually the incisional biopsy will be done, a frozen section made, and radical mastectomy performed immediately, if indicated.

It is imperative to remove the cancerous lesion as soon as possible to prevent spread. The more it is handled or biopsied, the more likely it is to spread. For this reason, it is not usually the practice to biopsy on one day and do surgery at a later time. It is the recommended medical practice to do biopsy, frozen section, and radical mastectomy at the same operation, to avoid further handling of the lesion.

BREAST PAP SMEAR. A new procedure has been devised to obtain secretions from the nonlactating breast which are then examined in much the same way as the cervical smear is examined. It is more difficult to obtain secretions from postmenopausal women. This procedure offers another means of diagnosing breast cancer early enough so that it can be successfully treated.

## Teaching Good Feminine Hygiene

The nurse is in an excellent position in the examining room or the hospital to teach the patient about good hygiene practices. Many women do not realize that after urinating or defecating, they should wipe from front to back, to prevent urinary tract infections. The nurse can also teach about feminine hygiene deodorant sprays and suppositories. Some patients will want to douche, and the nurse can assist with proper procedure. The practical nurse can teach the patient the procedure for breast self-examination and reaffirm the necessity of yearly cervical Pap smears, breast examination, and serology tests for venereal disease.

## Gynecologic Nursing Procedures

**Perineal Care.** Many patients will need instruction in perineal care. Be sure to teach the patient to wipe from front to back and to use each cotton ball or Zephiran sponge only once. She should be taught to wipe the outside areas first, saving the last sponges for the urethral area. Sometimes, the doctor will order sterile water or saline to be poured over the perineal area.

**Sitz Baths.** Sitz baths are frequently ordered for female patients. While the procedures involved have been described before, it is important to remember that the tub should be disinfected between each usage and that the patient should be instructed as to why the procedure is necesary, whether it be to cleanse the area, assist in the healing process, or make the patient more comfortable.

**Douche.** The douche is not as frequently prescribed as before, but should the doctor order it, the procedure and purpose should be explained to the patient—it is simply a vaginal irrigation. A douche is easiest to administer when the patient is lying in a bathtub. The solution is warm, not hot, and is placed in a douche bag, which is held about 12 to 18 inches above the perineal area. The nozzle is inserted gently and rotated while the solution is flowing into the vagina. The fluid is allowed to run out into the bathtub. Remember to clean the bathtub carefully after this procedure.

## FEMALE REPRODUCTIVE DISORDERS

### Disturbances of Menstruation

The most common menstrual disorders are amenorrhea, menorrhagia, metrorrhagia, dysmenorrhea, premenstrual tension, and extreme irregularity.

*Amenorrhea* is absence of or abnormal stopping of menses. If the menses have not been established (*menarche*) by the 15th year, the patient should be examined to determine the reason. The difficulty may be a hormonal problem, but in any case it should have the careful and wise attention of a specialist. Amenorrhea may be due also to nutritional or emotional causes or to malformations of the female organs. (The menses are normally absent in pregnancy and after menopause.)

*Menorrhagia* is excessive bleeding, both in amount and duration, at the menstrual time. If this irregularity occurs in the young girl it may adjust itself, but it should be watched. If it occurs during the menopause, it may be significant as an indication of pathology. Menorrhagia may also occur in the patient with an IUD (intrauterine device). For excessive bleeding which is unexplained by organic causes, endocrine therapy may be helpful. Curettage, which is scraping out the lining of the uterus, may be effective. Dilatation (stretching the cervical opening) and curettage (sometimes termed a "D & C") may be performed as a therapeutic treatment.

*Metrorrhagia* is bleeding between the menstrual periods. This is abnormal and should have the attention of a physician, since it may indicate cancer or retained placental tissue in the postpartum patient. Metrorrhagia is a fairly common side-effect of oral contraceptives and is referred to in this instance as *breakthrough bleeding*.

*Dysmenorrhea* is painful menstruation. Normal menstruation should not be a painful process. However, many times, through lack of information, a young girl has been led to expect menstruation to be difficult and painful. Consequently, the slight cramps and backaches which may normally accompany the menses may be magnified. Functional causes of menstrual pain may stem from constipation, insufficient exercise, poor posture and fatigue or improper placement of a tampon and can be remedied easily. If the pain is intense and consistent, a medical examination is indicated, followed by the appropriate treatment for any abnormal organic conditions which exist.

*Premenstrual tension* is associated with symptoms common to many women. Complaints of abdominal distention, headache, generalized edema, and occasional vomiting are typical, as are irritability and moodiness or depression. Recent information relates these symptoms to a disturbance of electrolyte balance. Some relief has been brought about by a salt-free diet for a week or so during the premenstrual cycle and by medications which increase the excretion of sodium ions. Menstrual headache in some instances is very severe and has been treated with medications.

*Extreme irregularity* should be evaluated, since it may be indicative of a hormonal deficiency which could result in later sterility.

**Management of Menstrual Flow.** The nurse is in a position to teach the patient about menstrual hygiene. Various means are available to absorb or catch the flow. The most common is the sanitary napkin, available in the long postpartum size and the regular size sold in stores. Minipads are also available for use on the days of lightest flow. Internal devices consist of cups to catch the flow or tampons which absorb the flow. The patient needs to understand that she must choose the method of protection which is most convenient and comfortable for her.

## Menopause Difficulties

The menopause is the cessation of menstruation which occurs in the woman, usually in her 50's, although it may occur earlier or later. Another name for the menopause is the *climacteric* or *involution*. This signifies that the production of progesterone has stopped and ovulation has ceased. The woman may no longer become pregnant, although in rare cases, it does happen.

Some women have difficulties during the menopause because of the hormonal changes which are taking place. A sign of this may be irregular menstrual cycles during which a woman may skip 2 or 3 periods. When a woman has not had a menstrual period for one year, climacteric is considered to be complete. An unpleasant symptom which occurs during this time is commonly called "hot flashes," in which the woman alternates between being hot and cold. This is due to a disturbance in the sympathetic nervous system's control of blood vessels and can usually be remedied by medication. Some women feel depressed or anxious during the menopause and can usually be treated with chemical therapy, such as estrogens. A commonly used estrogen is Premarin. The menopause has no effect upon sexual desire (libido), except that it may increase it.

The woman is encouraged to exercise, follow good diet patterns, and see her doctor if she has any severe difficulties.

**Premature Menopause.** A woman who has had a hysterectomy (removal of the uterus) or radiation therapy for cancer will experience an artificial menopause. If she is young, she will usually be maintained on estrogen therapy. She may also have more menopausal difficulties than the older woman who has undergone a normal menopause.

**Postmenopausal Difficulties.** Some women have vaginitis or pruritis; atrophy of urogenital structures which can cause uterine prolapse, rectocele, or cystocele; and progressive bone resorption leading to osteoporosis and loss of height. Atherosclerosis is also more likely to develop after menopause.

## Vulvitis

Inflammation of the vulva may be the result of improper cleansing or of irritating vaginal discharge; more often it is caused by a gonorrheal infection. Infection in this area usually involves the Bartholin glands and may result in an abscess. Pain during urination or defecation and swelling are usually associated with vulvitis or Bartholin gland infection. If treatment with antibiotics is not wholly effective, usually the gland is excised.

## Vaginitis

*Vaginitis* is an inflammation of the vagina. Normally, the secretions in the vagina protect it from infection. However, two organisms often do cause vaginal infection—*Trichomonas vaginalis* and *Monilia albicans*. The outstanding symptom of vaginitis is a whitish vaginal discharge called *leukorrhea*. The discharge is odorous and profuse, making the perineum and the urethra burn and itch. It may be frothy or thick and whitish. The usual treatment consists of a vaginal jelly or a suppository, douches, or the application of a sulfonamide cream. Women who tend to spill sugar in their urine, whether diabetic or not, are very difficult to cure.

Frequently the husband is infected and also needs treatment. Since this condition is most common in women whose husbands are not circumcised, circumcision may be the only way of successfully treating the disorder.

Vaginitis is hard to cure; early, persistent treatment is the only way to prevent the disease from becoming chronic. It can be extremely irritating and persists for a long time. Even when cured, the infection can return. Frequently the patient may feel that she is unclean or that she has a venereal disease. Changing the pad frequently and administering perineal care when necessary will help to prevent odor and irritation.

## Cervicitis

Inflammation of the cervix, *cervicitis,* is caused by any one of a number of organisms, notably the *staphylococcus* or the *streptococcus.* Small lacerations in the cervix during childbirth make such infections more likely. Formerly, gonorrhea was a major cause of cervicitis and sometimes still is the cause. Cancer also causes cervicitis. The main symptoms are leukorrhea and sometimes bleeding. Pain with sexual intercourse may also be a symptom. Unless cervicitis is treated promptly, if may be difficult to cure. Periodic vaginal examinations help to discover cervicitis.

The chief treatment consists of douching and taking antibiotics. Sometimes the cervix is cauterized. After this treatment, a watery discharge appears which later may become odorous. It takes about 6 to 8 weeks for the area to heal after cauterization.

## Pelvic Inflammatory Disease (P.I.D.)

Infection of the pelvic organs causes inflammation of the ovaries (*oophoritis*) and of the fallopian tubes (*salpingitis*); if pus forms in the tubes, the condition is called *pyosalpinx.* Infection may enter through the vagina, the peritoneum, the lymphatics, or the bloodstream. The *tubercle bacillus* often enters the pelvic organs through the bloodstream. The *gonococcus* is often the cause of pelvic infection, even though penicillin is effective in killing that organism.

**Symptoms and Treatment.** A foul-smelling, vaginal discharge is a common symptom of P.I.D. The patient may also complain of backache and pelvic pain, with fever, nausea and vomiting. Antibiotics are given, and the patient is usually placed in Fowler's position to encourage pelvic drainage. Sitz baths may be ordered to relieve the pain; douches may or may not be ordered. Precautions should be taken to wrap soiled pads well for safe disposal as soon as they are removed; always wash the hands thoroughly after handling the pads. If the infection is gonorrheal, the patient may be placed on isolation precautions, and the nurse will wear gloves when changing the pads and giving perineal care. If the discharge is profuse, the patient should have perineal care after removing the pad and after using the bedpan.

If P.I.D. is not treated, it may become a chronic condition and cause sterility. The husband is also examined, since he may be infected and need treatment. If he is not infected, sexual intercourse is discouraged as long as the wife has any trace of infection. Sometimes an abscess forms, and the surgeon institutes drainage through an incision in the abdomen. Dressings soiled with discharge from this wound should be handled with the same precautions as the perineal pads.

## Ectopic Pregnancy

An *ectopic* (extra-uterine) pregnancy occurs when a fertilized ovum does not reach the uterus but becomes implanted in the fallopian tube or, very rarely, in the abdominal cavity. The growing ovum distends the tube, and, if untreated, the tube eventually bursts, rupturing many blood vessels. Usually the patient has all the signs of pregnancy, but the first indication of its being an ectopic pregnancy is a sudden, sharp pain in the abdomen, followed by internal hemorrhage and shock when the tube ruptures. Surgery is necessary at once to tie off the ruptured blood vessels and remove the ruptured tube (*salpingectomy*). The patient is treated for shock and is given blood transfusions to replace the blood loss. Nausea, vomiting, and adbominal pain may be signs of peritonitis due to the bleeding or infection in the abdominal cavity.

If the condition is discovered before the tube ruptures, the situation is not nearly as serious. The same surgery is done, but without the accompanying shock and danger of peritonitis.

This may be an emotionally upsetting experience for the patient—she has lost her baby and may fear that she cannot have another, or she may feel that in some way it was her fault. She can be assured that there is no medical evidence whatsoever that a mother can do anything to cause an ectopic pregnancy. She also may be comforted to feel that she still has one tube left and therefore can become pregnant again, although she has a greater chance of having another ectopic pregnancy.

## Uterine and Ovarian Tumors

There are 3 chief types of uterine and ovarian tumors: the benign ovarian cyst, the benign uterine tumor, and the malignant tumor.

**Benign Ovarian Tumors.** Also known as *cysts,* these benign growths may form from fluid retained in the ovary or from other causes. Although they usually do not cause any trouble, cysts may enlarge and press on other abdominal organs and cause pain if they rupture or twist.

**Benign Uterine Tumors.** The *fibroid tumor* is the most common type of tumor of the uterus. These tumors are all sizes and usually grow slowly; many times the patient is not aware of the tumor at all. The first symptom to appear is vaginal bleeding, with a feeling of heaviness and pressure in the pelvic region. This type of tumor is called a fibroid or myoma, and it may prevent or interfere with pregnancy. Such a tumor may also become so large that it presses on the urethra and the bowel, causing retention of urine and constipation. The treatment depends somewhat on the patient's age—often a nonmalignant tumor can be removed from the uterus without removing the uterus itself. This is important for a woman during her childbearing years. A nonmalignant tumor usually tends to shrink after the menopause. Bleeding after this time is seldom caused by a myoma.

### Malignant Tumors.

CANCER OF THE OVARY. Cancer of the ovary is rare, but it is often detected after metastasis has occurred. It is treated surgically with *panhysterectomy* (the common name for panhysterosalpingo-oophorectomy, which means removal of the uterus, including the cervix, both tubes and both ovaries). If only part of one ovary is diseased, the undiseased part is left for hormonal reasons.

CANCER OF THE CERVIX. Cancer of the cervix (the neck of the uterus) is the second greatest cause of cancer in women (breast cancer is first). It would be impossible to emphasize too strongly the importance of the Papanicolaou test for women past their late teens, and certainly over age 30, because it is possible to cure cancer of the cervix if it is discovered early, before it has a chance to spread. *Bleeding* is the first symptom of cancer of the cervix, but bleeding does not occur in the early stages when a positive Papanicolaou smear would indicate cancer. Bleeding usually appears first as spotting, then a watery discharge appears that turns to a darker, more bloody one, with an unpleasant odor. If the cancer is confined to the cervix and has not spread, a *hysterectomy* may be done. However radiation is often the treatment of choice and is often done by means of implanting radon seeds or other radioactive material. (The nursing care of this patient was discussed in Chapter 43.)

Some doctors warn of the dangers involved in using female hormone drugs over long periods of time because of the possibility that they might cause cancer. However, this is essentially unproven.

*Classification of Cervical Cancer.* Several stages of cervical cancer have been identified in order to define the relative treatment of each. The earlier stages are most susceptible to radiation and are more easily localized and are therefore easier to cure. The later stages would be more likely to be treated surgically, by hysterectomy.

*Stage 0:* Carcinoma *in situ* (in place). The cancer is limited to the epithelial layer and shows no signs of invasion of deeper tissue or of surrounding areas. This may be treated by biopsy (the biopsy may obtain all the cancer tissue).

*Stage I:* The cancer is confined to the cervix and is often treated by implantation radiation.

*Stages II and III:* The cancer is infiltrated into the vagina or has spread to other areas. Stage III shows isolated pelvic metastases. It would most likely be treated surgically, probably by an abdominal-perineal resection, possibly combined with radiation or deep x-ray therapy postoperatively.

*Stage IV:* The cancer is widely spread throughout the pelvic region or throughout the body. This stage is generally inoperable.

CANCER OF THE FUNDUS OF THE UTERUS. The *fundus,* the body of the uterus, is not attacked as frequently by cancer as the cervix; however, malignant growths do occur in the fundus. They are most likely to appear during and after the menopause. Vaginal bleeding is the first symptom, which may begin as a watery, bloodtinged discharge. If it occurs before the menopause, it may be mistaken for a menstrual irregularity. A diagnostic curettage, to get scrapings from the uterus, is done if a Papanicolaou smear looks suspicious. If the condition is due to malignancy, a *hysterectomy* is performed, followed by radium and x-ray therapy in the pelvic cavity. Cancer of the fundus of the uterus is most likely to occur in women in their 50's or older, when diabetes or hypertension may be complicating factors, making surgery a greater risk for them.

The uterus may be removed by means of a vaginal hysterectomy or an abdominal hysterectomy. In a *vaginal hysterectomy,* the uterus is removed through the vagina, whereas in an *abdominal hysterectomy* it is removed through an abdominal incision. Sometimes the cervix is not removed in the abdominal procedure.

*Treatment and Nursing Care.* In addition to the usual preparation for abdominal or perineal surgery, the patient may have a vaginal irrigation (douche). She may be catheterized, since it is especially important that the bladder be empty to lessen the danger of damaging it while removing the uterus. Routine postoperative care is given to prevent complications.

The patient may have trouble voiding at first; often a Foley catheter is inserted in the bladder at the time of the operation in anticipation of this difficulty.

Nursing care must be planned according to the type of hysterectomy done. The patient who has had a vaginal hysterectomy wears a perineal pad and has frequent perineal care. The patient who has had an abdominal hysterectomy is treated as is any patient with an abdominal incision. Sometimes, an abdominal-perineal resection is done, in which case, the patient has both abdominal and perineal incisions.

*The Patient's Point of View.* Uterine disturbances can be very upsetting for a woman. Fear of cancer, sterility, or the disturbance of marital relations are worries that any patient may have. She may feel that she is not up to making some of the adjustments that will be necessary. A nurse who is sensitive to these worries can learn what they are by listening to the patient's questions and comments and by giving her some of the reassurance she needs.

ADVANCED MALIGNANCY. When a patient has an inoperable malignancy of the reproductive organs, only palliative measures can be taken, such as x-ray therapy or chemotherapy. The nurse should always provide as much support and reassurance as possible and should perform all the routine measures of good nursing care which apply to the terminally ill patient. If the patient is a mother with a growing family, a social worker may be helpful in planning for the family's needs.

PELVIC PERFUSION. In this comparatively new treatment for pelvic malignancy, cancer-destroying drugs, such as nitrogen mustard, are circulated through the pelvic bloodstream for about 2 hours, by means of a pump oxygenator. These drugs have toxic effects on the bone marrow and the spleen, and the patient must be watched for signs of infection or bleeding after the treatment. Pelvic perfusion seems to make some patients more comfortable, but it is still too new to know how effective it can be. However, it is palliative not curative.

## Vaginal Fistulas

A *fistula* is an opening between 2 organs which normally do not open into each other. It is the result of an ulcerating process, such as cancer, irradiation, or childbirth injury. A fistula may develop between the ureter and the vagina (ureterovaginal), between the bladder and the vagina (vesicovaginal), or between the bladder and the rectum (rectovaginal). It is a most troublesome condition. If the fistula is between the ureter or the bladder and the vagina, urine will leak into the vagina. If it is between the rectum and the vagina, it causes fecal incontinence. A long-standing fistula is difficult to repair successfully, because the tissues are eroded. Infection is an added problem. Efforts are made to assist the healing process by building up the patient's resistance and by keeping the patient as clean as possible with perineal irrigations. Heat-lamp treatments to the perineum are sometimes used. The patient with an unrepairable fistula is distressed by the odor and the constant drainage. Sitz baths and deodorizing douches are aids to cleanliness.

## Cystocele and Rectocele

Due to the improvement in obstetric care, cystocele and rectocele are not seen as frequently as they once were. *Cervical tears* that have not been repaired, *frequent childbearing* or *multiple births* may relax the pelvic floor, allowing the bladder to sag downward and protrude into the vagina (*cystocele*) or into the rectum (*rectocele*). The uterus may sag (*prolapse*) into the vagina or even outside it. This is more likely to be seen in postmenopausal women.

These conditions are the cause of nagging discomforts: pelvic pain, backache, fatigue, and a sagging weight in the pelvis. They may interfere with emptying the bladder or with bowel movements or cause a dribbling of urine if the patient coughs or strains. A protruding organ becomes irritated and sometimes infected.

**Treatment and Nursing Care.** The surgical repair of a cystocele is called *anterior colporrhaphy;* the repair of a rectocele is called *posterior colporrhaphy*. Repair of the *perineum* is called *perineorrhaphy*. Preoperative orders for these procedures are likely to include a cleansing douche. Postoperatively, the patient will be given sterile perineal care. With rectocele repair the diet will be liquid for several days, to avoid defecation until some healing has taken place. With a *cystocele*, a Foley catheter is inserted to keep the bladder from becoming overdistended. Sometimes a patient is afraid to try to urinate after the catheter is removed and needs assurance that it is safe to void naturally.

## The Displaced Uterus

A displaced uterus is usually a congenital condition, but it may be the result of childbearing. Backward displacement is called *retroversion* or *retroflexion*. Forward displacement is called *anteversion* or *anteflexion*. These terms mean that the uterus is *turned* or *bent* backward or forward. A displaced uterus may cause backache, dysmenorrhea, or sterility.

Uterine displacement can be corrected by surgery to suture the uterus back in place. If a complicating condition makes surgery inadvisable, a *pessary* will help to reduce the prolapse. A pessary is a device made of hard rubber or plastic which is inserted into the vagina to hold the uterus in place. If it is inserted correctly, it usually causes no discomfort. The patient is instructed to return to the doctor at the time he designates—this is usually in a week and about every 2 months after that. The pessary can be left in place for 6 weeks at a time. Usually, the patient takes douches several times a week and is instructed to make every effort to keep the pessary clean. Assuming the knee-chest position for a short time once or twice a day helps to keep the pessary in place.

## BREAST DISEASE

The breast is part of the reproductive system; it functions in relation to menstruation and fertilization and is affected by the hormones produced by the reproductive organs. The breast is a glandular organ filled with blood and lymph vessels. After pregnancy it manufactures milk from certain substances in the blood. This process is called *lactation*. Milk is carried to the nipple by numerous ducts distributed throughout the fatty tissue. Progesterone, an ovarian hormone, and prolactin, a pituitary hormone, stimulate lactation. Estrogen, another ovarian hormone, suppresses lactation.

### Symptoms of Breast Disease

Lumps in the breast are always a suspicious symptom. They may be harmless; again, they may not. Beginning cancer is not likely to be painful. A discharge that oozes from the nipple without squeezing is a suspicious sign. Sometimes a malignant growth makes a dimple in the skin or retracts the nipple, or breast tissue becomes fixed to the chest muscles. Lumps in the axilla are indications that cancer has spread to this area.

### Benign Disorders

**Chronic Cystic Mastitis.** Cystic disease is the most common breast disorder. Breast tissue cells mass together, shut off the ducts, and form cysts. These masses may form fibrous tumors (fibromas) or lumps in the breast, which should be biopsied to make sure that they are not cancerous. Most lumps removed from the breast are benign. The cyst may be excised without removing any of the surrounding tissue. If there are numerous cysts, the doctor may do a simple mastectomy, removing the breast only, as a palliative measure since the cysts are sometimes precancerous.

**Breast Abscesses.** A breast abscess may occur following acute cystic mastitis which is an inflammatory condition found at times in the nursing mother. If the inflammation becomes localized or confined, it forms an abscess. Treatment includes antibiotic therapy combined with measures designed to drain the abscess such as the application of warm, moist packs or the use of the breast pump. Sometimes the abscess must be incised and drained. Since the inflammation is often caused by the staphylococcus organism, the patient may be placed in isolation.

## Cancer of the Breast

Next to cystic disease, cancer is the second most common cause of breast disorders. In fact, cancer of the breast is the most common form of cancer in women. More than 60,000 women develop breast cancer every year. Over half of these women are cured, but the number would be higher if more cases were discovered and treated earlier. Breast cancer tends to appear in women who have a family history of this disease; it is not as common in women who have nursed babies.

**Breast Changes.** Breast changes may be evident before pain appears. Women are urged to consult a doctor if they notice a lump or any other changes in the breast. Prompt action may mean the difference between life and death. More than half of the women who consulted a doctor immediately after finding a lump in the breast were alive 5 years later; less than a third of those who delayed this visit lived that long.

**Diagnosis of Breast Cancer.** A biopsy should be taken of any breast lesion and sent to the laboratory for a frozen section. The pathologist studies the frozen section and then returns his findings to the surgeon.

**Radical Mastectomy.** If the pathologist's report following a biopsy shows that the growth is malignant, the surgeon will do a radical mastectomy (removal of the breast,

the overlying skin, the axillary channels, and the lymph nodes which drain the area). The nodes are also tested for cancer. If they contain cancer cells, the finding is referred to as "nodes positive," with the pathologist identifying the number of nodes involved. If the lymph nodes are not involved, then the patient's prognosis is good. However, if all the nodes are involved, the prognosis is very poor. Thus the fewer the nodes involved, the better the prognosis.

When the nodes are positive, follow-up treatment after surgery includes x-ray or cobalt therapy or chemotherapy as palliative measures. Even when the nodes are negative, these treatments may be used as a preventive measure.

Since a radical mastectomy involves removing an extensive amount of skin, it may be necessary to take a skin graft from the thigh to close the wound. The patient's arm may be bandaged against her body to avoid pull on the graft, with her elbow bent at a right angle and the arm supported by a pillow. If there is no skin graft, the arm is free. Sometimes, the patient has the radical mastectomy first and comes in at a later date for a *plastic revision* of *the wound.* (Plastic surgery or skin grafting is done to improve the looks or skin coverage of the wound.) This is often the treatment of choice, because the plastic surgery is more likely to be successful and is easier to do after the initial wound has healed and the edema has abated.

**The Patient's Point of View.** The patient who is going to have a breast operation is understandably apprehensive. Will she lose her breast? Will she hear the dread word "cancer"? Will she be repulsive? These questions and many more may be going through her mind. Be patient with her questions and worries. Show that you are willing to listen; encourage her to talk about the things that trouble her. Assure her that she was sensible to consult her doctor—thousands of women are doing this regularly.

**Preoperative Care.** It is important to set the stage preoperatively for rehabilitation after surgery. In addition to the routine preoperative teaching about turning, deep breathing, and early ambulation, the nurse should inform the mastectomy patient that she will be asked to do special exercises. She should also be aware that prostheses are available.

Because of the emotional attitudes associated with breast surgery, the nurse should not be surprised if the patient becomes angry, withdrawn, or cries. Such feelings are stirred because the breasts are closely related to femininity and motherhood.

EXERCISES. Postmastectomy exercises are necessary to prevent shortening of muscles, contractures of joints, and loss of muscle tone. They also assist the lymphatic circulation and reduce the edema of the arm on the affected side. Exercises to bring back the normal use of the arm are started as soon as the arm is freed, if the skin graft permits. Encourage the patient to keep her shoulders level and relaxed—patients tend to hunch the affected side. It may be difficult when the arm is first unbandaged from her side to get her to move it away from her body. However, it is important to keep the muscles from becoming permanently contracted. Steady, persistent exercise every day is necessary to stretch the muscles gradually. The exercises should be done for a *short time* 3 or 4 times a day to avoid fatigue. Meanwhile, the patient should be encouraged to use her other arm to do things for herself, such as washing her face and brushing her hair. She may not be able to cut her meat or butter her bread, but she can feed herself. The American Cancer Society publishes a booklet, *Help Yourself to Recovery,* telling how to do postmastectomy exercises at home. Some exercises can be combined with ordinary daily activities, such as sliding a towel back and forth over the back and reaching with the arms when making a bed. The patient has a good start in learning how to exercise the muscles before she goes home. Some hospitals have postmastectomy classes for patients to exercise together (see Fig. 51-1).

OTHER POSTMASTECTOMY TREATMENTS. Other treatments are designed to prevent complications and to rehabilitate the patient as soon as possible.

If drains or wicks are placed in the surgical wound to drain excess fluid and prevent edema, the nurse should be aware of this so that she does not become alarmed at the large amount of drainage.

Another possible method of drainage is to connect the suction tube to a suction machine or other device such as the Hemo-Vac, a plastic drainage box, which creates a slight vacuum when flattened and exerts a gentle suction on the wound catheter when expanded.

Elastic bandages are often applied to the affected arm in an effort to reduce edema. Even-pressure is used in wrapping the bandages from the fingers up to the axilla. Sometimes, the edema is so severe that an air-pressure cuff must be applied to the arm. The mastectomy patient may also be treated with antibiotics, a low-sodium diet, and diuretics.

COMPLICATIONS. Infection in the wound area is always a possible development. Edema in the arm sometimes follows a radical mastectomy; normally, this is temporary, but if it persists it may be a sign of infection. Edema does not disappear as rapidly in obese patients. In the case of infection, antibiotics will be given. Signs of infection in the arm or the hand should be reported immediately.

**The Prosthetic Breast.** A *prosthesis* answers the problem of disfigurement. It can be fitted to duplicate the remaining breast so there will be no change in the patient's appearance. Until the doctor decides that she is ready for the prosthesis, the patient can purchase a padded brassière (many of them are available), or she can pad her own brassière. Surgical supply houses and corsetières that carry prostheses usually have an experienced fitter. Ordinarily, the doctor will recommend the place where this can be done. One of the most adaptable types of a prosthetic breast is made of foam rubber which is light and washable. Another is filled with a heavy liquid which looks and feels much like the normal breast.

**Metastatic Cancer.** Metastases in another part of the body are always a threat with cancer. Periodic check-ups are routine for any patient who has had a malignant growth removed. X-ray therapy is usually employed as treatment following the removal of a malignant growth. If the patient is not yet past the menopause, a second operation may be performed to remove the ovaries so as to remove the source of the hormone, estrogen, which is

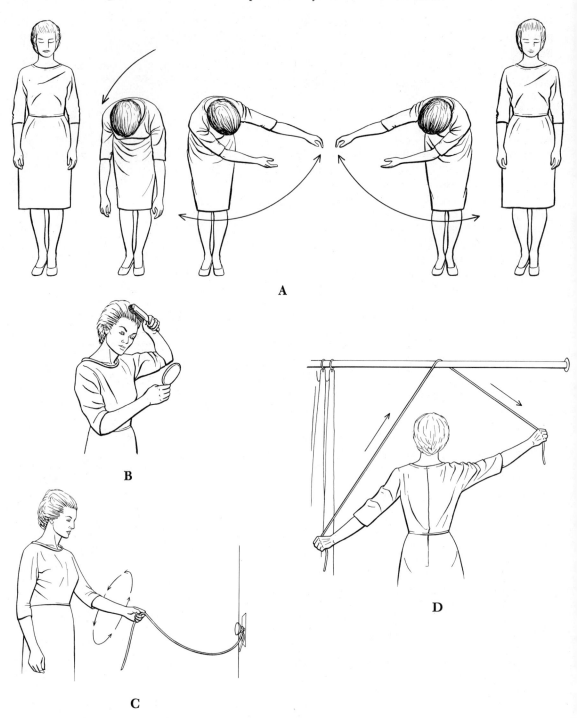

Figure 51-1. Exercises for the postmastectomy patient. (A) Pendulum-swinging exercise. (B) Hair-brushing exercise. (C) Rope-turning exercise. (D) Rope-sliding exercise. (E) Wall-climbing exercise. (Smith, D. W., Germain, C. P., and Gips, C. D.: Care of the Adult Patient, ed. 3. Philadelphia, Lippincott, 1971)

thought to stimulate tumor growth. The production of estrogen ceases with the menopause. In cases where metastasis has taken place, hormonal therapy may be used in the hope that it will make the patient more comfortable.

**Other Breast Surgery.** Sometimes corrective surgery is done on the breast. A plastic surgery revision of the breast is referred to as a *mammoplasty*. If the breast is to be made larger, the term *augmentation* mammoplasty is used; if the breast is to be made smaller, the appropriate term is *reduction* mammoplasty. Usually, these operations are not serious and do not have any side-effects. Occasionally, however, the materials implanted in the augmentation mammoplasty are rejected and must be removed.

Occasionally, the male breast enlarges, a condition called *gynecomastia*. These may be removed by plastic surgery. The male occasionally, though rarely, gets cancer of the breast or other diseases more common to women.

## THE MALE PATIENT

The male patient with a disease of the reproductive system is treated by the *urologist,* since his condition often is genitourinary in nature. Treatment usually involves many of the same procedures that are used in caring for the urologic patient. In reviewing some

organs of the male reproductive system, we see that they include the *testes,* which produce the male sperm cells (the spermatozoa), the male *hormones,* and the *semen,* the fluid that carries the cells; the *epididymis,* the *seminal ducts,* and the *ejaculatory ducts,* which are the passageways for the semen; the *prostate gland,* which adds a secretion to the semen; and the *penis,* in which the urethra provides the outlet for the semen. The male urethra is the passageway for both urine and semen. The tissues in the penis stiffen and fill with blood to hold the penis erect during sexual intercourse.

Spermatozoa are produced in large numbers and are extremely active. They are able to wiggle their way through the vagina into the uterus and on up into the fallopian tube to impregnate the ovum. Conception takes place only if an ovum is present in the tube.

## DISORDERS OF THE MALE REPRODUCTIVE SYSTEM

A male patient with a disorder of the reproductive system is frequently embarrassed because the nurse taking care of him is often a woman. He may also be worried about impotence or cancer and naturally feels hesitant to mention these fears. Thus it is difficult for him to relieve his worries by discussing them or asking questions. However, he should have an opportunity to talk with the doctor alone if

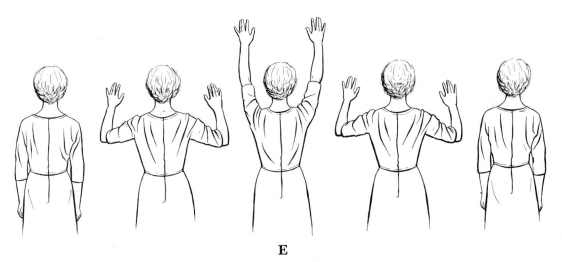

**E**

Figure 51-1. E—(*Caption on facing page.*)

he seems unduly worried or disturbed. Men at any age may be apprehensive about the loss of sexual powers.

## Prostatic Difficulties

We have already seen that an enlarged prostate can cause urinary difficulties (Chapter 50). As a man grows older, the prostate gland tends to enlarge and may constrict the urethra. This does not necessarily indicate cancer nor does it always mean that surgery is necessary. In 100 men, 65 of them will have some prostatic enlargement by the time they are 65 years old.

**Symptoms.** The first symptom to appear may be difficulty in urination. The patient does not empty his bladder completely when he voids, and he finds that he must void several times during the night. He may also find it increasingly difficult to start to void and may notice traces of blood in his urine. This may lead to cystitis. The doctor can find out the effects of prostatic enlargement on the urinary system by examining a catheterized specimen of urine and by cystoscopy; a blood chemistry test will also indicate how well the kidneys are functioning.

**Treatment and Nursing Care.** The usual treatment for *nonmalignant* prostatic enlargement (*benign prostatic hypertrophy*) is the surgical removal of the prostate. Before the operation the patient may have a catheter inserted for continuous drainage of urine, to prevent an accumulation of stagnant urine in the bladder. The patient is given plenty of fluids, with proper diet and rest to build up his resistance. The prostate can be removed in several ways. In a transurethral resection (TUR), which is a relatively safe procedure, the prostate is removed through the urethra by means of a cystoscope which has a cutting edge that slices the prostate away bit by bit. The prostate may also be dissected out through an incision over the bladder (a suprapubic prostatectomy or a suprapubic resection).

The suprapubic procedure may be done in 2 stages. First, a cystostomy (an incision into the bladder) is done to relieve retention of urine; secondly, the prostate is removed. After the 1-stage suprapubic operation, the patient returns with 2 in-dwelling catheters in place: one in the urethra and the other in the suprapubic wound. The wound catheter is attached to an irrigation apparatus, and the urethral catheter is attached to a bottle for drainage. This arrangement provides for bladder irrigation and urine drainage. The wound catheter is usually removed in 5 or 6 days; the urethral catheter stays in for about 10 days. Some urine will dribble onto the dressings after the wound catheter is removed, so attention must be given to keeping the skin clean and dry. It takes a while for the wound to heal, perhaps a month or more.

The prostate may also be removed through an incision in the perineum (*perineal prostatectomy*). In this case, catheter drainage is through the perineal incision only. Since the patient will find sitting up painful, a foam rubber pad should be provided. Sitz baths are usually ordered. Care to avoid contaminating the wound will be necessary after a bowel movement. Cleansing should not be left to the patient simply because a male nurse or orderly is not available.

The most commonly used procedure for older men, or for men who are poor surgical risks, is the TUR (transurethral resection). This procedure does not involve an incision so the risks of surgery are much less and the recovery period is much shorter. However, one possible postoperative complication is bleeding.

The patient who has had a TUR will, almost without exception, return from the operating room with a TUR irrigation set-up in place.

**TUR Irrigations.** Preoperatively, the patient often has an in-dwelling urinary catheter. In the operating room, a special catheter which has 3 lumens is inserted. One is used to inflate the bag; one allows fluids to run into the bladder; and the third is used for drainage from the bladder. The irrigation may be continuous after surgery or it may be intermittent.

The purpose of the postoperative TUR irrigation of the bladder is to prevent or remove clots. The continuous irrigation washes out blood before it can form clots. The intermittent irrigation, which is usually begun after a day or so, washes out clots, as well as building up the capacity of the bladder again. The nurse should realize that the new postoperative patient will show bloody drainage, but the amount of blood in the drainage should decrease. Any sudden increase of blood in the drainage should be reported at once. It is also important to record the amount of solution injected into the bladder, so that an accurate record of the patient's urinary output can be kept. The amount of the irrigation solution is subtracted from the total output to determine the patient's urine volume.

**Emotional Aspects of a Prostatectomy.** These patients are elderly and often lonely people, who become confused by the tubing arrangements and procedures; they feel unwanted and are without hope of ever being well again. They need to be noticed and encouraged often to let them know that someone cares about their recovery.

**Cancer of the Prostate.** *Cancer of the prostate* does not usually occur until after 50 years of age. Of the men who have prostatic difficulty after that age, 25 per cent have cancer. The symptoms may not appear for years, but when they do appear as the result of metastases to the nerves, they are in the form of pains in the back and sciatica. A rectal examination will show a hard mass which will not have caused pain until metastases had spread, which is one of the reasons why it is hard to discover cancer of the prostate early enough. Thus, every man should have a rectal examination at least once a year, especially after age 50.

A biopsy of the tumor will determine the diagnosis as cancer. A *radical prostatectomy,* removing the prostate gland, the seminal vesicles, and part of the urethra, will sometimes cure cancer of the prostate if metastases have not developed. A TUR is sometimes done to relieve symptoms of difficult urination if the lesion has metastasized. With metastasis, the most that can be done is to make the patient as comfortable as possible. The administration of female hormones (estrogens) and radiation therapy may help, but the relief is temporary. As the disease advances, sedatives are given, and sometimes bladder drainage is necessary.

The goals in management of the patient with inoperable cancer of the prostate are: (1) to eliminate urine either by catheterization or cystostomy, if the patient is unable to void, (2) to cause tumor atrophy by use of estrogens or radiation, which also control pain, and (3) to relieve pain.

## Other Disturbances

**Undescended Testicle (Cryptorchism.)** A small percentage of male babies are born with testicles that have not descended to their normal place in the scrotum. Sometimes the testicles descend without treatment; but if this does not happen before puberty, they should be brought into place or else sterility may result. After puberty, an operation for 2 undescended testicles will not be effective in preventing sterility.

**Orchitis.** *Orchitis,* inflammation of the testes, may be the result of an infection or an injury. *Mumps* after puberty may cause orchitis which results in sterility (gamma globulin may help to make mumps less severe). The symptoms of orchitis are pain and swelling in the scrotum and, sometimes, urethral irritation. A 4-tail bandage is used to support the testes, and an ice cap is applied. Heat is *never* used, because even a few degrees of heat may damage spermatozoa.

**Hydrocele.** A *hydrocele* is an accumulation of fluid in the space between the membrane covering the testicle and the testicle itself. It may be due to infection (orchitis) or to an injury. The scrotum enlarges but does not cause pain, unless the hydrocele is a sudden development, in which case there may be both pain and swelling. It is treated by aspirating the fluid or by injecting a substance that disposes of the sac in which the fluid collects. Sometimes the sac is removed surgically. The treatment includes applying cold packs, administering diuretics, providing support for the scrotum, and keeping the dressings changed to prevent skin irritation.

**Abnormal Placement of the Urethra.** If the urethral meatus is located on the lower wall of the penis, this condition is known as *hypospadias;* if the meatus is located on the upper surface, the condition is known as *epispadias.* These are congenital conditions and are usually repaired surgically at a young age.

**Epididymitis.** *Epididymitis* is an inflammation of the tube that carries the sperm cells away from the testes. It is usually due to gonorrheal, staphylococcic, streptococcic, or colon bacillus infection, and it often follows an infection of the urinary tract or prostatitis.

The symptoms are redness, pain, and swelling in the scrotum, which are sometimes accompanied by chills, fever, nausea, and vomiting. The treatment includes giving antibiotics for the infection and applying support and an ice cap to the scrotum. If an abscess forms, it usually is incised and drained surgically. Repeated or chronic infection will destroy the production of sperm.

**Varicocele.** A *varicocele* is caused by dilatation of the veins in the scrotum. It may be caused by an abdominal tumor which obstructs the spermatic vein. The symptoms of varicocele are swelling and a nagging pain in the scrotum. It is treated by removing the cause of the obstruction and sometimes by removing a mass of dilated veins. A snug suspensory is applied for support.

**Phimosis.** Many men who have not been circumcised at birth, develop a condition known as *phimosis* in which the foreskin becomes so tight that it will not retract over the glans penis. The condition is relieved by circumcision, which may also be done for aseptic reasons if the wife has a chronic vaginal infection.

The emotional aspects of adult circumcision are often greater than the discomfort of the operation itself. Although it is usually a quick and relatively painless procedure, it is difficult for the man to accept the fact that it is necessary, and he often will delay surgery as long as possible.

**Cancer of the Penis.** Cancer of the penis is relatively rare, especially in men who have been circumcised. It is treated locally, as a skin cancer, but occasionally amputation of the penis is necessary as a lifesaving measure.

**Emotional Aspects of Nursing Care.** As mentioned before, it is difficult for the man to tell his problems to a female nurse. It is, in fact, often difficult for him to discuss these problems with the male doctor, because many emotional and psychological factors are involved. The patient may be embarrassed, he may fear that he has a venereal disease, or he may be afraid that he will become impotent. The nurse should understand these feelings and try to give as much support as she can. However, she should also realize that a male patient will often appreciate being cared for by a male nurse.

## Fertility and Infertility

There are a number of causes for barren marriages. About 12 per cent of all marriages in this country are barren; although many of these couples want children, conception does not take place. Sterility in the man seems to be the cause in about one third of these marriages. It may be due to undescended testicles, orchitis after mumps, irradiation of the testes, obesity, internal adhesions, glandular disturbances, infection, or emotional tensions. Although 1 cc. of semen contains literally millions of sperm cells, the number of *normal* and *active* spermatozoa may be comparatively small, which lessens the chances of fertilization. Sterility in women may be due to many of the same systemic causes as in men. In addition, a woman may have a displaced uterus, obstructed fallopian tubes, or a cervical or a vaginal infection. She may have ovarian cysts or a fibroid tumor. A common cause of sterility in both sexes, especially in the female, is gonorrhea.

If conception has not taken place after a year or 2 of marriage, a doctor should be consulted. He will check on the general health of husband and wife; he will make tests of the semen and of the vaginal and cervical secretions. He may inflate the fallopian tubes with carbon dioxide (*Rubin test*). An x-ray determination may also be done (hysterosalpingogram). Sometimes a light curettage of the uterus is done to determine whether the lining of the uterus is undergoing the normal changes necessary to receive a fertilized ovum.

The woman can tell when she ovulates by an abrupt drop and rise in her body temperature. This is recorded on a chart and is known as *basal body temperature* (BBT).

The difficulties are treated symptomatically and, in many cases, are successful. Many states have fertility clinics, and Planned Parenthood of America assists people with fertility counseling.

## Sterilization Procedures

Since several permanent sterilization procedures are possible, the husband and wife usually make the decision together concerning which method they will employ.

The man may have a *vasectomy* done, in which case the vas deferens is ligated and sometimes removed. This procedure is relatively easy and painless and may even be done in the doctor's office under local anesthesia. There is only a small perineal incision, and the postoperative course is usually uneventful. Recently, efforts have been made to reanastomose the ligated vas, with some success. Of course, if the vas has been removed, the operation is irreversible, but if the vas is still in place, it is possible, through a very delicate procedure, to join the 2 ligated ends together. However, the man who chooses to have a vasectomy should anticipate that he will remain sterile, because the revision procedures are not often successful. The man should understand that he will not be impotent, just sterile.

A fallopian tube ligation or *tubal ligation,* as it is commonly called, is the most common and effective procedure for sterilization in women. This is done through an abdominal incision and involves ligating and sometimes removing all or part of the fallopian tubes. The results are usually permanent, although some recent attempts at revision have been successful. If the procedure is done immediately after delivery, while the woman is still on the delivery table, the tubes can be ligated through the uterus. This procedure, called an immediate puerperal ligation, is much safer since it does not involve an abdominal incision.

## Birth Control

For the couple who does not wish to have more children, permanent sterilization may be the answer. However, in many families, temporary birth control is desired. There are many methods of birth control or planned parenthood, most of which are used by the woman. They are discussed in this section because they involve the relationship between the partners.

**The Rhythm Method.** This involves limiting intercourse to the time of the month when the woman is infertile. The basal body temperature may be used as a gauge and is reliable for the woman who ovulates regularly and knows when she is fertile, but it is unreliable for many couples. (The fertile period lasts from 2 days before ovulation to one day after.) It may also cause emotional difficulties in the marriage relationship.

**Birth Control Pills.** These are used very commonly today in the United States. They are taken by the woman from the completion of her menstrual period for 20 to 28 days. (Recently, pills have been developed which are taken less often. They are still being studied.) She then stops taking the pills and has a period. The rationale behind the use of the pill is that since it is an estrogen, it simulates a pregnancy so the woman does not ovulate. If she does not ovulate, she cannot become pregnant. "The pill" is the most effective method now in use, other than sterilization. However, there are some side-effects, which can usually be regulated by changing the type of pill. Some women, for whom the prolonged estrogen level would be dangerous, should not take birth control pills. For example, the diabetic woman may experience some symptoms of eye change as a result of taking the pill. Women with high blood pressure, heart defects, or other blood disorders should not take the pill because a clotting tendency is one of the side-effects. However, even with its side-effects, the pill seems to be the most acceptable and effective method of birth control in use today.

BIRTH CONTROL PILLS FOR MEN. New research has developed pills which will cause temporary sterility in men, who would not need to take the pills daily. More research is being done, but this promises to be an effective method.

**Chemical Barriers.** There are several creams and douches as well as vaginal foams, jellies, creams, suppositories, and tablets, which offer protection to the woman. The foams are the most effective, especially when used with a diaphragm.

**Mechanical Barriers.** A man may use a condom, which is also a fairly good prevention against venereal disease. Mechanical devices for the woman include the vaginal cap and the diaphragm. They must be fitted by the physician and must be inserted each time prior to intercourse. They are more effective when used in combination with foams.

**Intrauterine Devices (IUD).** There are several types of devices which are inserted into the uterus to prevent pregnancy. It is believed that they either prevent ovulation or speed up ovulation to the point where the egg is not mature enough to be implanted and therefore does not develop into a pregnancy. The IUD is very effective, about 95 per cent of the time. The various devices include the spiral, the loop (which is most commonly used), and the spring ring. They are inserted into the uterus with a straight stylet and can remain in place indefinitely. If the nurse is asked to assist in the placement of the IUD, she should be aware that the patient may feel a sharp pain upon insertion. The patient may have cramps for a few days, but usually these do not continue. Often, menstrual flow becomes heavier in the patient with an IUD and may cause the patient to expel the device within the first few months. If she does not expel it within 2 to 3 months, the chances are that it will remain in place indefinitely. The device requires that the woman check it monthly to make sure that it is still in place. She should also be sure to have at least a yearly Pap smear and pelvic examination to make sure that there is no irritation from the IUD. Sometimes, the device is changed every 2 or 3 years.

## Abortion

The subject of abortion, the interruption of an estabished pregnancy, has been discussed elsewhere in this book but will be mentioned here, since it also serves as another means of birth control.

The term *abortion,* when used medically, denotes the termination of a pregnancy, for whatever reason or by whatever means. A "miscarriage" is known medically as an abortion (spontaneous) and has been discussed in Chapter 36. The *therapeutic abortion* is generally done to save the mother's life, although some states acknowledge other reasons. The term *criminal abortion* was used, until recently, to denote the illegal termination of a pregnancy. However, it is now legal in many states to perform an abortion upon a woman, whether the pregnancy is life-threatening or not. This is done by various means such as D & C, injection of hypertonic solution into the uterus, with various drugs, or by a "vacuum" method. Whatever procedure is used, it should always be done by a qualified physician under sterile conditions.

An abortion done under other than sterile conditions, is very dangerous, because a generalized septicemia may develop and lead to death. It has been estimated that unsterile abortion results in from 5,000 to 8,000 deaths per year in this country. If the patient with septicemia comes into the hospital for treatment, she is generally treated symptomatically. The patient receives massive doses of antibiotics, I.V. fluids, oxygen (in the hyperbaric chamber if it is available), and sometimes renal support in the form of dialysis. However, once the condition has progressed to the point where the patient is willing to come to the hospital and admit that she has had an illegal abortion, the prognosis is often poor.

## Venereal Disease

Venereal diseases occur generally in the urogenital tract and are contracted through sexual intercourse or sexual contact with an infected person. Venereal disease (VD) is one of the most acute health problems in the United States, its incidence increasing greatly every year. Other than the flu, it is said to be the most prevalent communicable disease in the country, affecting about 1 in 100 Americans. A report in the *National Observer* states that nearly 2 million Americans were treated in 1970 for gonorrhea. During that same year syphilis increased 8.1 per cent. Authorities believe that half of these cases will be cured, but half the victims will be seriously afflicted, with about 125,000 eventually dying from the disease.

The 2 most common venereal diseases are *gonorrhea* and *syphilis.* Gonorrhea is the number one communicable disease in this country, while syphilis is third. This is difficult to understand, since penicillin is effective in killing the organism in both diseases. The reluctance of the patient to go to the doctor for treatment and to report his or her contact is probably the reason for the large number of cases.

Another problem, which is just beginning to appear, is the development of penicillin-resistant organisms (especially gonococcus), which may cause these diseases to become more widespread.

It must be understood that venereal disease can be contracted by either heterosexual or homosexual relations. (There is a rising rate of VD among homosexuals in this country.) It may be contracted by kissing, although the infected person must have a lesion of the mucous membrane of the mouth in order to transmit the disease in this way.

The nurse must also remember that syphilis and gonorrhea are 2 different diseases. A person may have *both* diseases at the same time.

### Gonorrhea

*Gonorrhea* is the result of infection by the gonococcus organism and is the most common venereal disease (probably because of its shorter incubation period). It attacks the genital tract in men and women and can spread to other parts of the body. It is contracted through sexual intercourse. It is less serious to the life of the patient than syphilis, although it is more difficult to diagnose and to treat.

**Symptoms.** The symptoms may appear anywhere from 3 days to 2 weeks after intercourse with an infected person. Usually, the first symptom is pain and a burning sensation upon urination, followed by a yellowish discharge which contains pus. Without treatment, the disease progresses to infect the uterus and the fallopian tubes in women and the epididymis in men. In women, the tubes are filled with pus (salpingitis); strictures form and cause sterility. In men, prostatitis or an infection of the seminal vesicles and sterility may develop. In women, douches, sexual intercourse, and menstruation may spread the infection to the ovary and cause an abscess. This infection is also the cause of urinary difficulties in both men and women. The disease is difficult to diagnose in women. If the organisms enter the bloodstream, they can cause arthritis and heart disease. (Before antibiotics were known, many patients with gonorrhea became arthritics.)

**Diagnosis.** It is diagnosed by means of a smear test of the discharge.

**Treatment.** One dose of 1,200,000 U. of penicillin cures 95 per cent of the cases of gonorrhea in the early stage. If people delay treatment, the disease may spread to other parts of the body, and the infected person may continue to infect others. While the infection is active, soap and water should be used freely in washing the hands; toilet equipment should be isolated, and the toilet seat used by the patient should be disinfected after each use. Precautions to avoid touching the eyes are especially important, because the eye is particularly susceptible to gonorrheal infection. This is the reason for instilling silver nitrate into the eyes of the newborn; to prevent gonorrheal infection of the eyes, if the mother is infected. With an advanced infection, the patient is on bed care and may require sitz baths and douches. The nurse wears gloves in giving these treatments, or the patient may be on isolation precautions.

### Syphilis

*Syphilis* is a destructive disease that may result in many lesions throughout the body. It is known as "the great imitator" because its symptoms can and do resemble other diseases which involve all parts of the body. Syphilis *kills* over 4,000 Americans every year and infects 5 times that many. The increase in syphilis has been great in the last 10 years. Furthermore, only about 10 per cent of the cases are reported. Syphilis is caused by a spirochete (*Treponema pallidum*), which thrives in moisture and lives for a very short time outside the human body.

**Transmission.** Contact with a syphilitic lesion by kissing or by sexual intercourse transmits the spirochetes to mucous membranes, which they enter through cracks where they immediately multiply. From there, they enter the bloodstream and in about 3 weeks the first syphilitic lesion appears, the *primary lesion* or *chancre*. Syphilis is almost always contracted by sexual intercourse. Persons with untreated syphilis can infect others for about 3 years after the infection starts; after this time they are seldom infectious.

**Diagnosis.** Syphilitic infection can be detected by a blood test such as the Kahn, Wassermann, Massini, or Kolmar tests, or by a smear taken from a syphilitic lesion. A test, most commonly called the VDRL, is sometimes done routinely on all mature patients admitted to the hospital. This test is always done as part of prenatal care. Some states also require a blood test before marriage. (This blood test is not positive until at least 2 weeks after the infection.)

**Stages of Syphilis.** The primary lesion, *chancre,* may appear on the penis, inside the vagina, on the nipple, or in a crack at the side of the mouth. (This is not to be confused with a canker sore.) This chancre may not appear for 10 to 70 days after infection. It contains millions of spirochetes, but in 3 to 8 weeks this lesion will disappear spontaneously, whether the patient has received treatment or not. Sometimes enlarged lymph nodes also appear. The patient has no other symptoms. This is the *primary stage* of syphilis.

About 6 weeks after the initial infection, the *secondary stage* begins. Usually, the first sign is a skin rash which appears suddenly but soon disappears as quickly as it came. Wartlike spots may develop on the mucous membranes or around the anus. These spots are extremely infectious. Patches of the patient's hair may come out, and he may also have fever, headache, or sore throat; however, he may have none of these symptoms and feel normal and well. This stage also disappears spontaneously. During the first and second stages of syphilis, the patient is still highly *infectious*, even though he shows no symptoms. This is the main reason for the spread of the disease. The patient believes that he is "cured" or decides that he did not really have syphilis.

In the third, or *tertiary stage*, all the symptoms disappear. Half of the patients who reach this stage without having had treatment will have no more trouble; but for the other half, who live long enough, there is a different story. The disease may stay dormant anywhere from 1 to 20 to 30 years, but during that time, it has been invading the organs of the body, the heart, the liver, the brain, the bones, and all other parts of the body.

Eventually, the *tertiary stage* of syphilis begins to show overt signs of damage. The patient may have a heart attack, become blind, or suffer from severe bone or liver disease. He may suffer from severe brain damage (*paresis*), which makes him more or less helpless. It is important to realize that treatment may kill the organism at any stage of the disease, but it cannot reverse the damage which has already been done. The *damage is irreversible*.

**Effects of Syphilis.** Untreated syphilis in a pregnant woman may cause a miscarriage or the baby may be born with congenital syphilis or be deformed. Syphilitic lesions may affect the blood vessels or the heart valves. In the nervous system, they may cause meningitis. A common disturbance is *paresis,* which affects

the patient's personality—he becomes unable to concentrate or use judgment, is careless about his clothes, is irritable and, in the advanced stages, may become exuberant or depressed. His speech is slurred, and he may lose his sight and eventually become paralyzed and be a complete invalid.

Another manifestation of syphilis at this stage is *tabes dorsalis* (locomotor ataxia), a condition in which there is a loss of function in the legs. It is accompanied by a sharp burning pain in the legs; they feel numb, then cold or warm. The patient feels as if he cannot tell where his legs are, and acts as if he cannot manage them. He must watch them in order to walk, and his gait is jerky. He is unable to walk at all in the dark. Another complication is loss of function in a joint, such as the knee or the spine, which are affected most frequently.

**Treatment.** One injection of 2,400,000 to 4,800,000 U. of long-lasting penicillin will eliminate spirochetes in 85 to 90 per cent of the early cases of syphilis. This is not considered as a cure, and the patient must return to the doctor at 2-week intervals at first, then monthly for 6 months and then every 3 or 4 months for the next 3 to 5 years. If the patient is allergic to penicillin, he can be treated by *tetracycline,* or erythromycin. The organism is more difficult to kill in tertiary syphilis.

## Discussion About Venereal Disease

The nurse is in an excellent position to teach others about venereal disease. Since the number of young people being infected is growing by leaps and bounds, the nurse can encourage people to go to the doctor if they think they have the disease. A routine VDRL should be a part of the yearly physical examination. The nurse must be aware that VD is a special problem for a woman, because it is difficult to notice whether a woman has the disease. It should go without saying that the nurse should not be judgmental in her attitude toward the patient with VD.

**The Future.** It is hoped that a blood test as effective as the test for syphilis will be found for gonorrhea. This will make it easier to locate and control carriers of gonorrhea. It may also be possible to develop immunization against venereal diseases.

# 52

# The Patient With an Endocrine Disorder

---

### BEHAVIORAL OBJECTIVES

*The student successfully attaining the goals of this chapter will be able to:*

- *describe at least 5 tests for thyroid function and 5 tests for diabetes; discuss the special nursing and medical care involved in each; identify situations in which each might be done; and assist the doctor and patient in each instance.*

- *discuss at least 4 disorders of the pituitary gland; several disorders of the thyroid gland; describe the symptoms and medical management in each case; and assist the patient to meet special needs in each situation.*

- *briefly discuss conditions related to the parathyroid glands.*

- *briefly discuss at least 2 conditions related to the adrenal glands; identify symptoms and nursing and medical management of each.*

- *thoroughly discuss the condition of the pancreas known as diabetes mellitus, including a discussion of predisposing factors, types, common symptoms, and treatment such as diet, exercise, and medication; thoroughly discuss the types of insulin and their actions, as well as the procedure for administering the drug; discuss the oral hypoglycemic agents; differentiate between insulin shock and diabetic coma, discussing the symptoms of each and the emergency treatment of each; and demonstrate ability to perform special procedures related to the care of the diabetic patient, as well as to teach the patient to participate in his own care.*

---

The *endocrine* glands (ductless glands) are groups of cells that produce chemical substances called *hormones* (see Chapter 20). They secrete the hormones directly into the bloodstream, where they play a part in metabolism and influence the growth and the activity of cells and body systems. Normally, they produce, store, and release hormones as they are needed. It is known that many of the endocrine glands are sensitive to stimulation from each other, but even the authorities in this field do not wholly understand this relationship. Endocrine disorders are usually caused by the overproduction or underproduction of hormones, which sets up unfavorable reactions in the body.

## DIAGNOSTIC TESTS

Many routine blood and urine tests are done to diagnose an endocrine disorder. Since the endocrine glands usually cannot be felt or visualized, the components of the blood and urine are very important indicators of endocrine function. Direct observation also plays a part in the diagnosis of endocrine difficulties. Some endocrine disorders lead to defects in growth or appearance and can be identified by the physical appearance of the patient.

## Tests of Thyroid Function

**Basal Metabolic Rate (B.M.R.).** Although this test is not often done, it is a means of measuring the rate at which the patient uses oxygen when resting. The test is given after the patient has been without food for 8 to 10 hours. He lies quietly in bed and breathes into a tube. It is important to assure the patient that the test is not dangerous or upsetting. The only change in routine is that the patient must wait for breakfast and stay as quiet as possible until after the test. Precautions to prevent worry or excitement or activity are necessary because they can raise the metabolic rate temporarily and give an incorrect record.

**Radioactive Iodine Uptake Test.** This is also a test to determine how active the thyroid gland is. The patient is given a small amount of radioactive material (sodium iodide[131]) in distilled water. Twenty-four hours later, a scintillator (an instrument that measures radioactivity) is held over the thyroid gland to measure the amount of iodine that the gland has removed from the bloodstream. A normally active thyroid will remove 15 to 20 per cent in that time—in hyperthyroidism it may remove as much as 90 per cent. Some radioactive iodine is also excreted in the urine; the urine is saved during this period so that this amount of iodine also can be measured. Factors which can influence the accuracy of a radioactive test are pregnancy, oral contraceptives, iodine therapy, anticoagulants, salicylates, and propylthiouracil derivatives.

**Protein-bound Iodine (PBI).** The amount of protein-bound iodine (a component of the thyroid hormone) in the blood is measured by this test. The concentration above or below normal indicates either hyperthyroidism or hypothyroidism, respectively.

**T3 Red Cell Uptake.** This blood test also uses radioactive iodine, but since the radioactive chemical is added to the blood in a test tube, it is safer for the patient because he does not have to take radioactive iodine. This is called the *in vitro* method. (If a test is done within the body, this is called *in vivo*.)

**Thyroid Scan.** This test requires that the patient ingest I[131], after which a "scanogram" is taken to indicate the amount of radioactivity in the entire body. If a great deal of the radioactive iodine is taken up by the thyroid, this indicates that the thyroid is hyperactive. If a decreased amount is in the thyroid, a malignancy might be present. This test may also indicate where a thyroid malignancy has metastasized in other parts of the body.

**Blood Chemistry Tests.** Various blood chemistries are done to determine the hormone level and the hormone ratio in the blood.

Sometimes the amount of cholesterol in the blood is lowered in hyperthyroidism, but a test for this is not always reliable.

Any test done should be used in conjunction with other tests and other factors, since the thyroid is sensitive to outside influences.

## Tests for Diabetes

**Pancreatic Function.** The islets of Langerhans within the pancreas secrete the hormone, insulin. Tests of pancreatic function generally are aimed at determining insulin production. Lack of insulin indicates diabetes mellitus. The diabetic is not able to metabolize sugars and will spill sugar or acetone in the blood or urine. However, sugar in the urine does not necessarily mean that a patient has diabetes, nor does every diabetic excrete sugar in the urine. However, if sugar is consistently present in the urine (*glycosuria*) and if the patient's blood sugar level is above normal, there is a good probability that he has the disease. Tests of the blood and of the urine are routine for suspected diabetics.

**Fasting Blood Sugar Level.** This is the amount of sugar present in the blood when the patient has been fasting for a prescribed length of time.

**Glucose Tolerance Test.** The blood sugar level in the nondiabetic who has fasted goes up after sugar is eaten, but in about 2 hours it is back to normal again. This is not so with the diabetic. His blood sugar level is above normal with fasting and may not return to even that level for more than 2 hours after eating sugar. A glucose tolerance test will show whether or not sugar is accumulating in the blood. This is the procedure:

The patient is placed on a high-carbohydrate diet for 3 days preceding the test. The evening before the test, he is given nothing to eat or drink after supper.

Specimens for examination of both blood and urine are taken before breakfast.

The patient drinks about 100 grams of glucose in water (the amount is determined by his weight). He may also eat a specially prescribed breakfast.

Blood and urine specimens are taken at prescribed intervals, such as a half-hour, 1 hour, 2 hours, and 3 hours after the last swallow of glucose. The collection of specimens is timed from then.

The laboratory technician takes the blood specimens, and the nurse collects the urine specimens and labels the bottles, indicating the time when each was collected. The patient may have tap water to drink while the test is going on, but he is not permitted any food.

**Urine Tests for Sugar.** Normal urine is free from sugar or acetone, but both may be present in the urine of the diabetic. Excess sugar in the blood spills over into the urine; acetone appears as a by-product of faulty metabolism. Tests for sugar in the urine are easy to do and are not expensive, even on a large scale such as in a community diabetes detection program. The most commonly used tests are discussed here.

It is best to test freshly secreted urine rather than urine that has been in the bladder for some time. This means having the patient void, to empty his bladder, half an hour before you collect the specimen to be tested.

Clinitest. Add 5 drops of urine to 10 drops of water in a test tube and drop in the Clinitest tablet. Compare the result with the color chart. Readings may be done in percentage of sugar in the urine, but often are reported as negative trace, or +1 to +4.

Tes-Tape. Dip a strip of fresh Tes-Tape into urine. It will turn green or blue if sugar is present. Avoid touching the testing end.

Clinistix. Dip the test end in urine and read against the color chart.

Benedict's Test. This test is rarely done, because simpler methods are now available. The Benedict's solution is added to urine in a test tube and heated until it boils for 5

minutes. It is then compared with a color chart to indicate sugar content.

*Caution:* The nurse should be aware that some of these tests (such as the Clinitest) cause a chemical reaction which gives off heat.

The nurse must also remember that these substances are rendered ineffective by moisture. The lid should be kept on the bottle at all times. *Do not* use a tablet or tape if it has begun to change color. The tapes are also susceptible to light and should be kept in a closed, brown bottle.

**Test for Acetone.** Acetest tablets and acetone test powder are used most commonly to test for acetone in the urine. Place 2 drops of urine on the tablet or on a small heap of the powder. If the tablet or the powder turns purple, the test is positive. (In using these test materials it is important to keep the containers tightly covered. Otherwise, they absorb moisture from the air and are useless.)

The test for acetone is especially important if the patient is vomiting, if he has a fever, or if sugar is present in the urine. Acetone and sugar may show up in the urine at one time of the day and be absent at another.

**Test for Carbon Dioxide Combining Power.** This test measures the amount of carbon dioxide in the blood. A lower-than-normal amount indicates an excess of ketones (acetone) in the body.

**Self-Testing.** The diabetic must learn to do some of these tests in order to decide how to balance his insulin intake, exercise, and diet. Tes-Tapes or tablets have a decided advantage over Benedict's test because they are so convenient to carry around and to use. They are especially useful when traveling, and most drugstores carry the necessary supplies.

## THE PITUITARY GLAND (HYPOPHYSIS)

The pituitary gland is a tiny gland, but it has tremendous influence in the body and affects the operations of every other gland. For this reason it is sometimes called the *master gland.* It lies in the sphenoid bone at the base of the brain and has 2 parts—the anterior and the posterior lobes. It secretes at least 9 hormones, but only the most important ones will be mentioned here.

## The Anterior Lobe

To give some idea of the important activities of the pituitary gland, consider that the anterior lobe alone produces the following hormones: a growth hormone, the milk-producing hormones, ACTH, 2 hormones that stimulate the thyroid gland, and 2 hormones that regulate ovarian function. In men, one of these hormones stimulates the testes to produce the hormone testosterone.

**Giantism and Acromegaly.** Disturbances of the anterior lobe of the pituitary gland may cause overproduction of the growth hormone, *somatropin.* If this occurs in childhood, it causes prolonged growth of bones, or *giantism.* In an adult an excess of this hormone causes an overgrowth of other tissues (*acromegaly*). The victim's features coarsen, forming a massive lower jaw, thick lips, a bulbous nose, and bulging forehead; his hands and feet seem to be enormous. In women, facial hair also appears, and the voice deepens. Headaches develop, and the patient may become partially blind. The spleen, the heart, and the liver may enlarge; the muscles weaken, and pain and stiffness may appear in the joints. Impotence or amenorrhea may develop.

Treatment. Acromegaly is treated by irradiation of the pituitary gland; sometimes estrogens are given. Treatment can stop the progress of the disease, but it cannot undo the damage that has already been done.

**Simmonds' Disease.** This rare disease, also called *panhypopituitarism,* occurs when the pituitary gland is destroyed by a tumor, by surgery, or by postpartum emboli. The genitalia become atrophied, and the patient ages prematurely and becomes wasted. This disease can be treated by irradiation if a tumor is causing the difficulty. Hormones must be given to the patient once the pituitary gland is removed or destroyed.

## The Posterior Lobe

The posterior lobe of the pituitary secretes hormones that increase blood pressure, decrease urine volume (*vasopressin* or *ADH*), and stimulate uterine contractions (oxytoxin).

**Diabetes Insipidus.** *Diabetes insipidus* is a rare disease caused by underproduction of the hormone ADH, which regulates the passage of water through the kidneys.

*Primary diabetes insipidus* is caused by kidney dysfunction, because of a deficiency in ADH or a lesion in the midbrain. *Secondary diabetes insipidus* is a result of a brain tumor or pressure in the area of the pituitary.

As a result of the effects on the kidneys, the elimination of urine is copious. The patient may void as much as 15 to 20 quarts in 24 hours; he is constantly thirsty and restricting fluids has no effect. His urine is very diluted (low specific gravity, approaching 1.000) and contains no sugar or acetone. This condition makes him weak in spite of an abnormally large appetite and upsets his living patterns in general. The treatment consists of giving pituitary extract to control the output of urine in primary cases and removing or treating the causative tumor in secondary cases.

## Tumors of the Pituitary

Tumors of the pituitary can affect various aspects of body function. An overgrowth of eosinophilic cells in the pituitary can result in gigantism. A basophilic tumor in the pituitary can upset the production of the hormone which regulates the adrenals, leading to hyperadrenalism and Cushing's syndrome. A chromophobic tumor can destroy the pituitary and result in hypopituitarism. A patient with this disorder has fine, scanty hair, a lowered basal metabolism rate, a lowered body temperature, and a tendency to be slow and obese.

**Surgical Removal of the Pituitary (Hypophysectomy).** At times the pituitary is removed in an effort to arrest the metastasis of cancer, especially from the breast. It is not curative, but in about half of the cases of metastatic breast cancer, it causes a regression for a few months. This effect seems to be related to the hormonal influence of the pituitary upon the reproductive organs.

## THE THYROID GLAND

The thyroid gland has 2 lobes that lie in front and on either side of the trachea. It secretes the hormone *thyroxin,* which regulates metabolism. If it secretes too much thyroxin, the tissues burn oxygen rapidly; if it secretes too little, the reverse is true. The thyroid gland must have iodine to produce thyroxin; a pituitary hormone also contributes to the production of thyroxin.

## Hyperthyroidism

Hyperthyroidism is also called *Graves' disease* or *exophthalmic goiter*. It is a condition in which the metabolic rate is increased by an overproduction of thyroxin. The exact cause of this overactivity is not known, but it seems to develop as a result of physical or emotional strain, infection, or changes that take place during adolescence or pregnancy. It occurs most frequently in women.

**Symptoms.** Hyperthyroidism makes the patient highly excitable and overactive. She is unable to keep quiet, twists, and turns and moves her head and arms constantly. She may have tremors that make it impossible for her to feed herself. Her pulse is rapid, and she may have heart palpitations that cause heart damage if she does not have treatment. She feels hot; she eats voraciously but loses weight because her body burns calories at such a fast rate. Another common symptom is that of bulging eyes (*exophthalmos*), and frequently the neck is swollen due to the enlarged thyroid gland. Pressure from the gland may cause difficulty in swallowing or hoarseness. Tests reveal an increase in basal metabolism rate and an increase in uptake of protein-bound iodine and in $I^{131}$. This disorder, if untreated, may cause intense nervousness, delirium, and death from an exhausted heart.

**Treatment and Nursing Care.** The treatment for hyperthyroidism may be medical or surgical. Medical treatment consists of prescribing antithyroid drugs to block the secretion of the thyroid hormone. Propylthiouracil may be given either as a medical treatment or as a preparation for surgery. Medically, it is given daily, generally over a long period. Some of the toxic effects that may appear are fever, skin rash, and enlarged lymph nodes, with an increase in the white blood cells.

*Lugol's solution* (iodine and potassium iodide in water) is often given for a limited time (10 days to 2 weeks) before surgical removal of the thyroid. The patient must be

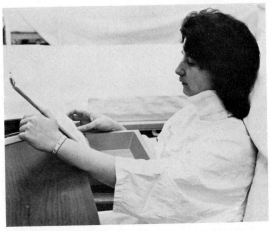

Figure 52-1. In making the thyroidectomy patient comfortable in a chair, the nurse sees that the head and neck are well supported with pillows. The overbed table enables the patient to reach frequently needed articles without turning her head. It is also convenient to use this table when inhalations are given.

observed for *iodism* or toxicity to the iodine, which is evidenced by rash, excessive salivation, and swelling of the buccal mucosa.

Thyroidectomy usually is not done until the basal metabolic rate has been reduced to normal by medical means.

## Thyroidectomy

*Thyroidectomy* is the surgical removal of the thyroid gland. Generally, about five-sixths of the gland is removed (*subtotal thyroidectomy*) so the patient will have some thyroid-hormone production postoperatively. Before the operation, the patient has a course of treatment with antithyroid drugs, a high-caloric, high-protein, and high-vitamin diet; her weight is checked every day. Radiation, generally in the form of radioactive iodine which will localize in the thyroid, may be given in an attempt to destroy part of the thyroid. The pulse is observed frequently, since the hyperthyroid patient's heart may be affected. In every possible way, the nurse should protect the patient from excitement or worry by maintaining a quiet environment, by controlling visitors, and by moving unhurriedly when giving care. Since many of these patients are exceedingly apprehensive, sedatives are often prescribed to help the patient rest. The nurse can help relieve anxiety by listening to the patient.

**Postoperative Care.** The patient is placed in semi-Fowler's position with the head elevated and supported by pillows in order to avoid strain on the suture line (Fig. 52-1). She will be given morphine or another narcotic for pain. Occasionally, a patient is given oxygen to make breathing easier. The patient should be told why this is being done, so that she will not be frightened. Her pulse and blood pressure are checked frequently, and the dressings are inspected for signs of excessive bleeding. Be sure to check for edema in the neck or bleeding at the back of the dressing, since the patient is sitting up. She may have sips of water as soon as nausea ceases. Noisy breathing or cyanosis must be reported immediately—a tracheostomy may be necessary. A tracheostomy set should *always* be at hand for a thyroidectomy patient. Observe signs of hoarseness, which may indicate injury to the laryngeal nerves. Suction may be used or inhalations given, usually in the form of the IPPB treatment, to relieve an excessive secretion of mucus.

Usually, the patient is allowed out of bed the day after the operation. She is first allowed to dangle her feet and then take a few steps with someone supporting her. Her head and neck should be supported when she sits in a chair. An overbed table makes it convenient for her to reach things without turning her head. The average patient is usually discharged from the hospital on about the fifth postoperative day. She must have thyroid function tests at periodic intervals. An occasional patient may be disturbed by muscle spasms if the parathyroid glands have been removed. Parathyroid hormone and calcium are remedies for this condition. A subtotal thyroidectomy usually prevents the recurrence of hyperthyroidism, since only enough of the gland is left to maintain normal function. If a total thyroidectomy is done, usually because of injury or malignancy, thyroid extract must be given to the patient for the rest of her life.

After discharge the patient should be encouraged to rest and avoid excessive physical activity. Usually, there is very little, if any, scar, because the incision is made carefully in the folds of the neck.

## Simple Goiter (Colloid)

Sometimes the thyroid gland, even though enlarged, does not cause toxic symptoms. If toxic symptoms (hyperthyroidism) occur, the goiter is referred to as a *toxic goiter*. Usually, the enlargement is caused by a deficiency of iodine in the diet. The thyroid gland must have iodine to produce the thyroid hormone; if a sufficient supply is not available, the gland enlarges in a greater effort to produce the hormone. In some localities the soil and the drinking water are deficient in iodine—this is especially pronounced in the Alps and other mountain areas. The Pacific Northwest, the Great Lakes region, Ohio, and Minnesota are areas in the United States which are deficient in iodine.

Colloid goiter affects more women than men and may appear during pregnancy, or adolescence or during an infection. Except for its appearance, a colloid goiter usually does not have a harmful effect on health, unless it becomes so large that it interferes with swallowing or breathing. It is treated by giving iodine for a period of 2 or 3 weeks, repeating the treatment 3 or 4 times during the year if the diet is deficient in iodine. Surgery may be necessary if the gland causes excessive pressure on the trachea. It is not difficult to reinforce the body's supply of iodine, because it needs such a very small amount. Since salt manufacturers have added iodine to table salt, enough salt is provided in most instances to prevent colloid goiter.

## Malignant Tumors of the Thyroid

If a thyroid tumor is cancerous, it must be removed surgically or treated by irradiation with radioactive isotopes. It usually appears in older persons as a small nodule on the gland. A biopsy will tell whether or not such a growth is malignant. Most common thyroid cancers are slow-growing, although a fast-growing adenocarcinoma, prone to metastasis and unresponsive to x-ray therapy, is possible.

## Hypothyroidism

Hypothyroidism (*myxedema*) occurs when a deficiency of the thyroid hormone slows down metabolic processes. This may be due to the removal of the thyroid gland or to a decrease in its activity for some reason. It is more likely to affect women than men. Symptoms of myxedema include slowing of physical and mental activity, accompanied by forgetfulness and chronic headache. The victim's expression becomes masklike, her skin is dry, her hair coarsens and tends to fall out, her voice is hoarse and low, and she gains weight. She may become chronically constipated and anemic, and her heart may be affected. Her basal metabolic or iodine uptake rate will be below normal.

**Treatment.** Oral thyroid extract is given to supply the hormone deficiency. The results are dramatic. The patient becomes more alert mentally and physically, and her appearance becomes normal again. This rapid change is not without danger; for example, her heart may show signs of strain from so much increased activity. Anyone with a thyroid deficiency is more than usually susceptible to respiratory depression from sedatives or hypnotics. Some people have to take thyroid extract all their lives, but with well-regulated treatment they stay normally well and healthy. Such a patient must see her doctor for periodic check-ups.

## THE PARATHYROID GLANDS

The parathyroids are tiny bean-shaped glands (4, 6, or 8 in number) located on either side of the underpart of the thyroid gland. They secrete the parathyroid hormone which, aided by vitamin D, regulates the amount of calcium and phosphorus in the blood and helps the bones to use these minerals.

### Hyperparathyroidism

Hyperparathyroidism occurs when there is an excess of the parathyroid hormone, which causes a calcium loss in bones and results in a softening of bone tissue or a loss of bone strength. This leads to skeletal tenderness, with the bones tending to break easily, even without pressure or injury (pathologic fractures). The patient's muscles become weak, and she is tired, nauseated, and constipated. She may also develop kidney stones and uremia. This condition is rare and may be secondary in chronic nephritis.

**Diagnosis.** Hyperparathyroidism is detected by a consistently high level of blood calcium and by x-ray indications of skeletal changes or pathological fractures.

**Treatment and Nursing Care.** Hyperparathyroidism requires surgery to remove some of the gland. If, after the operation, muscle spasm (*tetany*) appears, the patient is given calcium lactate to restore the calcium-phosphorus balance in the blood. The prescribed diet is high in fat and carbohydrate. This patient needs special care to prevent bumps and pressures that might cause a fracture.

### Hypoparathyroidism

This condition, as you might guess, is a deficiency in the parathyroid hormone. It is caused by lowered production of the hormone, with a consequent reduction of the amount of calcium available to the body in the blood and an accumulation of phosphorus. This causes tremors and muscle spasm (tetany), which is the outstanding symptom of hypoparathyroidism. This extreme muscular irritability may be so pronounced as to cause laryngospasm or convulsions. Other symptoms include loss of hair, coarsening of the skin, and brittle nails.

The treatment is to give oral parathyroid hormone extract and a preparation that is similar to vitamin D (A.T. 10 or Hytakerol). Calcium salts must also be given, usually intravenously. Calcium preparations are never given intramuscularly, because they would injure the tissues.

## THE ADRENAL GLANDS

The adrenals (suprarenals) are 2 small 3-cornered glands, one on the top of each kidney. Each has 2 parts. The medulla secretes the hormones, epinephrine and norepinephrine and is stimulated by the sympathetic nervous system. The cortex, or outer covering, secretes several hormones called *cortisones* and is stimulated by the pituitary hormone, ACTH. Epinephrine is secreted instantly to increase the flow of blood to the brain, the heart, and the muscles and to other vital organs when quick action is needed. The cortisones influence many vital functions, such as helping to regulate metabolism to supply quick energy, aiding in the control of fluid and electrolyte balance, and controlling the development of sex characteristics.

## Tumors of the Adrenal Medulla

A tumor on the medulla of the adrenal gland increases the secretion of the hormones epinephrine and norepinephrine. This, in turn, causes hypertension, tremor, headache, nausea and vomiting, dizziness, and increased urination (polyuria). The treatment for this condition is surgical removal of the tumor, a dangerous operation because it may cause sudden and extreme changes in blood pressure.

## Destruction of the Adrenal Cortex (Addison's Disease)

Destruction or degeneration of the adrenal cortex causes a condition called *Addison's disease*. It is comparatively rare and can be the result of tuberculosis, cancer, or a massive infection. It decreases the production of adrenal hormones, with the result that the fluid and electrolyte balance in the body is upset, and the level of sugar in the blood is lowered (hypoglycemia). In addition the basal metabolism rate is low and the blood chemistries are abnormal (low sodium, high potassium). The patient becomes dehydrated and anemic and loses weight. His skin has a dark, bronzed appearance and his hair becomes thin. He may develop tremors and be disoriented, finally going into coma and convulsions. Strain or stress of any kind may send him into adrenal shock, with abnormally lowered blood pressure, nausea and vomiting, diarrhea, headache, and restlessness.

**Treatment.** The treatment consists of supplying the needed hormones by giving cortisone, hydrocortisone, prednisone, or prednisolone in an effort to restore normal fluid and electrolyte balance. The patient must cooperate by seeing his doctor regularly and avoiding strain or excitement of any kind, such as overwork, infection, or exposure to cold. By protecting his health, the patient with Addison's disease can do very well. His outlook was gloomy before hormones became available. As added protection, he should always carry an identification card or tag. Instructions for dosage of cortisone as prescribed by his doctor should be included on the card in case his doctor cannot be reached. Time means everything to a patient in adrenal shock.

This patient's diet is usually high in protein and salt and low in fluid—sometimes 5 or 6 small meals a day are given instead of 3 meals, or he may be given between-meal snacks of milk and crackers. He should be watched for dizziness or lowered blood pressure and be protected from falling. An accurate record of food and fluid intake is vital, with the type and amount of all fluids and food being recorded, as well as urine volume and specific gravity of each voiding.

## Hyperfunction of the Adrenal Cortex (Cushing's Syndrome)

This disease is the opposite of Addison's disease and is not common. It is caused by the overproduction of the adrenal cortex hormone or of **ACTH** by the pituitary gland. It may be precipitated by cortisone therapy, by tumors of the adrenal glands or by tumors of the pituitary. Fat accumulates in spots, particularly on the face, giving a "moon face" appearance. As the disease progresses, the patient becomes weaker, his bones soften, and he may have backache. He also develops edema and has a reduced urinary output and hypoglycemic, as well as high blood sodium and low potassium levels.

If hyperadrenalism occurs in childhood, the child undergoes early puberty. The girl child becomes masculine, with emphasis upon masculine traits. If this disease occurs while the female is *in utero* (unborn), a true hermaphrodite may result. After birth, the condition causes *pseudohermaphroditism*. (A true hermaphrodite is one in which both male and female hormones and characteristics are present.)

The treatment involves surgical removal of the adrenal gland or x-ray therapy. Adrenal cortical hormones will be given as indicated. After surgery the patient will be treated as though he had Addison's disease.

## THE PANCREAS

The pancreas lies against the posterior abdominal wall behind the greater curvature of the stomach. As noted earlier the pancreas produces 2 secretions: the pancreatic juice which drains into the duodenum and is important in digestion in the gastrointestinal tract; and *insulin,* which is produced by the islets of Langerhans and is poured into the bloodstream to regulate glucose metabolism. Without insulin, glucose can neither be stored in the body nor used by the cells. This condition affects a large number of people. It is called *diabetes mellitus,* or more commonly, diabetes (not to be confused with diabetes insipidus).

## Diabetes Mellitus

It is estimated that at least 3 million people in the United States have diabetes. However, it is believed that only 55 per cent of these cases are recognized. The yearly increase (50,000) in the number of known diabetics may be due to the increase in the number of diabetic detection centers and clinics, and also to the fact that because people live longer, diabetes has more time to develop. These figures are not as depressing as they sound. The discovery of the hormone, *insulin,* in 1921, by Sir Frederick Banting and his colleague Dr. Charles Best, revolutionized the treatment of diabetes. Today most diabetics can control the disease and lead normal, or nearly normal, lives if they follow orders.

**What is Diabetes?** As was previously stated, diabetes mellitus is a condition which results from the inability of the body cells to use glucose due to a deficiency in the production of the hormone, *insulin,* by the pancreas. The body gets its supply of energy from glucose, a product of carbohydrate digestion. Normally, the liver stores glucose in the form of glycogen and releases it when the body needs it—that is, when the amount of glucose in the circulating blood falls below a normal level. (A glucose deficiency is called hypoglycemia.) If the cells are unable to use insulin or if insulin is not produced in adequate amounts, glucose accumulates in the blood (hyperglycemia) and spills over into the urine (glycosuria).

**Who Gets Diabetes?** There is a heredity factors in diabetes. Studies show that the person with diabetes almost always reports that some relative has had it. If both parents have diabetes, there is a good chance that their children will develop the disease. If one parent has it and the other has the gene, their

children have about a 50-50 chance of escaping it. If both parents have the gene but are not diabetics, the children's chances of escaping the disease are increased by 25 per cent. For some unknown reason diabetes is highly prevalent among Jewish people, while it is found less frequently among Orientals, who develop a less severe form. In general, women are more prone to the disease than men, with married women outnumbering single women.

Diabetes may also be caused by a tumor of the pancreas and other malfunctions in the body, such as renal shutdown or a severe cardiac vascular accident.

**Diabetes and Obesity.** There is a definite relationship between diabetes and obesity. More than 80 per cent of all diabetics were overweight before diagnosis. The exact reason for this is still unknown. One theory is that excessive food intake puts excessive strain on the pancreas because of overuse, which then results in exhaustion and possibly diabetes.

**Diabetes and Age.** Diabetes is a disease of the elderly, as it occurs much more frequently in older people than it does in younger people. People over 40 make up a very large percentage of all diabetics. The older a person becomes, the more likely he is to develop the disease.

**Types of Diabetes.** There are 2 types of diabetes: juvenile diabetes and maturity onset diabetes. In *juvenile diabetes,* there is a deficiency of insulin which requires that the patient be maintained on insulin injections. Because the blood glucose can fluctuate widely, juvenile diabetes may be hard to control, in which case the patient is referred to as a *brittle* diabetic. There is also a tendency for ketosis, which is an accumulation of excessive amounts of ketone bodies in the blood. (Ketone bodies are acid substances formed by the incomplete metabolism of fat.) While juvenile diabetes generally occurs in young people, it may also occur in adults.

In *maturity onset diabetes,* the synthesis, production, or release of insulin is below normal, possibly as a result of the islets of Langerhans not functioning up to capacity. Patients with this form of diabetes are often regulated by diet alone. In some cases oral hypoglycemic agents are used. Overweight patients with mild maturity onset diabetes compose about 80 per cent of all diabetics, with the highest incidence occurring between the ages of 40 and 60.

Other rare forms of diabetes, such as achrestic, alimentary puncture, and renal diabetes, also exist but will not be discussed in detail here.

**Symptoms.** Diabetes mellitus usually comes on more quickly in children than in adults, and in children it is more than likely to be severe, causing a loss of weight, sugar in the urine, copious urination, and a high level of glucose in the blood. In adults, diabetes often develops so gradually that it may not be noticed for months or even years, until it is discovered through a routine urine examination in connection with some other disorder. The most common and noticeable early symptoms are loss of weight and strength, general weakness and drowsiness, copious urination, excessive thirst and appetite, and itchy, dry skin. In cases where diabetes has gone untreated for a long time, additional symptoms include the presence of boils and carbuncles, arteriosclerosis and gangrene of the feet, retinal changes (hemorrhages), which cause visual blurring and other visual disturbances, cataract, neuritis, and coma.

## The Treatment of Diabetes Mellitus

**Diet.** One of the most important factors in controlling diabetes is the patient's diet. If he takes in more carbohydrates than his body can use or store, the diabetic will develop *ketosis* or *acidosis*. With too little food he will be undernourished, and if he is taking insulin, he will be threatened with insulin shock. Therefore, he must have the right kind of food as well as the right amount of food to prevent these complications from developing. The doctor calculates the diet for the individual diabetic in relation to his age, sex, activity, health, cultural background, and his usual dietary habits. Diabetics, like everyone else, must have the essential amounts of vitamins, minerals, and calories, but the amounts will vary with each patient.

A diabetic must accept the fact that he will have to observe dietary rules all his life. At first this may seem to be an impossible prospect, but once he understands that in other ways his life can be normal if he follows the doctor's orders, the diabetic can accept his disability and learn to live with it.

The patient does not have to worry about planning his diet while he is in the hospital. However, when the patient goes home, the picture changes, for then he (or she) or some member of the family must be able to calculate the diet. This means that the patient must have instructions before he leaves the hospital. The American Diabetes Association offers *Meal Planning With Exchange Lists* to help the diabetic to plan his diet. It gives 6 lists of food of equal value, showing possible food exchanges. Thus, if a patient does not want an egg, he can substitute an ounce of chicken without upsetting the calculated balance in his diet. The *ADA Forecast*, a magazine for diabetics, gives recipes for preparing food. Directions for portions or servings of food give cup or spoon measurements.

**Meals.** The dietary allowance is usually divided among 3 meals as well as snacks. The patient cannot have more than his food allowance, and he must eat all of it. Otherwise, he will upset the balance between his diet and his insulin dosage. The doctor may want him to spread the amount of carbohydrate in his diet throughout his meals in different proportions. He may also prescribe a vitamin supplement.

**Diabetic Foods.** Sugarless products are on the market in increasing numbers, but some doctors feel that a diabetic patient should learn to adjust his diet while using regular foods, since these special products are more expensive and have no special nutritional advantages. Patients are usually allowed to use saccharin or sucaryl in tea or coffee or to add them to foods. If they are added to foods during cooking they may have a bitter taste. No-Cal sugar-free beverages are available, as are cookies and candies made with artificial sweeteners. Patients should be cautioned to steer clear of products that do not spell out their sugar, fat, and protein content on the label. "Dietetic" alone is not enough. A diabetic has a lot to learn when he first takes over the routines that he must follow. The public health nurse can make follow-up visits after he goes home, to see how he is getting along and to help him and his family with any problems.

## TABLE 52–1.  INSULIN ACTIONS

| Action | Type of Insulin | Onset (hrs.) | Peak (hrs.) | Duration (hrs.) | Time when Hypoglycemia most Likely to Occur |
|---|---|---|---|---|---|
| Rapid-Acting* | Crystalline (regular or unmodified) | ½–1 | 3–4 | 5–8 | Before lunch |
| | Semilente | 1 | 6–10 | 12–16 | Before lunch |
| Intermediate-Acting† | NPH | 2–4 | 8–12 | 24–28 | Late afternoon |
| | Lente (semilente and ultralente combined) | 2–4 | 8–12 | 24–28 | Late afternoon |
| | Globin (globin zinc) | 2–4 | 6–12 | 18–24 | Late afternoon |
| Long-Acting§ | Protamine zinc (PTI) | 3–6 | 14–20 | 36+ | During night and early morning |
| | Ultralente (very slow) | 8 | 16–24 | 36+ | During night and early morning |

\* *Rapid-Acting:* These insulins may be mixed with longer lasting insulin to give all-day coverage.

† *Intermediate:* Patients must have a noon meal and a midafternoon snack to prevent insulin shock.

§ *Long-Acting:* These insulins must be mixed thoroughly before the syringe is drawn. The patient will often need a bedtime snack to avoid insulin shock.

**Exercise.** Because diabetes is a disorder in metabolism, it is imperative to provide a daily balance in diet, exercise, and insulin. Without this balance, serious problems will occur because the diabetic's body is not able to compensate for differences in daily exercise and diet. Therefore, the diabetic must regulate the balance himself. By exercising, the diabetic can reduce the amount of sugar in the body, strengthen his muscles, and improve circulation.

When the diabetic is in the hospital he most likely will not receive his usual amount of exercise. Thus the nurse should be alert for symptoms of insulin shock or diabetic coma.

**Insulin.** With luck, a diabetic 50 years ago might have expected to live 5 or 10 years, at the most, after the onset of diabetes. Insulin has changed that picture. Today insulin is available in many different forms, to meet the needs of individual patients. However, all forms of insulin must be given hypodermically, because the digestive juices destroy its effectiveness if it is taken by mouth. Table 52-1 lists the different forms of insulin and their side-effects.

FORMS OF INSULIN. *Crystalline insulin* is merely a slightly different form of *regular insulin* and has the same effects. Both of them are quick-acting and are given 15 to 30 minutes before a meal so that they will reach the bloodstream at about the same time as the glucose. Long-acting insulins are usually given 30 minutes before a meal. Quick-acting insulins usually have to be repeated during the day because their effects do not last as long as those of the other forms of insulin. Researchers found that by adding other substances to insulin the effects could be prolonged. Protamine zinc insulin (PZI), neutral protamine Hagedorn (NPH), and globin are examples of these combinations. These compounds have made it possible for many diabetics to get along with 1 insulin injection a day, since their effects last 20 hours or longer. *Lente insulin,* a combination, is both quick-acting and long-lasting. (See Table 52-1.)

Insulin is a liquid that comes in units of varying strengths—U 40, U 80 (U 40 means 40 units per cc.; U 80 means 80 units per cc.), which are marked on the bottle. Syringes for giving insulin are marked in units for measuring the dose of insulin. However, these unit scales are different for U 40 and U 80 insulin. Sometimes both scales are marked on one syringe, but it is simpler, and there is less chance of making a mistake, if separate syringes are used with each type of dosage. For example, a U 40 syringe should be used to give only U 40 insulin. The doctor specifies the type of insulin and the number of units to be given.

To preserve its effectiveness, insulin is kept in the refrigerator, but it should not be frozen. The diabetic who must travel can keep his supply of insulin cool in a thermos or an insulated bag.

PRECAUTIONS TO FOLLOW WHEN GIVING INSULIN. Since insulin is a drug which is so vital to metabolism, it is of the *utmost importance* that extreme care be used in its administration:

1. Be sure that you are giving the correct *type* of insulin.
2. Be sure that you are preparing the correct unit dosage (U 40 or U 80).
3. Be sure that you are using the appropriate insulin syringe. Do not substitute U40 for U80 syringe or vice versa and do not use a regular hypodermic syringe for giving insulin. The dosage is too delicate and cannot be measured in another type of syringe.
4. Be sure that the insulin is properly mixed and that regular or globin insulin is *not cloudy.*
5. Be sure there are *no* air bubbles in the syringe. One tiny bubble can displace 2 or 3 units of insulin.
6. Check your syringe and card before giving the injection and have another nurse double check before you give it. All nurses, whether graduates or students, should double check insulin before giving it.
7. Watch for the symptoms of insulin shock or diabetic coma.
8. It is important to test the patient's urine for sugar and acetone each day before giving the insulin. Insulin is usually given before breakfast.
9. Give the injection subcutaneously, rotating the injection sites.

ORAL MEDICATIONS (HYPOGLYCEMIC AGENTS). Insulin itself is not effective when given by mouth, but several products that can be given orally stimulate the pancreas to secrete more insulin. These agents are not insulin, but they are effective in the less brittle forms of diabetes; they are not effective in treating juvenile types. The agents most commonly used are tolbutamide (Orinase), chlorpropamide (Diabinese), phenformin (DBI), and tolazamide (Tolinase).

Orinase is the most widely used. It acts quickly, within an hour after it is given, with the effects lasting almost 24 hours. Orinase and Diabinese have few side-effects which are more common with DBI: the patient may have headache, gastrointestinal disturbances, skin irritation, and a lowered white blood count. Some persons have an increased sensitivity to alcohol.

INSULIN COVERAGE. Many diabetics experience difficulty when they become ill. For this reason, the hospitalized diabetic, no matter what the reason for hospitalization, will be on routine urine testing for sugar and acetone and will often be on "insulin coverage." This means that if he spills sugar or acetone in his urine he will be given insulin (usually regular) to prevent further *spillage.* He will receive this coverage in addition to his usual dosage in the morning. Many patients who are usually well-controlled on oral hypoglycemic agents must be controlled on insulin during the course of an operation, a pregnancy, or a systemic disease.

The procedure for the coverage is as follows: Have the patient void about ½ hour before you need the urine specimen. Collect the specimen and test it (usually done 4 times a day, before meals, and at bedtime). Then, follow the doctor's orders for the amount of insulin to be given. Usually, he will designate the amount and type of insulin to be given for each percentage of sugar and acetone spilled. If you are assigned to a patient who is on insulin coverage, but you are not giving medications, *be sure* to report to the team leader immediately after testing the urine. Even if the patient has not spilled sugar and acetone, report to the team leader so that she does not have to ask you.

INSULIN SHOCK. The dose of insulin is calculated to control an individual's diabetic condition. The purpose of giving insulin is to keep the sugar level in the blood at normal. Too much insulin in relation to the amount of glucose will reduce this level to below normal and will cause a reaction which is called *insulin shock*. The patient feels weak, cold, and suddenly exhausted; he is hungry and nervous, and he trembles and perspires. With the longer-acting insulins he may experience headache and drowsiness, nausea, and

## TABLE 52–2. INSULIN SHOCK VS. ACIDOSIS

| Insulin Shock (Hypoglycemic Reaction) | Acidosis (Diabetic Ketoacidosis) |
|---|---|
| Also known as "insulin reaction." | Also known as "diabetic coma." |
| REASON: too much insulin. | REASON: too little insulin. |
| ONSET: sudden. (Patient must be taking injected insulin.) | ONSET: slow—several hours to days. |
| CAUSES: omitted meal, overdose of insulin, overexertion, vomiting. | CAUSES: omitted dose of insulin, spoiled insulin, error in dosage, improperly mixed insulin, increased need for insulin due to stress of illness, exposure, or surgery. |
| SYMPTOMS: | SYMPTOMS: |
| *Skin:* pale, moist, cool, sweating | *Skin:* flushed, dry, hot |
| *Behavior:* nervous, irritable, trembling, confused, disoriented, strange actions. Later, unconsciousness. | *Behavior:* drowsy, lethargic, dizzy (*vertigo*), weak. Later, delirium and unconsciousness. |
| *Breath:* normal odor | *Breath:* fruity odor (acetone) |
| *Respirations:* normal, rapid, and shallow | *Respirations:* air hunger (Kussmaul breathing) |
| *Hunger:* great hunger | *Hunger:* anorexia |
| *Thirst:* none | *Thirst:* great thirst |
| *Vomiting:* absent | *Vomiting:* present, with abdominal pain |
| *Sugar in urine:* usually absent | *Sugar in urine:* present |
| *Urination:* small amount | *Urination:* frequent, copious |
| *Blood sugar:* low, below 60 | *Blood sugar:* high, over 130 |
| | *Chemistry:* blood electrolytes and BUN elevated |
| *Other:* blurred vision | *Other:* ringing in the ears |
| RESPONSE TO TREATMENT: rapid | RESPONSE TO TREATMENT: slow |
| TREATMENT: glucose. In more severe reaction, adrenalin may be given. | TREATMENT: insulin, forced fluids. |
| NURSING CARE: prepare to assist with blood samples, urine collection, I.V. administration of glucose. Remain with patient until he is fully conscious and watch for symptoms of recurrence. | NURSING CARE: prepare to insert catheter, assist with I.V., gastric lavage, EKG. Prepare to deal with circulatory or respiratory complications. Remain with the patient and observe. |

vomiting. Without treatment, other symptoms develop, such as dizziness, confusion, and loss of speech. The patient is unable to coordinate his movements; he sees double, and if he is still untreated, he may have convulsions and become unconscious. Without treatment, his brain may become permanently damaged, and he may die, although this rarely happens. This condition may develop so rapidly that the patient is having convulsions or becomes unconscious before anybody knows that something is wrong. The nurse should be quick to recognize the early symptoms of insulin shock.

*Treatment.* The administration of carbohydrates is the treatment for an insulin reaction. For a conscious patient this is sugar in some form, such as orange juice, candy, honey, sweetened warm tea or coffee. It is easiest and safest to give sugar in liquid form. The unconscious patient is given dextrose intravenously. An insulin reaction requires emergency treatment, which is followed by the adjustment of the patient's carbohydrate intake and his insulin dosage to regulate his disturbed metabolism. This is not easy in the first 24 hours following the reaction, and the patient needs close observation to notice unfavorable symptoms that may reappear.

ACIDOSIS. To make up for the loss of sugar as a source of energy, the body uses more fats and proteins, which are broken down into substances called *ketones* and sent to the muscles to provide energy. If an excess amount of these ketone bodies accumulate in the body (ketosis), it upsets the alkali-acid balance in body fluids and causes a condition called *acidosis*. In this process, a volatile substance called acetone is produced; it has a characteristic sweetish odor which can be detected on the breath. Any condition that interferes with the storage of glycogen in the liver and increases the body's need to burn fat for energy, such as lack of insulin, vomiting, surgery, or anesthesia, may increase the production of ketone bodies.

For a comparison of insulin shock and acidosis see Table 52-2.

KETOSIS AND DIABETIC COMA. The patient with ketosis experiences weakness, drowsiness, vomiting, thirst, abdominal pain, and dehydration, and has flushed cheeks and a dry skin and mouth. The patient's breath may have the sweetish odor mentioned above; his breathing may become slow, deep, and labored; his pulse may be rapid and weak, and his blood pressure low. This may lead to coma. Sometimes the comatose patient who is admitted to the hospital has not been aware that he has diabetes. Others have a diabetic condition that is hard to control and gets out of hand even when the patient follows rules faithfully.

*Treatment.* While the examination of blood and urine specimens is being completed, blankets are applied to the unconscious patient to keep him warm, and his pulse and respiration are checked frequently. If he has dentures, they are removed. As soon as the examinations show that he is a diabetic, insulin is given. Insulin, by lowering the production of ketones, makes more carbohydrate available to the tissues and builds up the glycogen supply in the liver. Regular insulin is given because it acts rapidly. Intravenous fluids help to relieve dehydration.

Sometimes insulin is given and the urine is tested every half-hour. Blood specimens are tested for sugar frequently, and a record is kept of the patient's fluid intake and output. In extreme cases, a stimulant may be necessary, such as epinephrine or caffeine. When the patient's metabolism is in balance again, he continues with the indicated routine.

**What the Patient Should Know.** Infection or severe emotional strain may upset well-regulated treatment after it has been established. Sometimes the patient does not understand how important it is to follow orders, or he becomes careless about his diet and then attempts to adjust his insulin dosage himself. Every diabetic should know that he should report loss of appetite, hunger, or any gastrointestinal upset that is severe enough to keep him from eating or causes diarrhea or vomiting. He should know that sugar-free urine is a sign that his treatment is progressing favorably, but when sugar is evident in his urine it is an unfavorable sign which should be reported at once to his doctor.

**Instructing the Diabetic.** The most important aspect in the long-term management of the diabetic is educating the patient and his family so that they will understand the disease and its treatment. A great part of this teaching is the responsibility of the practical and professional nurses.

POINTS TO REMEMBER. Do not assume that

the patient knows anything about his condition. He may be embarrassed to admit that he is not aware of some aspect of the disease, especially if he has had diabetes for some time. Explain everything to him in terms that he can understand. Remember that he may be upset about his condition, so do not give him too much information at one time. Give him ample opportunity to ask questions and be willing to repeat information given. Use booklets and pictures and give him materials which he can keep and look over again later. Include the patient's family, if at all possible.

DEFINING DIABETES TO THE PATIENT. It is easiest for the patient to understand his disease if it is explained to him in the following terms: "The body needs sugar for energy, and insulin is needed so that the sugar can be converted into energy. In diabetes, the body does not have enough insulin so the body gets weaker from lack of sugar. The result is you are hungry, but unable to use the food you eat. As you eat more, sugar accumulates in the blood and urine causing you to become thirsty because your body wants water to dissolve the sugar. Some of this sugar is spilled over into the urine."

TESTING THE URINE. The patient should be aware that his urine is to be tested to determine whether or not he is spilling sugar and acetone. Teach him to do the tests and assist him in comparing the results with the color charts. If the patient helps to test his urine in the hospital, he will be better prepared to do the tests when he goes home.

THE BLOOD TEST. The patient may be told that his blood will be tested at intervals by the doctor and that a blood sugar of 80 to 120 is within the normal range.

THE INJECTION OF INSULIN. The patient should learn to give the insulin injection to himself, if at all possible. Since the patient often has a great many fears about giving the injection to himself it may help if the nurse draws up the insulin the first time and immediately lets the patient inject it so that he may get over the initial fear of injection. Once he is rid of this anxiety, he will be better able to listen and learn about the method of drawing up the insulin. The patient must be taught about types of insulin and syringes and dosages. Use the type of syringe that he will be using at home.

THE ROTATION OF INJECTION SITES. The patient must learn that injection sites must be rotated to prevent infections or lumps from forming from the insulin. Injections should never be given within 1 inch of the same spot twice in 1 month. Possible sites include the arms, the thighs, the buttocks, and the back. The patient should be taught to make a chart showing where the last injection was so that he remembers to alternate sites.

THE DIET PLAN. The diet plan should be explained to the patient and his family in terms that he can understand and follow. Many children are allowed to eat foods which formerly were forbidden and are able to control their disease by insulin. The patient should understand the relationship between diet, insulin, and exercise.

SYMPTOMS OF ACIDOSIS AND INSULIN REACTION. The patient must understand what the symptoms are and be aware of the treatment. He should carry sugar with him in case of an insulin reaction. He should be aware that he must consult the doctor if he has frequent reactions.

PERSONAL HYGIENE. The patient must understand that since infection is harder to heal in a diabetic than in a nondiabetic, he should avoid infections and injuries as much as possible. Special care should be given to the feet, hands, and teeth. These are the places where difficulty is most likely to begin because of the circulatory problems which may go along with diabetes.

DENTAL EXAMINATION. It is important to have teeth checked regularly to eliminate possible source of infection.

EYE EXAMINATIONS. The diabetic must realize the importance of a yearly eye examination. Because of circulatory problems, the retinal arteries are often the first to show atherosclerosis, hemorrhage, or inflammation. Inflammation of the retina (*retinitis*) occurs 10 times more frequently in diabetics than in nondiabetics and may damage the retina permanently. Cataracts may develop and often do. A cataract may be removed surgically if retinal damage is not too great. The blind or almost-blind diabetic fears losing his independence, but there are devices which he can use to help him give himself insulin and test his urine. For example, special syringes are available (Tru-Set or Cornwall) with the plunger fixed at the correct dose. Furniture

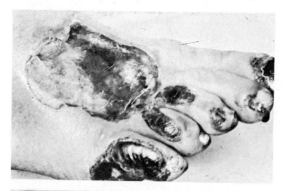

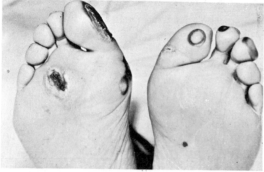

Figure 52-2. Gangrene of the feet in diabetes mellitus. (Dr. John R. Williams, North Carolina Med. J.)

can be placed where he is less likely to bump into it—a bump may cause a break in the skin.

INFECTIONS. Infections aggravate diabetes, and diabetics are susceptible to tuberculous infections and to carbuncles and furuncles. The common cold is another menace. If the diabetic has a stomach upset, he should go to bed, drink a glass of water every hour, take his insulin, test his urine, and call the doctor.

EXPOSURE. The patient should also be aware that exposure to extreme cold has the effect of slowing down circulation of blood, especially in the extremities.

FOOT CARE. The diabetic should be warned against injury. He should not cut out calluses or corns, dig out ingrown toenails, or walk barefoot. He should avoid burns from the sun and from excessively hot water. He should see a doctor at the first sign of any difficulty.

Because of the impaired circulation in the diabetic, gangrene of the feet is a possibility (Fig. 52-2). The patient should not be frightened, but should realize that he must take meticulous care of his feet to prevent this complication. There is no treatment for gangrene, other than amputation.

Painstaking care of the feet is so important to the diabetic that detailed directions for the treatment is given here and can easily be followed by both the nurse and the diabetic.

Soak feet in warm, soapy water for 5 minutes every day.

Dry thoroughly, especially between the toes.

Massage gently with cold cream or pure lanolin.

Exercise daily to improve circulation: sit on the edge of the bed, point toes upward, then downward. Do this 10 times. Make a circle with each foot 10 times.

Make sure that shoes fit well. Wear new shoes only for a short period each day for a few days.

Never wear circular garters.

Avoid sitting with crossed knees.

Cut nails straight across with sharp scissors. See a chiropodist for treatment of corns and calluses. Self-treatment in any form is dangerous and absolutely forbidden.

Never pick at sores or rough spots on the skin.

Do not walk barefooted.

Do not use adhesive tape on the skin.

Put lamb's wool between overlapping toes.

For cold toes, use warm socks and extra blankets at night. Heating pads and hot water bags are dangerous.

See a doctor for a cut, no matter how small it is. If first-aid treatment is necessary, cleanse the area gently with 70 per cent alcohol (no harsh antiseptics) and apply a dry sterile dressing. It is still essential to see a doctor as soon as possible.

Get the answers to your questions from the doctor or the nurse.

It is not enough to give the diabetic a list of the things he must do unless the reasons for these precautions are explained carefully. Some of them may seem to be trivial, and he may hesitate to bother the doctor with things that to him seem to be so trifling.

SMOKING AND DIABETES. Smoking is definitely contraindicated in the diabetic because of the vasoconstrictor effect of the nicotine, which will increase the possibility of circulatory disorders. The diabetic patient should be strongly urged to stop smoking.

THE PERSONAL AND SOCIAL FACTORS. The patient may have a great many questions about the effect diabetes will have on his lifestyle. He should be assured that he will not need to alter his life to a great degree and that he can easily adjust his diet to include foods which are common to his culture. He should also be assured that he can participate in

Figure 52-3. Identification card for diabetics. (American Diabetes Association, 1 East 45th Street, New York 17, New York)

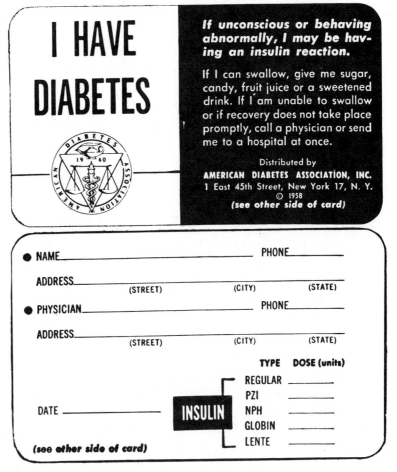

social activities, just keeping in mind the dangers of overexertion and fatigue. In terms of posterity, the patient should be aware of the hereditary characteristics of his disease.

The patient should realize that in general the outlook is good and that he can lead a normal and useful life. With determined effort and conscientious attention to the routines, he can contribute substantially to the successful management of his diabetes.

**Identification.** Every diabetic should carry an identification card, such as the one that is available from the American Diabetes Association (Fig. 52-3). It tells people what to do in an emergency, such as in an insulin reaction, and may prevent a diabetic's being considered drunk.

It is safer, however, for the diabetic who is prone to acidosis, to wear a tag, such as the Medic Alert tag, which gives immediate and positive identification of the problem. Many times, the card in the billfold is not found until it is too late. The tag worn on the body is readily identifiable to the nurse or doctor and gives immediate information.

**Surgery and Diabetes.** The diabetic is often considered a poor surgical risk because of the circulatory problems associated with diabetes, because of the difficulty in regulating the insulin balance during and after surgery, and because the patient is often older and may be more prone to postoperative complications. The diabetic is also more prone to infections from any wound, including the surgical incision, and has a more difficult time in healing because of sugar in the blood and impaired circulation. Because of the circulation difficulties, a local anesthetic is given if at all possible.

Nursing care includes frequent testing of the urine, watching for possible diabetic complications, forcing fluids, and general measures to prevent respiratory and circulatory complications.

# 53

# The Patient With a Disorder of the Sensory System

---

## BEHAVIORAL OBJECTIVES

*The student successfully attaining the goals of this chapter will be able to:*

- *identify and describe the major medical terms and at least 8 diagnostic tests related to the eye; describe the types and functions of corrective lenses; describe 5 common nursing treatments for eye disorders; and demonstrate ability to assist the patient with an eye disorder.*
- *describe the special pre- and postoperative care of the patient who has eye surgery.*
- *describe at least 10 common eye disorders, including cataract and glaucoma; and describe the major aspects of nursing and medical care.*
- *discuss the special needs of the person who is partially sighted or blind; and identify the roles of health workers in assisting these people.*
- *discuss the special needs of the person who has a hearing loss and identify the roles of health workers in assisting this person.*
- *describe the various types of apparatus used in hearing tests; discuss the various types of hearing loss; and discuss some of the predisposing factors in hearing loss.*
- *discuss at least 6 disorders of the external ear; at least 2 disorders of the middle ear; and the most common disorder of the inner ear; describe the symptoms of each disorder; discuss the major aspects of medical treatment; and demonstrate the ability to assist the patient to meet his needs in each case.*

---

As you know, the sensory system involves those organs and structures which give the person information about the world around him, as gathered through the senses of touch, smell, taste, sight, and hearing. The receptors for these senses are located in the peripheral areas of the body, from whence the impulses are transmitted to the brain, where they are interpreted. Any defect in the sensory organ, the transmission to the brain, or the brain itself can cause a defect in the sensory system. Specific disorders of the

nervous system and brain are discussed in Chapter 46. The present chapter will discuss primarily those disorders relating to the senses of sight and hearing—the disorders of the eye or ear.

## THE EYE
### Diagnostic Tests

**Refraction Test.** Refraction is the function which the lens performs in order to focus light rays on the retina; in this way, we can see objects clearly at different distances. To do this, the lens is constantly adjusting the curvature in its shape, a function called *accommodation*. Drops of the drug atropine or homatropine (which acts for a shorter time) instilled into the eye will temporarily paralyze the iris, the muscles of the eye which control the opening to the lens. This keeps the iris wide open (artificial dilation of the pupil), so that the ophthalmologist can see how effectively the lens focuses the light rays. Then he can correct a refractive error with the strength and the type of artificial lens necessary. He will try different lenses over the eye until he finds the one which will correct the error, so that he can prescribe the correction. The optician then grinds a lens to this prescription.

**Peripheral Vision.** A semicircular instrument, known as the *perimeter,* is used to measure side vision or peripheral vision by indicating how far up, down, in, and out each eye can see. This measurement of peripheral vision is called *perimetry.* The perimeter is also used to measure the curvature of the eyeball for fitting contact lenses.

**The Slit Lamp.** This is a special microscope which is used to see tiny parts of the eye.

**Tonometry.** *Intraocular pressure* (pressure within the eyeball) is measured by an instrument called a tonometer. The cornea of the eye is anesthetized by using a local anesthetic, such as proparacaine hydrochloride (Ophthaine). The sterile footplate of the tonometer is placed upon the cornea and indicates a pressure reading (normal is 12 to 22 mm. mercury). An electronic tonometer, which is also available, makes a graphic record of pressure changes within the eyeball. The applanation tonometer measures intraocular pressure without touching the eyeball.

**The Ophthalmoscopic Examination.** The ophthalmoscope is an instrument used to view the retina and other interior structures of the eye. The examination yields information about the blood vessels of the inner eye, especially those of the retina, as well as information as to the presence of tumors and the condition of the junction of the optic nerve. Because the blood vessels of the eyes can be visualized, they are often checked to determine the general condition of the blood vessels throughout the rest of the body. Atherosclerotic changes and hypertensive changes in

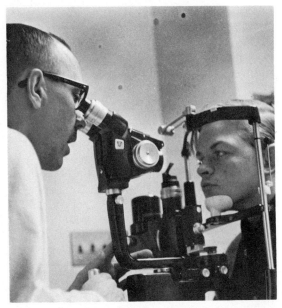

Figure 53-1. Eye testing equipment is very sophisticated. The eye doctor can determine if there are any eye disorders or diseases which may be dangerous to sight or to life. (Linda Berglin—Brookson-Broenen, Inc. and University of Minnesota Health Sciences Center)

the blood vessels of the eyes usually indicate that the same conditions exist elsewhere in the body.

**Fluorescein Dye.** This is a sterile astringent dye which is placed into the eye to delineate any scratch or injury. An injury will retain the dye longer than the rest of the eye and can be visualized with an ultraviolet lamp. The test will reveal any corneal ulceration and is also used to check the fit of contact lenses. The solution comes in a liquid preparation or is already impregnated on paper strips.

**The Electroretinogram (ERG).** This device records electrical impulses which the retina gives off when light strikes it. Computers may be used with the ERG to pick up very faint signals.

**Ultrasound.** The ultrasound echo is used to locate foreign particles and possible tumors in the eye. Because a foreign body is denser than normal eye tissue, the echo from a foreign particle is greater than that from the normal tissue of the eye.

**Radioactive Uptake Studies.** As with

other radioactive uptake tests, the method and theory are the same, i.e., a neoplasm or other defect will retain more radioactive material than normal eye tissue.

**Simple Eye Examinations.** The *Snellen eye chart* is perhaps the most commonly used means of determining gross errors in vision. Letters of the alphabet or E's pointing in various directions are presented on the chart. The chart for small children consists of pictures of familiar objects. The figures or letters are of differing sizes, depending upon the distance at which the normally sighted person can see the object. When a person stands 20 feet away from the chart, he should be able to read the line marked 20. This means that he has 20/20 vision (he *can* see at 20 feet what he *should* see at 20 feet). If he can only see at 20 feet what he should see at 100 feet, his vision is described as 20/100, and he is most likely "near-sighted." If the person can see at 20 feet what he should see at 15 feet, his vision is 20/15, indicating that he is most likely "far-sighted." (In a small room the person can stand 10 feet away from the chart and identify the direction of the E's while looking in a mirror.)

The *Ishihara chart* for determining color vision may also be used. The instructions for its use accompany the chart. Color blindness is a hereditary defect of the rods and/or cones in the eyes. It most often affects males (3 to 1), although females are often carriers of the defective gene. It rarely affects Black people. Most often, the person has an inability to distinguish red and green tones or, less frequently, yellow and blue. It is very rare that a person is totally color-blind.

Color blindness is a simple defect and is due either to the absence of one of the color sensitive pigments (red, green, or blue) or to the fact that 2 of the pigments overpower the third and cause a confused sensation. There is no cure for color blindness, but the patient should be educated so that he is aware of his limitations. For example, he will need to remember whether the red or green light is located on top of the semaphore in his state. (Many states have begun coloring the red and green lights with tones of yellow and blue, so that the color-blind person can distinguish them.) The person must also realize that he will have difficulty working in electronics or other occupations in which color discrimination is necessary.

**Eye Signs in Neurological Nursing.** While this subject is discussed at length in Chapter 46, it might be well to remind the reader at this point that changes in the pupils of the eyes reveal a great deal about the patient's brain status, such as in the case of increased intracranial pressure. In the normal patient both pupils should be round, regular, and equal and should react to light.

## Corrective Lenses

**Types of Lenses.** As people grow older, the lens loses some of its elasticity and does not adjust completely for near vision. This condition is called *presbyopia*—one can see evidences of presbyopia in people who hold their newspapers at arms' length. These people probably need *bifocals* (two lenses in one), which are ground to correct defects in both far vision and near vision. Trifocal lenses are also used; these add still another correction, making things sharper in the 27-inch to 50-inch range of vision.

**Contact Lenses.** The *contact lens* is a type of lens which fits directly over the eyeball instead of being placed in external glasses. Most contact lenses are made of plastic and are lightweight and paper thin. They fit over the eyeball (*corneal contact lenses*), where they *float* on the eyeball fluid. They are kept in place by capillary attraction and the upper eyelid. Contact lenses have a special appeal for people who dislike the looks of conventional glasses, for people who are engaged in active sports, or for people who make their living in the entertainment world where their appearance matters considerably to them. Contact lenses are not suitable for everyone—the shape of the eyeball may prohibit their use, and they are not recommended in conditions such as glaucoma, corneal infection, or iritis. Also, they are more expensive than conventional glasses, and getting used to them sometimes requires time and patience. However, they often prevent the cornea from changing shape, so that the lenses do not need to be replaced so often. Usually, the patient becomes accustomed to them gradually by wearing them for short periods of time at first. It is important to keep them clean and to avoid scratching them so that there is no interference with vision. They should be washed with special soap and water or a solution of benzalkonium chloride, dried carefully, placed in soaking solution overnight, and handled gently.

Soft, pliable contact lenses are now available, which are much easier to insert and easier to adjust to. They also reduce greatly the danger of ulceration of the cornea. *Scleral contact lenses* are larger than corneal lenses and cover the entire white of the eye, as well as the cornea. They are used in some eye conditions and in contact sports. They are much more difficult to insert and to adjust to than are corneal lenses.

### OTHER TYPES OF CONTACT LENSES

*Cataract Lenses.* Many patients have more success with contact lenses than with regular lenses, following cataract surgery. The contact lenses eliminate the need for the very thick eyeglasses which cataract patients formerly wore.

*Bifocals and Trifocals.* There are 2 forms of bifocal contact lens: one is weighted so the bifocal remains at the bottom, while the other has the bifocal lens all the way around so the lens can rotate. The weighted type of lens is not as comfortable because the lens does not rotate. In addition the patient will be unable to read while lying on his side, because the lens will be in the wrong position, due to the pull of gravity.

*Lenses for Astigmatism.* Astigmatism is marked by differences in curvature in different parts of the eyeball. Contact lenses for this condition must be fitted perfectly and must be weighted so the lens will conform exactly to the curvature of the eye at all times.

*Sunglass Lenses.* The person who is outside a great deal should wear sunglasses to protect his eyes. Contact lenses are available in various tints, from a slight shade of tint to regular sunglass tints.

COMPLICATIONS FROM WEARING CONTACT LENSES. It is dangerous to sleep with contact lenses in the eyes, even for a short time. When the eyes are closed, the fluids do not circulate freely, and *corneal ulcers* (the most common complication of contact lenses) can quickly form.

*Identification.* Many people do not realize the potential danger of wearing contact lenses. In the case of accident or unconsciousness, the person could become blind if the contact lenses are not removed. Any person who is wearing contact lenses should wear a Medic Alert or similar identification tag at all times (see Chapter 35).

*Emergency Removal of Contact Lenses.* The nurse in the emergency room may be called upon to remove contact lenses from the eyes of an unconscious person. Special tiny suction cups are available for this purpose and should be present in every emergency room. If they are not available, an eye doctor should be consulted. Be sure to wash your hands before doing this procedure. After the contacts are removed, they should be placed in a container with lens-soaking solution. If no solution is available, a weak solution of Zephiran may be used. Be careful to put the lenses into the correct sides of the container, so the right and left lens are marked. If the lenses have been in the eyes for some time, the patient should be checked for possible corneal ulceration.

The nurse must remember that the patient must remove contact lenses before going to surgery.

*Eye Injury While Wearing Contact Lenses.* If a person who is wearing contact lenses is hit in the area of the eye, he may sustain an injury to the cornea. It is almost impossible to break lenses while they are in the eye, because the eyeball will give with the blow and because the eye is protected by the bony structure surrounding it. However, in cases of severe swelling or infection of the eye the lens may need to be removed by the nurse.

**Eyeglasses.** Glasses have become so ornamental and glamorous, with a variety of attractive frames available, that most people scarcely mind wearing them. The wearer can choose a shape and colored frame to suit his or her face and personality, and also to fit different occasions. There are glasses for study as well as for business, with more elaborate types for social use.

People are sometimes concerned about wearing sunglasses. Sunglasses are not harmful if the lenses are carefully ground and do not distort vision. People who wear glasses all the time should have dark glasses ground to their prescription or wear clip-on dark lenses over their conventional glasses.

Questions have also been asked concerning the use of eyedrops which are advertised as effective in soothing or resting the eyes. Generally, these preparations are harmless unless they are used in cases of irritation caused by a condition requiring medical attention, such as eye infection or glaucoma.

## Common Nursing Treatments

**Patching.** There are many reasons for eye patching; the eyes may need to be rested after an operation or protected during special treatments, such as when an infant with jaundice is exposed to fluorescent light or when certain diseases or disorders require that the eyes be covered. If the nurse is asked to apply the patches she should be sure to use sterile eye pads and to apply them tightly enough so the eyelids cannot be opened but

not so tightly that they cause pressure. An elastic bandage may be wrapped around the eyes and head to hold the patches in place.

The nurse should explain to the patient why the patches are being placed on his eyes. Once the patches are in place the nurse must remember to speak to the patient before touching him so as not to frighten him, and she should assist him when necessary since he cannot see.

**Instillation of Eyedrops.** Eyedrops are instilled for various reasons—to contract or dilate the pupil of the eye, to treat an infection, or to produce local effects, such as anesthesia. It is often the nurse's responsibility not only to carry out the procedure herself but also to instruct others.

The lids and the lashes are wiped clean, and the patient lies down or sits with his head tilted backward. He keeps a tissue in readiness in case there is a slight overflow. The nurse rests the hand in which she is holding

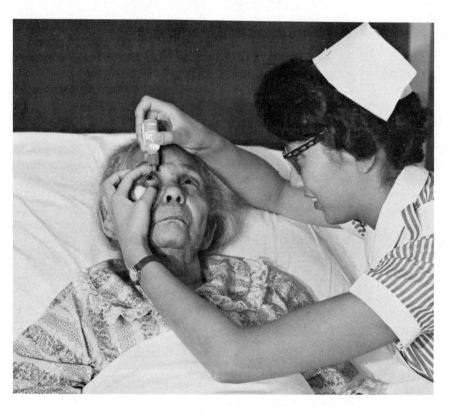

Figure 53-2. The nurse rests her hand against the patient's forehead, thus steadying her hand and controlling the movement of the bottle. The drop is placed inside the lower lid. (Smith, D. W., Germain, C. P., and Gips, C. D.: Care of the Adult Patient, ed. 3. Philadelphia, Lippincott, 1971)

the dropper against the patient's forehead and, with the other hand, depresses the lower lid (Fig. 53-2). The patient is asked to look up, and the prescribed number of drops is allowed to fall into the center of the everted lower lid. Then the patient is instructed to close his eyelids gently and to move the eye to distribute the solution.

Extreme caution should be heeded to prevent the drops from falling on the sensitive cornea. It is also important to remember that any unused solution cannot be returned to the stock bottle, so an effort should be made to avoid being wasteful when drawing the solution into the dropper.

**Eye Irrigations.** The eyes may be irrigated by means of a syringe containing warmed solution. The solution is instilled into the eye from the nose outward and is caught in an emesis basin. If possible, the patient should be allowed to assist in the procedure.

Continuous irrigations may be needed in cases of eye burns or when poisons have irritated the eye. In this case, a tiny catheter is inserted into the lacrimal duct to allow continuous irrigation. When this procedure is used, a great deal of explanation and support is needed.

**Eye Ointments.** When eye ointments are ordered, the ointment is usually applied to both eyes, even though only one eye is affected. The nurse must be very careful not to spread infection from one eye to the other. Usually, when one eye is infected, a separate tube is used to apply ointment to that eye and is clearly marked as such. The ointment is applied most often inside the lower lid, in a thin line without touching the eye, after which the patient is asked to blink a few times. The nurse may need to massage the eye gently to distribute the ointment.

**Warm or Cold Packs.** Packs are often ordered to relieve eye symptoms. Eye pads may be used or several layers of gauze can be cut to the size of the eye. For warm packs, the temperature of the fluid should be between 115 and 120° F. For cold packs, the pads are cooled on ice and then applied. In either case, the pads are changed every 15 to 30 seconds, usually for 10 to 15 minutes at a time. The skin around the eye may need to be protected from irritation during the procedure and the patient's eyes should be thoroughly dried after the procedure. The nurse must be very careful to keep the pads separated, to avoid spreading infection from one eye to the other.

**Everyday Eye Care.** Sound advice for daily eye care is the following:

Always work in a good light.
Rest the eyes at intervals when doing fine, intricate work.
Include sufficient vitamin A in a nutritious diet.
Get enough sleep.
Avoid touching or rubbing the eyes.
Never use eye cups (they help to spread infection).
Be careful about excessive exposure to sun lamps or strong sunlight—these can burn the eyelids and may harm the eyes.

## Pre- and Postoperative Nursing Care

**Before an Eye Operation.** The patient who comes into the hospital for an eye operation often cannot see very well, or perhaps not at all. You can help him to get his bearings and give him a sense of location, so that he will not feel as completely lost when he returns from the operating room with his eyes covered. While he is ambulatory, encourage him to find his way around the room and to the bathroom. Remember to tell him that both eyes may be covered for a short time after the operation and be sure that he can locate his call bell. His preoperative preparation might include an enema and a sedative to ensure a good night's sleep. Elderly patients sometimes become disoriented after taking sedations and may need special attention.

**Preoperative Care.** In addition to routine preoperative care, sometimes special preparation is done for the ophthalmic patient. If there is an order to clip the eyelashes, this should be done very carefully with a small, blunt scissors, which has been coated with petrolatum to catch the lashes. The patient's eyes are often patched prior to going to the operating room. If the patient is a man, his face should be shaved.

The nurse must remember that the eye is a very delicate organ of the body and that the surgeon is often working with the use of special magnifying glasses in order to perform the procedure. And deviation from orders, no matter how slight, can interfere with the success of the operations.

Eye operations on adults are usually performed under local anesthesia. The patient who is awake can be questioned by the surgeon, and there is less danger of nausea and vomiting afterward; the surgeon is anxious to avoid this strain after such delicate procedures. The patient should know that he will be awake during the procedure and that he will need to follow the surgeon's instructions.

**Postoperative Care.** The postoperative treatment is centered on preventing strain and hemorrhage. Special precautions are taken to keep the patient's head from moving or turning suddenly. He must be lifted gently from the operating table directly onto his bed while someone holds his head firmly and steady. He may have a small pillow on either side of his head; sandbags are not considered safe because they are too hard. Although the patient is awake, he may be drowsy and disoriented, especially since his eyes are covered. *He should not be left alone.* If he complains of nausea, it should be reported at once and he should be given nothing by mouth. The patient will have to be fed as long as his eyes are covered, and his head must be retained in one position. He is given oral care but is not allowed to brush his teeth. The doctor will decide how long this is to be. He may be allowed to get up in a day or 2, perhaps a week. After he begins to move around, he must be very careful not to stoop, to lift anything heavy, to cough, or to laugh heartily. When he goes home the doctor will tell him how much he is allowed to do.

The nurse must avoid surprising the patient by making loud noises or by touching him without first speaking to him. A radio often provides comfort and diversion to the patient.

**The Prosthetic Eye.** *Enucleation* (removal of an eye), may be done for cosmetic or for medical reasons when sight has been destroyed either by disease, often cancer, or injury. After the eye is removed, a metal or plastic ball (implant) is buried in the empty eye capsule. The ball is moved by the eye muscles attached to the capsule. After healing is complete, a glass or plastic "shell" is fitted over the buried ball. This shell, which is tinted to match the sighted eye, is the prosthesis familiarly known as a *glass eye.* Artificial eyes are so cleverly made today that they often are undetected. An artificial eye is usually fitted

8 weeks after an enucleation. The patient must learn how to insert and remove the eye and how to care for it. It is usually removed for the night and placed in a soaking solution. When the patient practices inserting and removing the eye, he should lean over a soft or padded surface to prevent breaking the eye if it should drop. Newer artificial eyes are made of plastic and are less breakable.

To insert a prosthetic eye, wet the eye and lift the upper eyelid; slip the eye under the lid by holding the eye with one hand and pulling down on the lower lid, slipping it over the edge of the eye. To remove a prosthetic eye, pull down on the lower lid and press inward under the eye. The eye will then slip out.

The doctor will instruct the patient about the care of the eye socket, if it is felt that this should be done. Rinsing with tap water or Zephiran solution is usually considered as adequate care for the artificial eye.

EMOTIONAL ASPECTS. The patient may often be very sensitive about the fact that he must wear an artificial eye. He may feel that it is disfiguring and embarrassing. In such instances, the nurse should be supportive and listen to the patient's feelings.

In the case of *exenteration* (removal of the eyelids, the eyeball, and all contents of the orbit, down to the bone), the patient is severely disfigured, and may wish to wear an eye patch. The nurse should help the patient to make the decision and support him in his decision, no matter what it may be. The patient must learn to live with his defect and cope with the situation in the way which is most helpful and supportive to his own self-image.

## Common Eye Disorders

**Errors in Refraction.** Refractive errors are a common type of eye disorder which can be inherited. *Myopia* (nearsightedness) is caused by an elongation of the eyeball, while *hyperopia* (farsightedness) is the result of a shorter than normal eyeball (see Chapter 21). An irregularly shaped cornea or lens produces *astigmatism* (distorted vision), causing objects to look wider or taller and blurred. *Presbyopia* was mentioned previously as a condition of old age in which the lens loses its ability to change focus readily. Holding objects at a distance, squinting, and headaches are some of the signs that may indicate refractive errors and the need for corrective lenses.

**Strabismus.** *Strabismus* (squint) is the condition commonly called "cross-eye." In looking at an object, one eye appears to be looking somewhere else and is turned either inward or outward. Strabismus frequently occurs in children. It can be caused by an injury, disease, or eye defects. The initial treatment usually consists of eye exercises; if this is not successful, properly fitted glasses may be effective. If both these measures fail, a surgical operation may be necessary to straighten the eyes.

**Hematoma Formation ("Black Eye").** A blow to the orbital area often causes hemorrhage into the orbit, resulting in the common "black eye." This is not a dangerous situation, because almost always, the bleeding stops spontaneously. For the first 12 hours, swelling and bleeding are lessened by application of cold packs. After that time, the coloration is absorbed faster by application of warm packs, which increases circulation.

**Acid or Alkali Burns.** If any foreign substance is accidentally splashed into the eye, the best emergency first-aid treatment is to rinse the eye with a large amount of warm water and seek immediate medical treatment. Do not attempt to neutralize the substance.

**Actinic Trauma ( Welder's Flash, Snow Blindness).** A very short exposure to the direct rays of the sun (less than 10 seconds) can cause permanent loss of central vision. The damage results when the pigment structures behind the retina are damaged as a result of exposure to infrared rays. There is no pain when the damage occurs and there is no treatment.

**Conjunctivitis.** *Conjunctivitis* is an inflammation of the conjunctiva, the membrane lining the eyelids and covering the front of the eyeball (except for the cornea). It causes pain, redness, and irritation and sometimes a discharge. A common name for conjunctivitis is *pink eye*. It may be caused by an infection, in which case it is treated with the appropriate antibiotic. Proper washing of the nurse's hands and the disinfection of the patient's linen are essential to prevent the spread of infection. Early medical care is important in order to prevent eye damage. Allergy may also cause conjunctivitis, in which case the treatment consists of avoiding the offending allergen, giving antihistamines, and desensitization (see Chapter 54). Boric acid or saline solution irrigations are given at frequent intervals to remove the discharge from the eye.

**Stye (Hordeolum).** A *stye* is an infection on the edge of the eyelid which starts in a hair follicle or a sebaceous gland. Styes are red, swollen, and painful and usually rupture, discharging pus. This drainage relieves the pain, after which the wound heals itself. Hot, wet compresses applied to the area will help to localize the infection, which is often caused by the staphylococcus. Antibiotics are usually given, and in some cases the swelling must be incised and drained. The infection is easily spread by unnecessary picking or squeezing. People with poor health and lowered resistance to infection may have a succession of styes. A better diet and rest, with relief from worry and tension, will help to improve the patient's resistance to infection.

**Ectropion, Entropion, and Ptosis.** *Ectropion* is the turning-out of the eyelid. This condition is often seen in older people. It is usually accompanied by tears because the lachrymal fluid cannot be excreted in the normal fashion.

*Entropion* is the turning-in of the eyelid, usually caused by a spasm.

*Ptosis* is a drooping upper eyelid. It can be caused by injury or a neurologic disorder, or it may be congenital. The usual treatment for these 3 conditions is surgery.

**Trachoma.** *Trachoma* is a highly communicable disease of the eyelids which is caused by a virus. The eyes become red and swollen, and small granulations appear on the conjunctiva. A scar forms on the eyelid, causing the lid to turn in. The eyelashes then scratch the cornea, infecting it. Trachoma may eventually lead to ulceration and blindness. Antibiotic treatment which is started early may control the disease. Trachoma is rarely seen in this country but is a serious health problem in some parts of the world where sanitation methods are poor.

**Glaucoma.** Glaucoma is a condition of increased pressure or tension of the aqueous fluid within the eye. The cause for *primary glaucoma* is not known, except that it usually occurs in people over 40 years of age and seems to accompany conditions such as emotional disturbances, endocrine imbalance, or allergies. It may also be inherited. (A steroid test is available which indicates predisposition to the disease.) *Secondary glaucoma* is usually associated with some other disturbance in the eye, such as iritis, tumor, hemorrhage, or trauma. The tonometer is the instrument used to measure pressure within the eye. If this pressure is not relieved, blindness results, because the nerve cells within the retina are destroyed. The symptoms are the impairment of side vision, blurred vision, pain in the eye, and the appearance of rainbowlike halos around lights or objects. (Everything looks blue-green.)

Glaucoma is a serious health problem. The Prevention of Blindness Society estimates that glaucoma has blinded almost 50,000 people and partially blinded 150,000 others. Early and continued treatment is highly important to preserve vision. A medical survey conducted in one state showed recommendations that a test for glaucoma be done in every routine physical examination.

TREATMENT. Many new drugs, such as Humorsol, Phospholine-iodine, and Epitrate, have been introduced in the treatment of glaucoma. Other miotic drugs used to contract the pupil are pilocarpine, eserine, and Carcholin. If drugs do not control the tension, then surgery is necessary. A procedure, called *iridectomy* (removal of a portion of the iris), is done to allow fluid to escape, thereby lowering intraocular pressure. Other procedures are also done to accomplish the same purpose.

The successful control of glaucoma depends on the patient's perseverance in following the doctor's orders, which usually consist of avoiding worry and tension, following good health practices, avoiding tight collars and belts (in order to keep circulation active), staying out of dark rooms as much as possible, and limiting any activities which strain or fatigue the eyes. The patient is also encouraged to avoid activities which increase intraocular tension, such as heavy lifting, or extreme physical exertion or excitement.

IDENTIFICATION. The glaucoma patient should wear a tag identifying his disorder so that he will be treated correctly in case of accident.

**Cataract.** A *cataract* is opacity of the lens of the eye. Since light entering the eye must pass through the lens in order to reach the retina, vision is impaired when the lens loses its transparency. This condition develops slowly, but eventually all sight will be lost in the affected eye. If cataracts develop in both eyes, the patient will become totally blind. A cataract usually occurs after middle age, but younger people may also be affected. Occasionally, a baby is born with a cataract, a condition called congenital cataract. It is believed that one cause for this condition is German measles during pregnancy. In this case, surgery is most effective if performed between the ages of 6 and 18 months. Cataracts are also common among patients with certain diseases, such as diabetes.

TREATMENT. The only remedy for cataracts is surgery to remove the lens. This may be done by simply removing the intact lens capsule. A new technic called *cryosurgery*, uses freezing technics to remove the lens more easily. Rupture of the lens during removal is a complication.

*Postoperative Care.* The patient does not usually have any pain after this operation, but if he does experience severe pain, it may be due to a serious complication, such as hemorrhaging, and must be reported immediately. After the operation, the affected eye or both eyes are covered with eye patches, which may cause the patient to become confused, especially if he is elderly and worried about the outcome of the operation. The patches are usually removed 5 to 10 days postoperatively. A pleasant "voice in the dark" will be most reassuring to him. The patient is urged not to cough or strain, so that he will avoid putting pressure on the suture line.

Six or 8 weeks after the operation, the patient will be fitted with glasses or a contact lens strong enough to take the place of the lens that was removed. After 6 months, the patient will be fitted with his permanent glasses or contact lenses. Because the power of accommodation is lost when the lens is removed, the patient will always have to wear corrective lenses, usually bifocals.

A cataract operation restores sight to many elderly patients and can be performed safely at any age. As a result, many a grandmother has been able to retain her independence and interest and keep up her contacts with others.

THE PROSTHETIC LENS. Sometimes, it is possible to insert a plastic lens in place at the time of surgery. At present this very difficult technic is still in experimental stages. But if it proves successful, it would remove the necessity of wearing contact or other lenses after surgery.

**Detached Retina.** A *detached retina* is a separation of the retina from the choroid, which deprives the layer receiving sight images of its blood supply. Separation of these layers usually follows a hole or a tear in the retina, the result of a blow or an injury, or degenerative changes. Whatever the cause, vision in the affected area is lost.

The symptoms may occur suddenly or gradually. If a large area of the central part of the retina is affected, the loss of vision is greater than if the outer edges are destroyed. The patient sees flashes of light, his vision is blurred, and he will see moving spots or experience gaps in his vision. There will be no pain, but the patient is likely to become bewildered and apprehensive. The usual treatment is surgery (usually with a procedure called *scleral buckling,* which makes the eyeball smaller, so the retina will fit), in order to put the separated layers back into place. Cryosurgery or the use of a laser beam (*photocoagulation*) has also proven useful. Liquid silicone may be injected to replace the vitreous fluid and hold the retina in place. After the operation, the patient must lie quietly, keeping his head still. Any sudden motion may loosen the retina again. The postoperative orders will vary with the individual operation and the ophthalmologist. The patient may be allowed out of bed the day after the operation, or on the other hand, he may have to stay in bed for 2 weeks. Surgical treatment of detached retinas has greatly improved, and patients today have a more favorable outlook for recovery.

**Sympathetic Ophthalmia and Enucleation.** Several weeks after a disease or an injury affects one eye, inflammation may develop in the other eye, a condition known as *sympathetic ophthalmia.* Nobody knows why this occurs, but it often follows a penetrating injury to the eyeball. To prevent the loss of sight in the unaffected eye, it is frequently necessary to remove a severely injured eye at once. The surgical removal of an eye is called an *enucleation.* The patient and his family may hesitate to consent to this operation, in the hope that the injured eye will recover. They will find it hard to believe that the injury could cause trouble in the untouched eye.

**Corneal Ulcers.** The cornea is transparent, thus allowing light to enter the eye. If anything causes the cornea to thicken or become scarred, vision will be affected, and blindness may result. Inflammation of the cornea (*keratitis*), resulting from injury or infection, may destroy corneal tissue and cause ulcers. If it invades the iris, it is more serious and is called *iritis* or *uveitis.* The main treatment for corneal ulcers is rest, with the administration of antibiotics and atropine drops to dilate the pupil. The symptoms of corneal ulcer are pain, tearing, and a marked inability to tolerate light (*photophobia*). The eye appears bloodshot. The treatment consists of eye irrigations with antibiotic solutions and warm compresses, along with tetracaine (Pontocaine) to relieve pain and *mydriatic drugs* to dilate the pupil. Frequently, fever therapy is used, or small doses of x-ray are given. The patient should wear dark glasses to relieve the photophobia. Fluorescein, a green dye, may be instilled into the eye in order to outline the ulcer. One of the important reasons that we are cautioned against rubbing or poking our eyes or removing foreign bodies without caution, is the danger of injuring the cornea. First aid to remove foreign bodies from the eyes is outlined in Chapter 35.

CORNEAL TRANSPLANTATION (KERATOPLASTY). If the cornea is so scarred that vision is affected seriously, it is sometimes possible to restore sight by transplanting a normal cornea in place of the affected one. Anyone who wants to help a blind person to see again can make provisions for donating his eyes for corneal transplants after his death. Each state has an agency for the blind which will provide information about the procedure to follow. Immediately after the donor's death, his eyes are removed and placed in the nearest eye bank. New technics allow the corneas to be stored for some time. The National Eye Bank for Sight Restoration is located in New York. After a corneal transplanation, the patient must remain flat in bed for about 1 week, without moving his head. Any sudden movement, such as coughing, sneezing, or vomiting, before the corneal graft has healed sufficiently, could tear it away from the eye. It is extremely necessary to preserve these grafts, since the supply of corneas for transplantation is limited. The problem of a rejection reaction has been attacked by the use of a transparent rubber membrane, which prevents the influx of fluid and the resulting edema and rejection of the graft. There is less danger of rejection of a cornea than there is of any other organ transplanted, because the cornea has no blood vessels and so is less likely to set up an immune reaction.

**Tumors of the Eye.** A neoplasm of the eye may lead not only to loss of vision but also to loss of life. Therefore, it is vital to diagnose the tumor early and to treat it as soon as possible. In some tumors, radiation therapy is effective (especially in retinoblastoma). Laser photocoagulation is effective in blood vessel tumors of the eye. Diagnosis has been aided in recent years by the use of fluorescent dyes, radioactive tracing methods, and ultrasound evaluations.

**Foreign Bodies in the Eye.** As previously mentioned, a foreign body may scratch or become embedded in the cornea or go even deeper into the eyeball. The ultrasound technic is a new method of locating an embedded foreign body. Some objects may be removed by use of the electromagnet or by surgery.

## Blindness

Sight difficulties are correctable for so many people that the need to wear glasses is considered as a minor inconvenience. Unfortunately, there are some people whose vision cannot be improved with the use of glasses or by any other means. The lives of these people, especially the elderly, are profoundly affected by the loss of sight.

**The Partially Sighted.** As was stated in Chapter 6, the needs of the partially sighted person are not the same as those of the blind. The partially sighted need a different kind of assistance. It is more difficult for these people to get assistance from agencies, since most of these organizations are set up to help the blind. Special lenses and magnifying glasses may help the patient's vision, and his opthal-

mologist will tell him how much he can use his eyes without harming them.

The kind of work he can do depends on his ability to see. He should not be doing work which would endanger him or others. In most states, the law governing automobile drivers includes a vision test.

**The Blind.** Blind people do not "live in darkness." Many of them can see light or "see" a grayness resembling a fog. Many people believe that the blind develop hearing and touch to a very sensitive degree, but tests have shown that this is not true. Probably what happens is that the blind learn to use these other senses more effectively *because they* cannot see. For instance, a blind person cannot see a person's angry expression, but he learns to detect anger in other people's voices. Assistance for the blind from the federal government and various organizations was discussed in Chapter 6.

**Where the Nurse Comes In.** Unfortunately, we are inclined to pity the blind and to do everything for them, when many times they would be far better off if we encouraged them to be more self-reliant. To make it easier for the blind person to feed himself, place his food on the plate in the same "clock positions" every meal. Always remember to tell him about changes—if a chair has been moved, or if he is having eggs instead of cereal for breakfast. Encourage him to shave himself and comb his hair and attend to the details of grooming himself. Be sure to keep his toilet articles in the same place and never disturb them without telling him. Guide him in his activities such as going out of doors or being seated in a chair. When walking with a blind person always let *him* take your arm, instead of propelling him along in your grasp. Be sure, too, to warn him of steps going up or down.

*Mistaken Kindness.* We are apt to overestimate a blind person's needs for assistance. More often than not, the blind person knows where he is going and how to get there, and he is perfectly capable of managing his own affairs. A blind person who seems to be bewildered or uncertain may be glad to accept a courteous offer of aid. Giving him directions or quietly offering him your seat on the bus is unobtrusive assistance that is not embarrassing.

Perhaps it is the little things that count most in helping a blind person. Speak to him by name—he cannot see that you are addressing him. Tell him what you have in your hand and what it looks like; tell him when you enter or plan to leave a room. If you want to shake his hand, you must grasp it yourself, since he does not know that you are extending your hand.

**Reading Aids.** One of the hardest things for a recently blinded person to get used to is his inability to read as he did previously. This handicap can be remedied if he learns to read in Braille. Braille is a system of raised dots which correspond to the letters of the alphabet and punctuation marks; the blind person discerns these characters with his fingertips. Obviously it takes patience to learn Braille, but it is well worth the effort since there are many books available in Braille. You can direct the blind person to agencies for the blind in his local area, so that he can find out how to get these books and where to find a teacher of the Braille system. Talking books, which are recordings on long-playing records of books and magazines, can be purchased or taken out on loan, and special typewriters that type in Braille are available. (Learning to type is no more of a problem to the blind person than it is to her sighted sister, since both use the touch system.)

**Traveling Aids.** Another problem for the blind person is getting around outside of his home and in his community. He is bound to encounter traffic, which today is difficult enough for those who can see. He probably cannot afford to employ a companion to guide him, and there may be no one in his family who is free or willing to undertake this service. One answer for this person would be the use of a Seeing Eye Dog; another would be a cane.

The Seeing Eye, Inc., Morristown, N. J., was the first center in the United States to train dogs to guide the blind. State agencies have additional information about similar centers. The guide dog is taught to recognize danger spots, such as curbs, obstacles or holes. The dog wears a harness, fitted with a U-shaped handle which the blind person grasps; dog and master can then communicate with each other through the movements of the harness. A Seeing Eye Dog is recognized almost anywhere and has special privileges. He is allowed to enter restaurants, subways, hotels, and other public places which might be off-limits to other pets. If his master is not moving, he will lie quietly nearby.

A blind person who wants a Seeing Eye Dog must live at these training centers for a period of time in order to learn how to use and take care of his particular dog. Sometimes, after a short trial period, dog and master find that they are temperamentally unsuited to each other. Then the trainer will exchange the dog for another, with no hard feelings! However, in many cases dog and master become devoted and inseparable companions. Some people are not able to use a dog, nor do they want to if they dislike dogs in general or are allergic to them.

The blind are taught to use their specially constructed cane to locate curbs and other obstructions in their progress. The cane is usually painted white as an indication to everyone that the user is blind.

## THE EAR

The branch of medicine concerned with diseases and disorders of the ear is called *otology*; the doctor in this specialty is known as an *otologist*. He tests hearing, examines the ear for signs of disease, and determines the treatment.

### Impaired Hearing

While hearing difficulties are more likely to occur as a person grows older, impaired hearing is a common difficulty that may occur at any age. Many a child has been scolded for poor marks in school or branded as dull when the real trouble was a hearing defect. Injuries to the hearing center in the brain, to the auditory nerve, or to the eardrum, as well as closed ear passages or poor conduction of sounds can affect hearing and cause deafness. Hearing may also be impaired by disease, by exposure to excessive noise, or by congenital factors which cause a person to be born deaf (congenital deafness). Hearing loss may vary from slight to moderate or may involve complete deafness.

There are 3 kinds of deafness: congenital

deafness, perceptive deafness (also called nerve deafness or sensorineural deafness), and central hearing loss. (It is possible for a person to have a combination of these hearing losses.)

*Conductive deafness* is an interference with the conduction of sound waves to the organs of hearing and may be caused by an accumulation of ear wax in the auditory canal or disease or injury of the vibrating bones, such as otosclerosis. In children, it is most often caused by excessive lymphoid tissue around the opening of the eustachian tube.

*Perceptive* or *sensorineural deafness* involves a disturbance of the organs of hearing and the transmission of sound. It may be caused by disorders of the inner ear which damage the eighth cranial nerve, the nerve pathways, or the auditory center in the brain. Such disorders may result from tumors, trauma, or injury from a toxic substance such as poison or alcohol. It may also be caused by senility, excessive noise, or congenital factors. A person who is losing his hearing because of impairment of the hearing organs has little chance of escaping deafness if the cause of the difficulty is not discovered before these organs are damaged.

*Central hearing loss* refers to the inability of the brain to interpret sounds once they are transmitted. This often occurs in atherosclerosis or after a cerebral vascular accident.

## Hearing Tests

Hearing tests will tell how well a person can hear and what type of deafness he has. A simple test involves determining at what distance a person can hear a watch tick. However, the *audiometry* test is much more accurate and reliable and has become a part of the modern school health program. An audiometer is used to test several children at a time, by means of individual earphones. Children who show defective hearing can then be tested again individually.

**Reflex Audiometry.** In this technic, which is used on very young children, a sound is presented to the child who then reacts, if he hears it, by blinking his eyes.

**Electrophysiologic Audiometry.** Since this type of testing does not require the cooperation of the subject, it is used in testing small children. Two chief types of response are checked to see if the child heard the sound presented. These are the *electrodermal* reflex (EDR) which measures perspiration and the *electroencephalographic* response (EER) which measures brain wave changes in response to sound and must be decoded by computer.

**Behavioral Audiometry.** In a child between the age of 2 and 5, the testing is disguised as a game, whereby the child is instructed to do something when he hears the sound.

**Tuning Fork Tests.** There are several tests which use the tuning fork to measure the degree and type of hearing loss. When air conduction hearing is tested, the tuning fork is held close to the ear meatus. When bore conduction is tested, the tuning fork is touched to the bone behind the ear or to the bridge of the nose.

THE WEBER TEST. The tuning fork is placed on the bridge of the nose or between the clenched teeth. If the hearing loss is conductive, the patient will hear the vibrations in both ears including the ear which has the greater loss. If the loss is sensorineural, he will hear the vibration only in his better ear.

THE RINNE TEST. This test compares air and bone conduction. If the patient hears better when the tuning fork touches the bone, he has a conductive hearing loss. If he hears better when the tuning fork is held outside the auditory meatus, he has either a sensorineural loss or normal hearing.

FOLLOW-UP AUDIOMETRY. If some type of hearing loss is indicated, an audiometry test is conducted to determine the exact magnitude of the hearing loss. Air conduction defects are measured by earphone, while bone conduction defects are measured by placing an oscillator on the mastoid process. If the results of the tests indicate that both air and bone conduction are about equal, a sensorineural loss is indicated. (In a person with normal hearing, sound is heard by air conduction about twice as long as by bone conduction.)

## Diagnostic Instruments

**The Otoscope.** The otoscope is a lighted, bell-shaped instrument which is used to examine the external auditory meatus, the eustachian tube, the eardrum and the middle ear. It helps when wax and foreign objects must be removed from the ear. The physician can also tell a great deal about the condition of the middle ear by looking at the *tympanic membrane* (eardrum).

For sanitary purposes, the otoscope must be sterilized after each patient is examined, and when a patient has an infected ear, it should be sterilized before the other ear is examined.

**The Otomicroscope.** When tiny structures are to be examined or operated upon, the otomicroscope is used to magnify the structures to be studied.

## The Patient With a Hearing Loss

A person with a marked hearing loss cannot hear sounds that warn him of danger, such as the horn of an approaching car or the hiss of escaping steam. He loses the thread of a conversation and may ask questions or make comments that have no relation to the discussion. This becomes embarrassing, and finally he lapses into a silence that makes him seem to be disinterested or inattentive. Because he is unable to hear his own voice he may talk very loudly or in a monotonous undertone. People are less tolerant of deafness than eye defects and become impatient when they are asked to repeat their words. Some people with impaired hearing stubbornly refuse to admit that they do not hear well, and they deny themselves the help of a hearing aid because they feel that there is something degrading about an honest admission of deafness, as if it were something of which to be ashamed.

**Helping the Hard-of-Hearing.** Hearing loss which is due to advancing age cannot be restored, but there are ways of helping a person to make up for it. He can learn *lip reading*—it is sometimes called speech reading because it includes watching facial expressions as well as lips. He can have the doctor look for and remove accumulations of ear wax. Others can help him by speaking slowly and distinctly in a moderately loud tone and by not allowing their voices to drop at the end of a sentence. Always try to include a patient who is hard-of-hearing in conversations as much as possible. We do not always realize how "left out" a deaf person feels. People with normal hearing often miss parts of an ordinary conversation because words are mumbled and voices are low; a deaf person is in complete silence.

As a nurse, you can be most helpful in dealing with a person who is hard-of-hearing, by calling the person by name, by talking while he is looking at you, by speaking distinctly and slowly, and by teaching him to turn his best ear toward the speaker.

HEARING AIDS. Hearing aids have renewed life for many deaf people. A hearing aid will not restore hearing loss to a normal level, but it will improve hearing. The doctor will determine whether or not a hearing aid will help, and which type of aid will be of the most benefit to an individual patient. No hearing aid will help deafness as effectively as glasses help sight. It takes time and patience to get used to wearing a hearing aid and to learn to adjust it.

Up-to-date hearing aids, like the midget radios, are operated on dry cells and transistors encased in a light-weight container. They may be in the form of earrings or bows of eyeglasses. They may operate on the principle of either bone conduction or air conduction. This device amplifies sounds and transmits them to a tiny receiver inserted in the ear. The wearer can regulate the volume and the intensity of sounds. One difficulty encountered when getting used to a hearing aid is that distracting sounds are amplified, as well as the ones the patient wants to hear. However, the difficulties can be overcome if the patient perseveres and wears the aid all the time, not just occasionally. The ear piece should be washed every day with mild soap and water and dried well; a pipe cleaner will help in cleaning the cannula.

If a person who is hard-of-hearing asks your advice about getting a hearing aid, tell him to consult an ear specialist. Do not make over-enthusiastic statements about what it will do for him just because a hearing aid has done wonders for your Aunt Ethel. If his doctor is prescribing a hearing aid for him, tell him not to be discouraged if it seems to be difficult to adjust to it, but that he should keep on trying.

**Preventing Hearing Loss.** The prompt treatment of infectious diseases, such as upper respiratory infections which can spread to the ear, helps to prevent deafness. It is also wise to avoid prolonged exposure to loud noise. Antibiotics and soundproof buildings have reduced these hazards. The American Hearing Society and its branches provide information about employment and social clubs which are helpful to the deaf and the hard-of-hearing.

## Ear Disorders

Disorders of the ear will be discussed according to the 3 parts of the ear—the outer ear, the middle ear, and the inner ear. The outer ear collects sound waves and transmits them to the eardrum (tympanum), a membrane between the outer and the middle ear. Vibrations from the eardrum are carried across the middle ear by 3 tiny bones (malleus, incus, stapes) to the inner ear, which contains the organs of hearing.

## External Ear Disorders

Most external ear disorders are more annoying than serious. If treated properly, they disappear. Unfortunately, many people attempt to treat difficulties themselves, or they turn to someone who is not qualified to give either advice or treatment. The good intentions of zealous amateurs often do more harm than good.

**Impacted Earwax.** Impacted earwax (cerumen) in the auditory canal is one example of a condition requiring a doctor's attention. He will generally remove the wax by irrigating the outer ear with a solution warmed to about 105 or 110° F. If a great deal of wax is present, the procedure may be very uncomfortable when the plug is loosened and air comes in contact with the eardrum. If the nurse helps in the procedure, she holds the external ear so that the meatus is as straight as possible. Free drainage must be present so the eardrum is not ruptured. The ear is then plugged with sterile cotton and the patient instructed to lie on that side until all the water has drained out.

It is not unusual for a patient to try and dig out the wax with a hairpin when he feels that his ear is stuffed up and he cannot hear. Or he may ask the nurse to wash it out for him. There are several reasons why an otologist should prescribe the treatment:

Impacted earwax may not be the cause of the trouble. Children are noted for putting things in their ears. If the object happens to be a pea, an ear irrigation will make it swell.

If the patient has a perforated eardrum, an irrigation might force the wax and the solution into the middle ear and cause infection.

Poking at the wax with a finger, a hairpin, or an applicator may injure the canal and cause infection, or it may push the wax further in. Sometimes the doctor advises a patient to put a few drops of warm olive oil in the ear occasionally, to soften the hardened wax so that it will come out by itself.

**External Otitis (Swimmer's Ear).** The most common cause of chronic external ear inflammation is prolonged exposure to water. The patient is usually given antibiotics and told to avoid swimming until the infection clears up. He should be advised to wear ear plugs when swimming in the future.

**Furuncles.** *Furuncles* (boils) are infections in the auditory canal; they often are the result of picking at the ear to remove wax. They are intensely painful, and codeine may be necessary to relieve the pain. Heat may be applied, and antibiotics are given.

**Fungous Infections.** These infections in the auditory canal occur in warm, damp climates, especially when the auditory canal has not been completely dried. Dead skin cells collect in the canal as a sort of mold. They can be treated with ear drops composed of copper sulfate, alcohol, and glycerin. They resist treatment, so that often it is necessary to continue treatment for a number of weeks.

**Insects.** Sometimes insects enter the auditory canal. If they remain they cause agonizing distress by their fluttering and buzzing. If a flashlight is held to the ear, the light may draw the insect out; sometimes a few drops of mineral oil or alcohol may kill it and it will float out if the patient's head is turned to one side. If none of these expedients works, the patient should see a doctor at once. It is dangerous to try to remove an insect with forceps; removing an insect from the ear is a delicate process which requires great skill.

**Foreign Objects.** Objects are often put in the ear canal by children or mentally retarded persons. As in the case of impacted wax, foreign objects must be removed by a doctor because pushing on the object may rupture the eardrum. If the object is a protein substance, such as a pea, irrigations are contraindicated because the object often swells, causing damage to the eardrum.

**Piercing the Earlobes.** This procedure should be done by a doctor, using the appropriate equipment to make the procedure quick and almost painless. After the procedure is done, the patient is advised to keep the original earrings in place for at least 2 weeks, to turn them frequently, and to cleanse the earlobes often with an antiseptic solution.

**A Punctured Eardrum.** A punctured or perforated eardrum is a serious threat to later hearing, as well as a possible source of middle-ear infection. While the perforation will often heal spontaneously, surgery is sometimes necessary. Occasionally, myringotomy (surgical puncture of the eardrum) is done for therapeutic reasons.

## Conditions That Affect the Middle Ear

**Otosclerosis.** *Otosclerosis* is a bony fixation of the stapes—one of the small bones in the middle ear which helps to transmit sound to the inner ear. This condition interferes with the vibration of the stapes and is usually slow in developing. No one knows exactly what causes otosclerosis, but it seems to have something to do with heredity, since it usually runs in families.

The patient may not notice that he is growing deaf until he begins to have difficulty in hearing ordinary conversation, especially when people speak in low tones, although if they speak loudly he can hear them. Another symptom is *ringing* in his ears (*tinnitus*), which is accentuated at night when everything around him is quiet. The patient with this condition may be aided by surgery or by a hearing aid.

STAPES MOBILIZATION. Surgery to restore vibration to the stapes (an operation known as stapes mobilization) may or may not be effective; therefore, it is usually left to the patient to decide whether or not he wants to take that chance. The operation is done under local anesthesia and frees the stapes so that it can vibrate. More often today, the stapes is removed (*stapedectomy*) and replaced by a metal prosthesis (tantalum wire), or a polyethylene prosthesis. The patient can often hear immediately after the prosthesis is placed.

The patient is usually allowed to be up out of bed following surgery and may be discharged in 2 days. He may feel dizzy and need assistance in walking, so precautions must be taken to prevent falls. He is told not to blow his nose violently for fear of spreading infection to the operative region through the eustachian tube, and he is warned not to get water in his ear. In about 2 weeks he can resume his normal activities. If this operation is not successful, a *fenestration* operation may be considered.

FENESTRATION OPERATION. Fenestration involves making a new window from the middle to the inner ear to let the vibrations through. This "window" is about as large as the head of a pin! The operation is more disturbing than the stapes operation, and the patient often experiences severe dizziness and nausea. He is cautioned to move slowly and to keep his head flat. Chewing is painful, so he is given soft foods and fluids. He may lie on his back or on the operative side—lying on the other side might allow drainage from the operative area to run into the inner ear. Usually, such patients remain in the hospital for 10 days to 2 weeks.

The patient's hearing may not be noticeably improved for a month to 6 weeks after the operation. He must avoid blowing his nose violently and be careful not to get water in his ears. Hearing tests will show how successful the operation has been.

EAR OPERATION PROCEDURES. In preparation for any ear operation, the patient must understand that the procedure may or may not be successful. He needs to understand how delicate the structures of the ear are and the skill needed by the surgeon.

Very little special preoperative preparation is done. The ear is usually packed with cotton, and eardrops are often instilled.

Postoperatively, the patient must understand that the dressings and packs in the ear cannot be removed for several days. He often is anxious to know if he can hear or not and needs explanation as to why the dressings must remain in place. The nurse should watch for signs of dizziness, a symptom of disturbance in the inner ear. Hemorrhage is also a possible complication and the nurse should be observant for obvious bleeding or complaints of pressure, pain, or lowered blood pressure.

**Ear Infections.** The ear is especially susceptible to upper respiratory infections because they spread to the ear through the eustachian tube from the nose and the throat. Children are the most vulnerable to these infections, but they also affect adults as the result of childhood infections. Before antibiotics became available, long, drawn-out ear infections did a great amount of damage and even caused death. Antibiotics changed this picture, but now we are faced with a new worry because some microorganisms are becoming resistant to antibiotics.

OTITIS MEDIA. *Otitis media* is an inflammation of the middle ear. There are 2 types: serous otitis media and purulent otitis media. In *serous* otitis media, fluid forms in the middle ear as a result of obstruction of the eustachian tube—a condition which may be caused by such things as infection, allergy, or growths, or by sudden changes in altitude. The symptoms are crackling sensations and fullness in the ear, with some hearing loss. If this condition is not treated promptly, the pressure of the fluid may rupture the eardrum. It is treated by puncturing the eardrum and aspirating the fluid, followed by treatment for the cause of the difficulty.

Acute *purulent* otitis media is caused by an infection spreading through the eustachian tube in upper respiratory infections. Pus forms and collects in the middle ear to create pressure on the eardrum. The symptoms are fever, earache, and impaired hearing. The eardrum is red and bulging and may rupture. Prompt treatment to puncture the eardrum prevents a rupture; a rupture heals slowly and leaves a scar which may interfere with the vibrations of the drum and damage hearing.

The puncture (*myringotomy*) releases the pressure and relieves the pain, and it heals quickly. The discharge from the ear is bloody at first and becomes purulent later. The ear should not be plugged tightly with cotton since this interferes with drainage; a small piece of cotton can be placed in the outer ear to absorb the drainage. This should be changed frequently. The appropriate antibiotics are given to fight the infection. Further treatment consists of rest, an adequate diet and the prevention of chilling.

Inflammation of the mastoid cells (*mastoiditis*) is a possible complication of acute otitis media, or meningitis may occur if the infection spreads to the meninges of the spine. Other complications include nausea and vomiting, dizziness, injury to the facial nerve causing facial paralysis, or a brain abscess: all this may start with a simple earache. If acute otitis media is neglected or is not treated properly, it may become chronic, inflicting the patient with a discharging ear, a noticeable hearing loss, and the danger of the infection spreading to the mastoid cells or to the brain.

MASTOIDITIS. Due to antibiotics, mastoiditis is rarely seen today. In acute mastoiditis the patient has fever, chills, and headache and experiences tenderness over the mastoid process. The treatment includes the administration of antibiotics and a mastoidectomy to remove the infected mastoid cells and to secure drainage. Usually, the patient's hearing is not affected.

Chronic mastoiditis often requires much more drastic treatment, which involves removing the eardrum and the 3 little bones in the middle ear, as well as removing the mastoid cells. An extensive operation causes a marked loss of hearing. Some of the newer surgical procedures reconstruct the middle ear to preserve vital parts, with less impairment of hearing.

## Disorders of the Inner Ear

Almost every disorder of the inner ear makes treatment difficult. In the first place, neither surgery nor hearing aids help inner ear deafness (perceptive deafness). Also, many drugs used to treat other conditions in the body may be injurious to the inner ear. Streptomycin, for instance, may injure the auditory nerve. Diseases such as measles, as well as the aging process, may also cause inner ear damage. Often, safe treatment consists merely in preventing further injury and training the patient in speech reading.

**Meniere's Syndrome.** Meniere's syndrome (also known as *Meniere's disease* or *labyrinthine hydrops*) is a disturbance of the semicircular canals in the inner ear, a body mechanism that is important in maintaining body balance. Although not fatal, it is not curable. There are many theories about how disease upsets this mechanism, but authorities have not been able to agree on any one cause.

The symptoms are devastating and alarming. The patient has sudden attacks of severe dizziness (*vertigo*), accompanied by nausea, vomiting, and a ringing sensation in the ears (*tinnitus*). If the condition is untreated, eventually hearing deteriorates. The attacks are violent; they may last only a few minutes or several weeks. The patient lives in constant fear of an attack, and he may have to give up his work because of his condition.

In Meniere's disease the normal amount of fluid in the spaces between the semicircular canals increases. The patient may be put on a low-sodium diet to reduce the amount of fluid; he may be given sedatives or tranquilizers to quiet his apprehension. Drugs, such as Dramamine and Bonamine, may be given to relieve dizziness and nausea. Nicotinic acid also may be given to relieve spasm of the auditory artery. The patient is advised to omit alcohol, coffee, and tobacco. Driving may be dangerous. Sometimes, when only one ear is affected, an operation to cut the auditory nerve is performed, which, of course, results in complete deafness in the affected ear.

When caring for these patients, every possible precaution is taken to avoid precipitating an attack by jarring the bed or making sudden movements. Everything must be done slowly and explained to the patient beforehand. If the dizziness is severe, the patient is in danger of falling. He should have side rails on his bed and assistance when he is up. If he is nauseated, he may be more willing to take food and fluids if they are given in small amounts. These attacks are so devastating that the patient is understandably apprehensive. He needs the reassurance that relief is possible if he keeps quiet and follows orders.

Persons with inner ear disorders are urged to bequeath their inner ears to the Temporal Bone Banks Program for Ear Research, so that studies which cannot be done on live subjects, can be carried out.

# 54

# The Patient With an Allergy

---

## BEHAVIORAL OBJECTIVES

*The student successfully attaining the goals of this chapter will be able to:*

- *define the word allergy and other medical terms related to allergies; and utilize these terms correctly in reporting patient care.*

- *describe methods by which allergies are diagnosed; and assist with these procedures.*

- *differentiate between different types of allergies.*

- *describe at least 3 treatments for allergy; describe the symptoms and treatment of a drug allergy; and demonstrate effectiveness in assisting the patient with an allergy to meet his special needs.*

- *discuss anaphylactic shock; describe the symptoms and list the 5 emergency measures which must be taken immediately.*

---

*Allergy* is an extreme sensitivity to one or more substances. When a foreign protein substance touches or enters the body, the body produces antibodies for protection against it. Later, contacts with this protein may set off a reaction with the antibodies that will cause unpleasant symptoms. This is called an *allergic reaction,* and we say that the person is sensitive or *allergic* to the foreign substance, which is called an *allergen* or an *antigen.* Some allergens are inhaled, such as pollens, dust, and animal dander; others are taken into the body in the form of drugs or foods, such as seafood, eggs, and chocolate. Allergens can also be skin contacts, such as cosmetics, hair dyes, or shoe dyes, and wool or nylon. Others enter the body through bee stings, immunizations, and blood transfusions.

Allergic reactions, which can occur at any age, may cause only minor discomforts, but they often can cause excessive irritation, and in certain severe instances death can result. Factors which influence the intensity and potential danger of the allergic response are the type of antigen, the type of antibody, the concentration of antigens and antibodies, and the part of the body which is involved.

## Causes of Allergy

It is not clearly known why certain proteins cause unpleasant symptoms. Since the antihistamine drugs bring relief, it is thought that the protein-antibody reaction may liberate an excessive amount of histamine in the body.

Scientists also believe that a general tendency toward allergic reactions may be inherited. However, this does not mean that a specific allergy is inherited. Estimates tell us that about 10 per cent of the population has allergic tendencies, including 1 child in every 10. There are many substances to which people are sensitive, but these people may not be equally sensitive to the same substance. Also, an individual's sensitivity to one substance may disappear while another takes its place, or an allergy may disappear entirely.

## Diagnosis of Allergies

It is not always easy to find out what is causing an allergy. In some cases the condition seems to have no relation to the substances tested or to anything in the air or in the victim's food. A person might be sensitive to a certain substance only when he is tired or upset. Sometimes he is only occasionally sensitive to it. The doctor should question the patient closely about his family history and any new substance with which he has been in contact.

There are 2 chief means of determining the cause of allergic reactions in the patient: taking a careful medical history and running a series of skin tests.

**The Medical History.** Aside from indicating the results of a general physical examination, the medical history includes data on past diseases, foods or substances which bother the patient in some way, and a family history of allergic type disorders.

**Skin Tests.** Skin tests are done to confirm suspected allergies or to determine the causes of allergic reactions. They are given in groups of several antigens, with each antigen injected intradermally or applied to a small scratch on the skin. These are then labeled or identified. After 20 minutes, the doctor reads the skin tests much as a Mantoux test is read. Erythema and edema indicate a positive skin test. The amount of edema is the indicator (measured in millimeters) and determines the severity of the reaction. In this way, the doctor can identify which substances are causing the allergic reaction in this particular patient and to what extent the patient reacts to each antigen. Sometimes, in spite of a positive skin test, an allergen does not cause an allergic reaction.

*Nursing Care.* The patient should be observed closely during a skin test, because occasionally a test will cause a severe reaction. Such a reaction is unusual, since the amount of allergen used is very small; however, it can happen if the patient is highly sensitive to the allergen.

## Kinds of Allergic Reactions

Allergic reactions most often affect the skin, the respiratory passages, and the gastrointestinal tract; they cause a rash (*erythema*), edema, and contractions of the smooth muscles and can result in total shock and death. Some examples of these reactions are:

*Asthma:* Spasms of the smooth muscles of the bronchi and edema create difficulty in breathing, which causes a cough, an accumulation of mucus, and wheezing. The patient may become cyanotic in a severe attack.

*Allergic rhinitis (pollinosis; hay fever):* The patient suffers from edema; his eyes and nose are inflamed and watery, and they itch.

*Urticaria (hives):* Reddened areas occur which itch and burn around swollen patches on the skin. They may appear suddenly and disappear after a few hours, or they may last for days (erythema).

*Eczema:* The skin is covered with tiny blisters that itch and ooze secretions, which usually appear in the folds of the neck, the elbows, and the knees. In chronic eczema, the skin becomes scaly and thickened.

*Poison ivy:* This is a contact allergy. The oils of the plant get on the skin and cause itching, redness, and blisters.

*Gastrointestinal allergy:* The patient experiences nausea, vomiting, diarrhea, and abdominal pain and tenderness.

*Angioneurotic edema:* Edema occurs in one part of the body, such as the lips and the eyelids. If the swelling presses on a vital organ, such as the larynx, it could have a dangerous effect on breathing.

*Anaphylactic shock:* This is a dangerous combination of erythema, edema, and contraction of smooth muscles.

*Transplantation of organs:* This elicits a special severe type of allergic reaction to the new organ or tissue and must be treated with very potent immunosuppressive drugs to prevent the body from rejecting the new organ. The same type of allergic response, coupled with a systemic infection, is elicited when a foreign object, such as a sponge, remains in the body after surgery. This is why the "sponge count" is so important and why surgical sponges now have *radiopaque* (x-ray indicator) strips so they may be detected, if a difficulty arises after surgery.

## Treatment of Allergies

Once the offending antigen is identified, treatment can begin. The type of treatment will depend on numerous factors, but generally includes the following:

**Avoidance of the Allergy-Producing Substance.** It is not always easy to avoid an allergen. For instance, while it is no problem to stop eating shrimp, it is more difficult to eliminate white flour from the diet. However, other types of allergens can be avoided. Foam rubber can be substituted for feather pillows, and cosmetics made especially for allergy sufferers are available. Some people are able to go to a pollen-free area during the heavy pollen season.

**Desensitization.** Desensitization consists of giving minute doses of the allergens subcutaneously to the patient. The doses are gradually increased to enable the patient to develop a gradual tolerance to the allergen. Sometimes this treatment eliminates the allergy with the injections being given weekly as long as the season lasts. If the allergy is not a seasonal one, the injections must be continued throughout the year. This treatment is fairly expensive, but it helps a great many people to find relief. Some of the newer preparations act more slowly and gradually so that fewer injections are required.

**Drug Therapy.** Drugs may be given (1) to specifically counteract the allergy or (2) to treat the symptoms of the allergy.

ANTIHISTAMINE THERAPY. Antihistamines are effective in the treatment of allergy because they are thought to inhibit the action of histamine within the body. However, they give only temporary relief and must be continued for the patient to remain free of symptoms. They should not be used for allergies which are not seasonal, since the prolonged use of antihistamines also causes side-effects. These drugs may cause drowsiness, and in asthma, they may dry out the secretions so much that the patient cannot cough up the secretions. The most commonly used antihistamines are Benadryl, Chlor-trimeton, Pyribenzamine, Decapryn, Phenergan (which may also be given for its sedative effects).

DRUGS USED TO TREAT SYMPTOMS. The type of drug used will depend, of course, on the symptoms. Adrenalin may be used to relax muscle spasms, to reduce congestion of bronchial mucosa, to constrict small blood vessels in the skin, or to counteract symptoms of shock.

Cortisone preparations and other anti-inflammatory agents may be given to reduce itching and inflammation in skin lesions. Lung symptoms may be relieved by bronchodilators and expectorants. External medications may be applied to the skin for their cooling, antiseptic effects and to reduce itching and other symptoms.

**General Nursing Care.** The nurse can do several things to make the allergic patient more comfortable while he is in the hospital. Suggestions include: eliminating excessive furniture (especially overstuffed furniture), covering pillows and mattresses with hypoallergenic cases and linens, and using hypoallergenic tape. The patient should avoid cigarette or other smoke and should use unscented hypoallergenic soap, face powder, and cosmetics. Very hot or very cold bath water should also be avoided. The nurse should suggest that the family avoid bringing flowers or foods which are known to cause allergic reactions. The hospital diet can be adjusted accordingly.

It is very important that the nurse report any allergies which the patient describes or exhibits. It is imperative that any drug allergies be noted in large letters on the front of the chart when the patient is admitted so that he will not be given one of these drugs by mistake.

The patient who is extremely allergic *must* wear an identifying tag so the hospital personnel will know instantly what is wrong. Immediate action must be taken to prevent irreversible damage to tissues and to prevent death.

The practical nurse must be aware that a person can be allergic to anything. Thus, allergic reactions may occur as possible side-effects when *any drug or immunization* is administered. While the effects will show up faster and more dramatically after a parenteral drug is given, they may also result from oral medications or foods. *No* large dose of penicillin or any other drug should be given without first making sure that the patient is not allergic to it. If there is any doubt, or if the patient has a history of allergies or asthma, a skin test (intradermal) should be given first. Even then, the nurse must be prepared to deal with possible anaphylactic shock.

## Drug Allergy

Drug allergy is common, especially for such drugs as penicillin, quinine, and Thiouracil. Aspirin, too may cause allergic reactions in some people. Symptoms of drug reaction may include urticaria, asthmatic breathing, gastrointestinal upsets, and anaphylactic shock. It takes only a small amount of the drug, to which a patient is sensitive, to cause an allergic reaction; this is quite a different matter from an overdose of a drug. A patient with an allergy is frequently given a small dose of a new drug first, in order to test his sensitivity to it. An allergic reaction may appear either immediately or some time later. Pay attention if a patient tells you that he is allergic to something. If he says he cannot take aspirin, do not force him to take it, even though it has been ordered. Instead, report the incident to the charge nurse.

## Bronchial Asthma

Bronchial asthma is a condition characterized by recurring paroxysms of dyspnea of the wheezing type, due to a narrowing of the lumen of the smaller bronchi and bronchioles. It is associated with an allergic reaction in the bronchioles. The *etiology* (origin) is unknown, but there seems to be an inherited allergic constitution and some relation to emotional upsets.

*Symptoms:* Symptoms include periods of dyspnea, a sense of tightness in the chest, wheezing, cough, tenacious sputum, cyanosis, and perspiration. 

*Treatment and Nursing Care:* Drug treatment is symptomatic and consists of adrenalin, aminophylline, expectorants, sedatives, and cortisone. Morphine is *contraindicated,* because it depresses respirations.

Nursing care includes IPPB treatments to assist in breathing, moist, warm humidity to liquify secretions, orthopneic positioning, and a calm, quiet atmosphere to reduce anxiety and stimulation. The asthmatic person should not eat heavy meals or drink carbonated beverages. He should be encouraged to walk slowly and not to overexert himself,

in order to avoid fatigue. After discharge, he should avoid overexposure to cold and may have to wear a face mask in extremely cold weather.

## Anaphylactic Shock (Serum Accident)

This is a sudden and severe allergic reaction perhaps to a drug, a foreign substance, a bee sting, or an animal serum. The patient first feels apprehensive and as though he is choking. He may then develop a rash; his blood pressure falls sharply, his pulse is rapid and weak, he perspires, he turns pale and feels faint, his pupils become dilated, and he may have convulsions and become unconscious. Symptoms of shock may appear quickly in severe asthma, urticaria, or vomiting and diarrhea when the patient has had a large dose of the substance causing his allergy, or after a small dose of an allergen to which he is sensitive.

This is what happens: the amount of circulating blood is decreased (*circulatory collapse*). Therefore, the heart cannot get enough oxygen to the tissues, and the patient may die because of the insufficient blood supply to the heart and the brain.

The usual first-aid treatment for shock is given; the doctor will hasten to give treatment to restore the volume of the circulating blood and to restore a normal blood pressure.

In very severe cases of anaphylactic shock, emergency treatment is essential to prevent death, which may occur in 5 to 10 minutes. Emergency treatment consists of:

*Opening the airway:* A tracheostomy or endotracheal tube may need to be inserted. Oxygen should be administered and excess mucus suctioned out.

*Supporting the circulation:* An intravenous infusion will be started, and plasma may be given. Vasopressors, such as Aramine or Levophed, may be given.

*Giving adrenalin:* This acts as a specific antidote. It is given intravenously in extreme emergency.

*Giving antihistamines:* Antihistamines are given to offset the antibody formation.

*Giving corticosteroids:* These are given to offset the inflammatory response after the emergency is over.

# Unit 11:
# Special Needs of the Aging Person

*55.   The Geriatric Patient*

# 55

# The Geriatric Patient

BEHAVIORAL OBJECTIVES

*The student successfully attaining the goals of this chapter will be able to:*

- *discuss the general concept of growing older and some of the emotional and physical implications which might affect nursing care.*
- *discuss special needs of the older person, including those related to nutrition, elimination, personal hygiene, safety, communication, and exercise; and describe ways in which the nurse can assist in meeting these needs.*
- *discuss the special emotional aspects of growing older; and identify ways in which the nurse might assist the older person to meet these special emotional needs.*
- *identify at least one local community resource designed to assist the older person; and discuss characteristics of a good nursing home or extended care facility.*
- *safely and compassionately assist the older person to meet his basic needs and to meet special needs due to his physical or emotional condition.*

Growing old can be rewarding or it can be a very frustrating and unhappy experience. Too often the older person feels useless and rejected because he is no longer earning money or because he is no longer needed by his family. As a result he is often lonely and afraid. Many psychiatrists believe that the greatest problem facing the aged is isolation from other people. Therefore, it is important that a person maintain his personal contacts and continue his life activities as he grows older.

Tantamount to this is the importance of developing many interests and hobbies while young in order to carry on with them later in life. It is this sense of continuity which seems to make it easier for a woman to adjust to growing older, although she may be faced with "the empty-nest syndrome" after her family has grown. For a man, adjustment is not so easy. He will most likely retire from his job and will need to have stimulating interests to occupy his spare time.

The proportion of older people in our country is increasing greatly. At this time, about 15 per cent of our total population is over the age of 65. In many instances, we have become a 4-generation society, so that a tremendous generation gap exists between the youngest and the oldest members of a family. At the same time, many families have found it impossible to keep the older person in the home. More than ever before, people are moving to retirement centers and nursing homes where practical nurses are needed to staff the facilities.

## The Aging Process

What is the aging process? It is a general slowing down of many body processes which affect hearing, vision, and other body functions.

In the words of one 94-year-old lady, "It seems to me they make the stairs steeper than they used to. They are using smaller print in newspapers and everyone speaks in a lower voice than when I was younger. I ran into an old friend the other day and she had changed so much, she didn't even know me. I don't know about all the other old ladies in this place, they are all so forgetful and crabby. I hope I don't ever get old like that."

Age is a relative sort of thing. Everyone feels that he or she is not getting old, but everyone else is. As one person put it, "Middle age is 10 years older than you are at the time."

The study of the aging process and the care of the aged is called *geriatrics*. Since you will meet many older people in the hospital, in the nursing home, and in your daily life, it is hoped that this chapter will give you some guidelines as to how you can assist the older person to meet his daily needs and face each day with new and renewed hope and enjoyment of life. While many of these suggestions cannot be carried out in the general hospital, the nurse should attempt to do as much as possible for the older person. (See Chapter 56 for a discussion of the disturbed senile patient.)

# SPECIAL NEEDS OF THE OLDER PERSON

## Nutrition

It is important for the older person to maintain a satisfactory nutritional status in order to prevent other body systems from breaking down. Often, the older person is not hungry, because he is not very active physically, or he finds it inconvenient to cook for himself, if he lives alone. While the nurse should encourage the patient to eat, she should not try to force him. He might be inclined to eat more if he is served the kinds of foods he likes and then is given some assistance. However, it is important to remember to let him do as much for himself as he can, no matter how long it takes.

**Teeth and Chewing.** Because many older people wear dentures or have no teeth at all, their food must be adapted so that they can chew and eat it. Yet at the same time, it must be nutritionally balanced. If the patient is reluctant to eat because of chewing problems, it may be helpful to serve his meals as attrac-

tively as possible so that he will want to eat.

**Swallowing Difficulties.** The nurse must be very careful to prevent the patient from aspirating his food or medicine. Be sure that the food is of a consistency which can be swallowed and then assist the patient to concentrate upon swallowing, so that he does not choke. It may be necessary to suction the patient, if he does choke. Usually the patient who has difficulty in swallowing is fed liquids, perhaps by syringe or by tube.

**Tube Feedings.** Since it is important that the patient receive the proper nourishment, tube feedings may be necessary. An accurate record of the intake and output of food and fluids may also be necessary to make sure the patient is receiving enough nourishment.

**Intravenous Therapy.** Although the patient may be given intravenous feedings for a short period of time, this method of feeding is not satisfactory over a long period of time.

**Vitamin and Mineral Supplements.** Many older people need to take vitamins and minerals to supplement their daily food intake and to maintain their body systems and their acid-base balance. The most usual vitamin is a general multivitamin tablet taken once a day. If other types of supplements are prescribed, the nurse must remember to assist the patient to take the medicine, perhaps by crushing tablets or by putting medicine into jelly to make the taste less disagreeable. If injections are given to the older person, the size of the person must be taken into consideration when selecting the size of the needle and the site of injection.

## Elimination

Frequently older people are preoccupied with their bowel function and need to be reassured that a daily bowel movement is not necessary if, for example, they have not been eating very much. If a patient needs help in eliminating wastes, the nurse should assist without making it seem like a very important event.

**Constipation.** Many older people need a stimulus to keep their bowels moving adequately. Often, bran flakes or prune juice is all that is needed. However, sometimes a laxative or stool softener may be required.

Unfortunately, many people become accustomed to taking a laxative daily and cannot do without it. To reduce this dependency, the patient should be encouraged to exercise regularly, to eat fruits and vegetables, and to drink plenty of water. This regimen will encourage regular and comfortable elimination.

**Bladder and Bowel Incontinence.** Older people frequently have difficulty in controlling their bladder or bowels. To overcome this problem, they can be retrained by following a regular schedule or by manually expressing the urine at designated times.

A bladder or bowel retraining program is accepted eagerly by almost any patient because he is usually embarrassed and ashamed by incontinence. At first the interval between trips to the bathroom or the time when he is given the urinal or bedpan is short and is then gradually lengthened. Within a few days, the patient will begin to feel the stimulus to go to the bathroom and will be able to make his needs known to you. You should heed this request as quickly as possible, so that he does not have an accident.

If the patient does soil himself, he should be cleaned up as quickly as possible and with as little fuss as possible, so that he can maintain his dignity and self-respect. He is very likely to be embarrassed and does not need to be reminded or scolded for his accident.

Catheters are not used, unless medically ordered for another reason. Occasionally, a vaginal prosthesis is inserted to assist with urinary control. The plastic prosthesis fits into the vagina and has a balloon which presses against the symphysis pubis and controls the leakage of urine. This simulates sphincter control in the patient with weak sphincter muscles.

Almost every patient can be retrained with effort and understanding on the part of the nursing staff. Although it takes time and patience, it pays off in nursing time and, most important, in the increased sense of self-esteem and worthwhileness felt by the patient.

## General Personal Hygiene

The patient should be encouraged to maintain personal hygiene, so that he or she will feel more presentable. Good hygiene is also important to prevent deformities or diseases from occurring.

**Special Skin Care.** The older patient often is more subject to skin breakdown than the younger person. Especially in the case of incontinence, it is vital to keep the patient clean and dry to prevent skin breakdown. It is also important to rub the skin with lotion to keep it soft and to restore circulation and to change the patient's position frequently.

**Oral Hygiene.** The patient must be encouraged to care for his mouth to prevent bad breath and dental difficulties. Sometimes, the nurse must assist with this care.

**Care of the Hair.** Although it is often difficult to shampoo the hair of an older woman, it must be done for reasons of cleanliness. In addition, a fresh hairdo will make the patient have positive feelings about herself. A trip to the beauty parlor is a great way to increase the patient's feeling of self-worth.

**Care of the Nails.** The fingernails and toenails of the older person are often hard and brittle and can become very difficult to care for. They should be soaked and then cut with a blunt scissor, although special care must be taken not to cut the patient. The nails should be cut straight across to prevent ingrown toenails. Sometimes, the nails become so hard and thick that they must be surgically removed.

**Clothing.** The nursing home resident should be allowed to wear his or her own clothing, if possible. Encourage the patient to look as nice as possible and compliment her when she is dressed up. A new dress once in a while can do a great deal for the morale.

## Safety

The older person may be unsteady on his feet or may use poor judgment as to what he can or cannot do safely. The nurse is responsible for making sure that the person is protected and does not become injured.

**Restraints and Bed Rails.** Do not restrain the patient unless it is absolutely necessary. Frequently a patient will fight to get out of the restraint and injure himself. However, the older person should be restrained while sitting up in a wheelchair or a regular chair, if their is any danger that he may fall out or try to get up without assistance. The restraint should be made as inconspicuous as possible, hidden under clothing or disguised, so the patient will not feel so "tied down."

Side rails should be up on the beds of an older patient at night, because he is more likely to become confused when it is dark. The patient should be instructed to ask for help if he wishes to get up to go to the bathroom. Some patients will need side rails all the time. Be sure that the patient does not endanger himself by trying to climb over the rails. Be sure all beds are in the low position when the patient is left alone, day or night.

**Adaptive Devices for Tub or Toilet.** The hospital or nursing home should be equipped with hand bars and rails to assist the patient in getting in and out of the bathtub or on and off the toilet. An antislip substance must be put into the bottom of bathtub or showers. The patient should not be allowed to shower or go to the bathroom alone, unless you are absolutely sure it is safe for him to do so. A patient lift may also be used to assist the patient into the tub.

## Communication

Many older people have difficulty in communicating because of failing sensory systems. However, they should be encouraged to communicate in any way that they can so that they won't feel isolated or rejected.

**Hearing Loss.** The patient who is hard of hearing should be fitted with a hearing aid, if at all possible. Since he may be reluctant to wear his hearing aid, the nurse should encourage him in a kind and gentle way. Special devices can be obtained for telephones or the television set to enable the hard-of-hearing person to hear better.

If the patient is unable to hear at all, he should be given an opportunity to write notes, so that he can still communicate.

**Aphasia.** A loss of speech often accompanies a stroke, a common affliction of older age. As indicated in a previous chapter, the nurse should remember to converse with the patient even if he is unable to speak. She should encourage him to communicate in other ways and to take part in a speech retraining program.

**Vision Impairment.** Although many older persons have difficulty in seeing because of cataracts or other eye disorders, they should be encouraged to participate in the things which they can do. To further facilitate matters, larger numbers can be placed on the telephone and the calendar and magnifying glasses made available for reading. For added diversion, these patients should be encouraged to listen to the radio or to communicate with other patients, even though their vision is failing.

These patients must be protected from falling, because they may not realize that they cannot see very well. They can be taught what dangers exist and how to avoid or deal with these situations.

## Physical Activity and Exercise

Physical rehabilitation is a very important part of the total health program for the elderly because it is vital to keep moving and exercising to maintain circulation, muscle tone, and general health, as well as to prevent deformities which may occur from disuse.

**Range of Motion Exercises.** The patient should be put through passive range of motion exercises, if needed. Active exercises should be instituted as soon as possible. If active exercise is not possible, the passive motion exercises must be continued to prevent deformities.

The patient should be encouraged to walk or to sit up in the chair as much as possible. No patient should be allowed to lie in bed day after day. The more activity the patient has, the more normal he will feel, which is the goal of all rehabilitation. If there is danger of accidents, the nurse should help the patient to move or walk.

## Emotional Support and Mental Stimulation

Psychological and mental rehabilitation is just as important as physical rehabilitation. The patient needs to be encouraged to become self-sufficient and mentally active. He also needs to be encouraged to participate in the activities around him. His mind must be kept active or he will disintegrate to a true senile state, marked by boredom and hopelessness.

**Remotivation Technics.** The remotivation technic is an important adjunct to therapy in the nursing home because it attempts to bring the patient back into the realm of reality as much as possible. It has proven very effective in nursing home care and has provided many patients with years of productivity and increased self-esteem, which they would otherwise have lost.

**Recreation.** Recreation programs are so important in a nursing home that there may be a recreation director or occupational or recreation therapist to plan or direct activities. If not, the nursing staff must assume the responsibility of giving the residents something interesting to do. Recreation not only occupies the patient's time, it also boosts his morale and gives him an opportunity to meet other people and make friends.

**Self-Esteem.** The recreational and social activities for residents of nursing homes need not be social events exclusively. Many residents are asking for educational programs, college courses, and other activities. This not only stimulates their minds and bodies, but it provides a means of maintaining dignity and personal self-worth. When the person begins to feel worthless, he begins to disintegrate in other ways.

**Social Life and Activities.** The patient should be encouraged to carry on a normal social life and to engage in as many of his previous activities as possible. The resident should be encouraged to visit home as often as possible, to attend ball games, and to go bowling, golfing, or shopping. The family should be included in the care plan and should be encouraged to visit and to take the older person with them on trips and outings. The older person loves to see his grandchildren or other young people. The student nurses are likely to be the favorite people in the nursing home. Enjoy these older people; they have a great deal to teach and to offer to you.

**Religious Support.** The patient should be encouraged to carry on his religious preferences as much as he can. Try to get him to church and be sure to allow him privacy when his clergyman comes to call on him. If religious services are conducted in the nursing home, the residents should be encouraged to attend if they can. If they cannot go in person, tape record the service or make other arrangements so that they can participate in their room.

**Confusion.** Older people frequently become confused. Sometimes, this confusion is general; sometimes, it concerns just one thing. When dealing with this kind of patient, the nurse should remember to be as explicit as possible and to try to make the patient understand what is going on, so that he will not become apprehensive. (See Chapter 56 for a more detailed discussion.)

**Senility.** The true senile state may be caused by lack of blood supply to the brain, although this can often be offset by specific medications. The true senile state is characterized by depression and feelings of worthlessness, hopelessness, insecurity, and fear. The patient often becomes very tired and bored and does not seem to care about anything. Eventually, he can lose contact with reality and can regress into infantile behavior. This process must be stopped as soon as possible and is often reversible, if treated energetically and with kindness and patience. Remotivation technics can play a big part in reversing this process. One source describes senility as the "period from birth to puberty in reverse." (See Chapter 56 for a further discussion of the acutely senile person and his nursing care.)

## COMMUNITY AGENCIES

There are many community agencies which are set up to assist the senior citizen meet the special demands of his life. Since the senior citizen club offers a good opportunity to meet other people and to take part in activities, such as concerts and trips, the older person should be encouraged to take part in these clubs. The practical nurse, as a member of the community, should be willing to give assistance to these clubs as a volunteer.

### Volunteers

Most nursing homes have a corps of volunteers, who help in the activity program of the agency. Since the nursing home cannot exist without the assistance of these volunteers, the nurse should encourage their activity. They provide many services, such as visiting patients who do not have visitors, taking residents on outings, helping with crafts and activities, providing parties and entertainment for the residents, and assisting with reading or writing letters.

Often, church groups or service clubs will take on a nursing home as a special project. The nurse should encourage this activity if she has a chance. Since the nursing home resident especially enjoys the company of younger people, the nurse should encourage high school groups to assist in the home's activities. This is not only good for the nursing home residents, but is also a rewarding experience for the students who participate.

Someone should work with the volunteers to make sure that they are helping and not disturbing the patient. They must be encouraged to keep confidences and to treat the patients with respect and dignity. If they promise to come on a certain day, it is important that they do so, because the resident will be very upset if they do not come, as promised. They should be taught to have *empathy* and not sympathy for the patients and to *help* the residents to do things, rather than to do things for the residents.

The nurse can make the volunteers feel welcome in the nursing home and should encourage their continued enthusiasm and support.

## THE NURSING HOME OR EXTENDED CARE FACILITY

### What are the Characteristics of a Good Nursing Home or Extended Care Facility?

The nursing home should provide the best possible nursing care in as homelike an atmosphere as possible. Nursing homes offer 3 general types of care:

1. *Residential care:* The patient is on his own, except that room and board, laundry, and some personal services are provided.

2. *Personal care:* The patient is given assistance in the activities of daily living, such as walking, getting to the bathroom, dressing, and being served a special diet.

3. *Nursing care or skilled-care home:* This type of home offers the care of a nurse who is able to give injections, treatments, and other procedures which are ordered by the physician. The extended care facility usually falls into this category.

Another type of residence is an apartment complex, purposely built for elderly people. However, they are not nursing homes and generally do not provide any services. The rent is usually quite low and the older person has the advantage of being near other people of his age group. Occasionally, a dining room or laundry service is provided.

A good nursing home is (1) licensed by the state or local agency, (2) is under the care of a physician who can be called in case of emergency, (3) has adequate nursing staff (licensed), (4) provides other services such as dental care, eye examinations, and beauty shop or barber services, (5) provides rehabilitation by trained personnel, (6) has an inservice program for new and continuing staff members, (7) maintains high standards of safety for the patients, (8) provides adequate food to the patients and special diets if needed, and (9) provides as homelike an atmosphere as possible. You can tell a great deal about a home by visiting and talking with some of the staff and residents. An attitude which fosters *rehabilitation* is most important.

### The Practical Nurse and the Nursing Home

Many practical nurses are employed in nursing homes. In some instances a practical nurse may be in charge of a floor or of the entire home. However, if you are offered such a post, be sure that you receive adequate instruction before undertaking the task.

The nursing home situation can be a very rewarding, challenging, and maturing experience for the practical nurse. Here, she will have an opportunity to put to use all of her nursing and rehabilitative skills, as well as all the skills of interpersonal relationships which she has learned during her practical nursing program.

# Unit 12:
## Assisting the Patient Who is Experiencing a Psychological Disorder

56. *The Person With a Psychiatric Problem*
57. *Drug Misuse*

# The Person With a Psychiatric Problem

## BEHAVIORAL OBJECTIVES

*The student successfully attaining the goals of this chapter will be able to:*

- *discuss the concept of mental health; describe ways in which a person may deviate from this totally healthy status.*
- *discuss the roles of various members of the health team in assisting the person with a psychiatric disorder; demonstrate competence in carrying out the role of the practical nurse in the clinical setting.*
- *thoroughly discuss the nurse-patient relationship as it relates to assisting any patient, including the patient in a psychiatric setting; demonstrate competence in these interpersonal skills in everyday life, as well as in the hospital.*
- *identify 6 general types of behavior and the best approach to each type of behavior.*
- *identify and describe at least 10 types of ward behavior which should be observed in relationship to the mental and emotional status of any patient, especially the patient in a psychiatric setting; demonstrate the ability to correctly observe and report such behaviors, utilizing the appropriate psychiatric-related medical terminology.*
- *assist the family of the hospitalized psychiatric patient to visit so that the visit is safe and therapeutic for the patient.*
- *assist the patient so that he does not injure himself or others, utilizing only as much restraint or protection as is absolutely necessary.*
- *assist with various therapies, such as recreation, occupational therapy, and psychotherapy, maintaining the appropriate role of the nurse, in a way which is most helpful to the patient.*
- *discuss at least 6 specific types of therapy used to assist patients with psychiatric disorders, including drug therapy.*
- *discuss the best ways to deal with specific behaviors such as suicidal behavior, the overactive or underactive person, and the hostile, confused, or regressed person; and demonstrate effectiveness in dealing with these behavior types in the clinical area, whether in the general or psychiatric area of the hospital.*
- *discuss the special needs of the person who is becoming senile; discuss the causes and treatment for senility; and demonstrate the ability to assist this person to meet his basic and special needs.*
- *discuss the rehabilitation of the person who has a psychiatric problem; identify community resources available to assist this person; and demonstrate effectiveness in assisting this patient and his family to seek the appropriate kind of assistance in the community or in the hospital.*

The principles of psychiatric nursing apply to the care of any patient. There are psychological aspects inherent in all illnesses, and all patients have emotional needs which must be met. Many patients with other illnesses also have psychiatric problems, and often these problems interfere with their recovery. A psychiatric problem does not necessarily mean that a patient is mentally ill to the extent that he needs care in a mental hospital. However, it may mean that his feelings and behavior are having a serious effect on his progress. If his attempts to handle his problems result in erratic or dangerous behavior, he is mentally ill.

## What is Mental Health?

In order to help the patient with a psychological problem, the nurse must first understand what mental health is. There are many definitions of mental health. Simple definitions are offered by the World Health Organization, which defines mental health as a state of physical and mental well-being, or by Glasser who defines the mentally healthy person as one who is "responsible." A more complex definition states that the mentally healthy person is able to adjust to new situations and can handle personal problems without severe discomfort, yet still have enough energy left to be a constructive member of society. Mabyl K. Johnston (*Mental Health and Mental Illness*) feels that the mentally healthy person must have intellectual insight into his strengths and weaknesses and must be able to live comfortably with those weaknesses and use the strengths constructively. In somewhat the same fashion, Lorraine Bradt Dennis in *Psychology of Human Behavior for Nurses* notes that a mentally healthy person must be able to accept frustration without resorting to harmful defense mechanisms and should be able to use life's problems to attain greater wisdom. Thus mental health is not a final state of being but a continuous process.

## What is Mental Illness?

Mental illness is a difference in degree of behavior, rather than a distinct difference in behavior. We all have some neurotic manner-isms or behaviors which we must learn to control or deal with. The person who is hospitalized because he deviates markedly from the cultural norm should be helped to master his emotions so that he can behave in a socially acceptable and safe way and function effectively outside the hospital situation.

**Signs of Mental Illness.** In certain instances, the following behavior patterns may be interpreted as symptoms of mental illness: a sudden change in behavior such as undue depression or inappropriate overexcitement, a sudden lack of concern about appearance, physical symptoms without any apparent medically related cause, or dependency on drugs or other medications. Of course any morbid talk of death or suicide is a cry for help and should be heeded.

**Minor and Major Mental Illnesses.** The degree of mental illness may vary considerably. Some of the minor abnormalities which do not completely incapacitate a patient are classified as *psychoneuroses,* or, simply, *neuroses,* the symptoms of which seem to be connected with anxiety. Psychoneuroses should be recognized as real illnesses because the patient suffers keenly from them. Many times the psychoneurotic patient remains in society without displaying marked personality changes. For example, people suffering from hysteria, compulsions, unreasonable fears, and hypochondriasis (a condition of extreme worry and concern about health) are frequently not in mental hospitals.

Marked deviations from normal behavior and seriously irregular conduct usually signify a *psychosis.* The psychotic person lacks insight and is unable to "see into himself." He has poor contact with reality and frequently is disoriented (does not identify the time, the place, or the people around him). His behavior is strange, and his thinking is disturbed. Psychoses can result from a physical cause, such as syphilis, brain tumors, or infection, or they may be functional disorders (maladjusted personalities which show no sign of tissue changes or disease). *Schizophrenia* and *manic depressive* psychoses are 2 major disorders of the latter type.

Toxic psychoses include alcoholism and certain stages of drug addiction. Also, a large group of people become mentally ill during the *involutional* period (those series of changes which take place during the menopause). This illness is sometimes spoken of as "agitated depression" or *involutional melancholia*. *Paranoia* is another psychosis; it is characterized by a system of well-organized delusions or false beliefs about persecution and grandeur. It can be a serious social problem, since paranoiacs may become quite dangerous.

## The Doctor's Responsibility

The psychiatrist is the doctor with special training in the treatment of mental disorders. However, every doctor has to consider the mental difficulties of his patients, as well as the physical ones. These difficulties may arise from a patient's everyday problems or from conditions around him which affect many other people, too—floods, hurricanes, plane and train disasters, fires, or wars. In a war, doctors are responsible for the selection of men for the armed services. They must decide on a man's physical fitness to serve; they also must decide on his ability to stand the emotional strains of training and combat. They must treat the mental disorders which develop as a result of training or war experiences.

## The Role of the Practical Nurse

The practical nurse functions as a member of the total psychiatric team in creating a therapeutic environment intended to help the patient return to as normal function as possible in the shortest time.

The special nursing skills required in a psychiatric setting include observing the patient's behavior as well as his physical symptoms, establishing rapport with the patient, giving emotional support, and dealing with specific types of behaviors exhibited by the patient.

In addition to performing these specialized nursing skills, the nurse also functions as a socializing agent, a counselor, a teacher, and a mother or friend substitute. The key word in all her dealings with the patient is *sensitivity*; she must be sensitive to both the physical and emotional needs of the patient, and she must remember to treat the patient as an individual who is simply coping with life as best he can.

## Changing Attitudes

Not long ago, a patient was sent to a mental hospital only when he was a danger to the community and when the community was no longer a safe place for him. Certainly, a patient who is potentially dangerous to himself and to others must be protected, and responsibility must be taken for him. However, to assume that a mental patient must reach this stage before he can be treated is as old-fashioned as to think that mental illness is a disgrace to be hidden away and denied.

Mental illness gradually is becoming recognized as being like any other illness; patients go to hospitals voluntarily for treatment, just as they might go to a general hospital for an appendectomy. Early hospitalization tends to shorten the illness, by removing the patient from the emotional stress often found in the home. In such instances the hospital provides a more suitable environment for the patient.

In many cases hospitalization is not necessary. A patient with beginning psychiatric difficulties may go to an out-patient clinic for treatment. Some psychiatric hospitals have established a service whereby a patient may spend his nights at the hospital and carry on with his regular job in the daytime. This plan assures him of the treatment he needs and removes him from a possibly disturbing home environment.

Changing attitudes toward mental illness and the discovery of the tranquilizing drugs have encouraged community hospitals to take care of mentally ill patients. These drugs are so effective in quieting agitated or disturbed patients that barred windows and restraining jackets are seldom necessary, and the fears of hospital personnel have largely been eliminated. More and more general hospitals are providing space for the in-patient care of psychiatric patients.

**Emergency Services.** In recent years many hospitals and medical centers in our larger cities have offered a special emergency service to the mentally disturbed. This is the *emergency psychiatric clinic,* which is a part of the hospital's emergency ward with a psychiatrist in charge around the clock. Disturbed people who reach a point where everything is too much for them may come here for help.

They find a sympathetic listener with whom they can discuss their troubles, and they can come back for help as often as they need it. Treatment may include antidepression drugs or a stay in the hospital's psychiatric ward, or periodic return visits to the clinic. The patients pay if they can; if not, the services of the psychiatrist are still available. One hospital reports that three fifths of the patients who come to this service can be taken care of adequately without being hospitalized, which is a great relief for the overcrowded mental hospitals.

The *Home Treatment Service* is another type of emergency service for disturbed people which sends a psychiatrist to the patient at home, giving the psychiatrist the advantage of seeing the patient in his home environment. Modern psychiatry recognizes the importance of working with the family of the mentally disturbed person, since his troubles often stem from his family environment. Home treatment also solves the problem of the patient who refuses to go to a psychiatrist, and it often seems to accomplish more than hospitalization, which many disturbed people fight and fear.

*Telephone services* are also available whereby a patient calls and talks to someone about his problems. If the patient cannot be helped over the phone, hopefully he can be persuaded to come to the hospital for treatment.

## THE HOSPITAL SETTING

### Admission to a Mental Hospital

The terms of admission to a mental hospital vary from state to state and even within a state. Generally speaking, one of 4 methods is followed: (1) voluntary admission, (2) admission on the certification of 2 physicians, (3) temporary care certificates, and (4) court commitments. The people who go into the hospital by voluntary admission often go to a private hospital and pay for their care and treatment. However, there are many state hospitals which admit patients voluntarily, sometimes for special treatment.

### The Patient's Security

The mentally disturbed patient needs a secure environment to protect him from himself, from other patients, and from the outside world. It is the hospital's responsibility to provide this protection, particularly when relatives and friends visit the patient. Often, with the kindest intentions, they will distress the patient by reminding him of things better left undiscussed. For the patient's sake, relatives and other visitors should be permitted to see him only with his consent. He may be uncommunicative, so that his consent cannot be obtained, but if he objects to any visitors, they should not be allowed to see him. The doctor must decide when exceptions should be made.

### Approach to Patients

**The Patient's Good Will.** The significance of the correct approach to patients cannot be overemphasized. This is the foundation on which all the nurse's work will rest. Her success or failure will, in a large measure, depend on her ability to understand how important the correct approach is and to adjust her own behavior accordingly. To be successful with mental or other patients, it is essential to have their good will. This does not mean bribing patients with favors, such as special privileges. The nurse must be kind but firm. A patient may appear to be out of contact, yet he may remember an unkindness, which he will hold against the nurse. This is bad for both the patient and the nurse. A calm, matter-of-fact attitude—friendly but not familiar—is important at all times. A nurse should *never* discuss her personal affairs with patients or have financial dealings with them.

**The Rights of the Mental Patient.** A nurse must realize that, although the patient may be psychotic, he is not necessarily demented; his opinions, wishes, and desires are as important to him as normal desires are to a well person. Even when a patient's expressions seem bizarre and out of harmony with reality, they still have meaning and significance *for him*. A nurse should never laugh at a patient's beliefs—this tends to destroy his confidence in the people who should be his protectors and has a demoralizing effect on other patients as well. She must be tolerant and kind to patients at all times, even in the face of abuse. An irritable or impatient attitude will only provoke the patient and lead to difficulties. A patient's request should be granted whenever possible. In many instances, the patient is a person who previously had attended to his own needs and affairs and may have been in a position to direct others. To go from this state of mind to utter dependence on others requires a considerable adjustment on his part. Everything possible should be done to help the patient to maintain his dignity as an individual during these trying times.

Even though he is not capable of being responsible for himself, a mental patient has certain rights which may not be violated. For instance, he may not be denied the privilege of seeing friends and relatives, except on the order of the doctor. He also has the right to receive all mail addressed to him and a right to send out mail. However, since the patient is not responsible, this must be supervised carefully, to prevent him from violating postal regulations by sending out obscene material, writing threatening letters, and so on. All communications should be reviewed by the doctor in charge or by his appointed representative.

**A Middle Road.** When it is necessary to refuse patients' requests or to control them, the nurse should explain that she is obeying hospital rules, rather than have the patient feel that *she* is trying to rule him. She must never punish the patient in any manner whatsoever or threaten him with punishment. His behavior and ideas must never be ridiculed. Neither should the nurse encourage and foster his peculiar patterns of thought and behavior. To agree with a patient's false beliefs is to reinforce them. It is equally useless to argue with him because it focuses attention on undesirable attitudes. It is better for the nurse to tell the patient that she cannot agree with him and then change the subject. The nurse must try to exercise self-control and always be cheerful. This is not so difficult when she realizes that nothing could be more worthwhile than helping mentally ill people get well or, at least, live more happily.

## The Nurse-Patient Relationship

These are the qualities that a nurse should have to establish a good relationship with any patient:

She should be polite and tactful, qualities which go hand in hand.

She should be skillful in handling situations.

She should be friendly to all patients. A nurse can show a warm feeling that reaches out to the patient and includes politeness, confidence, and institutional hospitality.

She should be truthful, but neither brutally so nor evasive. She demonstrates this by an earnest manner and sincerity.

She should be even-tempered and uncritical. Sometimes this is difficult, but she remembers that the patient is ill.

She should have poise—it gives her confidence in herself and lets the patient have confidence in her.

She should be an interested listener, always a desirable quality.

She should have empathy, which is an essential characteristic of effective interpersonal relationships. It is not enough for her to imagine how she would feel in the patient's situation; she must try to understand how the patient feels.

She should concentrate upon the patient's strengths and not upon his weaknesses.

On the other hand, some of the things that are likely to create an unsatisfactory relationship are:

A superior attitude
Overrating what the patient says
Intimate friendships with patients
Hurried contacts

**Adapting the Approach to the Situation.** The approach to the patient is influenced by the type of mental illness he has:

1. *The Excited Patient:* A quiet atmosphere is important in dealing with a restless person; the quieter the better. Use a calm voice. Avoid long discussions and do not force issues.

2. *The Retarded Patient:* This type of patient should be encouraged to talk. Encourage him to assist about the ward in any way that is possible.

3. *The Preoccupied Patient:* This patient may become annoyed because some pleasant fantasy is interrupted. By suggestion, divert his attention to some desirable action.

4. *The Hypochondriac:* The less you ask this patient about his condition, the better.

Physical complaints must not be disregarded entirely, but they should not be emphasized. Reassure the patient.

5. *The Withdrawn Patient:* Avoid stress and anxiety as much as possible.

6. *The Aggressive Patient:* Protect the patient.

## Observing the Patient

One of the most important roles of the practical nurse in psychiatry is that of observer of the patient's behavior. Observations, which are charted carefully, objectively, and accurately, can be of great help to the therapist working with the patient.

**Ward Observations.** The purpose of the ward observations and notes is to record, from time to time, the condition of the patient. They are mainly descriptions of the patient's conduct and behavior and are made without the patient's knowledge by observing him carefully on the ward. The following outline can be used as a guide:

APPEARANCE. Is the patient neat, clean, and tidy, or dirty and untidy?

SOCIABILITY. Does the patient associate freely with other patients? Or does he keep to himself? Does he associate only with the staff?

BEHAVIOR. Is the patient orderly or disorderly, still or restless, quiet or noisy, friendly or indifferent, interested or disinterested, destructive or violent? How does he spend his time? Is he bedridden? Is his conduct always the same, or does it change at times? Does he obey simple commands? Does he pay attention to what is said to him?

EMOTIONAL REACTION. Notice if and how the patient expresses emotions such as anxiety, depression, fear, suspicion, happiness, sadness, loneliness, and hostility. Is the patient irritable, angry, excited? Does he have sudden impulsive actions, unprovoked outbreaks of excitement, temper tantrums, assaultive tendencies? Is he depressed, distressed, perplexed, uneasy, fearful? Does he appear happy? Are his emotions relatively constant?

SPEECH. Does his speech seem natural or is it flighty, rapid, and disconnected or slow and retarded? Does his speech indicate that he understands what is said to him or what is wanted of him? Are his answers relevant and coherent? Are there any particular speech defects, such as stuttering, lisping, or stammering? Does he talk voluntarily or only when questioned? Does his conversation pass from one subject to another without order or apparent connection? Does he dwell on one subject or always return to the same subject? What does he like to talk about? Do his replies answer the questions asked? Does he repeat set words or phrases, use rhyming words, slang associations, or meaningless word salad sentences, or make new words? Is his language obscene?

NONVERBAL BEHAVIOR. What the patient does not say is often more important than what he does say. Such things as posture, facial expression, and personal hygiene tell you a great deal about the patient and how he views himself and his world. Does he react differently when you are with him as compared to when he does not know he is being observed? How does he react when he sees you or other staff members approaching? Does he have any characteristic and repeated gestures or mannerisms? Does he look at you and others when he is talking or interacting within the group?

BODY COMPLAINTS. Does the patient complain of pains in the stomach, pains and weakness in the legs, suffocation, difficult breathing, nausea, heart trouble, headache or dizziness?

PHYSICAL CONDITION. Note the general physical condition and anything unusual. Physically ill patients will have orders for medication and treatment in addition to other records.

SLEEP. Is the patient's sleep normal or does it appear disturbed? Does he talk or cry out during sleep? Does he walk in his sleep?

APPETITE. Note the patient's attitude toward food. Does he eat willingly or must he be urged and coaxed? Is he spoon-fed or tube-fed? Note any peculiar habits in relation to food or eating.

EXCRETIONS. Observe whether or not the normal functions occur; chart menstruation in female patients of reproductive age.

OTHER OBSERVATIONS. Any unusual occurrences, such as injuries or altercations between patients, should be recorded, with the names of witnesses. Overnight visits and long visits outside of the hospital should also be recorded.

## Observation Skills

1. Some people are naturally observant, but for those who are not, the art of observation can be cultivated.
2. Be alert with all the senses—report with absolute accuracy. It is better to turn in no report than a misleading one.
3. Nothing is too small or unimportant to mention; it may be just the small point or incident which throws light on the patient's behavior.
4. Tell only what you see or hear, without mentioning your own conclusion about it. Put quotation marks around the patient's statements, so the doctor will know it is a direct quote.
5. Do *not* say that the patient has delusions or hallucinations or is confused, excited, or incoherent. *Examples* of the patient's talk and descriptions of his actions and expressions give the information which the people who read the notes will use to judge mental and emotional disturbances.
6. Do not ask the patient leading questions; generally it is better to ask no questions unless the doctor tells you to.
7. It is important to report whether the patient seems to be absorbed in himself or takes no notice of his surroundings, or whether he seems to know what is going on.
8. Record in detail any attempt at self-injury or any accident involving a patient.
9. Choose your words carefully when writing notes.
10. Keep charts locked out of sight of the patients or their visitors.

**Medical Terminology Used in Observation.** The nurse must be aware of certain terms used in psychiatry, so that she can chart accurately.

**Affect:** a person's reaction; his feeling-tone; his prevailing mood.

**Ambivalence:** opposite feelings at the same time: e.g., love and hate.

**Anxiety:** a feeling of tension because of a real or imagined danger.

**Apathy:** state of indifference.

**Autism:** self-preoccupation and loss of interest in surroundings; daydreaming; fantasies.

**Blocking:** a sudden, involuntary stop in the person's train of thought.

**Catatonia, catalepsy (waxy-flexibility):** waxlike posture which is maintained. If the patient is moved from this position, he will maintain the position in which he is placed.

**Compulsion:** an uncontrollable urge to think or act in a certain way.

**Confabulation:** the act of filling in gaps in memory with imaginary statements.

**Delirium:** a state of confusion and disordered speech.

**Delusion:** a false belief, not subject to change by reasoning with the patient.

**Depression:** an uncontrollable feeling of sadness or hopelessness.

**Disorientation:** loss of recognition of time, place, or relationship of self to the environment.

**Euphoria:** an unrealistic sense of well-being.

**Exhibitionism:** exposure of the body or sex organs; the patient often derives erotic pleasure from this.

**Extroversion:** energies directed away from the self to other people.

**Fabrication:** stories or events made up to fill gaps in memory.

**Fantasy:** a product of imagination whether real or unreal, daydreaming.

**Fixation:** arrested development at an earlier emotional stage.

**Flight of ideas:** rapid change from one subject to another without logical sequence or reason.

**Grandeur:** delusions of great wealth, power, or fame.

**Hallucination:** a sensory perception, without a stimulus, which may occur in any of the senses, most commonly visual or auditory.

**Illusion:** misinterpretation of an actual stimuli.

**Insight:** awareness of self and one's problems.

**Introversion:** withdrawn behavior.

**Labile:** subject to rapidly shifting emotions.

**Masochistic:** inflicting pain upon one's self.

**Masturbation:** self-manipulation of one's genitals for sexual satisfaction.

**Narcissism:** love of self, extreme pride in one's body.

**Negativism:** a tendency to respond negatively to any suggestion or idea.

**Neologism:** a new word made up by the patient.

**Obsession:** urge to think thoughts against one's will.

**Phobia:** unreasonable fear of something.

**Regression:** infantile or withdrawn behavior.

**Sadism:** the derivation of pleasure from inflicting pain upon others.

**Suggestible:** easily accepts suggestions from others without any resistance.

**Voyeurism:** erotic satisfaction gained from secretly peeping at others or observing sexual objects.

## Visitors to Patients

**The Family and Friends.** Learning to receive the patient's visitors in an appropriate manner and understanding what to do and what not to do is most important. If a nurse is so unfortunate or tactless as to offend a visitor, she may work ever so hard for the patient's welfare and receive only criticism for her efforts. If, on the other hand, she can gain the relatives' good will and cooperation, it will help her to handle many of the patient's problems. Visitors take up much of the time of hospital personnel, but it is time well spent. The patient's relatives and other visitors are often greatly distressed by the patient's illness. Frequently, they are unable to appreciate his condition. Often they have the idea that mental hospitals are places where people are mistreated; with this prejudice, they are apt to exaggerate little things which otherwise would go unnoticed. Therefore, the nurse must show by word and deed that every possible consideration is being given to the patient. By thoughtful attention to the visitors who come to the hospital, she is establishing the reputation of the hospital in the community. In other words, every nurse is a representative of the hospital; if she has proper pride in her work and loyalty to her institution, she will do the things which will bring credit upon it and her.

**When Visitors Come.** To avoid overwhelming surprise, the patient should be told of the impending visit. He should be clean and neat, with hair combed and nails, teeth, and clothing clean. He should be fully dressed, if possible. Under no circumstances should the nurse give out information about his condition. All requests of this nature should be referred to the physician or the supervisor in charge.

## Preventing Injuries

Although, generally speaking, mental patients are not so dangerous as many people believe, in any hospital there are certain patients who are dangerous. The nurse's duty is to prevent injuries to herself, to other employees, and to other patients. Also, some patients are prone to attempt self-mutilation, such as scratching, biting, or beating themselves. It is difficult for persons unaccustomed to the behavior of mental patients to realize the kinds of things that they will do.

**Violent Patients.** Proper supervision will do much to prevent injuries. If certain patients tend to antagonize others, they should not be permitted to have close contact with other patients. If a patient is violently assaultive, the nurse should not attempt to handle him without sufficient help. Under no circumstances is a nurse to retaliate for any injury she receives. She must always remember that the patients are not responsible for their actions—that she is there as a leader, their protector, as it were, and not to enforce discipline. Patients are to be *helped* with their difficulties, not *punished*.

## Using Restraint

**Present Practice.** The practice of restraining patients has been more prevalent than is generally believed. The latitude in this respect is wide. At present, there are hospitals in America where restraint does not exist—where no mechanical devices for restraining a patient, even to a partial degree, can be found. In other hospitals, wristlets, camisoles (straight-jackets), and other restraining devices are being used. Such conditions need not exist.

**Substitutes for Restraint.** The substitutes for restraint are therapeutic treatments, such as the continuous bath, the wet pack, or seclusion. The last should be used with care, and no patient should be secluded without the written order of the physician. The patient should be observed carefully while in seclusion, and, when his condition permits, he should be released. The room temperature should be comfortable, and there should be fresh air. Patients should be given water to drink frequently while in seclusion. They should have exercise and frequent attention for toileting. The number of hours out of every 24-hour period that a patient spends in seclusion should be noted. The patient is secluded alone—never with another patient. There are hospitals in which the most acute cases are cared for with neither restraint nor seclusion. Where insufficient facilities and personnel make seclusion necessary, it should be carried out with every conscientious consideration for the patient.

**Restraint.** If it becomes necessary to restrain a patient to keep him from removing a dressing or interfering with a surgical treatment, certain precautions should be taken:

1. When restraining the arms and the legs, be very careful not to make the apparatus so tight as to impede the circulation. Stockinet or soft bandage should be used under the restraint to prevent injury.
2. Do not fasten the arms and the legs in an uncomfortable position. Remove the restraint every hour and allow the patient to exercise.
3. If it can be avoided, do not apply a restraint over the chest.
4. Never restrain only one side of the body. Even if it is unnecessary to restrain both hands or both feet, restrain the hand and the foot on the opposite side, too.
5. Frequently feel the pulse of the patient who is struggling against restraint and watch his general condition carefully. Death might result from exhaustion, from the extra work thrown on the heart.
6. Remove any patient in restraint every 2 hours for an alcohol or bathing-solution rub and powder. This reduces fatigue.

## Special Therapies

**Goals of Occupational and Recreational Therapy.** The goal of all therapy is to alter or modify the behavior of the patient so that he will be able to better meet the demands of life. Since the therapist and nurse will follow many of the same technics, the nurse must know what the goal of the therapist is so that the therapy can be continued by the nursing staff. These therapies can be of specific value in dealing with certain types of behaviors:

*The excited or manic patient:* The goal is to set limits for the patient in a consistent manner and to control him so that he does not harm himself or others. He should participate in large muscle activities, such as playing ball, hitting punching bags, and tumbling. He may also enjoy gardening, painting, or dancing. However, since his attention span is likely to be short, he should be able to see fast results.

*The depressed patient:* This patient requires warmth and acceptance, but not pity. He can benefit from routine activities which do not require him to concentrate or make decisions. He may need to work off guilt feelings by doing menial tasks. Whatever task he undertakes, be sure to protect him from injury or suicide attempts.

*The hostile patient:* Accept him as he is and do not argue with him. Set kind and fair limits. He can benefit from destructive activities, such as tearing rags or participating in competitive sports. However, be sure he does not hurt others.

*The withdrawn patient:* Welcome him to the group but do not force him to socialize. Gradually work him into the group. He needs to be stimulated by color or music and should participate in activities in which errors will not be noticeable.

*The paranoid patient:* Allow the patient to progress in the relationship at his own rate of speed. Avoid activities which involve competition with other patients. The patient should be given activities in which his chance of failure is slight. He will benefit from activities in which he can be creative or in which he can gain prestige. In all your dealings with this patient it is important to be honest.

**Hydrotherapy.** Usually, a large mental hospital will have a separate hydrotherapy department. Also, many wards, particularly in the admission and the disturbed services, are provided with continuous baths. Wet packs, both hot and cold, may be given to the patient on the wards or in the home. The effects of hydrotherapy on mental patients may be stimulating, sedative, or tonic.

**Individual and Group Psychotherapy.** Psychotherapy is the process of helping a mentally disturbed person by talking with him and letting him talk and by helping him with and sharing in his activities. Group psychotherapy takes in more than one patient and provides an opportunity for everyone to participate in introducing and discussing individual problems. Thus, the patient comes to know other people, becomes concerned with someone besides himself, and is drawn out of his little private world to become a part of the world around him. This type of therapy, directed by trained people, is helping many patients toward recovery from mental illness.

Psychotherapy depends on the personal relationship between the patient and the therapist. The aim of psychotherapy is to relieve the patient of his symptoms and to eventually free him of the disabling conflicts which caused the symptoms. The treatment encourages the patient to tell his story and to discuss his problems with an impartial adviser. Hypnosis and psychoanalysis are among the methods used to achieve this end.

**Therapeutic Environment (Milieu Therapy).** A *therapeutic environment* is one in which all aspects of the patient's surroundings, physical and social, are designed to promote health and to enable the patient to learn to meet the demands of life in such a way that he can live in the community after discharge from the hospital. The therapeutic environment concept involves forming a community within the hospital to encourage the patients to interact with one another and improve their interpersonal relationships. Hopefully they will gain insight into their actions and change undesirable behavior. The patients form a government and, with the help of the staff, set up rules and regulations. In this way, they are able to test out ways of coping with life outside the walls of the hospital. The therapeutic community can fulfill its therapeutic function only if the patients are encouraged to live in such a way as to prepare them for eventual discharge and life outside the hospital.

**Behavior Modification.** Also know as *operant conditioning* or *behavior shaping,* this technic is being used more and more frequently in dealing with mental patients, as well as retarded children and other types of patients. It is based on the theory that a person will respond to a *positive* reward for a task well done and will want to perform that activity again in order to win another reward. However, to be effective, the task or the behavior expected of the patient must be geared to his ability so that he will be able to succeed and will gain the reward.

The most effective reinforcers or rewards are food or other physical gratification, although almost any other reward can be reinforcing if used correctly. However, it is important to remember that what is rewarding to one patient may not necessarily be rewarding to another.

Negative reinforcement (punishment) is not as effective because it does not tell the patient what you want him to do, just what you want him *not* to do. He then must figure out for himself what is right. Thus, it is much more effective to reward "good" behavior and to ignore "bad" behavior.

When using this method, you should show the patient *what* you want him to do, *help* him to do it, and then *reward* him for a job well done. The reward is most effective if given immediately. Gradually let the patient assume more responsibility for doing the task alone.

**Remotivation Technic.** Many psychiatric units use a special method, called remotivation technic, to reorient the patient to the world of reality. Patients are placed in a group situation which is structured so that they can discuss things which are meaningful to them. Everyone is included in the discussion and all are encouraged to participate. The method and direction of the discussion are based upon the abilities of the group at hand. For example, in a group of severely regressed patients, the discussion would be very simple and the leader would need to ask many questions.

**Reality Therapy.** The goal of reality therapy is to help the patient face reality, reject irresponsible behavior, and learn new and more socially acceptable ways of behaving. Every person has a need to love and be loved and to feel worthwhile as a person to himself (self-esteem) and to others (acceptance). If a person is unable to meet these needs in a socially accepted way, he is considered by others to be irresponsible. Reality therapy attempts to get the patient to meet the demands of life and his individual needs within the framework of reality and within the context of dealing with other people.

Reality therapy does not necessarily accept the traditional approach to mental illness. It differs from conventional psychotherapy by concentrating on the "here and now" rather than on what happened in the patient's past. It contends that it is not as important to know why the patient is doing a certain thing or why he thinks in a certain way; what is important is to help him understand and solve his immediate problems.

The procedures of reality therapy include:

1. The patient must become personally involved with the therapist, so that he can begin to face reality.
2. The therapist must reject the patient's unrealistic behavior, while continuing to accept the patient as a person.
3. The therapist must teach the patient better ways in which to fulfill his needs within the confines of reality.

**Transactional Analysis.** Dr. Eric Berne and others have used this method in attempting to understand day-to-day interactions among people. All interactions between people have meaning and are based on the way the people involved feel at the moment. The goal of transactional analysis is to teach people to react in ways which will involve positive responses in other people instead of hostility.

The basic theory of transactional analysis states that all people react, at different times, as either the *child*, the *parent*, or the *adult*. At any one time, one of the 3 predominates. Two of these, parent and child, are actually from your own past. As parent, you will react as your parents did, and as child, you will react as you did when you were a child. The goal is to act as a reasonable adult in as many situations as possible. The purpose is to make everyone feel "I'm OK, You're OK."

**Shock Therapy.** Several types of shock therapy have been used in the treatment of mental illnesses. The treatment produces a convulsion which in some unexplained way helps the patient to improve. The drug, *metrazol*, can be given intravenously to cause a convulsion. Insulin may also be used for this purpose, although it is rarely used today. The great disadvantage of this therapy is the patient's fear before the treatment and the brief period of intense anxiety and distress between the moment of administration of the drug and the loss of consciousness.

*Electroconvulsive therapy* (also referred to as E.C.T. and electroshock therapy) causes a convulsion by sending an electric current through the brain. It has been used in the treatment of a very wide range of mental illnesses, but present opinion tends to restrict its use to a rather limited group of patients. When successful, this treatment can radically change nursing problems in connection with the patient's behavior.

*Regressive shock therapy* is undertaken with some patients, whereby the patient receives frequent EST treatments, until his behavior regresses to a stage in his emotional development before he began having difficulties. He is then allowed to rebuild his ego, hopefully, without the psychiatric problem. This method must be used in conjunction with active psychotherapy.

**Prefrontal Lobotomy.** Lobotomy is an operation which severs certain association tracts in the frontal lobes of the brain. Ordinarily, it is done only after the patient has failed to respond to other types of treatment. There is no doubt that it lowers tension greatly and makes the patient less difficult to care for. It is used *only* as a last resort.

**Drug Therapy.** The tranquilizing drugs have made a revolutionary change in the treatment of mental illness. These drugs arrest or greatly alleviate many mental disorders to the point where hospitalization is not necessary. The rate of patients discharged from mental hospitals is also greatly increased by their use. Tranquilizing drugs seem to decrease anxiety and disturbed behavior very quickly and make the patient more receptive to psychotherapy (see Chapter 33).

## The Suicidal Patient

From a nursing standpoint, suicide is probably the greatest single problem to handle in caring for mentally ill people. Any mental patient presents a potential risk, but certain types of patients are more likely to attempt suicide than others. Any attempt at suicide should be considered serious—*the nurse must report every attempt, however minor it seems.* Conversations which express the uselessness of life, the desire to die, and similar feelings should be noted on the chart and reported. The approach to this problem is to win the patient's confidence and to keep up a constantly hopeful attitude about his recovery. The method for preventing suicide is that of giving constant, continuous, and effective supervision.

**Attempts at Suicide.** Patients often attempt suicide with articles or material which are forbidden or restricted. Nurses should watch patients very closely while they are working in occupational therapy shops to prevent them from secreting tools, bits of metal and glass, or similar objects. Poisonous medications should also be kept under lock and key. If patients injure themselves or others with such forbidden articles, then there has been a slip in supervision somewhere. However, patients may commit suicide in other ways, such as diving to the floor from a window ledge or ramming the head into a wall. A mental hospital probably has barred windows, but there is no such protection in a general hospital or a home. Newspapers carry accounts every day of people falling or jumping from windows. In most instances, the more desperate and self-destructive type of patient chooses this method, but suicide should have been anticipated in such cases and thereby prevented.

Frequently, patients will plan their suicidal attempts to take advantage of a time when nurses change shifts. The early morning hours are a crucial time for depressed patients because they dread to face another day. Deeply depressed patients may not be alert enough to carry out a suicidal attempt or even to try. However, as they begin to recover and regain their will power, they become alert and may attempt suicide. The depressed patient who is recovering seems so much brighter that he may not be watched as closely. The greatest danger to depressed patients occurs in the early stages of illness and during convalescence. Some of the reasons for suicidal tendencies are:

A feeling on the part of the patient that his illness is a disgrace

Ideas of guilt and unworthiness and imaginary disease

Lingering or malignant disease

An overwhelming sense of failure

Loss of a motivating goal in life—"Nothing to live for"

Impulsive acts to seek attention

### SUICIDE METHODS RESORTED TO BY PATIENTS

1. Cutting arteries with glass or sharp instruments
2. Hanging by sheets, blankets, belts, ties, or other items
3. Standing on high places and falling on the head
4. Banging the head on such things as the floor or furniture
5. Turning chairs over backwards while sitting in them in hopes of breaking the neck
6. Drinking poison from dressing trays, cleaning solutions, or sterilizing solutions, saving up medications and taking them all at once
7. Biting and swallowing thermometers, glass, needles, nails
8. Bribing privileged patients to obtain destructive articles
9. Drowning in the bathtub

### TYPES OF PATIENTS NEEDING CLOSE OBSERVATION

1. New patients
2. Patients who have agitated depressions
3. Depressed patients—especially those going into and coming out of illness
4. Patients suffering from insomnia
5. Acute alcoholic patients
6. Patients with ideas of persecution, of being disgraced, of having an incurable disease; and those responding to nonexistent voices
7. Patients in confused states
8. Patients with sudden impulses—changes in mood
9. Patients undergoing special treatments
10. Hypochondriacs—particularly when they have a fixed idea about one organ or system
11. Patients who have made previous suicidal attempts
12. Patients who talk about suicide and express the wish to die

### PREVENTIVE MEASURES

1. Know where each patient is and what his condition is at all times.
2. Provide a sense of security for the patient.
3. Remove the utensils essential for his plans:
   a. Keep sharp instruments locked in the head nurse's office. They should be accounted for by each shift.
   b. Do not leave bottles or glassware of any sort on wards where there are suicidal patients.
   c. Collect and count all glass and silverware after each meal.
   d. Lock all doors carefully, including such outlets as laundry-chutes, dumbwaiter shafts, and elevators.

e. If some patients are allowed to smoke, make sure they do so under nursing supervision because of the danger of fire.

4. Provide a personal, understanding service which encourages the patient's confidence.

5. When possible, inject doubt into the patient's strange and bizarre ideas, his fears, or his delusions or hallucinations, but do not ridicule the patient or argue with him.

6. Actively suicidal patients should be "specialed" (be given a special nurse who takes care of one patient exclusively) during the full 24 hours of the day.

### TECHNIC OF "SPECIALING" SUICIDAL PATIENTS

This type of specialing is very different from that in a general hospital.

*A patient specialed in a mental hospital is never left alone for one second.*

1. Watch carefully every movement of the patient.
2. Remove from your person and from the patient any article which could be used for self-destruction.
3. Permit no strings, belts, or ties on the patient's clothing.
4. Do not permit the patient to use scissors, needles, or other sharp objects, even while the nurse is standing at his side (except by written order of the physician).
5. Do not leave the patient alone when reporting off duty; wait with the patient until relief arrives.
6. Occupy the patient with suitable games where possible. Encourage the patient to read, but do not read to him. Help the patient to gain a motive for living by interesting him in accomplishing something.
7. Anticipate the patient's behavior by being aware of changes in his mood. Occasionally, patients will pretend improvement to gain an opportunity for suicide.
8. Be sure that the patient receives any prescribed medication intended to help his condition.
9. See if remotivation technics are recommended since they often benefit the suicidal patient.

**Suicide Prevention Centers.** In some of our large cities suicide prevention centers have been established to help disturbed people who contemplate suicide. The person who calls the center to say that he is going to commit suicide can talk to a psychiatrist or other trained person who listens to his story, discusses his situation with him, and tries to persuade him to change his mind or at least to delay acting. Some centers may try to rush a psychiatrist to him to prevent him from carrying out his suicidal threat.

## Overactive Patients

Activity* is a characteristic of all forms of life and is therefore normal for people. However, certain people are by nature more animated and more forceful than others. Just as the degree of activity varies between normal people, so the behavior of mentally disturbed people varies among patients, from the person who is slightly agitated to the one who is in an extreme state of frenzy. Naturally, the nursing care for these 2 types of patients is not the same. Also, marked changes may occur in the same person from time to time, and the nursing care of the individual patient will have to be adjusted to meet them.

**The Hypomaniac Patient.** The person who is only slightly more active than normal falls into the so-called *hypomaniac* group. These patients can be more difficult to care for than the more acutely disturbed patients. Very often they are witty, breezy, and enterprising; because of their keen memory and quick repartee, they are not recognized as being the sick people they really are. This type of patient is also apt to be interfering, domineering, and irritable going quickly from one mood to another. He rarely accepts hospitalization willingly; as a rule, he makes many unreasonable demands. He is continuously busy, and the chief problem in his nursing care is how to use this activity.

The nurse should:

1. Be firm but kind.
2. Avoid familiarity.
3. Avoid arguments.
4. Keep the patient from irritating others.
5. Keep the patient occupied—if he cannot be permitted to participate in occupational activities off the ward, let him have writing or reading material for use in the ward.

This type of patient usually is fond of writing, particularly letters to important people, recording his history, or promoting schemes. This keeps him harmlessly occupied.

Along with this, there usually will be an active program of treatment, such as sedative hydrotherapy. Care should be taken to supply extra nourishment to an overactive patient because of the energy he expends, which consumes extra calories. His appetite is usually good, unless he is extremely overactive.

**The More Disturbed Patient.** Proceeding to the more disturbed patient, his management and nursing care include physical protection of himself and others, whereas, in the less disturbed or hypomaniac type, the patient is more apt to be a nuisance than a real danger. In theory, active patients should be allowed a wide scope of activity to work off this surplus energy. In actual practice, this is not always possible because of limited space and personnel. Therefore, seclusion may be used as a last resort. It should be used only for a stated period on written order from the physician. Under no circumstances should disturbed patients be placed in a mechanical restraint. This aggravates their condition, and they may die of exhaustion in attemptng to free themselves.

USEFUL ACTIVITIES. Every attempt should be made to direct the activities of the overly active patient toward useful ends. Even the most excited cases will sometimes tear rags for rugs. These patients are destructive, and for that reason should have a plain room. This does not mean that the environment is to be stripped of everything but bare walls and floors. Patients should be provided with every possible comfort under the circumstances. They should be bathed frequently, and their toilet habits cared for. Every measure to keep them clothed should be tried, but, if nudity is inevitable, they should not be exposed, in this condition, to other patients. When taken from their rooms, they should be covered by a robe, a sheet, or a blanket.

NURSING CARE. An abundance of fluids should be given, along with an adequate diet. When patients are too disturbed to take proper nourishment, they should be tube-fed or spoon-fed. Care of the mouth and the skin is important. The patient may have injuries, such as abrasions of the skin, which may become infected if not given attention. In general, hydrotherapy is the best treatment for the disturbed patient; it provides an opportunity for a much-needed rest. Warm milk at night may help to produce sleep—insomnia is one of the problems of these patients. They should be kept away from excitement and stimuli. When possible, disturbed patients should be taken for walks or allowed to play outdoor games. Outdoor activities should never be attempted without adequate help. In fact, it is important when giving any treatment to a disturbed patient to have adequate assistance at hand before attempting it.

Precautions for handling disturbed patients:

1. Know your patient.
2. Do not allow the patient to get behind you.
3. Approach a fighting patient from the rear.
4. Use a mattress as a protecting shield if the patient is threatening and has a weapon. In this manner, several nurses can approach safely to disarm him.
5. Never get between 2 disturbed patients to separate them.
6. Take the utmost care not to injure a patient, even so slightly as to inflict a scratch or a bruise.
7. Anticipate what you are going to do.
8. Avoid becoming excited.

Suicide is not so likely to be a problem here except with the so-called agitated type of patient. These patients are constantly in motion, pacing up and down, wringing their hands, picking at their fingernails, pulling their hair, or otherwise engaging in the small-type pattern of activities. They are resistive but rarely assaultive.

## The Hostile Patient

The hostile patient may be a threat to the people around him since he may attack, either verbally or physically. He may argue or be sarcastic, rude, and demanding. He may be physically violent and threaten verbally to injure the nurse or other patients. The first impulse of the nurse, as a person, is to defend herself. However, *the more defensive you are toward the patient, the less helpful you will be to him!* Thus you must control your emotions. A helpful response is one which recognizes the patient's feelings and allows him to discuss his concern. The nurse should not be judgmental or destroy the patient's self-esteem or dignity. Allow the patient to talk, to express his feelings, and to work out his own solutions. Do not tell him how to solve his problems. Rather, assist him to work out his own solutions.

## The Confused Patient

The patient who is confused needs a calm, quiet environment, regulated by routine and free from danger and anxiety. Since he may be disoriented as to time and place, the nurse can help by providing him with a calendar and a clock, so that he will know what month it is and what time it is. As a further reinforcement, you can mark off each day on the calendar and remind the patient about holidays or visiting days. To avoid confusion, speak in clear simple sentences and have the patient repeat if necessary. Question him about what he is saying to be sure of his meaning.

Don't forget that we are all a bit disoriented at times, so do not base all your observations upon one incident.

## Underactive Patients

Underactive patients are of 2 main types: (1) those who are withdrawn from reality and apparently unemotional, and (2) those who are depressed and think and act in a sluggish manner.

**The Withdrawn, Unemotional Patient.** As a rule, the patients in this group appear to be quite happy and content if they are left alone to think at leisure and enjoy their own fantasies. If they are permitted to do this, they will deteriorate to the point of merely existing like vegetables. Therefore, the aim of their nursing care is to hold these patients to reality. Stimulate them to respond to things about them; to take an interest in life. They are rarely suicidal and not usually assaultive; however, these 2 possibilities are to be kept in mind. When either occurs, it is apt to be sudden and without warning—the opposite of the threatening overactive patient.

Matters of the utmost concern to the normal person become completely unimportant to the patient who is no longer interested in the world or in keeping his place in it. He does not care about food, nor does he attend to his toilet habits, so that he frequently soils himself. He is not interested in conversation

with the people about him, although he may talk to imaginary people who are more real to him.

The nursing care varies widely from patient to patient and even with the same patient. However, the nurse should care for the *physical needs* of the withdrawn patient by:

1. Regularly bathing and otherwise keeping the patient clean—that is, keeping his nails cut, his hair combed, and his body clean. A lack of tidiness tends to hasten his disorganization.
2. Seeing that he receives an adequate diet, spoon-feeding him if necessary. If the patient does not eat, the physician should be notified.
3. Having an exercise routine, preferably out-of-doors.
4. Checking on physical functions, defecation, emptying of the bladder, and regularity of menstruation in women patients.
5. Weighing the patient at stated intervals.
6. Having the patient participate in remotivation sessions.

**The Inactive Depressed Patient.** The inactive patient who is depressed has some of the problems mentioned above as well as others. In this case, the main nursing objective is to prevent suicide. This patient requires much more constant observation than the patients previously referred to. As mentioned in relation to suicide, the period when the patient begins to improve but still has periods of returning depression is most dangerous (see page 752). The nursing care is essentially the same for all stuporous patients. Since depressed patients often eat too little, feeding is important, including nourishment between meals and at night.

Because all body processes are slowed up, constipation is a symptom to watch for. These patients should also be observed for symptoms of physical disease, for they rarely complain of pain.

Provide a cheerful, sunny room, but do not put depressed patients with groups of exuberant patients in an effort to cheer them up; this usually has the opposite effect and tends to make them more conscious of their own unhappiness.

Do not force them into activities too rapidly, although occupational therapy is of great value. When it does begin, it should be simple and for brief periods, since these patients tire quickly. As convalescence continues, reading, games, and amusements are helpful. Since indecision is a frequent symptom, the patient should not be asked to make decisions until he is well on the road to recovery. Continuous baths help to relieve tension and to produce sleep.

## The Regressive Patient

Regression is a return to infantile or childish behavior, such as eating with the hands instead of using a spoon or a fork, urinating on the floor, soiling the clothing instead of using the toilet, masturbating, or making homosexual advances to other patients. For some patients, this behavior is an attempt to recapture pleasurable childhood sensations; sometimes it is reviving methods that "worked" in childhood to get what they wanted. Regressive behavior is still another way the patient takes to escape from problems he finds too hard to handle. He disclaims all responsibility for himself by forgetting how to do the ordinary things that he once did automatically and considered acceptable.

It takes infinite patience to begin all over again to teach adult patients toilet habits and how to use a knife, a fork, and a spoon. It takes a great many people to provide enough service to have someone take care of such patients—teaching them proper eating habits at every meal, or taking them to the toilet at regular intervals (24 hours daily) to prevent them from soiling clothing or bedclothes. It takes planning and persistence in the face of the present personnel shortages in our mental hospitals to give this type of care, but we now know it is important and are gradually working toward it.

**Psychological Nursing.** The most important duty of the nurse in relation to the patient's mental state is to get him to focus on reality, to interest him in practical affairs, and to help him to keep in contact with his surroundings. To do this:

Encourage self-respect.

Do not try to show him that he is behaving foolishly; his behavior is more real to him than that of the people about him.

Do not scold the patient if he soils himself or behaves inappropriately. Often these patients are extremely sensitive, in spite of seeming oblivious to everything.

Be patient and kind during all contacts with him.

Occupation is most valuable. Useful work stimulates pride and gives the patient something to hold on to. Avoid stereotyped activities which can be performed without thought on the part of the patient.

Initiate games and participate in them along with the patients.

Use every opportunity to bring the patient into stimulating contact with others.

Strive to gain the confidence of the patient.

Be on the alert for outbursts of violence and suicidal attempts.

If the patient becomes inactive to the point of being stuporous, care for him in bed; also bathe him daily, with particular attention to the skin. Change his position frequently and give special care to proper feeding and elimination.

## Patients in Continued Treatment Services

All mental institutions of the state hospital type have many patients who are classified as being in the continued treatment group. In the main, they are the patients who have passed the acute stages of illness without improvement and are tending to deteriorate. Treatment is continued although there is little hope of recovery. They show a variety of symptoms, ranging from the actively disturbed to the emotionally dull or the bewildered senile cases. Many of them are untidy. Some who have been able to respond fairly well to life within the hospital cannot adjust to the outside world. In recent years more and more of the patients from this group have recovered. However, for those who remain, the problem is to establish a routine for the best possible hospital existence—many of them may remain patients for the rest of their lives.

**Nursing Care.** The program of nursing care should be approached from 3 angles: physical care, habit training, and occupation. Many of these patients will be unable to care for their physical needs, so soiling is one of the greatest problems. Therefore, at regular intervals they should be taken to the toilet. This does not mean that they should be herded into a toilet room and rapidly put through a process with unproductive results. Patients, although deteriorated, should be treated with *respect* and *consideration*. This requires time and personnel, but efforts have proved again and again that it is worthwhile. The entire atmosphere can be changed in this one way alone, besides the fact that odors disappear and linen is saved.

**Keeping Up Morale.** Patients should be bathed regularly, and suitable clothing should be provided. Even the most deteriorated patients often will respond in the most unexpected fashion to a treatment at the beauty parlor and a pretty, bright dress. Disregard for personal appearance hastens disorganization; therefore attention should be given to keeping these patients presentable at all times. Feeding is also a problem. Many eat too much and too rapidly; others take insufficient food. They should have a normal, well-balanced diet, with attention given to their eating habits. Many times, patients are given all of their food on tin plates and are expected to eat with only a spoon or even their fingers. When so little is expected, certainly little will be achieved. Never take it for granted that a patient cannot use a knife or a fork, but try again and again. Success often rewards persistence.

The value of recreation and occupation to this group is incalculable. Certain projects have been tried with whole wards of untidy patients; through simple activities such as walks, games, and crafts, they were kept busy all day, and untidiness disappeared. Such activities also tend to lessen combativeness and destructiveness; tensions are worked off in a healthy manner.

Grooming in general has been mentioned, but the nurse should pay daily attention to caring for the fingernails and the toenails, combing the hair, and brushing the teeth. Patients should be encouraged to do these things for themselves, but the nurse is responsible for seeing that they are done properly; she does them herself if the patient is unable to.

## The Senile Patient

The true senile state is characterized by a feeling of loneliness and rejection. The proponents of reality therapy feel that senility is really the emotional reaction of the older person to the isolation he feels when he is no longer able to get out with other people and when his loved ones die or leave home. He is further bothered by any loss of memory or hearing or control over body functions. Frequently, the senile person becomes apathetic, gives up, and decides that life is no longer worth living.

Chapter 55 discusses in detail the feelings of the older person and how the nurse can be helpful in restoring this person to a useful and active life.

The senile patient may present the same problems associated with many of the previously mentioned patients. However, there are other problems associated with the care of elderly people, such as the prevention of fractures due to falling. Because of physical frailty, older patients frequently have a tendency to seize either the nurse or the furniture when they are lifted or moved; therefore, it is essential to be extremely careful in handling them so that they will not feel rushed or harried. As an added precaution small rugs that may cause them to slip should be removed. Since old people get up frequently during the night, their beds should not be too high and, if possible, should be placed against the wall.

Since change confuses elderly people, they should not be moved from their accustomed place, nor should their possessions be rearranged. The same principle should apply in the assignment of personnel. Insofar as possible, senile patients should have the same nurses regularly. Even when they seem to be entirely out of contact, they often are soothed by a familiar voice or touch. Due to physical handicaps, the senile patient may not be able to do much in the form of occupational therapy. He may, however, enjoy learning new crafts. Occasionally an older patient can do very well at some work which he or she has learned and practiced years ago—knitting, for example. Even if she does it poorly, encourage her to keep on.

In general, the care and the management of the senile patient centers around these points:

*Temperament and Behavior:* The reactions of the senile patient are often unpredictable; these patients are subject to sudden changes in mood, varying from interest and co-operation to apathy or rebellion.

*Diet for Aged Patients:* It is necessary to provide a diet that includes the essential food elements for a person with limited activities and difficulties with chewing, elimination, and similar problems. Frequent light meals and night nourishment are desirable.

*Bathing:* Bathing is important for skin care and cleanliness—senile patients cannot be trusted to bathe themselves adequately and frequently are not able to do so. The nurse can use the bath procedure as a golden opportunity to make observations about the patient. The procedure should be done safely and without chilling the patient.

*Clothing:* Elderly patients need warmer clothing than other people; their garments should be comfortable and not irritating to the skin and should be easy to get into, durable, and easy to keep clean.

*Physical Care:* Adequate daily bowel and bladder elimination must be assured—elderly people are forgetful and may not remember when they last went to the bathroom. Cathartics or enemas may be necessary. Care must be taken to ensure an adequate amount of fluids for these patients.

*Prevention of Injuries:* Elderly people should never be hurried—they move with difficulty and fall easily. Senile patients frequently do not understand directions. They are also likely to stay in one position for long periods of time and may soil their clothing with urine or feces without being aware of or disturbed by their incontinence. Careful and frequent observations will prevent skin irritation. If any type of injury does occur, it should have prompt attention and should be reported at once to the proper authorities.

*Occupation and Exercise:* Most elderly patients have poor eyesight, so special attention must be given to helping them with daily routines and providing diversions which do not require that they use their eyes. They may be feeble, with impaired muscle control, and may tire easily; as a result they are inclined to make little effort. Thus, they should have as much exercise and diversion as possible.

(See Chapter 55 for a further discussion of the elderly person.)

## Convalescent Patients

**When the Patient Goes Home.** It is in the interest of the patient and the hospital to prepare the patient for discharge as soon as possible. Yet, there are certain responsibilities in this respect which the hospital cannot ignore. Both the patient and the community must have reasonable security. No one can be absolutely certain about whether or not a patient will have a relapse, yet everything possible must be done to help his adjustment when he is discharged, to prevent a relapse.

The care and treatment of the convalescent patient should be planned for certain definite purposes. We should think of convalescence as beginning early and encourage the patient to do as many normal things as he can. The keynote, then, is *normal activities leading to normal adjustment.* There may be times when the patient will be irritable and will fail to make progress. However, the nurse should not be discouraged. This is the time when she must endure, persist, and be ready to give reassurance to the patient. A hopeless attitude on her part will be reflected, most surely, in the behavior of the patient.

**The Patient's Feelings.** People often fail to realize how long it takes to recover from mental illness. Often no symptoms are evident, yet this must not be taken to mean that the patient is entirely well. Another important factor is that, while the physician and others who have been caring for the patient are always pleased and happy over his convalescence, to the patient it may be a period of intense suffering, possibly because he realizes what he has been through and sees the problems he faces, coupled with the insecurity that the future holds now that he has been a mental patient. Often this is so thwarting that he is unable to bring himself to face it and therefore continues to seek refuge in the hospital.

**Back to Independence.** Therefore, while the nurse must be sympathetic, she should not be oversolicitous, or else the patient will become too dependent on her as a nurse or upon the institution. From the moment he is admitted to the hospital, the patient should be encouraged to help himself in every way he can; as soon as possible, he should be permitted to resume the direction of his own affairs in accordance with his ability. However, patients should not be permitted to assume burdens that they are unable to carry.

**Community Resources.** There are a great many community resources available to help the person who is discharged from the mental hospital return to as normal a life as possible. It is important for the practical nurse to be aware of these resources, so that she may assist in making proper referrals.

THE DAY CLINIC. Often, the patient will benefit from living at home in the evening and coming into the clinic during the day when his family is working.

THE NIGHT CENTER. Other patients can benefit from going to work during the day, but return to the center at night since they cannot face the realities of living at home.

THE OUTPATIENT OR COMMUNITY MENTAL HEALTH CENTER. Many patients are seen daily, weekly, or less often in the counseling center. Here, they can receive guidance which will assist them to meet the continuing demands of life so that they can function normally on their own the rest of the time.

VOCATIONAL REHABILITATION. It is important for the discharged patient to become as self-supporting as possible. However, he may need to be vocationally retrained, so that he can obtain a job. Many agencies evaluate, train, and find jobs for these people. They may also need to reeducate employers to encourage them to hire people who have been discharged from a mental hospital and to treat them as capable individuals. If the patient is to put his illness behind him, he needs encouragement. To help in this endeavor, the employer should be encouraged to work closely with the vocational rehabilitation counselor.

## THE MENTAL ILLNESS PROBLEM

The awakened interest in the treatment of mental illness has come from the tremendous need to reduce the social and economic waste that it creates. The program starts with pre-

vention. Parents and teachers are informed about child training and learn how to recognize the symptoms of mental distress. Personnel departments in industry help with the adjustment problems of the workers. However, we need more psychiatrists, more professional and practical nurses, better trained psychiatric technicians, and better laws to provide the right kind of protection and care for the mentally ill.

**What is Being Done.** The American Psychiatric Association sets up standards for the care of mental patients and encourages psychiatric training for doctors and nurses. The National Mental Health Act of 1946 authorized the U.S. Public Health Service to set up a National Institute of Mental Health as a training and research center. Funds are available for research and education.

The National Association for Mental Health has been working since 1909 to prevent mental illness, to improve the treatment of mental patients, and to educate the public about mental disorders. On a nationwide basis, state mental health organizations are working to improve and expand care facilities, but these efforts must be doubled to give psychiatric services to the millions who need them.

**Where the Practical Nurse Comes in.** The care of the psychiatric patient provides a challenging opportunity for the practical nurse to use her abilities to the utmost. Because she works closely with the patient day by day, she is his source of stability—she is always there, will always listen, is always kind, does not condemn or punish, but believes in him and gives him hope. It is a rewarding experience to have had a part in his recovery. Special postgraduate training in the care of psychiatric patients is available, but the number of these courses is as yet limited.

Every nurse should know the facts about mental illness because she can use this information to understand the emotional problems of any patient. You will have endless opportunities in any hospital to use your knowledge of mental health and mental illness.

**Arthur James Morgan, M.D.**
*Director of Adult Services*
*Pennsylvania Hospital*
*Community Mental Health Center*
*Philadelphia*

# 57

# Drug Misuse

## BEHAVIORAL OBJECTIVES

*The student successfully attaining the goals of this chapter will be able to:*

- *clearly and precisely use the vocabulary that defines the relationship between a patient and a drug such as "addiction," "habituation," and "tolerance."*

- *discuss the various categories of drugs with respect to the physical dependence they can cause and the legal status of these drugs.*

- *demonstrate a working knowledge of the various drugs of abuse and distinguish the effects they cause, one from the other.*

- *recognize the drugged state and the habituated person in all settings based on the signs and symptoms of alleged drug misuse, differentiating similarly appearing psychotic and neurologic conditions.*

- *show an awareness of the dangers inherent in a general hospital setting for the habituated or addicted person.*

- *discuss the socioeconomic aspects of and the role of the health practitioner in the problems of drug misuse.*

- *demonstrate an understanding of the various treatment modalities that are available in cases of drug misuse and the basic treatment principles underlying them.*

The taking of drugs is presently quite popular, among young and old alike. This is not the first time in history that this phenomenon has happened, and undoubtedly it will not be the last. If present history follows the general trends of the past, we shall shortly go into a phase of "doing things naturally" again. That is, it will become popular to sleep without pills, study without stimulants, lose weight by eating less, and enjoy other people's company without being high.

Because of the growing sophistication of chemistry and pharmacology, however, each time that drugs have their day, they are more powerful and more specific and have greater ability to enhance life, and to diminish it. Also, each time a "drug culture" sweeps the civilized world it leaves behind both human casualties and victims and some residual customs attesting to its having been here.

As nurses you will have to quickly develop a great deal of maturity and wisdom to deal with very difficult problems—problems that involve matters of judgment as you will see.

The knowledge we have about the scientific aspects of nursing in drug misuse is rather clear and easy to learn. It is like a combination of medical-surgical practice and psychiatry. If someone comes into the Emergency Room obtunded from drugs (in a state of blunted alertness, marked by excessive sleepiness and dulled responses to stimuli), it is, of course, more important to establish a clear airway and assure respiratory exchange than to ponder what he took and why. If someone is suspicious, hostile, and feeling persecuted, it doesn't immediately matter whether he got that way from using "speed" or from being schizophrenic. The nursing aspects are essentially the same.

This chapter is not designed to prepare you for such specific tasks as nursing in a Methadone maintenance clinic, or in an alcoholic rehabilitation center, or an acute detoxification unit. These require experiences and information that go beyond the scope of a general textbook. It is designed to help you achieve a mature, thoughtful perspective to the problem of drug misuse, to make you aware of the professional hazards and the social implications of this problem, and to give you the basis for understanding the drug misuse you will undoubtedly encounter early in your nursing experience. Drug misuse is found on every floor of every hospital in every city in the country. The problem is, *it is usually not recognized.*

Let us begin by defining some basic terms. Because of the widespread use of these words, their meanings vary, and it is not always clear what a speaker or writer has in mind when he uses them. Quickly read through the list now, but as you study, feel free to return to it from time to time until the distinctions are quite clear.

**Addiction:** Habitual use of a chemical substance to the extent that *physiologic dependence* is established. The latter manifests itself as withdrawal symptoms (the abstinence syndrome) when the drug is withdrawn.

**Drug:** Any substance which by its chemical nature influences the structure or function of the living organism. Such a definition includes medicine, but it also includes household and industrial chemicals and pollutants. It must obviously also include less exotic substances such as coffee and tea, alcohol and tobacco.

**"Drug Abuse":** This is a popular term that has been so overused that it no longer conveys meaning. As a result, it is not used in this chapter.

**Drug Dependence:** This popular term is defined in the most recent edition of the official nomenclature of the American Psychiatric Association as "evidence of habitual use or a clear sense of need for the drug," including both physical and psychological dependence on drugs and drug addiction.

**Drug Misuse:** The use of any substance which affects mood or behavior to the extent that such use constitutes life-threatening behavior. By this we mean to include any physical, mental, and/or social harm to the *quality of life* of a person.

**Drug Use:** A general term to indicate the use by people of any substance previously defined as a drug. It is the most general term of all and does not distinguish between harmful and unharmful use. It also does not distinguish between prescription use and nonprescription use of drugs.

**Emotional Dependence:** This is the need that a person feels for a drug. This need may coexist with, but is distinct from physical dependence. There are no physical symptoms on withdrawal; however, withdrawal may result in a sense of loss or depression, or agitation, anxiety, and restlessness. An example would be a person, habituated to a large food intake, who decides to "crash diet." He may have many emotional symptoms while dieting, but no physical withdrawal. (See withdrawal symptoms).

**Habituation:** A habit is an acquired mode of behavior that has become more or less involuntary. Habituation to a drug implies an emotional dependence, need, desire, or compulsion to continue its use.

**Narcotic:** Any drug, natural or synthetic, that produces sleep or even stupor, and relieves pain. It is a term of convenience, of custom, and of law which generally refers to opium, cocaine, their derivatives, and the synthetic compounds that produce similar physiological results. It does not include psychostimulants such as Ritalin and amphetamines which have come, however, under the same restrictions as far as control and prescription writing are concerned.

**Narcotic Blockade:** Total or partial inhibition of the so-called euphoria ("high" feeling) produced by the narcotic drugs through the use of other drugs such as Methadone, which can be used as maintenance treatment without producing the peaks of elation, the withdrawal symptoms, and the demand for increasing dosage that characterize addiction to opiates.

**Tolerance:** An increasing resistance to the usual effects of a drug so that the user gradually requires larger doses.

**Withdrawal Symptoms:** The physical and mental effects which a person addicted to a drug experiences when the drug is withdrawn. The physical symptoms may include nausea, vomiting, tremors, abdominal pain, and convulsions. On the other hand, they may be no worse than a bad case of the flu.

Please note that the words "withdrawal" and "dependence" as used in psychiatric nursing have somewhat different meanings than the definitions given above. Withdrawal in psychiatry means pulling back from contact with people or the world

## TABLE 57–1.  COMPARISON OF DRUGS

| Legal Status | Drug Class | Physical Dependence |
|---|---|---|
| Unrestricted, except for age | Alcohol | Severe |
| | Tobacco | Moderate |
| | Caffeine | Mild |
| | Inhalants (airplane glue, gasoline, paint thinner) | None |
| Restricted to medical use (illegal without prescription) | Amphetamines and other psychostimulants ("ups, "speed") | Moderate (?) |
| | Barbiturates and others ("downs") | Severe |
| | Opiate narcotics (e.g., Morphine, Demerol) | Severe |
| | Inhalants (ether, nitrous oxide, amyl nitrate) | None |
| Illegal: importation, sale, possession, and use totally banned | Marijuana (THC) | None |
| | Hallucinogens (LSD, Mescaline) | None |
| | Cocaine | None |
| | Opiate narcotics (heroin) | Severe |

and implies going into one's own self as in a schizophrenic state. Dependence in psychiatry has to do with needs for mothering, love, affection, shelter, protection, security, food, and warmth. When such needs are unmet or are excessive in an adult, dependence may be a manifestation of regression.

People who become dependent on drugs are often manifesting a hidden desire to be psychologically dependent, as defined above.

## Legal Status

We live today on a steep slope of change. There are many inconsistencies in our laws, which require that they be constantly reviewed, lest they become too absurd. Such dangerous substances as tobacco and alcohol are freely available today because they became a part of our culture when drugs were not being scrutinized for their toxicity. We know from bitter experience that the prohibition of culturally accepted items is ineffective.

The lessons learned from the chronic toxicity of alcohol and tobacco are reason enough to slow down on the introduction of additional substances as "recreational chemicals." However, the pharmacologic error of calling marijuana a narcotic and treating it as if it were equivalent to heroin has been a serious mistake. Although the mistake has at last been corrected, the marijuana issue has confused us and has obscured what should have been a more sensible approach to the problem of serious drug misuse. It should be clear that laws and behaviors based upon defective information are themselves dangerous.

Table 57-1 compares legal status, drug class, and physical dependence for a variety of drugs. Be sure to remember that physical *dependence* and physical *damage* are entirely different. For example, amphetamines appear to have only moderate if any physical dependency, but cause considerable physical damage when used chronically. The opiate narcotics, both those that are restricted and those that are totally illegal, carry with them the danger of severe physical dependency; but if used in pure form under sterile conditions they cause relatively little physical harm.

## SPECIFIC DRUGS

### Alcohol

Approximately 100 million Americans (half of the population) ingest alcohol in some form. It is difficult to get statistics on the amount of misuse of this drug, but alcohol is directly involved in the majority of traffic deaths in America each year. It has been around about as long as recorded history in one form or another and is used by many people in many parts of the world as a relaxing beverage, as an aid to socialization, and as a household medicine for the "thousand shocks and heartaches flesh is heir to." However, misuse of alcohol is more common than is generally recognized. The noontime drinking businessman generally concedes that he should drink less but rejects the thought that he is an alcoholic.

Like most other psychiatric illnesses, alcoholism appears to consist of a hereditary predisposition combined with certain developmental experiences that together predispose the person to misuse alcohol and to become dependent upon it. We do not know at the time of this writing what factors constitute the genetic predisposition or what precise environmental factors lead to the development of this condition in one person and not in another, but work is being done in this field and the answer is very close indeed. Very recently it was found that mice could be made alcoholic by infusing a mist of ethyl alcohol into their cages which they would then inhale. Early reports indicate that the mice show much the same type of physical damage and psychological reactions as human beings. Until this break-through, it was very difficult to addict experimental animals to alcohol because its bad smell and taste caused most animals to recoil from it. Perhaps we are now on the verge of finding the biochemical basis for this disease.

It is a well-known fact that liver damage can result from the use of alcohol. Liver function tests are now performed more and more frequently on patients in general hospitals thanks to the use of such systems as SMA-12 (simultaneous multiple analysis), which usually includes several liver function tests. In some otherwise normal patients with no clinical evidence of liver involvement and no history of alcoholism, the values in the liver-sensitive test are mysteriously elevated. Studies underway indicate that many more patients than was previously realized come to the general hospital with their supply of alcohol (such as vodka because it doesn't smell). They may lace their morning orange juice or afternoon tomato juice with it, or just pour it into their water glass and drink it that way. Are such people alcoholic? Should they be treated? Should they at least be put on notice that their liver is not up to par and told by their physician why he expects that this is the case? The answers to these questions are not easy to find, and they are presented only for your thoughtful consideration.

### Tobacco

As early as the 17th century tobacco was described as the "lively image and pattern of hell." A recent statistic reported that 80 million Americans presently smoke cigarettes. Although these smokers would object to being called drugs misusers or drug dependent, there is no question but that they fall into both of these categories. If one is to believe even a portion of the evidence of physical harm caused by the habitual use of tobacco then it clearly follows that its use certainly constitutes life-threatening behavior. The clear sense of need for tobacco which exists among habitual users constitutes psychological dependence. Indeed there is also evidence of physical dependence in the form of withdrawal symptoms (physical) when the heavy use of tobacco is abruptly stopped. In terms of sheer numbers tobacco is clearly the number one drug of habituation in America.

### Caffeine

Caffeine, present in coffee and tea, is used quite widely in America and other parts of the world. Although it is a very mild psychostimulant, only a few persons use so much of it as to be classified as "misusers." It has been called the "think drink," because it tends to increase alertness and mental functioning in general. Too much of it, however, causes the familiar "coffee nerves" or mild agitation and insomnia that many people have experienced from time to time. It is included here primarily because it is a drug, by definition, which most of us use. It is also used medically as caffeine sodium benzoate generally administered parenterally in situations of lethargy and such special conditions as barbiturate overdosage. It should be noted here that the route of administration does not affect the definition of a drug.

## Common Inhalants

The term "common" is applied to this group of inhalants because they are easily accessible to most people, since they include many household substances, and because there is no restriction on their use.

Glue sniffing is one of the most publicized types of inhalation, but it is only one of many. Almost all volatile substances have been inhaled for their effect, at one time or another, including the solvents present in plastic cements and airplane glues (generally toluene and benzene), paint thinners, cleaning fluids, gasoline, and industrial solvents. All of these substances create a state of intoxication that is somewhat similar to that produced by alcohol. In high enough quantities, over a sufficiently prolonged time, most of these vapors can cause a toxic psychosis. The physical damage caused by their use includes lung disease, damage to nerve tissue, liver damage, and chromosomal damage.

Another common substance inhaled for its toxic effects is gasoline, which can lead to lead poisoning if the gasoline has a heavy lead content.

For this latter, rare condition, a determination of blood-lead level can be made, and evidence of plumbism (lead poisoning) may be seen in the bones. The most useful laboratory test for establishing a diagnosis of glue sniffing measures the level of hippuric acid in the urine. Liver biopsies are occasionally done along with liver function tests to determine the degree of damage done to this organ when severe vapor sniffing is suspected.

Much less commonly used inhalants include ether, nitrous oxide and amyl nitrite as well as most of the gases used for anesthetic purposes in hospitals. There is no known physical dependence to any of the inhalants although psychological dependence can be quite high depending on the patient's level of adjustment.

## Amphetamines and Other Psychostimulants

For many years this group of drugs, which includes several varieties of amphetamine and Ritalin, have been used for mental depression and weight reduction as well as to relieve fatigue and treat narcolepsy and certain hyperkenetic behavior disorders in children. Recently they have all come under federal control and are classified as dangerous drugs.

The use of amphetamines generally causes the person to experience elevation of mood and a sense of well-being. Continued use results in tolerance and habituation. With very heavy use, toxic effects appear, including profound behavioral changes and a characteristic "amphetamine psychosis" which clinically resembles an acute paranoid schizophrenic reaction. (Paranoid schizophrenia is a major mental illness in which the break with reality is characterized by unrealistic suspiciousness and feelings of persecution, as well as a lack of coordination between thoughts and feelings.)

There is a popular saying "speed kills" but there is much scientific disagreement as to whether or not this is the case. After the chronic use of amphetamines is stopped, physical and psychological depression often follows, accompanied by changes in the electroencephalographic sleep pattern. However, there are no characteristic withdrawal symptoms.

## Barbiturates and Other Sedatives

Although all of these drugs are restricted by law to medical use, they are still frequently misused. For the sake of convenience we include under this category both the long- and short-acting barbiturates and Doriden and Quaalude. The most common medical reason for using these drugs is to induce relaxation and sleep. Some short-acting barbiturates, such as sodium pentothal, are used for anesthetic purposes. Severe physical dependence develops with these drugs and seizures may occur if attempts are made to withdraw the patient from them. Whenever barbiturate, Doriden, Quaalude, or meprobamate addiction is suspected, the physician will withdraw the patient gradually, keeping a careful watch for any signs of couvulsive seizures. Because of this danger, withdrawal should generally be done in a controlled in-patient setting such as a psychiatric floor of a general hospital.

## Opiate Narcotics

This group of chemicals includes opium, all of its derivatives, and chemically related synthetic products. They are among the most valuable of medicinal agents. However, because of the severe physical dependence it is quite possible for an emotionally stable person to become addicted to these drugs. Heroin, a morphine derivative, has been totally banned from any type of legal use for years in the United States. It is known among other names as "H," "horse," "junk," "scag," and "smack." The use of raw opium is more indigenous to Eastern countries where it is usually eaten or smoked, but it can be used in any other way conceivable.

Most normal people, who are not in pain, find the effects of opiates quite unpleasant. Many persons who develop tolerance and physical dependence because they are given this drug for analgesic purposes, show little interest in the drug experience itself and tend not to resume after they are physically withdrawn.

There is little or no direct permanent physical damage as a result of chronic use of pure narcotics. Physical damage that does occur is the result of nonsterile injections and toxic additives. Tolerance is very likely to occur with chronic use, and the person may eventually use a dose as much as 30 times the quantity that would be lethal to normal persons. The physical effects of using opiates include: a reduction in respiratory and cardiovascular activity, a depression of the cough reflex, constriction of the pupils, warming of the skin, and a decrease in intestinal activity often causing constipation. In some people nausea and vomiting routinely occur. Overdosage causes coma, shock, respiratory arrest, and death.

The subjective or psychological effects vary widely with individuals and are influenced by the setting in which the drug is taken. In general they include mood changes, inability to concentrate, drowsiness, and lethargy. Higher doses produce withdrawal, a turning inwards, and sleep.

It is possible to lead a life addicted to opiates with little change in conventional habits. However, some people today who become addicted to these drugs (primarily heroin) live only to take the drug and engage in criminal activities to pay for it. Because these people lead a life centered around heroin, they are locked into a life without option. It is a chemical slavery in which free choice and autonomy have become irrelevant.

Withdrawal from opiates, although quite unpleasant, is not so life threatening as that of giving up barbiturates or even alcohol. Within 12 hours of the last dose of opiates the person begins to feel irritable, anxious, and weak. His eyes and nose become watery and he sweats and shivers. The reaction has been likened to a severe case of the flu. He then may have a few hours of uneasy sleep before beginning the "cold turkey" phase, so named because of the cold, clammy, goose-bumpy skin that occurs along with dilated pupils, nausea and vomiting, and severe abdominal cramps often with uncontrollable defecation, tremors, and occasionally convulsions. In some rare instances death results. The major symptoms may last a few days but noticeable recovery is almost certain within a week. Complete recuperation often takes up to 6 months. Tolerance is either abolished or very greatly reduced after withdrawal, and some dependent users voluntarily undergo withdrawal to reduce the size of their habit. Although chromosomal abnormalities and birth deformities are not known to be associated with this group of substances, the newborn infant of an opiate-dependent mother will also have withdrawal symptoms and may die if these are not recognized and properly treated.

There is considerable cross tolerance among the opiate family of drugs. Methadone is one synthetic form which has a longer lasting effect than heroin and, if substituted for heroin, can prevent withdrawal symptoms and psychological reactions when the patient is withdrawn from heroin. It is being increasingly used in chronic maintenance programs in which the person is intentionally addicted to Methadone which is legally dispensed in order to stop the addiction to heroin. Although this approach is still under investigation and is controversial, it is often seized upon by cities in their desperation to find a solution to the drug problem. Some recent studies have shown that after a year or 2 many patients on a long-term Methadone maintenance program are concurrently addicted to barbiturates, cocaine, amphetamines, or any of a number of drugs.

Another means of tackling this type of addiction is the administration of morphine antagonists. When these are injected into a person who has been taking opiates, withdrawal symptoms immediately occur. These antagonists are useful diagnostically and may serve as a therapeutic measure.

## Marijuana

Marijuana is most commonly known as "pot" or "grass" and is referred to as "tea," "Maryjane," and various other names at various times and places. It is prepared from the flowering tops and leaves of the Cannabis sativa (Indian hemp) plant. The products vary widely in potency depending on where they are grown and how they are prepared. There are several hundred varieties of this plant, differing somewhat in potency, one from the other. Marijuana may be smoked or cooked and eaten. Current studies are being conducted under controlled conditions to test the effects of measured doses of the active principal THC (tetrahydrocannabinol) on such factors as perception, awareness, and mental disorganization. Many investigators feel that studies which disregard the potency and dose of the drug used are worthless. None of these studies appears to have any information as yet regarding long-term or chronic use of marijuana. The acute effect of marijuana taken in small doses may range widely from nothing discernible to a feeling of euphoric detachment and relaxation. Perceptions of time and distance may be altered, and for almost everyone there is a heightened sense of well-being, self-confidence, and sociability. The occasional adverse effects of marijuana usage which have been reported have to do with panic states and mental disorganization in individuals who in retrospect had demonstrated emotional difficulties prior to taking the drug.

As most people are aware today, there is hardly a drug about which more dispute exists than marijuana. Its use has spread through colleges, high schools, and even grade schools. It is used by students in graduate schools, law schools, and medical schools and by young professionals throughout the Western world. Many users consider a little "pot" and a little wine a wonderful way to relax and enjoy the company of friends. While these people frequently consider heavy cigarette smoking or alcohol ingestion as being definitely dangerous to health, they feel that ordinary use of marijuana is harmless. There are other groups who feel that marijuana definitely leads to heroin addiction, and they claim to have statistics to prove it. There are yet others who believe that marijuana causes personality disintegration, severe anxiety, and depressive reactions. A group of Canadian psychiatrists concluded that high doses of tetrahydrocannabinol (THC), the active principal in marijuana, can induce a psychotic reaction in almost anyone.

Marijuana, in the form of "hashish," a concentrated tar of alkaloids such as THC and its close relatives, has been used for many years as part of the culture in some countries in the Middle East and Near East. It is reported that there is a high incidence of psychosis in such countries but it is very difficult to evaluate these findings. There are indeed many other causes for psychosis that have been identified in these cultures. Also, the dose of THC is many hundred times the dose used daily by American smokers of marijuana.

Like any other drug, it appears that the effects, both the ordinary effects and the toxic effects, are dose-related for the most part. However, just as there are some people who suffer "pathological intoxication" on very small doses of alcohol, there appears to be an identifiable group of persons who have a similar adverse reaction to very low doses of marijuana. These people are the exception rather than the rule.

There is no acceptable evidence at this time that marijuana results in the development of tolerance or addiction, nor has it been established that there is any association between its use and crime or violence.

With all of the discussion and the disagreement, there is very little scientific evidence at this point to substantiate either the dangers or the safety of using this drug. The pharmacology appears to be similar to that of other drugs in that side-effects and toxic effects increase proportionally to the amount of the drug taken. An average person taking a great deal of strong marijuana will almost surely experience feelings of fear or near panic, depersonalization, confusion, disorientation, depression, and paranoid feelings.

Habituation to either alcohol or marijuana is incompatible with the educational processes. The daily and/or excessive use of either definitely interferes with productivity, concentration, and intellectual endeavors.

## Hallucinogens (LSD, Mescaline)

A hallucinogen is a substance which produces an apparent sensory experience of something which does not exist outside the mind.

LSD ("acid"), lysergic acid diethylamide, was first synthesized in 1938. By 1965 it was outlawed because of the increasing number of psychiatric casualties which it produced. The hallucinogenic effects of this drug are fascinating and seductive. It has been and continues to be tested for use in the treatment of a variety of psychiatric conditions. However, follow-up studies of its use in alcoholic patients have failed to substantiate any significant lasting results.

LSD is colorless, odorless, and tasteless. An incredibly small amount of the chemical is able to cause far-reaching psychiatric changes that boggle the mind. Almost all persons who have taken this drug agree that it produces an intensely personal experience, involving, in great reverberations, the events of their lives, its joys and horrors, as they flash before them. All sensations seem to be more intense. There is extreme emotional lability in the sense that persons may experience simultaneously profound but opposite emotions. It is possible to be happy and sad, depressed and elated, all at the same time. Some persons, perhaps those who have been emotionally unstable to start with, undergo panic states and psychotic reactions that often require prolonged psychiatric hospitalization. In some instances LSD has resulted in suicide attempts, suicide, homicide, and deaths by misadventure. There have been spontaneous recurrences ("flashbacks") of the LSD experience sometimes up to 18 months after the last dose. It has been said that LSD "opens a window in the soul," and it seems that that window can never again be closed. In short it is a dangerous, frightening, and exciting chemical. It is also a herald of the psychopharmacology to come.

Another hallucinogen is mescaline, used either in its pure crystalline form or as peyote. Although tending to cause great sensory distortions, often of magnificent beauty and variety, the effect is less personal than that of LSD—it is somewhat as if the user is watching a heavenly light show. Little is known about the dangers of mescaline.

## Cocaine

Cocaine is a white crystalline alkaloid which was first used as a local anesthetic in Vienna in 1884 and became the first of a long series of drugs used for this purpose.

Cocaine is the active principal in the leaves of the coca plant, which is commonly found wild in Peru and Bolivia and cultivated in many other countries, including Indonesia. For many centuries the Indians of Peru and Bolivia have chewed the leaves of the coca plant either for pleasure or to help them withstand strenuous work, walking, hunger, and thirst. When taken by mouth it produces local anesthesia of the stomach so that hunger and thirst are not felt.

The cortex of the brain is first stimulated, mental powers increase, and the sensation of fatigue diminishes. Euphoria and pleasant hallucinations are also experienced. However, with larger doses and stimulation of the spinal cord, convulsions may result. Following the stimulation there is often a depression of the entire nervous system, which could result in death from respiratory failure.

Addiction can occur in a very short period of time, and a paranoid psychosis quite similar to amphetamine psychosis can develop.

Cocaine addicts are frequently fearful and may suffer from the belief that they are threatened. They are generally considered dangerous, and it is reported they may carry weapons which they are likely to use. The hallucinations may be auditory, visual, or tactile. Sometimes imaginary insects may be seen and felt crawling over the skin as in alcoholic hallucinosis.

Very recently cocaine addiction has been seen in large cities among former heroin addicts who are maintained on a Methadone maintenance program.

## NURSING SKILLS

As mentioned earlier, this chapter is aimed at giving the nurse an overall philosophy and background for dealing with the habituated or drugged person in all settings. For the nurse who is interested in specializing in the care of this type of patient certain additional information and basic skills must be acquired. However, recognizing the drugged state and the habituated person and being able to cope with drug misuse in a general hospital setting are basic and essential skills for every nurse to have.

### Recognizing the Drugged State

It is extremely important that the nurse develop the ability to recognize when a person is under the influence of drugs. Once you have learned to do this well, you will generally trust your own instincts despite the loud protests of the patient who insists that he has not taken anything at all. Indeed, any patient who has a secret "stash" of drugs which he is dipping into will invariably deny that he is taking drugs. Encountering such loud protestations early in the learning experience, can be somewhat disconcerting to the nurse and lead her to distrust her own impressions. However, after having your judgment confirmed positively several times, you will have no further difficulty.

Of course the signs and symptoms of drug use vary widely with the drug that is taken. However, the single most frequently recognized sign is some speech disturbance (dysphonia). Usually the speech is slurred when "downs" (tranquilizers and barbiturates) are used, and it has a somewhat brassy sound along with being somewhat indistinct when "ups" (amphetamines, Ritalin) are used. When a patient in a hospital or clinic is recognized as having some sort of speech disturbance, note should always be made of this for comparison later. The patient, of course, may have true speech pathology and certainly should not be accused of taking drugs on the basis of this sign alone. However, true speech pathology does not vary much from day to day but remains quite constant. The drug taker will speak quite clearly on some days and will be easy to understand, while on other days, he will mouth his words and speak indistinctly in a way that should alert you immediately to the possibility of drug misuse.

The second most common sign noted with drug taking is ataxia, i.e., the patient is clumsy, stumbles, and frequently acts like a "drunk." On the basis of this too, one must be very careful not to accuse a patient of drug taking. You may discover later to your embarrassment that he has a true neurologic condition. However, ataxia should, along with dysphonia, cause you to become alerted to the possibility of drug misuse. Again the most important aspect of this symptom is that it comes and goes with drug use. All of these signs and symptoms must be made note of and the patient observed longitudinally. (Longitudinal observance means that repeated observations of the patient are made over a period of time in order to determine a trend in his symptoms and condition.) There is nothing pathognomonic (pathologically characteristic) of drug taking except positive chemical identification of the drug in the blood or urine.

Other physical signs frequently noted are pupillary changes and injected conjunctiva (bloodshot eyes). With amphetamines the pupils are frequently large, although this is not always so. Large pupils are also seen in young people as compared with older persons. Small pupils are most often present with opiate use but also occur with the medical use of many of the major tranquilizers. Bloodshot eyes, of course, frequently occur with drinking and also with marijuana and the psychedelics. Nausea and vomiting is a frequent accompanyment of opiate use for many people, but not for all. Likewise mescaline makes a certain number of people sick to their stomach. Unusual drowsiness leading to stupor should, of course, always be noted, but great caution must be taken in the interpretation of this symptom. Unexplained drowsiness in any patient should not just be noted by the nurse, but should be reported to someone in higher authority because it frequently is a symptom of a very serious physical illness.

It is essential that the drug user not only be identified, but also be protected. This will only happen when medical and nursing personnel at all levels rid themselves of prejudicial thinking and develop the special skills necessary to handle persons with drug problems. It is inexcusable to ignore stupor in a known heroin addict with the glib presumption that heroin has caused the stupor. For example, the person could be poisoned or may have fallen and sustained a head injury.

When inspecting the body of a patient, regardless of the diagnosis, one should be aware of and alert to needle marks, called "tracks," over the veins of the arms or any part of the body. Also scars, abscesses, induration (hardening), and lumps under the skin are all suggestive of injection sites, but the cause must be carefully evaluated before any conclusions about drug misuse are reached.

Changes in the sympathetic-parasympathetic nervous systems should always be noted of course. These include such things as a dry or watery mouth, tachycardia or bradycardia, constipation or diarrhea, change in appetite, and blurred vision. These are all common side-effects of phenothiazine therapy and are common to most of the psychoactive drugs.

Suspiciousness, frank paranoid thinking, and strange behavior such as spending much time locked in the bathroom should always be noted and an attempt made to properly evaluate the behavior. The amphetamine type drugs and cocaine, as well as some of the psychedelics can make someone appear very paranoid. This must be very carefully distinguished from paranoid schizophrenia and other paranoid states.

There is at times the confusing combination of true paranoid schizophrenia and drug misuse. It is not easy to distinguish these conditions and to tell what effects are due to what cause, but the first step in discovery is to become aware of the possibilities and to keep an open, inquisitive, and reflective mind, with a nonjudgmental attitude.

## Recognizing the Habituated or Addicted Person

We have just discussed the signs and symptoms that the nurse should look for and be aware of in order to alert herself and the rest of the staff to the possibility that someone is under the influence of drugs. In this section, we will consider the person who is habituated or addicted to drugs and who comes to the attention of medical personnel for this or unrelated reasons. Detecting someone who is under the influence of drugs is not the same as detecting someone who is chronically habituated or addicted to their use. Not infrequently patients entering a hospital bring their own supply of drugs with them, not necessarily because they are addicted or habituated to their use, but because they may fear the entire hospital situation. They are experiencing fears associated with all of the procedures and with the possibility that severe and serious pathology will be found. There is a general distrust that hospital personnel will be able to respond to their needs because of the widespread belief among the public that hospitals are understaffed and that hospital personnel are overworked and unable to care for individual patients in an expeditious way. For these reasons, it is very common for private patients in particular to bring their own private supply of sleeping pills or minor tranquilizers to the hospital. These patients may hardly ever use such drugs outside the hospital or they may only use them in times of severe distress. They are not addicted or habituated. However, the strange surroundings, sights, and sounds of the hospital make it difficult for them to sleep, and so they attempt to take care of this problem. They do not mention their supply of drugs, for fear that they may be confiscated. The physician, on the other hand, frequently writes routine PRN orders for sleep medication or for mild tranquilizers in the event of anxiety attacks. The combination of the patient's supply and the doctor's orders can and, sometimes, does produce a state of drug intoxication. The nurse often is the first person to notice this state of affairs. Because she spends more time with the patient, develops better rapport, is neither feared nor venerated by the patient as the doctor often is, she is in a uniquely valuable position to gain the patient's confidence and to discreetly explore such possibilities as whether the patient is continuing to use medication that was prescribed for him outside the hospital. All such investigations and queries must be conducted with the utmost tact, politeness, and sensitivity to the patient's needs and with appreciation of his fears.

We now turn our attention to the patient who is not medicating himself because of anxiety or because of the strange and fearful surroundings of the hospital, but who is truly habituated or addicted and cannot "just stop" because he is entering the hospital. The diagnosis of addiction is of course the province of the physician. However, this diagnosis is often based as much on history as on physical examination. It is here that the alert nurse may obtain information which the physician is not in a position to readily discover. For example, families will frequently speak about a change in the personality of the patient over a period of several months to several years. They may mention something that sounds like transient paranoid episodes or inconsistencies in the patient's behavior; all of these should be made note of by the nurse, according to the practices of the institution in which she is working, and called to the attention of the attending physician.

Other such signs and symptoms which may be reported by the family are as follows: a change of habit and behavior; a change in the pattern of sleep and wakefulness; a tendency for the patient to be seclusive, to not relate to the family in as free and open a way as previously; a tendency to be away from the house suddenly without notice and without adequate explanation; the growing belief on the part of the family that valuables have begun to mysteriously disappear from the house and, perhaps, from the houses of neighbors and friends; a reluctance on the part of the patient to bring new-found friends home to visit the family; mysterious telephone calls in which the caller will not give his or her name but asks for the patient; spots of blood on shirt

sleeves, jackets, bed clothes; spoons found about the house, the bottoms of which are tarnished or covered with black soot; the discovery of needles, syringes, and eye droppers; the discovery of many colored pills in the patient's pocket or pocketbook; perhaps a sudden diminishing in the supply of prescribed medicine that the family had kept in the medicine cabinet; a loss of interest in work or school; and a loss of weight. There are many other signs and symptoms that often appear when a person becomes addicted or habituated to drugs of various types. To attempt to make a complete listing of them here would be impossible. Actual experience with a few persons habituated to drugs will teach far more than the crude outline presented above.

It is especially important in hospital practice that the possibility of drug addiction or habituation be recognized and acknowledged, especially in those patients who are scheduled for anesthesia or surgical procedures or those admitted for childbirth.

Giving anesthesia to a person who is taking drugs on his own becomes a tricky business. It is also fairly well known that children born to mothers addicted to opiates have a tolerance to these drugs and need to be carefully watched for withdrawal symptoms during the neonatal period.

As sophisticated and accurate laboratory procedures become more readily available it seems likely that hospitalized patients and those on out-patient care will be routinely tested for the presence of drugs in the blood or urine. This will help cut out much of the guesswork.

## Drug Nonuse and Hoarding

This is of course the other side of the coin and is certainly another type of drug misuse. With rising consumer interest and awareness, the sacrosanct position which the physician and the medical profession enjoyed for many, many years is being seriously challenged by the consumer public. Many patients today have copies of the _Physicians' Desk Reference_ at home; they look up the prescriptions that are written for them and read about the side-effects to make sure that the physician is not making a mistake and that they will not be hurt by the medication that he prescribed. There is no question but that certain aspects of this concern are healthy, but the fact that the patient may be altering his drug intake is all too often ignored by the medical profession instead of acknowledged and worked with.

Many hospitalized psychiatric patients have a tendency to adjust their own dosage by eliminating certain doses or, more dangerously, to hoard medications against the day when they decide that suicide is a reasonable alternative. To obviate this, many drugs can be given in a liquid concentrate form which the patient must swallow in front of the nurse; and assuming that he does not run to the bathroom and throw up immediately one can be relatively sure that he is getting the medication that is prescribed for him. Another advance is the present availability and use of long-acting injectable tranquilizing medication whereby the patient can be given an intramuscular injection once every week or 2 in a depot form, a dosage form which he cannot possibly manipulate himself. However, such things are not without their dangers. Patients suspected of mouthing pills and hoarding them or disposing of them, on the basis that a large dose of medication appears to be having no effect on his personality, should certainly not be switched to concentrate or intramuscular forms without the daily dose first being substantially reduced. If you truly believe that the patient is cheating by taking less medication than is given to him, then you must act as if he is not getting his full dosage and start at a much lower dose and build it up over a period of time. The problem of drug hoarding, of course, is not just that the patient is not receiving the medication on a daily basis as expected, or that he may be saving it against a rainy day to commit suicide, but that there is always the likelihood that the medication is being diverted to another patient. All of these considerations make the dispensing of medication in a hospital (any hospital) a procedure that needs a great deal of consideration and planning. With information such as we already have, it is very likely that courts could decide against hospitals on the basis of negligence, if the system is not quickly and thoroughly revised to take all of these factors into account.

## TREATMENT CONSIDERATIONS

This is a particularly thorny problem. First, little is known about the effectiveness of various treatment modalities for drug misuse. Second, a lot more money is needed for research and evaluation to assess present treatment methods and to stimulate the development of new ones. Third, in large measure the problem is a social rather than a medical one. These and other aspects will be covered in this section.

### Present Socioeconomic Aspects

At the time of this writing, society is just beginning to mobilize itself to deal in an effective way with the pressing social problems of drug misuse, especially in the military and among the young. For a variety of economic and political reasons, the government did not previously undertake any extensive study of the harmful effects of drug use. As previously noted, there still remains much debate and diversity of opinion regarding the harmful effects of marijuana and related chemicals. The harmful effects of morphine type narcotics, such as heroin, and opium, on the drug user are difficult to separate from harmful effects to the community. It appears to some investigators that the use of heroin alone— without the present legal complications involved in America, without the dangerous side-effects of unsterile injection, without the dangers of harmful contaminants and additives, without the necessary connection with the underworld to obtain the drug, and without the necessity to obtain large amounts of money by whatever means to secure the drug on a daily basis—results in very little physical harm or mental deterioration. For this reason various attempts have been made to separate the use of the drug from its dangerous setting.

One of the first attempts was made in 1923 when morphine clinics were established in the United States. Within a few years, these clinics were disbanded for several reasons, mostly political. In England, heroin clinics were set up in an effort to eliminate the underworld from the drug-delivery system. These efforts had varied success. In the United States more recently Methadone clinics have been established using a synthetic narcotic that has 2 advantages over the use of morphine and heroin: (1) the ease and effectiveness of oral administration, and (2) a longer lasting effect of the drug so that one dose in 24 hours is sufficient.

These measures have led to a wide diversity of opinion and much discussion. There are several facts which appear to be more certain than others and give us a point of view from which to examine these matters. Before heroin and other morphine type drugs were made illegal for free and general use in 1914 by the Harrison Narcotic Act, the problem of opium and heroin addiction in America was very large and growing rapidly. The legislation had several effects: (1) Within a relatively short time it very greatly reduced the number of persons using narcotic drugs. (2) There was a sharp increase in the involvement of organized crime in providing these drugs extralegally, because there was a great deal of money to be made in this market. (3) There was a great increase in costs for law enforcement measures to prevent organized crime from carrying out its business in this area. (These efforts by the government, by the way, have always appeared to be quite ineffective in stemming the illegal supply to any significant degree.) (4) The individual drug user, unable to obtain the drug by ordinary means, had to use the sources of the underworld and had to pay their price. This price today varies from $30.00 per day to several hundred dollars a day for heroin addiction. Women often make this money through prostitution, and men through stealing or robbery.

It is quite clear then, that the Harrison Narcotic Act had the dual effect of all such social legislation: (1) the absolute numbers of drug users was reduced; and (2) the harmful effects on society and the moral degradation of the individual user has been vastly increased.

Educational activities directed against drug misuse have been quite ineffective because there is not enough documented evidence about drug mechanisms and the effects of chronic use to make such educational activities meaningful and relevant. There has been a very recent effort to have short saturation advertising campaigns on television but there is much question as to whether these have any effect at all. People (fortunately) seem to be getting more and more immune to being told

how they should feel or what they should do without being given reasons that make sense.

## The Role of the Health Professional in Drug Misuse

In 1969, 202 million prescriptions for psychoactive drugs were filled in pharmacies for persons who saw their doctors first and obtained the prescription from them. These figures would be substantially higher, if they included hospital and clinic usage. Nonetheless, 202 million such prescriptions in a population of little over 200 million is staggering indeed, especially since these drugs are taken primarily to keep people *from* feeling. Although depression is clearly the most widespread psychiatric disorder, the most frequently prescribed drugs in the psychoactive category are tranquilizers, which are not designed for the treatment of depression. Anxiety and agitation are often difficult if not impossible to distinguish from one another. It has been shown in controlled studies, however, that pure anxiety is a relatively rare condition. Anxiety neurosis alone, occurs very seldom. Most of the time, one sees neurotic depression in which agitation is a significant feature. The use of tranquilizers in such a patient will not relieve his depression, but probably will increase it. The use of tranquilizers and sleeping pills in such a person (and difficulty in getting to sleep and early awakening are very frequent symptoms of depression) will not improve the circadian (daily) rhythm distortion of depression nor will it increase the amount of REM (rapid eye movement associated with dreaming) sleep, which causes such profound effects on the person's mental and emotional life. There is clearly a need for education among the medical profession to keep all health professionals up-to-date on the latest work that is being done in our fast moving world of powerful, valuable, and, at the same time, potentially dangerous chemicals.

Although the major tranquilizing drugs have transformed the practice of psychiatry, made possible the mental health center movement, and dramatically decreased state hospital populations, they are not without their danger. In some people, especially elderly females, a central nervous system disorder known as "tardive dyskinesia," (characterized by difficulty in performing voluntary muscular movements) which is possibly irreversible, has begun to make its appearance. We do not know who will succumb to this disease but a review of long-term prescribing practices in hospitals is urgently needed. We know enough already to realize that an elderly woman on a 1000 milligrams of Thorazine a day, for over 3 months is in clear jeopardy of succumbing to this condition. Whether or not the medical profession and nursing professions like the idea, it is essential that we devote much more energy to our understanding of biochemistry and pharmacology. Basic science is becoming less abstract and something we all live with day by day.

Fixing the blame in a difficult and extremely complicated problem such as drugs in America in the 1970's is a rather useless pastime which is indulged in by otherwise intelligent people because they really don't know what to do and are trying to get some kind of foothold or grasp on this subject. Among the people who have been blamed are psychiatrists, pharmacists, general practitioners, the church, the community, the war, the field of psychopharmacology, the role of the father in the American home, the role of the mother in the American home, the generation gap, communism, the black power movement, the white-backlash, the school system, a lack of moral fiber as compared to former times, urban crowding, the disease of the ghettos, organized crime, the police and the courts, and many, many others. Communities frequently say that the problem of drug addiction and drug misuse is the province of the mental health professionals. This is based on the view that these situations represent emotional disorders. Mental health professionals, weary and discouraged with attempting to work with drug takers who do not wish to be worked with, are beginning to say that it is not a psychiatric problem but a community problem. They cite as their chief example, the fact that we are a drug-taking culture and that the very mothers and fathers who complain about their child are themselves depending very heavily on psychoactive drugs.

When it comes to the matter of detoxification—that is, the drug user who wishes to stop, but is afraid to without medical support and requests admission to a hospital so that he can kick the habit in as painless and humane way as possible—mental health persons feel that this is primarily a medical problem requiring psychiatric support. They especially feel this way, when the drug problem in question has consisted of large and continuous use of barbiturate type drugs because there is a very great danger of convulsive seizures when the dose is reduced. Medical men, however, say that it is not in their province to handle such things but it is up to the psychiatrist to admit such patients to mental beds and take care of such problems that way with medical consultation, if necessary. Even today in large urban centers, there are few beds set aside specifically for the purposes of acute detoxification.

Another problem hardly ever touched is the fact that most general hospitals are a drug taker's dream. If injection is their thing, there are unattended carts in almost every hallway with sterile syringes, needles, and alcohol pledgets and most of the "goodies" that they want. The narcotic drugs, themselves, may be locked up, but the drug misuer can certainly get a running head start with the equipment that is readily available. Also, some hospitals allow nurses to leave medication doses on the patient's bedside table, if the patient is, at the time of dispensing, asleep or in the bathroom. This practice is, of course, frowned upon and not recommended, but in reality it happens very, very frequently, and a patient, interested in using whatever he can get his hands on, can without a great deal of difficulty step from room to room and in a few moments have quite a nice collection of sleeping pills, tranquilizers, and what-have-you. In the author's experience, and at the time of this writing, general hospitals are far from prepared to handle patients with a tendency to misuse drugs. Coupled with this is the fact that the majority of drug misusers are not even recognized throughout their entire period of hospitalization. They come in, they are treated for something entirely different, and they leave.

## "When They're Ready to Stop, They'll Stop"

This simplistic statement carries a great deal of truth, but does not, of course, tell the entire story. It means to imply that without a great deal of motivation on the part of the patient, all the effort and interest and energy on the part of the staff will mean very little, because the patient will be fighting the staff in much the same manner as he fights his own conscience. The civil rights issue is also very much a part of this attitude. Many people today feel that individuals have the "right" to use whatever drugs they choose, to take their own life if they wish, and to go insane if they are so inclined without interference from onlookers and "the helping professions." Such people say that so long as the person is not hurting anyone else or society, it is really nobody else's business how he conducts his life.

You will have to arrive at your own views by careful thinking, listening, and discussion with your peers and others. Let me bring one thing to your attention, however. Let us say a young man, age 17, has acquired some "speed" and is considering using it. Let us further say that he is quite sane and clear-headed and that, according to the information available to him from his friends and his reading, taking a little bit of "speed" is not a particularly harmful thing. Let us then say, that he takes about 30 milligrams of methamphetamine or its equivalent. We will call this young man person A. One hour elapses; person A, is no longer around. Person A, plus 30 milligrams of methamphetamine has resulted in the emergence of person B, a young man, with a distinctly different capacity to think and to make judgments and decisions about his life. Person B feels differently from person A. It may be better or worse but it certainly is different. Now person B is weighing the possibilities of taking more drugs. He may decide that he is tired and weary and should take more "speed"; he may decide that he is jittery and anxious and should take some "downs" to settle his nerves. He may decide that his thinking is getting a little "flaky" and he should take some Thorazine or something to keep from going crazy. And so, in his drug altered state of mind, he chooses one or another of these possibilties and takes some more drugs. Exit person B and enter person C. Let us suppose that person C got to be person C by taking additional "speed" in about double the quantity that person A took, and person C's state of mind includes a great deal of suspiciousness and paranoid thinking. It is so severe, let us say, that he pulls the blinds in the room where he is staying and gets out a gun that he has

kept in a drawer for years. He hides under the bed sheets and jumps at every sound and shuffle he hears in the house. *Question:* Should person A, B, and C all be looked upon as being equally capable of making judgments regarding themselves, their immediate circumstances, and their future? Should the civil rights of each of them include the right to make a decision about continuing or not continuing life? I offer this to stimulate your thinking about a very difficult and thorny question that is far from resolved. The help of all people is needed to clarify these questions for all of us.

## Drug Users are Liars: More Often True than Not

This statement is true enough of the time that it should be constantly kept in mind when dealing with persons who are known to be chronic drug users or habituated or addicted to drugs.

Persons who misuse drugs, persons who drink excessively, persons who take chances with their physical health in a variety of ways, compulsive gamblers, persons whose sexual behavior is contrary to the prevelant code of the majority of people—all have certain qualities in common:

1. They feel compelled to do what they are doing.
2. A part of them feels that they should stop because they feel it is dangerous or because they sense they are hurting themselves or they feel that there may be something really wrong with them for so urgently desiring to do whatever their particular "thing" is.
3. Unless they are insane or mentally defective they are aware that what they are doing breaks the law, and they realize that they could be arrested and forced to undergo all of the problems associated with arrest.
4. As a group they exhibit an almost universal tendency to get caught, one way or another.
5. At the same time, they do not wish to be thought of as bad persons but really wish to be understood as basically good people who feel compelled to do something that frightens them at least as much, if not more, than it frightens the onlookers.

Their chances of finding the understanding that they desire in this society are unfortunately rather slim. Therefore, they lie about what they are doing or they lie about the exact extent of their involvement in whatever it is they are doing, or they lie about exactly how motivated they are to do something about it, or they lie to avoid detection all together because they are afraid to stop and realize that detection may be the beginning of the end of the habitual pattern that has become such an intimate part of their daily lives.

Probably one of the oldest and most familiar examples of this is the alcoholic who voluntarily admits himself to the hospital in order to dry out and as he would say, "in order to save my life." However, he also brings a bottle of alcohol in his suitcase, "just in case." If you ask him whether or not he brought any alcohol or drugs he will say "no," in a most honest and convincing way. If you discover the bottle in his bag and discuss it with him, he may deny having anything to do with it; he may laugh and say, "I guess you caught me"; he may get angry and insist that his privacy has been invaded, and so on and on. It does not take long for the nurse to become familiar with this type of behavior in this patient. Even if you discover the bottle in his bag and remove it and report it to the proper authorities, and upon instructions confront the patient with the evidence, you can be fairly sure that whatever his reply is, he is already busy making plans to either recover that bottle or have another one brought in to him.

## TREATMENT MODALITIES

There are numerous types of drug misuse, as you have seen from the foregoing. There are also many treatment modalities that have been used and are being used in an attempt to combat drug misuse. There is far from universal agreement, however, on any of these measures, on their efficacy, on their safety, or on their applicability to the population at large. It seems most likely that there are as many different subcategories of drug misusers as there are subcategories of schizophrenia. Classifying people according to the drug that they are misusing has not led to any consistent and helpful conclusions. Nor have the traditional psychiatric categories been of much help. It is true that a certain number of drug misusers have what is classically known as a character disorder. It is also true that some of them are dependent, oral-type people. It is likely that some have a strong genetic or inherited predisposition toward drug misuse. It is clear in certain cases that the family environment has been a strong contributory factor in the development of drug dependence. In some, as mentioned previously, there is the coexistence of a definable major mental illness. In others there is the coexistence of a major physical illness.

Almost all workers in the field agree on 2 basic treatment principles: (1) that the drug misuse should stop immediately, and (2) that coexistent illnesses of any type should be treated as soon as possible. I say that most people agree on these things because unfortunately not even these 2 simple items meet with universal approval. The advocates of specific treatment modalities often exclude or disregard other modalities and concentrate on their special "thing." It should be the role of the nurse and supporting personnel to be quite open-minded in this regard. By that I mean, it is inappropriate for the nurse to be "for" a certain modality and "against" another. There is no way for her to tell, or for anyone else to tell for that matter, whether a particular patient will take to and be helped by Methadone maintenance, or Synanon, or psychotherapy, or whatever. For example, it may be a grave mistake for medical personnel to make every effort to help the patient avoid imprisonment. The legal system can be an aid to therapy. Some studies seem to indicate that imprisonment and enforced therapy under a closely controlled parole system offer some of the best results in the treatment of the drug misuser. It seems that for some people the pain of being in prison for a time satisfies some deep need so that they no longer have the overwhelming desire to continue to hurt themselves. In other persons, of course, imprisonment is disastrous. It is suggested that the nurse be familiar with the varieties of community resources and treatment methods that are available in her community. She should offer this information when it is asked for by the patient and when it is appropriate to do so. If the patient indicates an interest in a certain type of treatment, the nurse should be encouraging and supportive and, where possible, gain the family's support in backing the patient's endeavor to recover. Inquiries should be made and information gotten about the following types of agencies:

**Acute Detoxification Units.** Some hospitals only handle alcohol detoxification, some only heroin, some only barbiturate, etc. If local hospitals make this distinction this information should be known by the nurse.

**Self-Help Groups.** These vary from inspirational, religious, and supportive, to intensive group therapeutic efforts. They may operate strictly on an out-patient basis such as Alcoholics Anonymous, or they may have both out-patient and residential facilities available such as Synanon in California and Daytop Village in New York.

**Substitutive Chemotherapy.** Many big cities now have Methadone maintenance clinics and Methadone withdrawal programs. The pure opiate addicts who do not have the tendency to substitute other addictions while taking Methadone are sometimes helped by this approach.

**Group Psychotherapy and Family Therapy.** This type of therapy is available in many urban centers and appears to have a distinct advantage over individual therapy. Where these groups are available, the cost and the local reputation of the providers of service should be known by the nurse.

**Drug Antagonists.** Drug antagonists are available for both the opiate drugs and for alcohol. They have been used for diagnostic purposes and for preventing further misuse of the drug to which the patient has been addicted. They work by altering the normal metabolic pathways of the drug and usually cause violent physical reactions or immediate withdrawal symptoms when the drug of abuse is taken.

## CONCLUSION AND SUMMARY

The use of drugs to provide recreation, rest, and escape or to ease problems has been known since the dawn of civilization. Because of an (as yet) undetermined combination of genetic (physical) and acquired (psychological) factors, certain persons and families show the tendency to misuse drugs and/or to become dependent on them. Addiction requires, in addition, the use of a drug that has addictive potential (e.g., alcohol, opiates). No one questions the dangers and widespread misuse of alcohol and tobacco. These substances gained public acceptance long before the sciences of pharmacology and toxicology had begun testing drugs for harmfulness. Our experience with prohibition demonstrated dramatically the futility of opposing the established habits of the citizenry even "for their own good."

The development of powerful new psychotropic (mind-directed) drugs offers vastly increased medical potential, and the possibility that more refined recreational chemicals will be developed. It also opens further doors to misuse.

The nurse must be able to recognize the signs and symptoms of the drugged state and have a grasp of differential diagnosis (in order to determine what else might cause the symptoms and constitute a medical emergency). She must be prepared to recognize addiction, habituation, and drug dependency as indicated by the patient's history and signs regardless of the patient's socioeconomic status or his denials. She must learn to see the dangers in most hospitals through the eyes of the drug misuser and, if she is so inclined, work through professional groups, unions, and community organizations to press for every hospital to have a drug-safe zone where these patients can be helped. She must, most of all, develop mature perspective and an effective but nonjudgmental attitude toward the drug misuser who wants and needs help.

The nurse must be keenly aware that all health professionals who handle drugs run the added personal risk of drug misuse and addiction. If she finds herself becoming involved in drug misuse, she must seek help immediately from some knowledgeable and reliable source before her professional ethics become compromised or her professional standing or the welfare of the patients under her care becomes endangered. For some, nursing may prove to be too hazardous. It is best that this decision be made carefully and thoughtfully, by the nurse herself, with someone else in consultation, rather than by a board of inquiry or by a loss of license.

We are people too, not the mystical healers some would believe. Let us be as real, gentle, tough-minded, reasonable, and kind with ourselves and one another as we try to be with our patients.

# Unit 13:
## Bridging the Gap Between Student and Graduate

58. *Career Opportunities in Practical Nursing*
59. *The Legal Aspects of Practical Nursing*

# 58

# Career Opportunities in Practical Nursing

---

### BEHAVIORAL OBJECTIVES

*The student successfully attaining the goals of this chapter will be able to:*

- *define the specific role of the practical nurse in relationship to the total health team.*
- *list and discuss the types of health facilities in which the practical nurse might work; discuss the advantages and disadvantages of working in each type of facility; and discuss some of the special facilities in which the nurse might be employed, such as in the armed forces or industry.*
- *discuss some job opportunities for which more education might be needed, either as on-the-job training or in an educational institution.*
- *correctly apply for or resign from a job; conduct herself appropriately in a job interview; and write a professional résumé, a letter of application or resignation.*
- *describe the ways in which a nurse can keep abreast of new knowledge in the particular area of the country in which she lives; describe the advantages and importance of professional association membership; and put these ideas into practice by being a well-informed nurse and a contributing member of the professional and personal community.*

---

As the student practical nurse approaches the end of her nursing program, she realizes that soon she will be a graduate practical nurse. Suddenly, she is expected to have skills and knowledge expected of all licensed practical nurses. No longer will the instructor be available to give assistance. This chapter will attempt to introduce the student to some of the responsibilities and opportunities associated with a career in practical nursing.

## The Role of the Practical Nurse

The practical nurse is a valuable member of the total health care team. All members of that team work together to help the patient return to his optimum function as soon as possible. The practical nurse participates in and contributes to the activities of the team. This means assisting others when they are rushed, as well as offering suggestions or contributions, in either a formal team conference or the day-to-day work situation.

**Organize Your Work.** You will most likely find that as a graduate, you will be caring for more patients than you did as a student. Whatever the situation, you must learn to organize your work so that you are able to give adequate care to all of your patients. This comes with experience, but in the beginning your team leader or head nurse will be willing to assist you.

The most important things for the new graduate to remember are (1) to ask when in doubt about a technic or a procedure; (2) to know when to report significant symptoms and to whom, and (3) to know where to go to look up information about drugs and treatments.

## The Scope of the Field

There is a constant demand for the practical nurse today in hospitals, nursing homes, visiting nurse services, doctors' offices, private duty nursing, industry, and many other areas Practical nurses are also being called on more and more to work on committees with professional nurses, to speak to health and civic groups, and to participate in the recruitment of students for practical nursing programs.

The practical nurse has become a valuable member of the health team, and her opportunities for employment are virtually unlimited. Although graduation from an approved practical nursing program is always an asset when applying for a position, employers recognize as evidence presented by a *licensed* practical nurse that she has passed a state examination in which she has been required to demonstrate her competence to practice. (The licensing law, called the Nurse Practice Act, will be discussed in the next chapter.)

**In a Hospital.** By far the greatest number of practical nurses find positions in hospitals as staff nurses who give bedside care on the various nursing services. If a vacancy exists, consideration may be given to an applicant's preference for a specific service, such as pediatrics or obstetrics. The practical nurse works under the supervision of professional nurses as a member of the nursing team.

When she accepts a position she is entering into an agreement, so she should be fully informed about and understand the personnel policies of the institution. Personnel policies are concerned with such matters as the number of hours in the work week, the tour of duty (morning, afternoon, night), vacation and illness allowances, the salary and the possibility of salary increases, hospitalization coverage, and sometimes, living accommodations. Every hospital establishes its own policies, which vary somewhat from one hospital to another. Salaries vary with the size of the institution and its type and location; they are usually higher in large cities and in certain

parts of the country. Most hospitals today provide a cafeteria service where employees may purchase meals at a nominal cost, or nurses are permitted to bring their own lunches. Some institutions have living quarters available at a moderate price; but for the most part, nurses today live outside of the hospital in their own homes or elsewhere. Many hospitals require employees to carry hospitalization coverage; some provide it for their employees. These are items the nurse can ask about during a personal interview.

**In a Nursing Home.** There are many openings for positions on the nursing staff of nursing homes. A well-run nursing home establishes policies for employment similar to those of hospitals by stating its requirements for employees. The applicant should inquire about the amount of professional nurse supervision that is provided and the extent of her responsibilities in the care of patients. Patients in a nursing home offer a real challenge in that the practical nurse must encourage and help these patients to develop activities and maintain independence, in spite of their disabilities.

**As a Team Leader.** The practical nurse may be asked to be a team leader, or even a charge nurse, especially in nursing homes and extended care facilities. While she needs special postgraduate training in the skills needed for these posts, she also needs other knowledge and attributes. She needs information about legislation, such as Medicare; she needs assistance in planning and implementing patient care and in coordinating and directing other staff members; she must be able to evaluate the nursing care being given, as well as her own leadership abilities; and she should have someone to whom she can freely go for qualified assistance. She is usually responsible to the department supervisor, a professional nurse who provides guidance and assistance.

Some of the specific duties which the LPN in charge might be asked to do are reporting to the next shift, planning nursing care through care conferences, coordinating the services offered by other departments, and teaching other members of the nursing team. She must have leadership and administrative abilities, as well as a thorough knowledge of practical nursing. She must understand basic behavior of people and basic leadership technics. Not every LPN has the ability to be a good charge nurse or team leader, and she must be able to recognize and admit this fact.

**With a Visiting Nurse Service.** Many visiting nurse services or public health nursing services, throughout the country employ practical nurses on the nursing staff. The first requirements for such a position are graduation from an approved school and state licensure. In addition, an applicant is selected on the basis of her nursing ability, her ability to get along with people, and her personal maturity (which may have nothing to do with her age). She makes scheduled home visits to the patients assigned to her care, under the direction of her supervisor who is a professional nurse with special public health preparation. The practical nurse keeps records and makes reports of her visits, and she participates in conferences of the nursing staff. She wears the uniform adopted by the agency, or may wear street clothes, depending upon the agency.

**In a Doctor's Office.** A practical nurse may be employed in a doctor's office, to assist with physical examinations, dressings, and other procedures. Her duties may also include answering the telephone, making appointments with patients, and serving as a receptionist.

**Private Duty.** The private practitioner of nursing takes care of individual patients in a home, an institution, or wherever a patient may desire to go, as in a case when the patient is traveling. This is known as private duty nursing. The nurse is usually paid by the patient or his family, although in the hospital, she is directly responsible to the physician and the hospital administration for the performance of her duties. Private duty gives the practical nurse an opportunity to practice her basic bedside and teaching skills and to meet the total needs of her patient. Since it often includes the care of patients during a long-term illness, or of patients who are wholly or partially disabled, private duty nursing offers steady employment for long periods and may be especially desirable to the older nurse.

**In Industry.** Sometimes, a practical nurse is employed by an industry where she may serve as a preventive health teacher, a dispenser of first aid, or an assistant to the professional nurse or physician in that industry.

**In the Armed Forces.** There are opportunities in the Armed Forces for both male and female LPN's. The graduate and licensed person enters the Armed Forces at a rate higher than that of the usual enlisted man, after basic training. Usually, the nurse is assigned to a hospital or clinic in the United States or a foreign country.

**VISTA (Volunteers in Service to America).** This group gives care and education to those people in this country who need it.

**The Peace Corps.** To practical nurses who can qualify, the Peace Corps offers an opportunity to volunteer for services which are desperately needed in many parts of the world. An interested person can write to the Peace Corps, Washington, D.C., for detailed information.

**Headstart.** Headstart employs practical nurses as school nurses or as assistant instructors in their programs throughout the country.

## Other Opportunities

Some positions are available for practical nurses with special qualifications and the ability to meet the demands of a specialized job.

**Assistant Instructor in a Practical Nursing School.** Some practical nursing schools employ a practical nurse to assist with the supervision of practical nurse students. The qualifications for such a position include a good educational background, proficiency in carrying out nursing procedures, and the ability to get along with people. Previous experience in teaching is a valuable asset. It is not uncommon to find an occasional licensed practical nurse who was formerly a certified teacher.

As an instructor, her duties are to assist with the supervision of students as they practice nursing procedures in the classroom and carry out these procedures with patients in the hospital.

**In the Operating Room.** Many hospitals now employ practical nurses on the operating room staff. With special training they may assist in operating equipment, such as the heart-lung pump, or serve as surgical scrub nurses. The nurse is prepared for these functions by on-the-job training in the employing hospital or by a postgraduate course taken in operating room technics.

**The Dialysis Unit.** Many practical nurses are specially trained to work in the dialysis unit of the hospital. These nurses need special training in order to run the dialysis machines and to know about complications and emergency treatment associated with dialysis.

**Hyperbaric Medicine.** The practical nurse may be trained to work, either in the chamber itself or with the supporting team outside the chamber. A number of ex-Navy men with diving experience have found this a good career opportunity.

## Further Education

**Postgraduate Courses.** Approved postgraduate courses in the nursing specialties, such as pediatric and obstetric nursing, medical and surgical nursing, psychiatry, and operating room technics, are available to the licensed practical nurse in a number of centers. Information about approved courses can be obtained by writing to the National Association for Practical Nurse Education and Service, 535 Fifth Avenue, New York, N.Y. 10017.

**Becoming a Registered Nurse.** Some states have schools which are able to give advanced standing to the LPN who later decides to become a registered nurse. More and more schools are writing challenge examinations and are enabling people to acquire additional skills in education, without having to begin each program at the beginning. If you have questions about the practice of your state in this regard, contact your State Board of Nursing.

**Advanced Standing for Persons with Previous Training or Experience.** Some practical nursing programs are able to give advanced standing for previous medically related training or experience. If you are a corpsman or a former nurse's aide, contact your local practical nursing program or State Board of Nursing for information regarding advanced standing in a practical or professional nursing school.

## Volunteer Service

It is the responsibility of the graduate practical nurse to become involved in community affairs. She can be helpful by teaching others about health care or by assisting in time of disaster. She may be asked to assist with special health teaching by a school, a church group, or another organization.

## Employment

**Placement Services.** Many nurses, both registered and practical, get positions through placement services or registries. Nonprofit services usually require a flat fee on a yearly basis. A commercial registry is operated for profit and may charge a fee every time it places an applicant. However, some registries of this type have been known to be interested in only the fee when placing private duty nurses, disregarding the needs of the patient and the standards of the nurse as well as those of the employer. A good registry operates under policies established to serve the best interests of nurses and patients. Nonprofit registries are usually operated by the official district association of professional nurses, but they may also be operated by similar associations of practical nurses, or by individuals. Some local branches of the State Employment Service provide placement services for practical nurses.

When using a placement service, the nurse notifies the registrar when she is available for work. She also notifies the agency when she is no longer with a patient as a private duty nurse or when she leaves a position, and she indicates when she will be available again. This helps the registry to give better service to the community. At the present time, the demand for practical nurses is so much greater than the supply that many are directly employed as soon as they graduate.

A practical nurse may also obtain employment on the recommendation of a doctor or through personal contacts with the relatives and the friends of former patients. Many find positions by placing personal applications in a hospital, nursing home, or agency. In addition, a practical nurse can refer to many of the nursing journals which usually have large sections listing job opportunities.

**The Personal Interview.** The routine procedure for employment usually includes a personal interview with the prospective employer. When you go for the interview you want to make a favorable impression. This means that you will give careful attention to your appearance and grooming. Leave your tightest skirts, slacks, shorts, and toeless sandals at home. These garments all have their proper place in your life, but that place is not in a business interview. Whatever the prevailing style of hair-do, be sure that your hair is clean. Avoid extremes in make-up and nail polish. Employers are likely to take a dim view of glamor girls on the nursing staff. And surely, there is no need to mention *gum*.

Take your license and Social Security card with you and be prepared to furnish the names of people for references, should you be asked for them. Most employers prefer to get references this way, rather than accepting any letters you may present. Be sure that you have obtained prior permission from the people whose names you use as references. Naturally, you will not lounge in your chair or indulge in long-winded recitals of the nice things former employers have said about you—your references should reveal this. If you are asked why you left a previous position, tell the truth, since the reasons can be checked.

**Keeping a Résumé.** It is important for the nurse to keep a résumé or an up-to-date account of her education, previous employment, and any nursing experience which she has had. This résumé should include what schools you attended and when, whether or not you graduated, and what degree or diploma you received. All jobs should be listed with the dates of employment, whether it was full or part time, and the name of your immediate supervisor, as well as his or her address and telephone number. You may be asked to indicate your specific duties and the reason for leaving that job. You should also include any pertinent information about yourself including special skills, such as the ability to speak a foreign language or special art and craft skills. When applying for a job, take this information with you. It will give you an easy and fast way to fill out application forms, as well as assuring that you will not make mistakes on dates or forget any important information. Sometimes, the practical nursing organization will compile this sort of information for you and will keep it on file permanently.

**Aptitude and Interest Tests.** You will often be asked to take aptitude and interest tests when you are applying for a job. Do the best you can on these, but remember that there is no "right" answer to an interest test and that you cannot study for an aptitude test. Try not to panic when you are taking the test and try to finish as soon as possible. Gen-

erally, it is best not to change an answer once you have written it down.

**The Written Application or Letter of Application.** When you are applying for a position and a personal interview is not immediately possible, your application should include the kind of information that you would be asked to give in an interview. You state the name of your practical nursing program and the year of graduation, whether you are licensed and in what state or states, your age, your marital status, and what previous positions you have held and for how long. You should also mention any special preparation that you may have had in a postgraduate course. Use conservative stationery, and be sure to write legibly in ink—if you can type, so much the better. It is businesslike to include the names and the addresses of 2 or 3 persons to whom the prospective employer may write for references.

**Resigning From a Position.** When resigning from a position, it is honorable to give your employer advance notice of your intentions—at least 2 weeks in advance, and preferably, 1 month in advance. This enables him to find someone to replace you by the time you leave. The advance notice required varies with the position and is established in personnel policies. Customarily, if you leave before the designated time or leave without notice, you will be paid up to the time of your departure. If an employer asks an employee to leave because she is no longer needed or because her work is unsatisfactory, she may be asked to leave at the end of the time required for a notice. If she is discharged without notice, it is customary to pay an employee for the time required for giving notice.

**Preservice Orientation Programs.** Most hospitals have an orientation program for new employees. Be sure to take advantage of this. Don't be afraid to tell the instructor about procedures in which you feel you need more practice. She will be happy to assist you to gain this extra knowledge and experience. If you are applying for a job, be sure to ask about the orientation program; this might be your reason for accepting the position.

The new graduate must remember that she needs further education and experience to become a fully contributing LPN in today's health team.

## Other Considerations

**Keeping Abreast of New Knowledge.** As a student you were learning new things every day with your instructors to guide you, and you had a library to keep you informed and up-to-date on new developments in nursing and health care. As a graduate practical nurse you are on your own and must turn to other sources of information. These sources are all around you. Books and magazine articles will help to keep you informed about scientific discoveries which are improving the treatment of disease. Radio and TV programs discuss health problems. Workshops, conferences, and conventions will be available, through which you can learn how to improve your care of patients. Many hospitals maintain in-service education programs for employee groups to keep them informed about new developments in hospital and nursing procedures. The nurse who does not take advantage of these opportunities to improve her knowledge is in danger of finding herself bringing up the rear in the march of progress. It is vital to subscribe to nursing journals so that you can keep up-to-date.

**The State Practical Nurse Association.** Every licensed practical nurse has an obligation to support and participate in the activities of her state practical nurse association. She can join through the local division where she lives. The activities of these associations were discussed in Chapter 1. The state practical nurse associations have done and are presently doing a great number of things for their members. Everyone knows that a group working together can get things done which one person never could accomplish alone. A representative of the local division may be given an opportunity to tell your student group about the activities of the association in your area and how you can join. Your instructors will also have this information. *The National Association for Practical Nurse Education and Service (NAPNES), The National Federation of Licensed Practical Nurses (NFLPN),* and *The National League for Nursing (NLN)* are the national organizations with a special interest in the education and the activities of practical nurses. Practical nurses are eligible for membership in these organizations.

The NLN is an organization with its membership open to both individuals and agencies. In addition to professional nurses, practical nurses, and those in the paramedical professions, interested laymen may join. Agency membership includes organizations and groups involved in nursing service, and schools or departments which provide educational programs in nursing. Other organizations may join as allied agency members. Membership in the NLN gives the practical nurse a broad view of current areas of nursing education and service, by bringing her into contact with many people interested in community health problems. The test service offered to student practical nurses by the NLN was discussed in Chapter 1. It has also recently established a program of accreditation for schools of practical nursing.

**Alumnae Associations.** Many schools have an alumnae association. Among their many activities are student recruitment programs, the establishment of scholarship and loan funds, and fund raising events to purchase needed educational equipment for the school. Most schools today also have some form of student government. This group should work closely with the alumnae association and the faculty. Together they can do much to maintain high standards of nursing practice.

**Your Personal Plans.** Your work life is affected by your personal life. Plan recreation for yourself. Sir William Osler said: "No man is really happy or safe without a hobby . . . anything will do so long as he straddles a hobby and rides it hard." This is good advice because your personal satisfaction is reflected in your work.

Make a plan for financial security. Annuities and retirement plans can be budgeted through your best earning years. Apply for your Social Security account number. Invest in a health examination once a year; it is cheaper than being sick or disabled. Get hospitalization and medical care insurance with a reliable group plan—just in case! Widen your interests; do not wrap yourself up in your work so completely that you feel life is over when you reach the retirement age. All this is insurance for a safer and happier life when you are older, but it begins to pay dividends in peace of mind long before that time comes.

# 59

# The Legal Aspects of Practical Nursing

---

## BEHAVIORAL OBJECTIVES

*The student successfully attaining the goals of this chapter will be able to:*

- *discuss licensing laws for practical nursing; differentiate between a mandatory licensing law and a permissive licensing law and identify which law exists in the state in which the nurse lives.*

- *describe the procedure by which a nurse becomes licensed in the particular jurisdiction in which he or she lives; follow through on this by becoming duly licensed after graduation from an approved nursing program.*

- *describe the role of the State Board of Nursing; define the nurse practice act in the jurisdiction where the nurse lives; discuss interstate endorsement; and discuss actions which might cause the nurse's license to be revoked.*

- *discuss the legal responsibilities of the nurse as they relate to some of the more common situations which might arise; protect herself or himself by keeping current malpractice insurance; and practice nursing in such a way as to prevent any chance of legal action.*

- *discuss the particular role of the nurse in an emergency; determine whether or not there is a "Good Samaritan" law in the state where the nurse lives; and practice within the legal confines of the laws of that state.*

- *briefly discuss the importance of the written records kept by the nurse; and discuss the legal rights of the nurse in the place of employment.*

- *practice nursing at all times in such a way as to maintain professional and personal integrity and the highest possible standards of patient care.*

- *practice nursing in such a way as to be a good model for others.*

---

## The Licensing Law

The legal aspects of practical nursing begin with the licensing law, which gives the practical nurse the legal right to practice nursing; also, it defines her responsibilities. This was discussed previously in Chapter 1, where it was mentioned that every state, as well as the District of Columbia, Puerto Rico, Guam, Samoa, and the Virgin Islands, has a law for licensing practical nurses. It was also pointed out that in some states the law is *mandatory,* making it illegal for a practical nurse to practice nursing for pay without a license, while in other states, the law is *permissive,* making it illegal to use the title *Licensed Practical Nurse (L.P.N.)* or *Licensed Vocational Nurse (L.V.N.)* without a license. A mandatory law protects the practice of nursing, but a permissive law protects only the title. Some states have changed the licensing laws from permissive to mandatory; others are working toward such a change.

The practical nurse licensing laws vary in other respects from state to state in their requirements for licensure. It is hoped that eventually more uniform requirements can be established in order that a license issued in one state will be recognized in all other states. This is not true at the present time, but the situation is improving.

**The Licensing Examination.** *The graduate nurse's first responsibility* is to pass the licensing examination upon her successful completion of an approved practical nursing course and to obtain a license to work as a practical nurse.

Your school must send your application and a transcript of your records, and you must send the required fee to the State Board of Nursing, which is the authority responsible for giving the examination. Licensing examinations are given several times a year—the applicant will be notified of the time and the place. After passing the examination, she receives her license. If an applicant fails, she is given a chance to repeat the examination a limited number of times within a specified period, as stated in the law. After receiving her license, the practical nurse is responsible for renewing it according to the regulations, and for keeping the board informed about any changes in her address, her name, or her employment status.

**The Nurse Practice Act.** The licensing law is called the Nurse Practice Act. It defines the title and the regulations governing the practice of practical nursing. In some states one nurse practice act covers the regulations for both professional and practical nurses and is administered under one board. In other states practical nursing is regulated by a separate act under a separate board. In many of the states with a single board, the law demands that a specified number of practical nurses serve as board members; this gives practical nurses a voice in affairs concerning them. The state practical nurse association makes recommendations for these appointments.

PROVISIONS IN A NURSE PRACTICE ACT. The law defines the regulations for practical nursing, including:

A definition of practical nursing.

The requirements for an approved school of practical nursing (length of the course, the curriculum, admission requirements).

Requirements for licensure (age, graduation from an approved course, the licensing examination).

Conditions under which a license may be suspended or voided.

THE STATE BOARD OF NURSING. The authority for administering the nurse practice act is the State Board of Nursing (sometimes known by other titles, such as the Board of Nurse Examiners). As stated previously, in some states practical nursing may be under a separate board. The board is responsible for approving schools of practical nursing, visiting the schools, administering the licensing examinations, and issuing and renewing practical nurse licenses; it also has the authority to suspend or revoke a license. The board is subject to the conditions defined in the law, but it usually has some leeway in its interpretation of these conditions.

INTERSTATE ENDORSEMENT. Interstate endorsement or "reciprocity" enables the practical nurse who is licensed in one state in the United States to transfer her licensure to another state. This may be done if her scores on the state board examination were high enough to be acceptable in the other state and if her school meets the state's educational requirements. If you have obtained your licensure by waiver or "grandfather clause," it is often not acceptable in another state. If you have any questions about the requirements for practicing as a Licensed Practical Nurse in another state, contact the State Board of Nursing in that state.

**Cause for Revoking or Suspending a License.** The law defines the conditions under which a license may be revoked. These conditions include unbecoming conduct, such as habitual drunkenness; serious crimes, such as robbery or murder; serious negligence in caring for patients, or practices which might endanger patients, such as drug addiction.

## Legal Responsibilities in Nursing Service

In the course of her activities, the practical nurse encounters many situations which involve legal responsibilities. She will be held responsible for maintaining the standards of nursing care which are set up for practical nursing. She may be found negligent: if she performs nursing procedures that she has not been taught, or if she fails to meet established standards for the safe care of patients or for preventing injury to hospital employees and visitors (for which she may consequently be sued for damages).

**Negligence.** One of the most common causes of lawsuits instigated by patients is negligence. Negligence is defined as harm done to a patient as a result of neglecting the ordinary precautions expected of a responsible person.

Some common types of situations which might cause injury to a person and involve legal liability are: (1) burns—from hot-water bags, heating pads, contact with steam pipes or scalding water; from chemicals by either improper mixture or application; (2) sponges overlooked in surgical wounds; (3) falls on slippery floors; (4) falls from an unprotected bed or crib by an unconscious patient (children and adults must be protected by side rails or other means, according to age and physical and mental condition); (5) injury from the wrong medicine or from the wrong dosage; and (6) injury from visibly defective or improperly tested equipment.

A damage suit may be instituted against a nurse for any injury caused by her failure to observe hospital regulations established to protect the patient or to care for his belongings. The patient is likely to have certain property which must be protected from loss, theft, or damage, and proper safeguards must be observed in the care of money, jewelry, dentures, spectacles, and clothing. When the nurse or the hospital takes over the care of property, she and/or the hospital will be held responsible for it.

*Lack of sleep or overwork will not be accepted as legal reasons for carelessness about safety measures or mistakes in medicines.*

**Personal Liability.** Although a practical nurse works under the direction of professional nurses and physicians, she is personally liable for any harm a patient suffers as a result of her own acts. In a hospital, her employer may also be legally liable for her acts of negligence.

Legal actions involving negligent acts by a person engaged in a professional field are generally known as *malpractice suits*. Many people doing this type of work protect themselves from possible legal suits by carrying *malpractice insurance*. This insurance is available through private insurance companies or sometimes through the hospital or the professional organization. It is usually inexpensive and well worth the investment. Usually, the insurance covers legal fees and sometimes the judgment expenses, in the event the nurse is sued for malpractice. It generally covers only expenses involved in a suit for a nursing act. It will not cover other types of liability suits.

**Criminal Liability.** A crime involves the deliberate commission or omission of an act forbidden or required by law. As a citizen, a nurse knows that acts such as murder and robbery are illegal. There are other laws which she, as a nurse, must be equally careful not to violate. For example, the federal law requires that records be kept on dispensing narcotics. This law specifies that narcotics must be given under the direction and the supervision of a physician, a dentist, or a veterinarian and that all unused portions be returned to the physician, the dentist, or the veterinarian. In a hospital all narcotics are kept under lock and key, and every tablet must be accounted for (see Chapter 33).

**Intentional Invasion of a Patient's Rights.** A nurse may be held liable for damages arising from intentional acts which invade the personal rights protected by law. Civil suits may ask damages from assault and battery, false imprisonment, restraint of movement, slander, and libel.

When a patient enters the hospital, presumably he gives his consent to being treated. He may withhold his consent to certain acts. Surgery, the giving of certain medications or treatments, the administration of blood, and restraining a patient for his own protection involve a violation of his rights, if his consent is withheld. Consent may be given verbally, but in some cases (especially surgery) there *must* be a written permission. The practical nurse has an obligation to follow the policies of her hospital or employer in this matter; in cases where there is any doubt, she should notify her superior. Sometimes, the patient is asked to sign a "waiver" which states that he will not hold the hospital or doctor liable if the patient, for example, refuses surgery or a blood transfusion.

Every person has the right of protection of

his privacy, which is the right to withhold himself and his property from the public eye. For example, stories or photographs of a patient must not be given out without his written consent. Physical freedom is another personal right, unless it has been removed legally following the conviction for a crime or the declaration of mental incompetence. Therefore, if a nurse should confine a patient against his will, she could be liable to a suit for false imprisonment.

A patient's rights may be invaded in ways other than physical damage. If untrue and damaging statements are made about a person, the one who made such verbal statements may be sued for *slander;* if the statements were in writing, the suit would be for *libel.*

**Legal Responsibility in an Emergency.** In some states a person who is involved in an automobile accident is required by law to give aid to a person injured in that accident. This is on a par with the law which makes a hit-and-run driver liable to prosecution for leaving the scene of an accident. Other than areas where this law applies, no person is legally obligated to render aid during an emergency. However, when one voluntarily does so, he should act as a reasonably prudent person would.

In a true emergency situation, which involves saving a life, a medical act involving recognized first-aid practices *only* can be performed without being considered a violation of medical practice, whether it is performed by a professional nurse, a practical nurse, or a layman. However, it must be remembered that substantial proof must be presented in court which will attest that it was in fact an emergency situation. It must also be remembered that in such legal cases, the nurse, who has had more training and experience than the layman, will be considered as being more capable of evaluating an emergency situation and will be held *more* responsible for the consequences of her actions.

**Legal Advice.** A nurse should never attempt to advise a patient on his legal rights; he should be encouraged to confer with his family and to consult his attorney. The laws governing the personal and property rights of an individual are many and complex. Professional advice is essential to ensure proper protection.

**Gifts.** Sometimes an ill person will wish to transfer his personal property to his family or friends, if he has not already made a will. If this is done because he expects to die, the gift is known as a gift *causa mortis;* in the event that the donor does not die, the gift may be revoked. There are many technicalities in the law regarding gifts, which cover the intention to give, the delivery of the property, and its acceptance.

**Wills.** A nurse should never attempt to help a patient draw up a will. The law has very formal requirements which a will must meet to make it valid. The law generally requires 2 or more witnesses to the signing of a will; the number varies in the different states. Because of this variance, it is better to have at least 3 witnesses. Certain formalities govern the signing of a will; generally, the will must be declared to be a last will and must be signed in the presence of witnesses, who then must sign in the presence of each other. They must witness the signature of the patient making the will, as well as the affixing of the names, or the marks, of the other witnesses.

A nurse may be called upon to witness a will in the performance of her duties. The student nurse, however, should *never* witness any legal document. After the death of a patient, the nurse, as well as the other witnesses, may be called upon to testify to the mental competence of the testator or to other conditions prevailing at the time of the execution of the will. This will enable the court to determine whether or not all legal requirements were met in drawing up the document.

**The Importance of the Written Record.** We cannot emphasize too strongly the importance of keeping exact records of all treatments, medications and everything which is done for or which happens to the patient, as well as a record of the patient's behavior. The patient's chart is the written evidence of his treatment during his stay in the hospital, or of occurrences in the home. Be sure to state only facts, and *not* to make judgments.

**The Nurse's Legal Rights.** In employment, a nurse has a right to legal protection by contract (oral or written) which states the terms of her employment in relation to her duties and salary. If either party fails to live up to the terms, the contract can be terminated.

# Glossary

**Abdomen** (ab-do′men), that portion of the body lying between the chest and the pelvis.

**Abnormal** (ab-nor′mal), contrary to normal.

**Abrasion** (ab-ra′zhun), a scraping or rubbing off of the skin.

**Abscess** (ab′ses), a local collection of pus in the tissues.

**Absorption** (ab-sorp′shun), the taking up of fluids or other substances by the skin and the tissues.

**Acceleration** (ak-sel-er-a′shun), a quickening of rate, as of the pulse or respiration.

**Accreditation** (ah-kred-i-ta′shun), attaining standards approved by recognized authority.

**Acid** (as′id), a chemical compound having properties opposed to those of the alkalis.

**Acute** (ah-kute′), a sudden, poignant illness of short duration but with severe symptoms.

**Addiction** (ah-dik′shun), a compulsion to use drugs or stimulants habitually.

**Adenitis** (ad-e-ni′tis), inflamation of a gland.

**Adenoids** (ad′en-oids), glandular growths at the back of the nose, behind the palate.

**Adhesion** (ad-he′zhun), the abnormal joining of tissues by a fibrous band, usually resulting from inflammation or injury.

**Adipose** (ad′i-pose), fatty.

**Adolescence** (ad-o-les′ens), the period of development between childhood and adulthood.

**Aerosol** (a′er-o-sol), a solution of a drug or a bacteriocidal solution which can be atomized into a spray form.

**After-birth** (af′ter-berth), a mass of tissue, consisting of the membranes and the placenta with the attached umbilical cord, which is cast off after the expulsion of the fetus.

**Albolene** (al′bo-lene), an oily, white substance derived from petroleum.

**Albumin** (al-bu′min), a protein substance found in animal and vegetable tissues.

**Alimentary canal** (al-im-en′ta-re kan-al′), the passage leading from the mouth, the stomach and the intestines to the outer opening of the rectum.

**Alkali** (al′ka-li), a compound which neutralizes acids.

**Allergy** (al′er-je), a state in which the body is hypersensitive to some protein.

**Alleviate** (a-le′vi-ate), to lessen or make easier to endure.

**Alopecia** (al-o-pe′she-ah), loss of hair from skin where it normally appears.

**Ambulatory** (am′bu-la-to-re), walking or able to walk.

**Amenorrhea** (ah-men-o-re′ah), absence or abnormal stoppage of menses.

**Amnesia** (am-ne′se-ah), loss of memory.

**Amputation** (am-pu-ta′shun), cutting off of a limb or other part of the body.

**Analgesic** (an-al-je′sik), relieving pain.

**Anastomosis** (ah-nas-to-mo′sis), the joining together of 2 normally distinct spaces or organs.

**Anemia** (ah-ne′me-ah), a deficiency of the blood in quality or quantity.

**Anesthetic** (an-es-thet′ik), a substance which produces loss of feeling or sensation.

**Ankylosis** (an-ki-lo′sis), abnormal consolidation of a joint which prevents motion.

**Anodyne** (an′o-din), a medicine that relieves pain.

**Anomaly** (a-nom′ah-le), a deviation from the normal.

**Anorexia** (an-o-rek′se-ah), lack or loss of appetite for food.

**Anoxia** (an-ok′se-ah), a decrease of oxygen below the normal level in body tissues.

**Anthelmintic** (ant-hel-min′tik), an agent that destroys worms.

**Antibody** (an′ti-bod-e), a specific blood substance which neutralizes foreign bodies.

**Antidote** (an′ti-dote), a remedy that will counteract or remove the effect of poison.

**Antiemetic** (an-ti-e-met′ik), an agent that prevents or relieves nausea and vomiting.

**Antipyretic** (an-ti-pi-ret′ik), an agent that relieves or reduces fever.

**Antiseptic** (an-ti-sep′tik), a substance that inhibits the growth of microorganisms without necessarily destroying them.

**Antispasmodic** (an-ti-spas-mod′ik), an agent that relieves muscular spasm.

**Antitoxins** (an-te-tok′sins), substances found in the blood and other body fluids which counteract the harmful effect of the toxins or the poisons to which they are allied.

**Anuria** (an-u′re-ah), total suppression of urine.

**Anus** (a′nus), the outer opening, or outlet, of the rectum.

**Aortitis** (a-or-ti′tis), inflammation of the aorta.

**Aphagia** (ah-fa′je-ah), inability to swallow.

**Aphasia** (ah-fa′ze-ah), inability to express oneself by speech or writing.

**Aphonia** (ah-fo′ne-ah), loss of voice.

**Apnea** (ap′ne-ah), a temporary cessation of breathing.

**Apoplexy** (ap′o-plek-se), a paralysis commonly referred to as a "stroke," resulting from a cerebral vascular accident.

**Appendix** (ah-pen′diks), a slender wormlike tube, connected to the large intestines at the lower end of the cecum.

**Apprehension** (ap-re-hen′shun), anxiety or fear.

**Area** (a′re-ah), a limited surface.

**Arrhythmia** (ah-rith′me-ah), absence of rhythm, particularly in relation to the abnormality in the rhythm of the heart.

**Artery** (ar′ter-e), any one of the vessels through which the blood passes from the heart to all the different parts of the body.

**Artificial** (ar-ti-fish′al), not natural.

**Aseptic** (ah-sep′tik), free from disease germs.

**Asphyxia** (as-fix′e-ah), suffocation.

**Aspiration** (as-pi-ra′shun), withdrawal of fluid or gas from a cavity by means of suction.

**Assimilation** (ah-sim-i-la′shun), the process of changing food into living tissue.

**Asthma** (az′mah), a disease marked by difficulty in breathing due to spasmodic contractions of the bronchial tubes.

**Astringent** (as-trin′jent), an agent that causes contraction and arrests discharges.

**Ataxia** (ah-tak′se-ah), failure or irregularity of muscle coordination.

**Atomizer** (at′om-i-zer), an instrument for throwing a jet of spray.

**Atonic** (ah-ton′ik), lacking normal tone or strength.

**Atresia** (ah-tre′ze-ah), a closing or congenital absence of a normal anatomical opening.

**Atrophy** (a′tro-fe), a decrease in size or wasting away of a cell, tissue, organ or part.

**Audiometer** (au-de-om′et-er), an instrument to test the acuity of the hearing.

**Aura** (aw′rah), a subjective sensation experienced by a person prior to a seizure such as an epileptic attack.

**Aural** (aw′al), pertaining to the ear.

**Auscultation** (aw-skul-ta′shun), listening to sounds within the body to determine abnormal conditions.

**Autopsy** (aw′top-se), examination of the organs of a dead body.

**Auxiliary** (awk-sil′e-a-re), that which assists or helps.

**Axilla** (ak-sil′ah), the armpit.

**Bacteremia** (bak-ter-e′me-ah), the presence of bacteria in the blood.

**Bacteria** (bak-te′re-ah), disease germs or microbes.

**Benign** (be-nine′), doing no harm; not malignant.

**Biliary** (bil′e-a-re), pertaining to bile, the liver, the gallbladder and the associated ducts.

**Biopsy** (bi′op-se), removal of a piece of body tissue for diagnostic examination, usually microscopic.

**Blood pressure** (blud presh′ur), the pressure of the blood on the elastic walls of the arteries.

**Bradycardia** (brad-e-kar′de-ah), abnormally slow heart action.

**Bright's disease** (brites dis-eze′), a kidney disease accompanied by albumin in the urine.

**Bronchitis** (brong-ki′tis), inflammation of the bronchial tubes.

**Bronchoscope** (brong′ko-skope), a lighted instrument used for the examination of the interior of the bronchi.

**Buccal** (buk′al), pertaining to the cheek or mouth.

**Buttocks** (but′oks), the prominence of muscle and fat on the posterior part of the body at the hip line.

**Calculus** (kal′ku-lus), an abnormal concretion, usually composed of mineral salts, occurring within the body.

**Callosity** (kal-os′it-e), a hardening and thickening of the skin.

**Callus** (kal′us), a callosity; the bony material that makes the union between the ends of fractured bones.

**Calorie** (kal′o-re), a unit of heat.

**Capsule** (kap′sul), a small gelatinous case for holding a dose of medicine.

**Carbon dioxide** (kar′bon di-ok′sid), a colorless gas which is exhaled in respiration.

**Carbon monoxide** (kar′bon mon-ok′sid), a colorless poisonous gas which is found in coal gas, automobile exhaust, etc.

**Carcinoma** (kar-sin-o′mah), a cancer.

**Cardiac** (kar′de-ak), pertaining to the heart.

**Cardiograph** (kar′de-o-graf), an instrument for recording the action of the heart.

**Carrier** (kar′e-er), an individual who harbors in his body the specific organisms of a disease without manifesting its symptoms and thus acts as a distributor or transmitter of the infection.

**Cast** (kast), an appliance to render immovable displaced or injured parts.

**Cathartic** (kath-ar′tik), a medicine that causes the evacuation of the bowels.

**Cavity** (kav′it-e), a hollow space within the body or within one of its organs.

**Cell** (sel), the minute protoplasmic building unit of living matter.

**Cephalic** (se-fal′ik), pertaining to the head.

**Cervical** (ser′vi-kal), pertaining to the neck or cervix of any structure.

**Chancre** (shang′ker), the primary lesion of syphilis.

**Chemotherapy** (ke-mo-ther'ah-pe), the use of chemical agents to treat disease.

**Chest** (chest), the thorax; the part of the body which lies between the neck and the abdominal cavity.

**Chorea** (ko-re'ah), St. Vitus' dance; a nervous disease characterized by involuntary jerking muscular movements.

**Ciliated** (sil'e-a-ted), provided with a fringe of hairlike processes.

**Cirrhosis** (sir-ro'sis), chronic inflammation and degeneration of an organ, especially the liver.

**Clavicle** (klav'i-kil), the collar bone.

**Clinical** (klin'ik-al), pertaining to instruction at the bedside or actual treatment of the patient, as distinguished from theoretical or experimental.

**Coagulation** (ko-ag-u-la'shun), the changing of a liquid to a thickened, curdlike form.

**Colic** (kol'ik), acute abdominal pain.

**Colitis** (ko-li'tis), inflammation of the colon.

**Colon** (ko'lon), the main part of the large intestine, extending from the cecum to the rectum.

**Colostomy** (ko-los'to-me), an artificial opening into the colon.

**Colostrum** (ko-los'trum), the fluid secreted by the mammary (breast) glands a few days before or after childbirth.

**Coma** (ko'mah), profound stupor due to disease or injury.

**Communicable disease** (ko-mun'ni-ka-bil), a disease that can be transmitted from one person to another.

**Concentrated** (kon'sen-tra-ted), made stronger.

**Concurrent** (kon-kur'ent), happening at the same time.

**Congenital** (kon-jen'it-al), existing at or before birth.

**Congestion** (kon-jest'yun), an abnormal accumulation of blood in a part of the body.

**Conscious** (kon'shus), mentally awake.

**Consistency** (kon-sis'ten-se), the degree of firmness or stiffness.

**Constipation** (kon-stip-a'shun), difficult or infrequent movement of the bowels.

**Contagion** (kon-ta'jun), the communication of disease from one person to another.

**Contaminate** (kon-tam'i-nate), to make unsterile or unclean by contact.

**Contraindication** (kon-trah-in-di-ka'shun), any condition which makes a form of treatment undesirable.

**Contusion** (kon-tu'zhun), a bruise.

**Convalescence** (kon-val-es'ens), the return to health after an attack of disease.

**Convulsions** (kon-vul'shuns), involuntary contractions of the voluntary muscles.

**Copulation** (kope-u-la'shun), sexual intercourse between the male and the female.

**Cornea** (kor'ne-ah), the transparent front part of the eye.

**Coronary thrombosis** (kor'o-na-re throm-bo'sis), a clot in a coronary artery.

**Corrosive** (ko-ro'siv), destructive to the tissue.

**Coryza** (ko-ri'zah), a cold in the head with an acute inflammation of the nasal mucous membrane.

**Counterirritants** (kown-ter-ir'it-ants), agents used to produce a superficial irritation and thus to relieve irritation or inflammation existing elsewhere.

**Crisis** (kri'sis), the turning point of a disease.

**Cyanosis** (si-an-o'sis), blueness of the skin due to the deficiency of oxygen and the excess of carbon dioxide in the blood.

**Cyst** (sist), a sac containing liquid or soft material.

**Cystitis** (sis-ti'tus), inflammation of the urinary bladder.

**Debility** (de-bil'i-te), loss or lack of strength.

**Decompose** (de-com-poze'), to decay; to rot.

**Decubitus** (de-ku'bi-tus), a bed or pressure sore.

**Defecation** (def-e-ka'shun), the discharge of fecal matter from the intestines.

**Defect** (de'fect), an imperfection or failure.

**Degeneration** (de-jen-er-a'shun), deterioration from a higher to a lower form.

**Dehydration** (de-hi-dra'shun), the removal of water.

**Delirium** (de-lir'e-um), a mental disturbance, usually temporary, marked by cerebral excitement, wandering speech, illusions and hallucinations.

**Delusion** (de-lu'zhun), a false belief that cannot be corrected by reason.

**Dementia** (de-men'she-ah), deterioration of mental capacity.

**Demulcent** (de-mul'sent), a bland, soothing medication or application.

**Denture** (den'tur), an artificial set of teeth.

**Deodorant** (de-o'der-ant), an agent that destroys unpleasant odors.

**Depilatory** (de-pil'at-o-re), a preparation for removing superfluous hair.

**Depression** (de-presh'un), lowered mental and physical activity.

**Dermatitis** (derm-ah-ti'tis), an inflammatory condition of the skin.

**Desquamation** (des-kwa-ma'shun), the shedding or scaling of the skin or cuticle.

**Detergent** (de-ter'jent), a cleansing or purifying agent.

**Deviation** (de-ve-a'shun), a turning aside.

**Diagnosis** (di-ag-no'sis), the recognition of a disease by its signs and symptoms.

**Diaphoresis** (di-ah-fo-re'sis), profuse perspiration.

**Diaphragm** (di'af-ram), the muscular partition between the thoracic and the abdominal cavities.

**Diarrhea** (di-ar-e'ah), abnormal frequency and fluidity of discharges from the bowels.

**Digestion** (di-jest'yun), the process of converting food into materials which can be assimilated and absorbed by the tissues.

**Dilatation** (dil-ah-ta'shun), a stretching of a part beyond normal dimensions.

**Dilute** (di-lute'), to make weaker or more fluid by mixture.

**Disease** (dis-eze'), a condition which is a departure from the normal health of the body or the mind.

**Disinfectant** (dis-in-fek'tant), an agent that frees from infection by destroying germs.

**Disorientation** (dis-o-re-en-ta'shun), a state of mental confusion or loss of bearings.

**Distention** (dis-ten'shun), the state of being enlarged.

**Diuresis** (di-u-re'sis), increased secretion of urine.

**Divergence** (di-ver'jens), a spreading apart or deviation from the normal course.

**Dorsal** (dor'sal), pertaining to the back.

**Douche** (doosh), a stream of water or other fluid directed against a part of a body or into a body cavity.

**Dropsy** (drop'se), an abnormal accumulation of serous fluid in the tissues.

**Dysentery** (dis'en-ter-e), a disorder accompanied by inflammation of the intestines and marked by pain and frequent stools containing blood and mucus.

**Dysfunction** (dis-funk'shun), abnormal functioning of an organ.

**Dysmenorrhea** (dis-men-o-re'ah), difficult and painful menstruation.

**Dysphagia** (dis-fa'je-ah), difficulty in swallowing.

**Dyspnea** (disp'ne-ah), difficulty in breathing.

**Dystrophy** (dis'tro-fe), a disorder arising from impaired nutrition, usually referring to muscles.

**Dysuria** (dis-u're-ah), difficult or painful urination.

**Ecchymosis** (ek-i-mos'sis), bleeding into the tissues under the skin.

**Eczema** (ek'ze-mah), a skin disease, with itching and red scaly patches.

**Edema** (e-de'mah), swelling due to an accumulation of watery fluid in the tissues.

**Elimination** (e-lim-in-a'shun), the act of expelling from the body.

**Emaciation** (e-ma-se-a'shun), a wasting away of the flesh causing extreme leanness.

**Embolus** (em'bo-lus), any foreign substance or an air bubble brought to a vessel by the blood, and which partially or completely obstructs the flow of blood.

**Emesis** (em'e-sis), the act of vomiting.

**Emetic** (e-met'ik), an agent that causes vomiting.

**Emollient** (e-mol'e-ent), a soothing medicine.

**Emphysema** (em-fi-se'mah), an inflation or swelling of the tissues due to the presence of air.

**Empyema** (em-pi-e'mah), collection of pus in a body cavity.

**Enteritis** (en-ter-i'tis), inflammation of the intestines.

**Enucleation** (e-nu-kle-a'shun), the surgical removal of the eyeball.

**Enuresis** (en-u-re'sis), involuntary discharge of urine, usually referring to the hours of sleep.

**Environment** (en-vir'on-ment), the surroundings.

**Epidemic** (ep-i-dem'ik), widespread disease in a certain geographical region.

**Epidermis** (ep-i-der'mis), the outermost layer of the skin.

**Epilepsy** (ep'il-ep-se), a chronic disease marked by attacks of convulsions.

**Epistaxis** (ep-e-stak'sis), nosebleed.

**Eructation** (e-ruk-ta'shun), forceful expulsion of air from the stomach, known commonly as belching.

**Eruption** (e-rup'shun), a breaking out of the skin due to disease.

**Erythema** (er-i-the'mah), redness of the skin due to the congestion of the capillaries.

**Etiology** (e-te-ol'o-je), the sum of knowledge regarding the cause of a disease.

**Euphoria** (u-fo're-ah), a general feeling of comfort and well being.

**Eustachian tube** (u-sta'ke-an tube), the passage from the throat to the middle ear.

**Euthanasia** (u-thah-na'ze-ah), an easy or painless death, often referred to as mercy death.

**Evisceration** (e-vis-er-a'shun), the removal of the abdominal organs, or the protrusion of the intestines through an abdominal wound.

**Excoriation** (eks-ko-re-a'shun), the removal of pieces of skin as a result of scratching or scraping.

**Excreta** (eks-kre'tah), waste matter discharged from the body, such as feces, urine, vomitus, etc.

**Excreted** (eks-kre'ted), thrown off, as waste matter, by a normal discharge.

**Exhaustion** (eks-awst'yun), the loss of vital power.

**Expectoration** (eks-pek-to-ra'shun), spitting out mucus or other fluid from the lungs and the throat.

**Expiration** (eks-pi-ra'shun), exhaling air from the lungs; sometimes used to refer to death.

**Exudate** (eks'u-date), material that has escaped from blood vessels and is deposited in the tissues or on tissue surfaces.

**Fahrenheit** (far'en-hite), a thermometer scale in which the boiling point of water is 212° and the freezing point is 32°.

**Faint** (faint), loss of consciousness due to insufficient blood in the brain.

**Fatigue** (fah-tig'), weariness resulting from over-exertion of the body or the mind.

**Febrile** (fe'bril), pertaining to a fever.

**Fecal** (fe'kal), pertaining to feces.

**Feces** (fe'seze), the residue from digested food which is discharged from the intestines.

**Fester** (fes'ter), to suppurate superficially.

**Fetid** (fe'tid), having a disagreeable odor.

**Fever** (fe'ver), abnormally high body temperature.

**Fibrous** (fi'brus), composed of or containing fibers.

**Fimbriated** (fim'bre-at-ed), fringed.

**Flaccid** (flak'sid), weak, lax or lacking muscle tone.

**Flatus** (fla'tus), gas in the intestines or the stomach.

**Flex** (fleks), to bend.

**Fomite** (fo'mite), any object that may harbor or transmit pathogenic organisms without being corrupted itself.

**Foreign body** (for'in bod'e), any substance lodged in a place where it does not belong.

**Formula** (for'mu-lah), a prescribed method of preparation.

**Fracture** (frak'tur), a break in a bone.

**Friction** (frik'shun), rubbing.

**Fumigation** (fum-i-ga'shun), the use of disinfecting fumes to destroy living organisms.

**Function** (funk'shun), the normal action of a part of an organ.

**Fusion** (fu'zhun), the joining together of two adjacent parts or bodies.

**Gait** (gate), a manner or style of walking.

**Gall** (gawl), the bile.

**Gangrene** (gan'green), the death of a part or a tissue.

**Gargle** (gar'gul), a solution to rinse the mouth or throat.

**Gastric** (gas'trik), pertaining to the stomach.

**Gavage** (gah-vahzh'), passing food into the stomach through a tube.

**Geriatrics** (jer-e-at'riks), the branch of medicine that deals with old age and its related diseases, including the psychosocial problems of senility.

**Germicidal** (jer-mi-si'dal), destructive to germs.

**Germs** (jerms), bacteria; microbes.

**Gestation** (jes-ta'shun), the period of development of the individual from fertilization to birth.

**Gland** (gland), an organ by means of which a secretion is produced.

**Glossitis** (glos-si'tis), inflammation of the tongue.

**Glucose** (gloo'kose), a form of sugar.

**Gluteal** (gloo'te-al), pertaining to the buttocks.

**Goiter** (goi'ter), an enlargement of the thyroid gland, causing a swelling in the front part of the neck.

**Graft** (graft), a piece of skin or other tissue from one part of the body which is implanted on another part.

**Granulation** (gran-u-la'shun), the formation of fleshy tissue in healing wounds.

**Groin** (groin), the lowest part of the abdominal wall, where it joins the thigh.

**Gynecology** (jin-e-kol'o-je), the science that treats diseases of women, particularly those of the genital organs.

**Hallucination** (ha-lu-si-na'shun), seeing, hearing or feeling something when there is no objective stimulus.

**Heliotherapy** (he-le-o-ther'ah-pe), treatment of disease by exposing the body to the sun's rays.

**Hematemesis** (hem-at-em'e-sis), vomiting of blood.

**Hematocrit** (he-mat'o-krit), the volume percentage of red blood cells in whole blood.

**Hematuria** (hem-ah-tu're-ah), discharge of blood in the urine.

**Hemoglobin** (he-mo-glo'bin), the coloring matter of the blood.

**Hemoptysis** (he-mop'ti-sis), expectoration of blood or blood-stained sputum.

**Hemorrhage** (hem'or-aje), bleeding; an escape of blood from the arteries, veins or capillaries.

**Hemorrhoids** (hem'or-oids), a dilatation of the veins of the anal region.

**Hemothorax** (hem-o-tho'raks), presence of blood in the pleural cavity.

**Heredity** (he-red'it-e), the inheritance of physical or mental characteristics from ancestors.

**Herpes** (her'peze), fever blisters; cold sores.

**Hiccup** (hik'up), an involuntary spasmodic contraction of the diaphragm caused by the irritation of the phrenic nerve, which produces a sharp, inspiratory cough.

**Hirsutism** (her'sut-izm), abnormal hairiness, particularly in women.

**Homeopathy** (hom-e-op'ath-e), a system of medical practice which treats disease by the administration of small doses of medications which, if administered to a healthy person, would produce the symptoms of the disease being treated.

**Host** (host), a plant or animal which harbors or nourishes another organism.

**Humidity** (hu-mid'it-e), moisture in the atmosphere.

**Hydronephrosis** (hi-dro-ne-fro'sis), distention of the pelvis and calyces of the kidney with urine, as a result of obstruction of the ureter.

**Hydrotherapy** (hi-dro-ther'ap-e), the use of water in the treatment of disease.

**Hydrothorax** (hi-dro-tho'raks), collection of watery fluid in the pleural cavity.

**Hygiene** (hi'jene), the science and the preservation of health.

**Hyperalgesia** (hi-per-al-je′ze-ah), increased sensitiveness to pain.

**Hyperemia** (hi-per-e′me-ah), excessive blood in a part due to local or general relaxation of the arterioles.

**Hyperopia** (hi-per-o′pe-ah), farsightedness.

**Hypertension** (hi-per-ten′shun), chronic elevation of blood pressure.

**Hypertrophy** (hi-per′trof-e), a diseased enlargement of a part or an organ.

**Hypnosis** (hip-no′sis), an artificially induced passive state resembling a trance.

**Hypochondriac** (hi-po-kon′dre-ak), a person with a morbid anxiety about his health.

**Hypoglycemia** (hi-po-gli-se′me-ah), an abnormally low amount of sugar in the blood.

**Hypomania** (hi-po-ma′ne-a), mania of a mild type.

**Hypotaxia** (hi-po-tak′se-ah), diminished control over the will or the actions.

**Hypotension** (hi-po-ten′shun), chronic depression in blood pressure.

**Hypothermia** (hi-po-ther′me-ah), a low body temperature.

**Hysterectomy** (his-ter-ek′to-me), the surgical removal of the uterus.

**Hysteria** (his-ter′e-ah), lack of emotional control or actions.

**Idiosyncrasy** (id-e-o-sin′krah-se), a personal peculiarity.

**Illusion** (i-lu′zhun), a false impression or interpretation of a sensory image.

**Immobilize** (im-mo′bil-ize), to prevent motion.

**Immunization** (im-u-niz-a′shun), protection against infection from any particular disease.

**Impacted** (im-pak′ted), firmly wedged in place.

**Incise** (in-size′), to cut.

**Incontinence** (in-kon′tin-ens), inability to refrain from the urge to urinate or defecate.

**Incubation** (in-ku-ba′shun), the period of a disease between the implanting of the germs and the manifestation of the symptoms of the disease.

**Infection** (in-fek′shun), the invasion of the body by disease-producing agents with a resulting reaction to their presence and their toxins.

**Inflammation** (in-flah-ma′shun), a condition resulting from irritation in any part of the body, marked by pain, heat, redness and swelling.

**Inhalation** (in-hah-la′shun), drawing air, vapor or fumes into the lungs.

**Inherent** (in-her′ent), belonging to anything as a result of natural circumstances.

**Inhibition** (in-hi-bish′un), the partial or complete restraint of any process.

**Injection** (in-jek′shun), forcing a liquid into a part of the body or into a body cavity.

**Inoculation** (in-ok-u-la′shun), introduction of a virus or disease-producing microorganism into the body to give protection against certain diseases.

**Insanity** (in-san′i-te), the legal or lay term referring to a mental derangement or disorder.

**Insecticide** (in-sek′ti-side), an agent that is destructive to insects.

**Insomnia** (in-som′ne-ah), sleeplessness.

**Intellect** (in′te-lekt), thinking ability or understanding.

**Intermittent** (in-ter-mit′ent), occurring at intervals.

**Intubation** (in-tu-ba′shun), the insertion of a tube, as in inserting a tube into the larynx in diphtheria to introduce air.

**Intussusception** (in-tus-sus-sep′shun), the telescoping or prolapsing of one part of the intestine into an adjacent part.

**Inuction** (in-ungk′shun), application or rubbing of an ointment on the skin.

**Involuntary** (in-vol′un-ta-re), not under the control of the will.

**Irrigation** (ir-i-ga′shun), washing out by a stream of water or a solution.

**Irritant** (ir′i-tant), an agent that causes stimulation or undue sensitiveness to any part of the body.

**Ischemia** (is-ke′me-ah), decrease of blood to a part as a result of the obstruction or constriction of blood vessels.

**Isolation** (i-so-la′shun), the separation of persons having infectious diseases from others.

**Isthmus** (is′mus), a narrow structure connecting 2 larger parts.

**Jaundice** (jawn′dis), a yellowish discoloration of the skin due to bile.

**Jejunectomy** (je-joo-nek′to-me), excision of part or all of the jejunum.

**Jurisprudence** (joor-is-proo′dens), the application or study of legal principles.

**Juvenile** (joo′ve-nile), pertaining to childhood or immaturity.

**Keloid** (ke′loid), a scar on the skin consisting of dense tissue, found most often in the Negro race.

**Keratitis** (ker-a-ti′tis), inflammation of the cornea.

**Ketosis** (ke-to′sis), an increase in ketone bodies in the body tissues and fluids.

**Koplik's spots** (kop′liks spots), bright red spots in the mouth and throat found in the early stages of measles.

**Kyphosis** (ki-fo′sis), an abnormal increase in the thoracic curvature of the spine giving a "hunchback" appearance.

**Laceration** (las-er-a′shun), a wound produced by tearing.

**Lacrimal** (lak′ri-mal), pertaining to tears.

**Lactation** (lak-ta'shun), secretion of milk.

**Lactose** (lak'tose), a sugar found in milk, commonly called "milk sugar."

**Lanolin** (lan'o-lin), wool fat.

**Laryngitis** (lar-in-ji'tis), inflammation of the larynx.

**Latent** (la'tent), a condition that is concealed or not manifest.

**Lateral** (lat'er-al), pertaining to a side.

**Lavage** (lah-vahzh), washing out of an organ, such as the stomach or bowel.

**Laxative** (laks'ah-tiv), a mild cathartic which acts to promote evacuation of the bowel.

**Lens** (lenz), a transparent crystalline structure in the eye which converges or scatters light rays as they focus images on the retina.

**Lentigo** (len-ti'go), small brownish pigmented areas on the skin due to an increased amount of melanin, commonly known as freckles.

**Lesion** (le'zhun), a break in the body tissue, such as a sore or a wound.

**Lethargy** (leth'ar-je), a condition of sluggishness or mental dullness.

**Leukorrhea** (lu-ko-re'ah), a whitish or yellowish viscid discharge from the vagina.

**Ligate** (li'gate), to bind or tie with a ligature.

**Liniment** (lin'e-ment), an oily preparation for rubbing on the skin.

**Lipoma** (li-po'mah), a benign tumor made up of fatty tissue.

**Local** (lo'kal), limited to one part or place; not general.

**Lochia** (lo'ke-ah), the vaginal discharge occurring a week or two following childbirth.

**Lordosis** (lor-do'sis), an abnormal increase in the lumbar curvature of the spine, sometimes called "swayback."

**Lotion** (lo'shun), a liquid used on the skin to soothe, heal or cleanse.

**Lubricant** (lu'bri-cant), an oily substance that relieves friction.

**Lumbar region** (lum'bar re'jun), that part of the back between the pelvis and the thorax.

**Lumen** (lu'men), a tube or channel within a tube or tubular organ.

**Lymphoma** (lim-fo'mah), any malignant condition of lymphoid tissue.

**Malignant** (ma-lig'nant), deadly, tending to go from bad to worse.

**Malingering** (mah-ling'ger-ing), a deliberate feigning or exaggeration of the symptoms of illness or injury, usually to arouse sympathy.

**Malpractice** (mal-prak'tis), injurious or faulty treatment that results in injury, loss or damage.

**Mania** (ma'ne-ah), a disordered mental state of extreme excitement.

**Margin** (mar'jin), a boundary line; an edge.

**Massage** (mah-sahzh'), applying friction to or stroking and kneading the body tissues for therapeutic measures.

**Masticate** (mas'ti-kate), to chew food.

**Mastitis** (mas-ti'tis), inflammation of the breast.

**Mastoiditis** (mas-toid-i'tis), inflammation of the mastoid bone.

**Masturbation** (mas-tur-ba'shun), the handling of the genitals to obtain pleasant sensations.

**Maturation** (mat-u-ra'shun), the process of ripening or becoming fully developed.

**Meconium** (me-ko'ne-um), dark green or black fecal substance in the intestines of the full grown fetus or newly born infant.

**Membrane** (mem'brane), a thin layer of tissue covering a part or lining a body cavity.

**Menarche** (me-nar'ke), the establishment of menstruation.

**Meninges** (men-in'jeze), the membranes which cover the brain and the spinal cord.

**Meningitis** (men-in-ji'tis), inflammation of the meninges.

**Menopause** (men'o-pawz), cessation of menstruation in the human female.

**Menorrhagia** (men-o-ra'je-ah), an abnormally profuse menstrual flow.

**Mental** (men'tal), pertaining to the mind.

**Metabolism** (me-tab'o-lizm), the sum of all the chemical and physical processes involved in the building up and breaking down of protoplasm in living cells.

**Metastasis** (me-tas'tah-sis), transfer of disease from one body part to another, usually referring to malignant cells or the tubercle bacillus.

**Metrorrhagia** (me-tro-ra'je-ah), abnormal uterine bleeding occurring at completely irregular intervals.

**Microbe** (mi'crobe), a minute organism; a germ.

**Micturition** (mik-tu-rish'un), the passage of urine from the urinary bladder.

**Migraine** (mi'grane), severe periodic headaches, frequently unilateral, and often accompanied by nausea, vomiting and sensory disturbances.

**Mores** (mo'reze), fixed customs and habits of a group generally accepted as conducive to social welfare.

**Mucus** (mu'kus), the viscid secretion of the mucous glands.

**Mutism** (mu'tizm), refusal or inability to speak.

**Myopia** (mi-o'pe-ah), nearsightedness.

**Myositis** (mi-o-si'tis), inflammation of a voluntary muscle.

**Narcotics** (nar-kot'iks), drugs that produce sleep or stupor and relieve pain at the same time.

**Nasal** (na'zal), pertaining to the nose.

**Nausea** (naw'se-ah), an unpleasant, sick sensation in the stomach which often leads to vomiting.

**Necrosis** (ne-kro'sis), death of tissues, usually in a localized area.

**Negativism** (neg'ah-tiv-izm), resistance to outside suggestion, in which the person does the opposite of what is considered normal.

**Nephritis** (ne-fri'tis), inflammation of the kidney.

**Neuralgia** (nu-ral'je-ah), pain which extends along one or more nerves.

**Neurasthenia** (nu-ras-the'ne-ah), nervous exhaustion characterized by extreme fatigue and lack of energy.

**Neuritis** (nu-ri'tis), inflammation of a nerve or nerves.

**Neurosis** (nu-ro'sis), a mental or psychic disorder characterized by fears, anxieties and compulsions.

**Nevus** (ne'vus), a congenital circumscribed discolored area of the skin, either vascular or non-vascular.

**Nits** (nits), the eggs of lice.

**Nomenclature** (no'men-kla-tur), a classified system of names.

**Nutrition** (nu-trish'un), the process of using food for growth and development.

**Obese** (o-bese'), extremely fat.

**Obstetrician** (ob-ste-trish'un), a physician who specializes in the management of pregnancy, labor and the puerperium.

**Oculist** (ok'u-list), an old term for ophthalmologist.

**Ointment** (oint'ment), a greasy semisolid preparation for external use on the body.

**Oliguria** (ol-ig-u're-ah), deficient urinary secretion or too infrequent urination.

**Onset** (on'set), the beginning of an illness when the first symptoms of disease appear.

**Oophorectomy** (oo'fo-rek'to-me), the surgical removal of an ovary or the ovaries.

**Ophthalmologist** (op-thal-mol'o-jist), a physician who specializes in the treatment of disorders of the eye.

**Opiate** (o'pe-ate), a drug containing or derived from opium.

**Optician** (op-ti'shun), one who grinds lenses and fits eyeglasses.

**Optimum** (op'tim-um), the most favorable condition.

**Optometrist** (op-tom'e-trist), one who measures vision and prescribes glasses for visual defects.

**Oral** (o'ral), pertaining to the mouth.

**Orchitis** (or-ki'tis), inflammation of the testicles.

**Organ** (or'gan), a group of body tissues having a particular function.

**Orthopedic** (or-tho-pe'dik), pertaining to the correction of deformities.

**Orthopnia** (or-thop'ne-ah), difficult breathing relieved only by sitting or standing erect.

**Osseus** (os'e-us), bone-like; pertaining to bone.

**Osteoarthritis** (os-te-o-ar-thri'tis), a chronic degenerative form of joint disease.

**Osteoporosis** (os-te-o-po-ro'sis), a chronic bone disorder caused by a loss of minerals in the bone.

**Otosclerosis** (o-to-skle-ro'sis), a spongy bone formation in the labyrinth of the ear.

**Ovaritis** (o-vah-ri'tis), inflammation of an ovary.

**Oxidize** (ok'si-dize), to combine or bring about the combination with oxygen.

**Oxygen** (ok'si-jen), a colorless, odorless gas which is essential to all life and makes up about one fifth of the air.

**Pallor** (pal'or), absence of skin pigment; paleness.

**Palpitation** (pal-pi-ta'shun), an unduly rapid or throbbing heartbeat which can be sensed by the patient.

**Palsy** (pawl'ze), loss of motion (paralysis) in a part of the body.

**Papule** (pap'ule), a small, solid, circumscribed elevation of the skin.

**Paracentesis** (par-ah-sen-te'sis), a surgical puncture of a body cavity for the aspiration of fluid.

**Paralysis** (par-al'i-sis), loss of motion or impairment of sensation in a part.

**Parasites** (par'ah-sites), plants or animals which live upon or within another organism.

**Paresis** (pah-re'sis), slight or incomplete paralysis.

**Parietal** (pah-ri'e-tal), pertaining to the walls of a cavity.

**Paroxysm** (par-ok'sizm), a sudden periodic attack or recurrence of symptoms of a disease.

**Parturition** (par-tu-rish'un), the act of giving birth to a child.

**Passive** (pas'iv), submissive or not produced by active efforts.

**Pasteurization** (pas'tur-i-za-shun), the destruction of pathogenic bacteria and the inhibition in the growth of others by heating a solution without altering to any extent the chemical composition of the substance.

**Patency** (pa'ten-se), the condition of being freely open.

**Pediatrics** (pe-de-at'rix), the branch of medicine concerned with children's diseases.

**Pediculi** (pe-dik'u-li), lice.

**Pellagra** (pel-lag'rah), a deficiency disease or syndrome caused by the lack of niacin.

**Percussion** (per-kush'un), tapping a part of the body with short, sharp blows to elicit sounds or vibrations which aid in diagnosis.

**Peripheral** (pe-rif'er-al), pertaining to the outward part or surface.

**Peristalsis** (per-is-tal'sis), the wavelike contractions of the intestines by which they propel their contents.

**Pessary** (pes'ah-re), an instrument inserted into the vagina to support the uterus.

**Petechiae** (pe-te'ke-i), small, nonraised, hemorrhagic areas on the skin which occur in certain severe fevers, such as typhus.

**Petrolatum** (pet-ro-la'tum), a purified semisolid mixture of hydrocarbons from petroleum, used as a lubricant and a base for ointments.

**Pharmaceutical** (fahr-mah-su'ti-kal), pertaining to pharmacy or drugs.

**Pharyngitis** (far-in-ji'tis), inflammation of the pharynx.

**Phlebotomy** (fle-bot'o-me), incision of a vein.

**Phlegm** (flem), viscus mucus secreted by the mucous membrane of the nose and mouth.

**Phobia** (fo'be-ah), a persistent abnormal fear or dread.

**Physical** (fiz'ik-al), pertaining to the body.

**Placebo** (plah-se'bo), an inactive or nonmedicinal substance given in place of a medication to gratify a patient without his knowledge of its actual physiological therapeutic value.

**Pledget** (pled'jet), a small tuft of cotton or wool.

**Podiatrist** (po-di'ah-trist), one who diagnoses and treats foot disorders.

**Poliomyelitis** (pol-e-o-mi-e-li'tis), an acute viral disease involving the spinal cord, commonly known as infantile paralysis.

**Pollinosis** (pol-i-no'sis), an allergic body reaction due to air-borne pollen.

**Polymenorrhea** (pol-e-men-o-re'ah), abnormally frequent menstruation.

**Polyp** (pol'ip), a small protruding growth on a pedicle extending from a mucous membrane.

**Polyphagia** (pol-e-fa'je-ah), an abnormal craving for all kinds of food.

**Polyuria** (pol-e-u're-ah), the voiding of an excessive amount of urine.

**Postpartum** (post-par'tum), after childbirth or delivery.

**Poultice** (pol'tis), a soft, moist, hot mass applied to the skin.

**Premature** (pre-mah-tur'), before the proper time.

**Presbyopia** (pres-be-o'pe-ah), farsightedness associated with the impairment of vision due to the aging process.

**Prescription** (pre-skrip'shun), a written direction for the preparation and the use of a medicine.

**Process** (pros'es), a prominence or projection, as of the end of a bone.

**Proctoscope** (prok'to-skope), an instrument used for inspecting the rectum.

**Prognosis** (prog-no'sis), judging in advance the probable duration, course and termination of a disease.

**Prophylaxis** (pro-fi-lak'sis), prevention of disease.

**Prosthesis** (pros-the'sis), the replacement of a missing part by an artificial substitute.

**Prostration** (pros-tra'shun), extreme exhaustion.

**Psychiatrist** (si-ki'ah-trist), a physician who specializes in the treatment of disorders of the psyche or mind.

**Psychology** (si-kol'o-je), the science that deals with the mental processes and their effects upon behavior.

**Psychosis** (si-ko'sis), a mental disturbance in which there is a personality disintegration and an escape into unreality.

**Ptosis** (to'sis), a drooping or sagging of an organ or part from its normal position.

**Puberty** (pu'ber-te), the period in life when a person becomes sexually able to reproduce.

**Pubes** (pu'beze), the hairy region found in the lower part of the hypogastric region.

**Puncture** (punk'tur), a hole made by a pointed object.

**Purulent** (pur'u-lent), consisting of or secreting pus.

**Pus** (pus), a yellowish secretion formed in certain kinds of inflammation, consisting of albuminous substances, a thin fluid, and leukocytes or their remains.

**Pustule** (pus'tule), a small elevation of the skin filled with pus or lymph.

**Pyelitis** (pi-e-li'tis), inflammation of the pelvis of the kidney.

**Pyemia** (pi-e'me-ah), the presence of pus forming organisms in the blood.

**Pyloric** (pi-lor'ik), pertaining to the last portion of the stomach.

**Pyogenic** (pi-o-jen'ik), producing pus.

**Pyrosis** (pi-ro'sis), a burning sensation in the stomach and the esophagus, commonly known as heartburn.

**Pyuria** (pi-u're-ah), the presence of pus in the urine.

**Quack** (kwak), one who pretends to have medical skill and knowledge of remedies.

**Quarantine** (kwor'an-tene), a period of detention or isolation as a result of suspected contagion of a communicable disease.

**Quickening** (kwik'en-ing), the first movements of the fetus felt in pregnancy, usually occurring from the 16th to the 18th week.

**Radiate** (ra'de-ate), to diverge or spread from a common central point.

**Radium** (ra'de-um), a metallic element that gives off rays which are used in treating malignancies.

**Rapport** (rah-por'), a state of harmony or good relationship between 2 individuals.

**Rash** (rash), a superficial eruption of the skin.

**Reaction** (re-ak'shun), action in response to some influence or force.

**Rectum** (rek'tum), the distal portion of the large intestine between the sigmoid colon and the anal canal.

**Recumbent** (re-kum'bent), lying down.

**Recuperate** (re-ku'per-ate), to recover health or gain strength after an illness.

**Recurrence** (re-kur'ence), the return of symptoms after their remission.

**Regurgitation** (re-gur-ji-ta'shun), the return of food from the stomach soon after eating, without the ordinary efforts of vomiting.

**Relapse** (re-laps'), recurrence of former symptoms during convalescence.

**Relax** (re-laks'), to loosen up or make less stiff.

**Remission** (re-mish'un), the lessening in severity or subsiding of the symptoms of an illness.

**Research** (re-surch'), a careful and diligent hunting for facts, theories or laws.

**Resection** (re-sek'shun), excision of a portion of an organ or structure, such as bone.

**Resistance** (re-zis'tans), the power of the body to overcome the ill effects of injurious agents, such as pathogenic microorganisms, poisons or irritants.

**Retention** (re-ten'shun), holding or keeping within the body matter which is usually expelled, as retention of urine.

**Rhinitis** (ri-ni'tis), inflammation of the mucous membrane lining the nasal cavity.

**Rigor mortis** (ri'gor mor'tis), the stiffening of muscles after death.

**Rubeola** (ru-be-o'lah), measles.

**Sac** (sak), a baglike organ or structure; a pouch.

**Sanatorium** (san-ah-to're-um), an institution for the care of the chronically ill, especially those with mental illness or tuberculosis.

**Sarcoma** (sar-ko'mah), a type of tumor, often malignant, made up of a substance like the embryonic connective tissue.

**Saturated** (sat'u-ra-ted), pertaining to a solution in which no more of a substance can be dissolved.

**Sclerosis** (skle-ro'sis), a hardening of a part.

**Scoliosis** (sko-le-os'is), a lateral curvature of the normally straight vertical line of the spine.

**Sebaceous** (se-ba'shus), pertaining to sebum, the oily, fatty secretion of the sebaceous glands.

**Seborrhea** (seb-o-re'ah), an increase in the secretion of the sebaceous glands, causing an oily skin.

**Sebum** (se'bum), the oily, fatty secretion from the sebaceous glands.

**Secrete** (se-krete'), to separate from the blood.

**Secretion** (se-kre'shun), a substance secreted, as urine secreted by the kidneys.

**Sedative** (sed'ah-tiv), a remedy that has a quieting effect.

**Seizure** (se-zhur), a sudden attack or recurrence of a disease, as in an attack of epilepsy.

**Senescence** (sen-es'ens), the process of growing old.

**Senile** (se'nile), pertaining to old age.

**Septum** (sep'tum), a dividing wall between 2 cavities.

**Serum** (se'rum), the clear liquid which separates from the blood after clotting.

**Shock** (shok), depression of the body functions due to the failure of the circulation.

**Smear** (smere), a specimen for microscopic study made by spreading infected material on a glass slide.

**Soluble** (sol'u-bul), capable of being dissolved.

**Solution** (so-lu'shun), a liquid in which a substance has been dissolved.

**Somnambulism** (som-nam'bu-lizm), sleep-walking.

**Sordes** (sor'deze), the foul, dark matter that collects around the teeth and lips in low fevers.

**Spasm** (spazm), a sudden muscular contraction.

**Specialist** (spesh'a-list), a physician who devotes his services to a special class of disease.

**Specific** (spe-sif'ik), definite; particular.

**Specimen** (spes'i-men), a sample.

**Sphincter** (sfingk'ter), a ringlike muscle surrounding and closing an opening, as the sphincter muscle of the rectum.

**Splint** (splint), an appliance for holding parts of the body in place.

**Sputum** (spu'tum), matter ejected from the respiratory tract through the mouth.

**Stasis** (sta'sis), a stoppage or stagnation of the flow of fluid in any part of the body.

**Sterile** (ster'il), the absence of microorganisms.

**Stertorous** (ster'to-rus), characterized by a snoring sound, as stertorous breathing.

**Stethoscope** (steth'o-skope), an instrument used to listen to internal body sounds.

**Stimulant** (stim'u-lant), any agent that produces an increase in the activity of the body or one of its parts.

**Stoma** (sto'mah), a small opening on a free surface, such as a pore; an artificially created opening between a body cavity and the body's surface.

**Stool** (stool), feces.

**Stricture** (strik'tur), an abnormal narrowing of a passage.

**Stroke** (stroke), a sudden paralysis of one or more parts of the body, also known as apoplexy or cerebral vascular accident.

**Stupor** (stu'por), reduced responsiveness or partial unconsciousness.

**Subacute** (sub-ah-kute'), between an acute or chronic state, with some acute features.

**Subcutaneous** (sub-ku-ta'ne-us), beneath the skin.

**Substitute** (sub'sti-tute), an article or material with which to replace another.

**Suppository** (sup-oz'i-to-re), a cone-shaped mass to be introduced into the vagina, the rectum or the urethra.

**Suppuration** (sup-u-ra'shun), the formation of pus.

**Susceptible** (sus-sep'ti-bul), having little resistance.

**Suture** (su'tur), a surgical stitch.

**Symptoms** (simp'tums), a functional evidence of a disease or of the patient's condition.

**Syncope** (sin'co-pe), a temporary state of unconsciousness, commonly known as fainting.

**Syndrome** (sin'drome), a group of symptoms which occur together.

**Synthesis** (sin'the-sis), an artificial production of a compound.

**Tactile** (tak'til), pertaining to touch.

**Talcum** (tal'kum), a dusting powder with a soft mineral base.

**Taut** (tawt), tightly drawn.

**Temperature** (tem'per-a-tur), the degree of hotness or coldness of a substance.

**Tension** (ten'shun), a stretched or strained condition.

**Tepid** (tep'id), moderately warm.

**Terminal** (ter'min-al), at the end.

**Therapy** (ther'ap-e), the treatment of disease.

**Thoracotomy** (tho-rah-kot'o-me), a surgical incision of the wall of the thoracic cavity.

**Thorax** (tho'raks), the chest.

**Tibia** (tib'e-ah), the shinbone.

**Tissue** (tish'u), a group of similar specialized cells united to perform a special function.

**Tolerance** (tol'er-ans), the ability to endure the continued use of a drug.

**Tone** (tone), normal vigor and tension.

**Topical** (top'e-kal), pertaining to an external or local spot.

**Tourniquet** (toor'ne-ket), a device such as a bandage, used to stop hemorrhage from an external wound by the compression of one or more blood vessels.

**Toxic** (tok'sik), pertaining to a poison.

**Transection** (tran-sek'shun), a cross-section made by cutting across a long axis.

**Transmit** (trans-mit'), to pass on.

**Trauma** (traw'mah), a wound or injury.

**Tumor** (tu'mor), an abnormal new growth of tissue having no physiologic use, which grows independently of its surrounding structures.

**Tympanites** (tim-pah-ni'tez), distention of the abdomen due to the accumulation of gas.

**Ulcer** (ul'ser), an open sore on an external or internal surface of the body which causes the gradual distintegration of the tissues.

**Umbilicus** (um-bil-i'kus), a small scar on the abdomen which marks the former attachment of the umbilical cord to the fetus.

**Unconscious** (un-kon'shus), a lack of awareness of the environment with an incapability to react to sensory stimuli.

**Urea** (u-re'ah), the end product of protein metabolism in the body and the chief nitrogenous substance in the urine.

**Urinalysis** (ur-in-al'is-is), examination of the urine.

**Urticaria** (ur-ti-ka're-ah), hives; an allergic reaction of the skin characterized by wheals which are often attended by severe itching.

**Vaccination** (vak-sin-a'shun), the injection of killed or modified live microorganisms for the purpose of treating or producing immunity to certain infectious diseases.

**Valve** (valv), a membranous structure in an orifice or passage which allows the passage of contents in one direction only.

**Vapor** (va'por), steam; a gas given off by a liquid or a solid.

**Varicose veins** (var'i-kose vanes), enlarged and twisted veins, usually occurring in the legs.

**Venipuncture** (veni-i-punk'tur), a puncture of a vein.

**Venisection** (ven-i-sek'shun), an incision of a vein.

**Ventilation** (ven-til-a'shun), the circulation of air in a room or the supplying of oxygen to the body through the lungs.

**Vertigo** (ver'ti-go), a whirling sensation of oneself or of objects in the environment.

**Viscera** (vis'er-ah), the internal body organs, particularly referring to those in the abdominal cavity.

**Vitality** (vi-tal'it-e), the life force.

**Void** (void), to empty or cast out as waste matter.

**Volatile** (vol'ah-til), tending to vaporize rapidly.

**Voluntary** (vol'un-tar-re), controlled by the will.

**Vomitus** (vom'i-tus), matter forcibly expelled from the stomach through the mouth.

**Vulva** (vul'vah), the region of the external female genital organs.

**Wean** (ween), to substitute another method of feeding for breast feeding of an infant.

**Wen** (wen), a sebaceous cyst.

**Wheal** (wheel), a smooth, slightly elevated area on the skin, usually pale in the center with a reddened periphery, which is often attended by severe itching.

**Wound** (woond), an injury to any body structure caused by physical means.

**Xanthosis** (zan-tho'sis), a yellowish pigmentation of the skin, often the result of the ingestion of excessive carotene-rich foods, such as carrots and egg yolks.

**Xenophobia** (zen-o-fo′be-ah), an abnormal fear of strangers.

**Xeroma** (ze-ro′mah), an abnormal dryness of the conjunctiva.

**Xerosis** (ze-ro′sis), abnormal dryness of the skin, conjunctiva or mucous membranes.

**X-ray** (eks′ra), a ray which is able to penetrate most substances, used to make photographic plates of parts of the body and to treat disease.

**Zoomania** (zo-o-ma′ne-ah), a morbid love of animals.

**Zoophobia** (zo-o-fo′be-ah), an abnormal fear of animals.

**Zoopsia** (zo-op′se-ah), a hallucination in which a person thinks he sees animals.

**Zygote** (zi′gote), the cell resulting from the fusion of 2 mature germ cells, as an unfertilized egg and a mature sperm cell.

**Zymocite** (zi′mo-site), an organism which causes fermentation.

# Medical Terminology

## COMBINING FORMS AND PREFIXES

These forms, with a prefix or a suffix, or both, are those most commonly used in making medical words. G indicates those derived from the Greek; L, those from the Latin. Properly, Greek forms should be used only with Greek prefixes and suffixes; Latin, with Latin. Often a vowel, usually a, i or o, is needed for euphony.

**A-** or **Ab-** (L) *away, lack of:* abnormal, departing from normal.

**A-** or **An-** (G) *from, without:* asepsis, without infection.

**Acr-** (G) *an extremity:* acrodermatitis, a dermatitis of the limbs.

**Ad-** (L) *to, toward, near:* adrenal, near the kidney.

**Aden-** (G) *gland:* adenitis, inflammation of a gland.

**Alg-** (G) *pain:* neuralgia, pain extending along nerves.

**Ambi-** (L) *both:* ambidextrous, referring to both hands.

**Ante-** (L) *before:* antenatal, occurring or having been formed before birth.

**Anti** (G) *against:* antiseptic, against or preventing sepsis.

**Arth-** (G) *joint:* arthritis, inflammation of a joint.

**Auto-** (G) *self:* auto-intoxication, poisoning by toxin generated in the body.

**Bi-** or **Bin-** (L) *two:* binocular, pertaining to both eyes.

**Bio-** (G) *life:* biopsy, inspection of living organism (or tissue).

**Blast-** (G) *bud, a growing thing in early stages:* blastocyte, beginning cell not yet differentiated.

**Bleph-** (G) *eyelids:* blepharitis, inflammation of an eyelid.

**Brachi-** (G) *arm:* brachialis, muscle for flexing forearm.

**Brachy-** (G) *short:* brachydactylia, abnormal shortness of fingers and toes.

**Brady-** (G) *slow:* bradycardia, abnormal slowness of heartbeat.

**Bronch-** (G) *windpipe:* bronchiectasis, dilation of bronchial tubes.

**Bucc-** (L) *cheek:* buccally, toward the cheek.

**Carcin-** (G) *cancer:* carcinogenic, producing cancer.

**Cardi** (G) *heart:* cardialgia, pain in the heart.

**Cephal-** or **Cephalo** (G) *head:* cephalic measurements.

**Cheil-** (G) *lip:* cheilitis, inflammation of the lip.

**Chole-** (G) *bile:* cholecyst, the gallbladder.

**Chondr-** (G) *cartilage:* chondrectomy, removal of a cartilage.

**Circum-** (L) *around:* circumocular, around the eyes.

**Cleid-** (G) *clavicle:* cleidocostal, pertaining to clavicle and ribs.

**Colp-** (G) *vagina:* colporrhagia, vaginal hemorrhage.

**Contra-** (L) *against, opposed:* contraindication, indication opposing usually indicated treatment.

**Cost-** (L) *rib:* intercostal, between the ribs.

**Counter-** (L) *against:* counterirritation, an irritation to relieve some other irritation (e.g., a liniment).

**Crani-** (L) *skull:* craniotomy, surgical opening in skull.

**Crypt-** (G) *hidden:* cryptogenic, of hidden or unknown origin.

**Cut-** (L) *skin:* subcutaneous, under the skin.

**Cyst-** (G) *sac or bladder:* cystitis, inflammation of the bladder.

**Cyto-** (G) *cell:* cytology, scientific study of cells; cytometer, a device for counting and measuring cells.

**Dacry-** (G) *lacrimal glands:* dacryocyst, tear-sac.

**Derm-** or **Dermat-** (G) *skin:* dermatoid, skinlike.

**Di-** (L) *two:* diphasic, occurring in two stages or phases.

**Dis-** (L) *apart:* disarticulation, taking a joint apart.

**Dys-** (G) *pain or difficulty:* dyspepsia, impairment of digestion.

**Ecto-** (G) *outside:* ectoretina, outermost layer of retina.

**Em-** or **En-** (G) *in:* encapsulated, enclosed in a capsule.

**Encephal-** (G) *brain:* encephalitis, inflammation of brain.

**End-** (G) *within:* endothelium, layer of cells lining heart, blood and lymph vessels.

**Entero-** (G) *intestine:* enterosis, falling of intestine.

**Epi-** (G) *above or upon:* epidermis, outermost layer of skin.

**Erythro-** (G) *red:* erythrocyte, red blood cell.

**Eu-** (G) *well:* euphoria, well feeling, feeling of good health.

**Ex-** or **E-** (L) *out:* excretion, material thrown out of the body or the organ.

**Exo-** (G) *outside:* exocrine, excreting outwardly (opposite of endocrine).

**Extra-** (G) *outside:* extramural, situated or occurring outside a wall.

**Febri-** (L) *fever:* febrile, feverish.

**Galacto-** (G) *milk:* galactose, a milk-sugar.

**Gastr-** (G) *stomach:* gastrectomy, excision of the stomach.

**Gloss-** (G) *tongue:* glossectomy, surgical removal of tongue.

**Glyco-** (G) *sugar:* glycosuria, sugar in the urine.

**Gynec-** (G) *woman:* gynecology, science of diseases pertaining to women.

**Hem-** or **Hemat-** (G) *blood:* hemopoiesis, forming blood.

**Hemi-** (G) *half:* heminephrectomy, excision of half the kidney.

**Hepat-** (G) *liver:* hepatitis, inflammation of the liver.

**Hetero-** (G) *other* (opposite of homo): heterotransplant, using skin from a member of another species.

**Hist-** (G) *tissue:* histology, science of minute structure and function of tissues.

**Homo-** (G) *same:* homotransplant, skin grafting by using skin from a member of the same species.

**Hydr-** (G) *water:* hydrocephalus, abnormal accumulation of fluid in cranium.

**Hyper-** (G) *above, excess of:* hyperglycemia, excess of sugar in blood.

**Hypo-** (G) *under, deficiency of:* hypoglycemia, deficiency of sugar in blood.

**Hyster-** (G) *uterus:* hysterectomy, excision of uterus.

**Idio-** (G) *self, or separate:* idiopathic, a disease self-originated (of unknown cause).

**Im-** or **In-** (L) *in:* infiltration, accumulation in tissue of abnormal substances.

**Im-** or **In-** (L) *not:* immature, not mature.

**Infra-** (L) *below:* infra-orbital, below the orbit.

**Inter-** (L) *between:* intermuscular, between the muscles.

**Intra-** (L) *within:* intramuscular, within the muscle.

**Kerat-** (G) *horn, cornea:* keratitis, inflammation of cornea.

**Lact-** (L) *milk:* lactation, secretion of milk.

**Leuk-** (G) *white:* leukocyte, white cell.

**Macro-** (G) *large:* macroblast, abnormally large red cell.

**Mast-** (G) *breast:* mastectomy, excision of the breast.

**Meg-** or **Megal-** (G) *great:* megacolon, abnormally large colon.

**Ment-** (L) *mind:* dementia, deterioration of the mind.

**Mer-** (G) *part:* merotomy, division into segments.

**Mesa-** (G) *middle:* mesaortitis, inflammation of middle coat of the aorta.

**Meta-** (G) *beyond, over, change:* metastasis, change in the seat of a disease.

**Micro-** (G) *small:* microplasia, dwarfism.

**My-** (G) *muscle:* myoma, tumor made of muscular elements.

**Myc-** (G) *fungi:* mycology, science and study of fungi.

**Necro-** (G) *corpse, dead:* necrosis, death of cells adjoining living tissue.

**Neo-** (G) *new:* neoplasm, any new growth or formation.

**Neph-** (G) *kidney:* nephrectomy, surgical excision of kidney.

**Neuro-** (G) *nerve:* neuron, nerve cell.

**Odont-** (G) *tooth:* odontology, dentistry.

**Olig-** (G) *little:* oligemia, deficiency in volume of blood.

**Oo-** (G) *egg:* oocyte, original cell of egg.

**Oophor-** (G) *ovary:* oophorectomy, removal of an ovary.

**Ophthalm-** (G) *eye:* ophthalmometer, an instrument for measuring the eye.

**Ortho-** (G) *straight, normal:* orthograde, walk straight (upright).

**Oss-** (L) *bone:* osseous, bony.

**Oste-** (G) *bone:* osteitis, inflammation of a bone.

**Ot-** (G) *ear:* otorrhea, discharge from ear.

**Ovar-** (G) *ovary:* ovariorrhexis, rupture of an ovary.

**Para-** (G) *irregular, around, wrong:* paradenitis, inflammation of tissue in the neighborhood of a gland.

**Path-** (G) *disease:* pathology, science of disease.

**Ped.**[1] (G) *children:* pediatrician, child specialist.

**Ped.**[2] (L) *feet:* pedograph, imprint of the foot.

**Per-** (L) *through, excessively:* percutaneous, through the skin.

---

[1] **Ped**—from Greek *pais*, child.
[2] **Ped**—from Latin *pes*, foot.

**Peri** (G) *around, immediately around* (in contra-distinction to para): periosteum, sheath around bone.

**Phil-** (G) *love:* hemophilic, fond of blood (as bacteria that grow well in presence of hemoglobin).

**Phleb-** (G) *vein:* phlebotomy, opening of vein for bloodletting.

**Phob-** (G) *fear:* hydrophobic, reluctant to associate with water.

**Pneum-** or **Pneumon-** (G) *lung* (pneum—air): pneumococcus, organism causing lobar pneumonia.

**Polio-** (G) *gray:* poliomyelitis, inflammation of gray substance of spinal cord.

**Poly-** (G) *many:* polyarthritis, inflammation of several joints.

**Post-** (L) *after:* postpartum, after delivery.

**Pre-** (L) *before:* prenatal, occurring before birth.

**Pro-** (L and G) *before:* prognosis, forecast as to result of disease.

**Proct-** (G) *rectum:* proctectomy, surgical removal of rectum.

**Pseudo-** (G) *false:* pseudoangina, false angina.

**Psych-** (G) *soul or mind:* psychiatry, treatment of mental disorders.

**Py-** (G) *pus:* pyorrhea, discharge of pus.

**Pyel-** (G) *pelvis:* pyelitis, inflammation of pelvis of kidney.

**Rach-** (G) *spine:* rachicentesis, puncture into vertebral canal.

**Ren-** (L) *kidney:* adrenal, near the kidney.

**Retro-** (L) *backward:* retroversion, turned backward (usually, of uterus).

**Rhin-** (G) *nose:* rhinology, knowledge concerning noses.

**Salping-** (G) *a tube:* salpingitis, inflammation of tube.

**Semi-** (L) *half:* semicoma, mild coma.

**Septic-** (L and G) *poison:* septicemia, poisoned condition of blood.

**Somat-** (G) *body:* psychosomatic, having bodily symptoms of mental origin.

**Sta-** (G) *make stand:* stasis, stoppage of flow of fluid.

**Sten-** (G) *narrow:* stenosis, narrowing of duct or canal.

**Sub-** (L) *under:* subdiaphragmatic, under the diaphragm.

**Super-** (L) *above, excessively:* superacute, excessively acute.

**Supra-** (L) *above, upon:* suprarenal, above or upon the kidney.

**Sym-** or **Syn-** (G) *with, together:* symphysis, a growing together.

**Tachy-** (G) *fast:* tachycardia, fast-beating heart.

**Tens-** (L) *stretch:* extensor, a muscle extending or stretching a limb.

**Therm-** (G) *heat:* diathermy, therapeutic production of heat in tissues.

**Tox-** or **Toxic-** (G) *poison:* toxemia, poisoned condition of blood.

**Trache-** (G) *trachea:* tracheitis, inflammation of the trachea.

**Trans-** (L) *across:* transplant, transfer tissue from one place to another.

**Tri-** (L and G) *three:* trigastric, having three bellies (muscle).

**Trich-** (G) *hair:* trichosis, any disease of the hair.

**Uni-** (L) *one:* unilateral, affecting one side.

**Vas-** (L) *vessel:* vasoconstrictor, nerve or drug that narrows blood vessel.

**Zoo-** (G) *animal:* zooblast, an animal cell.

## SUFFIXES

**-algia** (G) *pain:* cardialgia, pain in the heart.

**-asis** or **-osis** (G) *affected with:* leukocytosis, excess number of leukocytes.

**-asthenia** (G) *weakness:* neurasthenia, nervous weakness.

**-blast** (G) *germ:* myeloblast, bone-marrow cell.

**-cele** (G) *tumor, hernia:* enterocele, any hernia of intestine.

**-cid** (L) *cut, kill:* germicidal, destructive to germs.

**-clysis** (G) *injection:* hypodermoclysis, injection under the skin.

**-coccus** (G) *round bacterium:* pneumococcus, bacterium of pneumonia.

**-cyte** (G) *cell:* leukocyte, white cell.

**-ectasis** (G) *dilation, stretching:* angiectasis, dilatation of a blood vessel.

**-ectomy** (G) *excision:* adenectomy, excision of adenoids.

**-emia** (G) *blood:* glycemia, sugar in blood.

**-esthesia** (G) *(noun) relating to sensation:* anesthesia, absence of feeling.

**-ferent** (L) *bear, carry:* efferent, carry out to periphery.

**-genic** (G) *producing:* pyogenic, producing pus.

**-iatrics** (G) *pertaining to a physician or the practice of healing* (medicine): pediatrics, science of medicine for children.

-itis (G) *inflammation:* tonsillitis, inflammation of tonsils.

-logy (G) *science of:* pathology, science of disease.
-lysis (G) *losing, flowing, dissolution:* autolysis, dissolution of tissue cells.

-malacia (G) *softening:* osteomalacia, softening of bone.

-oma (G) *tumor:* myoma, tumor made up of muscle elements.
-osis (-asis) (G) *being affected with:* atherosis, arteriosclerosis.
-(o)stomy (G) *creation of an opening:* gastrostomy, creation of an artificial gastric fistula.
-(o)tomy (G) *cutting into:* laparotomy, surgical incision into abdomen.

-pathy (G) *disease:* myopathy, disease of a muscle.
-penia (G) *lack of:* leukopenia, lack of white blood cells.
-pexy (G) *to fix:* proctopexy, fixation of rectum by suture.
-phagia (G) *eating:* polyphagia, excessive eating.
-phasia (G) *speech:* aphasia, loss of power of speech.

-phobia (G) *fear:* hydrophobia, fear of water.
-plasty (G) *molding:* gastroplasty, molding or reforming stomach.
-pnea (G) *air or breathing:* dyspnea, difficult breathing.
-poiesis (G) *making, forming:* hematopoiesis, forming blood.
-ptosis (G) *falling:* enteroptosis, falling of intestine.

-rhythmia (G) *rhythm:* arrhythmia, variation from normal rhythm of heart.
-rrhagia (G) *flowing or bursting forth:* otorrhagia, hemorrhage from ear.
-rrhaphy (G) *suture of:* enterorrhaphy, act of sewing up gap in intestine.
-rrhea (G) *discharge:* otorrhea, discharge from ear.

-sthen (ia) (ic) (G) *pertaining to strength:* asthenia, loss of strength.

-taxia or -taxis (G) *order, arrangement of:* ataxia, failure of muscular coordination.
-trophia or -trophy (G) *nourishment:* atrophy, wasting, or diminution.

-uria (G) *to do with urine:* polyuria, excessive secretion of urine.

# Bibliography

Abdellah, F., *et al.*: Patient-Centered Approaches to Nursing. New York, Macmillan, 1960.

AMA Drug Evaluations. Chicago, American Medical Association: Council on Drugs, 1971.

American Red Cross First Aid Textbook. Garden City, New York, Doubleday, 1957.

American Hospital Formulary Service: A Collection of Drug Monographs. Hamilton, Ill., American Society of Hospital Pharmacists, 1972.

The Anatomy of Sleep. Nutley, New Jersey, Hoffman-Laroche, 1966.

Anderson, L., *et al.*: Nutrition in Nursing. Philadelphia, Lippincott, 1972.

Anderson, M.: Basic Nursing Techniques. Philadelphia, Saunders, 1969.

Anthony, C.: Structure and Function of the Body, ed. 4. St. Louis, Mosby, 1972.

Anthony, C., and Kolthoff, M.: Textbook of Anatomy and Physiology, rev. ed. St. Louis, Mosby, 1971.

Arkoff, A.: Adjustment and Mental Health. New York, McGraw-Hill, 1968.

Armstrong, I., *et al.*: Armstrong and Browder's Nursing Care of Children. Philadelphia, Davis, 1970.

Asperheim, M.: Pharmacology for Practical Nurses, ed. 3. Philadelphia, Saunders, 1971.

Avila, D., *et al.*: The Helping Relationship Sourcebook. Boston, Allyn and Bacon, 1971.

Babcock, D.: Introduction to Growth, Development and Family Life, ed. 3. Philadelphia, Davis, 1966.

Baker, K., and Fane, X.: Understanding and Guiding Young Children, ed. 2. Englewood Cliffs, N. J., Prentice-Hall, 1967.

Barber, H., and Graber, E. A.: Quick Reference to OB-GYN Procedures. Philadelphia, Lippincott, 1969.

Becker, B., and Hassler, R.: Vocational and Personal Adjustments in Practical Nursing. St. Louis, Mosby, 1970.

Beers, C.: A Mind That Found Itself: An Autobiography, rev. ed. Garden City, New York, Doubleday, 1953.

Beeson, P., and McDermott, W. (eds.): Cecil-Loeb Textbook of Medicine. Philadelphia, Saunders, 1971.

Beland, I.: Clinical Nursing: Pathophysiological and Psychosocial Approaches, ed. 2. New York, Macmillan, 1970.

Bergerson, B.: Pharmacology in Nursing, ed. 12. St. Louis, Mosby, 1973.

Berne, E.: Games People Play: The Psychology of Human Relationships. New York, Grove Press, 1964.

Bethea, D. C.: Introductory Maternity Nursing, ed. 2, Philadelphia, Lippincott, 1973.

Bird, B.: Talking with Patients. Philadelphia, Lippincott, 1973.

Blake, F., *et al.*: Nursing Care of Children, ed. 8. Philadelphia, Lippincott, 1970.

Blake, T.: An Introduction to Electrocardiography. New York, Appleton-Century-Crofts, 1964.

Bleier, I.: Maternity Nursing, ed. 3. Philadelphia, Saunders, 1971.

Blumberg, J., and Drummond, E.: Nursing Care of the Long-Term Patient, ed. 2. New York, Springer, 1963.

Bookmiller, M., *et al.*: Textbook of Obstetrics and Obstetric Nursing, ed. 5. Philadelphia, Saunders, 1967.

Bordicks, K.: Patterns of Shock: Implications for Nursing Care. New York, Macmillan, 1965.

Borgstrom, G.: Too Many: The Biological Limitations of Our Earth. New York, Macmillan, 1969.

Brachman, L. (ed.): Encyclopedia for Medical Assistants, Including a Dictionary of Medical Terms. Milwaukee, Cathedral Square Publishers, 1965.

Branch, C. (ed.): Aspects of Anxiety. Philadelphia, Lippincott, 1968.

Breckenridge, M., and Murphy, M.: Growth and Development of the Young Child, ed. 8. Philadelphia, Saunders, 1969.

Broadribb, V.: Foundations of Pediatric Nursing, ed. 2. Philadelphia, Lippincott, 1973.

Brown, E.: Newer Dimensions of Patient Care. New York, Russell Sage Foundation, 1965.

———: Nursing Reconsidered: A Study of Change. Philadelphia, Lippincott, 1970.

———: Patients as People. New York, Russell Sage Foundation, 1964.

———: The Use of the Physical and Social Environment of the General Hospital for Therapeutic Purposes. New York, Russell Sage Foundation, 1961.

Brown, M., and Fowler, G.: Psychodynamic Nursing. Philadelphia, Saunders, 1971.

Brunner, L., *et al.*: Textbook of Medical-Surgical Nursing, ed. 2. Philadelphia, Lippincott, 1970.

Bullough, B., and Bullough, V.: The Emergence of Modern Nursing. New York, Macmillan, 1964.

Bullough, B., and Bullough V. (eds.): Issues in Nursing. New York, Springer, 1966.

Burt, J., and Miller, B.: Personal Health Behavior in Today's Society. Philadelphia, Saunders, 1972.

Burton, G.: Personal, Impersonal, and Interpersonal Relations: A Guide for Nurses, ed. 3. New York, Springer, 1970.

Bush, C.: Personal and Vocational Relationships for Practical Nurses, ed. 2. Philadelphia, Saunders, 1966.

A cancer guide for practical nurses. New York, American Cancer Society, 1960.

Carlson, C., *et al.*: Behavioral Concepts and Nursing Intervention. Philadelphia, Lippincott, 1970.

Chaffee, E., and Greisheimer, E.: Basic Physiology and Anatomy, ed. 2. Philadelphia, Lippincott, 1969.

Chapman, A.: Management of Emotional Problems of Children and Adolescents. Philadelphia, Lippincott, 1965.

Cherescavich, G.: A Textbook for Nursing Assistants, ed. 2. St. Louis, Mosby, 1968.

Clark, A., *et al.*: Patient Studies in Maternal and Child Nursing. Philadelphia, Lippincott, 1966.

Cleland, C., and Swartz, J.: Mental Retardation. New York, Grune and Stratton, 1969.

A Clinical Guide to the Menopause and the Postmenopause. New York, Ayerst Laboratories, 1968.

Closed Drainage of the Chest: A Programmed Course for Nurses. Washington, D.C., U.S. Public Health Service Publication No. 1337, U.S. Government Printing Office, 1965.

Cole, F.: The Doctor's Shorthand. Philadelphia, Saunders, 1970.

Combs, A., *et al.*: Helping Relationships: Basic Concepts for the Helping Professions. Boston, Allyn and Bacon, 1971.

Committee on Dietetics of the Mayo Clinic. The Mayo Clinic Diet Manual. Philadelphia, Saunders, 1971.

Conference on Identifying Suicide Potential: Teacher's College, Columbia University. New York, Behavioral Publications, 1971.

Conn, H. (ed.): Current Therapy 1972. Philadelphia, Saunders, 1972.

Cooper, P.: Ward Procedures and Techniques, New York, Appleton-Century-Crofts, 1967.

Crawford, A., and Buchanan, B.: Psychiatric Nursing, a Basic Manual, ed. 3. Philadelphia, Davis, 1970.

Craytor, J., and Fass, M.: The Nurse and the Cancer Patient: A Programmed Textbook. Philadelphia, Lippincott, 1970.

Creighton, H.: Law Every Nurse Should Know, ed. 2. Philadelphia, Saunders, 1970.

CRM Books Editorial Staff: Developmental Psychology Today. Del Mar, Calif., CRM Books, 1971.

———: Readings in Developmental Psychology Today, Del Mar, Calif., CRM Books, 1970.

Culver, V.: Modern Bedside Nursing, ed. 7. Philadelphia, Saunders, 1969.

Current Medical Information and Terminology. Chicago, American Medical Association, 1971.

Dean, W., *et al.*: Basic Concepts of Anatomy and Physiology: A Programmed Study. Philadelphia, Lippincott, 1966.

deGutierrez-Mahoney, C., and Carini, E.: Neurological and Neurosurgical Nursing. St. Louis, Mosby, 1965.

Dennis, L.: Psychology of Human Behavior for Nurses, ed. 3. Philadelphia, Saunders, 1967.

DeRobb, R. S.: Drugs and the Mind. New York, Grove Press, 1960.

Dick-Read, G.: Childbirth Without Fear: The Original Approach to Natural Childbirth, ed. 4. New York, Harper, 1972.

Dienhart, C.: Basic Human Anatomy and Physiology. Philadelphia, Saunders, 1967.

Dietz, L.: History and Modern Nursing. Philadelphia, Davis, 1963.

Dison, N.: An Atlas of Nursing Techniques, ed. 2. St. Louis, Mosby, 1971.

Dolan, J.: History of Nursing, ed. 12. Philadelphia, Saunders, 1968.

Dolger, H., and Seeman, B.: How to Live with Diabetes. New York, Norton, 1965.

Dorland's Illustrated Medical Dictionary, ed. 24. Philadelphia, Saunders, 1965.

Downey, J., and Darling, R. (eds.): Physiological Basis of Rehabilitation Medicine. Philadelphia, Saunders, 1971.

Dreikurs, R., and Grey, L.: A Parents' Guide to Child Discipline. New York, Hawthorn Books, 1970.

Drug Misuse: A Psychiatric View of a Modern Dilemma. Group for the Advancement of Psychiatry Report No. 80, June, 1971. Price $1.00. Order from: Publications Office, G.A.P., 419 Park Avenue South, New York 10016.

DuGas, B.: Kozier-DuGas' Introduction to Patient Care: A Comprehensive Approach to Nursing, ed. 2. Philadelphia, Saunders, 1972.

Duvall, E.: Family Development, ed. 4. Philadelphia, Lippincott, 1971.

Essentials of cancer nursing: a primer on cancer for nurses. New York, American Cancer Society, 1963.

Falconer, M., *et al.*: The Drug, the Nurse, the Patient, ed. 4. Philadelphia, Saunders, 1970.

Falconer, M., *et al.*: 1972-1974 Current Drug Handbook. Philadelphia, Saunders, 1972.

Farrow, R., and Forrest, D.: The Surgery of Childhood for Nurses, ed. 3. Baltimore, Williams and Wilkins, 1968.

A Federal Sourcebook: Answers to the Most Frequently Asked Questions about Drugs. National Clearing House for Drug Abuse Information, 1970. Order from: Superintendent of Documents, U.S. Government Printing Office, Washington, D.C. 20402.

Fielo, S., and Edge, S.: Technical Nursing of the Adult: Medical, Surgical, and Psychiatric Approaches. New York, Macmillan, 1970.

Finnie, N.: Handling the Young Cerebral Palsied Child at Home. New York, Dutton, 1970.

Fish, H.: Activities Program for Senior Citizens. West Nyack, N. Y., Parker Publishing, 1971.

Fitch, G.: The Role and Responsibilities of the Practical Nurse. New York, Macmillan, 1969.

Fitch, G., and Dubiny, M. (eds.): The Macmillan Dictionary for Practical and Vocational Nurses. New York, Macmillan, 1966.

Fitzpatrick, E., *et al.*: Maternity Nursing, ed. 12. Philadelphia, Lippincott, 1971.

Flint, T., and Cain, H.: Emergency Treatment and Management, ed. 4. Philadelphia, Saunders, 1970.

Fomon, S.: Infant Nutrition. Philadelphia, Saunders, 1967.

Food For Us All: Yearbook of Agriculture. Washington, D.C., United States Department of Agriculture, U.S. Government Printing Office, 1969.

Francis, G., and Munjas, B.: Promotion of Psychological Comfort. Dubuque, Iowa, Brown, 1968.

Freedman, M., and Hannan, J.: Medical-Surgical Workbook for Practical Nurses. Philadelphia, Davis, 1964.

Freeman, R.: Community Health Nursing Practice. Philadelphia, Saunders, 1970.

Frenay, M.: Understanding Medical Terminology. St. Louis, Catholic Hospital Association, 1969.

French, R.: Nurse's Guide to Diagnostic Procedues, ed. 3. New York, McGraw-Hill, 1967.

Frobisher, M., *et al.*: Microbiology in Health and Disease, ed. 12. Philadelphia, Saunders, 1969.

Fuerst, E., and Wolff, L.: Fundamentals of Nursing: The Humanities and the Sciences in Nursing, ed. 4. Philadelphia, Lippincott, 1969.

Garb. S.: Laboratory Tests in Common Use, ed. 5. New York, Springer, 1966.

Gardner, E.: Fundamentals of Neurology, ed. 5. Philadelphia, Saunders, 1968.

Gardner, E., *et al.*: Anatomy: A Regional Study of Human Structure, ed. 3. Philadelphia, Saunders, 1969.

Gartland, J.: Fundamentals of Orthopedics. Philadelphia, Saunders, 1969.

Gibson, A., with revisions by Manfreda, M.: The Remotivators' Guide Book. Philadelphia, Davis, 1967.

Gillies, D., and Alyn, I.: Saunders' Tests for Self-evaluation of Nursing Competence, ed. 2. Philadelphia, Saunders, 1968.

Ginott, H.: Between Parent and Child. New York, Macmillan, 1965.

———: Between Parent and Teenager. New York, Macmillan, 1969.

Given, B., and Simmons, S.: Nursing Care of the Patient with Gastrointestinal Disorders. St. Louis, Mosby, 1971.

Glasser, W.: Reality Therapy, a New Approach to Psychiatry. New York, Harper and Row, 1965.

Gondenson, R.: The Encyclopedia of Human Behavior. Garden City, New York, Doubleday, 1970.

Gordon, J. (ed.): Control of Communicable Diseases in Man. New York, American Public Health Association, 1965.

Greisheimer, E., and Wiedeman, M.: Physiology and Anatomy, ed. 9. Philadelphia, Lippincott, 1971.

Gross, V.: Mastering Medical Terminology. North Hollywood, Calif. Halls of Ivy Press, 1969.

Guyton, A.: Basic Human Physiology: Normal Function and Mechanisms of Disease. Philadelphia, Saunders, 1971.

Gyorgy, P., and Kline, O. (eds.): Malnutrition is a Problem of Ecology. New York, S. Karger, 1970.

Haas, K.: Understanding Adjustment and Behavior, ed. 2. Englewood Cliffs, N. J., Prentice-Hall, 1970.

Hadden, J., and Borgatta, M.: Marriage and the Family: A Comprehensive Reader. Itasca, Ill., Peacock Publishers, 1969.

Ham, A.: Histology, ed. 6. Philadelphia, Lippincott, 1969.

Hamilton, P.: Basic Maternity Nursing, ed. 2. St. Louis, Mosby, 1971.

———: Basic Pediatric Nursing. St. Louis, Mosby, 1970.

Harris, T.: I'm OK—You're OK: A Practical Guide to Transactional Analysis. New York, Harper and Row, 1969.

Hasler, D., and Hasler, N.: Personal, Home, and Community Health. New York, Macmillan, 1967.

Henderson, V.: The Nature of Nursing. New York, Macmillan, 1966.

Hill, M.: Food Choices: The Teen-age Girl. New York, The Nutrition Foundation, 1966.

Hirschberg, G., et al.: Rehabilitation: A Manual for the Care of the Disabled and Elderly. Philadelphia, Lippincott, 1964.

Hoffman, C., and Lipkin, G.: Practical Nursing Workbook. Philadelphia, Lippincott, 1969.

Hoffman, C., et al.: Simplified Nursing, ed. 8. Philadelphia, Lippincott, 1968.

Hofling, C., et al.: Basic Psychiatric Concepts in Nursing, ed. 2. Philadelphia, Lippincott, 1967.

Houchin, T., and DeLane, P.: How to Help Adults with Aphasia. Washington, D.C., Public Affairs Press, 1964.

Howe, P.: Basic Nutrition in Health and Disease, ed. 5. Philadelphia, Saunders, 1971.

Hurlock, E.: Child Growth and Development, ed. 4. New York, McGraw-Hill, 1968.

———: Developmental Psychology, ed. 3. New York, McGraw-Hill, 1968.

Hymovich, D.: Nursing of Children: A Guide for Study. Philadelphia, Saunders, 1969.

Hymovich, D., and Reed, S.: Nursing and the Childbearing Family: Guide for Study. Philadelphia, Saunders, 1971.

Ingalls, A., and Salerno, M.: Maternal and Child Health Nursing, ed. 2. St. Louis, Mosby, 1971.

Introduction to Asepsis: A Programmed Unit in Fundamentals of Nursing. New York, Teachers College Press, Columbia University, 1963.

Irving, S.: Basic Psychiatric Nursing. Philadelphia, Saunders, 1973.

Isolation Techniques for Use in Hospitals. Washington, D.C., United States Department of Health, Education and Welfare, U.S. Government Printing Office, 1970.

Jacob, S., and Francone, C.: Structure and Function in Man, ed. 2. Philadelphia, Saunders, 1970.

Jodais, J.: Personal Care of Patients: A Text for Health Assistants. Philadelphia, Saunders, 1970.

Johnston, D.: History and Trends of Practical Nursing. St. Louis, Mosby, 1966.

———: Total Patient Care: Foundations and Practice, ed. 3. St. Louis, Mosby, 1972.

Johnston, M.: Mental Health and Mental Illness. Philadelphia, Lippincott, 1971.

Keane, C.: Essentials of Nursing: A Medical-Surgical Text for Practical Nurses, ed. 2. Philadelphia, Saunders, 1969.

———: Saunders Review for Practical Nurses, ed. 2. Philadelphia, Saunders, 1972.

———: Study Guide and Workbook in Medical-Surgical Nursing for Practical Nurses. Philadelphia, Saunders, 1971.

Keane, C., and Fletcher, S.: Drugs and Solutions: A Programmed Introduction for Nurses, ed. 2. Philadelphia, Saunders, 1970.

Kempe, C. H., and Helfer, R. E.: Helping the Battered Child and His Family. Philadelphia, Lippincott, 1971.

Kempf, F., and Useem, R.: Psychology: Dynamics of Behavior in Nursing. Philadelphia, Saunders, 1964.

Kerr, A.: Orthopedic Nursing Procedures, ed. 2. New York, Springer, 1969.

Kerschner, V.: Simplified Nutrition and Diet Therapy for Practical Nurses. Philadelphia, Davis, 1969.

Kimble, G., and Garmezy, N.: Principles of General Psychology, ed. 3. New York, Ronald Press, 1968.

Kinsinger, R., and Arnold, W. M. (eds.): Career Opportunities: Health Technicians. New York, Doubleday, 1970.

Klinger, J., et al.: Mealtime Manual for the Aged and Handicapped. New York, Essandess Special Editions, 1970.

Kolb, L.: Noyes' Modern Clinical Psychiatry, ed. 7. Philadelphia, Saunders, 1968.

Krause, M., and Hunscher, M.: Food, Nutrition and Diet Therapy, ed. 5. Philadelphia, Saunders, 1972.

Kron, T.: Communication in Nursing, ed. 2. Philadelphia, Saunders, 1972.

———: The Management of Patient Care: Putting Leadership Skills to Work, ed. 3. Philadelphia, Saunders, 1971.

Krueger, E.: The Hypodermic Injection, a Programmed Unit. Philadelphia, Lippincott, 1966.

Kruse, H.: Nutrition: Its Meaning, Scope and Significance. Springfield, Ill., Charles C Thomas, 1969.

Kübler-Ross, E.: On Death and Dying. New York, Macmillan, 1970.

Larson, C., and Gould, M.: Calderwood's Orthopedic Nursing, ed. 7. St. Louis, Mosby, 1970.

Latham, H., and Heckel, R.: Pediatric Nursing. St. Louis, Mosby, 1967.

Leake, M.: A Manual of Simple Nursing Procedures, ed. 5. Philadelphia, Saunders, 1971.

Leifer, G.: Principles and Techniques in Pediatric Nursing, ed. 2. Philadelphia, Saunders, 1972.

LeMaitre, G., and Finnegan, J.: The Patient in Surgery: A Guide for Nurses, ed. 2. Philadelphia, Saunders, 1970.

Levine, M., and Seligman, J.: Your Overweight Child. New York, World Press, 1970.

Lingeman, R.: Drugs from A to Z. New York, McGraw-Hill, 1969.

Lockerby, F.: Communication for Nurses, ed. 3. St. Louis, Mosby, 1968.

Lockhart, R., *et al.*: Anatomy of the Human Body. Philadelphia, Lippincott, 1969.

Lowenberg, M., *et al.*: Food and Man. New York, Wiley, 1968.

Lowman, E., and Klinger, J.: Aids to Independent Living: Self-Help for the Handicapped. New York, McGraw-Hill, 1969.

Louria, D. B.: The Drug Scene. New York, Bantam, 1970.


MacBryde, C., and Blacklow, R.: Signs and Symptoms: Applied Pathologic Physiology and Clinical Interpretation, ed. 5. Philadelphia, Lippincott, 1970.

McCaffery, M.: Nursing Management of the Patient with Pain. Philadelphia, Lippincott, 1972.

McClain, M. Simplified Arithmetic for Nurses, ed. 3. Philadelphia, Saunders, 1966.

McDonald, J., and Chusid, J.: Correlative Neuroanatomy and Functional Neurology. Los Altos, Calif., Lange Medical Publications, 1970.

McGhie, A.: Psychology as Applied to Nursing. Edinburgh, Livingstone, 1969.

McKilligin, H.: The First Day of Life: Principles of Neonatal Nursing. New York, Springer, 1970.

McWilliams, M.: Nutrition for the Growing Years. New York, Wiley, 1967.

Mahoney, R.: Emergency and Disaster Nursing, ed. 2. New York, Macmillan, 1965.

Manfreda, M.: Psychiatric Nursing. Philadelphia, Davis, 1968.

Marlow, D.: Textbook of Pediatric Nursing, ed. 3. Philadelphia, Saunders, 1969.

Martin, E.: Nutrition in Action, ed. 3. New York, Holt, Rinehart and Winston, 1971.

Maslow, A.: Toward a Psychology of Being, ed. 2. New York, Van Nostrand-Reinhold Books, 1968.

Mason, M.: Basic Medical-Surgical Nursing, ed. 2. New York, Macmillan, 1967.

Mayer, J.: Overweight: Causes, Cost and Control. Englewood Cliffs, N. J., Prentice-Hall, 1968.

Meltzer, L., *et al.*: Concepts and Practices of Intensive Care for Nurse Specialists. Philadelphia, Charles Press, 1969.

———: Intensive Coronary Care: A Manual for Nurses. Philadelphia, Charles Press, 1970.

Memmler, R., and Rada, R.: The Human Body in Health and Disease, ed. 3. Philadelphia, Lippincott, 1970.

———: Structure and Function of the Human Body. Philadelphia, Lippincott, 1970.

Memmler, R., and Wood, D.: Workbook for the Human Body in Health and Disease. Philadelphia, Lippincott, 1972.

Mercer, L., and O'Connor, P.: Fundamental Skills in the Nurse-patient Relationship: A Programmed Text. Philadelphia, Saunders, 1969.

Merck Manual. Rahway, New Jersey, Merck, Sharp and Dohme, 1966.

Metheney, N., and Snively, W.: Nurses' Handbook of Fluid Balance. Philadelphia, Lippincott, 1967.

Mezer, R.: Dynamic Psychiatry in Simple Terms, ed. 4. New York, Springer, 1970.

Miller, B., and Burt, J.: Good Health, Personal and Community, ed. 3. Philadelphia, Saunders, 1972.

Miller, B., and Keane, C.: Encyclopedia and Dictionary of Medicine and Nursing. Philadelphia, Saunders, 1972.

Miller, N., and Avery, H.: Gynecology and Gynecologic Nursing, ed. 5. Philadelphia, Saunders, 1965.

Milliken, M.: Understanding Human Behavior. Albany, N. Y., Del Mar, 1969.

Mitchell, H., *et al.*: Cooper's Nutrition in Health and Disease, ed. 15. Philadelphia, Lippincott, 1968.

Modell, W., *et al.*: Handbook of Cardiology for Nurses, ed. 5. New York, Springer, 1966.

Mystification and Drug Misuse—Hazards in Using Psychoactive Drugs. San Francisco, Lennard and Associates: Jossey-Bass, Inc., 1971.


Nursing Procedures for the Practical Nurse: Learner's Manual. Columbus, Ohio, State Department of Education, Ohio Trade and Industrial Education Service, 1961.


O'Brien, M.: The Care of the Aged: A Guide for the Licensed Practical Nurse. St. Louis, Mosby, 1971.

O'Hara, F., and Reith, H.: Psychology and the Nurse, ed. 6. Philadelphia, Saunders, 1966.

Orem, D.: Nursing: Concepts of Practice. New York, McGraw-Hill, 1971.

Orlando, I.: The Dynamic Nurse-Patient Relationship: Function, Process, and Principles. New York, Putnam, 1961.


Pansky, B., and House, E.: Review of Gross Anatomy, ed. 2. New York, Macmillan, 1969.

Petrillo, M., and Sanger, S.: Emotional Care of Hospitalized Children. Philadelphia, Lippincott, 1972.

Peyton, A.: Practical Nutrition, ed. 2. Philadelphia, Lippincott, 1968.

Pfeiffer, J., *et al.*: The Cell. New York, Time-Life, 1964.

Physicians' Desk Reference (PDR). Oradell, N. J., Medical Economics Incorporated. Published yearly.

Pike, R., and Brown, M.: Nutrition: An Integrated Approach. New York, Wiley, 1967.

Pikunas, J., et al.: Human Development: A Science of Growth. New York, McGraw-Hill, 1969.

Pines, M.: Revolution in Learning: The Years from Birth to Six. New York, Harper and Row, 1967.

Plaut, T.: Alcohol Problems: A Report to the Nation. New York, Oxford University Press, 1967.

Plein, J., and Plein, E.: Fundamentals of Medications. Philadelphia, Lippincott, 1967.

Plumer, A.: Principles and Practice of Intravenous Therapy. Boston, Little, Brown, 1970.

Poland, R., and Sanford, N.: Adjustment Psychology: A Human Value Approach. St. Louis, Mosby, 1971.

Pollock, M., and Pollock, M.: New Hope for the Retarded: Enriching the Lives of Exceptional Children, ed. 3. Boston, Sargent, 1953.

Raffensperger, J., and Primrose, R. (eds.): Pediatric Surgery for Nurses. Boston, Little, Brown, 1968.

Rapier, D., et al.: Practical Nursing: A Textbook for Students and Graduates, ed. 4. St. Louis, Mosby, 1970.

Rasmussen, S.: Foundations of Practical and Vocational Nursing. New York, Macmillan, 1967.

Reed, G., and Sheppard, V.: Regulation of Fluid and Electrolyte Balance: A Programmed Instruction in Physiology for Nurses. Philadelphia, Saunders, 1971.

Reid, D., et al.: Principles and Management of Human Reproduction. Philadelphia, Saunders, 1972.

Reynolds, F., and Barsam, P.: Adult Health: Services for the Chronically Ill and Aged. New York, Macmillan, 1967.

Robinson, A.: Working with the Mentally Ill, ed. 4. Philadelphia, Lippincott, 1971.

Robinson, C.: Basic Nutrition and Diet Therapy, ed. 2. London, Collier-Macmillan, 1970.

———: Fundamentals of Normal Nutrition. New York, Macmillan, 1968.

Robinson, L.: Psychiatric Nursing as a Human Experience. Philadelphia, Saunders, 1972.

Rodman, M., and Smith, D.: Pharmacology and Drug Therapy in Nursing. Philadelphia, Lippincott, 1968.

Rosdahl, C.: Ages and Stages—the Ever-Changing Child. In McDermott, I. E., and Nicholas, J. L.: Homemaking for Teenagers, Book 2. Peoria, Ill., Bennett Co., 1972.

Ross, C.: Personal and Vocational Relationships in Practical Nursing, ed. 3. Philadelphia, Lippincott, 1969.

Routh, J.: Introduction to Biochemistry. Philadelphia, Saunders, 1971.

Routh, J., et al.: Essentials of General, Organic and Biochemistry. Philadelphia, Saunders, 1969.

Rusk, H., et al.: Rehabilitation Medicine: A Textbook on Rehabilitative Medicine, ed. 3. St. Louis, Mosby, 1964.

Sackheim, G., and Robins, L.: Programmed Mathematics for Nurses, ed. 2. New York, Macmillan, 1964.

Sanderson, R. (ed.): The Cardiac Patient: A Comprehensive Approach. Philadelphia, Saunders, 1972.

Sarner, H.: The Nurse and the Law. Philadelphia, Saunders, 1968.

Sawyer, J.: Nursing Care of Patients with Urologic Diseases. St. Louis, Mosby, 1963.

Schaefer, H., and Martin, P.: Behavioral Therapy. New York, McGraw-Hill, 1969.

Scheinfeld, A.: Your Heredity and Environment. Philadelphia, Lippincott, 1965.

Schifferes, J.: How to Understand, Help, Enjoy and Get Along Better with the Older People in Your Life. New York, Washington Square Press, 1962.

Schwartz, S.: Principles of Surgery. New York, McGraw-Hill, 1969.

Scott, L.: Programmed Instruction and Review for Practical and Vocational Nurses. New York, Macmillan, 1968.

Secor, J.: Patient Care in Respiratory Problems. Philadelphia, Saunders, 1969.

Seedor, M.: Aids to Nursing Judgment, ed. 2. New York, Teachers College Press, Columbia University, 1972.

———: Introduction to Asepsis: A Programmed Unit in Fundamentals of Nursing. New York, Teachers College Press, Columbia University, 1969.

———: Therapy with Oxygen and Other Gases: A Programmed Unit in Fundamentals of Nursing. New York, Teachers College Press, Columbia University, 1966.

Shackelton, A.: Practical Nurse Nutrition Education, ed. 3. Philadelphia, Saunders, 1972.

Shafer, K., et al.: Medical-Surgical Nursing, ed. 5. St. Louis, Mosby, 1971.

Sharp, L., and Rabin, B.: Nursing in the Coronary Care Unit. Philadelphia, Lippincott, 1970.

Shepard, R.: Human Physiology. Philadelphia, Lippincott, 1971.

Simmons, J.: The Nurse-Patient Relationship in Psychiatric Nursing. Philadelphia, Saunders, 1969.

Simpson, D.: Learning to Learn. Columbus, Ohio, Merrill, 1968.

Skelley, E.: Medications for the Nurse. Albany, Delmar, 1967.

Skipper, J., and Leonard, R. (eds.): Social Interaction and Patient Care. Philadelphia, Lippincott, 1965.

Smith, D., *et al.*: Care of the Adult Patient: Medical-Surgical Nursing, ed. 3. Philadelphia, Lippincott, 1971.

Smith, G., and Davis, P.: Medical Terminology. New York, Wiley, 1967.

Snively, W., and Beshear, D.: Textbook of Pathophysiology. Philadelphia, Lippincott, 1972.

Spock, B.: Baby and Child Care. New York, Duell, Sloan and Pearce, 1968.

Spock, B., and Lowenberg, M.: Feeding Your Baby and Child. New York, Pocket Books, 1956.

Springer, E. (ed.): Nursing and the Law. Pittsburgh, Aspen Systems, 1970.

Squire, J.: Basic Pharmacology for Nurses, ed. 4. St. Louis, Mosby, 1969.

Staton, T.: How to Study. Montgomery, Alabama, How to Study, 1968.

Stevens, M.: Geriatric Nursing for Practical Nurses. Philadelphia, Saunders, 1965.

———: Personal and Vocational Relationships of the Practical Nurse. Philadelphia, Saunders, 1967.

Stewart, I., and Austin, A.: A History of Nursing, from Ancient to Modern Times, ed. 5. New York, Putnam, 1962.

Stryker, R.: Rehabilitative Aspects of Acute and Chronic Nursing Care. Philadelphia, Saunders, 1972.

Sutton, A.: Bedside Nursing Techniques in Medicine and Surgery, ed. 2. Philadelphia, Saunders, 1969.

———: Workbook for Practical Nurses, ed. 3. Philadelphia, Saunders, 1969.

Tanner, J., and Taylor, G.: Growth. New York, Time-Life, 1965.

Thompson, E.: Pediatrics for Practical Nurses. Philadelphia, Saunders, 1970.

Travelbee, J.: Interpersonal Aspects of Nursing, ed. 2. Philadelphia, Davis, 1971.

———: Intervention in Psychiatric Nursing. Process in the One-to-One Relationship. Philadelphia, Davis, 1969.

Ujhely, G.: Determinants of the Nurse-Patient Relationship. New York, Springer, 1968.

———: The Nurse and Her Problem Patients. New York, Springer, 1963.

Verville, E.: Behavior Problems of Children. Philadelphia, Saunders, 1967.

Volk, W., and Wheeler, M.: Basic Microbiology, ed. 3. Philadelphia, Lippincott, 1973.

vonGremp, Z., and Broadwell, L.: Practical Nursing Study Guide and Review, ed. 3. Philadelphia, Lippincott, 1971.

Watson, J.: Medical-Surgical Nursing and Related Physiology. Philadelphia, Saunders, 1972.

Whittaker, J.: Introduction to Psychology, ed. 2. Philadelphia, Saunders, 1970.

Winters, M.: Protective Body Mechanics in Daily Life and in Nursing. Philadelphia, Saunders, 1952.

Wohl, and Goodhart (eds.): Modern Nutrition in Health and Disease. Philadelphia, Lea and Febiger, 1968.

Wood, L., *et al.* (eds.): Nursing Skills for Allied Health Services. Philadelphia, Saunders, 1972.

Worcester, A.: The Care of the Aged, the Dying and the Dead. Springfield, Ill., Charles C Thomas, 1940, reprinted 1961.

Worley, E.: Pharmacology and Medications for Vocational Nurses, ed. 2. Philadelphia, Davis, 1967.

Yablonsky, L.: Synanon: The Tunnel Back. Baltimore, Penguin Books, 1967.

Yost, E.: American Women of Nursing. Philadelphia, Lippincott, 1965.

Young, C.: Introduction to Medical Science. St. Louis, Mosby, 1969.

Young, C., and Barger, J.: Learning Medical Terminology Step by Step, ed. 2. St. Louis, Mosby, 1971.

Young, H., *et al.*: Lippincott's Quick Reference Book for Nurses, ed. 8. Philadelphia, Lippincott, 1967.

# Index

Abdomen, 103
Abdominal cavity, 84
Abduction, in body movements, 94
Abnormalities, congenital. See *Congenital Disorders*
Abortion, 411, 688
  criminal, 411, 688
  habitual, 411
  incomplete, 411
  inevitable, 411
  missed, 411
  spontaneous, 411
  therapeutic, 411, 688
  threatened, 411
Abrasions, in children, 469
Abruptio placenta, 412
Abscess(es)
  anal, 648
  brain, 558
  breast, 680
  liver, 652
  lung, 614
Absorption, in digestion, 135
Accommodation, visual, 157, 708
Acetone, 165
  in diabetes, 704
  test for, 693
Acetylsalicylic acid, 350
Acid-alkaline diet, 181
Acid-base balance, minerals in, 167
  urinary system in, 139
Acidosis, 666, 700, 704
  vs insulin shock, 703t
Acne vulgaris, 493, 518
Acoustic nerve, 156, 157
Acromegaly, 151, 694
ACTH, function and production of, 150, 694, 697
  in Cushing's syndrome, 698
Activities of daily living, 562
Adenoidectomy, 464
ADH (antidiuretic hormone), 151, 694
Addiction, drug, 761. See also *Drug misuse*
  signs of, 769
Addison's disease, 698
Adduction, 94
Adipose tissue, 86
Admission procedures, 204
Adolescent
  cardiovascular disorders in, 494
  emotional difficulties in, 496
  endocrine disorders in, 494
  gastrointestinal disorders in, 494
  genitourinary disorders in, 494

Adolescent (*continued*)
  growth and development of, 59-64
  infectious disease in, 495
  malignancies in, 495
  musculoskeletal defects in, 492
  nursing care of, 497-498
  skin problems in, 493
  suicide and, 497
Adolescent psychiatry, 497
Adrenal glands, 153
  disorders of, 697-698
  effect of ACTH on, 150, 697
Adrenalin, 153
Aerobic organisms, 42
Afterbirth, 399. See also *Placenta*
Agammaglobulinemia, 481
Aged. See *Elderly*
Aging process, 733
Agranulocytosis, 591
Air pollution, and respiratory disorders, 623
Airway, patency of, in first aid, 382
  in oxygen therapy, 299
  method for establishing, 300
Albuminuria, 657
Alcohol
  as depressant, 354
  as vasodilator, 358
  ethyl, 354
  methyl, 354
  misuse of, 763
Alcohol, sponge bath, 274
Alimentary canal, 131-136
Allergen, 726
Allergy, 726-729, 609
  causes of, 726
  diagnosis of, 726
  drug therapy in, 370, 727
  due to drugs, 729
  due to food, diet in, 181
  gastrointestinal, 727
  kinds of, 727
  skin reaction, 519
  treatment of, 727
Alveoli, 128
Ambu bag, 306, 579, 582
Ambulation, 238
  following surgery, 320
  in fracture, 538
  in puerperium, 423
Amebiasis, drugs for destruction of, 370
Ameboid movement, of cells, 75
Amenorrhea, 674
American Cancer Society, 515
American Nurses' Association, 9

American Psychiatric Association, 759
American Red Cross, 36
Amino acids, 165
Amniotic aspiration, 436
Amniotomy, 416
Amphetamines, 347
  misuse of, 764
Ampules, 323
  withdrawing drug from, 338
Amputation, 541-542
Amylase, 134
Amylopsin, 134
Amyl nitrate, 358
ANA (American Nurses' Association), 9
Anabolism, 76, 138
Anaerobic organisms, 42
Analgesics, 348
  coal tar, 350
  in labor, 419
  narcotic, 348
  non-narcotic, 349
Analysis, transactional, 751
Anaphylactic shock, 299, 729
  in allergy, 727
Anatomy, 73-84. See also specific body systems
Androgens, 154, 369
Anemia, 115, 481, 590
  aplastic, 591
  diet in, 180
  due to blood loss, 591
  due to folic acid deficiency, 173
  due to Vitamin $B_{12}$ deficiency, 174
  in children, 481, 494
  iron-deficiency, 481, 591
  oxygen needs in, 298
  pernicious, 591
  sickle-cell, 480, 591
Anesthesia, in labor, 419
  in surgery, 315
    stages of, 315
  personnel for, 315
Anesthesiologist, 315
Anesthetics, 315
  in cesarean section, 424
  in labor, 419
Aneurysm, 298, 560, 584
Angina
  decubitus, 577
  intractable, 577
  nocturnal, 577
  Vincent's, 635
Angina pectoris, 576
Angiocardiogram, 574

Angiography, cerebral, 547
Angioma, 522
Angioneurotic edema, 727
Ankylosing spondylitis, 531
Ankylosis, 529
Anomalous venous return, 483
Anorexia nervosa, 496
Antacids, 362
Antepartum, 402
Anthelmintics, 370
  in enemas, 251
Antibiosis, 44
Antibiotics, 44, 342-346
  action of, 342
  appropriate, selection of, 343
  characteristics of, 343
  for skin, 341
  for special use, 346
Antibody, 44
  formation of, thymus and, 154
Anticoagulants, 360
Anticonvulsant drugs, 353
Antidiarrheics, 365
Antidiuretics, 361
Antidiuretic hormone (ADH), 151, 694
Antiemetics, 363, 419
Antifungal drugs, 341
Antigens, 44, 726
Antihistamines, 370, 727
Antipruritics, 342
Antipyretics, 350
Antiseptics, 40, 366
  and disinfectants, 340
  for skin, 341
  urinary, 361
Antispasmodics, 370
Antitoxins, 44, 371
Antitiussives, 366
Anuria, 217, 657
Anus, 135
  abscess of, 648
  fissure of, 648
  imperforate, 438
Anvil, of middle ear, 156
Anxiety, drug treatment for, 772
Aorta, 118
  aneurysms of, 584
  coarctation of, 484
  stenosis of, 484
Apgar scale, 427
Aphasia, 551
  in children, 504
  in CVA, 561
  in elderly patient, 736
Apical pulse, 209
Apical-radial pulse, 209
Aplastic anemia, 591
Apnea, 298
Apothecaries' system of measurement, 328
Appendicitis, 135, 494, 643
Appendicular skeleton, 90
Appetite, factors influencing, 176
  loss of, as symptom, 188

Aqueous humor, 158
Areola, 148
Armed forces, practical nursing opportunities in, 781
Arms, structure of, 98
Arrhythmias, 581
Arterial pressure, mean, in blood pressure, 215
Arteries, 119-120
Arteriography, 547, 659
Arteriosclerosis, 575
Arthritis, 529-532
  body changes in, 529
  causes of, 529
  development of, 529
  exercise in, 530
  forms of, 529
    infectious, 529
    rheumatoid, 529
      juvenile, 486, 493
    of spine, 531
  traumatic, 529
  treatment of, 529
    drug therapy in, 530, 532
    long-term, 532
    physical therapy in, 532
    surgery in, 530
Ascorbic acid, 171
Asepsis, medical, 278-283
  surgical, 284-287
Asphyxia, 298
  first aid for, 381
Aspidium, 370
Aspiration, amniotic, 436
  of foreign bodies, 468, 607
  prevention of, in surgery, 313
Aspiration pneumonia, 615
Asthma, 210, 727
  bronchial, 729, 610
  drugs for, 370
Astigmatism, 714
  lenses for, 711
Ataractics, 354
Ataxia, in drug misuse, 768
Atelectasis, 598
  following surgery, 319
  in newborn, 436
Atherosclerosis, 575
  oxygen needs and, 298
Athlete's foot, 490, 519
Atoms, 74
Atresia, biliary, 473
  tricuspid, 483
Atrium, 118
  septal defects of, 483
Atrioventricular node, 119
Atrophy, yellow, 652
Audiometry, 720
Auditory canal, 156
Auricle, of ear, 156
Auricular fibrillations, 582
Autism, 491
Autoclave, 42, 284
Autograft, 525

Autonomic nervous system, 110
  drugs affecting, 355-356
Axial skeleton, 90
Axillary temperature, 212

Back rests, 234
Back rub, 237
Bacteria, 40
Bacterial endocarditis, 585
Bacterial pneumonia, 615
Bag of waters, 416
Ball-and-socket joints, 92
Ballard school, 5
Bandages, 391-393
  and binders, 276
  circular, 391
  elastic roller, 277
  figure-8, 392
  roller, 391
  spiral, 392
  spiral reverse, 392
  triangular or handkerchief, 393
Baptism, emergency, of neonate, 427
Barbiturates, 351, 352t
  misuse of, 764
Barium, in G.I. series, 626
Bartholin cysts, 148
Bartholin's glands, 148
  infection of, 675
Basal metabolic rate (BMR), 138, 166, 692
  thyroid and, 152
"Basic 4", in foods, 163
Bath
  alcohol, 274
  bed, 257
    partial, 260
    postpartum, 422
  for elderly, 758
  for infant, 453
  for newborn, 430, 432
  hip, 272
  shower, 257
  sitz, 272, 674
  sponge, 274
    in pediatrics, 453
  therapeutic, in skin disorders, 518
  tub, 256
"Battered child" syndrome, 470
Bed, 196-201
  circle, 196, 550
  equipment for, 201
  exercises in, 238
  making of, body mechanics in, 197
    closed, 197
    procedure for, 198
    purpose of, 197
    occupied, 197
    unoccupied, 197
  opening of, 199
  parts of, 201
  placing patient in, 205
  types of, 197

Bed bath, 257
  partial, 260
  postpartum, 422
Bed board, 201
Bedbugs, 521
Bed cradle, 200
Bedpan, 247
Bedrest, complications from, following surgery, 319
Bedside stand, 201
Bedsides, adjusting, 200
  for child, 448
  for elderly, 735
Bedsores, 264
Bed-wetting, 57, 480, 496
Behavior, 30
  of patient, observation of, 189
  problems of, in children, 491
  psychology and, 24
Behavior modification, 750
  in mental retardation, 501
Belching, 244
Bell's palsy, 560
Benedict's test, 693
Beriberi, 171
Bile, 134
Biliary atresia, 473
Bilirubin, in jaundice, 649
  in urine, 657
Binders, and bandages, 276
Binocular vision, 157
Biopsy, bone marrow, 590
  liver, 628
  of breast lesion, 673
  of cervix, 672
Biotin, 173
Birth certificate, for neonate, 428
Birth control, 149, 369, 687
Birth injuries, 436
  mental retardation due to, 501
Bites, dog, 469
Bladder, 141, 657
  catheterization and, 289, 661
  cystitis of, 662
  drainage of, 661
  drugs affecting, 361
  exstrophy of, 478
  incontinence of, in elderly patient, 735
    in neurologic patient, 550
  trauma to, 665
  tumor of, 666
Bladder retraining, for neurologic patient, 551
Bland diet, 179
Bleeding
  breakthrough, 674
  control of, in first aid, 380
  iron-deficiency anemia and, 591
  postoperative, 317
  shock due to, 317
Bleeding disorders, 594

Blindness, 36, 718
  color, 710
  partially sighted and, 36, 718
  reading aids in, 719
  rehabilitation in, 377
  snow, 715
  traveling aids in, 719
Blood, 81, 114-117
  circulatory route of, 122
  clotting of, 116
  communicable diseases of, 279
  culture of, 575
  disorders of, 590-595. See also *Blood disorders*
  drugs affecting, 359
  formation of, cobalt and manganese in, 169
  observation of, 189
  pH of, 598
  specimens of, 220
  sugar level of, fasting, 692
  tests of, 574, 692
    in diabetes, 705
    in urinary disorders, 658
  transfusion of, 326, 360
  types of, and hemorrhage, 117
  volume of, 574
Blood banks, 35
Blood cells, red, 114
  white, 115, 480
Blood count, complete (CBC), 575
Blood disorders, 480-482, 590-595
  agammaglobulinemia, 481
  agranulocytosis, 591
  anemia, 481, 590
  diagnosis of, 590
  hemophilia, 186, 480, 595
  hypogammaglobulinemia, 481
  in children, 480-482
  leukemia, 480, 592
  purpura (ITP), 481, 594
  sickle-cell anemia, 480, 591
  surgical treatment of, 595
Blood gas determinations, 598
Blood plasma, 114, 360
Blood pressure, 116, 214
  as symptom, 188
  diastolic pressure in, 215
  drugs for, 358
  in heart disease, 573
  in shock, 299
  kidneys and, 141
  mean arterial pressure in, 215
  measuring of, 215
  normal, 215
    child, 449
  pulse pressure in, 215
  systolic pressure in, 215
  taking of, 214
Blood proteins, 360
Blood types, 117
Blood urea nitrogen (BUN), 658
Blood vessels, 119-123
  drugs affecting, 357
Bloodshot eyes, in drug abuse, 768

Blow bottle, in respiratory disorders, 601
  following surgery, 319
BMR (basal metabolism rate), 138, 166, 692
Body
  alignment of, for neurologic patient, 549
    for prone patient, 236
Body, anatomy of, 73-84
  care of, following death, 296
    isolation technic in, 283
  cavities of, 83-84
  planes of, 83
Body directions, 82-83
Body fluids, 79
Body mechanics, 27
  in bedmaking, 197
  in moving helpless patient, 241
Body odor, in adolescent, 484
Body positions, changing of, 234
Body rub, 236
Body salts, urinary system in balance of, 139
Boils, 520
  of auditory canal, 722
Bolus, 132
Bone(s)
  and joints, tuberculosis of, 618
  disorders of, due to hypoparathyroidism, 697
  markings of, 93
  structure of, 91
  tumors of, 495, 528
Bone marrow, 92
  anaplastic anemia in disease of, 591
  biopsy of, 590
Bottle feeding, 433
Botulism, 387
Bowel, 134. See also *Intestines*
  function of, in burns, 523
  incontinence of, in elderly patient, 735
    in neurologic patient, 550
Bowel movement, 245
Bowel retraining, for neurologic patient, 550
Bowlegs, 527
Bowman's capsule, 140
Braces, for neurologic patient, 550
Brachial plexus palsy, 436
Bardycardia, 208, 581
Braille system, 36, 719
Brain, 110
Brain disorders, 555-560
  abscess, 558
  convulsive seizures, 558
  in children, 475-478
  craniostenosis, 477
  encephalocele, 475
  hydrocephalus, 476
  microcephalus, 477
  seizures, 477
  tumors, 478

Brain disorders (continued)
  injuries, 556
    in CVA, 561
    in syphilis, 690
  intracranial pressure, 555
  surgery in, 557
  tumors, 556
Brain scan, radioactive, 547
Braxton-Hicks contractions, 416
Bread-cereals, daily requirements, 163
Breakfast, importance of, 174
Breasts, 148
  care of, during pregnancy, 404
    in nursing mother, 433
    in postpartum, 422
  changes of, in breast cancer, 680
  disorders of, 679-683. See also Breast disorders
  examination of, 672
  prosthetic, 681
Breast disorders, 679-683
  abscesses, 680
  cancer, 511, 680
  lesions, diagnosis of, 673
  mastitis, chronic cystic, 679
    in postpartum, 425
Breast-feeding, 432
Breast milk, 422
Breathing, abdominal, 601
  difficult, 187
  mechanics of, 129
Breathing difficulty(ies), 209
  in dying patient, 295
  in heart disease, 573
  oxygen needs and, 298
  postural drainage in, 599
  relief of, 599
  signs of, 210
Breathing, exercises, 601
Breathing sounds, as respiratory symptom, 597
Breech presentation, 419
Bricker procedure, 661
Bright's disease, 479, 663
Bromides, 353
Bronchi, 127
Bronchial asthma, 610, 729
Bronchiectasis, 610
Bronchioles, 127
Bronchitis, 611
Bronchogram, 599
Bronchopneumonia, in newborn, 436
Bronchoscopy, 599
Buccal cavity, 131
Buerger's disease, 589
Bulbourethral glands, 145
BUN (blood urea nitrogen), 658
Bundle of His, 119
Burns, 522-525
  bowel function in, 523
  chemical, treatment for, 390
  cosmetic surgery in, 524
  debridement in, 524
  degree of, 389, 522

Burns (continued)
  dietary management in, 523
  dressings in, 524
  effects of, 522
  electrolyte balance in, 523
  emotional aspects of, 525
  first aid for, 389
  first degree, 522
  fluid intake in, 523
  fourth degree, 522
  in children, 467
  nursing care in, 523
  occupational therapy in, 525
  of eye, acid or alkali, 715
  pain control in, 524
  physical therapy in, 525
  preventing contractures in, 525
  preventing infection in, 524
  prevention of, 389
  renal function in, 523
  respiratory status in, 523
  "Rule of Nines" in, 468, 523
  second degree, 522
  skin grafts in, 525
  third degree, 522
  treatment for, 389
  vital signs in, 523
Bursae, 94
Bursitis, 527

C. A. (cancer), 509
Caffeine, as drug, 347, 763
Calciferol, 170
Calcium, 167
  and iron, daily dietary pattern of, 168t
  loss of, in hyperparathyroidism, 697
Calculi, urinary, 534, 664
Calories, 166
Cancer, 509-515
  cause of, 510
  chemotherapy in, 513
  diagnosis of, 511
  diet in, 515
  drugs for, 372-373
  infection in, 515
  intestinal obstruction due to, 646
  location of, 511
  metastatic, of breast, 681
  nursing care in, 514-515
  odor control in, 515
  of breast, 511, 680
  of cervix, 671, 677
  of colon, 647
  of esophagus, 638
  of gallbladder, 655
  of gastrointestinal tract, 635
  of larynx, 607
  of liver, 652
  of lung, 621
  of mouth, 637
  of ovary, 677
  of pancreas, 655
  of prostate, 685

Cancer (continued)
  of rectum, 648
  of reproductive system, test for, 671
  of skin, 522
  of stomach, 641
  of urinary tract, 666
  of uterine fundus, 677
  pain control in, 515
  Papanicolaou test for, 671
  radiation therapy in, 512
  skin care in, 514
  spread of, 510
  symptoms of, 510
  treatment of, 511
    chemotherapy, 513
    radiation, 512
    surgery, 511
Cancer quackery, 515
Cancer research, 515
Canker sore, 520, 636
Capillaries, 120
Caput succedaneum, 437
Carbohydrate diet, low, 180
Carbohydrates, 163
Carbuncle, 520
Carcinogens, 510
Carcinoma(s), 509, 510
  in children, 484
Cardiac arrest, 582
  oxygen needs and, 298
  ventricular fibrillation in, 582
Cardiac catheterization in, 574
Cardiac dyspnea, 298
Cardiac massage, closed-chest, 582
  opened-chest, 584
Cardiac muscle, 102
Cardiac orifice, 133
Cardiac sphincter, 133
  spasm of, 638
Cardiac tissue, 80
Cardinal symptoms, 207
Cardiopulmonary resuscitation, 582
Cardiospasm, 638
Cardiovascular disorders, 572-595. See also Heart disease
  aneurysms, 584
  arrhythmias, 581
  arteriosclerosis and atherosclerosis in, 575
  blood disorders in, 480-482, 590-595. See also Blood disorders
  cardiac arrest, 582
  congestive heart failure in, 580
  coronary artery disease, 576-584
  heart block in, 581
  heart disease, 573-576
  hypertension in, 575
  in school-age child and adolescent, 494
  infectious, bacterial endocarditis, 584
    heart diseases in, 584-585
    rheumatic fever, 584

Cardiovascular disorders (*continued*)
  peripheral vascular disorders, 586-590
    Buerger's disease, 589
    embolism, 587
      Raynaud's disease, 589
      thrombophlebitis, 586
      varicose veins, 588
Carditis, rheumatic, 466
Care plan, nursing, Kardex and, 224
Career opportunities, in practical nursing, 779-784
Caries, dental, 636
Carminatives, 363
  in enemas, 251
Carotene, 170
Cartilage, 86, 94
Cartilaginous joints, 92
Casts, in fractures, 534
    care of, 535
    petalling of, 535
    removal of, 535
    spica, 534
  in urine, 658
Cat scratches, in children, 469
Catabolism, 76, 138
Cataract, 716
  in diabetes, 705
Cathartics, 363
Catheter
  Foley, 290
  in-dwelling, 290
  nasal, in oxygen therapy, 302
  retention, 290
    patient, care in, 248
  types of, 289
  urinary, 660
    care of, 661
    irrigation of, 661
Catheterization, 289
  cardiac, 574
  following surgery, 318
  in labor, 419
  in premature infants, 440
  in puerperium, 423
  in urinary disorders, 660
  of female patient, 289
    precautions in, 290
    preparing patient for, 290
    procedure for, 290
    side-lying position for, 291
  of male patient, 291
  pediatric, 450
  reasons for, 289
  types of catheters in, 289
Catholic faith, in spiritual needs of patient, 266
Caudal block, in labor, 419
Cavities, of body, 83-84
  peritoneal, 137
  sinus, of skull, 95
CBC (complete blood count), 575
CCU (coronary care unit), 202
Cecum, 135
Celiac disease, glutin-induced, 474

Cell(s), 74, 76-82
  membrane of, 77, 79
  nerve, 107-109
  pattern of, 85-88
Cellulose, 163, 164
Central nervous system, 110-112
  drugs affecting, 347-355
Central venous pressure (CVP), 575
Centrioles, 77
Centrosomes, 77
Cephalic presentation, 419
Cephalohematoma, 437
Cephalopelvic disproportion, 420
Cerebellum, 111
Cerebral angiography, 547
Cerebral embolism, 561
Cerebral hemorrhage, 561
Cerebral palsy, 502, 566
Cerebral thrombosis, 561
Cerebral vascular accident (CVA), 561
  oxygen needs and, 298
Cerebrospinal fluid, 112
  lumbar puncture and, 545
Cerebrum, 110
Cerumen, 156
Cervical vertebrae, 96
Cervicitis, 676
Cervix, 147
  biopsy of, 672
  cancer of, 671
  cauterization of, 672
  dilatation of, in D&C, 672
  dilation of, in labor, 416
  effacement of, in labor, 418
  inflammation of, 676
Cesarean section, 413, 424
  hysterectomy and, 424
  postoperative care in, 424
  preoperative care in, 424
  reasons for, 424
Chadwick's sign, 402
Chalasia, 471
Chancre, in syphilis, 689
Chart, patient's, 224
    graphic, for TPR, 214
  in pediatrics, 452
Cheiloplasty, 487
Chemical changes, 74
Chemical reactions, 75
Chest
  injuries of, 622
  penetrating wounds of, 622
  surgery of, exercises following, 604
  thoracentesis of, 602
  x-ray of, 221, 599
    in tuberculosis, 619
Chest drainage, 603
Chest movements, uneven, 597
Cheyne-Stokes respirations, 210, 298
  in dying patient, 295
Chickenpox, 463
Child(ren). See also *Pediatric nursing*
    administering medications to, 340, 456

Child, admission of, to hospital, 448
  "battered child" syndrome, 470
  burns in, 467
  catheterization of, 450
  crib death in, 470
  death of, 457
  discharge of, from hospital, 456
  disorders of, 458-497. See *Childhood disorders*
  dog and cat scratches in, 469
  enema procedure for, 253
  forcing fluids in, 452
  foreign object trapped in body orifice in, 468
  fractures in, 469
  gavage feedings of, 452
  growth and development of, 51-56
  handicapped, 499-505
  hospitalization of, adjustment to, 446
    cultural differences and, 491
    emotional aspects in, 445
    family-centered care in, 446
    long-term, 456
    parents and, 447
    preparation of, 446
    safety measures for, 447
  needs of, 48
  oral hygiene in, 453
  oxygen therapy, for, 308
  physical examination of, 228
  poisoning in, 468
  pulse rate of, 208
  restraints for, 450
  resuscitation of, 455
  suffocation in, 469
  surgery for, special consideration of, 459
  urine specimen and, 450
  vital signs and, 449
  with diarrhea, 454
  with poor prognosis, 457
Childbearing stage, of family living, 67
Childbed fever, 424
Childbirth, emergency, 441
  natural, 409
Childhood diseases, communicable, 459-467. See also *Communicable diseases, childhood*
Childhood disorders, 458-497. See also under specific types of disorders and specific disorders and diseases
  behavior disorders, 490-491, 496
  blood defects, 480-482
  brain disorders, 475-478
  carcinomas and neoplasms, 484, 495
  cardiovascular, 494
  communicable diseases, 459-467, 495
  due to trauma, 467-470
  eyes, nose, and mouth disorders, 486-488

Childhood disorders (*continued*)
  gastrointestinal disorders, 471-472, 494
  heart and blood vessel defects, 482-484, 494
  metabolic disorders and nutritional deficiencies, 473
  musculoskeletal and orthopedic disorders, 484-486
  neurological or sensory disorders, 475-478
  parasitic infestations, 489-490
  skin disorders, 488-489
  urinary and reproductive disorders, 478-480
Childlaunching stage, of family living, 68
Chloramphenicol, 345
Chlorides, in dietary needs, 168
Chlorpromazine, 355
Choanal atresia, in newborn, 436
Cholecystitis, 137, 653
Cholecystogram, 653
Cholecystokinin, 137
Cholelithiasis, 137, 653
Cholesteatoma, 465
Cholesterol, formation of, 165
  in arteriosclerosis, 575
Choline, 174
Chorea, 565
  in rheumatic fever, 465
Chorionic villi, 398
Choroid, 157
Chromatin, 77
Chromosomes, 77
Chyme, 133
Cigarettes, and cancer, 510. See also under *Smoking*
Cilia, 85
Ciliary body, 157
Circle bed, 196, 550
Circulation, failing, in dying patient, 295
  fetal, 399
  pulmonary, 118
Circulatory disorders. See also *Cardiovascular disorders, Heart disease,* and *Peripheral vascular disorders*
  and kidney disease, 657
  in neurologic patient, 554
  oxygen needs due to, 298
Circulatory system, 81, 113-124
  and endocrine system, 150
Circulation time, determination of, 574
Circumcision, 145, 432
Circumduction, 94
Cirrhosis, 649
Cisternal puncture, 546
Clark's rule, for administering medications to children, 456
Clavicles, 98
Cleanliness, assisting patient with, 254

Cleansing enemas, 250
  procedure in, 252
Cleft lip, 486
  repair of, 487
Cleft palate, 486
  repair of, 487
Climacteric, 149, 675
Clinistix, 693
Clinitest, 693
Clitoris, 148
Closed water-seal drainage, 603
Clothing
  during pregnancy, 405
  for elderly, 735, 758
  for neurologic patient, 549
  patient's, care of, 206
    removal of, on admission, 205
Clotting, of blood, 116
Clotting time, 574
Clove-hitch restraint, 451
Clubfoot, 485
Clysis, in pediatrics, 456
Coagulants, blood, 360
Coagulation, 116
Coal tar analgesics, 350
Cobalt, manganese, body function and, 169
Cocaine, misuse of, 767
Coccyx, 97
Cochlea, 156
Code of ethics, for practical nurse, 9
Codeine, 349
Coitus, 146
Cold, common, 613
  remedies for, 367
Cold applications, 273-276
  alcohol bath, 274
  cold moist compresses in, 274
  cold sponge bath in, 274
  ice collar in, 273
Cold sore, 520, 636
Colectomy, 643
Colic, 475
Colitis, 642
  bland diet in, 179
  ulcerative, 494, 642
Collagen diseases, 465
Colon, 135. See also *Intestines*
  cancer of, 647
  irrigation of, 253
  irritable, 642
  removal of, 634
  sigmoid, and rectum, disorders of, 647
Color blindness, 710
Colostomy, 631
  and ileostomy, odor in, 634
    diarrhea in, 634
    differences between, 634
    skin care in, 634
    patient's reactions in, 634
  diet for, 634
  dressing changes in, 632
  irrigation of, 254, 632

Colostomy (*continued*)
  patient teaching in, 632
  regulated, 633
  stoma in, 631
Colostrum, 404, 422
Colporrhaphy, 679
Coma, diabetic, ketosis and, 704
  hepatic, 649
Comfort measures, 234-237
Commode, use of, 248
Communicable diseases, 42-43, 459-467
  aspesis in, 278
Communicable diseases, childhood, 459-467, 495
  chickenpox, 463
  croup, 460
  diphtheria, 464
  encephalitis, 467
  German measles, 462
  measles, 461
  measles encephalitis, 462
  meningitis, 467
  mumps, 463
  otitis media, 464
  rheumatic fever, 465
  roseola infantum, 462
  scarlet fever, 464
  streptococcal sore throat, 461
  tetanus, 467
  tonsillitis, 461
  upper respiratory infection, 460
  whooping cough, 461
  concepts of care in, 460
  control of, 34, 43
  gastrointestinal, 279, 460
  mononucleosis, 495
  of blood, 279
  of skin and mucous membrane, 460
  parenteral, 460
  respiratory, 460
  spread of, 42, 278, 460
Communications, as learning process, 15
  in elderly, 736
Community health, 32-36
Community resources, for handicapped, 505
  for psychiatric patient, 759
Compounds, chemical, 74
Compresses, cold moist, application of, 274
  warm-moist, application of, 270
Conchae, 125
Concussion, 556
Conductive deafness, 720
Cones, of retina, 158
Confused patient, 755
Congenital disorders, 23, 186, 437. See also under specific types and names of disorders
  gastrointestinal, 471
  genitourinary, 478-480
  heart defects, 482

Congenital disorders (*continued*)
hip dysplasia, 484
intellectual impairment, 500
neurological, 475
Congestive heart failure, 580
Conjunctiva, 157
injected, in drug abuse, 768
Conjunctivitis, 715
Connective tissue, 80, 86
Constipation, 254
atonic, diet and, 179
chronic or acute, 642
during pregnancy, 406
following surgery, 318
in adolescent, 496
in elderly patient, 734
in fractures, 534
in puerperium, 423
Contact lenses, 710
complications from, 711
emergency removal of, 711
eye injury and, 711
types of, 711
Contagious diseases. See *Communicable diseases*
Contraception, 369, 687
Contractility, 75
Contractions, 416
Braxton-Hicks, 415
Contractures, in burns, 525
in fractures, 534
in neurologic patient, 552
Convalescent diet, 178
Convulsive disorders, 558. See also
*Seizure disorders*
Copper, in body function, 169
Copulation, 146
Cord(s), spermatic, 145
spinal, 112. See also *Spinal cord*
umbilical. See *Umbilical cord*
vocal, 126
Cornea, 157
transplants of, 717
ulcers of, 717
in contact lenses, 711
Coronal plane, 83
Coronary arteries, 122
diseases of, 576-579
Coronary care unit, 202, 579
Coronary occlusion, 577. See also
*Myocardial infarction*
Corpus luteum, 146
Corti, organ of, 156
Cortisone, 153, 697
in arthritis, 532
secretion of, 697
side-effects of, 532
Coryza, 461
Cosmetic surgery, in burns, 524
Cough, as symptom, 187, 597
drugs for, 366
Cough reflex, 50
Cowper's glands, 145
Coxa plana, 493
Cradle, bed, 200

"Cradle-cap", 489
Cranial nerves, evaluation of, 545
Craniectomy, 557
Craniostenosis, 477
Craniotomy, 557
Cranium, bones of, 95
Cretinism, 152
Crib, making of, 448
Crib death, 470
Crib net, as restraint, 451
Cross-eye, 715
Croup, 460
Croupette, in oxygen therapy, 308, 454
"Crowning," 417
Crushing injuries, in children, 469
Crusts, skin, 517
removal of, 518
Crutch walking, 538-541
crutches in, 538
four-point, 540
swing or tripod walking, 540
technic for, 539
three-point, 539
two-point, 539
Crutches, 538
Crying, in neonate, 431
Cryosurgery, 716
Cryptorchidism, 478, 685
Crystalluria, 658
C-section. See *Cesarean section*
Culdoscopy, 672
Culture
blood, 575
gastric washing for, 598
in microbiology, 39
sputum, 598
throat, 598
urine, 658
Curare, 356
Curettage, of uterus, 672
Cushing's syndrome, 694, 698
CVA (cerebral vascular accident), 298, 561
CVP (central venous pressure), 575
Cyanosis, 299
as symptom, 187
in newborn, 435
Cylindruria, 658
Cyst(s)
Bartholin, 148
in mastitis, 679
of kidneys, 666
ovarian, 677
pilonidal, 648
sebaceous, 518
Cystic fibrosis, 474
Cystitis, 662
Cystocath, suprapubic, 661
Cystocele and rectocele, 679
Cystogram, 659
Cystoscopy, 659
Cystostomy, cutaneous, 661
Cystotomy, 665
Cytoplasm, 77

D&C (dilatation and curettage), 672
Daily needs of patient, assisting with, 230-266
Dandruff, 519
Deafness, conductive, 720
perceptive or sensorineural, 720
rehabilitation in, 377
Death
biological, 582
care of body following, 296
clinical, 582
crib, 470
occurrence of, 296
physical changes preceding, 294
psychology of, 292
sudden, 582
Debridement, of burns, 524
Decathexis, dying patient and, 293
Decubitus ulcers, 264
Deficiency diseases, 186
Deformities, prevention of, 264
Deglutition, 132
Dehydration, 139
in urinary disorders, 662
of newborn, 438
Delivery, 419-421
by instrument, 420
injury due to, 437
fear of, 407
fetal presentation in, 419
labor and, complications of, 420
precipitate, 420
Demand feeding, 435
Demerol, 349
Dendrites, 107
Dental care, 27-28. See *Oral hygiene*
Dental caries, 636
Dentifrices, 362
Dentures, 636
mouth care and, 255
removal of, before surgery, 314
Deoxyribonucleic acid (DNA), 78
Depressants, 348-355
heart, 357
respiratory, 366
Depressed patient, 749
Dermatitis, 517
seborrheic, 519
Dermatitis venenata, 517
Dermatologist, 516
Dermatology, 516
Dermis, 87
Desensitization, in allergy, 727
Detoxification units, in drug abuse, 776
Developmental tasks, 48
Diabetes insipidus, 694
cause of, 151
primary, 694
secondary, 694
Diabetes mellitus, 153, 699-707
age and, 699
brittle, 699
coma in, ketosis and, 704
diet in, 180, 700, 705

Diabetes mellitus (*continued*)
　exercise in, 700
　identification, 707
　in child, 475, 494
　infant of mother with, 438
　infection in, 706
　instructing, patient with, 704
　juvenile, 475, 494, 699
　maturity onset, 699
　obesity and, 699
　pregnancy and, 413
　rehabilitation in, 376
　smoking and, 706
　surgery in, 709
　symptoms of, 700
　tests for, 692
　treatment of, 700
　types of, 699
Dialysis, 667
Dialysis unit, 202
　career opportunities in, 781
Diaphragm, 103
Diaphragmatic hernia, 471
Diaphysis, 92
Diarrhea, 254, 642
　as symptom, 187
　bland diet in, 179
　caring for child with, 454
　following vagotomy, 641
　in colostomy or ileostomy, 634
　in newborn, 438
Diarthrodial joint, 92
Diastole, 116
Diastolic pressure, 215
Diet(s)
　acid-alkaline, 181
　as treatment, 179-181
　bland, 179
　charting of, for child, 452
　convalescent, 178
　daily, recommended, 167t
　during pregnancy, 403
　effects of, on teeth, 28
　following surgery, 320
　for aged, 758
　for neurologic patient, 554
　for nursing mother, 433
　full, 178
　high calorie, 179
　high fiber, 179
　high iron, 180
　high vitamin, 181
　in burns, 523
　in cancer, 515
　in colostomy, 634
　in diabetes, 700, 705
　in food allergy, 181
　in ileostomy, 634
　in peptic ulcer, 638
　in puerperium, 423
　in tuberculosis, 620
　light, 178
　liquid, 178
　low calorie, 180
　low carbohydrate, 180

Diet(s) (*continued*)
　low purine, 181
　low residue or residue-free, 179
　low sodium, 180
　Sippy, 179, 638
　soft, 178
　special, 177-181
　types of, 177-179
Diet planning, 169, 175
Digestants, 363
Digestive disorders, 244, 624-655. See
　　also *Gastrointestinal disorders*
　　and specific disorders
　colostomy and ileostomy, 631
　common, 625
　diagnostic tests for, 625
　esophageal disorders, 637-638
　gastrointestinal cancer in, 635
　intestinal disorders, 642
　mouth disorders, 635
　nursing procedures in, 628-635
　stomach disorders, 638-641
　suction drainage in, 628
　tube feeding in, 630
Digestive system, 81, 130-138, 625
　accessory organs of, 136
Digitalis, 356, 581
Dilaudid, 349
Dilatation and Curettage (D&C), 672
Diphtheria, 464
　immunity test for, 372
Diplopia, 488, 564
Disaster emergency, 232
Disc, herniated, 567
　intervertebral, 96
Discharges, body, disposal of, in iso-
　　lation technic, 282
Disease. See also types of diseases or
　　specific names of diseases
　acute, 186
　chronic, 186
　classification of, 186
　communicable, 42-43
　　childhood, 459-467
　congenital, 186
　course of, 186
　deficiency, 186
　hereditary, 186
　infectious, 186
　metabolic, 186
　neoplastic, 186
　occupational, 186
　organic and functional, 185
　signs and symptoms of, 185-189
　subacute, 186
Disimpaction, 631
Disinfectants, 40
　and antiseptics, 340
Disinfection, and sterilization, 284
　concurrent, 278
　of clinical thermometer, 214
　terminal, isolation technic in, 283
Dislocations, 533
　of hip, in children, 484
Distention, following surgery, 318

Diuretics, 361
Diverticulitis, 645
Diverticulosis, 645
Diverticulum, Meckel's, 471
DNA (deoxyribonucleic acid), 78
Doctor's orders, 224
　checking of, 207
　for drugs, 326
　transcription of, 340
Dog bites, in children, 469
Dorsal cavity, 83
"Double-bagging," in isolation tech-
　　nic, 282
Douche, 287, 674
Down's syndrome, 500
Drainage
　closed water-seal, 603
　following surgery, 320
　postural, 599
　suction, gastrointestinal, 628
　urinary, 660
Dressings
　changes of, following surgery, 320
　　in colostomy, 632
　　sterile technic and, 287
　in burns, 524
　moist, in skin disorders, 517
Drug(s), 323, 761
　abbreviations in prescription of,
　　326
　administration of, by injection, 330
　　by mouth, 330, 325
　　by rectum, 325
　　to children, 340
　allergic reactions to, 729
　and health, 34
　and individual patient, 324
　anticonvulsant, 353
　comparison of, 762t
　contraceptive, 369
　control of, 34
　dependence on, 761
　dosage of, 324
　effects of, on autonomic nervous
　　system, 355-356
　　on blood, 359
　　on blood vessels, 357
　　on central nervous system, 347-
　　355
　　in intestinal action, 363
　　on mouth, 362
　　on musculoskeletal system, 356
　　on reproductive system, 367-369
　　on respiratory system, 366
　　on urinary system, 361-362
　enzymes as, 372
　for arthritis, 530
　for allergies, 370, 727
　for asthma, 370
　for cancer, 372-373, 513
　for cough, 366
　for eye disorders, 369-370
　for gastrointestinal disorders and
　　disease, 362-365

Drug(s) *(continued)*
  for heart and blood vessel disorders, 356-359
  for psychiatric disorders, 751
  for skin and mucous membranes, 340
  for stomach conditions, 362
  for tuberculosis, 618
  forms of, 323
  immunosuppressive, 586
  in x-ray procedures, 363
  inhalation of, 325
  injection of, intradural, 325
    subcutaneous, 325
  intravenous, 339
  local application of, 325
  mental retardation due to, 500
  methods of giving, 325
  names of, 323
  nonuse and hoarding of, 770
  preoperative, 313
  prescription of, 326
  sources for study of, 323
  systemic, 325
  to destroy parasites, 370
Drug abuse. See *Drug misuse*
Drug allergies, 729
Drug antagonists, in drug abuse therapy, 776
Drug misuse, 760-776
  acute detoxification units in, 776
  chemotherapy in, 776
  group psychotherapy in, 776
  in school-age child and adolescent, 497
  legal aspects of, 762
  nursing skills in, 768-771
  role of health professionals in, 772
  signs of, 768
  socioeconomic aspects of, 771
  specific drugs in, 763-768
    alcohol, 763
    amphetamines in, 764
    barbiturates and sedatives, 764
    caffeine, 763
    cocaine, 767
    glue sniffing, 764
    hallucinogens, 767
    inhalants, 764
    LSD, 767
    marijuana, 766
    Mescaline, 767
    opiate narcotics, 765
    psychostimulants, 764
    tobacco, 763
  treatment considerations in, 771-775
  treatment modalities in, 775-776
Drug standards, 323
Dry heat, 268
Duct(s), ejaculatory, 145
  nasolacrimal, 125
Ductus arteriosus, 399
Ductus deferens, 145
"Dumping," in peptic ulcer, 641

Duncan presentation, of placenta, 417
Duodenum, 154
Dura mater, 112
Dwarfism, 151
Dying patient, 292-296
  family of, 292, 294, 296
  physical care of, 294
  psychological aspects of, 292
Dyskinesia, tardive, 772
Dyslexia, 504
Dysmenorrhea, 674
Dyspepsia, in stomach cancer, 641
Dysphagia, 597
Dysphonia, in drug use, 768
Dysplasia, hip, congenital, 484
Dyspnea, 129, 209, 298, 597
  as symptom, 187
  during pregnancy, 406
Dysrhythmia, in epilepsy, 558

Ear, 155-157
  disorders of, 719-725
    impaired hearing, 487, 719, 720, 736
    of external ear, 722
      external otitis, 722
      foreign objects in, 390, 469, 722
      fungous infections, 722
      furuncles, 722
      impacted earwax, 722
      insect infestation, 722
      punctured eardrum, 722
    of inner ear, 724
      labyrinthine hydrops, 724
      Meniere's disease, 724
    of middle ear, 723
      cholesteatoma, 465
      infection, 724
      otitis media, 724
      otosclerosis, 723
    hearing tests and, 720
Eardrum, 156
  punctured, 723
Earlobes, piercing of, 723
Earwax, impacted, 722
Eating habits, poor, 162
ECG (electrocardiogram), 573
Eclampsia, 410
Ecology, 33
Ectopic pregnancy, 147, 412, 676
Ectropian, 715
Eczema, 486, 489, 521, 727
  infantile, 489
Eczema herpeticulum, 489
Eczema vaccinatum, 463
Edema, 139, 181
  angioneurotic, 519, 727
  as symptom, 187
  in casts, 534
  in heart disease, 573
  in pregnancy, 407
  in skin disorders, 519
  pitting, 589

EEG (electroencephalogram), 547
  in epilepsy, 558
Ejaculatory duct, 145
EKG (electrocardiogram), 573
Elastic stocking, 277
Elastic tissue, 86
Elderly
  developmental tasks of, 69
  diet for, 758
  clothing for, 758
  communication in, 736
  community agencies for, 737
  elimination problems of, 734
  emotional support and mental stimulation of, 736
  nursing care of, 733-738
  occupation and exercise for, 758
  personal hygiene in, 735
  physical activity and exercise in, 736
  safety precautions for, 735, 758
  skin care in, 758
  special needs of, 734-737
  swallowing difficulties in, 734
  tube feeding in, 734
Electrical equipment, 194
Electric pad, 269
Electrocardiogram, 573
Electroconvulsive therapy, 751
Electrodermal reflex, in hearing, 720
Electroencephalography, 547
Electrolyte(s), 80
Electrolyte balance, 80
  following surgery, 320
  in burns, 523
  in skin disorders, 518
Electromyelogram, in musculoskeletal disorders, 527
Electroretinogram, 709
Elimination
  assisting patient with, 245-254
  habits of, in general health, 27
  disorders of, 254. See also under specific disorder
  in elderly patients, 734
  in observation of patient, 189
  in pregnancy, 404
  in traction, 538
  nutrition and, 245
  special procedures for, 630
Embolism, 587
  and thrombosis, in limb, 588
  cerebral, 561
  in fractures, 534, 535
Embolus, 117, 319
Embryo, 401
Emergency(ies)
  and first aid, 379-394
  disaster, 232
  enemas in, 251
  fire, 232
  in childbirth, 441
  legal responsibilities in, 788

Emergency(ies) (*continued*)
nursing care in, 379
oxygen therapy in, 305
psychiatric, services in, 743
Emergency room, 202
Emesis, 187, 244
Emetics, 363
Emollients, 340
in enemas, 251
Emotional disorders. See also *Psychiatric disorders*
in adolescents, 496
Emotions, 30
effect of, 24
of patient, in surgery, 311
observation of, 189
Emphysema, 612
Empyema (pyothorax), 614
Encephalitis, 467, 566
Encephalocele, 475
Encephalomyelitis, 467
Endocarditis, bacterial, 585
Endocardium, 117
Endocrine disorders, 691-707
diagnostic tests in, 691-693
in school-age child and adolescent, 494
of adrenal glands, 697-698
Addison's disease, 698
Cushing's syndrome, 698
pseudohermaphroditism, 698
tumors of adrenal medulla, 698
of pancreas, 698-707
diabetes mellitus, 699-707
of parathyroids, 697
hyperparathyroidism, 697
hypoparathyroidism, 697
of pituitary, 693-694
acromegaly, 694
diabetes insipidus, 694
gigantism, 694
panhypopituitarism, 694
Simmonds' disease, 694
tumors, 694
of thyroid, 694-697
exophthalmic goiter, 695
Graves' disease, 695
hyperthyroidism, 695
hypothyroidism, 696
myxedema, 696
simple (colloid) goiter, 696
tumors, 696
Endocrine system, 81, 150-154
Endometrium, 147
Endoscopy, 627
Endosteum, 92
Endotracheal tube, in opening airway, 300
in oxygen therapy during surgery, 306
Enemas, 249-253, 630
care of, equipment for, 253
doctor's orders concerning, 253
difficulties with, 253
emergency measures in, 251

Enemas (*continued*)
for child, 253, 454
kinds of, 250
anthelmintic, 251
carminative, 251
cleansing, 250
emollient, 251
medicated, 251
nutritive, 251
methods and equipment for, 249
patient's position for, 251
predelivery, 417
preoperative, 313
rectal tube in, 249, 252
solution in, 250
Energy, 75
and growth, food for, 161-174
Entropian, 715
Enucleation, 714, 717
Enuresis, 57, 480, 496
Enzymes, 130, 134t
as drugs, 372
pancreatic, 134
stomach, 133
zinc and, 169
Ephebiatrics, 59
Epidemic parotitis, 463
Epidermis, 87
Epididymis, 145
Epididymitis, 685
Epiglottis, 126, 133
Epilepsy, 558. See also *Seizure disorders*
Epinephrine, 153, 355, 357, 697
Epiphysis, 92
Episiotomy, 417
Episodic stupor, 649
Epispadias, 478, 685
Epistaxis, 482, 495, 605
Epithelium, 80, 85
Equipment, hospital
cleaning of, 195
enamelware, 195
glassware, 195
linen, 195
rubber, 195
stainless steel, 195
electrical, use of, 194
for bedmaking, 197
for patient unit, 195
for physical examination, 226
for traction, 201
in recovery room, 316
sterile, 285
ER (emergency room), 202
Erb-Duchenne paralysis, 436
Erepsin, 165
ERG (electroretinogram), 709
Erythroblastosis fetalis, 400
Erythrocytes, 114
Erythromycins, 345
Esophageal speech, 608
Esophagoscopy, 599

Esophagus, 133
disorders of, 637-638
atresia, 437
cancer, 511, 638
cardiospasm, 638
diverticulum, 637
varices, 588, 637
tubes for compression of, 630
Estrogen(s), 146, 154, 368
in lactation, 148
in menstruation, 149
preparations of, 368
secondary sex characteristics and, 144
Ethics, code of, for practical nurse, 9
telephone, 229
Ethyl alcohol, 354
Eupnea, 129
Eustachian tubes, 126, 156
Evening care, 232
Eversion, 95
Evisceration, following surgery, 320, 641
Ewing's sarcoma, 495
Examination
breast, 672
eye, 710
gynecologic, 227, 571
licensing, for practical nurse, 786
neurologic, 544
ophthalmoscopic, 709
pelvic, 671
physical, assisting with, 225-229
in pregnancy, 402
of neonate, 430
postpartum, 423
rectal, 228
in labor, 418
vaginal, 227
Exanthem sebitum, 462
Excoriations, 517
Excreta, disposal of, in isolation technic, 282
Excretory system, 139-141
Exenteration, 714
Exercise(s)
and rest, health and, 29
bed, 238
breathing, 601
during pregnancy, 404
following chest surgery, 604
for amputation, 541
for elderly, 736, 758
in arthritis, 530
in diabetes, 700
range of motion, 552, 736
Exophthalmia, 152
Exophthalmic goiter, 695
Exophthalmos, 695
Expansional dyspnea, 298
Expectorants, 366
Expectoration, as respiratory symptom, 597
Expiration, respiratory, 125, 597
Expirational dyspnea, 298

Extended care facility, 738
Extension, in body movements, 94
Exteroceptors, 108
Extracellular fluids, 79
Extremities, structure of, 97-99
Exudate, 188
    removal of, 518
Eye(s), 157-158
    bloodshot, in drug abuse, 768
    care of, 28
        in dying patient, 295
        in neonate, 431
        in neurologic patient, 553
    disorders of, 708-719. See also *Eye disorders*
    examination of, 710
        in diabetes, 705
        Ishihara chart in, 710
        Snellen chart in, 710
    foreign bodies in, 718
        in child, 469
        removal of, 390
    hematoma of, 715
    irrigations of, 713
    ointments for, 713
    prosthetic, 714
    silver nitrate prophylaxis for, 429
Eye blink reflex, 157
Eye disorders, 708-719
    acid or alkali burns, 715
    actinic trauma, 715
    blindness, 718
    cataract, 715
    common, 714
    conjunctivitis, 715
    corneal transplants, 717
    corneal ulcers, 717
    corrective lens for, 710
    detached retina, 717
    diagnostic tests for, 708
    drugs for, 369-370
    ectropian, 715
    entropian, 715
    enucleation, 717
    glaucoma, 715
    hematoma formation (black eye), 715
    in children, 488
    nursing care in, 712
        preoperative and postoperative, 713
    pink eye, 715
    ptosis, 715
    refraction error, 714
    strabismus, 715
    stye, 715
    sympathetic ophthalmia, 717
    trachoma, 715
    tumors of, 718
Eye signs, in neurological examination, 544
Eyeball, 157
    pressure within, 709
Eyedrops, instillation of, 712

Eyeglasses, 711
Eyelid, 157
    ptosis of, 488, 715
    trachoma of, 715
    bones of, 95

Face mask, in oxygen therapy, 303
Facet, of bone, 93
Fainting, first aid for, 387
Fallopian tubes, 147
    ectopic pregnancy in, 412
    inflammation of, 676
    ligation of, 687
Family, 66
    as unit, 65
    changes within, 65
    developmental tasks of, 66
    life cycle of, 66
    needs of, 19
    of dying patient, 292, 294, 296
    of hospitalized child, 447
        in cerebral vascular accident, 563
    of patient, in rehabilitation, 377
        in surgery, 315
    patient as part of, 70
    stages of, 66
Family-centered care, 408, 446
Family living, 65-70
Farsightedness, 158, 714
Fascia, 100
    renal, 140
Fascial membrane, 86
Fatigue, as symptom, 187
Fat-soluble vitamins, 170
Fatty acids, 165
Fats, 163, 164
Feces, 136
    collecting specimen of, 246
    digital removal of, 254, 631
    observation of, 245
Feeding(s)
    in cerebral palsy, 503
    in cleft lip and palate, 486
    in gastrostomy, 630
    intravenous, 243
    nasogastric, 630
    of elderly patients, 734
    in infant, 432-435
    of premature infant, 440
    of semiconscious patient, 554
    tube, 630
        nasogastric, in laryngectomy, 608
Femur, 97
    epiphysis of, slipped, 493
Fenestration operation, in otosclerosis, 723
Fertility and infertility, 686
Fertility drugs, 369
Fertilization, 147, 398
    timing of, 149
Fetal heart tones, 403
Fetus, 401
    abortion of, 411
    circulation of, 399

Fetus (*continued*)
    development of, 401
    presentation of, in delivery, 419
        abnormal, 420
        breech, 419
        cephalic, 419
Fetuscope, 417
Fever, 211
    as symptom, 187
    childbed, 424
    continued, 211
    crisis in, 211
    glandular, 495
    in leukemia, 593
    intermittent, 211
    lysis in, 211
    remittent, 211
    rheumatic, 465, 495, 584
Fever blister, 636
Fibrillation, auricular and ventricular, 582
    oxygen needs and, 298
Fibrin, 116
Fibrinogen, 116
Fibrosis, cystic, 474
Fibrous joints, 92
Fibrous membrane, 86
Fibula, 98
Films, as learning aids, 12
Fingernails, care of, 260
Fire emergency, in hospital, 232
First aid, 379-394
    bandages in, 381
    cardiopulmonary resuscitation in, 380
    in asphyxiation, 381
    in bleeding, 380
    in burns, 389
    in chest injuries, 622
    in fainting, 387
    in fractures, 380, 388
    in frostbite, 388
    in head injuries, 390
    in heat exhaustion, 389
    in hemorrhage, 380, 382
    in myocardial infarction, 578
    in poisoning, 386
    in removing foreign body from eye, 390
    in shock, 380
    in sunstroke, 389
    legal aspects of, 393
    principles of, 380
    procedures and follow-up in, 380
    pulmonary resuscitation in, 380
    tourniquet use in, 384
    transporting patient and, 388
    wound dressing in, 380
Fission, 40
Fissure, anal, 648
    skin, 517
Fistula, 188
    anal, 648

Fistula (*continued*)
  tracheo-esophageal, 437
  vaginal, 678
Fixation, internal, 535
Flatus, relief of, 248
  following surgery, 318
Flexion, 94
Fluid(s), body, 79
  cerebrospinal, 112
  synovial, 94
Fluid intake, 243
  health and, 27
Fluid therapy
  following surgery, 320
  for neurologic patient, 554
Fluid therapy, in burns, 523
  in skin disorders, 518
  in pediatric nursing, 452, 455
Flukes, 490
Fluoridation, water, and dental
  health, 28
Fluorine, body needs and, 169
Fluoroscopy, in digestive disorders,
  626
  in respiratory disorders, 599
Folacin, 173
Folic acid, 173
Folic-acid antagonists, in cancer
  therapy, 513
Follicles, graafian, 146
Follicular hormone, 368
Fomites, 42
Food(s), 130, 161-174
  and energy, 166
  and fluids, assisting patient with,
    243-244
  and health, 27, 162
  basic 4, 163
  before operation, 313
  carbohydrates in, 163
  diabetic, 700
  diet planning and, 169
  during pregnancy, 403
  fats in, 164
  following surgery, 320
  for growth and energy, 161-174
  for neonate, 431
  illness and, 189
  minerals in, 167
  proteins in, 165
  serving of, in hospital, 176
  special diets and, 177-181
  supplementary, for infant, 435
  vitamins and, 169
Food ellergy, diet in, 181
Food and Drug Administration, 34,
  323
Food poisoning, first aid for, 387
Food tray, serving of, 243
Foot, structure of, 98
Foot care, in diabetes, 706
Foot-and-mouth disease, 636
Footboard, 201
Footdrop, in fractures, 534
  in traction, 537

Footling, 419
Footprints, infant, 428
Foramen ovale, in fetal circulation,
  399
Forceps delivery, 420
  injury due to, 437
Forceps transfer, in handling sterile
  supplies, 285
Formulas, premixed, 435
  preparation of, 434
Fossa, 93
Fowler's position, 227
Fracture(s), 533
  casts in, 534
  causes of, 533
  complications of, 533
  during birth, 436
  first aid for, 380, 388
  in children, 469
  of hip, 538
  of jaw, 636
  of ribs, 622
  of skull, depressed, 556
  splinting of, 388
  symptoms of, 533
  treatment of, 533
  types of, 533
Frontal plane, 83
Frostbite, first aid for, 388
Fructose, 164
Fruits, daily requirements, 163
FSH (follicle-stimulating hormone),
  368
Fulguration, 659
Functional diseases, 185
Fundus, of uterus, 147
  cancer of, 677
  in postpartum care, 421
Fungi, 40
Furuncle, 520
  of auditory canal, 722
Furunculosis, 520

Gag reflex, 50
Galactose, 164
Gallbladder, 134, 136
  disorders of, 653-655
    cancer, 655
    cholecystitis, 653
    cholelithiasis, 653
    gallstones, 653
    inflammation, 653
Gallstones, 137, 653
Ganglion, 107, 528
Gargles, and mouthwashes, 362
Gas, relief of, 248
Gastrectomy, in peptic ulcer, 640
  in stomach cancer, 641
Gastric analysis, 625
Gastric lavage, for culture, 598
  in poisoning, 468
Gastrin, 154
Gastroenterostomy, 640
Gastrointestinal decompression, 628

Gastrointestinal disorders. See also
  *Digestive disorders*, specific
  name of disorder and disorders
  of specific part of gastrointestinal tract
  allergy, 727
  cancer, 635
  communicable diseases in, 279, 460
  congenital, 471-472
    chalasia, 471
    hernias, 471
    Meckel's diverticulum, 471
    phenylketonuria (PKU), 472
    pyloric stenosis, 471
  diagnostic series in, 626
  drugs affecting, 362-365
  in adolescent, 494
  in children, 471-472, 494
  in newborn, 437
  of esophagus, 637-638
  of gallbladder, 653-655
  of intestines, 642-647
  of liver, 649-653
  of pancreas, 655
  of sigmoid colon and rectum, 647-
    648
  of stomach, 638-641
Gastrointestinal tube, insertion and
  removal of, 629
Gastrostomy, 630
Gavage feedings, in pediatrics, 452
Genes, 77
  in Down's syndrome, 500
Genetic code, 78
Genetic counseling, in handicapped
  conditions, 505
Genitalia, external, of female, 148
  of male, 145
Genitourinary disorders. See also
  *Urinary disorders* and *Reproductive disorders*
  acute glomerulonephritis, 479
  Bright's disease, 479, 663
  congenital, 478
    cryptorchidism, 478
    epispadias, 478
    exstrophy of bladder, 478
    hermaphroditism, 478
    hypospadias, 478
    polycystic kidney, 478
  enuresis, 57, 480, 496
  hydrocele, 478
  in children, 478-480, 494
  nephritis, 478, 664
  nephroblastoma, 479
  nephrosis, 479
  pyelonephritis, 478, 663
  renal failure, 479, 666-668
  urinary obstruction, 479, 664
  Wilms's tumor, 479
Geriatric nursing, 733-738. See also
  *Elderly*
German measles, effects of, on newborn, 438
  in child, 462

G.I. series, 626
Giantism, 694
Gifts, and tips, nursing ethics and, 222
  legal aspects of, 788
Gigantism, 151
Gingivitis, during pregnancy, 407
Girdle pain, 555
Glands, 85
  adrenal, 153
    disorders of, 697-698
  Bartholin's, 148
  bulbourethral, 145
  Cowper's, 145
  ductless, 150, 691
  endocrine, 150, 691
  lacrimal, 157
  mammary, 148
  of Montgomery, 148
  parathyroid, 153
    disorders of, 697
  pineal, 154
  pituitary, 150
    disorders of, 693-694
  prostate, 145
  salivary, 132
  sebaceous, 88
    disorders of, 518
  suprarenal, 153
  sweat, 88
  thyroid, 151
    disorders of, 695
Glandular fever, 495
Glans penis, 145
Glaucoma, 715
  drugs for, 370
Gliding joint, 92
Glomerulonephritis, 663
  chronic, 664
  in children, 479
Glomerulus, 140, 663
Glove restraint, 452
Gloves, rubber, cleaning of, 195
  sterile, 286
Glucagon, 153
Glucose, 164
Glucose tolerance test, 692
Glue sniffing, 764
Gluteal muscles, 104
Glutin-induced celiac disease, 474
Glycogen, 164, 166
Glycogenesis, 153
Glycosuria, 657, 692
Goiter, 152
  colloid, 696
  exophthalmic, 695
  simple, 696
  toxic, 696
Gonads, 153
Gonorrhea, 689
  douches and, 288
  effects of, on infant, 438
  in urinary system, 664
  silver nitrate prophylaxis and, 429

Gout, 531
  diet for, 181
Gowns, in isolation technic, 280
  sterile, in surgical asepsis, 286
  in pediatrics, 452
Graafian follicles, 146
Grafts, skin, in skin disorders, 522
Grand mal seizures, 558. See also *Seizure disorders*
"Grandfather clause," in licensing laws, 7
Graphic chart, for TPR, 214
Grasp reflex, 50
Graves disease, 152, 695
Growth, and development, 47-58
  and energy, food for, 161-174
  and learning, 48
  stages of, 49-56
Growth hormone, 151
Guiac test, 625
Gynecologic examination, 227, 671
Gynecologic nursing procedures, 673
Gynecomastia, 683

Habituation, in drug use, 761
Hair, 88
  care of, 261
    for neurologic patient, 554
    in elderly patient, 735
  covering of, in surgical asepsis, 286
Hallucinogens, 767
Handicapped child, 499-505
  nursing care of, 504-505
  with intellectual impairment, 499-502
  with special learning needs, 502-504
Handicapped conditions, genetic counseling in, 505
  rehabilitation in, 374-378
Hand, structure of, 99
Handwashing technics, 233
  for patient, 254
  in isolation technic, 280
Harelip, 486
Hay fever, 609
Head, injuries of, first aid for, 390
Headache, as neurologic symptom, 547
  migraine, 547
Headboard, emergency, 201
Health, 23
  and personality, 25-31
  body mechanics and, 27
  community, 32-36
  dental, 27-28, 636
  drugs and, 34
  effect of heredity on, 23-24
  elimination habits and, 27
  exercise and rest and, 29
  food and, 27, 162
  mental, 742
  positive, 24

Health (*continued*)
  posture and, 25, *26*
  prenatal and postnatal, 35
  total, 24
Health agencies, 32
Health services, 35
Health test, 599
Hearing, 155
  impaired, 719
    in cleft lip and palate, 487
  loss of, central, 720
    in elderly, 736
    prevention of, 721
  tests of, 720
Heart, 117-119. See also under *Cardiac* and *Cardiovascular*
  disease of, 482-483, 573-576. See also *Heart disease*
  drugs affecting, 356-359
  surgery on, closed, 585
    open, 585
    nursing care in, 586
    types of, 586
  transplant of, 586
Heart disease, 482-483, 573-576
  aneurysms, 584
  angina pectoris, 576
  aortic stenosis, 484
  arrhythmias, 581
  auricular and ventricular fibrillation, 582
  bacterial endocarditis, 585
  breathing difficulties in, 573
  cardiac arrest, 582
  coarctation of aorta, 484
  congenital defects, 482-483
    anomalous venous return, 483
    aortic stenosis, 484
    atrial septal defects, 483
    coarctation of aorta, 484
    patent ductus arteriosus, 483
    pulmonary stenosis, 484
    tetralogy of Fallot, 483
    transposition of great vessels, 483
    tricuspid atresia, 483
    ventricular septal defects, 483
  congestive heart failure, 580
  coronary artery disease, 576-579
  coronary occlusion, 577
  cough in, 187
  diagnostic tests in, 573
  diet in, 180
  drugs for, 356-359
  functional, 579
  heart block, 581
  in children, 482-484
  infectious, 584-585
  ischemic, 576
  myocardial infarction, 577
  oxygen needs in, 298
  predisposing factors in, 575
  pregnancy and, 413
  restriction of activity in, 466
  rheumatic carditis, 466

Heart disease (continued)
  rheumatic fever, 584
  signs and symptoms of, 573
  surgical aspects of, 585
Heart block, 119, 581
Heartburn, 244
Heat
  application of, 268
    compresses and packs in, 270
    dry, 268
    electric pad and, 269
    lamp treatments in, 269
    moist, 270
    sitz bath in, 272
    soaks in, 271
    warm-water bag and, 268
  excessive, effects of, 388
  sensitivity to, 268
Heat exhaustion, first aid in, 389
Helminths, 42
  drugs for destruction of, 370
Hemangiomas, 488
Hematoma, of eye, 715
Hemiplegia, in CVA, 561
Hemodialysis, 667
Hemoglobin, 115, 359
  copper and, 169
  iron and, 168
  lack of, oxygen needs and, 298
  vitamin C and, 171
Hemoglobinuria, 657
Hemophilia, 186, 480, 595
Hemoptysis, 597
Hemorrhage
  and blood types, 117
  as symptom, 187
  cerebral, 561
  control of, by pressure, 382
  first aid in, 380, 382
  following gastrectomy, 641
  following hemorrhoidectomy, 647
  following nasal surgery, 605
  following surgery, 317
  from artery, 382
  from vein, 382
  in peptic ulcer, 640
  in tuberculosis, 621
  intracranial, due to birth injury, 437
  postpartum, 421, 424
  vitamin K and, 171
Hemorrhoidectomy, 647
Hemorrhoids, 588, 647
  external, 647
  in pregnancy, 407
  internal, 647
Hemostatics, 360
Henle, loop of, 140
Hepatic coma, 649
Hepatitis, 651
Heredity
  and environment, in growth and development, 49
  cancer and, 510

Heredity (continued)
  diseases due to, 186. See also specific names of diseases
  health and, 23-24
Hermaphroditism, 478
Hernia
  abdominal, 645
  congenital, 471
  diaphragmatic, 471
  inguinal, 145, 471
  strangulated, 646
  umbilical, 471
Herniorrhaphy, 646
Heroin, misuse of, 765
Herpes simplex, 520, 636
Herpes zoster, 520, 560
Hexylresorcinol, 371
Hinge joints, 92
Hip
  congenital dysplasia, 484
  coxa plana and, 493
  dislocation of, in children, 484
  fractures of, 538
  prosthesis for, 538
Hip bath, 272
Hirschsprung's disease, 473
Histoplasmosis, 617
  test for, 599
History, medical, 225
  in pregnancy, 402
Hives, 519, 727
Hodgkin's disease, 511, 594
Home care, of patient, 193, 232
Homeostasis, urinary system and, 139
Homograft, 525
Hood, surgical, surgical asepsis and, 286
Hookworms, 490
Hordeolum, 715
Horizontal plane, 83
Hormone(s), 150, 691
  antidiuretic, 151, 694
  changes in, during climacteric, 675
  extract of, affecting sex glands, 368
  follicular, 368
    from posterior pituitary, 367
  growth, 151
  menopause and, 149
  ovarian, 368
  placental, 368
  secondary sex characteristics and, 144
Hospital, 193-202
  admitting patient to, 204
  career opportunities for practical nurse in, 780
  departments of, 201
  discharge of patient from, 221
  electrical equipment in, 194
  intercommunication system in, 195
  introducing patient to, 203-221
  mental, 744-751. See also Mental Hospital

Hospital (continued)
  personnel and services of, 201
  ventilation in, 194
  ward order in, 195
Hostile patient, 749, 754
Household Nursing School, 5
HS medications, 330
Humerus, 98
Hunchback, 96
Huntington's disease, 565
Hyaline membrane disease, 436
Hydatidiform mole, 413
Hydrocele, 478, 685
Hydrocephalus, 476
Hydronephrosis, 665
Hydrotherapy, 749
Hymen, 148
Hyperactive child, 490
Hyperadrenalism, 698
Hyperbaric medicine, career opportunities in, 782
Hyperemesis gravidarum, 409
Hyperglycemia, 699
Hyperkinetic child, 490
Hyperopia, 158, 714
Hyperparathyroidism, 697
Hyperpnea, hysterical, 598
Hypersomnia, 496
Hypertension, 215
  essential, 576
  in heart disease, 575
  malignant, 576
  treatment and nursing care in, 576
Hyperthyroidism, 152, 695
Hyperuricemia, 531
Hyperventilation, 298, 597
Hypnotics and sedatives, 351
Hypochondriac, approach to, 745
Hypodermoclysis, 325
Hypogammaglobulinemia, 481
Hypoglycemia, 699
Hypokinetic child, 491
Hypomaniac patient, 753
Hypoparathyroidism, 697
Hypophysectomy, 694
Hypophysis, 150. See also Pituitary gland
Hypopituitarism, 694
Hypospadias, 478, 685
Hypostatic pneumonia, 538, 554, 615
Hypotension, 116, 215
Hypothalamus, 111
Hypothermia, 211
Hypothyroidism, 152, 696
Hypoxia, following surgery, 318
Hysterectomy
  abdominal, 678
  cesarean section and, 424
  vaginal, 678

Icecap, 273
Ice collar, 273
Icterus, 649
Icterus gravis, 652
ICU (intensive care unit), 202

Identification, of patient
  in diabetes, 707
  in glaucoma, 716
  in laryngectomy, 608
  in seizure disorders, 560
  on admission, 206
Ileocecal valve, 135
Ileal conduit, 661
Ileostomy, 631
  and colostomy, differences between, 634
  odor in, 634
  patient's reaction in, 634
  skin care in, 634
  diet for, 634
  in ulcerative colitis, 643
Ileus, paralytic, 318
Ilium, 97, 135
Illness, individual's response to, 19
  signs and symptoms of, 185-189
Immersions, 271
Immobilization, in fractures, 533
  casts, 534
  internal fixation, 535
  splints, 536
  traction, 536
Immunity, 44
  tests for, 372
Immunization, 495
Immunology, 38
Immunosuppressive drugs, 586
Impaction, fecal, digital removal of, 631
Imperforate anus, 438
Impetigo contagiosa, 519
  in newborn, 438
Incontinence, 141, 218, 662
  in dying patient, 295
  in elderly patient, 735
  in neurologic patient, 550
  in ulcerative colitis, 643
  retraining in, 550
Incubation period, in communicable diseases, 459
Incubator, in oxygen therapy, 308
  premature infant and, 440
Incus, 156
In-dwelling catheter, 290
Infant. See also *Neonate*
  bathing of, 453
  characteristics of, 50
  death of, 414
  developmental tasks of, 51
  disorders of. See *Childhood disorders* and specific names of disorders
  initial care of, 426
  physical examination of, 228
  postmature, 441
  premature, 439-440
  supplementary foods for, 435
Infantile eczema, 489
Infarction, myocardial, 577. See also *Myocardial infarction*

Infection, 185
  as cause of mental retardation, 501
  as postpartum complication, 424
  body's defenses against, 43
  fungous, of ear, 722
  in burns, prevention of, 524
  in diabetes, 706
  microorganisms in, 43
  of ear, 722, 724
  of eyes, drugs for, 369
  of skin, 519
  of umbilical cord, 439
  prenatal, in congenital intellectual impairment, 500
  puerperal, 424
  secondary, in cancer, 515
  staphylococcal, newborns and, 439
  susceptibility to, 44
  upper respiratory, 460
  urinary, 142
  wound, following surgery, 320
    in fractures, 534
Infectious diseases, 186, 495. See also *Communicable diseases*
Infertility, 686
Infiltration, in intravenous therapy, 321
Inflammation, as symptom, 188
Influenza, 613
Infrared rays, 269
Infusion, intravenous
  following surgery, 320
  in pediatrics, 455
  observing patient during, 339
  subcutaneous, in pediatrics, 456
Inguinal hernia, 471
Inhalants, misuse of, 764
Inhalation, of drugs, 325
  steam, 272
Injection(s), 330
  complications of, 338
  intradermal, 325, 331
  intramuscular, 326, 331, 335
    dangers of, 335
  intravenous, 326, 331
  location of, 333
  of insulin, 339, 705
  parenteral, 331
  subcutaneous, 325, 331
Injury(ies)
  birth, 436
    retardation due to, 501
  crushing, in children, 469
  prevention of, in elderly, 758
  to brain, 556
  to chest, 622
  to head, first aid for, 390
  to liver, 652
  traumatic, 186
Innominate bones, 97
Inositol, 174
Inspiration, respiratory, 125, 597
Inspirational dyspnea, 298
Instrument delivery, 420

Insulin, 699
  crystalline, 701
  forms of, 701
  in diabetes, 180
  injection of, 339, 705
  Lente, 701
  precautions in use of, 702
  production of, tests of, 692
  secretion of, 137, 153
Insulin coverage, 702
Insulin shock, 703
  vs acidosis, 703t
Intake, record of, 246
Integumentary system, 87
Intellectual impairment. See *Mental retardation*
Intensive care, 202, 232
Intercellular fluids, 79
Intercommunication system, in hospital, 195
Intermediate care, 232
Intermittent positive pressure breathing (IPPB), 309, 319, 601
Interoceptors, 108
Interstitial fluids, 79
Intervertebral discs, 96
Intestine(s), 134, 135. See also *Colon*
  action of, drugs affecting, 363
  disorders of, 642-647
    abdominal hernia, 645
    acute constipation, 642
    appendicitis, 643
    cancer, 646
    colitis, 642
    diarrhea, 642
    diverticulitis, 645
    irritable colon, 642
    obstruction, 472, 646
    peritonitis, 645
    ulcerative colitis, 642
Intracellular fluids, 79
Intracranial pressure, 555
Intrauterine device (IUD), 687
Intravenous feedings, 243
Intravenous therapy, in pediatrics, 455
  observing patient during, 339
  in elderly patient, 734
  indications for, 320
  infiltration in, 321
  methods of, 320
  observing patient in, 321
Intrinsic factor, in pernicious anemia, 591
Intussusception, 472, 646
Inversion, 95
Involuntary muscle, 86, 102
Involuntary nervous system, 110
Involution, menopausal, 423, 675
  melancholia during, 743
Iodine
  body needs for, 169
  goiter and, 696
  protein-bound, test for, 692

Iodine (*continued*)
　radioactive, uptake test for, 692
　thyroid function and, 152
Iodism, 695
IPPB (intermittent positive pressure breathing) therapy, 601
　following surgery, 319
　methods for, 309
Iridectomy, 715
Iris, 157
Iritis, 717
Iron, administration of, 591
　blood and, 359
　body need of, 168
　preparations of, 359
Iron-deficiency anemia, 591
　in children, 481
Irrigation
　colonic, 253
　colostomy, 254, 632
　eye, 369, 713
　nasal, 607
　of nasogastric tube, 629
　of urinary catheter, 661
　throat, 601
　TUR, 684
　vaginal, 287
Irritability, as characteristic of protoplasm, 75
Irritable colon, 642
Irritants, and counterirritants, 276
　and stimulants, for skin, 342
Ischium, 97
Ishihara chart, 710
Islets of Langerhans, 137, 153
Isolation, 34, 459
　emotional aspects of, 460
　masks in, 282
　protective, 283
　reverse, 283
Isolation technic, 278
　care of body after death, 283
　care of dishes in, 282
　disposal of body discharges in, 282
　"double-bagging" in, 282
　gown technic in, 280
　handwashing in, 280
　linen care in, 282
　medications in, 282
　specimen collection in, 283
　"scrubbing-out" in, 280
　taking vital signs in, 283
　terminal disinfection in, 283
　transporting patient in, 283
Isolette, 308
Isotopes, radioactive, in cancer therapy, 373
ITP (ideopathic thrombocytopenic purpura), 481
IUD (intrauterine device), 687

Jacket restraint, 451
Jacksonian seizures, 559

Jaundice, 649
　as symptom, 187
　homologous serum, 651
Jaw, fracture of, 636
Jejunum, 135
Jenner, Edward, 38
Jewish faith, spiritual needs of patient and, 266
Joints, 92
　and bones, tuberculosis of, 618
Juvenile diabetes, 475, 494, 699
Juvenile rheumatoid arthritis, 493, 496

Kardex, 340
　and nursing care plan, 224
Keloids, 522
Keratitis, 717
Keratoplasty, 717
Kerolytics, 342
Ketone bodies, 165, 657, 699
Ketonuria, 657
Ketosis, 700
　and diabetic coma, 704
Kidney(s), 140, 657
　acid-base balance and, 139
　artificial, 667
　blood pressure and, 141
　Bright's disease and, 479, 663
　cysts of, 666
　disease of, and circulatory disorders, 657. See also *Urinary disorders*
　　diet in, 180
　　surgical procedures in, 668
　failure of, 666-668
　function of, in burns, 523
　glomerulonephritis, 479, 663
　hydronephrosis of, 665
　nephritis of, 478, 663, 180
　nephrosis of, 180, 478
　nephrosis, 180, 479
　polycystic, 478
　pyelonephritis, 478, 663
　transplant of, 669
　trauma to, 665
　tumor of, 479, 666
　uremia and, 666
Kidney stones, 534, 664
Knee-chest position, 227
Knee-jerk, 544
Koplik's spots, 461
Kwashiorkor, 473
Kyphosis, 96, 492

Labia majora, 148
Labia minora, 148
Labor, 415-419
　and delivery, complications of, 420
　induction of, 416
　precipitate, 420
　relief of pain in, 419
　signs of, 415
　stages of, 416
Labor room, 417

Laboratory, diagnostic, 201
　pathology, 201
　research, 201
Labyrinth, of ear, 156
Labyrinthine hydrops, 724
Lacerations, in children, 469
　of lips, 636
Lacrimal glands, 157
Lactation, 148, 679
Lactose, 164
Laennec's cirrhosis, 649
Laminectomy, in spinal cord injuries, 567
Lamp treatments, 269
Laryngectomy, 608
Laryngitis, 607
Larynx, 126
　cancer of, 607
　laryngitis and, 607
Laws, licensing, 7, 785
Learning, and growing, 48
　effective, guides to, 11-17
　processes used in, 15
Leeuwenhoek van, Anton, 38
Leg, structure of, 97
Leg cramps, in pregnancy, 406
Legg-Perthes disease, 493
Lens(es), of eye, 157
　contact, 710
　corrective, in eye disorders, 710
　prosthetic, 717
Leukemia, 115, 480, 511, 592
　acute, 592
　chronic, 593
Leukocytes, 115, 480
Leukocytosis, 115
Leukopenia, 115, 591
Leukoplakia buccalis, 637
Leukorrhea, 675
LH (luteinizing hormone), 368
Liability, in nursing, 787
Lice, 521
License(s), for nurses, 7-8, 785
　examination for, 786
　law in, 7, 785
　revoking or suspending of, 786
Life, definition of, 74
Lifting, and moving, 27
Ligaments, 94
"Lightening," 406, 416
Linea negra, 402
Lip, cleft, 486
　lacerations of, 636
Lipase, 133, 134
Liquid diets, 178
Lithiasis, 664
Litholapaxy, 665
Lithotomy position, dorsal, 227
Liver, 136
　abscess of, 652
　biopsy of, 628
　cancer of, 652
　cirrhosis of, 649
　disorders of, 649-653
　failure of, 649

Liver (*continued*)
  injuries to, 652
  jaundice and, 649
  massive necrosis of, 652
  transplants of, 653
  viral hepatitis, 651
Living matter, 75-76
Lobectomy, in cancer of lung, 622
Lobotomy, 555
  prefrontal, in psychiatric disorders, 751
Lochia, 421
Loop of Henle, 140
Lordosis, 96, 492
Lotions and solutions, 341
LPN (licensed practical nurse). See *Practical nursing*
LSD, 767
LTH, 368
Lumbar puncture, 545
  pediatric, 450
Lumbar vertebrae, 96
Lungs, 128
  abscess of, 614
  benign tumors of, 622
  cancer of, 621
  surgery of, nursing care in, 622
  tuberculosis and, 618
Lupus erythematosus, 521
Luteal hormone (LH), 368
Lymph, 123
Lymph disorders, 590-595
Lymph nodes, 124
  in radical mastectomy, 680
Lymphangiomas, 489
Lymphatic leukemia, 592
Lymphatic system, 123-124
Lymphocytes, thymus and, 154
Lysis, 211

Macules, 517
Magnesium, in diet, 168
Malignancies, 495. See also *Cancer* and *Tumors*
Malleus, 156
Malnutrition, 473
Malpractice insurance, 787
Maltose, 164
Mammary glands, 148. See also *Breasts*
Mammography, 673
Mammoplasty, 683
Mandible, 131
Manic patient, 748
Mantoux test, 599, 618
Marasmus, 473
Marijuana, 766
Marriage, developmental tasks in, 66
Marrow, bone, 92. See also *Bone marrow*
Mask
  face, administration of oxygen by, 303
  in isolation technic, 282
  sterile, surgical asepsis and, 285

Massage, 236
Mastectomy, radical, 680
"Master gland", 150. See also *Pituitary*
Mastication, 132
Mastitis, chronic cystic, 679
  postpartum, 425
Mastoidectomy, in otitis media, 464
Mastoiditis, 724
Masturbation, in children, 56
Maternity clothes, 405
Matter, definition of, 74
  living, 75-76
Maturity, 30
Maxilla, 131
Meals. See also *Food*
  planning and preparing of, 175-176
  preparing the patient for, 176
  serving of, 176
Measles, German, effects of, on newborn, 438
  in child, 461
Measles encephalitis, 462
Measuring systems, 328
Meat, daily requirements of, 163
Meatus, urinary, 141, 148
Meckel's diverticulum, 471
Meconium, 431
Mediastinum, 84, 129
  shift of, in closed water-seal drainage, 604
Medic alert tag, 381
Medical asepsis, 278-283
Medical history, 225
  in pregnancy, 402
Medication(s), 322-373. See also *Drug*
  administration of, 327, 329
    errors in, 330
    in isolation technic, 282
    to child, 456
      Clark's rule in, 456
      Young's rule in, 456
  effects of, 189
  external, in burns, 524
  for pain relief, following surgery, 318
    in cancer, 515
    in labor, 419
  HS, 330
  in arthritis, 532
  measuring of, 328
  preoperative, in surgery, 313
  preparation of, 326
  PRN, 330
  STAT, 330
Medicine card, 328
Megacolon, 473
Melancholia, involutional, 743
Melanoma, malignant, 522
Membranes, 81, 86
  rupture of, in labor, 416
Memory, 15
Menarche, 149
Meniere's disease, 724

Meninges, 112
Meningitis, 467, 565
Meningocele, 476
Meningomyelocele, 476
Menopause, 149
  difficulties of, 675
  premature, 675
Menorrhagia, 674
Menstruation
  after delivery, 424
  difficulties of, in adolescence, 494
  disturbances of, 774
  health habits in, 29
  mechanism of, 149
Mental health, 742
Mental hospital, 744-750
  admission to, 744
  nurse-patient relationship in, 745
  rights of patient in, 744
  safety measures in, 744
Mental illness, 24, 742. See also *Psychiatric disorders*
  approaching patient with, 745
  minor and major, 742
  signs of, 742
  postpartum, 425
  problem of, 759
Mental retardation, 499
  acquired, 501
  congenital, 500
  drug-induced, 500
  extent of, 499
  in cerebral palsy, 502
  in handicapped, 499
  nursing care in, 501
  prevention of, 501
Meprobamate, 355
Mescaline, 767
Metabolism, 39, 75, 138, 166
  basal, 138, 166, 692
  thyroid and, 152
  disorders of, 186, 473-475
    biliary atresia, 473
    colic, 475
    cystic fibrosis (collagen disease), 474
    diabetes, 475. See also *Diabetes mellitus*
    glutin-induced celiac disease, 474
    megacolon (Hirschsprung's disease), 473
Metastasis, 186, 510, 681
Metatarsals, 98
Methadone, 765
Methyl alcohol, 354
Metric system, 328
Metrorrhagia, 674
MI. See *Myocardial infarction*
Microbes, 37-44
Microbiology, 38
Microcephalus, 477
Microorganisms, 37
  antibiotics and, 342
  characteristics of, 39-40
  communicable diseases and, 42

Microorganisms (*continued*)
  growth of, 39
  infection due to, 43
  sterilization and, 284
Microscope, invention of, 38
Micturition, 141
Midbrain, 111
Midsagittal plane, 83
Midwives, 397
Migraine headaches, 547
Milieu therapy, 750
Milk
  breast, 422
    expression of, 422
  calcium content of, 168
  daily requirements of, 163
Minerals, 163
  in daily diet, 167
Miscarriage, 411. See also *Abortion*
Mitochondria, 77
Mitosis, 76, 77
Mitral stenosis, 584
Mitral valve, 118
Mixtures, 75
Molding, in birth, 437
Molds, 40
Molecule, 74
Moles, skin, 522
Mongolian spot, 488
Mongolism, 500
Mononucleosis, 495
Mons pubis, 148
Montgomery, glands of, 148
Morning care, 231, 232
Morning sickness, 406
Morphine, 348
  synthetic substitutes for, 349
Morula, 398
Mother, divorced or widowed, 414
  unwed, 414
Motility, as characteristic of proto-
  plasm, 75
Motion sickness, drugs for, 370
Motor function, loss of, 548
Mouth
  administration of drugs by, 325,
    330
  care of. See *Mouth care*
  disorders of, 635-637
    cancer in, 637
    canker sores, 636
    dental caries, 636
    due to injuries, 636
    foot-and-mouth disease, 636
    herpes simplex infection, 636
    leukoplakia buccalis, 637
    stomatitis, 636
    Vincent's angina, 625
  drugs affecting, 362
  role of, in digestion, 131
Mouth care
  general, 254
  in children, 453
  in dying patient, 295
  in elderly, 735

Mouth care (*continued*)
  in neurologic patient, 554
  in leukemia, 593
  special, 256
Mouth-to-mouth resuscitation, 306
  in newborn, 429
Mouth-to-nose resuscitation, 306
Mouthwashes and gargles, 362
Movement(s), loss of, 548
  of skeleton, 94
Moving and lifting technic for, 27
Mucous membranes, 86
  application of drug to, 325
  drugs for, 340
Mucoviscidosis, 474
Multipara, 415
Multiple sclerosis, 564
Mummy restraint, 451
Mumps, 463
  orchitis and, 685
Muscle(s), 81, 100-105
  abdominal, 103
  cardiac, 102
  characteristics of, 101
  gluteal, 104
Muscle, of arm and chest, 103
  of back and chest, 104
  of extremities, 104
  of eye, 158
  of neck and shoulders, 103
  of respiration, 103
  power source of, 102
  rehabilitation of, 103
  types of, 102
Muscle tissue, 80, 86
Muscle tone, 102
Muscular dystrophy and atrophy,
  504
Musculoskeletal disorders, 484-486,
  492, 526-542
  arthritis, 528-532. See also *Arthritis*
  bone tumors, 495, 528
  bursitis, 527
  diagnostic procedures in, 527
  ganglion, 528
  in children, 484-486, 492
    clubfoot (talipes), 485
    congenital hip dysplasia or dis-
      location, 484
    juvenile rheumatoid arthritis
      (Still's disease), 486
    Legg-Perthes disease, 493
    osteogenesis imperfecta, 485
    postural defects, 492
  rickets, 486
    wry neck, 485
  injuries, 533-538
    dislocations, 533
    fractures, 533
    sprains, 533
  osteomyelitis, 528
  rickets, 527
  tenosynovitis, 527

Musculoskeletal system, 89-105
  disorders of, 526-542. See also
    *Musculoskeletal disorders*
  drugs affecting, 356
Myasthenia gravis, 564
Mydriatics, 369
Myelin sheath, 109
Myelogenous leukemia, 592
Myelography, 547
Myocardial infarction, 577
  complications in, 578
  first aid in, 578
  oxygen needs and, 298
  symptoms of, 577
  treatment and nursing care in, 578
Myocardium, 118
Myometrium, 147
Myopia, 158, 714
Myotics, 369
Myringoplasty, 465
Myringotomy, 464, 724
Myxedema, 696

Nails, 88
  care of, in elderly, 735
  for neurologic patient, 554
NAPNES, 8, 784
Narcolepsy, 496
Narcotic, 761
  in analgesic, 348
  antagonists to, 350
  for cough relief, 366
  opiate, misuse of, 765
Narcotic blockade, 761
Nasal septum, 125
  deviated, 605
Nasogastric tube
  insertion of, 629
  irrigation of, 629
  removal of, 629
  feeding by, 630
    in laryngectomy, 608
Nasolacrimal ducts, 125
Nasopharynx, 126
National Association for Mental
  Health, 759
National Association for Practical
  Nurse Education and Service, 4,
  8, 784,
National Federation of Licensed
  Practical Nurses, 8
*National Formulary,* 323
National Institute of Mental Health,
  759
National League of Nursing, 8
Nausea, following surgery, 318
Nearsightedness, 158, 714
Needle, hypodermic, 333
  in injections, 331
Needs
  basic, 18-19
  cognitive, 19
  ego, 19
  esthetic and consistency, 19
  of children, 48

Needs (*continued*)
  of community, 19
  of family, 19
  of individual, 18
  of patient, basic, 231
    daily, 230-266
    special, 267-296
  of preadolescent, 60
  physiological, 18
  safety, 19
  self-fulfilling, 19
  sex, 18
  social, 19
Negligence, in nursing, 787
Neonate. See also *Infant*
  Apgar scale in evaluation of, 427
  baptism of, in emergency, 427
  bathing of, 430, 432
  birth certificate for, 428
  birth injuries of, 436
  body temperature of, 430
  care of, 426-441
    initial, 426
    daily, 430-432
    of body, 430
    of cord, 429
    of ears, nose, and eyes, 431
    of skin, 431
  characteristics of, 427
  congenital deformities of, 437
  crying and, 431
  disorders of, 435-439. See also
    *Childhood disorders* and specific
    name of disorders
  gastrointestinal, 437
  respiratory, 435
  effects of coincidental diseases of
    pregnancy on, 438
    gonorrhea, 438
    rubella, 438
    syphilis, 438
  examination of, 430
  feeding of, 432
  identification of, 428
  normal, 49, 427
  of diabetic mother, 438
  PKU testing in, 435
  protection of, 430
    from disease, 429
  respiratory status of, 429
  responses of, 431
  resuscitation of, 428
  silver nitrate prophylaxis in, 429
  sleep needs of, 431
  stools of, 431
  urination and, 431
  warmth needs of, 429
  weight of, 430
Neoplasms, 186. See also *Tumors*
  in children, 484
  of lung, 621
Nephrectomy, 666, 668
Nephritis, 478, 663
  chronic, 664
  diet in, 180

Nephroblastoma, 479
Nephron, 140
Nephrosis, diet in, 180
  in children, 479
Nephrostomy, 661
Nephrotomy, 665, 668
Nerve(s)
  acoustic, 156, 157
  cranial, evaluation of, 545
  disorders of, 560. See also *Neuro-logical disorders*
  injury to, in fractures, 533
  of heart, 119
  olfactory, 158
  ophthalmic, 158
  optic, 158
Nerve cell, 107-109
Nervous system, 82, 106-112, 544
  and endocrine system, interaction
    of, 150
  autonomic, 110
    drugs affecting, 355-356
  central, 110-112
    drugs affecting, 347-355
  disturbances of, 543-571. See also
    *Neurological disorders*
  peripheral, 112
Neuralgia, 560
Neurilemma, 109
Neurological disorders, 543-571
  aphasia in, 551
  cerebral palsy, 566
  congenital, 475
    craniostenosis, 477
    encephalocele, 475
    hydrocephalus, 476
    microcephalus, 477
    spina bifida, 476
  degenerative, 563-565
    Huntington's disease, 565
    multiple sclerosis, 564
    myasthenia gravis, 564
    Parkinson's disease, 563
  diet and fluid requirements of, 553
  diversional activities in, 555
  examination for, 544-547
  in children, 475
  incontinence in, 550
  inflammatory, 565-566
    encephalitis, 566
    meningitis, 565
  nerve disorders, 560
    Bell's palsy, 560
    neuralgia, 560
    shingles (herpes zoster), 560
    trigeminal neuralgia (Tic dou-
      loureaux), 560
  nursing care in, 548-555
  of brain, 555-560
    abscess, 558
    convulsive or seizure disorders,
      558
    injuries, 556
    intracranial pressure, 555
    tumors, 556

Neurological disorders (*continued*)
  of spinal cord, 566-571
  emotional adjustment in, 554
    paralysis, 567
    poliomyelitis, 566
  pain in, 554
  personality changes in, 552
  physical inactivity and, 554
  physical problems in, 552
  rehabilitation in, 376
  symptoms of, 547-548
  unconscious patient with, 555
  vascular, 560-563
    aneurysms, 560
    cerebral vascular accident, 561
Neurons, 107
Neuroses, 742
Neutropenia, malignant, 591
Nevi, 488
Newborn. See *Neonate*
N.F. (*National Formulary*), 323
NFLPN, 8, 784
Niacin, 171
Nicotinic acid, 171
Nipples, retracted, 422
Nitroglycerin, 358
NLN, 8, 784
Nodes, lymph, 124, 680
  of heart, 119
Norepinephrine, 153, 356, 697
Nose, 125
  care of, in dying patient, 295
    common treatments for, 606
  disorders of, 605-607
    deviated septum, 605
    epistaxis, 482, 495, 605
      following surgery, 605
    nasal irrigation in, 607
    nasal spray in, 606
    nose drops in, 607
    polyps, 605
    rhinitis, 605
    sinusitis, 605
  plastic surgery of, 605
  removing foreign body from, 390
    in child, 469
Nose drops, 607
Nosebleed, 482, 495, 605
Note taking, 13
Nucleolus, 77
Nucleus, 77
Nurse
  licensing for, 7-8
  practical. See *Practical nursing*
  registered. See *Registered nurse*
Nurse practice act, 786
Nursing, nature of, 3
  oncologic. See *Oncologic nursing*
    and *Cancer*
  pediatric. See *Pediatric nursing*
Nursing care plan, Kardex and, 224
Nursing care study, 16
  practical nursing opportunities in,
    780

Nursing home, or extended care facility, 738
Nursing organizations, 8-9
Nursing schools, 5-6
Nutrients, essential, 162
Nutrition, 162
    and elimination, 245
    deficiencies in, 473
    in elderly patients, 734

Obesity, 164, 180, 244, 473
    and diabetes, 699
Observation skills, 11, 188
    in psychiatric nursing, 747
Obstetrics, 397
Obstetrician, 397
Obstipation, 642
Occupational therapy, 202, 265
    in burns, 525
    in psychiatric disorders, 749
    for elderly, 758
Oculist, 28
Odor, control of, in cancer, 515
    in casts, 534
    in colostomy or ileostomy, 634
Olfactory nerve, 158
Oliguria, 217, 657
Omnopon, 349
Omphalocele, 472
Oncologic nursing, 509-515. See also *Cancer*
Oophoritis, 676
Operating room, career opportunities in, 316, 781
    transporting patient to, 314
    staff of, 202
Operation. See *Surgery*
Ophthalmia, sympathetic, 717
Ophthalmic nerve, 158
Ophthalmologist, 28
Ophthalmoscopic examination, 709
Opiate narcotics, in drug misuse, 765
Opium, 348
Opium tincture, 349
Optic chiasm, 158
Optic nerve, 158
Optician, 28
Optometrist, 28
OR (operating room), 202
Oral cavity, 131
Oral hygiene, 27-28
    dental caries and, 636
    in children, 453
    in elderly, 735
Oral temperature, 211, 213
Orchitis, 685
Organ of Corti, 156
Organic disease, 185
Organisms, 39-42
Organizations, nursing, 8-9, 784
Orientation program, preservice, 783
Oropharynx, 126
Orthodontic care, in school-age child and adolescent, 493

Orthopedics, 527
    disorders in, in children, 484-486
Orthopedists, 527
Orthopnea, 187, 210, 298, 597
Orthopneic position, 601
Osmosis, 79
Ossicles, 156
Osteoarthritis, 530
Osteogenesis imperfecta, 485
Osteogenic sarcoma, 495
Osteomyelitis, 528
OT (occupational therapy department), 202
Otitis, external, 722
Otitis media, 724
    in child, 464
Otology, 719
Otomicroscope, 721
Otosclerosis, 723
Otoscope, 720
Output, record of, 246
    for child, 452
Ova, 146
Oval window, of ear, 156
Ovaries, 146
    cysts of, 677
    hormone extract affecting, 368
    hormone production and, 154
    inflammation of, 676
    tumors of, benign, 677
Overactive patient, 753
Overbed table, 201
Overeating, 244, 473
Overnutrition, 473
Ovulation, 146
    timing of, 149
Ovum, fertilization of, 147
Oxygen. See also *Oxygen therapy*
    administration of, by face mask, 303
        by nasal catheter, 302
        by oxygen tent, 304
        in drug therapy, 309
        in emergency, 305
        to child, 308
    basic need for, 298
    needs for, due to breathing difficulties, 298
        due to lack of hemoglobin, 298
        in circulatory disorders, 298
        in respiratory disorders, 298
        in shock, 299
        oxygen therapy and, 299
        reasons for, 298
        special, 297-309
        symptoms of, 298
    regulation of, in oxygen therapy, 301
Oxygen tent, 304
Oxygen therapy, 299-309
    administration of, methods of, 300
        face mask, 303
        nasal catheter, 302
        oxygen tent, 304
        rules for, 300

Oxygen therapy (*continued*)
    Ambu bag in, 306
    concentration of oxygen in, 300
    conditions requiring, 299
    drugs administered in, 309
    during surgery, 306
    for child, 308
    for newborn, 436
    for premature infant, 440
    in emergency, 305
    in hypoxia following surgery, 318
    in respiratory disorders, 306, 599
    mouth-to-mouth resuscitation in, 306
    mouth-to-nose resuscitation in, 306
    oxygen cylinders in, 301
    oxygen wall outlet in, 301
    oxygen tent in, 304
    patency of airway in, 299
    patient-tripped respirator in, 305
    precautions in, 300
    regulation of oxygen in, 301
    retrolental fibroplasia due to, 440
Oxytocics, 367
Oxytoxin, 151, 694

PABA (para-aminobenzoic acid), 174
Pacemaker, electric, 582
Pain
    appetite and, 176
    following surgery, 318
    general, 189
    girdle, 555
    illness and, 188
    local, 189
    management of, in burns, 524
        in cancer, 515
        in dying patient, 295
        in labor, 419
        in leukemia, 593
        in neurologic patient, 554
        in spinal cord injury, 554
        in urinary disorders, 662
    measurement of, 188
    referred, 189, 555
Palate, cleft, 486
Palatoplasty, 487
Palsy, Bell's, 560
    brachial plexus, 436
    cerebral, 502, 566
Pancreas, 134, 137, 153
    disorders of, 655, 698-707
    test for functioning of, 692
Pancreatectomy, 655
Pancreatitis, 655
Panhypopituitarism, 694
Panhysterectomy, 677
Pantothenic acid, 174
Pap test, 671, 673
    of breast, 673
Papanicolaou test (Pap test), 671
Papaverine, 349, 358
Papoose board, 452
Papules, 517

Para-aminobenzoic acid, 174
Paracentesis, 602
  abdominal, 627
Paraldehyde, 353
Parallel play, 52
Paralysis, Erb-Duchenne, 436
  facial, in forceps delivery, 437
  spinal cord injury and, 567
Paralysis agitans, 563
Paralytic ileus, 318
Paranoia, 743, 749
  and drug misuse, 768
Paraplegia, 569
Parasites, 40, 489
  drugs for destruction of, 370
Parasympathetic nervous system, 110
Parathormone, 153
Parathyroid, 153
  disorders of, 697
Parents. See also *Family*
  of dying child, 457
  of hospitalized child, 447
Parenthood, preparation for, 408-409
Paresis, 690
Parkinson's disease, 563
Paroxysmal dyspnea, 298
Paroxysmal tachycardia, 581
Pasteur, Louis, 38
Patella, 98
Patent ductus arteriosus, 483
Patch test, 619
Patching, for eye disorders, 712
Pathogens, 39
Pathology, definition of, 185
Patient(s)
  as people, 17
  chart of, 224
  dying, assistance to, 292
  helpless, moving and lifting of, 240
  needs of, daily, 230-266
  special, 267-296
  point of view of, 17
  unconscious, 555
  unit of, cleaning of, 196
PBI (protein-bound iodine), 692
  thyroid function and, 153
Pediatric nursing, 445-457. See also
    *Child*
  administering medications in, 456
  catheterization in, 450
  charting in, 452
  crib making in, 448
  croupette and humidity in, 454
  death of child and, 457
  diarrhea technic in, 454
  discharging child in, 456
  enema technic in, 454
  forcing fluids in, 452
  gavage feedings in, 452
  gowning technics in, 452
  infant bath in, 453
  long-term patient in, 456
  mealtimes in, 452
  oral hygiene in, 453
  parenteral fluids in, 455

Pediatric nursing (*continued*)
  preoperative and postoperative
    care in, 455
  procedures in, 448
  restraints in, 450
  resuscitation in, 455
  safety measures in, 447, 450
  urine specimen in, 450
  veni-puncture and lumbar punc-
    ture in, 450
  vital signs in, 449
  weighings in, 453
Pediculidides, 341
Pediculosis, 263, 490, 521
Pellagra, 171
Pelvic cavity, 84
Pelvic examination, 671
Pelvic inflammatory disease (P.I.D.),
  676
Pelvic perfusion, 678
Pelvis, 97
Penicillin, 342
  action of, 343
  method of giving, 343
  preparations of, 344t, 345
  side-effects of, 344
  types of, 344
Penis, 145
Peperazine preparations, 371
Pepsin, 133, 165
Peptic ulcer, 638
Pericardial cavity, 83
Pericardium, 86, 117
Perimetry, 709
Perineal care, 673
  postpartum, 422
Perineorrhaphy, 679
Perineum, 148
Periosteum, 91
Peripheral nervous system, 112
Peripheral vascular disorders, 586-
  590
  Buerger's disease, 589
  embolism, 587
  Raynaud's disease, 589
  thrombophlebitis, 586
Peristalsis, 133, 318
Peritoneal cavity, 137
Peritoneum, 86, 137
Peritonitis, 137, 645
Pernicious anemia, 591
Personality, 29-31
  changes in, in neurologic patient,
    552
  health and, 25-31
Petit mal seizures. See also *Seizure
    disorders*
pH, of blood, 598
  of urine, 657
Phagocytes, 44
Phagocytosis, 44, 115
Phalanges, 98
Pharmacology, 323. See also *Drugs.*
*Pharmacopeia of the United States
  of America,* 323

Pharynx, 126, 132. See also *Throat*
Phenosulfonphthalein test, 658
Phenylketonuria (PKU), 435, 472
Phimosis, 432
Phosphorus, hypoparathyroidism
  and, 697
  in body functions, 168
Photocoagulation, 717
Photophobia, 717
Physical examination, 225-229
  body positions in, 226
  in pregnancy, 402
  of adult, 225
  of infant, 228
Physical therapy, 202
  in arthritis, 532
  in burns, 525
Physiology, of body, 73-84
Pia mater, 112
P.I.D. (pelvic inflammatory disease),
  676
Pilonidal cyst, 648
Pineal gland, 154
Pink eye, 715
Pinna, 156
Pinworms, 490
Pitting edema, 589
Pituitary gland, 150
  disorders of, 693-694
    of anterior lobe, 694
    of posterior lobe, 694
  hormone extract and, 367
  removal of, 694
  tumor of, 694
PKU (phenylketonuria), 435, 472
Placenta, 154
  delivery of, 417
  fetal circulation and, 399
  hormones of, 368
  marginal, 412
  premature detachment of, 412
  presentation of, 417
Placenta previa, 412
Planes, of body, 83
Planogram, 599
Plantar warts, 520
Plasma, 114, 360
Plastic surgery, of nose, 605
Platelets, 115
Pleura, 86, 129
Pleural cavities, 83
Pneumoconioses, 612
Pneumoencephalography, 546
Pneumonia, 615
  aspiration, 615
  bacterial, 615
  following surgery, 319
  hypostatic, 538, 554, 615
  in children, 460
  "walking," 616
Pneumothorax, artificial, in tubercu-
    losis, 620
  in closed water-seal drainage, 604
  spontaneous, 598, 621
Pleurisy, 616

Plumbism, 764
Poisoning
as cause of mental retardation, 501
emergency treatment for, 386, 387
in children, 468
opium or morphine, 348
symptoms and treatments of, 384-385t
Poison ivy, 727
Poliomyelitis, 566
rehabilitation in, 376
Pollution, 33
and respiratory disorders, 623
Polycythemia, 115
Polyps, nasal, 605
Polyuria, 217, 657
Pons, 111
Porro's operation, 424
Portal system, 122
Port-wine stain, 489
Position(s)
change of, for dying patient, 295
dorsal lithotomy, 227
dorsal recumbent, 227
for enema, 251
Fowler's, 227
horizontal recumbent, 226
in physical examinations, 226
knee-chest, 227
observation of, 189
orthopneic, 601
prone, 227
side-lying, 234
Sims's, 227
sitting, 235
Trendelenburg, 299
Postanesthesia recovery room (PAR), staff, 202
Postmature infant, 441
Postnatal health, services for, 35
Postoperative complications, 317-318
Postoperative nursing care, 316-317
in pediatrics, 455
Postpartum, 421
after-pains in, 422
care in, 421
complications in, 424
postpartum blues in, 425
Postural drainage, 599
Posture, and health, 25, *26*
defects in, 492
during pregnancy, 405
Potassium, dietary needs, 168
Practical nursing, 4
as career, 1-5, 779-784
associations for, 8, 9, 784
code of ethics in, 9
legal aspects of, 785-788
nursing skills in, 4
role of nurse in, 779
training in, 6-7
Preadolescence, 59-61
Pre-eclampsia, 410

Pregnancy, 398-413
abruptio placenta in, 412
and diabetes, 413
breast care during, 404
clothing for, 405
complications in, 409-413
constipation during, 406
diet during, 403
discomforts of, 406
dyspnea during, 406
eclampsia in, 410
ectopic, 147, 412, 676
edema during, 407
effects of coincidental diseases of, on infant, 438
elimination during, 404
exercise during, 404
fears in, 407
fetal circulation in, 399
fetal development in, 401
full-term, calculation of, 401
gingivitis during, 407
health practices during, 404
heart conditions in, 413
hemorrhoids and, 407
hydatiform mole in, 413
hyperemesis gravidarum in, 409
leg cramps in, 406
morning sickness in, 406
multiple, 420
parenthood preparation during, 408
placenta previa in, 412
posture during, 405
pre-eclampsia in, 410
prenatal care and, 402-408
rest during, 404
Rh factor in, 117, 399, 403
seizure disorders and, 413
sex determination in, 399
sexual relations during, 405
signs of, 401
positive, 402
presumptive, 402
skin care in, 404
stretch marks and, 407
tests for, 402
toxemia in, 410
tubal, 147, 412, 676
vaginal discharge during, 407
varicose veins in, 407
weight gain during, 404
Premature infant, 439-440
Prenatal care, 402-408
Prenatal classes, 408
Prenatal health services, 35
Preoperative nursing care, 311-315
in pediatrics, 455
Prepuce, of penis, 145
Presbyopia, 710, 714
Prescription, for drugs, 326
parts of, 327
Presentation, fetal, 419. See under *Fetus*

Pressure, blood, 116. See also *Blood pressure*
central venous, 575
intracranial, 555
intraocular, measurement of, 709
Pressure points, for hemorrhage control, 382
Pretease, 134
Primigravada, 415
Primipara, 415
PRN medications, 330
Proctocylsis, 251
in pediatrics, 456
Proctologist, 250
Proctoscopy, 228
Progesterone, 146, 154, 368
effects of, on secondary sex characteristics, 144
in lactation, 148
in menstruation, 149
preparations of, 369
Premature infant, 440
Pronation, 95
Prostate, 145, 684
Prostatectomy, 684
Prosthesis
breast, 681
hip, 538
in amputation, 542
lens, 717
removal of, before surgery, 314
Prophylaxis, 43
Protein(s), 163, 165
blood, 360
Protein-bound iodine, 692
thyroid function and, 153
Proteinuria, 657
Protestant faith, in spiritual needs of patient, 266
Prothrombin, 116
Vitamin K and, 170
Prothrombin time, 574
Proprioceptors, 108
Protoplasm, 74, 75
Protozoa, 40
Protraction, 95
Pruritis, 516, 593
Pseudohermaphroditism, 698
Psoralens, 521
Psoriasis, 521
PSP, in urinary disorders, 658
Psychiatric disorders, 741-759
behavior modification in, 750
changing attitudes toward, 743
doctor's responsibility in, 743
drug therapy in, 751
emergency service in, 743
hospital setting in, 744-759
hydrotherapy in, 749
milieu therapy in, 750
occupational and recreational therapy in, 749
patient in
confused, 755
convalescent, 758

Index / 835

Psychiatric disorders, patient in (continued)
depressed, 749
hostile, 749, 754
hypochondriac, 745
hypomaniac, 753
manic, 748
overactive, 753
paranoid, 749
regressive, 756
senile, 757
suicidal, 751
underactive, 755
withdrawn, 749
practical nurse in, 743
prefrontal lobotomy in, 751
preventing injuries in, 748
psychotherapy in, 749
reality therapy in, 750
remotivation technic in, 750
restraints in, 748
shock therapy in, 751
transactional analysis in, 751
Psychiatry, 24
child and adolescent, 497
Psychomotor seizures, 559
Psychoneuroses, 742
Psychosis, 742
childhood, 491
Psychotherapy, 749
group, in drug misuse, 776
PT (physical therapy department), 202
Ptosis, of eyelids, 488, 564, 715
Ptylin, 132
Puberty, sexual development and, 143
Pubis, 97
Pubic safety, 35
Pudendal block, in labor, 419
Puerperal infection, 424
Puerperium, care during, 421-424
Pulmonary circulation, 118
Pulmonary function test, 598
Pulmonary resuscitation, in first aid, 380
Pulmonary stenosis, 484
Pulse, 120, 207-209
and respiration, rate of, in fever, 187
apical, 209
apical-radial, 209
in heart disease, 573
of hospitalized child, 449
pressure of, in blood pressure, 215
in shock, 299
radial, 208
rate of, 208
in shock, 299
rhythm of, 208
volume of, 208
Pulse deficit, 209
Puncture, cisternal, 546
lumbar, 545
sternal, 590

Puncture wounds, 469
Pupil, of eye, 157
changes in, in drug abuse, 768
drugs affecting, 369
Purine, 181
Purpura, 481, 594
Pustules, 517
Pyelogram, intravenous, 659
Pyelonephritis, 478, 663
Pyloric stenosis, 471
Pyosalpinx, 676
Pyothorax, 614
Pyrexia, 211
Pyridoxine (vitamin $B_6$), 174
Pyuria, 658

Quadraplegia, 569
Quarantine, 34, 459
"Quickening," 402
Quinacrine, 371
Quinine, 356

Radial pulse, 208
Radiation dermatitis, 517
Radiation treatment, in cancer, 512
in Hodgkin's disease, 594
in leukemia, 593
Radical neck dissection, 608, 637
Radioactive isotopes, 373, 513
Radius, 98
Rale, 597
Range of motion exercises, 238, 552, 736
Rash, in infants, 489
Rauwolfia drugs, 354, 358
Raynaud's disease, 589
Reading skills, 13
Reality therapy, 750
Receptors, 108
Records, information on, 206
of intake and output, 246
written, legal importance of, 788
Recovery room, 316
Recreational therapy, for elderly, 737
in psychiatric disorders, 748
Rectal examination, 228, 418
Rectal temperature, 212
Rectocele, and cystocele, 679
Rectum, 135
administration of drugs by, 325
cancer of, 648
parenteral fluids administered by, 456
sigmoid colon and, disorders of, 647
Red blood cells, 114
Red Cross, 36
Reduction, in breast surgery, 683
in fractures, 533
Referred pain, 189, 555
Reflexes, 109
electrodermal., in hearing, 720
gag, 50
grasp, 50

Reflexes (continued)
in musculoskeletal disorders, 527
in neurological examination, 544
knee-jerk, 544
of eye, 157, 544
of neonate, 50
rooting, 50
Refraction, errors of, 488, 708, 714
Registered nurse, 4, 7
Regressive patient, 756
Regurgitation, 244
Rehabilitation, 374-378
family of patient and, 377
following laryngectomy, 609
following surgery, 376
in blindness, 377
in cardiac conditions, 376
in CVA, 562
in deafness, 377
in diabetes, 376
in nervous system disorders, 376
in paraplegia, 571
in polio, 376
in psychiatric disorders, 759
in rheumatic fever, 466
in tuberculosis, 621
limitations of patient in, 376
long-term care in, 232
nurse's attitude in, 375
patient's attitude in, 375
patient's interests in, 375
planning in, 376
rehabilitative aids in, 378
restorative nursing care in, 374
Rejection, in transplants, 586
Religious support, of patient, 266, 736
Remotivation technic, in psychiatric disorders, 750
Renal arteries, 140
Renal dyspnea, 298
Renal failure, 480
Rennin, 133
Renogram, 659
Renoscan, 659
Reproductive system, 81, 143-149
disorders of, 670-690. See Reproductive disorders
in children, 478-480
drugs affecting, 367-369
female, 146-149, 671
male, 144-146, 683
Reproductive disorders, female, 674-683
breast disease, 679-683
cervicitis, 676
cystocele and rectocele, 679
displaced uterus, 679
ectopic pregnancy, 147, 412, 676
menopause difficulties, 675
menstrual disturbances, 674
pelvic inflammatory disease, 676
tumors of uterus and ovaries, 677
vaginal fistulas, 678

Reproductive disorders, female
  (*continued*)
    vaginitis, 675
    vulvitis, 675
  male, 683-686
    cryptorchism, 685
    epididymitis, 685
    epispadias, 685
    hydrocele, 685
    hypospadias, 685
    orchitis, 685
    prostatic difficulties, 684
Reserpine, 354
Residue-free diet, 179
Respiration(s), 209, 244
  rate and depth of, 209
  rate of, in hospitalized child, 449
  Cheyne-Stokes, 210, 295, 298
  control of, 209
  difficulty in, 209
  in burns, 523
  muscles of, 103
  organs of, 597
  shallow, 209
  sounds of, 209
  taking of, 209
Respirator
  external, 306
  negative-pressure, 306
  patient-tripped, 305
  positive-pressure, 306
Respiratory arrest, 298, 306
Respiratory disorders, 595-623
  air pollution and, 623
  allergic rhinitis (hay fever), 609
  blow bottles in, 601
  breathing exercises in, 601
  bronchial asthma, 610
  bronchiectasis, 610
  bronchitis, 611
  care of child with, 454
  chronic, 609-613
  common cold, 613
  cough as symptom of, 187
  diagnosis of, 598-599
  emphysema, 612
  empyema (pyothorax), 614
  following surgery, 319
  hay fever, 609
  histoplasmosis, 617
  in dying patient, 295
  in newborn, 429, 435
  infectious, 279, 460, 613-617
  influenza, 613
  IPPB therapy in, 601
  lung abscess in, 614
  neoplasms of lung in, 621-622
  nursing procedures in, 599-605
  of nose, 605-607
  of throat, 607-609
    throat irrigation and gargle in,
      601
  of upper respiratory tract, 460
  oral-nasal suctioning in, 602
  oxygen therapy in, 298, 599
  paracentesis in, 602

Respiratory disorders (*continued*)
  pleurisy, 616
  pneumoconioses, 612
  pneumonia, 615
  pyothorax (empyema), 614
  symptoms of, 597-598
  thoracentesis in, 602
  tuberculosis, 617
  turning, coughing, and hyperven-
    tilation in, 601
Respiratory system, 81, 125-129
Respiratory system, disorders of. See
    *Respiratory disorders*
  drugs affecting, 366
  lower respiratory tract, 127-129
  upper respiratory tract, 125-127
  waste removal and, 139
Restlessness, following surgery, 319
Restorative nursing care, 374-378
Restraint(s)
  board, 452
  clove-hitch, 451
  crib net, 451
  for children, 448, 450
  for elderly, 735
  glove, 452
  in psychiatric disorders, 748
  jacket, 451
  mummy, 451
  of infant, in examination, 228, 451
Resume, 783
Resuscitation
  cardiopulmonary, 582
  in first aid, 380
  mouth-to-mouth, 306
  mouth-to-nose, 306
  of child, 455
  of neonate, 428
  provisions for, 232
  pulmonary, in first aid, 380
Retardation, mental. See *Mental re-
    tardation*
Retention, urinary, 218
Retina, 157, 158
  detached, 717
Retraction, in body movement, 95
Retrolental fibroplasia, 440
Rh factor, 117, 399, 403
Rheumatic carditis, 466
Rheumatic fever, 465, 495
  heart disease and, 584
Rheumatoid arthritis, 529, 531
  juvenile, 486, 493
Rhinitis, 605
Rhinitis, allergic, 609, 727
Rhinoplasty, in cleft lip and palate,
    487
Rhythm method, 149, 687
Ribs, 97
  fractures of, 622
Riboflavin ($B_2$), 171
Ribonucleic acid (RNA), 77
Rickets, 170, 486, 527
Rickettsiae, 42
Rinne test, 720
R.N. See *Registered nurse*

RNA (ribonucleic acid), 77
Rocking, 57
Rods, of retina, 158
Role playing, learning by, 12
Rooting reflex, 50
Roseola infantum, 462
Rotation, in body movements, 94
Roundworms, 490
Rubber equipment, cleaning of, 195
Rubella, 462
  effects of, on infant, 438
Rubeola (measles), 461
Rubin test, 686
Rule of Nines, 468, 523

Sacral vertebrae, 96
Sacrum, 96
Safety provisions, in hospital, 232-
    233
    for disaster emergency, 232
    for elderly patient, 735
    for fire emergency, 232
    for resuscitation, 232
    in tub bath, 257
  in mental hospital, 744
Salicylates, 350
Salivary glands, 132
Salk vaccine, 567
Salpingectomy, 676
Salpingitis, 676
Salts, body, role of urinary system in
    balance of, 139
Saprophytes, 40
Sarcoma, 510
  Ewing's, 495
  osteogenic, 495, 528
Saturated fats, 165
Scabicides, 341
Scabies, 520
  drugs for, 341
Scales, 517
Scapulae, 98
Scarlatina, 464
Scarlet fever, 464
Schick test, 372
Schizophrenia, 491, 742
Schools, of nursing, 5-6
Schultz's presentation, of placenta,
    417
Sclera, 157
Scleral buckling, 717
Sclerosis, multiple, 564
Scoliosis, 96, 492
  functional, 493
  structural, 493
Scratches, cat, in children, 469
Scrotum, 145
"Scrubbing-out" technic, in isola-
    tion, 280
Scurvy, 171, 186, 473
Sebaceous cysts, 518
Sebaceous glands, 88
  disorders of, 518
Seborrhea, 519
Seborrheic dermatitis, 519
Secretin, 154

Sedatives, misuse of, 764
Sedimentation rate, 574
Seeing eye, 719
Seizure disorders, 558
  hospital precautions in, 559
  in children, 477
  pregnancy and, 413
  treatment of, 559
  types of, 558
Self-care, 232
Self-study programs, 12
Semen, 145
Semi-circular canals, of ear, 156
Seminal vesicles, 145
Seminiferous tubules, 145
Senility, 737, 757
Sensory system, 82, 155-158
  disorders of, 708-725
    of ear, 719-725. See also *Ear disorders*
    of eye, 708-719. See also *Eye disorders*
Septum, nasal, 125
  deviated, 605
  of heart, 118
Serous membranes, 86
Serum, 116
  as drugs, 371
Serum accident, 729
Sex
  as basic need, 18
  determination of, 399
  secondary characteristics of, 143
    effects of hormones on, 153, 154
Sexual development
  abnormal, 494
  and adrenocortical secretions, 153
  hypothyroidism and, 152
  puberty and, 143
Shampoo, method for giving, 262
Shaving, method of giving, 263
Shingles, 520, 560
Shock, 299
  air hunger in, 299
  anaphylactic, 299, 729
    in allergy, 727
  blood pressure in, 299
  first aid for, 380, 384
  following surgery, 317
  insulin, 703
    vs acidosis, 703t
  lack of oxygen and, 299
  signs of, 299
  supportive measures for, 318
  symptoms of, 317
  treatment of, 299
Shock therapy, in psychiatric disorders, 751
Shoulder, structure of, 98
Show, in labor, 416
Shower bath, 257
Sickle-cell anemia, 480, 591
Sicklemia, 480
Side-lying position, 234
  for catheterization, 291
Side rails, in hospitalized child, 448

Sigmoid colon, and rectum, disorders of, 647
Silicosis, 612
Silver nitrate, as prophylaxis, for neonate, 429
  in burns, 524
Simmonds' disease, 694
Sims's position, 227
Sinoatrial node, 119
Sinus, 188
Sinus bradycardia, 581
Sinus cavities, of skull, 95
Sinus tachycardia, 581
Sinusitis, 605
Sippy diet, 179, 639
Sitz bath, 272, 674
Skeletal membrane, 86
Skeletal muscle, 102
Skeletal system, 81
Skeletal tissue, 80, 86
Skeletal traction, 536
Skeleton, 90-99
  appendicular, 90
  axial, 90
Skin, 87-88
  and mucous membrane, communicable diseases of, 280
  application of drugs to, 325
  care of, during pregnancy, 404
    for elderly, 735, 758
    for neurologic patient, 552
    in cancer, 514
    in ileostomy and colostomy, 634
    in traction, 538
    in neonate, 431
  color and temperature of, in neurologic examination, 545
  color of, in shock, 299
  disorders of, 516-525. See *Skin disorders*
  drugs for, 340-342
  grafting of, 522, 525
    in burns, 525
  parasitic infestations of, 520
  preparation of, for surgery, 311
  tuberculosis of, 618
Skin clamps, removal of, 287
Skin disorders, 516-525
  acne vulgaris, 518
  allergy, 519
  boils, 520
  burns, 522-525
  cancer, 522
  cold sore, 520
  dandruff, 519
  disfigurement in, 522
  eczema, 521
  herpes simplex, 520
  herpes zoster, 520
  hives, 519
  impetigo contagiosa, 519
  in adolescent, 493, 496
  in children, 488-489, 496
  infection, 519
  lupus erythematosus, 521
  moist dressings in, 517

Skin disorders (*continued*)
  nursing procedures in, 517-518
  pediculosis, 521
  psoriasis, 521
  scabies, 520
  sebaceous gland disorders in, 518
  seborrhea, 519
  seborrheic dermatitis, 519
  terminology in, 516
  tumors, 521
  urticaria, 519
  vitiligo, 521
  warts, 520
Skin tests, in allergies, 727
  in respiratory disorders, 599
Skull, bones of, 95
  depressed fracture of, 556
Sleeping sickness, 566
Sleeplessness, following surgery, 319
Sleep walking, 496
Slit lamp, 709
Smallpox, 463
Smegma, 432
Smell, sensation of, 158
Smoker's patch, 637
Smoking, and diabetes, 706
  and lung cancer, 621
  and vascular diseases, 590
Smooth muscle, 102
Snellen eye chart, 710
Snow blindness, 715
Soaks (immersion), 271
Sodium, in daily diet, 168
Sodium diet, low, 180
Soft diet, 178
Solutions, lotions and, 341
Somatotropic hormone, 151
Somnambulism, 496
Specimen(s)
  blood, 220
  feces, collecting of, 246
  sputum, 598
  stool, 625
  urine, 218
    collection of, in isolation technic, 283
    pediatric, 450
Speech
  effective, as communication process, 15
  esophageal, following laryngectomy, 608
  in cerebral palsy, 503
  aids for, in cleft lip and palate, 486
  difficulties in, 504
  disturbance of, in drug abuse, 768
Speech therapy, in cerebral vascular accident, 563
  in cleft lip and palate, 487
"Speed", in drug misuse, 764
Sperm, 146
Spermatic cord, 145
Spermatozoa, production of, 145
Sphincter, of bladder, 142
Sphygmomanometer, 215
Spica cast, 534

Spina befida, 476
Spinal block, in labor, 419
Spinal cord, 112
    disorders of, 566-571
    injury to, pain control in, 554
    poliomyelitis, 566
    pressure on, 567
    trauma to, 567
Spinal fusion, 567
Spine, 96
    rheumatoid arthritis of, 531
Spiritual needs of patient, 266
Spleen, 124
Splenectomy, 595
Splints, 536, 550
Spondyloitis, ankylosing, 531
Sponge bath, 274, 453
Spores, 40
    sterilization of, 284
Sprains, 533
Sprue, 474
Sputum, as respiratory symptom, 597
Sputum culture, 598
Sputum specimen, 598
Squamous epithelium, 85
Squint, 488
Stapedectomy, 723
Stapes, 156
    mobilization of, 723
Staphylococcal infections, in new-
    born, 439
Starch, 164
Starvation, 473
Status epilepticus, 559
STAT medications, 330
Steam inhalation, 272
Stenosis, aortic, 484
    pulmonary, 484
    pyloric, 471
Sterile technic, 284-287
    sterile supplies, 285
        gloves, 286
        gown, in surgical asepsis, 286
        handling of, 285
        package, opening of, 286, 287
        tray, 285
Sterility, due to mumps, 463
Sterilization, and disinfection, 284
    methods of, 284, 686
    terminal, 434
Sternal puncture, 590
Sternocleidomastoid, 103
Sternum, 97
Steroids, 153
STH (somatotropic hormone), 151
Still's disease, 486, 493
Stimulants, 347
    and irritants, for skin, 342
    heart, 356
    respiratory, 366
Stirrup, of middle ear, 156
Stitches, removal of, 287
Stocking, elastic, 277
Stoma, in colostomy, 631
    in ileostomy, 634

Stomach, 133
    cancer of, 511, 641
    disorders of, 638-641
        drugs affecting, 362
    gastric analysis of, 598, 625
    irrigation of, in poisoning, 468
    peptic ulcer of, 638
Stomatitis, 636
Stool(s), 245
    of neonate, 431
    specimens of, 625
Strabismus, 488, 715
Strawberry mark, 489
Streptomycins, 345
Stress, emotional, and personality, 30
Stretcher, transfer to, 240
Striae gravidarum, 407, 424
Striated tissue, 80, 86
Stryker frame, for neurologic pa-
    tient, 549
Study skills, 12
Stump care, in amputation, 541
Stupor, episodic, 649
    in drug misuse, 769
Stuttering, 504
St. Vitus dance, in rheumatic fever,
    465
Stye, 715
Stylet, 333
Subcutaneous injection, 331, 332
Submucous resection, 605
Sucking reflex, 50
Sucrose, 164
Suction, chest, 603
    oral-nasal, 602
    gastrointestinal, 628
Sudoriparous glands, 88
Suffocation, of child, 469
Sugars, 164
    absorption and digestion of, 164
    blood, 692
    urine tests for, 693
Suicide, 751
Suicide, adolescent, 497
Suicide, attempts at, 751
Suicide, methods of, 752
    patient inclined to commit, 751
    "specialing" of, 753
Suicide prevention, centers for, 753
Suicide, preventive measures in, 752
Sulfonamides, 346
Sulfur, body needs for, 169
Sunburn, treatment for, 390
Sunstroke, 389
Supination, 95
Suppository, 249
    in pediatrics, 454
    vaginal, 289
Suppression, 218
Suprarenal glands, 153
Surgery. See also specific surgical
    procedures
    anesthesia in, 315
    asepsis in, 284-287

Surgery (continued)
    atelectasis following, 319
    bedrest complications following,
        319
    brain, 557
    catheterization following, 318
    circulatory complications follow-
        ing, 319
    constipation following, 318
    distention following, 318
    drainage following, 320
    dressing change and, 320
    electrolyte balance following, 320
    embolus following, 319
    evisceration following, 320
    flatus following, 318
    food restrictions preceding, 313
    hemorrhage following, 317
    hypoxia following, 318
    in burns, 524
    in diabetes, 709
    intestinal preparation for, 313
    IPPB therapy following, 319
    nausea following, 318
    nursing care in, 310-321
        postoperative, 316
        preoperative, 311-315
    nutrition following, 320
    pain following, 318
    parenteral replacement therapy
        following, 320
    patient's family and, 315
    patient's feelings in, 311
    plastic, of nose, 605
    pneumonia following, 319
    postoperative complication and
        discomforts of, 317-319
    preoperative medication in, 313
    preparing patient for, 311
    rehabilitation following, 376
    respiratory complications follow-
        ing, 319
    restlessness and sleeplessness fol-
        lowing, 319
    shock following, 317
    skin preparation in, 311
    thirst following, 318
    thrombophlebitis following, 319
    transporting patient for, 314
    turning, coughing, and deep
        breathing following, 319
    urinary retention following, 318
    wound infection following, 320
Swallowing difficulties, in aged, 734
Swayback, 96, 492
Sweat glands, 88
Swelling. See Edema.
Swimmer's ear, 722
Symbiosis, 44
Sympathectomy, 589
Sympathetic nervous system, 110
Sympathetic ophthalmia, 717
Symphysis pubis, 97
Symptoms, 186
    cardinal, 207

Symptoms (*continued*)
　general, 186
　local, 186
　objective, 186
　subjective, 186
Synapse, 108
Synovial fluid, 94
Synovial joint, 92
Synovial membranes, 86
Syphilis, 689
　chancre in, 689
　congenital, 186
　douches and, 288
　effects of, on newborn, 438
Syringe, disposable, 324
　in subcutaneous injections, 332
　sterile, handling of, 333
Systole, 116
Systolic pressure, 215

Tabes dorsalis, 690
Tachycardia
　paroxysmal, 581
　pulse rate in, 208
　sinus, 581
Talipes, 485
Tapeworms, in children, 489
Tardive dyskineasia, 772
Tarsal bones, 98
Tasks, developmental, 48
Taste, 158
Taste buds, 158
TB. See *Tuberculosis*
T binders, 276
Teaching machines, 12
Tear ducts, 125
Teeth, 132
　care of, during pregnancy, 404
　decay of, 636
　deciduous, 132
　effects of diet on, 28
　eruption of, in infant, 50
　fluorine and, 169
　function of, in digestion, 131
　malocclusion of, 493
Telephone ethics, for nurse, 229
Temperature, body, 210-214
　　axillary, 212
　　elevation of, 211
　　　following surgery, 320
　　　sponge baths in, 453
　　lowered, 211
　　of child, 449
　　of neonate, 430
　　oral or mouth, 211
　　normal, 211
　　rectal, 212
　　regulation of, 210
　　skin and, 87
　　taking of, 212
Tendons, 100
Tenosynovitis, 527
Tes-tape, 693
Testis, 144
　hormone extracts affecting, 368

Testis (*continued*)
　hormone secretion and, 153
　undescended, 685
Testosterone, 153
　preparations of, 369
　secondary sex characteristics and, 144
Tetanus, 467
Tetany, 153
Tetracyclines, 345
Tetralogy of Fallot, 483
Thalamus, 111
Thermometer, clinical, 211
　cleansing and disinfection of, 214
Thiamine (B$_1$), 171
Thompson Practical Nursing School, 5
Thoracentesis, 602
Thoracic vertebrae, 96
Thoracoplasty, 620
Thorax, structure and function of, 97
Three-man lift, 242
Throat
　culture of, 598
　disorders of, 607-609
　　aspiration of foreign bodies in, 607
　　laryngitis, 607
　irrigation of, in respiratory disorders, 601
　removing foreign body from, 390
　sore, 461
Thrombin, 360
Thromboangiitis obliterans, 589
Thrombocytes, 115
Thrombophlebitis, 319, 586
　following surgery, 319
　postpartum, 425
Thromboplastin, 116
Thrombosis, 298
　cerebral, 561
　embolism and, in limb, 588
Thrombus, 117
Thrush, in newborn, 438
Thumb-sucking, 57
Thymus, 154
Thyroid, 151
　disorders of, 694-697
　　exophthalmic goiter, 695
　　Graves' disease, 695
　　hyperthyroidism, 695
　　hypothyroidism, 696
　　myxedema, 696
　　simple (colloid) goiter, 696
　　tumors, 696
　function of, tests of, 692
　iodine needs and, 169
　removal of, 695
　tumors of, 696
Thyroid scan, 692
Thyroidectomy, 695
Thyrotomy, 608
Thyroxin, 151, 694

Tibia, 98
Tic douloureaux, 560
Tidal volume determination, 598
Tine test, 599
Tinea pedis, 490
Tinnitus, 725
Tips or gifts, ethics regarding, 222
Tissues, 80, 85-86, 92, 109
Tissue fluid, 79
Tobacco, as drug, 763. See also *Smoking*
Toenails, care of, 261
Toilet equipment, 205
Toilet-training, 57
Tolerance, in drug use, 761
Tongue, function of, in digestion, 132
Tonometry, 709
Tonsillitis, in child, 461
Tooth decay, 636
　fluoridation in, 28
Torticollis, 485
Touch, sense of, 158
Tourniquet, in first aid, 380, 386
Toxemia, during pregnancy, 410
Toxins, 43
Toxoid, 372
TPR (temperature, pulse, respiration), 207
　graphic chart for, 214
Trachea, 127
Tracheo-esophageal fistula, 437
Tracheostomy, assisting with, 307
　care of tube in, 308
　nursing care in, 308
Tracheotomy tube, in opening airway, 300
Trachoma, 715
Traction, 536
　equipment, 201
　in spinal cord injury, 567
　nursing care in, 537
　skeletal, 536
　skin, 537
　skull or head, 536
Tranquilizers, 354
　misuse of, 772
Transactional analysis, 751
Transferring, of patient, 221
　　for surgery, 314
　　in emergency, 388
　　isolation technic for, 283
　　to recovery room, 316
Transfer forceps, in handling sterile supplies, 285
Transfusion, 326, 360
Transplants
　corneal, 717
　heart, 586
　kidney, 669
　liver, 653
Transurethral resection (TUR), 684
Transverse plane, 83
Trauma
　as cause of mental retardation, 501

Trauma (*continued*)
  in children, 467-470
    abrasions, 469
    "battered child" syndrome, 470
    burns, 467
    crib death, 470
    crushing injuries, 469
    dog bites and cat scratches, 469
    fractures, 469
    lacerations, 469
    poisoning, 468
    puncture wounds, 469
    suffocation, 469
  injuries due to, 186
Tray, food, serving of, 243
  sterile, 285
Trench mouth, 635
Trendelenburg position, 299
Tricuspid atresia, 483
Tricuspid valve, 118
Trigeminal neuralgia, 560
Tripod walking, 540
Trypsin, 134
Tub bath, 256
Tubal pregnancy, 147
Tube(s)
  eustachian, 156
  fallopian, 147
  for compression of esophageal or
    gastric varices, 630
  gastrointestinal, 629
  nasogastric, 629
  tracheostomy, care of, 308
Tube feedings, 630
  in aged patient, 734
  in laryngectomy, 608
Tubercle bacillus, 617
Tuberculosis, 617-621
  chemotherapy in, 620
  chest roentgenograms in, 619
  complications of, 621
  detection of, 618
  drug therapy in, 618
  hemorrhage in, 621
  immunity test for, 372
  in urinary system, 664
  Mantoux test in, 599, 618
  nursing care in, 621
  of lungs, 618
  of skin, 619
  Patch test in, 619
  recurrence of, 621
  rehabilitation in, 621
  spontaneous pneumothorax in, 621
  spread of, 618
  symptoms of, 619
  Tine test in, 599
  treatment of, 620
  tubercle bacillus in, 617
  vaccination against, 618
Tuberosity, 93
Tubules, of kidney, 140
  seminiferous, 145
Tumors, 81, 186
  benign, 186, 510
  Ewing's, 495

Tumors (*continued*)
  malignant, 186
  of adrenal medulla, 698
  of bone, 495, 528
  of bladder, 666
  of brain, 556
    in children, 478
  of cervix, 677
  of eye, 718
  of kidney, 479, 666
  of lung, 622
  of ovaries, 677
  of pituitary, 694
  of skin, 522
  of thyroid, 696
  of urinary tract, 666
  of uterus, 677
  Wilms's, 479
Tuning fork tests, 720
TUR irrigations, 684
Turbinates, 125
Turning, coughing, and hyperventi-
    lation, 601
  following surgery, 319
Tympanoplasty, 465
Tympanum, 156

Ulcer(s), 188
  bland diet in, 179
  corneal, 717
    in contact lenses, 711
  decubitus, 264
  peptic, 638
  skin, 517
Ulcerative colitis, 494, 642
Ulna, 98
Ultrasound, in eye disorders, 709
Ultraviolet rays, 269
Umbilical cord
  care of, in emergency childbirths,
    441
  fetal circulation and, 399
  infection of, 439
  prolapsed, 420
    and respiratory distress in new-
      born, 436
  stump of, care of, 429
Umbilical hernia, 471
Unconscious patient, 555
Underactive patient, 755
Undernutrition, 473
*United States Dispensatory*, 323
Unsaturated fats, 165
Unwed mother, 414
Upper respiratory infections, 460
Urea clearance tests, 658
Uremia, 666
Uremic frost, 666
Ureterostomy, 661
Ureters, 141, 657
Urethra, 141, 657
  abnormal placement of, 685
  strictures of, 665
URI (upper respiratory infections),
    460
Urinal, use of, 247

Urinalysis, 217, 658
Urinary bladder, 141, 657. See also
    under *Bladder*
Urinary catheter, 660. See also *Cath-
    eter*
Urinary disorders, 656-669. See also
    *Genitourinary disorders*
  common problems of, 659
  complications of, 662
  diagnosis of, 657-659
  dehydration in, 662
  in children, 478-480
  infectious, 662-664
    chronic nephritis, 478, 664
    cystitis, 662
    nephritis (Bright's disease), 479,
      663
    pyelonephritis, 478, 663
    tuberculosis, 664
  hydronephrosis, 665
  kidney failure, 478, 666-668
  kidney stones, 534, 664
  laboratory procedures in, 658
  noninfectious, 664-666
  nursing care in, 660-662
  pain in, 662
  surgical procedures in, 668-669
  trauma to kidney or bladder, 665
  tumors of urinary tract, 666
  urethral strictures, 665
  urinary obstruction, 479, 664
Urinary system, 81, 139-141, 657
Urinary system, drugs affecting, 361-
    362
Urinary diversion, types of, 661
Urinary incontinence, 141, 662
Urinary meatus, 141, 148
Urine
  amount of, 217
  bilirubin in, 657
  blood in, 657
  characteristics of, 142
  color of, 217
  culture of, 658
  in diabetes insipidus, 694
  in diabetes mellitus, 692, 705
  in observation of patient, 189
  odor of, 217
  observation of, 217
  pH of, 657
  production of, 140
  protein in, 657
  residual, 657
  retention of, 218
    following surgery, 318
  specific gravity of, 246
  specimen of, 218, 283
    accumulated, 219
    midstream, 219
    pediatric, 450
    single, 218
  sugar in, 657
    in diabetes, 692
  suppression of, 218
  tests of, 658
    for sugar, 693

Urine, tests of (*continued*)
in diabetes, 705
Urticaria, 519, 727
U.S.P. (*United States Dispensatory*), 323
Uterine tubes. See *Fallopian tubes*
Uterus, 147
cancer of fundus of, 677
contractions of, 416
drugs causing, 368
timing of, 418
curettage of, 672
displaced, 679
drugs affecting, 367
inertia of, 420
involution of, 423
prolapse of, 679
retroversion of, 679
ruptured, 420
tumors of, 677
Uveitis, 717

Vaccines, 372
Vaccination, against tuberculosis,618
smallpox, 463
Vagina, 148
inflammation of, 675
discharge from, during pregnancy, 407
examination of, 227
fistulas of, 678
irrigation of, 287
suppository for, 289
treatments for disorders of, 287
Vaginitis, 675
Vagotomy, 640
Valve(s), ileocecal, 135
of heart, 118
van Leeuwenhoek, Anton, 38
Varicella, 463
Varicose veins, 588
esophageal, 637
tubes for suppression of, 630
in pregnancy, 407
Variola, 463
Vascular disorders, 560-563
peripheral, 586-590. See also *Peripheral vascular disorders*
smoking and, 590
Vas deferens, 145
Vasectomy, 687
Vasoconstrictors, 357
Vasodilators, 358
Vasopressin, 151, 694
VD (venereal disease), 688
Vectors, 42, 278
Vegetables, daily requirements of, 163
Veins, 121
varicose, 407, 588
Venereal disease, 688. See also under specific name of disease
and adolescence, 494
Venipuncture, and lumbar puncture, in pediatric nursing, 450
Venous pressure, central, 575

Ventral cavity, 83
Ventricles, of heart, 118
Ventricular fibrillations, 582
Ventricular septal defects, 483
Ventriculography, 547
Vertebrae, division of, 96
structure and function of, 96
Vertigo, 725
Vesicles, 517
seminal, 145
Vestibule, of ear, 148
Vials, ampules and, 323
withdrawing drug from, 338
Villi, 135
chorionic, 398
Vincent's angina, 625
Virus(es), 42
cancer and, 510
filtrable, 38
Visceral tissue, 80
Vision. See also *Eye*
accommodation in, 157, 708
binocular, 157
impairment of, in elderly, 736
mechanism of, 157
peripheral, 709
Visiting nurse service, practical nurse in, 781
Vital signs, 207
in burns, 523
in isolation technic, 283
of child, 449
Vitamin(s), 163, 169
A, function and source of, 170
B complex, 171
B$_1$ (thiamine), 171
B$_2$ (riboflavin), 171
B$_6$, 174
B$_{12}$, 174
in pernicious anemia, 591
injections of, 359
C, function and source of, 171
D, 170
deficiency of, in rickets, 486
E, 170
K, 170
fat-soluble, 170
water-soluble, 171
Vitamin diet, high, 181
Vitiligo, 521
Vitreous humor, 158
Vocal cords, 126
Voice box, 126
Voiding, mechanism of, 141
difficulties in, in puerperium, 423
Voluntary muscle, 86, 102
Volvulus, 646
Vomiting, 187, 244
as symptom, 187
in newborn, 438
pernicious, during pregnancy, 409
projectile, 244
Vomitus, observation of, 244
Vulva, 148
Vulvitis, 675

"Walking pneumonia," 616
Ward order, 195
Warm-water bag, application of, 268
Warts, 520
Waste elimination, urinary system and, 139
Water
chemical structure of, 74
in body fluids, 79
in body processes, 163
in daily diet, 169
Water-seal drainage, closed, 603
Water-soluble vitamins, 171
Weber test, 720
Weight
excessive, food habits and, 162, 244, 273
low calorie diet and, 180
gain in, during pregnancy, 404
loss of, after delivery, 423
of child, 449
of neonate, 430
Weighing(s)
in pediatrics, 453
of patient on admission, 217
Welder's flash, 715
Wharton's jelly, 399
Wheals, 517
White blood cells, 115
in leukemia, 592
Whooping cough, 461
Wills, nurse as witness of, legal aspects of, 788
Wilms's tumor, 479
Wind pipe, 127
Withdrawal, in drug use, 761
Withdrawn patient, 749
Wood alcohol, 354
Worms, parasitic, 42
drugs for destruction of, 370
Wound(s)
dressing of, in first aid, 380
infection of, following surgery, 320
in fractures, 534
penetrating, of chest, 622
puncture, in children, 469
Writing skills, in nursing, 15
Wry neck, 485

X-ray
and fluoroscopy, in respiratory disorders, 599
chest, 221, 599, 619
drugs in, 363
in digestive disorders, 626
in gallbladder disorders, 653
in musculoskeletal disorders, 527
in urinary disorders, 658

Yeasts, 40
Young's rule, 456

Zinc, in body function, 169
Zygote, 398